FOURTH EDITION 4

MOSBY'S
FUNDAMENTALS
OF THERAPEUTIC
MASSAGE

KU-592-802

SANDY FRITZ, MS, NCTMB

Founder, Owner, Director, and Head Instructor
Health Enrichment Center
School of Therapeutic Massage and Bodywork
Lapeer, Michigan

**FOREWORD BY LEON
CHAITOW, ND, DO**

Honorary Fellow
University of Westminster, London
United Kingdom

**CONTRIBUTION BY W.
RANDY SNYDER, DC, MS
NCTMB, CHCQM**

Owner/Director, College of Integrative Healthcare
Oceanside, California

MOSBY

ELSEVIER

1953989

LIBRARY

ACC. No.   DEPT.
3606 1531

CLASS No.

UNIVERSITY
OF CHESTER

11830 Westline Industrial Drive
St. Louis, Missouri 63146

MOSBY'S FUNDAMENTALS OF THERAPEUTIC MASSAGE   ISBN: 978-0-323-04861-3
Copyright © 2009, 2004, 2000, 1995 by Mosby, Inc., an affiliate of Elsevier Inc.   ISBN: 0-323-04861-7

All rights reserved. No part of this publication may be reproduced or transmitted in any form or by any means, electronic or mechanical, including photocopying, recording, or any information storage and retrieval system, without permission in writing from the publisher. Permissions may be sought directly from Elsevier's Rights Department: phone: (+1) 215 239 3804 (US) or (+44) 1865 843830 (UK); fax: (+44) 1865 853333; e-mail: healthpermissions@elsevier.com. You may also complete your request on-line via the Elsevier website at http://www.elsevier.com/permissions.

Notice

Neither the Publisher nor the Author assume any responsibility for any loss or injury and/or damage to persons or property arising out of or related to any use of the material contained in this book. It is the responsibility of the treating practitioner, relying on independent expertise and knowledge of the patient, to determine the best treatment and method of application for the patient.

The Publisher

ISBN-13: 978-0-323-04861-3
ISBN-10: 0-323-04861-7

Vice President and Publisher: Linda Duncan
Senior Editor: Kellie White
Senior Developmental Editor: Jennifer Watrous
Editorial Assistant: April Falast
Publishing Services Manager: Julie Eddy
Project Manager: Rich Barber
Designer: Teresa McBryan

Working together to grow
libraries in developing countries

www.elsevier.com | www.bookaid.org | www.sabre.org

ELSEVIER   BOOK AID International   Sabre Foundation

Printed in China

Last digit is the print number: 9   8   7   6   5   4   3   2   1

MOSBY'S
FUNDAMENTALS
OF THERAPEUTIC
MASSAGE

FOURTH EDITION DEDICATION

To my family, for their support in extraordinary
circumstances—my kids, my mother, my pa,
my brother, and especially my sister
and brother-in-law.

THIRD EDITION DEDICATION

To the students, especially the young ones,
learning in the present—our hope for the future.

SECOND EDITION DEDICATION

To both of my Dr. G's, who were
and are my teachers and my support.

FIRST EDITION DEDICATION

To my kids—Greg, Laura, and Luke—for doing
without me for so long.

To my mother, who kept the house together
and worried about me.

To all my dogs, who spend countless hours by my
side and in my lap, and especially
to my old bulldog, Ethan, who died quietly at my
feet while I worked on rewrites.

To Eric and Christine, for "making it happen."

To my special staff, who are my friends and family,
for giving me the space to write.

To all the wonderful people who teach with me.

To every client and student I have had
the opportunity to touch;
thank you for teaching me.

To all my teachers.

To those who listened.

To those who love me anyway.

Reviewers

Ken Alford, PhD
Department Head, Health and Human Performance
Texas A&M University-Commerce
Commerce, Texas

Julie Burroughs, BA
St. Louis, Missouri

Laura Cochran, BS
Certification, Secondary Education in Psychology and Biology
Flint, Michigan

Lorena Haynes, LMT
Department Chair, Massage Therapy Program
Westside Tech
Winter Garden, Florida

Bruce Froelich, JD, NCTMB
Member, American Massage Therapy Association
Program Director for Therapeutic Massage
Baker College
Auburn Hills, Michigan

Robin Jillson, LMT
Instructor, Healing Hands Institute
Westwood, New Jersey

Edward G. Mohr, MSIE, CPE, CSP, NCTM
Certified Professional Ergonomist
Certified Safety Professional, Engineering Aspects
Member, American Massage Therapy Association
Lake Orion, Michigan

Jessica L. Smith, NCTMB
Member, American Massage Therapy Association
Instructor, Health Enrichment Center for Therapeutic Massage
Lapeer, Michigan

Leann Zalasky, LMT, NCTMB
Owner, Serenity Massage and Bodywork
Owner, Hand-to-Paw Bodywork
St. Louis, Missouri

William Zalasky, LMT, NCTMB
Owner, Serenity Massage and Bodywork
St. Louis, Missouri

Foreword

Books appear to have lives of their own. As time passes, knowledge grows, new ideas emerge, research evidence alters our understanding of particular topics and issues, social and legal factors evolve, and subjects that previously seemed relatively unimportant begin to assume greater importance. In these, and other, ways, textbooks demand to grow, to expand on what only a few years ago seemed comprehensive.

For example, in this fourth edition, the author has increased the material on body mechanics and ergonomics (Chapter 7) as well as widening the information regarding shiatsu, Thai massage, hydrotherapy, thermotherapy, stone massage, color therapy, and aromatherapy (all in Chapter 11). In addition, there is more on career tracks and special populations, as well as spa applications (Chapter 12).

Instead of being an appendix, research literacy is now a core element of the book. This is an increasingly important area of knowledge for therapists, as massage moves into mainstream settings. New topics, such as nutrition, have been added in this new edition, in order for therapists to be better able to discuss these key issues with their clients in an informed manner.

This continuous process of revision, updating, and expansion therefore helps massage therapists to be up-to-date and well informed, as they commence their careers. This rapidly emerging profession, with its long and illustrious history, has for too long been a Cinderella in the healthcare community. This has changed, and change continues apace, as research shows the true value of appropriately applied massage, whether in its basic "wellness" format, or involving a variety of specifically applied therapeutic manual modalities and methods.

I recently conducted a data search of the clinical use of massage worldwide. What emerged did not surprise me, although it was almost overwhelming in its volume. Taking account of obvious contraindications and cautions (which are more than adequately dealt with in this excellent textbook), what emerged from my data search was evidence of massage being used beneficially in treatment of patients/clients with conditions and pathologies of almost every sort.

The fact that there appear to be opportunities for some aspect of "touch" therapy to be useful in almost all conditions of ill-health may give skeptics pause, in order to reflect on what other form of healthcare can be said to provide virtually universal usefulness.

In the Foreword to the previous edition I said:

"This is no longer just a fine entry-level book for prospective massage therapists, but one that addresses the needs of these times in which integration of health care approaches is advancing rapidly. As massage therapy grows into a major health care profession, society (as well as official agencies) insists that the level of training and the excellence of delivery, as well as the ethical standards of its graduates and practitioners, continue to improve. The demands of the present are that what is offered in health care be evidence based. This is as it ought to be, since without a solid training in the ethical, theoretical, and practical components of massage and bodywork, based on what is known and not just on what is believed, confidence would erode.

The public and other health care professions, as well as government agencies and insurance companies, expect and demand no less from the massage therapy profession than any other, in order to feel safe on all levels in the hands (literally) of its professionals.

If this confidence is to continue to grow, as it deservedly should, the broad spectrum of knowledge, so eloquently incorporated into this book, should be seen as a foundation on which to build. Its title is therefore a precise description of what it offers—the principal elements, the primary knowledge, the fundamentals."

I stand by these words, and congratulate the industrious lead author, and the contributors, on producing a fine text that will inevitably help to take the massage profession forward to a new level of excellence.

Leon Chaitow, ND, DO
Honorary Fellow
University of Westminster
London

Preface

Almost 30 years ago, when I was exploring a career in therapeutic massage, there were very few schools. Because none were readily accessible to me, I taught myself. I took a course of fewer than 100 hours, which at least provided basic skills. The rest of my massage therapy training has come from reading a multitude of books, attending hundreds of hours of workshops, undergoing apprenticeship training, taking college courses in related subjects, teaching more than 4000 beginning students, and providing more than 30,000 massage sessions. Since the publication of the first edition, I completed my bachelor's degree at Central Michigan University and master's degree at Thomas Edison State College. Becoming a student again in the university environment had a great influence on my perspective about education, as well as on my professional development.

For more than 10 years, I have been involved in an advanced sports massage program with an entire NFL team, as well as individual athletes from many different types of sports and fitness environments. What a learning experience this endeavor has been! An educational program between my Health Enrichment Center School of Therapeutic Massage and the Veterans Administration Hospital continues to remind me about the importance of touch. One of the veterans spoke at the Health Enrichment Center graduation and said that because of the student massage program, he has fewer bad days and more good ones. What better support for massage can we get than this? The Massage Outreach Program with Hospice brings its own unique rewards and learning. I am still learning the importance of the fundamental concepts upon which all bodywork methods are based. I learn more about the elegant simplicity of massage each time I teach or do massage, and I have learned a great deal through researching and writing textbooks as well. More than ever, I am convinced that a strong understanding of the fundamental concepts of therapeutic massage and the ability to reason effectively through a decision-making process are essential for proficient professional practice.

WHO WILL BENEFIT FROM THIS BOOK?

The fourth edition of *Mosby's Fundamentals of Therapeutic Massage* is intended to be used by skilled therapeutic massage educators, and beginning and advanced students, in the classroom setting. It will also be used as a continuing education resource by practitioners and as a reference text for health professionals and massage and bodywork practitioners.

CONCEPTUAL APPROACH AND WHY THIS BOOK IS IMPORTANT TO THE PROFESSION OF MASSAGE THERAPY

The changes and additions to the fourth edition reflect how much therapeutic massage has evolved as a profession over the past few years. *Mosby's Essential Sciences for Therapeutic Massage: Anatomy, Physiology, Biomechanics, and Pathology*, third edition, is a comprehensive anatomy, physiology, pathology, and clinical application text written to complement and support the body of knowledge of *Mosby's Fundamentals of Therapeutic Massage*. What a thrill it is for me to have participated in the development of "real" textbooks written specifically for the students I serve.

Today, the profession of therapeutic massage is in the process of standardizing and organizing. Major advances in the acceptance of therapeutic massage have occurred since the first edition of this text was published in 1995. This is primarily because valid research is now available to support the value of the simple work we do. Many highly respected schools are now teaching students therapeutic applications of nurturing, safe touch that stimulates the body's various physiologic processes.

A well-rounded education includes learning the following: how to perform massage manipulations and bodywork techniques; the anatomy and physiology of why the methods work; and the importance of structure, intent, and purpose of touch. It is as important to touch the whole person as it is to skillfully apply techniques. The massage professional must do both. In addition, the student needs to understand the importance of sanitation, hygiene, body mechanics, research literacy, business practices, and ethics and apply this knowledge through effective decision-making to build a well-balanced, professional massage career.

The fundamentals of massage methods are relatively simple. A well-planned school curriculum, as developed in this textbook and its instructor resources (TEACH Lesson Plan Manual and instructor resources), combined with a comprehensive science curriculum as presented in *Mosby's Essential Sciences for Therapeutic Massage* and its various ancillaries, will teach the basics in a program of 500 to 1500 class hours. The education should be competency-based, meaning all information in the educational setting is relevant to the actual professional practice of therapeutic massage. The design of this textbook, combined with the extensive content on the companion DVDs and Evolve website, support various applications of distance learning in web-enhanced education.

Once students learn the fundamental core body of knowledge for all therapeutic massage and bodywork methods, the essential learning begins. The uniqueness of our profession is not dependent on the methods or the technical application of massage techniques. The massage therapy profession offers skilled, structured, and safe touch in a nurturing environment. This relationship joins people in a healing partnership. The final chapter in this book containing 20 case studies helps the student appreciate the complexities of a therapeutic relationship in a competency-based format.

Therapeutic massage is a labor-intensive therapy that requires time to perform, with an emphasis on ergonomics and correct body mechanics. The fourth edition has been expanded with this information, and the new content has been evaluated by an ergonomics expert.

Our knowledge base is unique. Other licensed healthcare professionals are often too busy to do this work. Our work can be effectively done at a paraprofessional level that is more cost-effective for the public. This is the special gift our profession has to give.

Licensed medical professionals need a standardized basis of training proficiency before they can routinely incorporate therapeutic massage into their team healing approaches. Currently, the medical community cannot trust the expertise level of the massage profession because of the divergence in educational standards. Although a program length of 500 to 1000 hours will prepare the graduate to work effectively in general applications of therapeutic massage to the general public outside the healthcare environment, this level of classroom instruction may not include enough pathology, medical terminology, evaluation skills, or specific application of methods to effectively support a medical healing team approach. Ontario and British Columbia, Canada, have developed therapeutic massage as part of the healthcare system. Their standards of education exceed 2200 class hours, equivalent to a typical associate's degree. Many medical technicians are trained at this level, and it is an accepted paradigm.

I believe that massage has the most to offer in the realm of general service for the public at large, such as found in the spa environment and wellness massage clinics, and paraprofessional support in the healthcare environment. In this fourth edition, content on all of these career tracks has been expanded, especially the information for professional practice in the spa industry.

I do not see the formal educational requirements increasing beyond this level unless the practitioner wishes to teach in some capacity. I believe that proprietary private education and highly focused community college programs best serve the needs of therapeutic massage education. I also believe that an increasing number of healthcare professionals will learn more about therapeutic massage so that they can work more effectively with the massage professional and provide knowledgeable supervision in the healthcare setting.

The level of knowledge in the fourth edition of this text has been increased to reflect the skills necessary to work effectively with supervision. Although my love for this profession lies in humble service to the general public in the support of their wellness and compassion and help for the daily aches and pains of life, I recognize the importance of being able to also work within the healthcare system. My work over the past several years with a clinical physiologist, numerous physicians, athletic trainers, and physical therapists supports this observation. Because of the development of comprehensive textbooks, more schools will be better able to expand their curricula for those who wish to pursue the more complex approach to therapeutic massage applications.

Schools that offer training programs of 500 to 1000 hours adequately prepare students for the general wellness personal service approach of therapeutic massage. Everyone can benefit from massage, not just those who are under medical care. This level of education is an entry-level point for those who wish to serve the general public and provide wellness and health-enhancing massage and bodywork. In my opinion, fewer than 500 class hours is insufficient time to cover the necessary body of knowledge to meet the emerging educational standards. I also believe that 500 class hours is barely sufficient to present the necessary information and allow adequate time for integration of the information. Programs of 1000 to 1500 hours as a standard more effectively serve the student and the profession as a whole.

TERMINOLOGY

Because the profession has not yet reached consensus on any one term used to describe the massage and bodywork professional, the following terms are all currently used: *massage therapist, massage practitioner, massage technician, bodyworker, touch therapist, bodywork practitioner, bodywork therapist, myomassologist, neuromuscular therapist,* and *massagist.* All these terms describe a person who uses structured touch of some type to create physiologic response in the client. The use of the terms *masseuse* and *masseur* are discouraged in the United States, although these terms are still used in other countries. As an educator of therapeutic massage, I prefer the terms *massage practitioner, massage therapist, massage professional,* and *massage technician.* These terms are used interchangeably throughout this text. Early chapters tend to use the words *massage technician* and *massage professional;* middle chapters tend to use the words *massage professional* and *massage practitioner;* and end chapters tend to use the words *massage therapist.* This shows how the progression of knowledge corresponds with professional development.

Therapeutic application of massage (structured touch) is not a new phenomenon. Very little of the information presented in this text is my original creation. The foundation for therapeutic massage was laid centuries ago and will not change as long as human physiology remains constant. It is virtually impossible to acknowledge everyone who has contributed to the knowledge base. Our observations of the natural world are a good starting point for this basic knowledge. For example, animals know the value of rhythmic touch. Just watch a litter of puppies and observe the structured application of touch. The base of information goes beyond us to an innate need to rub an area that is hurt and to touch others to provide comfort, pleasure, and bonding.

ORGANIZATION

Chapters 1 through 5 build the theory base and decision-making skills for the reader. Chapter 1 begins with an exploration of touch and builds to the historical foundations of massage. Chapter 2 introduces the clinical reasoning problem-solving model for ethical decision-making. It also covers professionalism and legal issues. Chapter 3 builds on Chapter 2 to teach readers how to develop effective record-keeping skills. Appropriate medical terminology is presented to support this process. Chapter 4 explains the scientific basis for therapeutic massage and research literacy, and Chapter 5 begins the process of decision-making in terms of indications and contraindications to massage. Chapters 6 through 8 present information concerning sanitation, hygiene, safety, body mechanics, massage equipment and supplies, positioning and draping procedures, various massage environments, and other information ancillary to a successful massage practice. Chapters 9 through 11 are the technical skills chapters. Each chapter builds on the previous one, beginning with the basics and expanding to therapeutic applications while providing an introduction to complementary bodywork systems. As the methods and techniques of therapeutic massage and bodywork are presented, the reader learns how and why they work and when to use them to obtain a particular physiologic response.

Content in these chapters includes palpation and differential assessment, lymphatic drainage massage, Asian and Eastern massage therapy and application, and conflict resolution. Specifically in Chapter 10, illustrations and text explain gait assessment procedures and muscle firing patterns, two important areas of concern to a massage therapist. This content increases students' assessment skills to prepare them for advanced-level learning.

Chapter 12 focuses on three main career tracks and on providing massage to particular populations, whereas Chapter 13 explores the issues of wellness and nutrition, which has been expanded for this edition. Chapter 14 discusses business considerations for a career in massage, and it has been completely revised for this edition to better reflect the skills needed for current trends in the business of massage.

Finally, Chapter 15 sets the stage for integration of all the material through the use of comprehensive case studies based on the clinical reasoning model and outcome-based massage and treatment plan development. Chapter 15 presents 20 original case studies that integrate the information from both this textbook and the student's science studies, such as the content covered in *Mosby's Essential Sciences for Therapeutic Massage*. The case studies cover at least 90% of the common conditions seen by massage professionals in day and destination spas, as well as in wellness, health, fitness, sport, and medical settings. If students study the process of clinical reasoning carefully, through these case examples they should be able to address almost all other conditions encountered in professional practice. The entire book focuses on developing clinical reasoning skills for this profession.

Helpful appendices are located at the end of the book. These include *Appendix A: Indications and Contraindications to Massage; Appendix B: Skin Pathology*; and *Appendix C: Basic Pharmacology for Massage*. These appendices provide at-a-glance information that is supplemental to the content within the chapters.

The text can be taught in a sequential manner, or the more technical chapters (6 through 11) can be presented simultaneously with Chapters 1 through 5, so that the student learns "hands-on skills" in conjunction with "head or thinking skills." Chapters 12 through 15 can then act as integration chapters to be presented after other chapters are covered. Many of the exercises provided throughout the text support introspection and self-understanding to encourage "heart" learning as well.

DISTINCTIVE FEATURES OF THIS BOOK

- The full-color presentation that was implemented in the second edition continues to greatly enhance the clarity of both the text and illustrations.
- Content within the book and the companion Evolve website is applicable to certification exam test questions.
- New overall design: The internal design corresponds directly with the internal design of *Mosby's Essential Sciences for Therapeutic Massage*, also written by Sandy Fritz, so that if you are using both books in your curriculum, it will be a smooth transition.
- Continues to support COMTA requirements: There is a trend in COMTA toward competency-based education, and this new edition continues to be highly focused on students achieving competency.
- Chapter 10: Assessment Procedures for Developing a Care Plan: This chapter increases students' assessment skills to prepare them for advanced-level learning.
- Chapter 15: Integration—Case Studies: The interactive case studies help the reader understand and apply concepts from the book, and this tool supports student-directed learning. If students study the process of clinical reasoning carefully, from these case examples they should be able to address almost all other conditions encountered in professional practice.

NEW TO THIS EDITION

- Brand new photos throughout! All photos throughout the book have been replaced.
- 2 new DVDs in the back of the book include 4 hours of video, including techniques, expanded body mechanics section, full body general protocol, case studies, and scientific animations.
- Replaced line art in Chapters 8 and 9 (Draping and Massage Manipulations and Techniques) with photos for a more realistic depiction of procedures.
- Addition of two full body massage General Protocols in full color photos, and one full body massage General Protocol in video on a DVD at the back of the book.

- Brand new pet massage section.
- Added insurance reimbursement information.
- Common Medications appendix revised, adding more on pharmacology.

UPDATED IN THIS EDITION

The fourth edition of this book has been extensively expanded and revised, using recommendations from many of my teaching colleagues, into an even more highly effective work-text format.

Content has been significantly increased in the following areas:

- Chapter 7, Body Mechanics, with the help of an ergonomics consultant.
- Chapter 11, Complementary Bodywork Systems: expanded content on shiatsu, Thai massage, hydrotherapy, thermotherapy (including stone massage), color therapy, and aromatherapy, with new full color photos to demonstrate the techniques.
- Chapter 12, Massage Career Tracks and Massage for Special Populations: A new section on spa applications and techniques, as well as increased sports massage and fitness and clinical massage content has been added to this edition. Spa, sports massage, and clinical massage content has been increasingly showing up on licensing and certification examinations in massage therapy, and they are also popular career possibilities for massage therapists upon graduation.
- Chapter 14, Business Considerations for a Career in Therapeutic Massage: completely re-worked to expand on professional skills necessary for both employer and employee career focus.
- Research literacy: moved from an appendix into Chapter 4 of the core text—providing updated research findings supporting massage and demonstrating how to read, understand, and conduct research.
- Chapter 13's nutrition and wellness content, in response to reviewer and market feedback.

Throughout every chapter, content has been upgraded to cover new educational method research and curriculum standards. The new content and upgrades coincide with the Commission on Massage Therapy Accreditation (COMTA) standards. Specifically, the case studies chapter, conflict management section, information on prenatal and postnatal massage techniques, and added content on research in Chapter 4, which aids the student in analyzing and using the research compiled by others, all comply with COMTA standards. This compliance prepares students for competency-based questions that are being incorporated into the certification examination.

LEARNING AIDS

The work-text format of this book is highly interactive and enables the reader to learn and understand the information presented more easily.

Proficiency Exercises and Think it Over exercises are provided to enhance the reader's learning experience. For many of these the reader is encouraged to answer directly in the book. Examples are often provided to help guide the student in processing the exercises.

In addition, Workbook Sections at the end of the chapter help readers test their knowledge through short answer questions, labeling exercises, and various other activities. Answers are provided at the back of the book for those questions that have correct answers. In other cases the student is asked to use the clinical reasoning model to develop an answer to a question. In these situations, no single correct answer exists. Competencies can be determined by the effective justification of the answer that the student develops in response to the exercise. For each chapter in the fourth edition, specific competency-based activities have been added.

Although all of the exercises and activities throughout the chapters and workbook sections are valuable, not all of them need to be completed by every student. In support of various learning styles, offering the students a choice among the various exercises is appropriate.

At the beginning of each chapter are chapter outlines, chapter objectives, and key terms.

Although complex terminology is defined within the body of the text, a specific massage glossary is included at the end of the book. Each discipline has its own language, and therapeutic massage is no exception. This common language facilitates effective communication within the field of therapeutic massage, as well as between massage practitioners and other disciplines.

ANCILLARIES

Two brand new DVDs, bound into the back of the book, contain more than 3 hours of video, including techniques, body mechanics, lymphatic drain examples, a full body General Protocol, and case studies that take the viewer from the pre-session interview through application of massage techniques on the table. Several scientific animations are also included that feature biologic functions and medical procedures for enhanced student learning. Each video clip and animation on the DVDs are referenced in the textbook through double-numbered DVD icons, directing the students to where they can find particular clips on the two DVDs. These DVDs are playable on both set-top DVD players and in PCs and MACs with DVD drives.

ONLINE RESOURCES

The Evolve website that supports this text is extensive, with additional learning activities listed at the end of each chapter in a special box after the summary. Activity resources include certification and licensure exam review questions, critical thinking questions, mini image collections, electronic flashcards, computer-simulated programs to build business cards and resumes, drag 'n' drop labeling exercises, and crossword puzzles.

evolve

2-1 Electronic flashcards for key terms in this chapter aid in information retention.

2-2 Complete an ethical behavior matching exercise.

NOTE TO THE STUDENT

As the author, my intent is to make reading this textbook an enjoyable learning experience; I hope my purpose is reflected in the personal, conversational tone in which I have written the text. My personal conviction is that *Mosby's Fundamentals of Therapeutic Massage* effectively presents the information and reflects both the heart and the art of therapeutic massage. After all, no one cares how much you know until they know how much you care.

Sandy Fritz

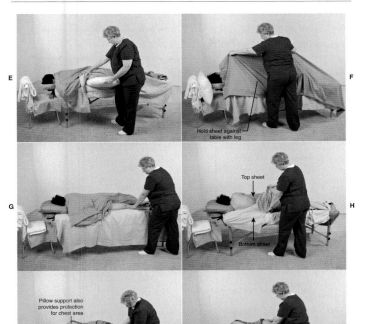

E
F
Hold sheet against table with leg

G
Top sheet
H
Bottom sheet

Pillow support also provides protection for chest area
I
Bolster under bottom sheet
J

FIGURE 8-13, cont'd **E,** Preparation to place client in the side-lying position: re to allow client to roll. **G,** Side-lying: Draping for leg. **H,** Side-lying: Draping for back. U **I,** Side-lying: Draping for leg. **J,** Move drape to provide access to upper thigh and glu

- ■ All new **photos** are high quality and in full color to add visual impact and reinforcement of concepts.

- ■ **Outlines** and **Objectives** at the beginning of each chapter help students organize their study material.

- ■ **Key Terms** are identified at the beginning of each chapter, and bolded throughout the text.

CHAPTER **8**

Preparation for Massage:
Equipment, Supplies, Professional Environment, Positioning, and Draping

■ **CHAPTER OBJECTIVES**

After completing this chapter, the student will be able to perform the following:

- Construct a massage setting in different types of environments
- List the equipment, supplies, and setup procedures required to prepare for a massage session
- Explain massage procedures to a client
- Effectively drape and position a client

■ **CHAPTER OUTLINE**

EQUIPMENT
  Care of the Massage Practitioner's Hands and Body
  The Massage Table
  The Massage Chair
  The Massage Mat
  Body Supports
  Draping Materials
  Lubricants
  Additional Equipment
THE MASSAGE ENVIRONMENT
  General Conditions
  A Typical Massage Room, Home Office, or Clinical
    Setting
DETERMINING A NEW CLIENT'S EXPECTATIONS
FEEDBACK
  Client Feedback
  Practitioner Feedback
  Client Conversation
GENDER CONCERNS
PREMASSAGE PROCEDURES
  Orientation Process
  Focus/Centering
POSITIONING AND DRAPING THE CLIENT
  Positioning
  Draping

AFTER THE MASSAGE
  Helping the Client off the Massage Table
  Closing the Session, Collecting the Fee, and Making the
    Next Appointment
SUMMARY

■ **KEY TERMS**

Body supports
Draping
Draping material
Feedback
Focus/centering
Lubricants
Massage chair
Massage mat
Massage table
Positioning

The massage practitioner must make certain preparations before beginning the massage. The room must be set up, and all necessary supplies must be gathered. The type of lubricant used and how it is dispensed, the temperature of the massage room, and the warmth of the practitioner's hands are all considerations. Massage professionals benefit from developing a method, referred to as *centering*, to help them focus on the client and the session to come. Client positioning and modest, appropriate draping procedures also must be considered. The practitioner then uses history taking and assessment procedures to identify client outcomes and to formulate the approach for the massage. The plan is discussed with the client, and informed consent is obtained. All this is done before the massage begins. This chapter is designed to help the student develop these important premassage

249

- **Workbook sections** at the end of each chapter encourage critical thinking through short answers, fill-in-the-blank questions, matching and labelling exercises, and more.

- Three **appendices** conclude the book with valuable resources for the student.

- **Glossary of terms** in the back of the book provides a quick reference for the terms that appear throughout the textbook.

357

Workbook Section

Answers for the Workbook Section for Chapter 9 are provided on p. 767.

■■■ SHORT ANSWER

1. What are the three effects that massage methods and techniques have on the body? Explain each one.

2. Which massage methods seem more mechanical?

3. Which methods seem more reflexive?

4. What are the seven aspects of quality of touch?

5. What is the importance of varying the quality of touch with regard to speed, rate, rhythm, and duration?

6. Why do you think that similar trends, applications, and methods continue to make up the body of knowledge of therapeutic massage?

10. What is the distinguishing characteristic of gliding?

11. Why should deeper applications of gliding always move slowly?

12. What are some specific uses of the gliding massage manipulation?

13. What are the distinguishing qualities of kneading?

14. Why should the massage professional use kneading sparingly?

15. What conditions interfere with the use of kneading?

16. What are the physiologic effects of compression?

17. What are some things massage practitioners should remember to protect their hands and arms while doing compression?

18. Where are the best anatomic locations to do vibration? Why?

APPENDIX C

Basic Pharmacology for the Massage Therapist

OVERVIEW*

Any chemical that affects the physiologic processes of a living organism can broadly be defined as a drug. The study or science of drugs is known as pharmacology. Pharmacology encompasses a variety of topics, including the following:

- Absorption
- Biochemical effects
- Biotransformation (metabolism)
- Distribution
- Drug history
- Drug origin
- Excretion
- Mechanisms of action
- Physical and chemical properties
- Physical effects
- Drug receptor mechanisms
- Therapeutic (beneficial) effects
- Toxic (harmful) effects

Pharmacology is an extensive science that incorporates several interrelated areas: pharmaceutics, pharmacokinetics, pharmacodynamics, pharmacotherapeutics, pharmacognosy, and toxicology. The various drugs discussed in each chapter of this text are described from the standpoint of one or more of these five areas.

Throughout the process of development, a drug will acquire at least three different names. The chemical name describes the drug's chemical composition and molecular structure. The generic name, or nonproprietary name, is given to the drug by the United States Adopted Names (USAN) Council. It is often much shorter and simpler than the chemical name. The generic name is used in most official drug compendiums to list drugs. The trade name, or proprietary name, is the drug's registered trademark and indicates that its commercial use is restricted to the owner of the patent for the drug. The owner is usually the manufacturer of the drug. Trade names are generally created by the manufacturer with marketability in mind. For this reason, they are usually shorter and easier to pronounce and remember than generic drug names. The patent life of a newly discovered drug molecule is normally 17 years. This is the length of time from patent approval until patent expiration. Because the research processes for new drug development normally require about 10 years, a drug manufacturer generally has the remaining 7 years for sales profits before patent expiration. A significant amount of these profits serves merely to offset the

multimillion-dollar costs for research and development of the drug.

After the patent expires for a given drug, other manufacturers may legally begin to manufacturer generic drugs with the same active ingredient. At this point, the drug price usually falls substantially, which offers many patients and third-party payers the benefit of savings on the generic (vs. the original brand name) drug.

Three basic areas of pharmacology—pharmaceutics, pharmacokinetics, and pharmacodynamics—describe the relationship between the dose of a drug given to a patient and the activity of that drug in treating the patient's disorder. Pharmaceutics includes the study of how various dosage forms (e.g., injection, capsule, controlled-release tablet) influence the way in which...

748

GLOSSARY

Abbreviation: Shortened forms of words or phrases.

Abuse: Exploitation, misuse, mistreatment, molestation, neglect.

Acquired immunodeficiency syndrome (AIDS): A dysfunction in the body's immune system, which defends the body against disease.

Active assisted movement: Movement of a joint in which both the client and the therapist produce the motion.

Active joint movement: Movement of a joint through its range of motion by the client.

Active range of motion: Movement of a joint by the client without any type of assistance from the massage practitioner.

Active resistive movement: Movement of a joint by the client against resistance provided by the therapist.

Acupressure: Methods used to tone or sedate acupuncture points without the use of needles.

Acupuncture point: Asian term for a specific point that correlates with a neurologic motor point.

Acute: A term that describes a condition in which the signs and symptoms develop quickly, last a short time, and then disappear.

Acute illness: A short-term illness that resolves by means of the normal healing process and, if necessary, supportive medical care.

Acute pain: A symptom of a disease condition or a temporary aspect of medical treatment. Acute pain acts as a warning signal because it can activate the sympathetic nervous system. It usually is temporary, of sudden onset, and easily localized. The client frequently can describe the pain, which often subsides without treatment.

Adaptation: A response to a sensory stimulation in which nerve signaling is reduced or ceases.

Aerobic exercise training: An exercise program focused to increase fitness and endurance.

Allied health: A division of medicine in which the professional receives training in a specific area of medicine to serve as support for the physician.

Anatomic barriers: Anatomic structures determined by the shape and fit of the bones at the joint.

Antagonism: Occurs when massage produces the opposite effect, such as with medications.

Antagonists: The muscles that oppose the movement of the prime movers.

occur passively with movement of the joint and are not under voluntary control.

Aseptic technique: Procedures that kill or disable pathogens on surfaces to prevent transmission.

Asian approaches: Methods of bodywork that have developed from ancient Chinese methods.

Assessment: The collection and interpretation of information provided by the client, the client's family and friends, the massage practitioner, and referring medical professionals.

Asymmetric stance: The position in which the body weight is shifted from one foot to the other while standing.

Athlete: A person who participates in sports as an amateur or a professional. Athletes require precise use of their bodies.

Autonomic nervous system: The body system that regulates involuntary body functions using the sympathetic "fight-flight-fear response" and the restorative parasympathetic "relaxation response." The sympathetic and parasympathetic systems work together to maintain homeostasis through a feedback loop system.

Autoregulation: Control of homeostasis through alteration of tissue or function.

Ayurveda: A system of health and medicine that grew from East Indian roots.

Bacteria: Primitive cells that have no nuclei. Bacteria cause disease by secreting toxic substances that damage human tissues, by becoming parasites inside human cells, or by forming colonies in the body that disrupt normal function.

Balance point: The point of contact between the practitioner and client.

Beating: A form of heavy tapotement involving use of the fist.

Bending forces: A combination of compression and tension. One side of a structure is exposed to compressive forces, while the other side is exposed to tensile forces.

Benign: A term that describes the type of tumor that remains localized within the tissue from which it arose and does not undergo malignant changes. Benign tumors usually grow very slowly.

Body mechanics: Use of the body in an efficient and biomechanically correct way.

Body/mind: The interaction between thought and physiology that is connected to the limbic system, hypothalamic influence on the autonomic nervous system, and the endocrine system.

EHNANCED LEARNING EXPERIENCE

FIGURE 1-5 Diversity in massage therapy.

FIGURE 1-6 A bright future: the teaching of the next generation.

wellness massage are becoming commonplace, as are massage professionals in the corporate setting.

Research into genetics, stress responses, neuroendocrine influences, and environmental hazards, as well as support for the whole person in coping with a world that seems to be moving too fast, encourages the development of massage as a counterbalance to a stressful lifestyle, stressful world events, and a persistent state of ambiguity that promotes anxiety states. The current trends supported by research seem to indicate that manual therapies are gaining recognition. Dr. Field of the Touch Research Institute is a major contributor to the growth of massage therapy because of her dedication to touch research.

As the world becomes a global community, the ever-increasing exchange of information will enrich the knowledge base of therapeutic massage. Exploration of ancient healing methods will reveal the wisdom and scientific validity of a body/mind/spirit approach to well-being.

Hopefully, the abundant massage and bodywork methods will combine into a consolidated system of therapeutic massage without losing the rich diversity of professional expression. Terminology and education will standardize, although the integrity of the individual applications of massage and body-work will be maintained. Two tracks of massage service probably will standardize: wellness massage outside the health care system and medical massage within the health care system. These trends will allow easy access for all to both types of services.

The future is very bright and promising, especially if we pay attention to our past and remember the words and wisdom of an old Russian physician, who says, "massage is massage." We ourselves constitute one of the biggest threats to the future of massage. All bodywork professions must come together to work for the common good. As the massage profession moves forward and reclaims its heritage as an important health service, it is important to look back. In retrospect, we can see

It also is important to honor those who have dedicated so much of their lives to developing the body of knowledge of therapeutic massage. Many today are dedicating a significant portion of their lives to the professional advancement of therapeutic massage. When the history of massage is written in the future, these names will appear with the information they have organized and contributed. We are all contributors to the future of massage, and we all will become part of its history.

THINK IT OVER

- What do you want the future of massage to bring?
- How are you going to assist in the development of that future?

■■■ SUMMARY

This chapter began with questions and ended with questions. The importance and nature of touch in the professional setting were discussed. The reader should now be aware of the ways in which culture, gender, age, life events, spirituality, and diversity all influence the experience of touching and being touched. Inappropriate forms of touch were identified, and appropriate forms of professional touch were explored. An understanding of the subjective experience of touch was addressed personally.

The history of massage from ancient times to the present presented, as were projections for the future. A time line lighted many key dates. The foundation has been laid study of therapeutic massage.

evolve

1-1 Explore the Evolve Web site that accompanies this book.
1-2 Complete an interactive order exercise by placing massage historical events on a timeline.
1-3 Answer true or false for a list of appropriate or inappropriate touching examples.

Don't forget to study for your certification and licensure exams! Review questions for this chap

---

Wellness Education **CHA**

PROFICIENCY EXERCISE 13-14

During a learning experience, one or two people may emerge who teach us more than we expected to learn. Often the learning has nothing to do with the courses we are studying. This is a love sharing. Go to those who have shared their love with you and say "Thank you."

■■■ SUMMARY

Wellness comprises more than the components discussed in this chapter. Wellness is living life in a simple, gentle, respectful way for ourselves, with others, and in the environment. Wellness is the result of the healing that takes place on multiple levels when we take care of ourselves, which then extends to caring for others and the planet in general. A competent massage professional practices self-care and educates clients about the basic components of wellness. This chapter has addressed methods for managing the physical, emotional, and spiritual stress in our lives.

Someone once said, "When half the world is receiving a massage and the other half is giving a massage, we shall have peace." Wellness is peace within and sharing that peace in simple ways. Sharing this peace consistently with respect and compassion can support the wellness of us all, and with faith, hope, and love provide peace for our world.

evolve

13-1 Additional wellness and nutritional available on the Evolve Web site.
13-2 Find comprehensive vitamin and the Evolve Web site.

Don't forget to study for your certi licensure exams! Review question are located on Evolve.

REFERENCES

1. Chaitow L: *The body/mind purification prog* Fireside.
2. Selye H: *The stress of life*, ed 2, New York,
3. Kisner C, Colby LA: *Therapeutic exercise: niques*, ed 5, Philadelphia, 2007, FA Davis.
4. Lippert L: *Clinical kinesiology and anatomy* 2006, The Author.

- **Think it Over** boxes add interest and reinforce the relevance of the material.

- **Proficiency Exercises** review material within the chapters as you work through the textbook.

- **General Protocol Photo Atlas** gives students a go-to resource when learning how to provide a comprehensive massage for clients.

GENERAL MASSAGE PROTOCOL—cont'd

3. Glide on back. Vary speed, drag, and depth of pressure.

4. Shift position. Glide/compress.

5. Knead.

6. Move underwear.

7. Glide lumbar and gluteal region.

8. Compression to gluteal area.

ELECTRONIC SUPPORT

- Two **bind-in DVDs,** one at the front of the book, and one at the back of the book, include video clips, scientific animations, and case studies, all referenced within the textbook by DVD icons.

- Special features of the **Evolve website** include brochure, business card, and resume writing activities, certification and licensure exam review questions, critical thinking questions following case studies, drag 'n' drop labelling exercises, categorizing and matching activities, and more!

MOSBY'S FUNDAMENTALS
OF THERAPEUTIC MASSAGE

→ **Chapter 3**
Medical Terminology for Professional Record Keeping

Chapter 9
Massage Manipulations and Techniques

Chapter 15
Case Studies

FRITZ

PROFICIENCY EXERCISE 13-14

During a learning experience, one or two people may emerge who teach us more than we expected to learn. Often the learning has nothing to do with the courses we are studying. This is a love sharing. Go to those who have shared their love with you and say "Thank you."

SUMMARY

Wellness comprises more than the components discussed in this chapter. Wellness is living life in a simple, gentle, respectful way for ourselves, with others, and in the environment. Wellness is the result of the healing that takes place on multiple levels when we take care of ourselves, which then extends to caring for others and the planet in general. A competent massage professional practices self-care and educates clients about the basic components of wellness. This chapter has addressed methods for managing the physical, emotional, and spiritual stress in our lives.

Someone once said, "When half the world is receiving a massage and the other half is giving a massage, we shall have peace." Wellness is peace within and sharing that peace in simple ways. Sharing this peace consistently with respect and compassion can support the wellness of us all, and with faith, hope, and love provide peace for our world.

evolve

13-1 Additional wellness and nutritional guidelines are available on the Evolve Web site.

13-2 Find comprehensive vitamin and mineral charts on the Evolve Web site.

Don't forget to study for your certification and licensure exams! Review questions for this chapter are located on Evolve.

REFERENCES

1. Chaitow L: *The body/mind purification program*, New York, 1991, Fireside.
2. Selye H: *The stress of life*, ed 2, New York, 1978, McGraw-Hill.
3. Kisner C, Colby LA: *Therapeutic exercise: foundations and techniques*, ed 5, Philadelphia, 2007, FA Davis.
4. Lippert L: *Clinical kinesiology and anatomy*, ed 4, Portland, Ore, 2006, The Author.

Acknowledgments

My thanks to the following professionals who have influenced the content and clarity of this text to ensure the accurate presentation of information:

  Patricia J. Benjamin, PhD
  Leon K. Chaitow, ND, DO
  Emily Edith Safrona Cowall, Reg MT
  Karen Craig, LMT, NCTMB
  Peter A. Goldberg, DIPL AC (NCCA), LMT
  Lucy Liben, MS, LMT
  Jean E. Loving, BA, LMT
  Karen B. Napolitano, MS
  Kathleen Maison Paholsky, MS, PhD
  Cherie Marilyn Sohnen-Moe, BA
  Mary Margaret Tuchscherer, DC, PhD
  Richard van Why
  Sherri Williamson, LMT
  Ed Wilson, PhD, LMT

In addition to these people, there are several people who also deserve special recognition for their efforts in the publication and promotion of the first, second, and third editions:

  Don O'Connor and Beverley Ransom for their terrific artwork.

  Jim Visser, for the incredible photos and for his energy and enthusiasm during the photo shoots.

  Chuck LeRoi and Chris Roider, for a perfect video shoot and editing process.

And a special thank you to:

  All of the individuals on my support team at Elsevier—especially Kellie White, Jennifer Watrous, April Falast, Linda Duncan, Rich Barber, Teresa McBryan, Kim Wingett, and Julie Burchett.

  My staff, Roxanne, Dianne and the kids, and Dennis, who put up with me during this revision, and to Amy, my assistant, who worked so hard, but even more important, can read my writing.

  The athletes I work with for constantly challenging me to figure out what to do with all of their assorted bumps, bruises, sprains, strains, breaks, performance stresses, and personalities.

  The Detroit Lions organization supporting the educational partnership with Health Enrichment Center, the University of Michigan Athletic Department, the VA Hospital in Detroit, Michigan, and all of the veterans there, and all of the residents and staff at Hospice.

  Kelly Challis for her great assistance on the material for the spa environment; Michael McPharlin, BSN, NCBTMB, for his review of the muscle firing patterns; and Ed Mohr, for his excellent consulting work on body mechanics. Glen Hymel and his wonderful work and research and its importance to the massage profession. Dr. Leon Chaitow for being my teacher, mentor, and supportive friend.

  It truly has been a team effort.

Contents

Detailed Contents

Foundations of Therapeutic Applications of Touch

CHAPTER OBJECTIVES

After completing this chapter, the student will be able to perform the following:

- Describe professional touch
- Identify personal interpretations of touch and their influence on professional interactions
- Explain the rich heritage and history of therapeutic massage
- Explain the influence of historical events on the current development of therapeutic massage

CHAPTER OUTLINE

PROFESSIONAL TOUCH
Touch
Touch as Communication
Professional Classifications of Touch
Touch Intention During Massage
The Uniqueness of Touch
HISTORICAL PERSPECTIVES
The History of Massage
Recent Trends
The Future of Massage: 2008 and Beyond
SUMMARY

KEY TERMS

Culture
Expressive touch
Healing
Mechanical touch
Occupation
Patterns
Profession
Professional
Professional touch
Professionalism
Service
System
Therapeutic applications
Touch technique

E ducation is just as much about asking questions as it is about seeking answers. Consider the possibility that information dispensed during an educational process, coupled with the ability to formulate insightful and productive questions, gives students the opportunity to make thoughtful decisions. Are decisions answers? Do answers come from thoughtful situational decisions? Are answers the truth? Some questions seem to have easy answers. For example, "What is the color of grass?" Quickly we jump to the answer "green," but is that always the answer? Because many questions have several answers, the truth can be difficult to determine. In what way is the professional application of touch influenced by the practitioner's ability to make thoughtful decisions and to find answers that best serve the situation at a particular moment?

In massage, which is professional, structured, therapeutic touch, education begins with questions: What is the significance of touch? What is professional touch? What motivates me to study therapeutic massage? What is therapeutic? How am I served by touching others? How do the connections with others created through touch influence the professional practice of therapeutic massage? When did touch become professional? Why did touch become professional? Do therapeutic forms of touch have to be provided by a professional? In what way is professional therapeutic touch different from casual touch, friendship touch, family touch, intimate touch, or erotic (sexual) touch? How do different individuals, social groups, or cultures view touch? In what way does the past affect the present and provide guidance for the future development of the profession of massage therapy? Questions continue to arise, and the answers are not necessarily simple.

As we seek to serve our clients, eventually we are faced with these questions and many others. Some of the questions mentioned previously are explored in this text, especially as they relate to the professional practice of therapeutic massage. Some are not explored directly; rather, both the questions and the answers evolve for each student as the individual's information base and experience increase and the journey through education continues. This text does not provide definitive answers to any of these questions, but it does provide information to help you find your own answers to questions you may face. What will your questions be? How will your answers influence those you touch? How will your answers touch you?

These are huge issues to consider at the beginning of any course of study. As you begin to think about them, you might feel interested, excited, overwhelmed, or maybe even frightened as you come to realize how necessary, beneficial, complex, and powerful touch can be. Remember that understanding evolves. These important questions are posed at the beginning of this study and possibly before you have sufficient information to develop effective answers. Your awareness of these questions during your course of study will help you make decisions and find answers as you progress in your study of therapeutic massage. You will come to understand the process of developing your answers to the previously mentioned questions and many others that will arise by embracing the importance of respect—for yourself and for all those with whom you interact, both personally and professionally (Proficiency Exercise 1-1).

PROFESSIONAL TOUCH

SECTION OBJECTIVES

Using the information presented in this section, the student will be able to perform the following:

- Distinguish between professional and nonprofessional forms of touch
- List factors that influence the communication of touch
- Identify factors that constitute appropriate and inappropriate touch in the professional setting

Dictionaries define a **profession** as an **occupation** requiring training and specialized study. An *occupation* can be defined

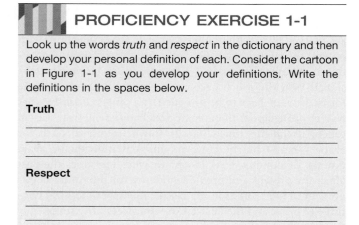

POT-SHOTS NO. 855.
Ashleigh Brilliant

History records no more gallant struggle than that of humanity against the truth.

©BRILLIANT ENTERPRISES 1975.

FIGURE 1-1 Pot-Shots. (Courtesy Ashleigh Brilliant, Santa Barbara, Calif.)

as a productive or creative activity that serves as one's regular source of livelihood. A **professional** is a person who engages in a profession. **Professionalism** is the adherence to professional status, methods, standards, and character (this idea of professionalism is explored further in Chapter 2 in the discussion on ethics).

To understand the concept of professional touch, we look at specialized training that allows a person to provide a service to another. Professionals may sell a product, but a profession usually is built around a skilled ability to provide a service, such as therapeutic massage. A **service** is something done for another that results in a specific outcome; for example, the car is fixed, the garden is tended, communication skills are taught, emotional problems are sorted out, changes are perceived in an unpleasant physical sensation, bodily functions are restored, and spiritual or life paths are discovered. In return, income (livelihood) is received for that service.

When a professional relationship exists, certain agreed-upon criteria apply. The person providing the service is skilled (educated) and operates within certain standards of practice, including technical application and ethical conduct. **Professional touch**, then, is skilled touch delivered to achieve a specific outcome, and the recipient in some way reimburses the professional for services rendered.

The aspect of skilled or schooled touch leads to the idea of structured touch. Professional touch is not random, but purposeful. It is organized according to systems and patterns. A **system** is a group of interacting elements that functions as a complex whole. Professional touch, such as that provided by a massage practitioner, requires education in the many systems of the body; the application of massage and other forms of soft tissue methodology; and an understanding of the influence of massage on body systems. Communication and interpersonal skills, including systems of social and cultural interaction, also are part of the education of the therapeutic massage professional.

Patterns are created by the replication of structures or functions that intertwine and influence each other. Patterns can be identified if we can see a big enough picture. The pattern may be missed if the focus is too small. For example, muscle tension can be identified in an individual muscle of

PROFICIENCY EXERCISE 1-1

Look up the words *truth* and *respect* in the dictionary and then develop your personal definition of each. Consider the cartoon in Figure 1-1 as you develop your definitions. Write the definitions in the spaces below.

Truth

_____

_____

_____

Respect

_____

_____

_____

the arm, or it can be seen as part of an interacting pattern of movement during walking. The ability to see both the individual segments or pieces, as well as the ways the pieces interact in patterns, is a necessary skill for the individual application of professional touch.

Inherent in the understanding of skilled and structured touch is the idea of therapeutic application of touch. The term **therapeutic applications** pertains to healing or curative powers. Something that is therapeutic provides the structure for beneficial change or support for current healing practices. A walk in the woods or a conversation with a compassionate friend can be therapeutic, just as are the application of various bodywork modalities, medical and mental health practices, and empowering spiritual rituals. **Healing** is the restoration of well-being, and therapeutic applications promote a healing environment.

Touch

Before discussing the historical perspectives of therapeutic massage (professional, structured, therapeutic touch), we need to consider the nature of touch so as to understand the role of professional touch and the evolution of therapeutic massage throughout history. It is important to look at the idea of professionalism in the physical, emotional, social, cultural, and, in some instances, spiritual dimensions of touch. The roots of the word *massage* (Box 1-1) concern touch and the various applications of touch. It is important to explore the ideas behind the structure of touch. We must differentiate the therapeutic value of touch in the professional sense from forms of touch shared between people in life circumstances outside the professional environment. These themes are expanded upon throughout this chapter, and in some instances the information is further developed in future chapters.

The Science of Touch

Anatomically and physiologically, touch is the collection of tactile sensations that arise from sensory stimulation, primarily of the skin but also of deeper structures of the body, such as the muscles.

The skin is an amazing organ. It has many functions, but the most notable one for this discussion is its function in touch. The skin is the largest sensory organ of the body. From the outside we are always touched first on our skin, and in many ways, through the skin, we touch ourselves from the inside. Many internal somatic soft tissue structures (e.g.,

muscles, connective tissue) and visceral structures (e.g., the lungs, heart, and digestive organs) project sensation to the skin (see Chapter 5 for a discussion of viscerally referred pain patterns). The autonomic nervous system (Chapter 3), which regulates the visceral and chemical homeostasis of the body, is highly responsive to skin stimulation in support of well-being. Mood (the way a person feels) often is reflected in the skin as we touch ourselves from the inside. We blush with embarrassment, flush with excitement, or grow pale with fear.

The anatomy of the skin is described in most comprehensive anatomy texts.* The anatomic parts that make up the skin—the epidermis (top layer), the dermis (inner layer), and the interlacing connective tissues of these layers—and the massive network of nerves both receive and relay information from the central nervous system. This vast network combines with the rich complex of circulatory vessels that supply the skin. Yet, even in their complexity, the anatomy and physiology of the skin cannot explain the experience of touch. In some way, the pressure, vibration, temperature, and muscle motion that move the skin enliven us with sensations and experiences of pleasure, connectedness, joy, pain, sadness, longing, and satisfaction.

We must be touched to survive. Touch is a hunger that must be fed; it is the very essence of our survival, not simply a matter of well-being. The importance of touch has been well described in the books of Ashley Montagu, particularly *Touching: The Human Significance of the Skin,* which is recommended reading for all students of therapeutic massage. Dr. Tiffany Field conducts scientific research on touch at the Touch Research Institute at the University of Miami's Miller School of Medicine, and additional research has been done at various locations (see Chapter 4). Initially much of this research was devoted to infant development, primarily in premature babies. However, Dr. Field has greatly expanded our understanding of the importance of touch by studying many different groups of people, including infants, elderly people, people currently well but under stress, and very ill people. Research supports the belief that touching in a structured way is a very important if not absolute need of all living beings.

Scientific study and technology have enabled us to describe some of the physiologic responses to touch, such as changes in the concentration of hormones, alterations in the activity of the central and peripheral nervous systems, and regulation of body rhythms (these mechanisms are discussed more extensively in later chapters). However, even this explosion of information falls short in helping us understand the experience of touch. For all its scientific interpretations, the experience of touch is much more than the sum of its parts.

The Experience of Touch

Touch often is the concrete experience of more abstract sensations. For example, something that can be seen may not necessarily be real, as is the case when watching a movie, but when

---

BOX 1-1

How Massage Got Its Name

The word *massage* is thought to be derived from several sources. The Latin root *massa* and the Greek roots *massein* and *masso* mean "to touch, handle, squeeze, or knead." The French verb *masser* also means "to knead." The Arabic root *mass* or *mass'h* and the Sanskrit root *makeh* translate as "to press softly."

---

*Further study of the anatomy and physiology of the skin is included in *Mosby's Essential Sciences for Therapeutic Massage* (Mosby, 2008), by Sandy Fritz.

something can be touched, it is tangible. When the first edition of this text was written, I certainly touched all the reference books and the keyboard of the computer, but these were not the book. Even the finished manuscript that I sent away to the publisher did not feel real to me. Not until I received the first copy of the text and held it in my hands, felt the size and weight of it, and experienced the pages turning between my fingers, did the experience become real to me.

It is the same when I am touched or when I touch someone. I can listen to clients tell me their history, and I can observe during a physical assessment, but it is not until I touch the client and feel the person that I begin to understand that individual's body. In a reciprocal sense, when I lay my hands on a person's body, the understanding that I, as the practitioner, have received from the client is conveyed back to the client. Touch is a fundamental, multilayered, and powerful form of communication. It is the most personalized form of communication we know.

Touch as Communication

Touch in many ways is a more emotionally powerful form of communication than speech. Verbal communication uses specific words with specific meanings to relay a message. Touch communication is more ambiguous, relying on interpretation of its meaning through past experience and current circumstances. Delivering a clear, concise verbal message is difficult enough when both parties—the one delivering the message and the one receiving it—agree on the meaning of the words. How much more challenging it is to deliver a touch message, in which many factors are involved in the interpretation of the message. The potential for misunderstanding increases. Often, with both verbal and touch communication, the message intended is not the one received.

The communication of touch is influenced by personal, family, and cultural contexts. Each person defines an area around himself or herself as personal space, and the distance encompassed by this personal space differs from person to person and culture to culture. Therapies of touch enter this personal space, therefore the professional must be sensitive to the various factors that influence people's responses when their personal space is entered. Understanding each person's culture and subculture, personal experiences in that culture, and genetically predetermined tendency to have a large or a small amount of personal space often becomes mind-boggling in designing individual interactions of touch.

Cultural Influences

A culture is defined by the arts, beliefs, customs, institutions, and all other products of human work and thought created by a specific group of people at a particular time. It is stereotypical to say that people of a certain culture act a certain way; individuals always vary. Yet, tendencies can be defined by culture, and this may provide a way at least to begin initial touch interaction, until the person's uniqueness is better understood.

Exploring the vast diversity of cultural norms and traditions is beyond the scope of this text. However, you, as a professional, are responsible for developing an understanding of the social, cultural, and spiritual ways of the client population you serve (Figure 1-2). You can do this by doing research at the library about a particular culture or by taking a class. In your practice, observe how clients act and model from them (follow the client's lead). Ask questions and let your clients teach you about themselves and their culture.

The following personal experience demonstrates one of the ways people can teach you about their culture.

After a lecture I had given, a group of people came up to greet me and ask questions. By nature and through years of conditioning in professional practice, when someone approaches me, I reach out to take the person's hand or touch the individual's shoulder. A gentleman approached, and I offered my hand, but he crossed his hands over his chest and nodded slightly. I reached out to touch his arm, and at that moment, he very gently became my teacher. He backed away just a bit and said, "In my country this is how we greet a woman with respect," and he again crossed his arms over his chest and nodded slightly. So I asked, "How would I respond in your country?" He replied, "You would nod back and then avert your gaze so you do not look me directly in the eyes." I asked the reason for averting my eyes, and he gently explained that touching with one's eyes is a very sacred act and not for casual contact. A meeting of the eyes is a meeting of the souls. He again crossed his arms over his chest and nodded, and I nodded in return and then turned my gaze just below his eyes. It was a very poignant moment for me.

Gender Issues

My experience in greeting the gentleman from another country points out not only cultural but also gender issues in touch. Women and men may have different concepts of the appropriateness of touch. The patterns of gender custom in touch are complex. Biology, survival behaviors, social learning, and cultural customs are some of the influences that affect the development of these patterns.

For example, women generally require a somewhat smaller and more permeable personal space for comfort. Until recently, childrearing was the responsibility primarily of women, and child care requires caregivers to enter another's personal space or allow someone to enter theirs without restriction. Men, in general, establish territories with distant boundaries. Personal space is entered by invitation, because the territory must be protected. A man's personal space often is larger and more structured, involving rules for behavior.

Although these gender trends can be viewed from biologic and survival behavior perspectives, the patterns do not necessarily hold true when cultural customs or other influences that affect gender roles or behavior patterns are factored into the equation. It is stereotypical to state that women always act this way, and men always act that way; it simply is not true. Diversity of expression will forever exist within biologic influences and the cultural or gender rules of behavior.

The Influence of Age on Touch

Age differences can be a factor in the interpretation of touch. Some may consider touching very young people appropriate

FIGURE 1-2 The beauty of diversity.

but may be more cautious about touching older people. A younger person touching an elder may be acceptable, yet when two people of the same age touch, the dynamics are different. The touch of a young practitioner may be interpreted differently from the touch of an older practitioner, even if the skill and experience levels are equivalent.

The Influence of Life Events and the Interpretation of Touch

Life events can influence the response to touch experiences. People who have undergone painful and extensive medical interventions, especially at a young age, may process touch differently from what might be expected. People who have experienced touch trauma are influenced by those events, and individuals who have experienced isolation respond uniquely to touch. People who grew up with excessive touch stimulation outside the context of trauma (e.g., being part of a large family in small living quarters or being an only child with many adoring family members) may develop certain touch responses. Having a healthy, appropriate touch history also influences a person's interpretation of touch. Any of these experiences and many more not listed affect the way in which a person understands another's experience of touch.

Spiritual Touch

Touch also can have a spiritual context. Many spiritual rituals incorporate touch, especially those that involve concepts of healing of the body (that which is organic), the mind (that which is of thought), or the spirit (that which is transcendent and sacred). Each person deserves respect for his or her personal truth and individual spiritual path.

Diversity and Touch

Generalities are useless in discussing cultural orientations to touch, and it is stereotypical to imply that all people from a specific culture hold to similar customs. The same difficulties with stereotyping occur with regard to gender, age, and life or spiritual path. Gender and age probably influence the interpretation of professional touch, but in just what way varies considerably.

On any given day or even at any given moment, the need, desire, interpretation, and appropriateness of touch given and received can change. These changes occur because a person is in a constant state of flux in responding and adapting to encountered events. The type of relationship between people and its duration influence touch. For example, a first-time client may not be receptive to the deeper pressure required in some applications of massage, especially if the goal of the session does not indicate this type of work. However, if that same client, 12 sessions later, is experiencing a tight muscle pattern in the back, he may be responsive to touch in that particular form. A client may be ticklish to light touch initially in the session, but after she relaxes somewhat, she may find light stroking pleasurable.

A person's response to and need for the delivery of touch cannot be predetermined. However, each individual, including you, has been influenced by many factors regarding the appropriate procedure for touch and ultimately the interpretation of the meaning of a touch.

As professionals, it is important that we be aware, sensitive, and open to an appreciation of the wide variety of influences that affect professional touch, and also that we diligently seek an understanding of our own desires, motivations, and responses to touch (Proficiency Exercise 1-2). After all, it is impossible to touch clients without them in turn touching us. A touch given is at the same time a touch received.

Professional Classifications of Touch

Various models have been developed for classifying touch. Touch involves many nuances, forms, and intentions. We will discuss two models for framing professional touch. In the professional world, touch can be inappropriate or appropriate.

Forms of Inappropriate Touch—Model 1

Hostile or Aggressive Touch. Hostile or aggressive touch occurs when a potential for conflict or a power struggle exists. Professionals who use touch need to be aware of the underlying energy directed toward the client to prevent this intention in the touch. The obvious is easy: if you are angry with a client, it is best not to touch at that moment; likewise, if a client is angry with you, it is best not to touch until the energy changes. A more subtle aspect is the undercurrent of conflict. For example, the client may arrive late for the appointment, or the massage therapist may be hurried or angry about something at home. In these cases, the practitioner inadvertently may be more aggressive than necessary during the massage.

The perception that one holds power over another underlies hostile or aggressive touch. Careful attention must be paid to this idea of power in the therapeutic relationship between the professional and the client. In the professional relationship, a power difference between the professional and the client exists simply because of the knowledge base that defines the profession. Knowledge is power, and most of the time the professional knows more about the service rendered than the client does. In body therapies such as therapeutic massage, the client's physical position often creates an environment that fosters a power differential. Clients usually lie down or are seated, and the professional is physically above the client, generating the impression of authority.

Touching is an action energy focused outside the body that has the ability to exert power. When a person is touched, energy is received and internalized; touch is not overtly an act of exerting power. Although the ability to receive touch is powerful, the difference in the power base between those who give touch and those who receive it must be considered. This interplays with the appropriateness or inappropriateness of touch. Careful attention must be paid during professional touch if the issue of power is to be managed appropriately (see Chapter 2 for more information).

Erotic (Sexual) Touch. The intention of erotic, or sexual, touch is sexual arousal and expression. The issue of erotic touch cannot be sidestepped in the study of massage therapy

PROFICIENCY EXERCISE 1-2

My Touch History

On a separate piece of paper, write a brief touch history of yourself; then, explain the ways your history may influence your delivery of professional touch. The following example is provided as a model.

Culture

I grew up in the United States in Michigan. I lived in a small town that was primarily Caucasian.

Subculture

My family was a blue collar, working class family.

Genetic predisposition

I am most comfortable with a large personal space and plenty of time alone.

Gender

Female

Age

Mid-50s

Life events

I experienced touch trauma from a grandfather and uncles, who would tickle me until I could not stand it.

I gave birth to three children and am a single parent.

I had a special friend who was blind.

Spiritual path

I initially had an unstructured Protestant focus. I developed a specific fundamentalist path in early adulthood. I embraced many paths as truth in later years as I evolved from the practice of religion to the development of personal spirituality.

Ways my touch history may influence my delivery of professional touch

I had to learn a lot about different cultures because my exposure to a diverse population was limited while I was growing up. I have to be careful to understand a person's culture before I approach to touch him or her. I am most comfortable with blue collar, working class people. I am more relaxed and find myself willing to spend more time when I touch someone from this population. I feel overwhelmed if I am touched too much and tend to limit initiated touch from the client. I am a woman, and I learned during my gender role development to fulfill others' needs before my own. I often overextend myself for a client instead of setting time limits. I am hypersensitive to light touch and tend to avoid giving light touch when I give a massage. I am understanding of the numerous demands on a single parent and tend to touch one in similar circumstances with sympathy instead of empathy. I have to be careful of boundaries when I touch stressed, overwhelmed, single parents. I am casual when touching someone with a disability. I seek to understand various spiritual paths and deeply wish to respect issues of touch within each discipline. I tend to assume that one must actually make physical contact during spiritual healing and must remind myself that this is not everyone's truth.

Your Turn

Culture

Subculture

Genetic predisposition

Gender

Age

Life events

Spiritual path

Ways my touch history may influence my delivery of professional touch

---

or any other body-oriented treatment in which touch is a primary aspect of the therapy. Complex physiologic, mental, and spiritual aspects of both the client and the practitioner influence the ideas of erotic touch.

Inherent in many forms of massage and bodywork is the pleasure of being touched. Pleasure is an important therapeutic tool. In later chapters you will learn that chemicals in the body create pleasure moods and that feelings of connectedness increase during massage. These chemical responses to massage are one of the main reasons for the therapeutic benefit of the methods. Constant attention must be paid to the appropriate understanding and interpretation of the feelings generated during professional touch so that pleasurable touch does not evolve into or become misinterpreted as erotic touch.

Not only in body-oriented therapies, but also in psychotherapy and other health care disciplines, it is not uncommon for professionals occasionally to have sexual feelings in the context of the professional environment. Professionals are people with complex, intertwined needs, desires, and means of expressing themselves. However, it is inappropriate for professionals to foster any type of erotic feelings with a client, either within the therapeutic environment or outside that environment. Erotic feelings should never be expressed with clients.

Body Areas of Touch Sensitivity. Different areas of the body reflect different tactile issues. Research literature shows some agreement about areas of the body that are more sensitive, or "charged," in terms of emotion or erotic interpretation. The more emotionally or physically charged a body area is, the more the person may feel insecure, anxious, fearful, threatened, connected emotionally, intimate, or aroused when touched in that area.

Some body areas are considered taboo or "do not touch zones" in terms of professional therapeutic massage touch. Orifices, including the anus, genitals, mouth, ears, and nose, have the highest level of taboo in most societies. The ventral, or front, surfaces of the body, including the breasts, are more charged than the dorsal surfaces. We see this pattern in massage; much of the massage session is devoted to the back of the torso and the legs while the client is lying face down, with the front of the body "protected" by the massage table. Therapeutically, this creates difficulties, because most areas of dysfunction occur in the front of the body, where sensations of touch are more apt to elicit emotional responses and feelings of vulnerability.

The trunk of the body is more charged than the limbs. For this reason, a client may feel more comfortable having the legs and arms massaged than the torso. However, this does not always hold true; often the least intrusive form of touch is laying a hand on a person's upper back near the shoulder, whereas having the hands massaged can feel very intimate and connected.

The head also is an area sensitive to touch. Although children often are touched on the head and face, adults seldom are touched casually in these areas. Adults often respond emotionally to touching of the face and head.

Areas of a person's body that have undergone trauma, such as through accidents or surgery, carry more emotional charge and therefore are more sensitive to interpretation of the appropriateness of touch.

The appropriateness or inappropriateness of touch, then, is about when, the way, and with what intent we touch.[1]

Forms of Appropriate Touch

Nontherapeutic forms of touch that people often encounter include inadvertent touch, such as touch that occurs when people are jostled together in an elevator, and socially stereotyped touch, which involves highly ritualized touch that carries a consensual meaning within a culture, such as a handshake.

Therapeutic forms of touch involve touch that communicates information or that expresses feeling as part of the therapeutic relationship. This form of touch is not so much about creating a specific outcome as it is about delivering information or expressing comfort or understanding.[2] Some examples of this type of touch are touching a client's shoulder to direct him to the massage room or holding a client's hand as she thanks you for the session.

Touch Technique. **Touch technique** is the basis of therapeutic massage methods. Touch is the tool for massage. Massage is the use of various forms of touch to achieve a specific outcome. This type of touch can be considered technical touch. In terms of touch technique, a therapeutic intent exists. The intention of touch therapy can be classified in two ways:

- **Mechanical touch,** which is used to achieve a specific anatomic or physiologic outcome (e.g., using massage to increase the range of motion of the shoulder).
- **Expressive touch,** which is used to support and convey awareness and empathy for the client as a whole person (e.g., using massage for general relaxation and pleasure to comfort a client after a particularly hard day at work).[1]

The professional's choices of the type of therapeutic intention influence the interpretation of touch. A client with a mechanical restriction in the shoulder might find a more expressive form of touch uncomfortable because it might feel too intimate for the circumstances. Stressed, overworked clients may find a mechanical approach distant and impersonal because they are seeking empathy and understanding along with physical changes.

As we develop as professionals, both forms of touch technique must be perfected. Mechanical touch skills increase as we learn anatomy, physiology, record keeping, and effective delivery of specific forms of massage (these topics are covered in Chapters 3 and 6 through 11).

Development of the expressive form of touch technique is more complex and involves the professional's personal growth, interpersonal and communication skills, and understanding of his or her own life experiences (this information is explored in this chapter and in Chapters 2, 4, 5, and 12 through 14).

Consciousness Levels—Model 2

The second model describing the concepts of touch appropriateness is based on consciousness levels; this model is represented by the theory of the Eastern chakra system. Seven chakras, or energy centers, are located along the trunk of the body (Figure 1-3). This particular model demonstrates how historical, cultural, and spiritual factors dictate appropriate touch. The physical location of the chakras correlates with the autonomic nervous system plexuses. As you will learn later, the autonomic nervous system is involved with the expression of behavior. This connection begins to identify the physical (body) and emotional (mind) influence of function.

Traditionally, the base, or first, chakra pertains to survival, security, and safety. The second chakra concerns pleasure experiences of sensuality and sexuality. The third chakra involves power and control. These lower chakras are transcended by the fourth, or heart, chakra, which is the center of nonjudgmental love. The heart chakra is the pivot point between the lower three chakras and the upper, more spiritual chakras. The fifth chakra is the throat center, which is concerned with communication and creativity. The sixth, or brow, chakra concerns the reflection of the total or essential self, and the seventh, or crown, chakra reflects the transcended and spiritual self.

According to the chakra model, the intention of professional touch does not come from the lower chakra energies and needs because the energies of these chakras can be equated with types of inappropriate touch (hostile, aggressive, and erotic), and the potential for misinterpretation and manipulation is greater. The intention of professional touch projects from the fourth through seventh chakras, which support nonjudgmental love and respect for each person's individual mode of expressing the sense of self and sacredness.[2]

Touch Intention During Massage

The touch intention of therapeutic massage closely fits with both models except in the area of pleasure and safety. Many seek massage because it feels good, and these pleasure needs project from the second chakra. The importance of this pleasure factor and the interpretation of the meaning of the expe-

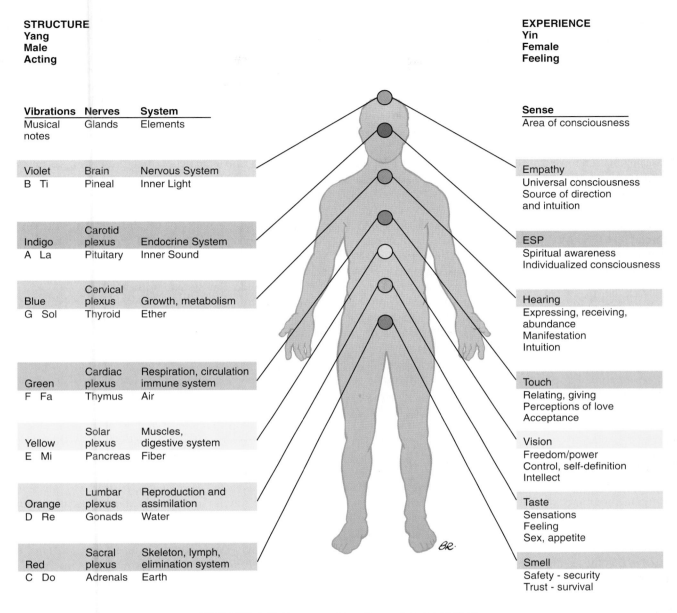

STRUCTURE
Yang
Male
Acting

Vibrations	Nerves	System
Musical notes	Glands	Elements
Violet	Brain	Nervous System
B Ti	Pineal	Inner Light
Indigo	Carotid plexus	Endocrine System
A La	Pituitary	Inner Sound
Blue	Cervical plexus	Growth, metabolism
G Sol	Thyroid	Ether
Green	Cardiac plexus	Respiration, circulation immune system
F Fa	Thymus	Air
Yellow	Solar plexus	Muscles, digestive system
E Mi	Pancreas	Fiber
Orange	Lumbar plexus	Reproduction and assimilation
D Re	Gonads	Water
Red	Sacral plexus	Skeleton, lymph, elimination system
C Do	Adrenals	Earth

EXPERIENCE
Yin
Female
Feeling

Sense
Area of consciousness
Empathy Universal consciousness Source of direction and intuition
ESP Spiritual awareness Individualized consciousness
Hearing Expressing, receiving, abundance Manifestation Intuition
Touch Relating, giving Perceptions of love Acceptance
Vision Freedom/power Control, self-definition Intellect
Taste Sensations Feeling Sex, appetite
Smell Safety - security Trust - survival

FIGURE 1-3 Names and locations of major chakras.

rience for clients can blur the boundaries of the professional relationship. It is important to recognize the value of therapeutic massage in meeting nonsexual pleasure goals, because pleasure sensation supports a balance of neuroendocrine functions that affect mood. As massage therapists, we also need to consider a client's sense of safety and security, projected from the first chakra. We can make sure a client feels secure on the massage table by demonstrating that the table is strong and stable. We need to assure clients of privacy and a touch that does no harm to them.

It also is important to consider the touch intention projected from the sixth and seventh chakras. Interacting professionally with the essential self (the sixth chakra) requires extensive training in mental health, which can provide expertise in the development of the essential self. Touch that influences the transcendent or spiritual self requires the discipline

to walk any of the many spiritual paths. Commitment to this training prepares one to provide support that leads to understanding of the transcendent self.

Professional energy focused from these areas can lead to dual roles for the massage professional. Dual or multiple roles occur when a professional operates from many bases of knowledge in interacting with clients therapeutically. The main concern with dual roles is the distribution of power in the therapeutic relationship. The more roles a professional plays with a client, the more power the professional acquires in the therapeutic relationship. A client can easily come to feel disempowered with professionals who work from dual or multiple roles. This disempowerment can manifest in various forms, including anger ("You're the expert, so you should have known"), a submissive attitude ("The professional knows best"), or excessive admiration ("No one is as gifted as you").

In addition, the development of professional expertise in more than one role requires devotion to acquiring the knowledge encompassed by several areas. As you begin to study massage, you soon will realize that you could study for a lifetime just within the massage knowledge base and not absorb all the information available. Expecting a person to operate effectively as a professional in several areas may be unrealistic, because each of those areas also reflects a lifetime of experience and study.

A generalized knowledge of different areas of expertise and several forms of intervention adds to professional development. It can be helpful in fostering professional relationships with other professionals and in recognizing when a client can best be served by another discipline. However, developing expertise in several areas can become overwhelming. Professional touch provided through therapeutic massage, coupled with an understanding of the various needs and the diversity of the population we serve, is complex enough in itself. I often feel as if there is too much to know, and I can imagine the feeling of being overwhelmed that frequently besets a beginning student. It is important in professional development to honor personal and professional limits and to set appropriate personal and professional boundaries. When touch is the primary treatment method, it is even more important to understand the interpersonal dynamics of the therapeutic relationship. (Professional boundaries are discussed further in Chapter 2.)

The Uniqueness of Touch

A specific touch experience is difficult to replicate, because it is extremely multifaceted. The interaction between two individuals is unique. Students often ask instructors to demonstrate a method on them so that they know how it feels. Although this is a good learning experience, it is somewhat limited in that the feeling cannot be replicated with a different touching pair.

Students or fellow practitioners may tell an instructor about a client's situation and ask for recommendations. Often this is difficult for the instructor. Although instructors usually can give information about the pathology or a technical description of various methodologies, they really do not know in what way they would do a massage until they touch that particular client. If the instructor actually touches the student's client in a professional teaching session, the client's experience of the instructor's touch and the student's touch does not end up being the same, even if both use the same method. The instructor's interaction through touch is no more right than the student's; rather, the unique quality of the touch experience makes the difference.

When an instructor demonstrates a method of massage, this touch often is developed through experience. The person receiving the massage probably notices the difference in the touch, not the method, when the student attempts to replicate the instructor's actions because the experience level is different. The confidence of experience is displayed not so much in the expert execution of the methods as in the quality of the touch in delivering those methods.

The Subjective and Objective Qualities of Touch

Writing a textbook is mostly the dispensing of objective (fact based) information and is separate from the author's personal, subjective experiences. Each person who reads the information in a textbook incorporates the skills and information as tools and resources in his or her own experience. Most of this text is written objectively, and that is as it should be; however, ideas on the experience of touch are so subjective in interpretation and experience that presenting concepts of touch only through objective data seems impossible. The authors of the books used as references in this section have not been able to accomplish this objectification of touch, either. Something expansive and abstract about the simple, concrete experience of touch transcends technical writing. The experience of touching and being touched seems to extend beyond words and verbalization, beyond the skin, nervous system, and endocrine system, to the soul.

As this section concludes and building the foundation for using touch in a therapeutic and professional way begins, reflecting personally on touch needs seems appropriate.

I know that I need to be touched, and I know what happens to me when I am not touched enough or when the touch does not satisfy me because it is not safe touch or because it is needy touch that requires me to extend energy to someone else. When those with whom I can share or experience safe touch (my close family and friends, my pets, my woods, and my massage therapist) are unavailable, I become out of sorts and moody, my back hurts, I don't sleep as well, and I find myself involved in substitute behavior, such as eating, that attempts to feed my touch hunger.

When I'm alone, on good days I experience my own sense of touch through exercise and the enjoyment of tactile sensation, such as with my flannel sheets, or listening to music. However, these forms of self-touch lack body contact with another, and often touch longings are not satisfied unless they are shared with another living being, such as holding my dogs in my lap.

On not so good days, I overeat or use other excessive and detrimental forms of sensory stimulation. The excessiveness of the behavior is somewhat like trying to be satisfied with a carrot stick when you really crave vanilla pudding. It takes lots of carrots to fill me up, but I am still not satisfied. Then, when I finally give in to the vanilla pudding, I eat the whole box instead of the indicated serving. It is because I feel starved, beyond physical need, and I am operating in realms of emotional and maybe spiritual longing. Even more, this substitution behavior never really fulfills the desire. I still feel touch deprived and unsatisfied after the physiologic effects of the behavior (substituting food) wear off. No matter how many times I try to use them as substitutes, neither food nor exercise can replace the real need to be touched by someone who cares.

The desire for physical contact is an instinctive and physiologic need for well-being. Professional therapeutic touch often feeds touch hunger for people in a safe, professional environment. Massage professionals serve others by providing touch. If we are going to be able to provide this type of touch experience for others, how do we take care of our personal touch needs? What happens to you if your hunger for safe, nurturing (nutritious) touch is not met?

PROFICIENCY EXERCISE 1-3

In the space provided, answer the following questions.
1. What do I do when I am touch hungry?

2. Who and what touches me in a safe, respectful, and healing way?

It is important for massage professionals to embrace the expansive, abstract experience of touch. No one really cares how much you know until they know how much you care. The concrete experience of caring most often is conveyed through touch. That knowing, or "felt sense," experienced by both the client and the practitioner often is internalized through professional touch. We must show our willingness as practitioners to be open personally to sharing the experience with the client, at the same time being professional enough to respect the client and maintain the focus of the experience for the individual. To do this, each of us who uses touch professionally must be aware of self-care, and we must develop resources and support people (as well as pets and plants) who touch us in a safe, respectful, and healing way (Proficiency Exercise 1-3).

HISTORICAL PERSPECTIVES

SECTION OBJECTIVES

Using the information presented in this section, the student will be able to perform the following:

- Trace the general progression of massage from ancient times to today
- Relate historical information to current events

To understand professional, structured, therapeutic touch, the student must explore historical influences and the evolution of massage from its ancient foundations through projections for the future (Figure 1-4).

A knowledge of history helps massage therapists develop a sense of professional identity and pride in their profession. Historical perspectives help members of a profession identify the profession's strengths and weaknesses. As students of massage read historical books about massage, they discover that the fundamental body of knowledge has changed little over the centuries. The most prevalent concepts in massage today were in fact written about many years ago. Massage has stood the test of time, proving itself a vital, health-enhancing technique and a rehabilitative discipline. Currently the profession is at a defining moment; it is growing in acceptance and scientific rigor but is still paying for grave mistakes made long ago. As we move forward, we will also make mistakes. In the future, beginning massage professionals will learn from our historical events.

Many people have played important roles in tracing the historic journey of therapeutic massage and bodywork methods. Many of these resources and people are listed on the

Evolve Web site. Specific acknowledgment must be given to Richard van Why, who compiled the Bodywork Knowledgebase, a collection of more than 100 historical books and more than 4,000 research and journal articles on therapeutic massage and related methods. Much of the information in this chapter comes from this work. If it were not for van Why's diligence, much of the history of massage would be scattered in research libraries and would be unknown to us today. Another who deserves mention is Fran Tappan, a true master of massage. She wrote respected textbooks about massage that include a historical perspective, and she was a part of that history.

This chapter consolidates the historical information. Because the references used overlap extensively, text citation has been kept to a minimum. With gratitude and respect for those who have devoted their lives to this work, the many mentioned and the many more who are not, let us begin the journey by looking to the past.

The History of Massage

Identified animal behavior, such as the application of pressure, rubbing, and licking, indicates that massage is used instinctively to relieve pain, to respond to injury, and for comfort. Massage has always been one of the most natural and instinctive means of relieving pain and discomfort. When a person has sore, aching muscles, abdominal pain, or a bruise or wound, the instinctive impulse is to touch and rub that part of the body to obtain relief.

Touch as a method of healing appears to have numerous cultural origins (see Box 1-1). Therapeutic massage has strong roots in Chinese folk medicine, but it also has many aspects in common with other healing traditions, such as Indian herbal medicine and Persian medicine. The art of massage is believed to have been first mentioned in writing about 2000 B.C.,[3] and it has been discussed extensively in books since about 500 B.C. The historical medical literatures of Egypt, Persia, and Japan are full of references to massage. The Greek physician Hippocrates advocated massage and gymnastic exercise. Asclepiades, another eminent Greek physician, relied exclusively on massage in his practice.

Throughout history, many different systems and supporting theories have come and gone regarding the management of musculoskeletal pain and dysfunction. The scientific thinking of the day provided the validation for massage. Over the years, scientific research has changed the philosophy of massage theory. Current research continues to define the physical effects of therapeutic massage.

The endurance of massage through the centuries has been amazing. Current trends suggest an increase in the popularity of massage and body-related therapies used to reduce stress and to treat chronic musculoskeletal problems (see Chapter 4).

Manual medicine, which has always been part of the art of medicine, is the use of the hands in the treatment of injury and disease. Its therapeutic value derives from changes in soft tissue and structure rather than from surgery or pharmaceuticals.[4] Massage can be considered a part of manual medicine, although throughout history it also has functioned indepen-

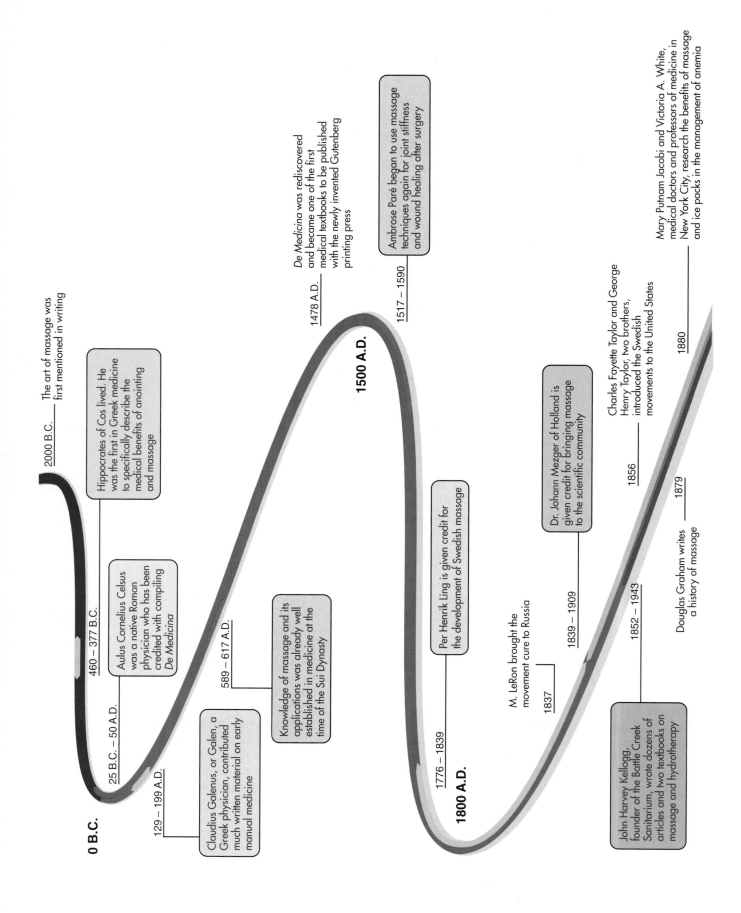

0 B.C.

2000 B.C. — The art of massage was first mentioned in writing

460 – 377 B.C. — Hippocrates of Cos lived. He was the first in Greek medicine to specifically describe the medical benefits of anointing and massage

25 B.C. – 50 A.D. — Aulus Cornelius Celsus was a native Roman physician who has been credited with compiling *De Medicina*

129 – 199 A.D. — Claudius Galenus, or Galen, a Greek physician, contributed much written material on early manual medicine

589 – 617 A.D. — Knowledge of massage and its applications was already well established in medicine at the time of the Sui Dynasty

1478 A.D. — *De Medicina* was rediscovered and became one of the first medical textbooks to be published with the newly invented Gutenberg printing press

1500 A.D.

1517 – 1590 A.D. — Ambrose Paré began to use massage techniques again for joint stiffness and wound healing after surgery

1776 – 1839 — Per Henrik Ling is given credit for the development of Swedish massage

1800 A.D.

1837 — M. LeRon brought the movement cure to Russia

1839 – 1909 — Dr. Johann Mezger of Holland is given credit for bringing massage to the scientific community

1852 – 1943 — John Harvey Kellogg, founder of the Battle Creek Sanitarium, wrote dozens of articles and two textbooks on massage and hydrotherapy

1856 — Charles Fayette Taylor and George Henry Taylor, two brothers, introduced the Swedish movements to the United States

1879 — Douglas Graham writes a history of massage

1880 — Mary Putnam Jacobi and Victoria A. White, medical doctors and professors of medicine in New York City, research the benefits of massage and ice packs in the management of anemia

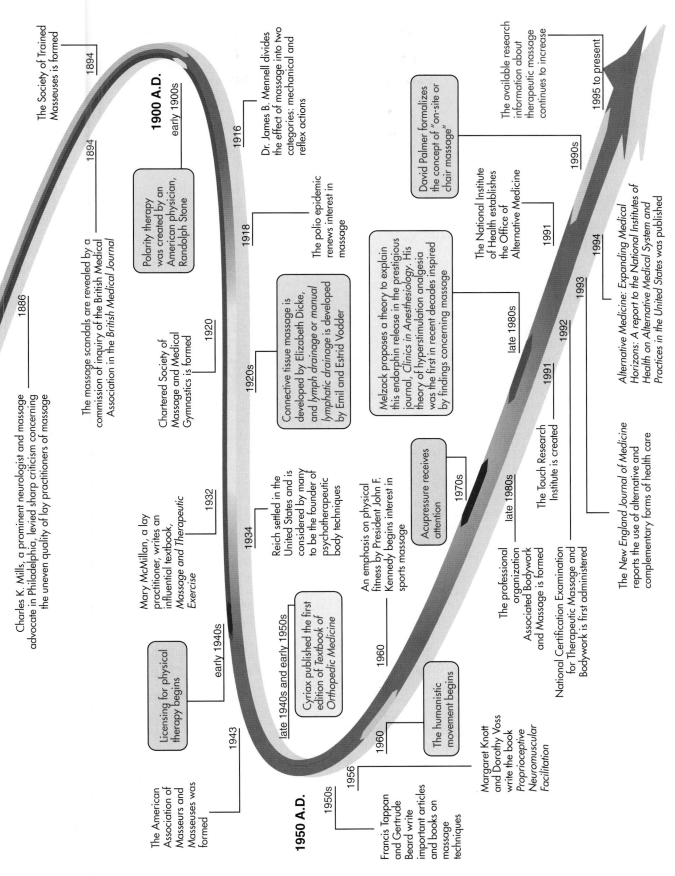

Charles K. Mills, a prominent neurologist and massage advocate in Philadelphia, levied sharp criticism concerning the uneven quality of lay practitioners of massage

The Society of Trained Masseuses is formed

1894

1886

1894

1900 A.D.

The massage scandals are revealed by a commission of inquiry of the British Medical Association in the *British Medical Journal*

Polarity therapy was created by an American physician, Randolph Stone

early 1900s

Dr. James B. Mennell divides the effect of massage into two categories: mechanical and reflex actions

1916

1918

The polio epidemic renews interest in massage

Chartered Society of Massage and Medical Gymnastics is formed

1920

1920s

Connective tissue massage is developed by Elizabeth Dicke, and *lymph drainage* or *manual lymphatic drainage* is developed by Emil and Estrid Vodder

Mary McMillan, a lay practitioner, writes an influential textbook, *Massage and Therapeutic Exercise*

1932

1934

Reich settled in the United States and is considered by many to be the founder of psychotherapeutic body techniques

Melzack proposes a theory to explain this endorphin release in the prestigious journal, *Clinics in Anesthesiology*. His theory of hyperstimulation analgesia was the first in recent decades inspired by findings concerning massage

An emphasis on physical fitness by President John F. Kennedy begins interest in sports massage

Acupressure receives attention

1970s

David Palmer formalizes the concept of "on-site or chair massage"

1990s

The National Institute of Health establishes the Office of Alternative Medicine

1991

The available research information about therapeutic massage continues to increase

1995 to present

1994

1993

1992

1991

late 1980s

late 1980s

The professional organization Associated Bodywork and Massage is formed

The Touch Research Institute is created

National Certification Examination for Therapeutic Massage and Bodywork is first administered

The *New England Journal of Medicine* reports the use of alternative and complementary forms of health care

Alternative Medicine: Expanding Medical Horizons: A report to the National Institutes of Health on Alternative Medical System and Practices in the United States was published

Licensing for physical therapy begins

early 1940s

1943

The American Association of Masseurs and Masseuses was formed

late 1940s and early 1950s

Cyriax published the first edition of *Textbook of Orthopedic Medicine*

1960

1960

The humanistic movement begins

1956

Margaret Knott and Dorothy Voss write the book *Proprioceptive Neuromuscular Facilitation*

1950s

1950 A.D.

Francis Tappan and Gertrude Beard write important articles and books on massage techniques

FIGURE 1-4 Historical time line.

dently to promote health. Manual medicine has grown to become the foundation of osteopathy, chiropractic, and physical therapy.[5]

THINK IT OVER

- If you were going to rename massage, what would you call it?
- If touch is so instinctive, why do you have to go to school to learn to do it?
- Why do you think every culture has had some form of massage?
- What do you think is the difference between massage and manual medicine?

Ancient Times

According to research reports, most ancient cultures practiced some form of healing touch. Often a ceremonial leader, such as a healer, priest, or shaman, was selected to perform the healing rituals. The healing methods frequently used were herbs, oils, and primitive forms of hydrotherapy. Archaeologists have found many prehistoric artifacts depicting the use of massage for healing and cosmetic purposes. Some speculate that massage used for pain relief incorporated concepts of counterirritation, such as scraping, cutting, and burning of the skin, as part of the process. Massage may have been used as a cleansing procedure, along with fasting and bathing, in preparation for many tribal rituals.

In China, massage has been known by three names: *anmo* and *amma*, the ancient names, meaning "press-rub," and *tui-na*, of more recent origin, meaning "push-pull." These Chinese methods were administered by kneading or rubbing down the entire body with the hands and using a gentle pressure and traction on all the joints.[6]

The practice of acupuncture involved the stimulation of specific points along the body; this usually was done by inserting tiny, solid needles, but massage and other forms of pressure also were used. Such practices were also found in traditional Eskimo and African medicine, in which sharp stones were used to scratch the skin's surface. Today, scientists are able to give physiologic reasons for the value of these ancient practices.

Knowledge of massage and its applications already was well established in Chinese medicine at the time of the Sui Dynasty (A.D. 589-617). The Japanese came to know massage through the writings of the Chinese. Massage has been a part of life in India for almost 3,000 years. The Chinese introduced the methods in India during trading forays. Like Chinese acupuncture, hatha yoga, which was developed in India, has reappeared in modern forms of body therapy, with its energy concepts of prana, chakras, and energy balance.

The ancient Egyptians left artwork showing foot massage. Before Greek athletes took part in the Olympic games, they underwent friction treatment, anointing, and rubbing with sand. The use of touch as a mode of healing is recorded in the writings of the Hebrew and Christian traditions. The "laying

on of hands" was particularly prominent in first-century Christianity. Massage with oils (anointing) goes back even farther in Jewish practices. The ancient Jews practiced anointing for its ritual, hygienic, and therapeutic benefits. The Jewish culture honored rubbing with oils to such an extent that the root word for rubbing with oils and for the Messiah is the same (*Ma-shı-ah*).[6]

The ancient Mayan people of Central America, the Incas of South America, and other native people of the American continent also used methods of joint manipulation and massage.

Hippocrates of Cos (460-377 B.C.) was the first physician in Greek medicine specifically to describe the medical benefits of anointing and massage, along with the chemical properties of oils used for this purpose. He called his art *anatripsis*, which means "to rub up." Of this art he said, "The physician must be acquainted with many things and assuredly with anatripsis, for things that have the same name have not always the same effects, for rubbing can bind a joint that is too loose or loosen a joint that is too hard."[6] Hippocrates' methods survived, virtually unchanged, well into the Middle Ages. Many techniques similar to those methods, especially traction and stretching principles, are still in use today.[5]

Claudius Galenus, or Galen, another Greek physician (A.D. 129-199), contributed much written material on early manual medicine, including many commentaries on Hippocrates' methods.[5]

Massage came to the Romans from the Greeks. Julius Caesar (100-44 B.C.) had himself "pinched all over" daily to relieve his neuralgia and prevent epilepsy attacks.[3] Aulus Cornelius Celsus (25 B.C.-A.D. 50), a Roman physician, has been credited with compiling *De Medicina*, a series of eight books covering the body of medical knowledge of the day. Seven of the books deal extensively with prevention and therapeutics using rubbing, exercise, bathing, and anointing. This work was rediscovered during the late Middle Ages by Pope Nicholas V (1397-1455). In 1478 *De Medicina* was one of the first medical textbooks to be published with the newly invented Gutenberg printing press. It was one of most popular medical textbooks during the Renaissance.

THINK IT OVER

Why do you think ancient people started sticking things into the skin and scratching the skin to produce healing?

The Middle Ages

Massage developed differently in the East and the West. In the East, as part of the Islamic empire, it represented a continuation of Greco-Roman traditions. In the West, the Greco-Roman traditions disappeared, but massage was kept alive by the common people and became part of folk culture. In this form, massage was an important part of the healing tradition of the Slavs, Finns, and Swedes. As massage was integrated into the health practices of the common people, it often was associated with supernatural experiences and observances.

This association alienated massage from what little scientific approach there was during this time. Practitioners of folk medicine often were persecuted, and the Church claimed that the practitioner's healing powers came from the devil.[6]

Not until the sixteenth century did massage regain its respectability in Europe. One of the founders of modern surgery, the French physician Ambrose Paré (1517-1590), began to use massage techniques again for joint stiffness and wound healing after surgery. In his work Paré described three types of massage strokes: gentle, medium, and vigorous. His ideas were passed down to other French physicians who believed in the value of manual therapeutics.

The Nineteenth Century

Per Henrik Ling. Per Henrik Ling (1776-1839) is credited with developing Swedish massage, but he did not invent it. He learned massage from others and through persistent experimentation put the information together in a workable form.

Ling proposed an integrated program for the treatment of disease using active and passive movements and massage. Legend has it that Ling's interest in these methods was sparked by the gout in his own elbow. He developed a system of massage that used many of the positions and movements of Swedish gymnastics. Combining these strokes with exercises, he healed his diseased elbow. Ling's program was based on the newly discovered knowledge of the circulation of the blood and lymph. (It is interesting to note that the Chinese had been using these methods for centuries.)

While teaching fencing, Ling observed that habitual movements interfered with the development of desired movements. He determined that the development of a skill depended on the mental mastery of habit; therefore he began teaching bodily movements systematically. He developed his medical gymnastics in 1814, but his methods were bitterly opposed by the Swedish medical establishment for almost 20 years. He was not trained in medicine, and his tendency to use poetic and mystic language in his writings on gymnastics was thought to interfere with wider acceptance of his ideas.[7] Current experts in massage would be wise to take note of Ling's experience; it is essential that massage be explained in the medical and scientific terminology of the day.

With the support of influential clients, Ling was granted a license to practice and teach his method, and he established the Royal Gymnastic Central Institute. The primary focus of Ling's system, especially in his later writings, was gymnastics applied to the treatment of disease. This position was a change from his earlier educational and military gymnastics, which were intended only for healthy people.

In his system, Ling divided movements into active, duplicated, and passive forms. Active movements were performed by the person's own effort; these movements correspond to what commonly is called *exercise*. Duplicated movements were performed by the person with the cooperation of a gymnast (therapist); they involved active effort by both parties in which the action of the one was opposed by the action of the other. Duplicated movements correspond to what today is commonly called *resistive exercise*. Passive movements were performed for the person by the active effort of the gymnast

alone. They consisted of passive movements of the extremities, which today we call range of motion work and stretching. Movement therapy was not separated from massage, and the two were considered integral to the system.

Ling taught many physicians from Germany, Austria, Russia, and England, who spread his teachings to their own countries. He was recognized by his contemporaries and later followers not so much as a great innovator, but as a keen observer who adopted methods only after testing their effectiveness. He combined many techniques into one coherent system. By the time of Ling's death in 1839, his system had achieved worldwide recognition.[6] Ling's teachings endured because he developed a school to continue teaching medical gymnastics, or the Swedish movement cure, as it became known in the United States in the late nineteenth century.

 THINK IT OVER

Why do you think Ling's development of a school was so important?

The Modern Revival of Massage. Per Henrik Ling and others who practiced the Swedish movement cure deserve credit for reviving massage after the Middle Ages. Initially, nonprofessionals spoke to physicians in a language they did not share, making communication difficult. Dr. Johann Mezger of Holland (1839-1909) is credited with bringing massage to the scientific community. He presented massage to fellow physicians as a form of medical treatment. The French terms *effleurage*, *pétrissage*, and *tapotement* did not come from Ling. Mezger's followers in Holland began to use these names, although historical references do not explain why French terms were chosen. So often history is confusing, and the issue of who deserves credit for what becomes clouded.[7]

As physicians talked to one another about massage, its popularity began to grow. The physicians sought common ground between their methods and massage, both to justify their current view of massage and to expand it. Lay magazines and medical journals published manuscripts on massage. The successful experience and testimony of distinguished people, especially monarchs and diplomats, further bolstered the image of massage and increased public and medical acceptance. Many physicians were drawn to study massage because they had a strong scientific interest in its effects. They conducted animal studies and well-designed clinical trials, which further persuaded physicians of the value of the method and increased the interest of the medical community. The same situation has held true for massage in this century; it currently is bolstered by the work of Dr. Tiffany Field at the Touch Research Institute and by studies conducted under grants from the National Institutes of Health (NIH).

The Swedish movement cure quickly spread to the other countries of Europe; the first institute outside Sweden was established in Denmark. In 1837, 2 years before Ling's death, his disciple, M. LeRon, brought the movement cure to Russia, establishing a clinic in St. Petersburg.

Massage in the United States. In the United States the first waves of European immigration came from Northern Europe, which had accepted massage earlier because of its therapeutic benefits. The immigrants provided many great writers and teachers of massage, as well as eager, trusting clients.[6]

Two brothers, Charles F. Taylor and George H. Taylor, introduced the Swedish movement system to the United States in 1856. They had learned the skills from Dr. Mathias Roth, an English physician who studied directly with Ling. Roth, also a leader in the homeopathic movement, felt that massage worked on the same principles as homeopathy: the law of similars and the concept of "like cures like."

Dr. John Harvey Kellogg (1852-1943), founder of the Battle Creek Sanitarium in Michigan, wrote dozens of articles and two textbooks on massage and hydrotherapy and edited and published a popular magazine, *Good Health.*

In 1879 Douglas Graham, in his history of massage, described the lomi-lomi of the Hawaiians as a hygienic measure used to relieve fatigue or for the pure pleasure of it. Graham continued to write on massage and its use in almost every area of medicine until his death in the late 1920s.

In 1889 a letter from a physician in Kansas appeared in a New York medical journal; the physician said that he had thought massage was but "a novel method of therapeutics" until he had read a passage from Captain James Cook's diary of his third voyage around the world near the end of the eighteenth century. Cook had described how his pseudosciatic pain was relieved in an elegant and generous ritual by a Tahitian chief and his family, using a type of massage method called *romee.*

The Massage Scandals of the Late 1800s. In a very real sense, massage was a victim of its own success. In 1886 Dr. Charles K. Mills, a prominent neurologist and advocate of massage in Philadelphia, sharply criticized the uneven quality of lay practitioners of massage and their often unsubstantiated and unethical claims. In 1889 British physicians, who were just beginning to view massage favorably because Queen Victoria supported the methods, became increasingly aware of patterns of abuse, including false claims about lay practitioners' education or skills, client stealing, and the charging of high fees. The massage scandals of 1894, revealed by a British Medical Association commission of inquiry in the *British Medical Journal,* eroded the public's and the medical profession's confidence in massage as a legitimate medical art.

An inconsistent system of education, which encompassed private trade schools, hospitals, and physicians who took private students, appeared to be a major contributor to the loss of confidence in massage. Courses in technique, anatomy, physiology, and pathology varied immensely, as did the teachers' experience and capability. Some held that they could teach with minimal training in massage or directly after graduation from programs of questionable quality. Students often were encouraged to have grand expectations of career opportunities, only to find a difficult job market in which many of them

were inadequately trained to compete. Richard van Why provides an example of the problem[6]:

> Many schools used improper student recruitment tactics. The worst involved young women from poor neighborhoods, who were approached by recruiters claiming that extraordinary career opportunities awaited masseuses or medical gymnasts upon graduation from schools of professional training. The recruiters offered to defer payment of tuition until a reasonable time had elapsed after their graduation, so that the women could build resources to pay their living expenses and still pay the loans back. They were typically trained in short programs and then were released to a marketplace full of lay practitioners. As they found no work, they could not pay the loans back. Soon the recruiters returned, demanding payment. The women were told that if they did not pay, they would be thrown into debtors prison until they did. To work off the debt, they would have to work at a clinic attached to the school or for a friend or a colleague of a school administrator. The best of these "clinics" offered incompetently performed classical massage. The worst of the "clinics" were pretexts for houses of prostitution. In the scandals that followed in British cities and in Chicago and New York, the "massage parlor" caught on, and the lay practice of massage became associated with vice.

Another notorious abuse involved "certification," which some physicians who supported massage considered merely a receipt for money paid. Still another problem concerned advertising. The medical profession and the well-trained, classical lay practitioners of massage and medical gymnastics did not make false claims in their advertisements. Conversely, many entrepreneurs and poor massage practitioners, seeking publicity to increase enrollment at their schools and attendance at their clinics, did make such claims, which often flew in the face of the principles of anatomy, physiology, and pathology.

In 1894, the same year that the massage scandals were revealed in Britain, eight women who envisioned massage professionals as "well-trained, properly equipped masseuses serving those in need" formed the Society of Trained Masseuses. Before this time, the quality of lay practitioners of massage was inconsistent. Recognizing the need for rigorous standards, the founders modeled their standards after those used in the medical profession. They set academic prerequisites for the study of massage. Training could be given only in recognized schools, which were to be inspected regularly to ensure that standards were maintained. Only qualified instructors could teach classes. Examinations for teachers and graduates of basic massage training were conducted by a board, which included a physician. Examinations were to include both written tests and a demonstration of clinical achievement.

Problems arose within the Society of Trained Masseuses during a period of sustained growth, and another, competing association was established. This weakened both organizations. In 1920 the society assembled an advisory committee to aid reorganization and to reconcile with the opposing association. The two groups joined as the Chartered Society of Massage and Medical Gymnastics.

In 1909, before the reorganization, the society had 600 members; by 1939 the membership had grown to 12,000.

Certificates of competence were granted to individuals who had passed a rigorous examination. To be admitted to the Chartered Society of Massage and Medical Gymnastics, prospective members had to pledge not to accept clients unless they had been referred by a physician. Members were forbidden to advertise in the lay press. The organization worked to provide a central registry of well-trained massage practitioners and to provide referrals for inquiries from the medical profession or the public, based on location and any special needs. However, membership in the association was voluntary, and many ill-trained, unscrupulous practitioners continued to thrive.

THINK IT OVER

- How is the success of the massage profession today similar to the success of massage practice in the early and mid-1800s?
- Do you think the darker history of massage could be repeated in our times? If so, what factors would contribute to this development?
- What can members of the massage profession do to prevent a situation similar to that which arose in the late 1800s?

Massage as Health Care. Even during the difficult time of the late 1800s, massage endured. Institutes of massage appeared in France, Germany, and Austria by the middle of the nineteenth century. Between 1854 and 1918, the practice of massage developed from an obscure, unskilled trade to a field of medical health care, from which the profession of physical therapy began. Treatments consisted of massage, mineral baths, and exercise.[6]

Dr. David Gurevich, a Russian physician and instructor of Russian medical massage, believed that the long-standing interest in massage and its continuing development are strong proof of its usefulness and necessity.[8] According to Dr. Gurevich, massage was practiced by ancient Slavic tribes, especially in combination with therapeutic bathing, or hydrotherapy. Beginning in the eighteenth century, many great Russian scientists and doctors (Mudroff, Manasein, Botkin, Zakharin, and others) contributed to the development of the theory and practice of massage. I. Z. Zabludovski wrote more than 100 books, textbooks, and scientific articles devoted to the methods of massage and its physiologic basis in therapy, postsurgical care, and sports.

An institute of massage and exercise was founded in Russia at the end of the nineteenth century, and many courses in massage also were started. Massage gradually progressed from an auxiliary method of therapy to an independent therapeutic method that was used effectively with other types of treatment. The practice of massage became widespread in Russia, and most medical clinics used massage therapy. Massage used with therapeutic exercises has been adapted for the management of the viscera, the nervous system, and gynecologic disorders, as well as for orthopedics, posttraumatic care, and

postoperative care. Prospective students of massage must have some medical education. The change in Russia's economy in the late 1980s and early 1990s to a market system made it possible for private massage clinics, which charge fees, to open.[8]

The Historical Influence of Women. Women made early and important contributions to the development of massage and medical gymnastics, primarily in the United States. Contemporary massage has been influenced extensively by women, and 70% to 75% of practicing massage professionals today are women. Two women physicians conducted the first controlled clinical trial of the benefits of massage in the management of disease. Dr. Mary P. Jacobi and Dr. Victoria A. White were professors of medicine in New York City in 1880. Their research addressed the benefits of massage and ice packs in the management of anemia.

Broad licensing for physical therapy began in the early 1940s. Louise L. Despard's *Text-Book of Massage and Remedial Gymnastics* was one of a handful of textbooks on massage recommended in 1940 as essential reading for all students of massage by the Massage Round Table of the American Physical Therapy Association.

Mary McMillan, an English lay practitioner of massage, wrote an influential textbook, *Massage and Therapeutic Exercise,* in 1932. She had extensive experience in the field. From 1911 to 1915 she was in charge of massage and therapeutic exercise at the Greenbank Cripples Home in Liverpool, England, and from 1916 to 1918 she served as director of massage and remedial gymnastics at the Children's Hospital in Portland, Maine. During World War I she served in the military as a rehabilitation aide.[3]

In the west, Eunice Ingham formalized the system of reflexology derived from ancient Chinese roots. Dr. Janet Travell's work with myofascial pain and trigger points is unsurpassed. Bonnie Prudden popularized trigger point work. Fran Tappan's outstanding contributions to massage and physical therapy are formalized in her textbook, *Healing Massage Techniques.* Sister Kenny used massage in the treatment of polio. Ida Rolf's massage system grew to become the technique of Rolfing. Dr. Dolores Krieger has made major contributions to the more energetic approaches through her system of therapeutic touch. Because of the extensive influence of women in massage today, it is likely that when massage history is written in 20 years, many women will be listed as vital contributors to the continued development of massage.

The Twentieth Century

Sigmund Freud (1856-1939), an Austrian neurologist and theorist who developed the system of psychoanalysis, experimented with the use of massage in the treatment of hysteria, a form of mental illness common in his day. This condition is characterized by a paralysis that has no physiologic basis. Freud's *Studies on Hysteria,* published in 1895, explained his methods.

Wilhelm Reich, an Austrian psychoanalyst who was a clinical assistant to Freud for 6 years, became interested in the physiologic basis of neurosis. In 1934 Reich emigrated to the

United States. He is considered by many to be the founder of psychotherapeutic body techniques. Reich gradually moved the emphasis of his therapeutic approach away from the psychologic and toward the realm of the physical, the body. Reich developed many somatic techniques to dissolve what he saw as the muscular armor. Because of his controversial techniques, he came into conflict with the medical establishment and eventually was investigated by the U.S. Food and Drug Administration (FDA). He was convicted of fraudulent medical practices and died in 1957 while serving his sentence in federal prison.

Reich's earlier ideas and therapies have greatly influenced contemporary bodywork. Bioenergetics, a popular somatotherapy, evolved directly from his system. Bioenergetics was founded by Alexander Lowen, an American psychiatrist who was Reich's student for 12 years.

1900 to 1960. In the early 1900s Dr. Randolph Stone, an American physician, devised polarity therapy. Stone studied many body systems, both ancient and modern, including acupuncture, hatha yoga, osteopathy, chiropractic techniques, and reflexology. From his investigations he concluded that magnetic fields regulated and directed the physiologic systems of the body. Influenced by Eastern philosophy and medicine, Stone believed that all aspects of the universe were expressed in opposite poles (e.g., male and female, positive and negative electrical charges); therefore he called his therapeutic method *polarity.*

In 1907 Edgar F. Cyriax began a distinguished publishing career that spanned almost 40 years. He was the last great proponent of Ling's Swedish movement cure, which Cyriax called *mechanotherapeutics.*

At the turn of the nineteenth century, the United States and England looked to Japan for innovation in the vocational rehabilitation of the blind. The British Institute for Massage by the Blind was established in 1900. Other European nations tried to develop their own models of the Japanese and British institutions, but failed.

A textbook published in 1900 by Albert Hoffa and revised in 1913 by Max Bohm describes the more classic massage techniques, such as effleurage, pétrissage, tapotement, and vibration. Most therapists still learn these methods as standard massage techniques in entry level programs. However, many massage professionals of the time disregarded this type of massage, considering it too basic to be included in the realm of advanced manual therapy. Others warned against leaving behind traditional massage techniques, believing that fundamentals could not be replaced with more modern forms of bodywork.

In 1916 Dr. James B. Mennell divided the effects of massage into two categories: mechanical actions and reflex actions. Mennell showed that massage exerts a mechanical effect in four ways:

- By aiding venous return of blood to the heart
- By promoting lymph movement out of the tissues
- By stretching the connective tissue (e.g., tendons, scar tissue)

- By stimulating the stomach, small intestine, and colon

Mennell also maintained that certain forms of tactile stimulation, such as stroking and light touch, stimulated reflex arcs, causing muscles to relax or contract according to the type of stroke. He theorized that both smooth and skeletal muscles were under the control of such reflexes. Experimental research now supports the theories of Ling, Mennell, and others that massage has mechanical and reflex effects.

The polio epidemic of 1918 sparked a more widespread interest in massage because victims and their families were desperate for any remedy that offered any promise at all. Research on the benefits of massage in preventing the complications of paralysis began at this time.

Connective tissue massage (CTM) was developed in the 1920s by German physiotherapist Elizabeth Dicke and later was expanded upon by Maria Ebner. CTM was first used because Dicke herself suffered from a prolonged illness caused by an impairment of the circulation in her right leg. As with Ling, her search for self-healing added much to the development of massage.

During this time Emil Vodder, a Danish physiologist, and his wife, Estrid, developed a technique of light massage along the course of the surface lymphatics; this technique was called *lymph drainage* or *manual lymphatic drainage.* It was and still is used to treat chronic lymphedema and other diseases of the lymphatic and peripheral vascular systems.

The American Association of Masseurs and Masseuses was formed in Chicago in 1943. It subsequently was renamed the American Massage Therapy Association. Another professional organization, the International Myomassetics Federation, was formed later through the efforts of Irene Gauthier, a notable massage instructor, and others.

James H. Cyriax, the son of Edgar Cyriax, became an orthopedic surgeon at St. Thomas Hospital, a prestigious teaching institution in London. The younger Cyriax gained fame through his development of transverse friction massage. In the late 1940s and early 1950s, he published the first edition of his now classic *Textbook of Orthopedic Medicine.* His work is especially significant in the area of massage because it recognized, categorized, and provided differential diagnoses for pathology of the body's soft tissues. The fact that pain can be caused by dysfunction of soft tissues, including periarticular connective tissue, is the foundation of soft tissue manipulation today. Cyriax also was the first to introduce the concept of *end feel* in the diagnosis of soft tissue lesions.

Dr. Herman Kabat researched neuromuscular concepts based on the work of neurophysiologists and Pavlov's conditioning of reflexes. Sherrington's law of successive induction provided the foundation for the development of rhythmic stabilization and slow reversal techniques. By 1951 research had begun on a new method, which was formalized in 1956 in the book *Proprioceptive Neuromuscular Facilitation,* written by Margaret Knott and Dorothy Voss (see Chapter 9).

Frances Tappan and Gertrude Beard also wrote important articles and books on massage techniques during the 1950s.

Their texts are still available, and serious students of massage can benefit from reading these classic works. Fran Tappan influenced the profession of massage through interviews, conferences on the future of massage, and consultation with many leaders in the field.

1960 to the Present: The Most Recent Revival of Massage. The most recent revival of massage began around 1960 and has continued to this day. Recognition of chronic diseases that are resistant to surgical or drug treatment has increased. Neither the acute care concept nor a single solution approach seems to work with these cases. A more complex way of envisioning and treating these diseases has had to be developed, and massage is one approach that has proven effective over time.

The humanistic movement that began during the 1960s spilled over into medicine and allied health. Concerns about "bedside manner," "genuineness," and the benefits of touch again raised the issue of the legitimacy and value of massage for its nurturing effect alone. Later, the Esalen movement and Gestalt psychology inspired psychologists and psychotherapists to explore massage and other movement therapies. Many controlled clinical studies in medicine, nursing, physical therapy, and psychology inspired more academic and clinical interest in massage.

In 1960 increased medical awareness that lack of exercise contributed to cardiovascular disease and other disorders prompted President John F. Kennedy to emphasize physical fitness, especially for children. This new interest grew into the physical fitness movement of the late 1960s and led the health sciences into a movement toward preventive medicine. The benefits of sports were rediscovered, and as a result, historic literature in the field of massage was brought to light, such as Albert Baumgartner's book, *Massage in Athletics*, which discussed the relationship between massage and exercise and the value of massage in conditioning and stress control.

Acupressure received more attention than any other bodywork method during the 1970s and 1980s. The medical, physical therapy, and nursing literature examined it closely on the basis of controlled clinical trials. In writings on nursing and rehabilitation medicine, a body of knowledge arose concerning the benefits of massage in preventing and treating decubitus ulcers and in the overall management of heart rate and blood pressure in people suffering from acute and chronic manifestations of cardiovascular disease.[6]

Richard van Why has said, "It was in the field of pain research and pain management that the greatest gains for massage were made."

Ronald Melzack, a professor of psychology in the anesthesiology department of McGill University Medical School and one of the initial proponents of the gate control theory of pain, published the results of several controlled clinical trials on the value of ice massage and manual massage for the relief of dental pain and low back pain. Melzack not only found these techniques effective in preventing or reducing pain, he also proposed the neural mechanisms by which they operated. Other researchers picked up on this theme and began to examine the role of massage in the liberation of endorphins, pain-killing chemicals more potent than morphine that are produced by the brain in response to certain stimuli, including massage.

In the late 1980s, in the prestigious journal *Clinics in Anesthesiology*, Melzack proposed a theory to explain endorphin release. His theory of hyperstimulation analgesia was the first in recent decades inspired by findings concerning massage. It argued that certain intense sensory stimuli, such as puncture with a needle or exposure to extreme cold or pressure, when applied near the site of an injury, sent a signal to the brain by a faster channel than that used by the pain signal it was attempting to treat, thereby disrupting the pain.[6]

Recent Trends

In the late 1980s the professional organization Associated Bodywork and Massage Professionals was formed to serve the needs of a growing and diverse group of bodywork therapists. Additional professional organizations are likely to form in the future.

In 1988 the American Massage Therapy Association spearheaded a proposal for the development of a national certification process. The proposal stirred up much controversy and was hotly debated. With the participation of other professional massage and bodywork sources, the National Certification Examination for Therapeutic Massage and Bodywork was devised in 1992. Since its inception, the examination has had a positive influence on the professional development of therapeutic massage.

The trend toward state licensure of massage continues. Educational requirements set through state licensure average 500 to 1,000 hours and show signs of increasing in the future. European and Canadian standards range from little or no training to extensive educational requirements (2,200 to 3,500 hours).

The University of Westminster in England offers bachelor's and master's degrees in massage and bodywork. This program was developed by Dr. Patrick Peitroni, Dr. Leon Chaitow, and others. Schools of massage therapy have begun to work with colleges and universities to develop articulation agreements that allow graduates of their program to complete degrees in massage. The first of these articulation agreements was reached in 1995 between the Health Enrichment Center in Lapeer, Michigan, and Siena Heights University in Adrian, Michigan, to grant both associate's and bachelor's degrees in applied science in massage therapy.

Some private massage schools have increased their educational requirements to enable them to grant associate's degrees. More community colleges are developing certificate programs in therapeutic massage, and some of these programs can lead to an associate's degree in applied or general science.

Those who have experienced the revival of massage from 1960 to the present may wonder if this success carries with it mixed blessings. Before 1985 massage professionals worked primarily in independent settings with little or no supervision. The very best of this situation was the freedom to serve clients' needs without the constraints of regulation. The worst was the lack of consistent training and the confusion among other professionals and the public about what constituted therapeutic massage.

Frustration with massage parlor regulations enacted to control prostitution and the desire of many massage professionals to enter the mainstream of public awareness pushed the massage therapy profession to begin seeking an alliance with the existing health care structure to justify the validity of massage. In some instances this movement into the existing health care world created turf battles over which profession would provide massage therapy. Questions and concerns, both legitimate and reactionary, were expressed by the physical therapy and nursing professions.

The public's desire for physical fitness had reached its peak during this time, and the concept of "sports massage" provided an avenue for mainstreaming massage therapy. During the 1990s the mainstream approach shifted from sports to corporate America. David Palmer can be given credit for formalizing the concepts of on site and chair massage. These two trends allowed the public to see massage in a way much different from the preconceived notions of a "feel good" luxury of the wealthy or a front for prostitution.

As research continues to validate massage therapy and as massage evolves into a distinct professional course requiring a credible, standardized education, the turf battles in the health care system seem to be quieting down. Health care is moving in the direction of using multidisciplinary teams in which many different professionals work together. As this process continues, nurses and physical therapists probably will find themselves supervising massage paraprofessionals and working as partners with more comprehensively trained massage therapists who have earned a degree.

In 1991 the Touch Research Institute at the University of Miami opened under the direction of Dr. Tiffany Field. More than any other single development in the 1990s, the research produced by the institute has moved massage into the mainstream and into accepted health care practice.

Also in 1991 the NIH established the Office of Alternative Medicine. Two years later, the *New England Journal of Medicine* reported on a national survey on the use of alternative and complementary forms of health care. Massage was the third most used treatment. In line with this trend, *Alternative Medicine: Expanding Medical Horizons: A Report to the National Institutes of Health on Alternative Medical Systems and Practices in the United States* was published in 1994.

The credibility and acceptance of natural approaches to health and illness are developing, and knowledge bases are beginning to overlap. Three areas in osteopathic medicine that currently are applicable to massage are muscle energy techniques, positional release and strain/counterstrain techniques, and neuromuscular techniques. The most noteworthy educator and author in these methods is Dr. Leon Chaitow, who, like Ling, is a master synthesizer of the best of many concepts. Dr. Chaitow developed a strong foundation in manual medicine working as an assistant to his uncle, Dr. Boris Chaitow, the codeveloper of neuromuscular technique along with his cousin, the legendary Dr. Stanley Lief.[9] Dr. Leon Chaitow has written many books that have enriched the body of knowledge for soft tissue methods, including therapeutic massage.

Other authors worthy of mention include Ida Rolf, developer of the Rolfing system; Dr. Milton Trager, developer of Trager; and Dr. Janet Travell, coauthor with David Simons of the most comprehensive texts written on the subject of trigger points.* Since 1995 the amount of information available on therapeutic massage has increased dramatically. Many new and exciting books are on the market, and Web sites for therapeutic massage have been created on the Internet. All forms of media, including television, magazines, and newspapers, carry supportive stories about the benefits of massage.

Research continued to validate the benefits of massage through the 1990s. After years of struggle for acceptance and validation, massage in the mid-1990s moved into the mainstream, and as the new millennium progresses, the next century of massage will evolve. (See the Evolve Web site for a list of individuals who have contributed to the evolution of massage.) What the future will bring depends on our commitment to the ideals of massage.

The Future of Massage: 2008 and Beyond

The role of massage and related bodywork methods is expanding at an accelerated rate. Massage now has enough validation to justify its use by the public as well as health care professionals. An explosion of information and awareness has occurred. The future will determine the way the profession responds to the needs created by this success.

The massage therapy profession is changing. It is becoming more sophisticated, requiring education not only in technical skill development but also in pathology, medications, record keeping, and communication skills, as well as in the important area of professional ethics. The more massage professionals work with other health care professionals, the more they need to know to be able to understand the world of health care. As we blend our world of professional touch with theirs, it will be interesting to watch the exchange of information. We hope that the best of both worlds will emerge and that the lessons of the past will temper and soften the process (Figure 1-5).

More and more employment opportunities are becoming available in the area of health care. Mental health interventions that use massage are becoming commonplace. Some health care insurance plans and managed care systems are beginning to look at ways to include massage therapy among their covered services. Sports massage for amateur and professional athletes is becoming the norm, with massage therapists working side by side with athletic trainers and coaches.

In the wellness and personal service areas, day spas are bringing the art of pampering to the general public. No longer does a person have to travel to some far-off place and spend thousands of dollars to experience the pleasure of a day of luxury. The spa industry is one of the fastest growing employers of massage professionals. Massage clinics that focus on

---

*The two texts by written by Travell and Simons are *Myofascial pain and dysfunction: the trigger point manual* and *myofascial pain and dysfunction: the trigger point manual: the lower extremities*, vol. 2.

FIGURE 1-5 Diversity in massage therapy.

FIGURE 1-6 A bright future: the teaching of the next generation.

wellness massage are becoming commonplace, as are massage professionals in the corporate setting.

Research into genetics, stress responses, neuroendocrine influences, and environmental hazards, as well as support for the whole person in coping with a world that seems to be moving too fast, encourages the development of massage as a counterbalance to a stressful lifestyle, stressful world events, and a persistent state of ambiguity that promotes anxiety states. The current trends supported by research seem to indicate that manual therapies are gaining recognition. Dr. Field of the Touch Research Institute is a major contributor to the growth of massage therapy because of her dedication to touch research.

As the world becomes a global community, the ever-increasing exchange of information will enrich the knowledge base of therapeutic massage. Exploration of ancient healing methods will reveal the wisdom and scientific validity of a body/mind/spirit approach to well-being.

Hopefully, the abundant massage and bodywork methods will combine into a consolidated system of therapeutic massage without losing the rich diversity of professional expression. Terminology and education will standardize, although the integrity of the individual applications of massage and bodywork will be maintained. Two tracks of massage service probably will standardize: wellness massage outside the health care system and medical massage within the health care system. These trends will allow easy access for all to both types of services.

The future is very bright and promising, especially if we pay attention to our past and remember the words and wisdom of an old Russian physician, who says, "massage is massage." We ourselves constitute one of the biggest threats to the future of massage. All bodywork professions must come together to work for the common good. As the massage profession moves forward and reclaims its heritage as an important health service, it is important to look back. In retrospect, we can see the strengths and weaknesses of the professional journey (Figure 1-6).

It also is important to honor those who have dedicated so much of their lives to developing the body of knowledge of therapeutic massage. Many today are dedicating a significant portion of their lives to the professional advancement of therapeutic massage. When the history of massage is written in the future, these names will appear with the information they have organized and contributed. We are all contributors to the future of massage, and we all will become part of its history.

THINK IT OVER

- What do you want the future of massage to bring?
- How are you going to assist in the development of that future?

■ ■ ■ SUMMARY

This chapter began with questions and ended with questions. The importance and nature of touch in the professional setting were discussed. The reader should now be aware of the ways in which culture, gender, age, life events, spirituality, and diversity all influence the experience of touching and being touched. Inappropriate forms of touch were identified, and appropriate forms of professional touch were explored. An understanding of the subjective experience of touch was addressed personally.

The history of massage from ancient times to the present was presented, as were projections for the future. A time line highlighted many key dates. The foundation has been laid for the study of therapeutic massage.

1-1 Explore the Evolve Web site that accompanies this book.

1-2 Complete an interactive order exercise by placing massage historical events on a timeline.

1-3 Answer true or false for a list of appropriate or inappropriate touching examples.

Don't forget to study for your certification and licensure exams! Review questions for this chapter are located on Evolve.

REFERENCES

1. Lederman E: *Fundamentals of manual therapy physiology, neurology, and psychology,* New York, 1997, Churchill Livingstone.
2. Smith EWL, Clance PR, Imes S: *Touch in psychotherapy,* New York, 1998, Guilford Press.
3. Tappan FM, Benjamin PJ: *Tappan's handbook of healing massage techniques: classic, holistic, and emerging methods,* ed 4, 2004, Prentice Hall.
4. Greenman PE: *Principles of manual medicine,* ed 3, Baltimore, 2003, Williams & Wilkins.
5. Cantu RI, Grodin AJ: *Myofascial manipulation: theory and clinical application,* Gaithersburg, Md, 1992, Aspen Publishers.
6. van Why RP: *History of massage and its relevance to today's practitioner,* the Bodywork Knowledgebase, New York, 1992, self-published.
7. van Why RP: *Notes toward a history of massage,* ed 2, New York, 1992, self-published.
8. Gurevich D: Historical perspective, 1992 (unpublished article).
9. Chaitow L: *Soft tissue manipulation,* Rochester, Vt, 1988, Healing Arts Press.

Workbook Section

■ ■ ■ SHORT ANSWER

1. What is the skin's significance in touch?

2. What factors can influence an individual's experience of touch?

3. What are the forms of inappropriate professional touch?

4. What are the forms of appropriate professional touch?

5. In what way and where did massage originate? Why is this answer important?

6. What has provided the validation for massage?

7. What methods did the ancient Chinese massage system use? In what ways are the methods of today different?

8. Why was massage associated with folk medicine and connected with supernatural experiences during the Middle Ages in Europe?

9. Why is credit given to Per Henrik Ling for the development of the Swedish movement cure and Swedish massage?

10. In what way did problems with terminology interfere with the acceptance of Ling's work?

11. Who or what was one of the main contributors to the massage scandals in the late 1800s?

12. What aspect of massage remained active outside the medical establishment from the 1940s to the present?

13. What research has provided the current validation of massage?

14. In what way has massage brought the best of the East and West together?

■ ■ ■ REVIEW QUESTIONS

Write your personal definition for each of the following words.

1. Professional
2. Structured
3. Therapeutic
4. Touch

■ ■ ■ ESSAY QUESTIONS

1. What does "touch intention" mean to you?
2. How would you describe your professional touch intention?

Workbook Section—cont'd

■ ■ ■ MATCHING

Match the person or information in the first column with the best response in the second column.

1. Massage in the Eastern world
2. Massage in the Western world
3. Ambrose Paré
4. Per Henrik Ling
5. Followers of Johann Mezger
6. Duplicated movements
7. Active movements
8. Passive movements
9. Charles F. Taylor and George H. Taylor
10. Mathias Roth
11. Sister Kenny
12. Ida Rolf
13. Dr. Dolores Krieger
14. Dr. John Harvey Kellogg
15. Dr. Charles K. Mills
16. Wilhelm Reich
17. Alexander Lowen
18. Elizabeth Dicke
19. Margaret Knott and Dorothy Voss
20. *Esalen and Gestalt*
21. Autonomic approach
22. Mechanical approach
23. Movement approach
24. Dr. Boris Chaitow and Dr. Stanley Lief
25. Dr. Milton Trager

a. known as exercise
b. proposed an integrated program of active and passive movements based on Swedish gymnastics
c. an English physician who studied with Ling
d. developed Rolfing
e. a neurologist and massage advocate who criticized the uneven quality of practitioners
f. founded bioenergetics
g. inspired psychotherapists to explore massage and movement therapies
h. changes abnormal movement patterns into optimal ones
i. used French terms such as *effleurage* and *pétrissage*
j. a continuation of Greco-Roman traditions
k. commonly called *resistive exercises*
l. cofounders of the neuromuscular technique
m. developed therapeutic touch–energetic approach
n. range of motion and stretching that are performed by a therapist
o. a Battle Creek, Michigan, physician who used massage and hydrotherapy
p. attempts mechanical changes in soft tissue
q. introduced Swedish movements in the United States
r. used massage for joint stiffness and wound healing after surgery
s. kept alive as part of folk culture
t. founded psychotherapeutic body techniques
u. developed the Trager system
v. developed connective tissue massage
w. wrote the first major book on proprioceptive neuromuscular facilitation
x. used massage in the treatment of polio
y. exerts a therapeutic effect on the autonomic nervous system

____ d. Julius Caesar has himself pinched all over to relieve pain.
____ e. A cave dweller stubs his toe and instinctively rubs it.
____ f. Per Henrik Ling combines massage and Swedish gymnastics into a new system.
____ g. Dr. Mary P. Jacobi and Dr. Victoria A. White research massage benefits.
____ h. The massage scandals occur in England.
____ i. Charles F. Taylor and George H. Taylor introduce Swedish movements in the United States.
____ j. Galen writes on early manual medicine, supporting the methods of Hippocrates.
____ k. Albert Hoffa publishes a textbook on classic techniques of massage.
____ l. The polio epidemic sparks widespread interest in massage.
____ m. Elizabeth Dicke develops connective tissue massage.
____ n. The Royal Gymnastic Central Institute is established.
____ o. Celsus compiles *De Medicina*.
____ p. The American Association of Masseurs and Masseuses is formed.
____ q. Hippocrates encourages physicians to use massage.
____ r. Dr. James H. Cyriax writes the classic *Textbook of Orthopedic Medicine*.
____ s. Dr. Charles K. Mills criticizes the uneven quality of the practice of massage.
____ t. Margaret Knott and Dorothy Voss write *Proprioceptive Neuromuscular Facilitation*.
____ u. The National Certification Examination for Therapeutic Massage and Bodywork is developed.
____ v. Dr. Tiffany Field researches massage.

■ ■ ■ ASSESS YOUR COMPETENCIES

Now that you have studied this chapter, you should be able to:

1. Explain the meaning of professional touch.
2. Identify personal interpretations of touch and their influence on professional interactions.
3. Explain the rich heritage and history of therapeutic massage.
4. Explain the influence of historical events on the current development of therapeutic massage.

■ ■ ■ TIME LINE EXERCISE

Number the following events, activities, and people in chronologic order. For example, (e) is no. 1.

____ a. The art of massage is first mentioned.
____ b. Ambrose Paré uses massage to aid postsurgical recovery.
____ c. M. LeRon introduces the Swedish movement cure in Russia.

■ ■ ■ PROFESSIONAL APPLICATION EXERCISE

You are asked to present a brief lecture on the history of massage at a meeting of the local historical society. Develop a presentation outline.

Professionalism and Legal Issues

CHAPTER OBJECTIVES

After completing this chapter, the student will be able to perform the following:

- Define professionalism
- Define therapeutic massage
- Define a scope of practice for therapeutic massage
- Develop and explain a code of ethics and the standards of practice for therapeutic massage
- Complete an informed consent process
- Take ethics into consideration in maintaining professional boundaries and the therapeutic relationship
- Use basic communication skills to listen effectively and deliver an I-message
- Identify and resolve conflict in the professional setting
- Use a problem-solving approach to enhance ethical decision making
- Identify legal and credentialing concerns of the massage professional
- Identify and report unethical conduct of colleagues
- Become familiar with the Health Insurance Portability and Accountability Act (HIPAA) and its requirements and training

CHAPTER OUTLINE

Continued.

KEY TERMS

Active listening	Mentoring
Aspirational ethics	Needs assessment
Confidentiality	Peer support
Conflict	Power differential
Countertransference	Principles
Credentials	Reciprocity
Defensive climate	Reflective listening
Dual role	Right of refusal
Ethical behavior	Scope of practice
Ethical decision making	Standards of practice
Ethics	Supervision
Informed consent	Supportive climate
Initial treatment plan	Therapeutic relationship
Mandatory ethics	Transference

The student of therapeutic massage must be able to define therapeutic massage, identify the types of professional services a massage practitioner legally and ethically can provide, and establish guidelines for conduct in the professional setting. This chapter cannot give specifics for all these issues, because the massage community itself is unclear in many areas, and professionalism in many ways evolves as a profession evolves. What this chapter can do is provide content that enables students to intelligently begin asking the necessary questions and formulating effective processes for answering these questions for themselves. The following professional development issues and skills are addressed in this chapter:

- The definition of massage
- The scope of practice for massage professionals
- Ethical conduct and standards of practice for massage professionals
- The therapeutic relationship
- Communication and conflict management skills to support professional interaction
- Professional record keeping to support professional achievement
- Provisions of the Health Insurance Portability and Accountability Act of 1996
- Credentialing, licensing, and other legal concerns of the massage professional
- Peer support, supervision, and mentoring

This information provides the structure for professional and ethical decision making. This chapter is intended to encourage the student to develop the level of professionalism essential to the successful practice of therapeutic massage.

First we will explore the name of our profession. What do we call ourselves? The student will discover that this is more complicated than it might seem at first. Then we will look at what we do—the definition of therapeutic massage. Armed with these two pieces of information, we will discuss the scope of practice for therapeutic massage and the appropriate training for the practice of therapeutic massage.

The chapter further describes professional services and the various forms of therapeutic massage services, ranging from wellness massage to medical/clinical rehabilitative massage.

PROFICIENCY EXERCISE 2-1

The following questions should be answered regarding professional services and the various forms of therapeutic massage services, ranging from wellness massage to medical/clinical rehabilitative massage.

- What is ethical conduct for the massage professional, and how does one make ethical decisions?
- What communication and record-keeping skills are necessary to support a professional practice and fulfill legal responsibilities?
- What are the legal requirements for practice?
- What professional organizations represent the profession?
- How does one identify and report unethical conduct in peers?
- What is the importance of peer support, supervision, and mentoring?
- What is your question? Write it here.

Ethics and professionalism have a unique language. The following definitions clarify some of the terminology used in this chapter.

- *Countertransference* is an inability on the part of the professional to separate the therapeutic relationship from personal feelings and expectations for the client; it is personalization of the professional relationship by the professional.
- A *dual role* results when scopes of practice overlap, with one professional providing support in more than one area of expertise.
- *Ethics* is the science or study of morals, values, and principles, including the ideals of autonomy, beneficence, and justice. Ethics comprises principles of right and good conduct.
- **Ethical behavior** is right and correct conduct based on moral and cultural standards as defined by the society in which we live.
- **Ethical decision making** is the application of ethical principles and professional skills to determine appropriate behavior and resolve ethical dilemmas.
- *Informed consent* is a consumer protection process; it requires that clients be informed of the steps of treatment, that their participation be voluntary, and that they be competent to give consent. Informed consent is also an educational process that allows clients to make knowledgeable decisions about whether to receive a massage.
- *Mentoring* is a professional relationship in which an individual with experience and skill beyond those of the person being mentored provides support, encouragement, and career expertise.
- *Peer support* is the interaction among those of similar skill and experience to encourage and maintain appropriate professional practice.
- A *principle* is a basic truth or rule of conduct.
- The *scope of practice* is the knowledge base and practice parameters of a profession.
- *Standards of practice* are principles that serve as specific guidelines for directing professional ethical practice and quality care, including a structure for evaluating the quality of care. They are an attempt to define the parameters of quality care.
- *Supervision* involves a person who oversees others and their professional behavior. The supervisor may be from a different discipline (e.g., a nurse) or may be a massage therapist who has more skill and experience than those supervised. Supervisors usually are in a position of authority. They are actively involved in such areas as the development and approval of treatment plans, review of clarity, scheduling, discipline, and teaching.
- A *therapeutic relationship* is created by the interpersonal structure and professional boundaries between professionals and their clients.
- *Transference* is the personalization of the professional relationship by the client.

PROFESSIONALISM AND THERAPEUTIC MASSAGE

SECTION OBJECTIVES

Using the information presented in this section, the student will be able to perform the following:

- Compare therapeutic massage with professional development criteria
- Describe the two professional development trends in therapeutic massage

The subjects of ethics and professionalism are very important to the therapeutic massage profession. In any professional practice, the ambiguity of ethics and the concreteness of professionalism and standards of practice converge to form a basis for ethical decision making. A profession is different from a job, and a professional does more than go to work. Expanding on the definition of a professional that was presented in Chapter 1, we could say that a professional is one who has the following characteristics:

1. A specialized body of knowledge
2. Extensive training
3. An orientation toward service
4. A commonly accepted code of ethics
5. Legal recognition through certification or licensure by a professional organization
6. Membership in a professional association

Specialized Body of Knowledge

Massage therapy methods are grounded in a specialized body of knowledge (some of this knowledge base is presented in this textbook). Historical foundations and current research validate this body of knowledge. As we discussed in Chapter 1, a lifetime of study easily could be devoted to therapeutic massage methods.

Extensive Training

Questions have arisen about the duration of massage training and the information and technical skills that should be included in that training. The area of professional development for therapeutic massage requires elements of standardization to allow continued progress toward professionalism. Currently, no agreement has been reached on the difference between a wellness orientation to massage and a medical or rehabilitative orientation.

Three distinct career tracks are emerging for massage:

- Spa setting
- Sports and fitness setting
- Medical/clinical/rehabilitation setting

Spa Setting

The evolving spa environment encompasses a range of massage services for wellness- and pleasure-based massage; these services can overlap with sports and fitness massage and massage directly related to health care in the so-called medical spa. This text provides the skills necessary to develop a successful career in the spa environment, especially with supervision in the fitness-focused spa or medical spa.

Sports and Fitness Setting

The sports and fitness career track covers a spectrum of massage outcomes, ranging from wellness to medical intervention typically (but not exclusively) based on issues related to environments that support exercise and sports performance. The importance of exercise in the management of most lifestyle-related diseases, such as diabetes, obesity, cardiovascular, mental illness, and many more, is well documented. Massage can support physical changes related to exercise and can help manage the discomfort related to physical activity and injury for those beginning an exercise program. Massage can also be beneficial for the extensive performance demands required of entertainers and professional athletes. Information in this text, presented in the appropriate scientific context, provides the foundation for working in this setting. However, continuing education is necessary to provide the information that enables a practitioner to be confident and proficient in this area.*

The common thread of the medical/clinical/rehabilitation career path is integration with health care systems. This type of massage treatment may focus on stress management and prevention, management of chronic disease and pain, acute care palliation, presurgical and postsurgical care, prenatal care, elder care, and hospice care. This text provides the necessary foundation for general massage in this area, and continuing education provides the information that enables the practitioner to be confident and proficient providing this type of massage therapy. (Chapter 12 describes this content in depth.)

The current standard of 500 to 750 contact hours (10 to 15 credit hours) may be sufficient for basic wellness massage methods, but judging from data collected from actual job duties and current trends in licensing requirements, 1,000 contact hours (20 to 24 credit hours) probably is more appropriate for supporting professional development in the wellness realm. It does not seem reasonable to expect that programs of 500 to 1,000 contact hours provide sufficient time for integration of clinical reasoning methods; extensive physical assessment procedures; and the study of pathophysiology, pharmacology, and psychology, as well as other information the massage professional needs to work effectively with other health care professionals and with complicated, multifaceted health concerns. The same can be said for sports massage or working with athletes. To work effectively with athletes, the professional must have an in-depth education in the dynamics of sports activity, the injury process, and rehabilitation.

Current educational trends are moving toward the development of two professional tracks in therapeutic massage: (1) vocationally trained wellness massage service professionals and paraprofessionals in the health care area and (2) degree-holding professionals in the allied health care system.

The current model for service professionals (e.g., those working in the field of cosmetology) and for paraprofessionals (those trained to assist a professional) in health care and sports and fitness calls for 300 to 1,800 contact hours (7 to 40 credit hours) of vocational training in technically based programs, after which the student is granted a certificate or diploma. Obviously, training standards vary widely.

A professional usually is considered to be a person who has a degree in his or her chosen field. It may be an associate's degree (usually requiring 64 credits); a bachelor's degree (usually requiring 124 credits); or a master's or doctoral degree, such as those held by teachers, physicians, athletic trainers, and mental health professionals.

Most educational models for therapeutic massage in the United States fall into the vocational services professional or paraprofessional realm. However, more massage programs have begun offering programs leading to an associate's degree or higher. Some Canadian provinces, as well as Australia, England, New Zealand, Poland, Russia, and other countries, require or offer training that meets the current definition of a professional degree. Individuals who already have professional degrees are obtaining massage therapy training and combining the two skills to function effectively in the health and athletic worlds; some examples of these combinations are nurse/massage therapist, athletic trainer/massage therapist, respiratory therapist/massage therapist, physical therapy assistant/massage therapist, occupational therapist/massage therapist, and social worker or psychologist/massage therapist.

The level of information in this text supports training programs of 500 to 1,500 contact hours (10 to 34 credit hours) in the service and paraprofessional realms. The greatest employment potential for therapeutic massage probably will follow this career orientation. The training level of this text is sufficient to allow those with other degrees (i.e, nursing, athletic training) to integrate massage therapy into their professional worlds. In longer programs (i.e., those requiring more than 2,000 contact hours), the information in this text can serve as the foundation on which clinical or more specific forms of therapeutic massage approaches are built.

Orientation Toward Service

The definition of service that best applies to this discussion is "to meet a need." An additional concept in a service orientation is that, although reimbursement is expected for services rendered, the desire to meet a need takes precedence over financial return. Observation of those who practice massage professionally and of the attitudes of current students indicates that providers of therapeutic massage definitely have an orientation toward service, sometimes to the detriment of sound business practices. Although it is important to care for the people we serve, it is just as important to generate the necessary and appropriate income base to support the professional practice and a reasonably comfortable lifestyle for the professional.

---

*Comprehesive content is available in Fritz: *Sports & exercise massage: comprehensive care in athletics, fitness, & rehabilitation* and Fritz; *Clinical massage in the healthcare setting*, St. Louis, 2006, Mosby.

Commonly Accepted Code of Ethics

As you study the rest of this chapter, you will see that although general agreement exists about what a code of ethics entails, no agreement has been reached on a specific code of ethics to serve the entire massage profession.

Legal Recognition Through Certification or Licensure by a Professional Organization

Licensure and certification for therapeutic massage are not standardized, therefore this area of professional development remains ambiguous. About one third of the U.S. states and half of the Canadian provinces have formal licensing or legislated certification for massage professionals. Legal recognition in various other countries ranges from extensive licensing requirements to no legal control. The United States now has a voluntary national certification process, which eventually may clear up the confusion in the eyes of the public and other professionals over the practice parameters of therapeutic massage methods. It will be interesting to watch this whole issue unfold in the next few years. (See the Evolve Web site for a list of states in which licensing is offered.)

Membership in a Professional Association

Several organizations attempt to represent the therapeutic massage profession. In addition, each of the various bodywork methods (e.g., reflexology, shiatsu, polarity) has its own professional organization. Although diversity is good for a profession and supports professional development, the lack of coherence in the field of therapeutic massage confuses the public, ourselves, and other professionals. Developments in this area also will be interesting to watch (Proficiency Exercise 2-2).

FINDING A NAME

SECTION OBJECTIVE

Using the information presented in this section, the student will be able to perform the following:

- Distinguish between a technician, a practitioner, and a therapist

 PROFICIENCY EXERCISE 2-2

In the space provided, answer each of the questions with your opinion. Exchange and compare your opinions with others.

- How would you rate massage therapy against the six criteria listed previously on pp. 27–29?

- What areas of the massage profession do you think are well developed, and what areas need development?

- What do you think is required to enable the therapeutic massage profession to continue to evolve?

- What can you do to contribute to this evolution?

The therapeutic massage profession has not yet agreed on a professional career name. It is difficult to establish a unique professional identity when we do not know our name. The lack of a single name also makes the creation of standardized textbooks somewhat frustrating. What do we call ourselves? Are we technicians, practitioners, or therapists?

A technician is perceived differently from a therapist, particularly in terms of educational level. A *technician* can be defined as one who has expertise in a technical skill or process. A technician has the least training and the most limited scope of practice in a professional group.

The next educational level is the practitioner. A *practitioner* can be defined as one who practices an occupation or a profession. A practitioner operates from a greater knowledge base and within a larger scope of practice than a technician.

A *therapist* can be defined as one who treats illness or disability. A therapist requires the highest educational background and has the broadest scope of practice.

The massage profession currently does not use these designations as they are defined in this text, but the public and the health care professions often do. What is the public's perception, then, if *massage therapist* becomes our name? Although all forms of massage are therapeutic, perhaps the names *technician* and *practitioner* are best suited to the massage profession as it is currently practiced outside the health care system. *Massage therapist* might be more fitting when massage is practiced in the health care environment and the person has a more extensive education.

The confusion continues. Are we massage professionals, myomassologists, neuromuscular therapists, or soft tissue practitioners? Are we bodyworkers, and is massage a form of bodywork? Are we massage professionals, with other forms of bodywork becoming subcategories of massage?

As is explained in the Preface, for the purposes of this text, the terms *massage technician, practitioner, therapist,* and *professional* are used interchangeably (Proficiency Exercise 2-3).

 PROFICIENCY EXERCISE 2-3

Write the name you prefer for a therapeutic massage professional and justify your choice. An example is provided.

Example

Preferred name: Massage practitioner

Justification: The name "practitioner" indicates a level of training that meets the definition of professional but does not indicate the function of therapy, which is the treatment of illness or disability.

Your Turn

Preferred name:

Justification:

THE DEFINITION OF THERAPEUTIC MASSAGE

SECTION OBJECTIVES

Using the information presented in this section, the student will be able to perform the following:

- Develop a definition of massage
- Explain the differences and similarities of various approaches to therapeutic massage
- Clarify the eight basic approaches to therapeutic massage
- Classify a massage method according to its fundamental physiologic basis

In Chapter 1 we began to trace the development of the term *massage*. The roots of the word *massage* mean to touch, handle, squeeze, knead, and press softly (see Chapter 1); therefore we defined massage as professional, structured, therapeutic touch. Over the past few years, as the popularity of therapeutic massage has grown, the profession has seen an expansion in styles and systems (Box 2-1). The term *bodywork* has been used to cover the scope of these developments. As individual systems have emerged, a difference in styles has developed. However, the overlap of these methods reveals a fundamental sameness in all the work, and this core could become the foundation for professional standards and definitions. These similarities should not detract from the devotion, training, and expertise of the various practitioners in specific disciplines. Unification of the profession around these shared aspects should not threaten individual practice of specific disciplines.

Research has shown that the application of systematic touching for health purposes (i.e., therapeutic massage) is valid (see Chapter 4). By carefully examining any style or system of massage, the student can see that basic methods are used to stimulate sensory receptors. These methods either stimulate a rhythmic order in body functions or disrupt an existing pattern in the central nervous system control centers, resulting in a shift in nerve and chemical patterns to re-establish homeostasis (reflexive methods). The very same methods can be applied in a different way to change the consistency or position of connective tissue or to shift pressure in the vessels to facilitate blood and lymph circulation (mechanical methods). Although most of the systems have been developed over the centuries, a few new massage approaches have come into their own over the past few years (Figure 2-1).

Technology and research probably will prove that massage methods share the same physiologic basis in their effectiveness. All massage approaches have the same basis because the people they serve share the anatomy and physiology of the human form. No one particular style of massage is better than another if the fundamental components are included along with the methods purposefully used by a trained professional to serve the client's needs. The profession must begin to standardize terminology to avoid confusion about the various styles and systems of massage. The explanations of anatomy and physiology given in Asian styles of massage may be different from those of Western science, but the human body is the same, and the effects of these styles are the same as those of systems developed in Polynesia, India, Europe, Africa, the United States, and around the world. Various massage systems (e.g., Swedish massage, deep tissue techniques, reflexology, sports massage, and body/mind integration) work through the same anatomic and physiologic mechanisms, but each has developed a language unique to that approach. The study of various systems becomes confusing only when so many different names are used for similar methods. A core body of knowledge exists from which therapeutic massage approaches have evolved, and a skilled practitioner should be able to identify and explain any approach based on physiologic effects.

The different systems and styles presented in this text are variations on a theme. To become skilled practitioners, students learn the theme and explore the variations. Any of these systems can be explained in anatomic and physiologic terminology (Figure 2-2).

Defining Massage

A definition of *massage* (Box 2-2) must encompass all the methods used by various systems. Massage cannot be considered a single skill; a more appropriate concept is that of a collection of skills. In addition, the definition of therapeutic massage depends on individual laws and the definition of massage included in those laws. Members of the profession itself have not agreed on a definition. This text offers a general definition of *massage*. Defining massage accurately and completely is difficult because of the many forms of massage currently practiced. An attempt is made to include items from the many definitions found in historical literature, from guidelines provided by state and local laws and professional organizations, and from individual styles and approaches to massage.

SCOPE OF PRACTICE

SECTION OBJECTIVES

Using the information presented in this section, the student will be able to perform the following:

- Understand the scope of practice of various health and service professionals
- Explain what constitutes the practice of medicine
- Explain the difference between medical or rehabilitative massage and wellness massage
- Develop a scope of practice for massage that respects the scope of practice of other professionals

As mentioned earlier, the scope of practice of a profession defines the knowledge base and practice parameters of that profession. Each health and service profession has a unique information/knowledge base, yet members of many professions share a common knowledge and methodology. Because of this shared information, the lines defining a profession's scope of practice are not always clear, and overlap can occur.

BOX 2-1

Popular Methods of Massage

This list of styles, systems, founders, and developers is not meant to be all-inclusive because the information changes almost daily. Rather, it is meant to show the great variety of therapeutic massage approaches.

Asian

■ *Amma, acupressure, shiatsu, jin shin do, do-in, hoshino, tui-na, watsu, Tibetan point holding, Thai massage*

These methods derive from original Chinese concepts and from offshoots of the Chinese base. These compressive manipulations and stretches, which focus on specific areas of the body, elicit responses in the nervous and circulatory systems. The efficient use of the therapist's body and the performance of these techniques on a clothed client have many benefits. The philosophy of these systems is grounded in ancient concepts that have stood the test of time. The effects are both reflexive and mechanical.

Structural and Postural Integration

■ *Bindegewebs massage, Rolfing, Hellerwork, Looyen, Pfrimmer, Soma, Bowen therapy*

These techniques focus more specifically on the connective tissue structure to influence posture and biomechanics. The approaches are systematic and effective because they are grounded in the fundamentals of physiology and biomechanics. Practitioners of these styles have received an extensive education.

Neuromuscular

■ *Neuromuscular techniques, muscle energy techniques, strain/counterstrain, orthobionomy, Trager, myotherapy, proprioceptive neuromuscular facilitation, reflexology, trigger points*

These are the European approaches based on the work of Dr. Stanley Leif and Dr. Boris Chaitow and the Western methods based on the work of Dr. Janet Travell, Dr. John Mennell, Dr. Raymond Nimmo, Dr. Lawrence Jones, Dr. Milton Trager, Eunice Ingham, William Fitzgerald, Arthur Lincoln Pauls, Bonnie Prudden, and others. Dr. Leon Chaitow has written extensively on these concepts and currently teaches in the United States and Europe. Many of the techniques are similar to those found in Rolfing, Asian methods, and Swedish massage and gymnastics. As the name implies, the approach is a nervous or reflexive method. Observation of the systems reveals that connective tissue also is affected. The common threads running through all the styles are the basic concepts of activation of the tonus receptor mechanism, reflex arc stimulation, positional receptors, and applications of stretching and lengthening.

Manual Lymphatic Drainage

Vodder Lymphatic Drainage

Emil Vodder developed an excellent system that uses the anatomy and physiology of lymphatic movement with both mechanical and reflexive techniques to stimulate the flow of lymphatic fluid. Others have contributed to the understanding of lymphatic drain procedures, including Brian Chickly and Lyle Lederman. The variations of this system sometimes are called *systemic massage.*

Energetic (Biofield)

Polarity, Therapeutic Touch, Reiki, Zero Balancing

These systems, which are based on ancient concepts of body energy patterns, recently were formalized by Dr. Randolph Stone, Dr. Dolores Krieger, Dr. Fritz Smith, and others. Subtle energy medicine is under study by Dr. Elmer Green at the Menninger Foundation in Topeka, Kansas, and elsewhere by other researchers. Polarity and similar energetic approaches use near touch or light touch to initiate reflexive responses, often with highly effective results.

Craniosacral and Myofascial

■ *Craniosacral therapy, myofascial release, soft tissue mobilization, deep tissue massage, connective tissue massage*

These systems focus more specifically on the various aspects of both mechanical and reflexive connective tissue functions. Dr. William Garner Sutherland was the first to formalize the concept of minute movement of the cranium and dura. Dr. John Upledger and John Barnes, PT, have expanded upon and formalized his work. Both light and deep touch are used, depending on the method. Dr. James Cyriax's cross-fiber friction methods fall into this category.

Applied Kinesiology

Touch for Health, Applied Physiology, Educational Kinesiology, Three-in-One Concepts

Dr. George Goodheart formalized the system of applied kinesiology within the chiropractic discipline. The approach blends many techniques but works primarily with the reflexive mechanisms. A specific muscle testing procedure is used for evaluation; this process acts somewhat like a biofeedback mechanism. Some of the corrective measures use Asian meridians and acupressure; others rely on the osteopathic reflex mechanisms defined by Chapman, Bennett, and McKenzie that seem to correspond to traditional Chinese acupuncture points. Dr. John Thie and others modified these techniques for use by massage professionals and the public.

Integrated Approaches

■ *Sports massage, infant massage, equine/animal massage, on site or seated massage, prenatal massage, geriatric massage, massage for abuse survivors, Russian massage*

Many styles of massage that focus on a specific type of population use combinations of methods based on physiologic interventions. Founders and teachers of integrated methods include every massage professional who designs a massage specifically for an individual client and every devoted massage instructor who attempts to combine and explain methods to students.

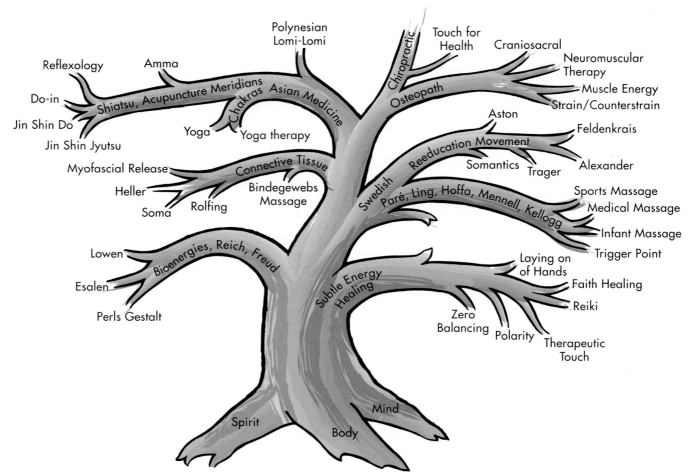

FIGURE 2-1 The therapeutic massage tree. Although massage encompasses a wide diversity in its uses and applications, all forms of therapeutic massage methods stem from the same roots.

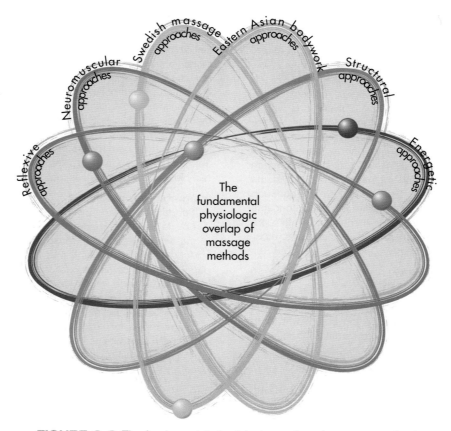

FIGURE 2-2 The fundamental physiologic overlap of massage methods.

BOX 2-2

Definition of Therapeutic Massage

Therapeutic massage is the scientific art and system of assessment and systematic, manual application of a technique to the superficial soft tissue of the skin, muscles, tendons, ligaments, and fascia, as well as to the structures that lie within the superficial tissue, by means of the hand, foot, knee, arm, elbow, and forearm. The manual technique involves systematic application of touch, stroking (effleurage), friction, vibration, percussion, kneading (pétrissage), stretching, compression, or passive and active joint movements within the normal physiologic range of motion. Also included are adjunctive external applications of water, heat, and cold for the purposes of establishing and maintaining good physical condition and health by normalizing and improving muscle tone, promoting relaxation, stimulating circulation, and producing therapeutic effects on the respiratory and nervous systems and the subtle interactions among all body systems. These intended effects are accomplished through the physiologic, energetic, and mind/body connections in a safe, nonsexual environment that respects the client's self-determined outcome for the session.

Each member of a particular profession acquires a specific knowledge base and must define her personal scope of practice. A professional must be able to evaluate his acquired body of knowledge and skills realistically to determine the parameters of ethical practice within the scope of practice. True professionals understand the limits of their technical skills and scopes of practice and choose to work with other professionals for the best possible outcome for the client.

Currently much of the literature defines the scope of practice of massage by what cannot be done, to avoid infringing on the scope of practice of other health and service professions (Boxes 2-3 and 2-4).

The scope of practice authorized by a medical or surgical degree is broad and extensive. It authorizes the physician to use drugs and medical preparations and the surgeon to sever and penetrate human tissue during treatment. It further authorizes physicians to use other methods to treat disease, injuries, deformities, and other physical and mental conditions. The law grants such a broad authorization to physicians because the education and testing requirements for a physician's license ensure that the individual is qualified to act as a healer.

BOX 2-3

Occupational Definitions and Scopes of Practice

The scope of practice described for the following professions is derived from regulations typically established to govern these occupations. The regulations predominantly used for these descriptions are the administrative rules of the Michigan Occupational Regulations' Department of Licensing and Regulation and the Occupational Regulations section of the Michigan Public Health Code.

Acupuncture
Acupuncture is a form of primary health care based on traditional Chinese medical concepts. It uses acupuncture diagnosis and treatment, as well as adjunctive therapies and diagnostic techniques, to promote, maintain, and restore health and prevent disease. Acupuncture includes but is not limited to the insertion of acupuncture needles and the application of moxibustion (medicinal herbs burned on or near the skin) to specific areas of the human body.

Athletic Training
Athletic training is the study of athletic performance, injury prevention, and rehabilitation. It includes training regimens; evaluation and assessment of injury, treatment, rehabilitation, and reconditioning of athletic injury, therapeutic exercise, and use of therapeutic modalities.

Chiropractic
Chiropractic is the discipline within the healing arts that deals with the nervous system, its relationship to the spinal column, and its interrelationship with the other body systems. Chiropractic uses radiography to detect spinal subluxation and misalignment and adjusts related bones and tissues to establish neural integrity through techniques that use the inherent recuperative powers of the body to restore and maintain

health. Examples of these techniques include the use of analytic instruments, the provision of nutritional advice, and the prescribing of rehabilitative exercise. Chiropractic does not include the performance of incisive surgical procedures or any invasive procedure that requires instrumentation or the dispensing or prescription of drugs or medicine.

Cosmetology
Cosmetology is a service provided to enhance the health, condition, and appearance of the skin, hair, and nails through the use of external preparations designed to cleanse and beautify. It includes the application of beautification processes, such as makeup and skin grooming.

Dentistry
Dentistry is the discipline of diagnosis, treatment, prescription, and surgery for disease, pain, deformity, deficiency, or injury of human teeth, alveolar processes, gums, jaws, and dependent tissues. Dentistry is also concerned with preventative care and the maintenance of good oral health.

Esthetics
An esthetician is a person who works to clean and beautify the skin.

Medicine
Medicine is the diagnosis, treatment, prevention, cure, or relief of human disease, ailment, defect, complaint, or other physical or mental condition by attendance, advice, device, diagnostic test, or other means.

Naturopathy
Naturopathy is the combination of clinical nutrition, herbology, homeopathy, acupuncture, manipulation, hydrotherapy,

Continued

BOX 2-3

Occupational Definitions and Scopes of Practice—cont'd

massage, exercise, and psychological methods, including hypnotherapy and biofeedback, to maintain health. Naturopathic physicians use radiography, ultrasound, and other forms of diagnostic testing but do not perform major surgery or prescribe synthetic drugs.

Nursing

Nursing is the systematic application of substantial specialized knowledge and skill, derived from the biologic, physical, and behavioral sciences, to the care, treatment, counsel, and health education of individuals who are experiencing changes in the normal health process or who require assistance in the maintenance of health and the prevention or management of illness, injury, and disability.

Osteopathic Medicine

Osteopathic medicine is an independent school of medicine and surgery using full methods of diagnosis and treatment in physical and mental health and disease, including the prescription and administration of drugs and vitamins; operative surgery; obstetrics; and radiologic and electromagnetic diagnostics. Osteopathy emphasizes the interrelationship of the musculoskeletal system with other body systems.

Physical Therapy

Physical therapy is the evaluation or treatment of an individual by the use of effective physical measures, therapeutic exercise, and rehabilitative procedures, with or without devices, to prevent, correct, or alleviate a physical or mental disability. It includes treatment planning, the performance of tests and measurements, interpretation of referrals, instruction, consultative services, and supervision of personnel. Physical measures include massage, mobilization, and the application of heat, cold, air, light, water, electricity, and sound.

Podiatric Medicine

Podiatric medicine is the examination, diagnosis, and treatment of abnormal nails and superficial excrescences (abnormal outgrowths or enlargements) on the human feet, including corns, warts, callosities, bunions, and arch troubles. It also includes the medical, surgical, or mechanical treatment and physiotherapy of ailments that affect the condition of the feet. It does not include amputation of the feet or the use or administration of general anesthetics.

Psychology

Psychology is the rendering to individuals, groups, organizations, or the public service involving the application of principles, methods, and procedures of understanding, predicting, and influencing behavior for the purpose of diagnosis, assessment, prevention, amelioration, or treatment of mental or emotional disorders, disabilities, and behavioral adjustment problems. Treatment is by means of psychotherapy, counseling, behavior modification, hypnosis, biofeedback techniques, psychological tests, and other verbal or behavioral methods. Psychology does not include the prescription of drugs, performance of surgery, or administration of electroconvulsive therapy.

BOX 2-4

Defining the Scope of Practice for Massage

The scope of practice for many types of bodywork has been defined by a number of professional organizations and by state law.

American Massage Therapy Association (AMTA)

Massage or massage therapy is any skilled manipulation of soft tissue, connective tissue, and/or body energy fields with the intention of maintaining or improving health by effecting change in relaxation, circulation, nerve responses, or patterns of energy flow. Massage or massage therapy may be accomplished manually with or without the use of the following: movement, superficial heat or cold, electrical or mechanical devices, water, lubricants, or salts.[1]

Associated Bodywork and Massage Professionals (ABMP)

Massage, bodywork, and somatic therapies are defined as the application of various techniques to the muscular structure and soft tissues of the human body.

- *Massage:* The application of soft tissue manipulation techniques to the body, generally intended to reduce stress and fatigue while improving circulation. The many variations of massage account for several different techniques.
- *Bodywork:* Various forms of touch therapies that may use manipulation, movement, and/or repatterning to effect structural changes to the body.
- *Somatic therapies:* The term *somatic* means "of the body." Many times this term is used to denote a body/mind or whole body approach, as distinguished from a physiology-only or environmental perspective.

More than 200 variations of massage, bodywork, and somatic therapies exist, and many practitioners use multiple techniques. Application of these techniques may include but is not limited to stroking, kneading, tapping, compression, vibration, rocking, friction, and pressure to the muscular structure or soft tissues of the human body. The techniques may also include nonforceful passive or active movement and/or application of methods intended to affect the energetic systems of the body. Oils, lotions, and powders may be used to reduce friction on the skin.

Note: Massage, bodywork, and somatic therapies specifically exclude diagnosis, prescription, manipulation, or

BOX 2-4

Defining the Scope of Practice for Massage—cont'd

adjustment of the human skeletal structure, as well as any other service, procedure, or therapy that requires a license to practice orthopedics, physical therapy, podiatry, chiropractic, osteopathy, psychotherapy, acupuncture, or any other profession or branch of medicine.

Proposed Michigan State Law

Michigan House Bill 5218 was introduced on September 22, 2005 to provide for state licensure of massage therapists. The bill also would establish the Michigan Board of Massage Therapy. If enacted into law, it would go into effect when funding is appropriated.

The bill defines the practice of massage therapy as "the application of a system of structured touch, pressure, movement, and holding to the soft tissue of the human body in which the primary intent is to enhance or restore the health and well-being of the client. Practice of massage therapy includes complementary methods, including the external application of water, heat, cold, lubrication, salt scrubs, or other topical preparations; and electromechanical devices that mimic or enhance the actions possible by the hands."

In the section on definitions and principles of construction, the bill provides the following:

1. As used in this part: "Practice of massage therapy" means a scientific discipline of manual therapy that provides assessment, education, consultation and treatment of and with an individual through applying manual therapy techniques, for the purpose of relieving stresses to the human body. Massage therapy includes treatment planning and delivery of therapy by use of hands on technique or manual physical practices. The practice of massage therapy does not include medical diagnosis or identification of diseases or causes of diseases. The practice of massage therapy does include:
   (a) The assessment of soft tissue tension and hyperesthesia for the purpose of relaxing connective and muscle tissues, normalizing circulation, reducing inflammation, and promoting soft tissue healing, and the maintenance of general good physical and mental well-being.
   (b) The use of mechanical soft tissue vibratory devices or manual vibration, thermal heat, cupping and cold applications and stretching.
   (c) Therapeutic assistance, coordination, and delivery of manual therapy in conjunction with medical and chiropractic physicians, physical therapists, occupational therapists, nurses, and other approved allied medical personnel.

Missouri State Code

The Missouri state code defines massage therapy as "a health care profession which involves the treatment of the body's tonus system through the scientific or skillful touching, rubbing, pressing or other movements of the soft tissues of the body with the hands, forearms, elbows, or feet, or with the aid of mechanical apparatus, for relaxation, therapeutic, remedial or health maintenance purposes to enhance the mental and physical well-being of the client." The code specifies that "[it] does not include the prescription of medication, spinal or joint manipulation, the diagnosis of illness or disease, or any service or procedure for which a license to practice medicine, chiropractic, physical therapy, or podiatry is required by law." http://www.sos.mo.gov/

National Institutes of Health: National Center for Complementary and Alternative Medicine (NCCAM)

The term *massage therapy* (also called *massage*, for short; massage also refers to an individual treatment session) covers a group of practices and techniques. There are more than 80 types of massage therapy. In all of them, therapists press, rub, and otherwise manipulate the muscles and other soft tissues of the body, often varying pressure and movement. They most often use their hands and fingers but may also use their forearms, elbows, or feet. Typically, the intent is to relax the soft tissues, increase delivery of blood and oxygen to the massaged areas, warm them, and decrease pain.

NCCAM Publication No. D327
Created: September 2006

No one but the physician has the legal right to perform any act that falls within the parameters of a medical license. The principle underlying this is simple: a person may not dispense therapeutic or medical advice about the effect of his or her services on a specific disease, ailment, or condition unless that person has adequate training, knowledge, and experience to ensure that the advice given is sound and reliable.

All the professionals listed in Box 2-3 must meet educational standards that far exceed the currently accepted requirements for massage in most areas. Professionals with more education are allowed to do more within their specialized fields. Those with less education work under supervision or within a limited scope of practice. The scope of practice for therapeutic massage should complement but not infringe upon the boundaries of the work of these professionals. Hopefully, the future will allow more flexibility and overlap of professional practice for the benefit of clients. The trend toward integrated health care appears to support cooperation in health care delivery and will likely provide career opportunities for massage therapists.

The Unique Scope of Practice Parameters for Therapeutic Massage

As mentioned previously, therapeutic massage is unique in that it can be used in two distinct professional worlds: wellness and personal services, and health care and sports massage services. Massage professionals are involved in various levels of care and support, each requiring more education and higher levels of competence.

Wellness and Personal Services

In the professional world of wellness services, clients seek massage for pleasure, relaxation, and general health maintenance. Wellness approaches enhance and maintain the functioning of the person. They usually focus on education and methods that encourage normal balance and the activation of self-regulating mechanisms of the mind and body. In addition to massage skills, the massage professional must be educated and skilled in teaching prevention measures and encouraging a general wellness lifestyle for clients. When presenting this type of information in the educational context, the professional must make general recommendations rather than specifically tell clients what to do, because the latter can be interpreted as diagnosing and prescribing, both of which are out of the scope of practice for massage.

In the personal services world of wellness massage, the key is enhancing the client's health or providing massage for individuals who already are healthy and who want to maintain or improve their health. It also is important not to infringe upon the cosmetology scope of practice by working with cosmetic applications to the skin through the use of oils, wraps, or other preparations. A major growth industry for wellness is the spa (see Chapter 12).

The wellness and personal services professional track allows the therapeutic massage professional to work most independently, with the broadest spectrum of people (and in some instances animals), and to share the gifts of professional touch with the general population, many of whom need support in managing stress so that they do not become ill and require medical attention. This world of wellness services is a wonderful place for a professional. It will be important to make sure that wellness services are not abandoned as the professional development of therapeutic massage progresses.

Taking a wealth of information into account, this textbook determines the scope of practice of wellness massage to be a nonspecific approach that focuses on assessment procedures for detecting contraindications to massage, as well as the need for referral to other health care professionals, and on the development of a health-enhancing physical state for the client. The plan for the massage session is developed by combining information, desired massage outcomes, and directions from the client with the skills of the massage practitioner to provide an individualized massage session aimed at normalizing the body systems. This normalization is accomplished (1) through external manual stimulation of the nervous, circulatory, and respiratory systems; connective tissue; and muscles to achieve generalized stress reduction, a decrease in muscle tension, symptomatic relief of pain related to soft tissue dysfunction, increased circulation, and other benefits similar to those of exercise; or (2) through other relaxation responses produced by therapeutic massage to increase the client's well-being.

Health Care and Sports Massage Services

The professional world of health care requires specific training for the skilled application of massage to promote rehabilitation and performance and to manage pathologic conditions (sports massage comes under this definition).

Currently, health care professionals do not receive extensive education in massage therapy. The time and labor intensity required for massage make it difficult for physicians, physical therapists, nurses, occupational therapists, and athletic trainers to include therapeutic massage with their other interventions and responsibilities. These considerations support the development of massage therapy as a distinct health practice and an adjunct to these other professions.

Physical therapy and athletic training are the professions most likely to be compared with the practice of rehabilitative massage, and care must be taken to respect the professional boundaries of these disciplines. This is particularly important because as massage training increases, the massage professional will become qualified to work with more complicated situations involving rehabilitation and the management of chronic conditions. Nevertheless, even the most comprehensive massage training programs do not compare with the extensive training of the physical therapist or other professionals, such as nurses and athletic trainers. Yet this does not invalidate the expertise of the therapeutic massage professional. A higher level of education allows the massage professional to work effectively with the physician, physical therapist, or other health professional in the health care setting, with these professionals supervising an overall treatment program of which massage is a part.

The scope of practice for clinical massage delivered within the health care setting and massage in conjunction with specific athletic training protocols is as follows: Massage therapists develop, maintain, rehabilitate, or augment physical function; relieve or prevent physical dysfunction and pain; and enhance the well-being of the client. Methods include assessment of the soft tissue and joints, as well as treatment by soft tissue manipulation, hydrotherapy, remedial exercise programs, and client self-care programs. The Canadian provinces of Ontario[2] and British Columbia have this type of scope of practice for therapeutic massage. The educational requirement in the two provinces currently exceeds 2,200 class hours and is rising.

The information in this text will carry the student from the service world of wellness massage into the world of health care services (Figure 2-3), primarily working to manage dysfunctional conditions, such as pain and chronic disorders, and to support those who may benefit from a generalized approach to massage, such as an athlete. Chapter 15 presents a series of case studies and treatment plans that provide a model of massage applications in both professional worlds. This text does not attempt to develop specific protocols for the precise intervention measures needed for serious illness and trauma. As presented here, massage can provide supportive care using stress and pain management for those who are ill if the massage professional is supervised by qualified medical personnel.

Normal Functions

Client displays resourceful functioning with good ability to respond to and recover from stress.

Massage Professional

Technician — 500+ hours of education.

Health Care Supervision Required?

No.

Support Professionals

Fitness trainers, cosmetologists, wellness educators, prevention and healthy lifestyle focused health care and mental health professionals.

Dysfunctional and Complex Athletic Patterns

(Scope of practice encompasses Technician Level)

Client displays ability to function with effort and reduced ability to respond to and recover from stress. Recovery time is increased. Client demands extraordinary function of body.

Massage Professional

Practitioner — 1000+ hours of education.

Illness/Trauma

(Scope of practice encompasses technician and practitioner levels)

Client displays function breakdown — substantially reduced ability to respond and recover or extensive healing period required such as with surgery and trauma.

Massage Professional

Therapist — 2000+ hours of education.

Health Care or Athletic Trainer Supervision Required?

Possibly. No for wellness service and mild dysfunctional patterns. Moderate to identifiable dysfunctional pattern — Yes, but indirect; attention to referral needs is important.

Support Professionals

Athletic trainers — exercise physiologist, health care and mental health professionals — spiritually based support.

Health Care Supervision Required?

Yes. Direct supervision for all clients in this category; Possibly for dysfunctional category; No for wellness clients.

Support Professionals

Entire multidisciplinary team — health care/mental health professionals — spiritually based support.

▮ Comprehensive scope of practice for therapeutic massage
☐ Wellness personal service scope of practice for therapeutic massage
▯ Dysfunctional and athletic patterns scope of practice for therapeutic massage
▨ Illness/trauma scope of practice for therapeutic massage

FIGURE 2-3 The most expansive scope of practice for therapeutic massage is represented by the entire box (outlined in dark purple). Within this scope of practice are levels of professional function based on training and experience. The entry level position, or technician, for a therapeutic massage scope of practice is found in the Normal Functions box *(white box)*. The next higher level of professional practice, the massage practitioner, is depicted in the Dysfunctional and Complex Athletic Patterns box *(light violet box)*. The third and highest level of professional practice, massage therapist, requires the most education and experience; it is depicted in the Illness/Trauma box *(light purple box)*. Note that each level encompasses the one next to it. As the model shows, a massage therapist can work effectively with all groups: normal function, dysfunctional and athletic patterns, and illness and trauma; the practitioner works only with the normal function and the dysfunctional and athletic patterns groups; and the technician works only with those displaying normal functioning. Most people who seek therapeutic massage can be served effectively by professionals trained to the practitioner level.

The distinction between wellness massage and medical rehabilitative approaches to massage used for illness and trauma may seem subtle, but the difference is simple. Wellness massage practitioners do not work with sick or injured people unless directly supervised by licensed and qualified professionals, such as physicians, nurses, and physical therapists. Rather, they help most of the population, who are not sick but are stressed and uncomfortable, to feel better and cope with stress. This benefit of massage may help prevent more serious, stress-induced illness.

Consider this metaphor: The owner's manual for a car recommends regularly scheduled maintenance. According to this schedule, a technician regularly and frequently changes the oil and filter and checks the fluids. A mechanic's assistant performs tune-ups. If the preventive maintenance schedule is followed, the car will be maintained in good running condition for a long time. It is a good idea to have a qualified mechanic do a complete evaluation of the car annually to catch problems while they are small and can be corrected easily. If this is not done, serious problems may arise, and a skilled mechanic may have to correct them.

The wellness massage technician is similar to the technician who keeps the car in order, changes the oil, and checks the fluids. Complete tune-ups by a qualified mechanic's assistant reflect the increased skill levels of the more comprehensively trained massage practitioner or massage therapist. The skilled mechanic represents the physician, athletic trainer, or physical therapist. However, lest you think that the technician is the least important person in the chain, remember that if prevention is done well, a serious problem is less likely to develop. If the car is involved in an accident or if something breaks down, it certainly goes straight to the mechanic and other specialists for repair, in just the same way that a person who suffers trauma or illness should see a physician for evaluation and treatment.

All professionals have specialized training, certain responsibilities, and positions in which they function best. Respecting each professional's strengths is the ethical thing to do. While therapeutic massage waits for a formalized scope of practice, knowing the definition and scope of practice of other health and service professionals helps the massage practitioner respect these professionals and maintain appropriate boundaries.

The Limits of Practice

Each professional has legal limits to the ability to practice massage. A scope of practice that has been legally adopted through legislation defines as well as limits the ability to practice massage. Respectful practice of therapeutic massage limits the scope of practice so that the practitioner does not encroach on the scope of practice of other professionals.

Each professional also has personal limits to the scope of practice. These limits involve the type and extent of the person's education, as well as personal biases, life experiences, specific interests in terms of the type of client served, and any physical limitations, such as size and endurance levels (Proficiency Exercise 2-4).

 PROFICIENCY EXERCISE 2-4

Write a scope of practice statement for therapeutic massage that fits your level of practice on graduation from your training program. If possible, talk with other professionals about this scope of practice and ask how it compares with their own.

Investigate the scope of practice defined by licensed professionals in your community for the listed health and service professions in this section. This information can be obtained from the state agency that oversees licensing and regulation.

Professional limits are valid and valuable. They allow us to set and maintain boundaries that support each professional in the most successful professional practice structure. Limits of practice free us from falling into the trap of believing we must be all things to all people; we cannot be, and it is ethical to acknowledge the limits of practice and to work together with other professionals.

Functioning realms also impose limits on practice. The three functioning realms are normal functioning, dysfunction or complex circumstances, and illness/trauma and breakdown. These functioning realms are related to the scope of practice (see Figure 2-3).

Normal Functioning

A person who is functioning well is able to be involved with work that is satisfying in both an intrinsic and extrinsic sense. For example, a woman may not love her work, but she may appreciate that the job supports her family (extrinsic value); or, she may love her work even if it does not financially provide for all wants (intrinsic value). A person responds normally when play balances work in such a way that the result is self-regulation and support for mental and physical functions.

Another example of normal functioning is a person who can share with others or who has a passion for a mission, a cause, or a vision, be it as simple as gardening or as complex as an encompassing environmental or political cause, and who receives intimacy, support, and fulfillment from the process.

A person who can make choices to regulate and cope with exterior influences internally and who can be resourceful and flexible in life situations displays normal functioning. The ability to love and be loved supports normal functioning. The supportive balance of these factors and the ability to exert an internal control to accommodate less than ideal situations, as well as to develop realistic and attainable goals and a plan to alter situations, indicate normal functioning.

Wellness approaches enhance and maintain normal functioning. Professional support can assist in the general maintenance of normal functioning through wellness support, education, and preventive care. Therapeutic massage plays a definitive role in general health maintenance. These clients use massage on a regular basis as part of a health and wellness program, comparable to the daily hygiene activities of bathing or brushing the teeth or to daily or weekly house cleaning. These clients want to maintain their current normal functioning status.

Massage professionals who provide services at the level of supportive wellness care require fundamental information about general wellness processes. Massage professionals should be able to teach general methods of stress management, including effective breathing, progressive relaxation, and quieting responses (meditation-type activities); they should be able to give general dietary recommendations; and they should emphasize the importance of appropriate exercise programs. Most people do better with the discipline required to maintain these activities when they have the support of a professional acting as a coach. A well-trained massage technician can provide this type of service.

Massage professionals need not always be supervised directly when working within a wellness scope of practice. A properly trained massage professional can recognize a client who is not functioning effectively, not recovering from the stress of daily activities, and beginning to fall into dysfunctional patterns. As the client's problems become more complicated, the support and expertise of the health or training professional become more important, and referral or supervision is indicated.

Dysfunction, Complex Circumstances, and the Athlete

People who are functioning with effort and are beginning to break down fall into the dysfunctional category. Physical or emotional strain may indicate the need for more focused and specific complex interventions.

Performance strain, which is seen in optimally functioning people who rely on fine motor skills and coordinated physical action (e.g., athletes, musicians, and dancers), requires a more complex massage interaction than that provided for wellness and preventive care. Such cases require a level of professional support similar to that used for dysfunctional patterns.

A multidisciplinary team approach may be needed, one that uses a defined care and treatment plan to reduce the level of physical stress and to re-establish or teach internal coping methods. A massage professional who works with dysfunction or deals with the complexities of fine motor functioning and performance strain needs a broader base of education and the supportive supervision of other health care or training professionals, such as coaches and athletic trainers. The broader-based education should encompass stress response, the origin of physical and mental difficulties, methods of improving functioning, standard health care interventions, and training protocols.

As mentioned, clients in this category benefit from a specifically designed treatment or care plan that includes a means of measuring the outcomes of care objectively. Realistic and attainable short- and long-term goals are developed, and time frames are set for the achievement of these goals. The general goals of the massage professional are to help the client move toward normal functioning, regain personal control of the body/mind/spirit systems, and achieve and maintain optimal functioning. This approach is different from that of massage used for wellness or preventive care. The methods and information provided may be the same or similar, but the focus and goals are different. Clients dealing with dysfunction or complex circumstances or who demand high levels of performance want to change where they are in life, not maintain the status quo.

Because massage temporarily helps take the edge off physical discomfort and reduces arousal levels, allowing people to feel or perform better under less than desirable circumstances, massage intervention may or may not be appropriate in these circumstances. People tend to be less motivated to change if their circumstances seem tolerable. Massage may diminish the client's motivation to change, interfering with the process being worked through with other health care or training professionals. For example, appropriate flexibility programs are important in athletic performance. Athletes need to participate in flexibility programs. If massage provides the flexibility and reduces the uncomfortable sensation of restricted mobility, these clients may not be motivated to warm up and stretch out as they should.

Massage can help support stress management in clients who find themselves faced with extraordinary stress loads. If the person cannot alter the situation causing the dysfunctional stress, massage can serve as a means of easing physical stress and a beneficial coping measure when combined with other medical, behavioral, and emotional coping techniques. Massage does not deal directly with the physical, emotional, or spiritual state contributing to the stress; rather, it supports the physical system so that the person can better withstand stress.

Illness/Trauma and Breakdown

A person experiencing a traumatic breakdown or illness requires a comprehensive intervention process. Often little distinction can be made between dysfunction and breakdown or illness. During acute illness or breakdown, massage is not likely to be part of therapy, at least initially. The client cannot handle any additional demand created by massage. Even the most subtle forms of massage involve a controlled physiologic stress to the system that requires a physical adaptation response. These individuals may need very specific professional intervention to re-establish some level of functioning before they can cope with the adaptation strain of massage.

A massage therapist working with a person facing illness, trauma, or a breakdown must be monitored carefully and supervised by a health care professional, especially if the client is taking medications (see Appendix C and the Evolve Web site). In such cases massage intervention supports health care approaches; a comprehensive treatment and care plan is developed with massage as one of the treatment approaches. Often massage is used primarily for palliative (comfort) care, and supervision by the primary health care professional is necessary. The massage professional needs additional training in pathology, pharmacology, psychology, and clinical reasoning skills to be able to help integrate massage into an overall health care plan.

Body/Mind/Spirit Connection

The body, mind, and spirit share a definite link. The physical biologic (body) functions involve all the anatomy and physiology, including the body's chemical responses. Feelings are body functions.

The cognitive process (the mind) interprets physical sensations and sets physical responses in motion. Emotions seem to be the result of the interplay between body and mind. Behavior is the action that results from the physical, emotional, and cognitive combination.

The spirit provides the strength, hope, faith, and love that create a reason for being. Each of these areas of functioning influences and interacts with the others.

In reality, the body, mind, and spirit cannot be separated, yet together they involve too much information to allow a professional to become an expert in all areas of human function. Professional skill levels, the parameters of the scope of practice, and avoidance of dual and multiple roles in the professional relationship artificially divide the functioning of the person seeking assistance. This is undesirable, yet many times unavoidable. An excellent solution is for professionals to work together. A multidisciplinary, integrative approach to care is best, with each professional showing a cooperative spirit and supporting a comprehensive care plan that addresses all the client's needs. Most hospice programs are excellent models for multidisciplinary teams.

Determining the Limits of Practice

As a massage professional, you can determine whether you are within your scope of practice by making sure your responses to the client are from a body and massage perspective. When a client expresses distress, shares personal information, or requests specific information, first determine whether the issue is most specifically a body, mind, or spirit issue. If it is a mental or spiritual issue, use listening skills and acknowledge the situation but do not attempt to problem solve or provide professional intervention. If the situation presented is a physical concern (i.e., affects the body), decide whether the information falls within the scope of therapeutic massage and respond accordingly.

The severity or complexity of a situation determines whether simple listening, without advice being given, is sufficient or whether a professional referral is indicated. Often the physical stress of the circumstances can be managed by massage approaches while the client seeks additional help from supportive resources and professionals who can deal more specifically with the source of the problem.

Health care, training, coaching, and cosmetology professionals have committed a significant part of their lives to formal schooling, licensing procedures, and continual experiential and formal education. The information they possess is specific to their professional discipline, yet is also quite broad. Although massage techniques may not be common knowledge among many professionals, the importance and power of touch are. Many of these professionals understand that massage professionals use touch skills that they may be unable to provide because of the nature of their therapeutic relationship with the client. To develop and support a cooperative, multidisciplinary philosophy of care, massage professionals must respect the dedication of the professionals with whom they work by maintaining the appropriate scope of practice for therapeutic massage.

Massage professionals benefit from being able to adapt massage therapy to various health care, training, and personal service needs; in doing so they are best able to serve both the professionals with whom they work and the clients they serve. In a multidisciplinary team setting (such as the spa environment, which may employ wellness professionals, fitness and sport professionals, and medical professionals), it is important to be able to communicate effectively with any professional with whom you work; this requires you to be familiar with the language and terminology used in that profession. It is important to be able to explain massage therapy intervention in terms familiar to the professionals on the team and also to be able to explain the ways you, as a massage professional, intend to support spa, health, or training professionals in providing appropriate care.

Understanding the functioning realms of people and the scope of practice of therapeutic massage helps the professional establish an ethical practice and begin the discovery of the therapeutic process.

ETHICS AND STANDARDS OF PRACTICE

SECTION OBJECTIVES

Using the information presented in this section, the student will be able to perform the following:

- Develop a personal and professional code of ethics using the eight ethical principles
- Explain the standards of practice for therapeutic massage

Ethics

Culture, time, location, events, politics, religion, scientific knowledge, and many other factors affect the way we interpret behavior. Ethics defines the behavior we expect of ourselves and others and society's expectations of a profession. A simplified definition of ethics is "what is right." Our society determines that a person has acted ethically when the right thing has been done. But what is the right thing? No one individual or group has the answer. Often the best that can be offered in discussions of ethics are questions and guidelines based on principles of conduct established by a group.

Ethics has social, professional, and personal dimensions. Separating these elements is not easy, in theory or in practice. We behave according to a complex and continually changing set of rules, customs, and expectations. Because of this, ethical behavior must be a dynamic process of reflection and revision.

Ethics is not just a varied collection of do's and don'ts; rather, it is a system of principles that tie together in a reasonable, coherent way to make our society and our lives as civilized and happy as possible. Conflicts and uncertainties are inevitable. For this reason, in applying ethics we must learn more than a list of guidelines, more than just what to do in this or that particular case; we must also develop a set of priorities and a way of thinking about them. To use ethics in decision making, we must be able to reason about what we have learned in order to capture the spirit of being ethical. Although morals and values ultimately are a personal concern, ethics is a reflection of one's professional and social character.

The purpose of practicing our profession ethically is to promote and maintain the welfare of the client. Laws often reflect the minimal standards necessary to protect the safety and welfare of the public, whereas codes of ethics represent the ideal standards set by a profession. Through their behavior, professionals can comply both with the law and with professional codes. If compliance with the law is the only motivation in ethical behavior, the person is said to be practicing mandatory ethics. If, however, the professional strives for the highest possible benefit and welfare for the client, the professional behaves with aspirational ethics.[3]

As professionals we must constantly be alert not only to gross violations of ethical principles, but also to the more subtle ethical violations that occur when the client's welfare is not the primary determining factor of professional behavior. An example of the latter is hesitating to refer a client to a more qualified massage professional because referral means the loss of a paying client. Often this type of unethical conduct goes unnoticed, yet the client's welfare is compromised. This situation is further complicated because the professional often does not recognize the breach in ethical behavior. Mentoring (career support by someone more experienced), supervision (monitoring by one with more expertise), peer support (interaction and exchange of information among fellow professionals), and meticulous objective personal reflection on professional behavior can bring to light these more subtle types of ethical violations. Professionals can monitor their own behavior by asking themselves often if they are doing what is best for the client and if their behavior is ethical.

Professional growth involves change in our knowledge, skills, attitudes, and beliefs. A professional code of ethics is a set of norms adopted by a professional group to direct choices and behavior in a manner consistent with professional responsibility. Many elements in the profession of massage enhance the lives of its practitioners, such as respect, authority, and prestige. In return, professionals must be willing to adjust their personal behavior for the professional good. We have to gauge our personal and professional behavior not only by what is right and good for us as individuals, but also by what is appropriate for the client and the profession as a whole.

Ethical Principles

The following eight principles guide professional ethical behavior:

1. *Respect:* Esteem and regard for clients, other professionals, and oneself
2. *Client autonomy and self-determination:* The freedom to decide and the right to sufficient information to make the decision
3. *Veracity:* The right to the objective truth
4. *Proportionality:* The principle that benefit must outweigh the burden of treatment
5. *Nonmaleficence:* The principle that the profession shall do no harm and prevent harm from happening
6. *Beneficence:* The principle that treatment should contribute to the client's well-being
7. *Confidentiality:* Respect for privacy of information
8. *Justice:* Equality

These broad concepts direct the development of standards of practice.

Standards of Practice

Standards of practice provide specific guidelines and rules that form a concrete professional structure. For example, in standards of practice, the ethical principle of respect translates into professional behavior, such as maintaining the client's privacy and modesty, providing a safe environment, and being on time for appointments. The principle of client autonomy and self-determination requires informed consent and ready access by clients to their files.

Standards of practice guidelines direct quality care and provide a means of measuring the quality of care. They usually are more concrete than ethical principles.

Code of Ethics and Standards of Practice for Therapeutic Massage

Because the massage therapy profession is not yet united in terms of professional affiliation and techniques, presenting a code of ethics or providing agreed-upon standards of practice for the massage professional is difficult (Proficiency Exercise 2-5). Because each professional group within the massage profession has developed its own code of ethics and standards of practice, this text offers a comprehensive compilation of many ethical codes and standards of practice, developed through professional organizations, licensing requirements, and the standards of practice of other health professions (Box 2-5). An attempt has been made to include all points presented in the various ethical conduct codes and standards of practice statements.

INFORMED CONSENT

SECTION OBJECTIVES

Using the information presented in this section, the student will be able to perform the following:

- List and explain the nine components of informed consent (Box 2-6)
- Determine whether a client can provide informed consent for a massage
- Prepare written client information materials to support the informed consent process
- Complete two different types of informed consent forms

Informed consent is a protection process for the consumer. It requires that clients understand what will occur, that they participate voluntarily, and that they be competent to give consent. Informed consent is also an educational procedure that allows clients to decide knowledgeably whether they want to receive a massage, whether they want a particular therapist to work with them, and whether the professional structure, including client rules and regulations, is acceptable to them. Informed consent supports professional ethical behavior. It reflects the ethical principle of client participation and self-determination in a client-centered approach.

Clients must be able to provide informed consent and demonstrate that they understand the information presented to them (Proficiency Exercise 2-6). Parents or guardians must provide informed consent for minors. Guardians must provide informed consent for those unable to do so, such as clients with dementia. Ethical decision making becomes important in "gray areas," such as when a language barrier exists and the massage professional is not sure the client understands him or her, or when any form of intoxication or prescription drug use is involved that alters the client's judgment.

PROFICIENCY EXERCISE 2-5

Given each point of the code of ethics and standards of practice statement presented in Box 2-5, consider this question: "How will I implement this ethical principle or standard of practice in my professional practice?" Then, in the space provided, develop a personal code of ethics and standards of practice statement.

Personal Professional Code of Ethics and Standards of Practice Statement

SCHOOL OF HEALTH & SOCIAL CARE
Library
2 5 JUN
Arrowe Park Site
UNIVERSITY OF CHESTER

BOX 2-5

Massage Code of Ethics and Standards of Practice

Ethical Principles

The four basic principles that constitute the code of ethics for massage professionals are as follows:

- *Respect for the dignity of people*—Massage professionals will maintain respect for the interests, dignity, rights, and needs of all clients, staff, and colleagues.
- *Responsible caring*—Competent, quality client care will be provided at the highest standard possible.
- *Integrity in relationships*—At all times the professional will behave with integrity, honesty, and diligence in practice and duties.
- *Responsibility to society*—Massage professionals are responsible and accountable to society and shall conduct themselves in a manner that maintains high ethical standards.

Standards of Practice Based on Ethical Principles

In compliance with the principles of the code of ethics, massage professionals will perform the following:

1. Respect all clients, colleagues, and health professionals through nondiscrimination regardless of age, gender, race, national origin, sexual orientation, religion, socioeconomic status, body type, political affiliation, state of health, personal habits, and life-coping skills.
2. Perform only those services for which they are qualified and honestly represent their education, certification, professional affiliations, and other qualifications. The massage professional will apply treatment only when a reasonable expectation exists that it will be advantageous to the client's condition. The massage professional, in consultation with the client, will continually evaluate the effectiveness of treatment.
3. Respect the scope of practice of other health care and service professionals, including physicians, chiropractors, physical therapists, podiatrists, orthopedists, psychotherapists, counselors, acupuncturists, nurses, exercise physiologists, athletic trainers, nutritionists, spiritual advisors, and cosmetologists.
4. Respect all ethical health care practitioners and work with them to promote health and healing.
5. Acknowledge the limitations of their personal skills and, when necessary, refer clients to an appropriately qualified professional. The massage professional will require consultation with other knowledgeable professionals when:
   - A client requires diagnosis and opinion beyond a therapist's capabilities of assessment
   - A client's condition is beyond the scope of practice
   - A combined health care team is required

   If referral to another health care provider is necessary, it will be done with the informed consent of the client.
6. Refrain from working with any individual who has a specific disease process without supervision by a licensed medical professional.
7. Be adequately educated and understand the physiologic effects of the specific massage techniques used to determine if any application is contraindicated and to ensure that the most beneficial techniques are applied to a given individual.
8. Avoid false claims about the potential benefits of the techniques rendered and educate the public about the actual benefits of massage.
9. Acknowledge the importance and individuality of each person, including colleagues, peers, and clients.
10. Work only with the informed consent of a client and professionally disclose to the client any situation that may interfere with the massage professional's ability to provide the best care to serve the client's best interest.
11. Display respect for the client by honoring a client's process and following all recommendations by being present, listening, asking only pertinent questions, keeping agreements, being on time, draping properly, and customizing the massage to address the client's needs.

    NOTE: Draping is covered in Chapter 8. The Ontario guidelines[2] specify these requirements for draping:
    - It is the responsibility of the massage professional to ensure the privacy and dignity of the client and to determine whether the client feels comfortable, safe, and secure with the draping provided.
    - The client may choose to be fully draped or clothed throughout the treatment.
    - The female client's breasts are not undraped unless specified by referral from a qualified health care professional and the massage professional is working under the supervision of such a health care professional.
    - The genitals, perineum, and anus are never undraped. The client's consent is required for work on any part of the body, regardless of whether the client is fully clothed, fully draped, or partly draped.
12. Provide a safe, comfortable, and clean environment.
13. Maintain clear and honest communication with clients and keep client communications confidential. Confidentiality is of the utmost importance. The massage professional must inform the client that the referring physician may be eligible to review the client's records and that records may be subpoenaed by the courts.
14. Conduct business in a professional and ethical manner in relation to clientele, business associates, acquaintances, governmental bodies, and the public.
15. Follow city, county, state, national, and international requirements.
16. Charge a fair price for the session. Gratuities are appropriate if within reasonable limits. (Similar to percentages for other service providers, i.e., 10% to 20%.) A gift, gratuity, or benefit that is intended to influence a referral, decision, or treatment may not be accepted and must be returned to the giver immediately.
17. Keep accurate records and review the records with the client.

Continued

BOX 2-5

Massage Code of Ethics and Standards of Practice—cont'd

18. Never engage in any sexual conduct, sexual conversation, or any other sexual activities involving clients.
19. Avoid affiliation with any business that uses any form of sexual suggestiveness or explicit sexuality in advertising or promoting services or in the actual practice of service.
20. Practice honesty in advertising, promoting services ethically and in good taste and advertising only techniques for which the professional is certified or adequately trained.
21. Strive for professional excellence through regular assessment of personal strengths, limitations, and effectiveness and through continuing education and training.
22. Accept the responsibility to oneself, one's clients, and the profession to maintain physical, mental, and emotional well-being and to inform clients when the professional is not functioning at full capacity.

23. Refrain from using any mind-altering drugs, alcohol, or intoxicants before or during professional massage sessions.
24. Maintain a professional appearance and demeanor by practicing good hygiene and dressing in a professional, modest, and nonsexual manner.
25. Undergo periodic peer review.
26. Respect all pertinent reporting requirements outlined by legislation regarding abuse.
27. Report to the proper authorities any accurate knowledge and its supportive documentation regarding violations by massage professionals and other health or service professionals.
28. Avoid interests, activities, or influences that might conflict with the obligation to act in the best interest of clients and the massage therapy profession and safeguard professional integrity by recognizing potential conflicts of interest and avoiding them.

BOX 2-6

Informed Consent

The following questions should be answered at the outset of the professional relationship:

- What are the goals of the therapeutic program?
- What services will be provided?
- What behavior is expected of the client?
- What are the risks and benefits of the process?
- What are the practitioner's qualifications?
- What are the financial considerations?
- How long is the therapy expected to last?
- What are the limitations of confidentiality?
- In what areas does the professional have mandatory reporting requirements?

 PROFICIENCY EXERCISE 2-6

Gather in groups of three and write about a specific situation in which informed consent is difficult to obtain from a client. The groups should then exchange responses and role play some of the situations, with one student acting as the massage practitioner, one being the client, and the third evaluating the way the situation was handled. Try different situations until each student has had a chance to play each role.

True informed consent presents the opportunity to evaluate the options available and the risks involved in each method and requires the massage professional to include information about the inherent and potential benefits and hazards of the proposed treatment, the alternatives available, and the probable results if treatment is not provided. Clients have the legal right to choose from a range of suggested options and to receive enough information to allow them to pick the most appropriate approach for them. Credentials and personal and professional limitations that may affect the client-therapist relationship must be disclosed and validated. Clients also need information about recourse options if the outcomes of the massage are undesirable. As professionals, we are ethically bound to ensure that the client makes choices based on a solid understanding of the information presented. The professional is responsible for providing the client with this information.

Intake Procedures

A comprehensive intake procedure, including an informed consent process, is necessary when defined outcomes span a series of sessions. A **needs assessment,** which is based on the client's history and a physical assessment, is used to devise an initial treatment plan. The **initial treatment plan** states the therapeutic goals, duration of the sessions, number of appointments needed to meet the goals agreed upon, cost, general classification of intervention to be used, and an objective progress measurement method for identifying when goals have been reached (the forms used for these procedures are presented in Chapter 3).

Single or random massage sessions usually do not necessarily require a full needs assessment or a treatment plan. Instead, possible contraindications to massage are identified. The informed consent process informs the client of the limita-

LIBRARY, UNIVERSITY OF CHESTER

tions of a single massage session and describes the approaches used in the single-session massage experience.

A form with all the pertinent information is signed by the client and kept in the massage practitioner's files. Maintaining a record of signed informed consent forms is an important legal issue; in many jurisdictions, touching a person without the person's consent is an action that can be prosecuted as assault.

The following is a possible sequence for obtaining informed consent.

1. The massage professional provides a general explanation of massage, supported by written information (often in the form of a brochure) about indications, benefits, contraindications, and alternative approaches that provide benefits similar to those of massage.
2. The massage professional informs the client about the scope of practice for massage; reporting measures for professional misconduct and recourse policies; the professional's training, experience, and credentials; and any limiting factors that may affect the professional relationship, including lack of training in a particular area and any special circumstances of the massage professional (e.g., hearing or vision difficulty) that may need to be considered. The client is given written information covering these topics, often in the form of a brochure, to enhance his or her understanding of this discussion.
3. The massage professional then discusses business and professional policies and procedures, including the logical

consequences of noncompliance on the part of the client. These policies include handling of payment, returned checks, additional charges, gratuities, late arrival, scheduling, sexual impropriety, draping, hygiene, sanitation, and confidentiality and limits of confidentiality. The client also is given pertinent written information about these topics, such as a professional policy statement (Box 2-7).

4. After these procedures have been followed, the client signs an informed consent form (see the sample in Box 2-9). The client should not be overwhelmed with extensive, detailed information, but it is important to provide enough information for the individual to make an informed choice. Informed consent is a continual process, and client education and involvement in the therapeutic approach are always supported and encouraged.

Needs Assessment and the Initial Treatment Plan

As mentioned previously, if the client is working toward specific outcome goals that will require several appointments, a needs assessment and an initial treatment plan are completed (Box 2-8). Specific details on completing this process are provided in Chapter 3.

The process of assessing needs, identifying goals, and developing a treatment plan takes 30 minutes to 1 hour and constitutes the initial intake procedure. In complex circumstances, this process can extend over the first two or three sessions. It is appropriate to charge for the intake session, which is an

---

BOX 2-7

Developing a Client Brochure and Policy Statement

A massage professional should cover the following important points in developing a client brochure and policy statement.

Type of Service
- Explain the type of work you provide.
- Explain the benefits and limitations of this particular style of massage.
- Specify whether you specialize in working with a particular group, such as elderly people, athletes, or people with specific problems such as headaches or back pain.
- Indicate any situations or conditions with which you do not care to work, such as pregnancy or certain medical conditions.

Training and Experience
- If your state requires licensing or if you are nationally certified, provide documentation.
- State how long you have been in practice, what school you attended, whether the school was approved by any state or accrediting body, and how many classroom hours were required for graduation.
- Provide information about continuing education you have pursued.
- Provide information about any additional education; for example, that you are also an athletic trainer.

- Provide the names of any professional organizations of which you are an active member.

Appointment Policies
- Specify the length of an average session.
- Inform the client of the days you work and your hours and whether you do on site residential or business work.
- Inform the client that the first appointment for intake will be longer than subsequent appointments; also state whether you take emergency appointments and how often you suggest that clients come for massage sessions.
- Be clear about the cancellation policy and your policy for late appointments.
- Explain to the client any change in or restriction on physical activity before or after the session.

Client/Practitioner Expectations
- Explain in detail what happens at the first massage session (i.e., paperwork, medical history, other preliminaries).
- Make sure that clients know they can partly undress or undress down to their underclothes and that they are always covered and draped during the session.
- Explain the order in which you massage (face up or face down to begin), the parts of the body on which you work

Continued

BOX 2-7

Developing a Client Brochure and Policy Statement—cont'd

and in what order, whether you use oils or creams, if a shower is available before or after the massage, and if bathing at home before the massage appointment is expected.

- Make sure the client understands whether talking is appropriate during the session and that you should be informed if anything feels uncomfortable.
- If you have low lighting and music during the session, be sure the client is comfortable with that atmosphere.
- Make sure the client understands when a reaction might be expected, such as tenderness over a trigger point when direct pressure methods are used.
- Tell clients that before the session you will discuss with them the goals for the massage, as well as the proposed styles and methods of massage, and that consent must be given for all massage procedures.
- Inform the client that your profession has a code of ethics and explain your policy on confidentiality.
- Let clients know that if they are uncomfortable in any way, a friend or relative may accompany them.

Fees

Make sure your fee structure is clearly defined regarding the following:

- How often you raise your fees
- Whether you have a sliding fee scale

- Whether you take only cash or will accept money orders, checks, or credit cards
- Whether you bill
- Whether you accept insurance
- How often insurance covers your services
- Different fees for variations in the length of a session
- Whether a series of sessions can be bought at a discount
- Whether you pay any referral fees for new clients

Sexual Appropriateness

Sexual behavior by the therapist toward the client or by the client toward the therapist is always unethical and inappropriate. It is always the responsibility of the therapist or health professional to ensure that sexual misconduct does not occur.

Recourse Policy

If a client is unhappy or dissatisfied, do you offer a refund or a free session? Let the client know that if the matter is not handled satisfactorily, a professional organization or licensing board is available where complaints can be registered.

NOTE: Some professionals send out client policy and procedure booklets before the scheduled appointment. If this is done, include a personalized cover letter asking the client to read the booklet carefully and stating that you will discuss it with him or her at the first appointment.

BOX 2-8

Needs Assessment and Development of the Initial Treatment Plan

First, the client's goals and desired outcomes for the massage sessions are determined. The client agrees to proceed with the next part of the session, which consists of history taking using a client information form, and a physical assessment using an assessment form. The information is evaluated to develop a care plan for the client; this is called a *needs assessment*. Care plans usually envision a series of sessions.

A care/treatment plan is developed that spells out the following:

- Specific outcomes (i.e., the therapeutic goals)
- Frequency of visits (number of appointments per week or month) and duration of visits (e.g., 30, 45, or 60 minutes)

- Estimated number of appointments needed to achieve the therapeutic goals (e.g., 10 sessions, 15 sessions, ongoing with no time limit)
- General methods to be used (e.g., Swedish massage, muscle energy methods, neuromuscular methods, trigger point techniques)
- Objective progress measurements (e.g., pain decreased on a scale of 1 to 10, 50% increase in range of motion, sleep improved by increasing 1 hour per night, episodes of tension headache reduced from four per week to one per week, feelings of relaxation maintained for 24 hours)

The client provides (informed) consent for the care/treatment plan by signing the appropriate form.

important part of the professional interaction. The treatment plan may evolve or change during subsequent sessions as the client's needs change during the therapeutic process. The initial treatment plan is the massage practitioner's best educated guess as to how the therapeutic relationship will proceed.

When massage is used in a very nonspecific way, especially if the client will be seen only once or if a series of massage sessions is not appropriate, the massage professional need not

perform an extensive needs assessment or develop a comprehensive treatment plan. Instead, the practitioner should predetermine the outcome of the session by informing the client that, under these circumstances, no specific work can be done and that massage can provide a general normalizing of the body. A short history and physical assessment are done to detect any contraindications to massage. A condensed version of the client policy statement is prepared and provided in written form. The client always provides formal written consent for the massage. An example of an informed consent process is presented in Box 2-9.

CONFIDENTIALITY

SECTION OBJECTIVES

Using the information presented in this section, the student will be able to perform the following:

- Establish and maintain client confidentiality
- Complete a release of information form

Confidentiality is the principle that the client's information is private and belongs to the client. It is built on respect and trust. In professional terms, confidentiality concerns client information and files. Client information is never discussed with anyone other than the client without the client's written permission. During peer counseling or supervision, client confidentiality extends to the professionals we consult. Even when the client's name is withheld, the situational uniqueness often is enough to breach confidentiality requirements.

Client files must represent information accurately and only as it relates to the service offered. Personal information about a situation that involves a muscle or skeletal complaint need not be recorded. For example, a client describes her headache and says that a coworker is disruptive and the manager does nothing about it, which she feels contributes to the tension

---

BOX 2-9

Informed Consent Process

A new client arrives for a massage.

The massage professional shows the client an informational brochure explaining massage, why it works, the procedures and process of massage, the benefits of massage, and the general contraindications. The client is asked to read the information. The massage professional then discusses the information with the client. In general terms the massage professional explains alternatives to massage, such as exercise and self-hypnosis, that provide benefits similar to massage.

The massage professional then tells the client about his or her professional background: that he or she graduated from a state-licensed massage therapy school 2 years ago, after a training program of 1,000 hours; that he or she has been nationally certified by the National Certification Board for Therapeutic Massage; that he or she has been in professional practice part time for 2 years and averages eight massages a week; and that he or she has taken additional training in myofascial approaches and massage for elderly people (approximately 100 hours for each). The client also is given information on methods of reporting misconduct of the massage therapist to state agencies, national professional organizations, and the police.

The client is given the policy and procedures booklet or statement and is asked to read it. After the client has done so, the massage professional goes over the booklet with the client, point by point, so that he or she understands the rules and requirements of the massage therapist. The massage professional makes sure that the requirements to report abuse and threat of deadly harm, as well as the release of files by court order, are discussed.

The massage professional hands the client a form that states the following:

I, (client's name) _____, have received a copy of the rules and regulations for Massage Works operated by Sue and John Grey. I have read the rules and regulations, and I understand them. The massage procedures, information about massage in general, general benefits of massage, contraindications to massage, and possible alternatives have been explained to me. The qualifications of the massage professional and reporting measures for misconduct have been disclosed to me.

I understand that the massage I receive is for the purpose of stress reduction and relief from muscular tension, spasm, or pain and to increase circulation. If I experience any pain or discomfort, I will immediately inform the massage practitioner so that the pressure or methods can be adjusted to my comfort level. I understand that massage professionals do not diagnose illness or disease or perform any spinal manipulations, nor do they prescribe any medical treatments, and nothing said or done during the session should be construed as such. I acknowledge that massage is not a substitute for medical examination or diagnosis and that I should see a health care provider for those services. Because massage should not be performed under certain circumstances, I agree to keep the massage practitioner updated as to any changes in my health profile, and I release the massage professional from any liability if I fail to do so.

Client's signature _____ Date _____

Therapist's signature _____ Date _____

Consent to Treat a Minor

By my signature I authorize (therapist's name) to provide therapeutic massage to my child or dependent.

Signature of Parent or Guardian _____ Date _____

For clients who will have several sessions, the next step is completion of the needs assessment and initial treatment plan (presented in detail in Chapter 3).

Continued

BOX 2-9

Informed Consent Process—cont'd

Modified Informed Consent Form for Single Session
For clients who will be seen only once (as might occur if the professional is working on a cruise ship, doing sports massage at an event, or doing promotional chair massage at a health fair), the following modification in informed consent can be made.

I, (client's name) _____, have received a copy of the rules and regulations for (name of business) _____, operated by (owner) _____. I have read the rules and regulations, and I understand them. The general benefits of massage and contraindications to massage have been explained to me. I have disclosed to the therapist any condition I have that would contraindicate massage. Other than to determine contraindications, I understand that no specific needs assessment has been performed. The qualifications of the massage professional and reporting measures for misconduct have been disclosed to me.

   I understand that the massage I receive is for the purpose of stress reduction and relief from muscular tension, spasm, or pain and to increase circulation. If I experience any pain or discomfort, I will immediately inform the massage practitioner so that the pressure or methods can be adjusted to my comfort level. I understand that massage professionals do not diagnose illness or disease or perform any spinal manipulations, nor do they prescribe any medical treatments. I acknowledge that massage is not a substitute for medical examination or diagnosis and that I should see a health care provider for those services.

   I understand that a single massage session or massage used on a random basis is limited to providing a general, nonspecific massage approach using standard massage methods and does not include any methods to address soft tissue structure or function specifically.

Client's signature _____ Date _____

Therapist's signature _____ Date _____

Consent to Treat a Minor

By my signature I authorize (therapist's name) to provide massage work to my child or dependent.

Signature of Parent or Guardian _____ Date _____

---

aggravating her headache. The only part recorded in the client's file is her belief that emotional tension is contributing to the headache. Including more of the story would be considered a breach of confidentiality, because it makes a permanent record of an event that may be made public if the client's files are ordered released to the court.

Clients must be told during initial informed consent procedures that files may be ordered released to the court. Massage therapists have no professional exemptions. Clients must be made to understand these limits to confidentiality during informed consent procedures.

Confidentiality also pertains to public recognition. Massage practitioners should not acknowledge a client in public unless the client recognizes and greets the professional first; to do so puts clients in the position of having it revealed that they were seeking professional services, a fact they may want kept private.

Clients also must be informed that confidentiality will be breached under laws that require professionals to report abuse and threat of deadly harm. If information is disclosed to you that a child, an elderly person, or a person who may be physically or mentally unable to report abuse or to protect himself is being harmed, as a professional you must report this alleged abuse to the appropriate government agencies. If a client threatens deadly harm to another person or to himself or herself, a professional must report this information to the police or other appropriate agency. Because the massage professional is not specifically trained to identify or diagnose those who may harm themselves or others, all threats must be taken seriously. In these most difficult situations, the massage professional should seek legal counsel on ways to proceed.

To allow professionals to exchange information, the client must sign a release of information form (Box 2-10).

A copy of the information release form is kept in the client's file, and the original is sent to the consulting professional. The use of the term "exchange information" in the form allows each professional involved to share pertinent information; otherwise, each professional must obtain a release of information form from the client to share information about that client.

HEALTH INSURANCE PORTABILITY AND ACCOUNTABILITY ACT OF 1996

SECTION OBJECTIVE

Using the information presented in this section, the student will be able to perform the following:

Explain the purpose of HIPAA and list the three primary areas it covers

The Health Insurance Portability and Accountability Act was signed into law by President Bill Clinton on August 21, 1996.[4,5] Conclusive regulations were issued on August 17, 2000, to be instituted by October 16, 2002. HIPAA requires that the transactions of all patient health care information be formatted in a standardized electronic style. In addition to protecting the privacy and security of patient information (Box 2-11), HIPAA includes legislation on the formation of medical savings accounts, the authorization of a fraud and abuse control program, the easy transport of health insurance coverage, and the simplification of administrative terms and conditions.

HIPAA encompasses three primary areas, and its privacy requirements can be broken down into three types: privacy standards, patients' rights, and administrative requirements. The following Web sites present a comprehensive discussion

---

BOX 2-10

Release of Information Form

The following is an example of a release of information form:

I, (client's name) _____, grant permission for _____ (therapist's name), a massage practitioner, to provide or exchange information with (other professional's name) _____ about the following conditions _____ for the time frame beginning _____ and ending _____ (dates). This permission may be revoked at any time either verbally or in writing.

Client's signature _____ Date _____

BOX 2-11

Training in the Requirements of the Health Insurance Portability and Accountability Act (HIPAA)

Who Should be Trained?

The Privacy Rule established by the Health Insurance Portability and Accountability Act of 1996 stipulates that all members of the enterprise workforce receive training that is appropriate to their organizational roles. The "workforce" includes employees, volunteers, trainees, and other persons who work for a covered entity, whether or not they are paid by it. Some staff members will need to be trained in applying specific policies and procedures, such as provision of the notice of information practices or obtaining authorizations. Others, such as those who rarely have access to protected health information (PHI), may require only an overview of HIPAA's background, objectives, principles, and general regulatory requirements.

New employees who join the organization must receive training within a reasonable period of time. It is often practical to include HIPAA privacy training in new employee orientation programs, particularly because privacy principles easily fit into discussions of the organization's mission and infrastructure. Workforce members who change jobs or receive new responsibilities must receive additional training if their new job duties include new patient privacy-related responsibilities. Further, the Privacy Rule requires retraining for each member of the covered entity's workforce whose functions are affected by a material change in the policies or procedures.

Covered entities also must document that privacy training has been provided. Although there is no requirement that members of the workforce sign a certificate after training, it is useful to document training completion by each worker for future verification purposes.

What Should Your Training Program Cover?

The privacy provisions do not prescribe the nature of the required training; the Department of Health and Human Services has left the design, approach, and specific content to the discretion of the covered entity. However, at the very least, it is recommended that the following topics be covered with all members of the workforce. In addition, more specialized training on detailed HIPAA requirements and internal procedural changes must be tailored for workforce groups that will be directly affected by them in the course of their work.

- Principles and objectives of HIPAA's Privacy Rule
- Background (e.g., what constitutes PHI)
- Need for privacy of PHI
- Overview of HIPAA privacy regulations, including penalties
- Individual's rights regarding privacy
- Individual's rights regarding control of uses and disclosure of PHI
- Individual's right to request access, accounting, and amendment
- New organizational privacy policies and procedures
- Sanction policy
- Notice of privacy practices
- Authorizations for use and disclosure
- Privacy Officer's role and contact information
- Complaint policies and procedures
- Cooperating with investigations or audits
- Reporting of violations and the whistleblower policy
- The organization's commitment to patient privacy

Modified from D'Arcy GG: The first and last word in privacy compliance, Phoenix Health Systems, 2003. http://www.hipaadvisory.com/regs/compliancecal.htm, accessed July 10, 2007.

of these terms and requirements and a complete list of HIPAA policies and procedures:

- U.S. Department of Health and Human Services, Office of Civil Rights: www.hhs.gov/ocr/hipaa
- Work Group on Electronic Data Interchange: www.wedi.org/SNIP
- Phoenix Health: www.hipaadvisory.com
- U.S. Department of Health and Human Services, Office of the Assistant Secretary for Planning and Evaluation: http://aspe.os.dhhs.gov/admnsimp/

PROFESSIONAL BOUNDARIES

SECTION OBJECTIVES

Using the information presented in this section, the student will be able to perform the following:

- Develop strategies for maintaining professional boundaries with clients
- Explore personal prejudices, fears, and limitations that may interfere with the ability to provide the best care for a client
- Help a client recognize personal boundaries in the massage process

Needs and Wants

People have needs and wants. *Needs* sustain life; when needs are not met, people become ill and die. Needs include air, water, food, shelter, and sensory stimulation. *Wants* lead to a sense of satisfaction. Some examples of wants are a certain type of car or home, a particular job, a piece of chocolate cake, or a relationship with a particular person. We all need shelter, but I want a cabin in the woods. We all need food, but I want home-baked, whole grain bread hot from the oven. We all need to be touched, but I want to be hugged by my children.

When massage provides sensory stimulation in the form of touch, it meets a need for clients. A client may want only a particular professional to provide the massage to meet the need of sensory stimulation.

When a need or perceived need (want) is met for someone by another, it is very easy to feel bonded to that other person. Needs and wants often become confused in the mind of the client; therefore the more unsettled or dysfunctional a client is, the more important it becomes to maintain boundaries in the professional relationship. This type of connection and interaction can lead to transference or countertransference (discussed later in the chapter), and it can happen with therapeutic massage. The massage professional should have a clear understanding of personal motivation in the therapy setting and should carefully maintain professional boundaries.

A *boundary* can be defined as the personal space within an arm's length perimeter. It also can be thought of as the personal emotional space designated by morals, values, and experience. Some people are not very good at defining personal boundaries or respecting others' boundaries. Certainly boundaries are defined by more than physical space, but for our purposes, a respect for personal boundaries simply begins with staying an arm's length away from another until invited to come closer. Personal space can be defined by extending the arm directly in front of the body and turning in a circle;

BOX 2-12

Determining a Client's Boundaries

An effective way to determine a client's boundaries is to ask. For example, the massage professional might ask the client the following questions:

- Is there any part of your body that you would rather not have massaged?
- Do you prefer any particular kind of music?
- I am a smoker, and I know the smell lingers. Will that bother you? (What will you do if the client says "Yes"?)
- I have three different massage lubricants. Which would you prefer?

---

the area within that space is that individual's personal space. Cultural differences may change this boundary, but for therapeutic massage, we will consider this a person's personal space range (see Touch in Chapter 1). No one should ever enter this space uninvited (i.e., without informed consent). It is important that students practice this policy while in school. They should ask whether another person may be approached, wait for the response, and act accordingly. This practice may seem silly at first, but it teaches an awareness of boundaries.

Sometimes people who have been emotionally, physically, or sexually abused have not had the chance to define or recognize personal boundaries. Practitioners should be especially respectful in their approach and should explain professional therapeutic boundaries carefully to the client (Box 2-12). It is just as important for those who have boundary difficulties to learn to define their own personal boundaries. Setting limits during a massage session may be a safe way to begin this process.

What is acceptable for us may be offensive for someone else. We may offend someone unintentionally because of differences in our personal and moral value systems. It is important for the massage therapist to help the client define a personal boundary. Once a client's boundaries have been defined, we must respect them. If a professional cannot respect a client's boundary needs, the professional should refer the client to a massage practitioner better able to deal with those needs. The massage professional should tell the client, "I will not be offended if you share with me things that you do not like about the massage. I will be happy to refer you to someone else if a different massage approach will serve you better. There are as many different ways to give a massage as there are people giving massage. I am here to help you achieve your outcomes from massage, as long as any activity does not conflict with my professional and personal standards."

It is equally important that the client understand the therapist's personal and professional boundaries; therefore the therapist must be honest in creating a personal code of ethics and must clearly communicate the professional boundaries to the client. Boundaries are discussed with the client during the initial informed consent procedures and are included in writing in the client policy statement. (Communication skills are presented later in this chapter.) Even when a massage professional is conscientious about establishing boundaries with the client during the initial intake procedure, those boundaries can become blurred as the professional interaction progresses, or something may occur that the professional had not considered. When this happens, the situation must be dealt with immediately; waiting only allows the problem to escalate and conflict to develop.

Boundaries are difficult to define. We bring to our adulthood varying experiences that shape what we feel is correct and define our personal boundaries. As professionals we are responsible for finding the client's comfort zone. This responsibility begins with learning our personal and professional comfort zones.

Anything that prevents us from being able to touch a person in a respectful, nonjudgmental way must be considered so that we can decide whom we may best serve as massage professionals. Hindrances include personal prejudices regarding body size, color, gender, and attitude. For example, some people do not relate well to children. It is ethical for such professionals to refer children to someone else for professional care. Others may be uncomfortable with those of the opposite gender, and again, it is best to refer such clients elsewhere. We may be uncomfortable with the prospect of working with people who have certain types of diseases. If this is the case, our touch may be uncomfortable for these people. A potential client may have a behavior that drives us crazy (e.g., sniffing). The behavior interferes with our ability to be the best massage professional for that particular client.

It is important, therefore, to explore professional boundaries by looking honestly at our fears, frustrations, prejudices, biases, and personal and moral value systems (Proficiency Exercise 2-7). These emotions and beliefs are very personal and often deeply held. The anchors for many of these beliefs may not be easily understood at a conscious level. Acknowledging factors that define and limit our personal and professional boundaries does not necessarily involve changing or even understanding why we feel a certain way. Changing belief systems is a complex process that often requires professional help. Although personal growth is encouraged, the expectation that we can overcome all our limitations is unrealistic. Instead, it is important to recognize when our personal boundaries will affect the professional relationship, because massage professionals work very closely with their clients. We touch our clients. (The essential quality of touch communication was explored in Chapter 1.) We must be honest with ourselves and about ourselves to be able to respect the individual needs and space of our clients.

Right of Refusal

Clients have the right to refuse the massage practitioner's services; this is called the **right of refusal**. The client has the right to refuse or to stop treatment at any time. When this request is made during treatment, the therapist must comply even though prior consent was obtained.

Professionals also have a right of refusal. Massage professionals may refuse to massage or otherwise treat any person if a just and reasonable cause exists. Obviously, lack of appropriate knowledge or skills is a reason for refusal and referral; it is

 PROFICIENCY EXERCISE 2-7

The following exercise may be the most difficult one you will have to do. On a separate piece of paper, write at least one page about your personal prejudices and fears about people and honestly list the physical and behavioral aspects of others that are difficult for you to deal with.

Here are some examples:

- Old people frustrate me. I cannot make myself listen to the same stories over and over.
- I hate ragged toenails. I do not know if I can rub anyone's feet if the nails are not well trimmed.
- People who are fat are undisciplined. They should exercise more.
- People who are skinny are obsessed with their appearance and are exercise addicts.
- When someone sniffs all the time, it makes me crazy.
- I am afraid of men with mustaches because of something that happened to me when I was young.
- I am afraid of people with the human immunodeficiency virus (HIV). I do not want to catch it.
- Women are so bossy; I hate it when they tell me what to do.
- As a man, I am uncomfortable with giving another man a massage.
- I am uncomfortable working with someone who is physically disabled. I especially feel squeamish with amputations.

It is important that you be very honest with yourself. Only by accepting that we have these areas of challenge will we be able to best serve potential clients.

the more ambiguous situations that cause concern. The next few paragraphs provide some direction for determining what constitutes "just and reasonable cause" for refusing to provide professional massage services to a client. Massage professionals also are bound by a nondiscrimination code of conduct. You may refuse to work with anyone as long as you explain the reasons and the fact that these reasons ultimately would affect the quality of care for the client; this is called *disclosure*.

Say, for example, that a person with multiple sclerosis (MS) wants to be your client. Your mother had multiple sclerosis, and you have bitter feelings about the ways her illness interfered with your childhood. You find it difficult to be with anyone who has MS because of your memories. Here are your choices:

- Tell the prospective client that you have limitations that prevent you from effectively working with MS and offer to refer her to a therapist who can provide the work needed. Make sure that at least three different qualified individuals are given as referrals so that the client has a choice.
- Be very honest with the client. Explain that you are uncomfortable working with MS and that you are concerned that the way you feel may interfere with doing what is best for her. Leave out all personal details. Knowing this up front, if the client still wants to work with you, you may decide to give it a try, as long as the quality of care for the client is not compromised and you are in a space where the challenges of the interaction can be professionally addressed.

Either way, the massage practitioner has taken responsibility for personal attitudes, and the client has the information necessary to make an informed choice. Remember, touch tells the truth. Touching someone with whom you are uneasy is difficult, whatever the reasons. By honestly telling the person about the situation, the client can make the decision. If the professional's touch seems strained, the client may realize that it is the practitioner's issue.

A massage professional has the right to refuse to treat any area of a client's body and to terminate the professional relationship if she feels that the client is sexualizing the relationship or if the professional feels adversely influenced in any way by the client.

Refusal becomes more difficult when clearly defined discrimination issues are involved. This might occur if a professional limits his practice to a particular ethnic group or refuses to provide services to someone with a legally classified disability. In these cases the professional is wise to seek legal counsel to determine the extent of professional liability.

Blurred boundaries create an environment conducive to the development of ethical dilemmas. Professional boundaries are situational and must be identified and established with each client. Clear professional boundaries support an effective therapeutic process for both the client and the professional.

THE THERAPEUTIC RELATIONSHIP

SECTION OBJECTIVES

Using the information presented in this section, the student will be able to perform the following:

- Define and recognize potential transference and countertransference issues
- Explain the professional power differential
- List factors that create dual or multiple roles
- Explain to clients feelings of intimacy between them and the massage professional
- Diffuse sexual feelings during the massage session
- Recognize and avoid sexual misconduct activities

In the therapeutic setting, specific parameters define the professional relationship between the client and the massage professional. As was explained in Chapter 1, the **therapeutic relationship** has an inherent **power differential**, which stems from the difference in knowledge and skills between the client and the professional. Even when services are exchanged between peer professionals, the power differential exists because one is placed in the position of controlling the situation. This power imbalance must be minimized as much as possible without denying its existence (Proficiency Exercise 2-8).

Transference

Issues of transference and countertransference diminish the effectiveness of the therapeutic relationship. **Transference** is the personalization of the professional relationship by the client. When a person seeks out a professional, very important

 PROFICIENCY EXERCISE 2-8

Working with a partner, follow the directions provided so that each of you plays the role of strength and of vulnerability.

1. The person playing the role of strength stands up. The person playing the role of vulnerability sits on the floor. The person who is standing looks down at the person sitting on the floor and says in a robust voice, "I am so strong, I am as strong as I have ever been. I am very strong." The person sitting on the floor looks up at the one standing and replies in a fragile voice, "I am so vulnerable. I have never been this vulnerable before. I am very vulnerable."

2. The two people remain in the standing and seated positions, but this time the person sitting on the floor says, "I am so strong, I am as strong as I have ever been. I am very strong." The person standing says, "I am so vulnerable. I have never been this vulnerable before. I am very vulnerable."

3. The two people change positions so that the one standing now sits on the floor, and the one sitting on the floor now stands. They then repeat the exercise.

Now, discuss what occurred. Possible experiences to explore include the following:

- Did a particular role cause discomfort?
- What was it like to be strong or vulnerable?
- How did the position influence the feelings?
- Which statement did you prefer to make?
- What position was most comfortable?
- In what way does this exercise relate to the therapeutic relationship?

Discuss what you learned about power differentials in the therapeutic relationship.

issues of power, trust, and control in the therapeutic relationship become the professional's responsibility. The more disorganized a person is, the stronger is the feeling of disempowerment. Clients often seek a sense of control outside themselves to help re-establish or replace their internal sense of control. The client is in a vulnerable state when doing this.

This situation is more common with people who are ill or under considerable stress, but even the well client is vulnerable in the therapeutic setting. The reality of today's society is that although most people cannot be diagnosed as sick, most have not achieved true wellness, either. Although we ideally speak of wellness massage to help a client maintain or achieve optimal wellness, the truth is somewhat different. Unfortunately, very few people seek massage for pure pleasure and to enhance their health. Most of the clients we serve, even outside the health care setting, are not optimally well. They just are not sick yet. Most seek massage services because they do not feel good and want to feel better.

The more disorganized, disempowered, and lacking in internal resources clients are, the more susceptible they will be to transference. Manifestations of transference include demands for more of the therapist's time, bringing the therapist personal gifts, attempting to engage the professional in personal conversation, proposals of friendship or sexual activity, and expressions of anger and blame. Transference occurs when the client sees the therapist in a personal light instead of a professional manner. This usually is a distorted view, because the professional is displaying a specific role and not letting her whole self be involved with the client. If the client becomes dependent on the professional, instead of re-establishing his or her personal functioning, unrealistic expectations may develop. If the client's expectations are not met, the person may blame the professional. If the client's expectations are met, the person may project the credit to the therapist instead of acknowledging his or her own efforts. In both cases the professional takes on a superhuman image that sooner or later crumbles, often leaving the client disillusioned and disempowered.

The massage professional must understand and separate the client's appropriate, genuine feelings from the transference issues. For example, a client may be angry if the therapist continually arrives late for the appointment; this is a justified feeling, not transference. Also, the client may truly appreciate the massage therapist's skill and may express that appreciation, but this does not constitute transference unless it interferes with the boundaries of the therapeutic relationship.

The professional has the ultimate responsibility for the therapeutic relationship and the direction of the therapeutic process. Managing transference is a common ethical dilemma.

Countertransference

Countertransference is the inability of the professional to separate the therapeutic relationship from personal feelings and expectations for the client; it is the professional's personalization of the therapeutic relationship. Countertransference presents itself in feelings of attachment to the client, such as sexual feelings, excessive thinking about a client between visits, a feeling of professional inadequacy if the client does not make anticipated progress, or a sense of the client as being special; it also can manifest as favoritism, anger, or revulsion toward a client. Countertransference often is fed by the following personal needs of the therapist:

- The need to fix people
- The need to remove pain and discomfort
- The need to be perfect
- The need to have the answer
- The need to be loved

The client's problems may serve as a reflection of the professional's personal life experiences. The massage professional is wise to consider his or her own personal needs and develop a reliable sense of self-awareness. Without a high level of self-awareness on the part of the professional, the focus of the massage session may shift from meeting the goals of the client to meeting the needs of the therapist. The massage therapist may begin to treat himself or herself while treating the client and lose objectivity and empathy in the therapeutic relationship (Proficiency Exercise 2-9).

Another way this can be stated is that the massage professional gives the client the kind of massage the professional

PROFICIENCY EXERCISE 2-9

Work with a partner. Face each other and look at each other. Decide who is A and who is B. A asks B the following questions, and B quickly answers. Then reverse roles.

- When do you need to fix people?
- When do you need to remove pain and discomfort?
- When do you need to be involved in a dual role?
- When do you need to be perfect?
- When do you need to have the answer?
- When do you need to be loved?

Now talk for a moment with your partner about the experience and discuss the areas in which you feel you may have the most difficulty with countertransference.

Go through the exercise again and substitute the word *want* for *need*. Discuss the feelings that arise with the word *want* and the ways they may be different from those produced by the word *need*.

would like to receive instead of the massage appropriate for the client. This situation actually occurs quite often. For example, the massage professional prefers to lie on his stomach when receiving a massage and enjoys deep work on his back. Because this position and level of pressure feel good to the massage practitioner, he may have a tendency to keep clients in the face down position and to use deep pressure on the back, even if this is not what the client would choose. Also, a massage professional may avoid using a method that she does not enjoy but that the client may like.

If the client's personal situation is similar to that of the massage practitioner, especially with regard to life challenges, the practitioner may give subconsciously based advice to the client in an attempt to solve the massage practitioner's personal problem. For example, both the professional and the client may be facing difficult marital issues, or struggling with managing menopause, or dealing with the recent loss of a parent or relocation to a new city. This dynamic can be detrimental to the client because it breaches the professional relationship and fosters psychologically unhealthy behaviors between the massage practitioner and the client. An environment of sympathetic dependence often results, and this dynamic is a basis for countertransference.

Practitioners personalize the professional relationship when they assume too much responsibility for the outcome of the session for the client or when they project a personal situation onto the client process. Countertransference issues often reflect unresolved issues on the part of the professional. Identifying countertransference in the therapeutic relationship can point out areas the practitioner may wish to explore and resolve with a qualified professional in order to remain objective and increase effectiveness as a massage professional. The goal is not for the massage professional to be faultless before beginning practice; rather, the goal is for the therapist to be aware of personal challenges that could interfere with the therapeutic relationship and thus the therapist's ability to maintain professional boundaries.

Managing Transference and Countertransference

Transference can be expected in some form in the therapeutic relationship. As it arises, it is the massage professional's responsibility to reinforce the boundaries of the professional relationship. The practitioner should explain to clients why these feelings may occur and help them redirect the transference activity to the appropriate people or situations in the client's life. This becomes difficult when the client does not move through the transference stage toward more self-directed resources and coping strategies or when the client has extremely limited resources and coping mechanisms. Such clients may need to be referred to another professional, with appropriate disclosure for the reason for referral, to help them understand that the boundaries of the professional relationship are being breached and that the existing situation is inappropriate.

The professional is always responsible for self-monitoring for the development of countertransference issues and for seeking supervision or professional support, such as problem solving with peers and/or a mentor or counselor, if necessary, to resolve personal issues. When the professional faces the realization that countertransference has occurred, the first step in resolving these issues has been taken. It is a breach of professional boundaries to allow countertransference issues to develop and linger or be acted upon. In extreme cases the client may need to be referred to a different therapeutic massage professional, with appropriate disclosure on the part of the therapist, so that the client does not take the need for referral personally.

Peer support, supervision, and mentoring are important for the massage professional dealing with transference and countertransference. Seeking information from more experienced professionals, which supervision and mentoring encourage, supports professional development. Those mentoring the massage professional do not necessarily need to be massage therapists. Various health care professionals grapple with similar issues. Mental health professionals in particular must consider transference and countertransference issues frequently. If supervision and mentoring are not part of your professional practice, it may be helpful to seek out a qualified mental health professional and establish a professional relationship with that person to sort out these particular issues.

Peer support is important as well. Interacting regularly with other massage practitioners creates an environment that promotes healthy work practices through both technical information and guidance on solving interpersonal dilemmas. When sharing with peers, be attentive to the confidentiality of your clients. It is important not to allow yourself to become isolated, with no regular sources of fresh information and perspectives.

Dual or Multiple Roles

A **dual role** exists when scopes of practice overlap and one professional provides support in more than one area of expertise. Dual or multiple roles develop when professionals assume more than one role in their relationship with their clients. These roles develop in many different ways. Providing massage in the professional environment for family members is a classic example of a dual role, as is providing professional services for a personal friend.

Dual and multiple roles are difficult to manage in the professional relationship and can be a breeding ground for ethical dilemmas. As soon as one professional assumes professional authority with the body and the mind, the body and the spirit, or the spirit and the mind, the therapist can be said to be assuming a dual role (or multiple roles if the authority is assumed in all three areas). In this situation the professional holds more power in the relationship than is appropriate, and the client begins to become disempowered. The power differential is increased. This allows a very dangerous power shift that supports the development of transference and countertransference. It often leads to enmeshment and dependence on the part of the client and burnout on the part of the therapist. Managing the inherent power differential of the therapeutic relationship is difficult enough without increasing the likelihood of transference and countertransference or the breach of professional boundaries by assuming dual and multiple roles.

In the professional therapeutic massage relationship, mental and spiritual issues need not be dealt with directly. The focus of massage is the body. When interacting with your client, maintain the focus of the work on the body while using attentive listening, acknowledging the client's circumstances, and always being alert to the possible need for referral. Interacting professionally in the area of the mind or spirit may breach the professional contract for services, which focuses on the body. Always recognize and appreciate the wholeness of the person while staying within the scope of massage therapy, and work with other professionals to deal with other areas so that the client remains empowered in the process of achieving wellness.

A dual role can arise in more subtle situations as well. The sale of products to a client, bartering of services, excessive personal disclosure by the therapist to the client, shared social interaction, or shared professional services all create situations in which the power balance of the therapeutic relationship can become problematic. As in all ethical dilemmas, decisions about conduct are gauged against the welfare of the client.

Massage Therapy and Intimacy

To dispel in advance any sexual innuendo associated with many of the terms used in the following paragraphs, definitions are included at this point for clarification.

The dictionary[6] defines *intimacy* as "the state or fact of being intimate"; *intimate* is defined as "inmost, essential, internal, most private or personal; closely acquainted or associated; very familiar." *Essential* means "intrinsic, fundamental, basic, and inherently primary." *Sensory* is defined as "connected with the reception and transmission of sense impressions" through the nervous system. *Stimulation* is defined as "the act of exciting or increasing activity."

The work of a massage practitioner is sensory stimulation; therefore by its very definition, body stimulation is sensual and may become intimate.

The massage professional must understand the physiologic aspects of therapeutic massage and recognize that the same massage techniques that alleviate stress and promote relaxation also stimulate the entire sensory mechanism, which may include a sexual arousal response. Within the parameters of professional ethics, it is always considered unethical for the client or the practitioner to interact on a sexual level, whether verbally or physically. However, it is essential that both client and practitioner understand why the urges and sensations of sexuality may present themselves. A more thorough knowledge of the physiologic and psychological network leads to a better understanding of the responses by both client and practitioner. The practitioner then is better able to alter the session to maintain a proper professional relationship.

The lumbar nerve plexus and the sacral nerve plexus conduct sensory information to and from the abdominal area, the lower extremities, and the buttocks, as well as to and from the genital area. Stimulation of a nerve plexus area is not confined to local perception, but rather is diffused throughout the area. For example, when the lower abdominal area is stroked, the nerve signals of the genital area are influenced as well. The entire sexual arousal response is part of the relaxation response via the output from the parasympathetic autonomic nervous system. Therefore each time a client relaxes out of the fight-or-flight responses of the sympathetic autonomic nervous system into the more relaxed response, the predisposing physiologic factors are present for sexual arousal. This reaction is possible not only for clients but also for practitioners as they begin to relax and entrain with the massage.

On a physiologic level, parasympathetic stimulation activates most of the benefits of massage for stress reduction. This neuralgic state also is favorable to sexual arousal. These physical responses are all connected, but it seems that the sexual response is short-lived and quickly replaced by feelings of deep relaxation as the massage continues. Responses vary with each client, and the sexual response may be totally bypassed. However, physical sexual arousal may occur (e.g., engorgement of erectile tissue with blood and shifts in breathing), and the massage practitioner needs to understand both the physiology of this situation and how to deal with it ethically.

The practitioner is responsible for putting the whole issue of sexuality into perspective, understanding it clearly, and explaining the "feelings" to the client on a physiologic level. The practitioner also is responsible for monitoring the client's responses and acting appropriately to adjust the physiology and change the pattern of the massage to diffuse the sexual energy (Box 2-13). This is easily accomplished by altering the approach of the session. It is common knowledge that sexual arousal is not purely physical and depends on both psychological and tactile responses; in these ways the practitioner can modulate the client-practitioner responses.

Intercourse is defined as "connection or reciprocal action between persons or nations; the interchange of thought, feelings, products, services, communication, commerce, and association."[6] Massage becomes an intercourse in the purest sense. *Essential intimacy* is the circle that begins to develop between practitioner and client. People want this type of intimacy; it is the type of interaction that promotes survival and

---

BOX 2-13

Diffusing Feelings of Sexual Arousal

1. Recognize the physiology and interrupt it; change what you are doing.
2. Be aware of your own psychological state and change it; become more alert.
3. Adjust the intent of the session to stimulate a more sympathetic output response by using stretching, compression, joint movement, and active participation by the client.
4. Change the music, lighting, and conversation and the client's position.
5. Stop working with your hands and use your forearms.
6. Explain the feelings in a professional manner using clinical terminology.

---

health. *Essential touch* is vital, fundamental, and crucial to well-being. It is the touch of a litter of puppies sleeping in one big pile. It is combined with the sexual interchange between lovers. However, it does not require sexual expression to be considered essential intimacy.

When a person encounters the essential touch that a sensitive and confident massage practitioner provides, that person's whole system responds. For many, the closest thing to essential touch ever experienced is parenting activities and sexual interaction. Because our bodies constantly react to new situations through comparison to past experience, a client's response system understandably might interpret these feelings as sexual arousal or as maternal or paternal. Furthermore, for many adults, the only familiar routine they have for expressing these feelings is a sexual one. It is easy to see why the client might misinterpret the sensations and feelings associated with massage, confusing them with sexual responses or a parenting role.

Remember, as massage professionals, when we touch, we also are being touched. The exchange is unavoidable, and we also need to monitor our own feelings and expressions of intimacy. If we do not deal effectively with these responses, the feelings associated with them could become very uncomfortable. The client may react by discontinuing the massage sessions, or the therapist may effectively detach from the client and possibly stop seeing the client altogether. In the latter case, the client may feel abandoned.

As the therapist closes the session and leaves the client's space, it is important to change both physiology and body language. When greeting a client and providing the massage, the therapist's body language is open, inviting, connecting, and moving toward the client (Figure 2-4). When it is time to close the session, the therapist's body language moves away from the client, pulls in toward the therapist, separates, and indicates that the session is finished (Figure 2-5). Separating well from the client is a skill that gives both the client and the massage therapist a sense of closure. It often helps to establish a "time to go" ritual by always saying good-bye the same way. Clients who linger at the door may not know how to leave or may not recognize that it is time to leave. A "time to go" ritual helps considerably.

One example of a leaving ritual is to keep a box labeled "A thought to take with me" that contains fun, empowering quotes on note cards. Have the client pick a card from the box. Put the information for the next appointment on the back of the card, hand it to the client with a warm handshake, and say good-bye. When the session is finished, the therapist should let the client go physically and emotionally as the room is prepared for the next person.

FIGURE 2-4 The body language of greeting. When greeting a client, the massage professional leans toward the person and gently draws the individual into the space of the massage session.

Touch Intimacy

Remember that, as was explained in Chapter 1, the intention of a touch is a determining factor in the interpretation of the touch. The touch of the massage professional is not focused on sexual arousal and release, nor are we the client's parents. The psychological aspect of this topic is another matter. Here the practitioner can set the stage and monitor responses. Keep discussions light. Change the topic. This is where the interpersonal communication skills of the practitioner come into play.

The moments of intimacy must be dealt with very carefully. Misunderstanding the psychological or physiologic responses, the client may interpret them as an indication of feelings of love or that the therapist is a new best friend. Clients manifest this response in different ways. Usually clients want to bring the professional into their lives, perhaps through invitations to lunch, a desire for more frequent sessions, or a proposal for a relationship. Do not allow this to happen. The practitioner must maintain professional space and monitor personal feelings. Keep the balance by confining the intimacy of massage to the therapy room.

Having little or no understanding of all these subtle interactions, the client cannot be blamed for wanting more attention from the massage practitioner. The moments of togetherness that are shared are special and can range from a great deal of laughter to sharing work-related experiences. The session can accomplish something as simple as relieving the day's tension or as complex as overcoming years of pain. Make no more and no less of the interaction.

Clients may look to the professional for emotional support beyond the ethical scope of practice for massage. Encourage them to find the support they require from another source. If a client needs assistance with coping skills, refer the person to someone who is qualified to help. Credit counselors, minis-

FIGURE 2-5 The body language of closure. When the massage is complete, the massage professional gently withdraws from the client by using body language that moves away from the person.

ters, rape crisis counselors, marriage counselors, counselors for sexual dysfunction, chiropractors, physicians, and many other caregivers can provide the help clients may need. The massage practitioner's intention is to support and accept the client in a nonjudgmental manner, listen, and blend touch skills to benefit the client.

Sexual Misconduct and Sexual Harassment

Sexual misconduct is any type of sexual activity that occurs between the professional and the client. Although sexual misconduct has been relatively well defined (Box 2-14), conduct that is invasive but not blatantly sexual remains a gray area.

A joke told between friends may be totally inappropriate in the professional setting. A statement about appearance may be taken as a compliment or could be interpreted as a sexual remark. Something that is appropriate with one client may not be acceptable with another. Practitioners can find it overwhelming to try to second-guess what is appropriate for clients. The best defense against confusion is communication. Ask questions and provide clients with information about acceptable behavior in the professional setting (Proficiency Exercise 2-10).

Sexual harassment occurs in the work setting between peers or with supervisors. Unwelcome sexual interaction (physical or verbal) in conjunction with employment status or work environment constitutes sexual harassment. Sexual harassment is clearly defined by law, whereas sexual misconduct often is more subtle and difficult to prosecute unless clearly coerced sexual acts have been committed.

Maintaining the Professional Environment

The therapeutic relationship is a unidirectional focus in which the knowledge and skills of the professional are used to assist the client in achieving therapeutic outcomes. To preserve the unidirectional focus, certain crucial professional boundaries must be maintained. For example, it is important to maintain professional space (Proficiency Exercise 2-11). Some simple ways to accomplish this are presented in Box 2-15.

Managing Intimacy Issues

Effectively managing intimacy issues can seem like an overwhelming task. However, do not be afraid of the special professional intimacy of therapeutic massage. Instead, educate

---

BOX 2-14

Guidelines on Sexual Misconduct

Guidelines developed for practitioners in Ontario, Canada, provide the following criteria for determining what constitutes sexual misconduct.

Sexual Impropriety and Sexual Abuse
1. The therapist will respect the integrity of each person and therefore not engage in any sexual conduct or sexual activities involving clients.
2. The therapist will not date a client.
3. The therapist will not commit any form of sexual impropriety or sexual abuse with a client.
4. Whatever the behavior of the client, it is always the responsibility of the massage therapist not to engage in sexual behavior.
   Sexual impropriety includes the following:
   - Any behavior, gestures, or expressions that are seductive or sexually demeaning to a client
   - Inappropriate procedures, including but not limited to:
     - Disrobing or draping practices that reflect a lack of respect for the client's privacy
     - Deliberately watching a client dress or undress
   - Inappropriate comments about or to the client, including but not limited to:
     - Sexual comments about a client's body or underclothing
     - Sexualized or sexually demeaning comments to a client
     - Criticism of the client's sexual orientation

- Discussion of potential sexual performance
- Conversations about the sexual preferences or fantasies of the client or the massage therapist
- Requests to date
- Kissing of a sexual nature

Sexual abuse includes the following:
- Therapist-client sex, whether initiated by the client or not
- Engaging in any conduct with a client that is sexual or reasonably may be interpreted as sexual, including but not limited to:
  - Genital to genital contact
  - Oral to genital contact
  - Oral to anal contact
  - Oral to oral contact (except cardiopulmonary resuscitation [CPR])
  - Oral to breast contact
  - Touching or undraping the genitals, perineum, or anus
  - Touching or undraping the breasts
  - Encouraging the client to masturbate (unless there is a specific therapeutic outcome) in the presence of the massage therapist
  - Masturbation by the massage therapist while the client is present
  - Masturbation of the client by the massage therapist

Modified from Regulated Health Professions Act and the Massage Therapy Act, Ontario, Canada, 1992.

PROFICIENCY EXERCISE 2-10

1. Working in groups of three, write down specific situations in which sexual misconduct or feelings of intimacy may develop. Exchange responses with other groups and role play a situation, with one student acting as the massage practitioner, one playing the client, and the third evaluating the way the situation was handled. Try different situations until each student has had a chance to play each role.
2. Develop a "time to go" ritual and discuss it in your group.

 PROFICIENCY EXERCISE 2-11

In the space provided, list three things you will do to maintain professional space. Choose from the list in Box 2-15 or make up your own.

1.

2.

3.

BOX 2-15

Maintaining Professional Space

1. At the beginning of a professional relationship, a formal informed consent process must be completed.
2. In most instances the time frame for working with a client should not exceed 90 minutes, with 45 to 60 minutes being the norm. If more time is spent with the client, it becomes difficult for both the professional and the client to maintain the original intent and focus of the session, and the result is an environment that fosters transference and countertransference.
3. Professionals should wear clothing that sets them apart from clients; this is one of the benefits of a uniform. A name tag that identifies one as a massage therapist also is helpful. Wearing a uniform or maintaining a professional style of dress that is different from casual clothing gives visual stimulation that reflects professionalism. The clothes do not have to be white but must be nonrevealing and present an understated and neutral appearance. Therapists must be conscious of their appearance and make sure it is kept as nonsexual as possible.
4. The therapist should avoid assuming a dual role and multiple scopes of practice. The professional contract is for a specific type of intervention. General information about lifestyle, health, or spiritual issues can be provided, but the contract is for massage. This is a consideration even if the professional is credentialed in more than one area or discipline. Often the therapist needs to decide which professional hat to wear.
5. The professional environment should be neutral and must not indirectly imply any content other than therapeutic massage. Choices made in decorating the space or in reading material can be seen as creating an environment that fosters a dual role by promoting a specific mental, spiritual, nutritional, or exercise approach.
6. Selling products to clients can become an issue because of the perceived authority influence and power differential of the professional. Closely related products, such as self-massage tools that are made available for the client's convenience, as opposed to products sold for profit making, often present less of a problem than

something like nutritional products. The client may like the services of the massage therapist but does not want to feel pressured into buying products. These situations must be managed with careful reflection, because ethical dilemmas often result from the sale of products.
7. Privacy can be preserved by using an answering machine or service and returning calls within set hours. If it is financially possible, have a receptionist or secretary monitor phone calls.
8. Maintain regular appointment hours. Begin and end sessions on time.
9. If you go to clients' homes, be extra cautious about entering a home alone. It is important to screen your clients carefully. The initial intake interview is a good opportunity to do this. Have the client come to your location, where you have more professional control over the screening process. Individual circumstances dictate when the following recommendations are necessary; however, remember: it is better to be safe than sorry.
   - An on site massage session for a bedridden elderly person will have a different level of concern than a female massage therapist providing on site massage to a single male client, or vice versa. At the very least, make sure someone always knows where you are and check in with someone periodically throughout the day. If you are anxious about doing an on site massage session, consider referring the client to someone else or team up with a fellow massage practitioner and both perform the massage.
   - Hire someone to go with you to the client's home. This person does not need to be a massage professional but should be able bodied in case the need arises to leave the home in a hurry. This person remains within hearing distance of the place where the massage is given and can act as a witness should the client claim inappropriate behavior by the massage professional. This person also provides protection from any type of entrapment or illicit advances against the massage practitioner. It is appropriate to charge for this protection, and it is reflected in the fee structure.

BOX 2-15

Maintaining Professional Space—cont'd

■ It is also important to use the phone when entering a home or other location where less control is available to the massage practitioner. Call a prearranged number and give an associate the name, address, and phone number of the client, the time of arrival, and the expected time of departure. Tell this person that you will call just before you leave. Leave instructions to call the authorities should you not call at the agreed time. Make sure that your client hears this conversation.

10. Think carefully before setting rules about client conduct, rescheduling, and payment methods. Make sure you are willing to enforce your policies. If you are not, do not make them. Record this information clearly and concisely and make sure the client reads it. Posting it on the wall provides additional reinforcement.

11. Do not spend personal time, such as lunch, with clients. In rare situations the professional may choose to forgo the professional relationship to develop a personal relationship. This decision can be considered a breach of professional ethics and is almost always a professional and personal mistake. The initial relationship structure was built on the basis of one who serves and one who is served. It is very rare that an effective transition is made to a relationship of mutual support. Both people usually end up hurt.

---

clients by answering their questions intelligently, basing your answers on the facts of physiology, and encourage them to use this information to interact more resourcefully with others. If you begin to feel physically and emotionally receptive to a client, take steps to diffuse the response (see Box 2-13). Later, review the session to evaluate your personal feelings. Was it a fleeting warm feeling? Is there just something about this particular person? Could it have been a hormonal response? Oxytocin, the bonding chemical, may be a big influence in couples bonding and parental feelings. This hormone is stimulated during skin contact such as massage. Therapists should also be aware that some women become more sexually responsive during certain times of their monthly cycle. Were you feeling alone and needing to be connected? If the problem arises from something lacking in life, empower yourself to search out the cause and change circumstances so that personal reactions are kept out of the therapy room.

If a professional relationship cannot be maintained with a client, stop providing therapeutic massage and refer the client to someone else. Give an honest, simple explanation so that the client understands it was not something he or she said or did that prompted the referral. Professional ethics cannot safeguard us from being human; however, behavior becomes unethical when the problem is not acknowledged and resourceful action is not taken to solve it.

If a client refuses or is unable to change an inappropriate response to the massage, the client must be refused further treatment. Explain to the client that the situation is uncomfortable and massage therapy can no longer be provided. The dismissal must be done gently but assertively, and the client must be told the decision is final.

A client who immediately asks for sexual release is a different case. If this occurs, the massage professional explains succinctly that neither sexual release nor any other kind of sexual interaction is provided and then dismisses the person immediately.

Care must be taken in situations that could become difficult, and any situation in which behavior could be questioned must be avoided. One such situation concerns male therapists who wish to do home-based appointments for women who are alone in the house. A good solution is to pair up with a female practitioner and do these massages as a team. It is important that a parent or legal guardian be in the room when massage services are given to a child under 18 years of age. A practitioner should never work behind a locked door, because this may be construed as entrapment. Instead, a sign should be posted indicating that a massage is in session and the room should not be entered without knocking.

Maintaining the delicate professional balance between client and practitioner is especially difficult with long-term clients. The nurturing approach of the massage practitioner fosters an environment in which friendships can form. Regular clients do become important as people, as well as in their roles as clients. Massage practitioners must always be honest with themselves about the development of personal feelings for a client. Remember, this is a relationship, and professional relationships can last a very long time. These people become important to us. When clients move away, we miss them. When a client dies, we grieve. When clients rejoice, so do we. And when clients do not need us anymore, we celebrate. Clients touch our lives. They are our best teachers. How can we not care about them?

The touch of a massage professional is safe touch. According to the dictionary definition, *safe* means not apt to cause danger, harm, or hurt; to be free of risk.[6] Physiologically, *safe* means a state of homeostasis rather than the alarm of the fight-or-flight responses of the sympathetic autonomic nervous system or the intense retreat and withdrawal responses of the parasympathetic autonomic nervous system (see Chapter 4). Being *safe* means having the ability to maintain well-being in a situation and to alter responses easily to cope resourcefully with the inevitable change and demands of everyday life. The therapeutic massage professional must consider everything, including personal beliefs and fears that may make touch unsafe for clients.

By using this educational experience to explore these issues, more safe places can be found for the practitioner, which will influence professional touch and make the massage environment a safe place. The essence of this work is human touch. By dealing with personal intimacy issues, not only can the massage professional provide essential touch for the client, the client also learns to establish proper boundaries. It must always be kept in mind that each individual massage practitioner represents the entire massage therapy profession. Demonstrating respect for the self demonstrates respect for the profession as a whole.

Consider all the dynamics of the therapeutic relationship, but if an error in judgment is to be made, err on the side of compassion, connection, and caring, which is no error at all. Learn from the experience. Do not become so "professionally detached" that the client does not connect with you, the person, and you with him or her.

ETHICAL DECISION MAKING

SECTION OBJECTIVES

Using the information presented in this section, the student will be able to perform the following:

- Implement an eight-step decision-making process

When ethical dilemmas are difficult to resolve, massage professionals are expected to engage in a conscientious decision-making process that is explicit enough to bear public scrutiny.

Decisions are thought-out responses based on principles, information, and the complexities of the situation. Decision making requires a person to consider the facts, possibilities, logical consequences of cause and effect (pros and cons), and impact on people. Each decision is unique. A few rules in the professional setting are absolutes: A professional does not breach sexual boundaries with a client; clients are to be referred when the skills required are out of the scope of practice or training of the professional; all care must focus on giving help and avoiding harm; and clients are to be given complete information about the treatment. However, most ethical dilemmas revolve around more ambiguous situations and require a thoughtful approach to decision making. These situations often are difficult to identify, and solutions may require objective input. Where does a professional go for help?

As stated previously, mentoring, supervision, and peer support are very helpful to a professional grappling with ethical dilemmas that fall into the more common situational gray areas. A mentor is concerned with the successful career growth of those they mentor. A mentor is usually one in the profession of therapeutic massage with a greater career experience. The relationship with a mentor does not have the hire, fire, and discipline role; therefore the relationship is more individually focused, with freedom to discuss issues without fear of inadequacy. Supervision involves periodic review of a professional's actions by one in authority in the work setting. This can be direct supervision, in which the supervising professional actually observes the professional at work, or reflective supervision, in which the supervisor discusses the professional practice with the practitioner. Supervision can help identify potential ethical concerns and assist in ethical decision making.

Peer support provides a format for discussion, brainstorming, and reflection on the professional practice. Two or three heads are better than one when working with ethical decision making.

Ethics is not just about answers; it is also the willingness to ask the questions. It is said that professionals do not let personal judgments interfere with professional care, but what do we do, for example, when we can't keep our mind on our work because of a client's body odor? What do we do when a client schedules appointments more frequently than necessary because the client likes being with us? How do we handle a client who refuses to seek medical intervention when indicated? And the questions continue . . .

The professional may wish to ask himself or herself the following questions:

- Can I handle the professional power differential from a position of respect and empowerment for the client?
- Do I have the knowledge and skills to respond effectively to the situation?
- Am I avoiding dual or multiple roles with the client?
- Am I maintaining the boundaries of the therapeutic relationship?
- Am I within the established scope of practice for therapeutic massage?
- Am I respecting the scope of practice of other professionals?
- Do I have the highest good of the client in mind?
- Is what I am doing supporting the highest good of the profession?
- Are my professional and communication skills effective?
- Would I want anyone else to know what I am doing?

A problem may be developing if the answers to these questions become ambiguous or inconsistent. When openly answered, these questions help us recognize the need to use a problem-solving approach to make ethical decisions.

The Problem-Solving Approach to Ethical Decision Making

Problem solving to reach an effective decision is not an easy task. A generic model created from many different problem-solving methods is presented here for the purpose of ethical decision making. This model is expounded on throughout the text in regard to what may be called clinical reasoning, which involves taking the client's health history, performing a physical assessment, developing a treatment plan, choosing methods to implement the treatment plan, and charting. Most of this information is presented in Chapter 3, with additional refinement of the material throughout this text.

We are most comfortable believing that our decision-making abilities are comprehensive, objective, intuitive, and workable. For some this actually may be the case, but years of teaching and self-exploration have shown that most people have never learned comprehensive decision-making skills. To complicate matters, different people, when gathering information, are naturally attracted to certain types of information and are influenced by certain types of criteria when evaluating possible solutions. Some experts believe that this attention focus is a genetic predisposition, and others believe that it is learned behavior. Regardless, most people, unless specifically trained, effectively consider only about half of the relevant and available information when making a decision. No wonder many of the decisions we make do not serve us well.

A problem-solving model not only leads us through the steps we more naturally would take, but also reminds us to take note of important information we might tend to overlook when making a decision (Proficiency Exercise 2-12). When this process is followed diligently, it eventually becomes a habit. In the beginning the process may feel cumbersome and uncomfortable. The parts of the process that we do not understand or with which we become impatient or frustrated often are the areas on which we do not naturally focus. These are the areas, then, that need the most practice.

The decision-making process presented in Box 2-16 acknowledges the importance of factual data; intuitive insight; concrete and objective cause and effect; and the feelings, experiences, and influences of the people involved.

 ## PROFICIENCY EXERCISE 2-12

NOTE: Learning this process can be difficult, but it is very important. It is okay to be confused and frustrated, but practice eventually will result in understanding. Proficiency exercises are important to do. In the beginning it is okay if you just attempt to do them. In time, they get easier.

Decision Making Using the Problem-Solving Model with Peer Support
Identify an ethical dilemma with which you are dealing or make up a dilemma that you believe you will deal with in the future. Describe the dilemma by answering the questions below on a separate piece of paper.

Step 1: Identify and define the situation.
 Key questions:

What is the problem?

What happened in factual terms?

What caused the situation?

What was done or is being done?

What has worked or not worked?

Who is involved and what responsibilities do they have?

Step 2: Divide into groups of four. Choose who will present the facts of his or her dilemma to the group. This presentation should not take longer than 5 minutes. Each of the other three group members will play a role in the decision-making process.

One of the three remaining group members now provides input from step 2 of the problem-solving model by suggesting possible solutions, using the following questions as a guide. For the purpose of this exercise, limit the possibilities to three or four. Spend 3 to 5 minutes on this portion of the exercise, and remember to stay within your role; it confuses the process when you bounce between steps 3 and 4.

Key questions:

What are the possibilities?

What does my intuition suggest?

What are the possible contributing factors?

What are possible approaches for corrective action?

What might work?

What are other ways to look at the situation?

What do the data suggest?

 Provide possible solutions to the dilemma.
1.

2.

3.

Step 3: The next person uses logic to evaluate each of the possible solutions presented in step 2, using the following questions as a guide. Spend 3 to 5 minutes on this part of the exercise. Again, stay in your role; do not work with steps 2 or 4.
 Key questions:

What are the costs, resources needed, and time involved?

What is the logical progression of the pattern, contributing factors, and current behaviors?

What are the logical causes and effects of each solution identified?

Continued

PROFICIENCY EXERCISE 2-12—cont'd

What are the pros and cons of each solution suggested?

What are the consequences of not acting?

What are the consequences of acting?

Step 4: The last person evaluates each of the possible solutions generated in step 2 in terms of the people involved, using the following questions as a guide. Spend 3 to 5 minutes on this part of the exercise. Stay with the process; do not become chatty or conversational.

In terms of each possible solution being considered in step 2, what is the impact on the people involved: client, practitioner, and other professionals working with the client?

Key questions:

How does each person involved feel about the possible solutions?

Does the practitioner feel qualified to work with such situations?

Does a feeling of cooperation and agreement exist among all parties involved?

Step 5: Now, the person who originally presented the ethical problem chooses a solution and develops an implementation

plan. Again, spend 3 to 5 minutes on this part of the exercise. Write the solution with the implementation plan on a separate piece of paper.

Step 6: Rotate the roles so that each member of the group plays all four roles. It will take 1 hour to complete the entire exercise with all participants playing all four roles. After the entire process has been completed, answer the following questions:

What was the easiest part of the process for me?

What was the hardest part of the process for me, and what made it difficult?

What was the most difficult part of the process for the group?

What might help the group problem solve more effectively?

How would I implement the process by myself without a peer support group?

BOX 2-16

Problem-Solving Model for Decision Making

Learning how to make good professional decisions is very important—therefore, practice, practice, practice.

Step 1: Gather the facts to identify and define the situation.
Key questions: What is the problem? What happened in factual terms?
- What are the facts?
- What has happened?
- What caused the situation?
- What was done or is being done?
- What has worked or not worked?
- Who is involved and what responsibilities do they have?

Step 2: Brainstorm possible solutions.
Key questions: What might I do? or What if?
- What are the possibilities?
- What does my intuition suggest?
- What are the possible contributing factors?
- What are possible approaches for corrective action?
- What might work?

- What are other ways to look at the situation?
- What do the data suggest?

Step 3: Logically and objectively evaluate each possible solution identified in step 2; look at both sides and the pros and cons.
NOTE: This objective analysis of the possible solutions generated in step 2 is very important. It has been my experience that most people drawn to learn massage therapy are not naturally attuned to this type of analysis and therefore tend to bypass this vital step in evaluating information to arrive at the most appropriate decision. The ability to analyze objectively is an essential skill for effective professional practice. In addition, this area of processing becomes important in dealing with conflict situations that may arise from ethical dilemmas because the focus of this information is a process. Processes can be evaluated and altered; people's feelings usually cannot. A professional who has not developed the ability to evaluate a situation logically and objectively will have difficulty identifying where processes have broken down. Remember, change an action and people's feelings change.

BOX 2-16

Problem-Solving Model for Decision Making—cont'd

Key question: What would happen if I . . . ? (Insert each brainstormed idea from step 2.)

- What are the costs, resources needed, and time involved?
- What is the logical progression of the pattern, contributing factors, and current behaviors?
- What are the logical causes and effects of each solution identified?
- What are the pros and cons of each solution suggested?
- What are the consequences of not acting?
- What are the consequences of acting?

Step 4: Evaluate the effect of each possible solution on the people involved.

Key question: How would each person involved feel if I . . . ? (Insert each brainstormed idea from step 2.)

- In terms of each possible solution being considered, what is the impact on the people involved: client, practitioner, and other professionals working with the client?
- How does each person involved feel about the possible interventions?
- Does the practitioner feel qualified to work with such situations?
- Does a feeling of cooperation and agreement exist among all parties involved?

Step 5: Choose a solution and develop an implementation plan after carefully processing steps 1 through 4.

Implementation plans are step-by-step procedures that detail what must be done to carry out the decision. For example, a solution arrived at using the previous steps might be: I will learn more about asthma so that I can work with my client better. The implementation plan would be as follows:

- Use the Internet to research asthma
- Look up asthma at the library
- Contact the local asthma support group for information
- Contact the client's physician for specific recommendations
- Talk with my friend who is a respiratory therapist
- Compile the information into a massage benefit report to develop the massage approach
- Discuss the report with my client

Step 6: Implement the plan and set a date for re-evaluation.

This is sometimes the hardest part—doing it.

Step 7: Determine the logical consequences if the plan is not followed.

It is important to determine what will happen if one of the parties in a decision that affects more than one person does not meet his or her commitment. Make sure to document this (write it down). For example, a decision is made between a massage therapist and a chronic no-show client that the client will be charged for the full session unless she calls 24 hours in advance to cancel the appointment. Both parties agree, but the very next session, the client does not show and does not call. Because the consequence has been agreed on in advance (i.e., the client will be charged for the full session), the possibility of escalation of the conflict is diminished.

Step 8: Re-evaluate and make necessary adjustments; then implement the refined plan.

Remember, decisions are not static; re-evaluation procedures can alter, refine, or change them.

COMMUNICATION SKILLS

SECTION OBJECTIVES

Using the information presented in this section, the student will be able to perform the following:

- Identify a person's preferred communication pattern
- Develop and use an I-message to deliver information and listen reflectively
- Follow a suggested communication pattern for resolving ethical dilemmas and conflict
- Identify three barriers to effective communication

Communication is the act of exchanging thoughts, feelings, and behavior. Many ethical and professional dilemmas result from communication difficulties. To make ethical decisions and resolve ethical dilemmas, we must communicate effectively.

Effective communication often is a difficult process for both the professional and the client. Without a direct communication approach, ethical dilemmas tend to escalate, and both parties suffer in the process. Professionals seek to establish genuine positive regard for all clients and to relate to each with sensitivity to that person's uniqueness. Professional ethics demands that when we have a feeling of criticism and negative judgment of a client, we must be aware of it and work to prevent it from interfering with our commitment to compassionate, quality care. Direct, honest communication that focuses on the concrete facts of the situation rather than the person's emotional behavior, as well as a gentle, respectful approach, opens the door for resolution.

As was described in Chapter 1, touch is a powerful mode of communication. The intent of professional touch may be influenced by many factors, including countertransference and the thought process of the therapist at the moment of the touch. The way touch is interpreted by the client often is influenced by the unspoken intent of the therapist; therefore it is important to monitor thoughts and feelings while professionally communicating through touch.

Putting ethical principles into action requires some basic communication skills. Communication skills are required to retrieve information, maintain charting and client records, and provide information effectively so that the client can give informed consent. Using the following communication skills will assist the professional in maintaining ethical practices in the therapeutic relationship.

The strongest message is delivered through the kinesthetic mode, or body language. As we express ourselves through our bodies, others visually receive the messages and feel our touch. It is important that congruence exist between what is heard, what is seen, and what is felt. When lack of continuity is a problem, the kinesthetic message seems to have the strongest effect.

The tone of voice is more important than the words spoken. Tone is kinesthetic and auditory because of the pressure waves emitted. We hear and feel the sound waves from the tone of voice.

The words are the least effective part of the communication pattern. Words can have mixed meanings, depending on each person's definition of a particular word (Proficiency Exercise 2-13). It is important to make sure that each of the people communicating is working from the same definition of a word. For example, the massage practitioner's definition of the word *disrobe* may be different from the client's definition. To a massage professional, *disrobe* may mean to remove external clothing but keep underwear on; the client interprets the same word as meaning to take off all clothing. During the informed consent process, the massage professional may say, "It is out of my scope of practice to diagnose or treat any specific condition." The massage practitioner defines the word *treat* as meaning to provide remedial or rehabilitation procedures. The client interprets the word *treat* as any type of method used.

Preferred Communication Patterns

Each person has a preferred method of delivering and receiving information in a style that is most comfortable for that individual. This is determined by genetic predisposition and conditioning (learning).

- People who prefer the visual mode make pictures in their mind and use many descriptive words as they paint word pictures during conversation. They tend to use "see" words and want to make eye contact when conversing. Others prefer the auditory mode. These people use "hear" words during conversation and are very attentive to the tone and rhythm of speech. They often hum, talk to themselves, and listen with their eyes closed.
- Some people operate primarily from the feeling, or kinesthetic, mode of communication. These people may find talking and listening fatiguing. When speaking they use a lot of body language and "feel" words. Often they find that they have to touch something or someone to understand.
- Almost everyone processes visual and auditory messages through the kinesthetic mode. The most common pattern is visual/kinesthetic, and the second most common is auditory/kinesthetic. People see and feel or hear and feel.
- The way information is delivered and received also depends on fundamental processing styles. Some people prefer facts and sequence, whereas others prefer concepts and ideas. Some people make decisions based primarily on processes of cause and effect, and others structure decisions in terms of people and social structure. No one way is better than another, only different.

When providing information, it is important to deliver the message in the style the person receiving it prefers. This often requires massage professionals to communicate in a way that is different from their preferred style, and it takes practice.

Listening

Effective listening involves the development of focusing skills. You cannot listen effectively if you are distracted, planning what you will say next, or preparing your response. Reflective listening involves restating the information to indicate that you have received and understood the message. Active listening may clarify a feeling attached to the message but does not add to or change the message.

Listening does not involve giving advice, resolving the problem presented, or in any other way interjecting information about what was said. Effective listening occurs when we listen to understand instead of to respond. Understanding the message and agreeing with the content of the message are not the same thing; the basis for this confusion most likely evolved from our feeling of being most understood when someone agrees with us. Understanding can occur regardless of whether agreement exists. Much time is wasted and conflict is encouraged when people equate understanding with agreement.

For example, while studying this chapter, the student may not agree with the position on wearing a uniform in the professional setting. Because the student has a different opinion does not mean that the textbook is wrong or that the student

PROFICIENCY EXERCISE 2-13

Write what each of the words below means to you and in what way you would behave if you were experiencing these words.

Joy

Love

Peace

Competence

Compare your list with those of three other students and identify the similarities and differences. What did you learn about the interpretation of a word?

BOX 2-17

I-Message Pattern

The steps for creating an I-message are as follows:
- Describe the behavior or problem you find bothersome (facts)
- State your feelings about the situation (impact on people)
- State the consequence (logical cause and effect)
- Request the preferred behavior or action (possibilities)

The pattern is:

When _____ happens, I feel _____.
The result is _____, and what I would prefer is
_____.

When delivering I-messages, remain pleasant, respectful, and honest. Be aware of your body language, tone of voice, and quality of touch.

 PROFICIENCY EXERCISE 2-14

Construct an I-message about a piece of information in this chapter that you feel is important.

Example: When I read about I-messages to enhance communication, I felt relieved. The result is that I will practice this pattern with my family, and I prefer that the communication between my family members improves.

Sit in a circle with at least three other people (more is better). Turn to your left and deliver your I-message to the person sitting next to you. That person repeats the I-message to you using the same format. Note what pieces are left out or how the pieces of the message become confused; or, on the other hand, note the clarity of the I-message when it is understood. Also note the preferred communication.

Now the person who just listened and repeated the message turns to the person on her left and delivers an I-message, which that person repeats to her. Continue this way around the circle.

is wrong; the two positions are simply different. The student can understand that the author is basing her information on the existing standards of professionalism and her prior experience but can choose not to follow the recommendation. I, as the author of the text, can understand that a valid case can be made for not visually creating distinction (a uniform) between the professional and the client, but I do not agree with the student's decision not to wear a uniform. Sometimes this is called "agreeing to disagree," but this approach still seems to hold to the context of right or wrong, whereas simply being understood feels nonjudgmental and essential.

Delivering Information with I-Messages

I-messages share feelings and concerns. You-messages put a person down, blame, criticize, and provoke anger, hurt, embarrassment, and feelings of worthlessness. I-message patterns require the four components of information used in effective decision making (Box 2-17):
- Describe the behavior or problem you find bothersome (facts)
- State your feelings about the situation (impact on people)
- State the consequence (logical cause and effect)
- Request the preferred behavior or action (possibilities)

It takes practice to use the simple I-message communication pattern well (Proficiency Exercise 2-14). Just as in problem solving, each individual attends to certain parts of the information and ignores other parts. If you are a person who naturally attends to people's feelings and you attempt to deliver a message to someone who views the world through logical outcomes, the two of you will seem to be on different wavelengths or speaking different languages. If a message is to be understood, it must be delivered on the wavelength most easily received by the person attempting to understand.

The following exercise may help you understand the importance of delivering information the way the receiver (listener) is most apt to understand.

A father enjoys jazz music and keeps the car radio tuned to a jazz station. His daughter, a teenager, likes contemporary rock. Whenever the teenager drives her dad's car, she changes the radio station. On the few occasions the two find themselves in the car at the same time, a battle begins over which station will be on, jazz or rock. Now, if the father has something important to say to his daughter or wants to connect with her, he would be wise to put the radio on the rock station, even though he prefers jazz music and may even find rock difficult to listen to. It may be that the father can have the radio on rock only for a short time before it becomes too difficult for him and he changes to the jazz station. If he insists on jazz music to begin with, his daughter will tune him right out, and the opportunity for connection is lost.

To encourage effective communication, begin by identifying a person's communication pattern; that is, the words used, tone of voice, and body language. Use neutral topics to generate general discussion. During this time adjust your communication pattern to meet the person's communication style. Shift your body language, word choice, and tone to match the client's before attempting to deliver a message.

When communicating feelings, be specific. Words such as *upset* are too ambiguous; instead, use words such as *afraid, angry, annoyed, discouraged, embarrassed, irritated, rejected, accepted, appreciated, capable, determined, compassionate, glad, grateful, proud, loved,* and *trusted.* Define the words you use. Do not assume that what you mean by a word is what your listener understands it to mean.

After an I-message has been delivered, request a response using open-ended questions. *Open-ended questions* encourage the sharing of information and cannot be easily answered in one word. Open-ended questions begin with *where, when, what, how,* and *which.* Avoid *why* questions because they encourage defensive reactions. When listening to the response, use active and reflective listening.

The I-message format also can be an effective listening tool. While listening, organize the information using the following questions:

- What happened or what are the facts?
- What feelings are being expressed?
- What was the logical outcome?
- What are the possibilities?

When listening reflectively, repeat the information as follows:

"What I heard you say was: When happened ___, you felt ___. The result was ___, and what you prefer is ___. Did I understand correctly?"

If a person leaves out information (as commonly occurs), you will not be able to fill in that blank. In that case a clarifying question can be formed, such as, "What would you prefer?" or "What was the logical outcome of the situation?"

Conflict and Conflict Resolution

Conflict is an expressed struggle between at least two interdependent parties who perceive incompatible goals, scarce resources, and/or interference from the other party in achieving their goals. There is perhaps nothing more common than conflict. Conflict arises from a number of factors, such as:

- Varied perspectives on a situation
- Differing belief systems and values, which have arisen from the involved parties' accumulated life experience and conditioning
- Differing objectives and interests

Conflict and conflict resolution play important roles in individual and social evolution and development. Many cultures value harmony, compatibility, satisfaction, and independence. Because of these values, there has been a tendency in the past to avoid conflict. Conflict arises when one or more people view the current system as not working. At least one person is sufficiently dissatisfied with the status quo that he or she is willing to own the conflict and speak up in the hope of being able to influence the situation to arrive at an improved condition. Through conflict we have opportunities to do things differently in the future.

Conflict should also be recognized as existing at two levels. In addition to the typically obvious interpersonal dispute among individuals, some measure of intrapersonal conflict almost always exists within ourselves. This inner conflict may be evidenced by confusion, inconsistency, or lack of congruity.

People in conflict share common ground as well as differences. These areas of common ground include:

- Overlapping interests
- Interdependence
- Points of agreement

The common ground can serve as the starting point for conflict resolution.

Conflict resolution does not necessarily resolve tensions between people. Conflict resolution may simply align matters sufficiently to allow each person to make progress toward his or her goals rather than stall in an uncertain and stressful state of disagreement.

Many people have long operated by the myth that the best way to resolve conflict is to "do battle," and the one who "wins" ends the conflict. This approach is more about power and control than conflict resolution. Doing battle and winning or losing supports a corresponding belief that every situation involves a "right" and a "wrong." If we respond to conflict this way, we have limited our awareness and understanding of the nature of conflict and of alternative means of responding to conflict, such as mediation and negotiation.

Factors and influences necessary for mediation and negotiation include the following:

- Concern about the impact of the dispute on the relationship
- Time concerns
- Expense
- Impact on affected others
- Lost opportunities
- Stress
- Lack of closure
- Uncertain compliance
- Areas of existing common ground

Types of Conflict

The decision-making process in this text presents a format for mediated and negotiated types of conflict resolution. Various types of conflict exist. If we can pinpoint the type of conflict, we are more likely to be able to resolve it.

Relationship Conflicts

Relationship conflicts, often called personality conflicts, occur as a result of strong negative emotions, misperceptions or stereotypes, poor communication or miscommunication, or repetitive negative behaviors. Relationship problems often lead to an unnecessary escalation in destructive conflict. Conflict resolution supports the safe and balanced expression of the perspectives and emotions of each person involved, leading to acknowledgment and understanding of that individual's point of view. Gaining a broader perspective of diversity of culture and individual operational style is very helpful. Evaluations exist for identifying different personality styles, and using these evaluation tools can be helpful. One of the most researched methods is the Myers-Briggs Type Indicator. These evaluations help individuals with opposite perspectives to interact well rather than allowing conflict to develop. The more we personalize a person's operational style, the more likely it is that conflict will develop.

Data Conflicts

Data conflicts occur when people lack information necessary to make wise decisions, are misinformed, disagree on which data are relevant, interpret information differently, or have collected data differently. Some data conflicts may be unnecessary because they are caused by poor communication between the people in conflict. Other data conflicts may be incompatibilities associated with data collection, interpretation, or communication. Most data conflicts have "data solutions," and once the information has been corrected, the conflict will resolve unless it has developed into a relationship conflict.

Interest Conflicts

Interest conflicts are caused by competition over perceived incompatible needs. Conflicts of interest result when one or more people believe that in order to satisfy their needs, the needs and interests of an opponent must be sacrificed. This often occurs during times of scarcity or when it is perceived that there is not enough to go around. Interest-based conflicts may occur over such things as money, physical resources, or time; over procedural issues, such as the way a dispute is to be resolved; or over psychological issues, such as perceptions of trust and fairness and the desire for participation and respect. For an interest-based dispute to be resolved, those involved need to define and express their individual interests so that all these interests may be addressed jointly. Interest-based conflict is best resolved through maximum integration of the parties' respective interests, positive intentions, and desired experiential outcomes. A third person, such as a mediator, is often necessary to successfully resolve this type of conflict.

Value Conflicts

Values give meaning to our lives. Values explain what is "just" or "unjust." Differing values need not cause conflict. People can live together in harmony with different value systems. Value disputes arise only when people attempt to force one set of values on others or lay claim to exclusive value systems that do not allow for divergent paths. It is no use to try to change values and systems during relatively short and strategic mediation interventions. However, supporting each participant's expression of his or her values and beliefs for acknowledgment by the other party can be helpful. Belief systems are more amiable to change. Values are like the ethical principles described earlier, whereas belief systems are like standards of practice. Belief systems are often superimposed on us during our developmental childhood years. We are taught what is right or wrong, good or bad. Because we learn our belief systems, we can change them through education and a willingness to be open to new possibilities.

Ways of Dealing with Conflict

There are five common ways of dealing with conflict. Learning about the alternative means of handling conflict gives us a wider choice of actions to use in any given situation and makes us better able to respond to the situation. Although the following methods are the common ways of increasing the chance of success, the reality is that we use each of these ways of dealing with conflict at least some of the time. We approach conflict in the way we believe will be most helpful to us. Our style for dealing with conflict changes with the circumstances. Conflict-handling behavior is not a static procedure; rather, it is a process that requires flexibility and constant evaluation to be truly productive and effective.

Denial or Withdrawal

With denial or withdrawal, a person attempts to eliminate conflict by denying that it exists and refusing to acknowledge it. Usually, however, the conflict does not go away, but rather grows to the point that it becomes unmanageable. When the issue and the timing are not critical and the issue is short-lived and will resolve itself, denial may be a productive way to deal with conflict. The effectiveness of this approach depends on knowing when to use denial.

Suppression or Smoothing Over

A person using suppression plays down differences and does not recognize the positive aspects of handling the conflict openly. Instead, the situation is acknowledged (unlike with denial), but it is glossed over. The source of the conflict rarely goes away. However, suppression may be used when preserving a relationship is more important than dealing with a relatively insignificant issue.

Power or Dominance

Power is often used to settle differences. Power may be inherent in one's authority or position. Power may take the form of a majority (as in voting) or a persuasive minority. Power strategies result in winners and losers. The losers do not support a final decision in the same way the winners do. Future meetings of a group may be marred by the conscious or unconscious renewal of the struggle previously "settled" by the use of power. In some instances, especially when other forms of handling conflict are not effective, power strategies may be necessary. Parents often say to children, "Because I said so." This use of power works in the short term, but over time results in deeper relationship conflict.

Compromise or Negotiation

Compromise (i.e., "You give a little, I'll give a little, and we'll meet each other half way") has some serious drawbacks. Such bargaining often causes both sides to assume initial inflated positions, because they are aware that they are going to have to "give a little" and want to reduce the loss. The compromise solution may be watered down or weakened to the point that it will not be effective. There may be little real commitment by any of the parties. Still, in some cases compromise makes sense, such as when resources are limited or a speedy decision needs to be made.

Integration or Collaboration

The integration or collaboration approach suggests that all parties to the conflict recognize the interests and abilities of the others. Each individual's interests, positive intentions, and desired outcomes are thoroughly explored in an effort to solve the problems in a maximizing way. Participants are expected to modify and develop their original views as work progresses. This sounds like the ideal way to manage and resolve conflict; however, for collaboration to be successful, those involved need a nonthreatening and collectively supportive system. This process takes time, openness, and energy.

Conflict Climate: Defensive or Supportive

A **defensive climate** reflects the type of atmosphere characteristic of competition—an atmosphere that inhibits the mutual trust required for effective conflict management. A supportive climate reflects collaboration—an environment that leads to mutual trust and to an atmosphere conducive to managing differences. Participants in conflict resolution hopefully come to appreciate that the apparent presenting problem does not need to limit their discussions. Participants are encouraged to express the full breadth and depth of their interests, with each participant seeking to identify a "value" that he or she can bring to the discussion and the maximized satisfaction of underlying interests and intentions.

Conflict is important. If managed well, it identifies and supports effective change. Conflict can foster avoidance, or it can expand our experiences. Making good decisions about managing and resolving conflict can pave the way for greater understanding and well-being.

During the process of resolving a conflict, written documentation should be maintained about the nature of the conflict, the type of resolution attempted, the success of the conflict resolution, and the outcome. Because conflict already exists, interpretation of the requirement for resolution can become confused. Objective documentation that is agreed upon by the parties helps maintain clarity. If the conflict cannot be resolved independently, documentation of the nature of the conflict is extremely important, in case the situation escalates to legal action.

Communicating When Dilemmas Arise

The following pattern can be used to resolve ethical dilemmas.

1. Carefully examine the facts, possibilities, logical causes and effects, and your feelings about the situation (see Box 2-16).
2. Speak with a mentor, a peer, or a supervisor about the situation in a peer review or support context.
3. Plan a time to talk about the situation with the other person or people involved.
4. Begin the conversation by identifying the problem as you see it.
5. Use the standard I-message format to provide information and professional disclosure about your inability to work with or be comfortable with the situation.

In the following example, a massage professional uses an I-message to talk with a client about the client's body odor:

"When a client seems to have a distinctive body odor that I am aware of (facts), I feel distracted from my work (impact on people). As a result, because of my inability to focus, the client does not receive the best massage (logical cause and effect). I would like to see if we can resolve this difficulty, and if I can't deal with the situation better, I may find it to your benefit to refer you to someone who is not as sensitive to odors as I am (possibilities)."

The client's body language and tone of voice may indicate embarrassment. The therapist then uses another I-message: "When I find it necessary to speak with someone about issues as personal as this (facts), I feel uncomfortable and embarrassed because I am afraid I will embarrass or hurt the person (impact on people). It is very difficult for me, but I truly want

you to have the best possible care (logical cause and effect). What information do you have that can help me (possibilities and open-ended question)?" Ending with an open-ended question encourages a problem-solving discussion.

It is essential to determine *who has the problem*. This can be done easily by deciding who will have to implement the solution to resolve the problem. Sometimes both parties own a part of the problem, with each needing to implement a portion of the solution for total resolution.

Continuing with the example of body odor, the therapist identifies and owns the problem by saying, "The difficulty is in my sensitivity to odors."

Next, information is gathered and possible solutions are devised. The client continues to express embarrassment through body language and states that he was aware of the problem. He tells you that body odor has been a problem since he began taking medication for a health problem but that he had just showered before he came to the session and thought the odor was gone.

The massage practitioner responds using reflective listening: "If I understand correctly, you are taking a medication that causes the body odor (facts), and others are aware of the odor (impact on people), but you felt the odor was gone since you showered before coming to the session (logical cause and effect)."

The therapist asks, "Do you have any suggestions?" The client replies, "Could you use a scented oil or a room scent?" The client also says that he can speak to his physician and continue to shower just before coming for the session (generating possible solutions).

The therapist explains that using a scented oil may be a problem because she has sensitive skin and that using a room scent bothers other clients. The therapist asks, "Would it bother you if I wore a mask treated with a scented oil?" The client indicates that would be fine (evaluating possible solutions in terms of logical outcomes and pros and cons, as well as people's feelings).

The therapist says, "How about if I try the mask next time you are here, and we will talk about it after the massage? If this doesn't work, we will see if we can come up with another solution. If nothing works, I will help you find a good therapist who can better serve your needs and is not so sensitive to odors." The client agrees (deciding on and implementing a plan, setting a date for re-evaluation, and agreeing on logical consequences).

After a decision has been made and agreed upon, it should be well defined and all parties should be in agreement about what will happen if the solution to the problem is not implemented effectively. The plan and the agreed-upon consequences should be written down.

The therapist closes with an I-message: "When I am able to work so well with a client about my sensitivity to odors (facts), I feel relieved (impact on people). This conversation has encouraged me to be more honest with myself and my clients (logical cause and effect). I hope that I will be able to continue to communicate effectively with you (possibilities). Thank you for being open with me."

A week later the plan is carried out, and the therapist finds that using the mask is distracting but effective. A sense of humor and understanding on the part of both the therapist and the client continue to support an effective solution (re-evaluate and make the necessary adjustments).

Barriers to Effective Communication

Effective communication is a skill. It can be learned. Effective communication is essential in the therapeutic relationship. Professionals diligently seek to improve their communication skills.

Time

It takes time to communicate effectively. This is why writing is sometimes a more effective form of communication. When writing, we should make time to consider the words and reflect on what is being said. The person responding to the written message also has time to reread and reflect on the message.

Old Patterns

Falling into old patterns and old conditioning limits effective communication. It is important to "know thyself," and we must recognize personal triggers to old reactionary patterns in communication (Proficiency Exercise 2-15). Sometimes we need to leave a situation and come back to it so that we can respond instead of react.

Avoidance

People generally avoid communicating about conflict until it is unavoidable, and they avoid people who display strong emotion because it makes them feel uncomfortable.

CREDENTIALS AND LICENSING

SECTION OBJECTIVES

Using the information presented in this section, the student will be able to perform the following:

- Describe the difference between governmental and private credentials
- Determine whether a credentialing program is valid
- Explain the basic roles of local and state laws and legislation and their influence on therapeutic massage
- Describe the two levels of practice for therapeutic massage
- Contact local, state, or provincial governments to obtain information about laws pertinent to the practice of therapeutic massage

 PROFICIENCY EXERCISE 2-15

In the space provided, evaluate your communication skills against the criteria presented in this section. Identify at least one area in which your communication skills currently are effective and one area that needs improvement.

Example: My communication skills generally are effective when I am not stressed. I remember to listen in a focused way and use the I-message pattern often. However, when I have many things on my mind, I become distracted, do not listen effectively, and tend to interrupt people.

Your Turn

Credentials

Credentials are a form of official verification, earned by completing an educational or examination process, that confirms a certain level of expertise in a given skill. Governmental and private professional credentialing processes are found in the massage profession. Standardization of the profession has resulted in different methods of proving one's skills in order to practice therapeutic massage. The massage professional should understand the various credentialing processes and the requirements of practicing legally.

The only credentials required for the practice of therapeutic massage are those specified by governmental bodies (Box 2-18). All others are voluntary. Because of some confusing and difficult local laws, special legislative concerns need to be addressed by the massage professional.

Many massage organizations and training programs have developed their own types of credentials. These credentials are valid only insofar as they indicate a level of professional achievement. A school diploma, which is granted on completion of a course of study, is an example. This is a very important document for a massage professional, but it is not a legally required credential unless stipulated by the law. For instance, a massage professional may need a diploma from a state-regulated school to take licensing examinations in states that license massage therapists.

Anyone can offer private certification. Therefore it is important to make sure that any educational program or examination you take is sanctioned and administered by a reputable, regulated provider. As an example, state-licensed schools, recognized national and state professional organizations, and classes approved for continuing education credits have had to undergo a review process that validates their educational offerings. Approval by the National Commission for Certifying Agencies (NCCA) validates certification processes.

The National Certification Examination for Therapeutic Massage and Bodywork has been available since 1992. The examination covers human anatomy, physiology, kinesiology, clinical pathology, massage and bodywork theory, assessment, adjunct techniques, business practices, and professionalism. It continues to be refined to reflect the skills and knowledge base needed to meet the current job market for massage professionals. Periodically a job analysis survey is used to upgrade and improve the examination. The examination is meant to evaluate the entry level knowledge base and skills. The educational requirement for taking the examination is equivalent to 500 hours in class, which must cover the information base and competencies required as indicated by the most recent job survey. The examination is computer generated and is administered regularly in convenient locations. It does not include a practical demonstration of skills. The questions are multiple choice. Most of the questions are not answered with a regurgitation of factual data but rather require effective decision-making skills to identify the best answer.

This examination is not a government-regulated test. It is a voluntary, privately administered examination unless an individual state decides to use it for a licensing examination. Some states have done this, and some have also required addi-

BOX 2-18

Governmental Credentials and Regulations

Licensing
- Requires a state or provincial board of examiners
- Requires all constituents who practice the profession to be licensed
- Legally defines and limits the scope of practice for a profession
- Requires specific educational courses or an examination
- Protects title usage (e.g., only those licensed can use the title of massage therapist)

Governmental Certification
- Administered by an independent board
- Voluntary but required for anyone using the protected title (e.g., massage therapist); others can provide the service but cannot call themselves massage therapists
- Requires specific educational courses and an examination

Governmental Registration
(Not to be confused with private registration processes)
- Administered by the state Department of Registry or other appropriate state agency

Voluntary Verification
- Does not necessarily require a specific education, such as a school diploma; often other forms of verification of professional standards, such as years in practice, are acceptable
- Does not provide title protection

Exemptions
- Means that a practitioner is not required to comply with an existing local or state regulation
- Excuses practitioners who meet specified educational requirements from meeting current regulatory requirements
- Does not provide title protection

 PROFICIENCY EXERCISE 2-16

1. Investigate the legal requirements to practice massage in your area.
2. Collect information to create an educational packet about massage for government officials and the public.
3. Attend a local government board meeting and observe the process.

tional test components, such as a practical demonstration of skills. In the future, other reliable tests may be developed and become an option for voluntary certification or government regulation.

Passing national certification exams is a concrete means of validating professional achievement. The Evolve Web site provides review questions for studying for certification and licensing exams.

Laws and Legislation

State and Local Regulation

The types of legislative controls massage therapists most often encounter are state or provincial controls and local controls. A province is a political unit of some countries, such as Canada. It typically is a large area made up of many small local units of government. In the United States, states are the equivalent of provinces. States are further subdivided into counties, local townships, and cities. The Federation of State Massage Boards has developed an exam specifically for state licensing of massage professions. Launched in 2007, this exam will support states in legislative development.

The main purpose of a law or an ordinance is to protect the safety and welfare of the public. When a governing body decides to enact regulations, the regulations must meet this criterion. Laws and ordinances are not passed to protect the interests of a small group, also known as a *special interest group*.

Many but not all health professionals are regulated at the state level through licensing (Proficiency Exercise 2-16). If the government feels that a particular activity could cause harm to the public, it seeks to control and limit the individuals who can participate in the activity. (For example, physicians, nurses, chiropractors, physical therapists, dentists, builders, electricians, cosmetologists, and plumbers are all licensed.) Requirements for a knowledge base and the amount and type of education are determined. Tests, often called *boards,* are given. The scope of practice is described in the law that governs the licensed professional.

If the state does not choose to license a particular profession (occupational licensing), local governments (usually townships and cities) can choose to regulate activities within their jurisdiction. Again, local laws, usually called *ordinances,* are in place to protect the public's safety and welfare. Local governments are most concerned with what types of activities go on in their region and the way the land is used (zoning).

If the state licenses a professional, the local government does not feel the need to regulate the actual practice of the professional by setting educational standards and administering competency tests. The local government does regulate where the professional may work. This is done through zoning ordinances. Professionals such as physicians, lawyers, and accountants often are required to locate their place of business in a particular zone or area of land use. Land use usually is determined on a master plan that directs the way the local government wants to see the area grow and develop. It is important to designate areas as residential (living), industrial (manufacturing), retail business districts (commercial), professional offices (office), parks (recreational), and farming (agriculture). Without such zoning, a loud industrial operation could disturb the quiet living in a residential area. Local governments are also concerned with the safety of the buildings in their areas. Monitoring the safety of buildings is the responsibility of the building inspector.

A case could be made for licensing massage therapists as a means of protecting the public, with the profession's need for formal training in sanitation, contraindications, and necessary referrals to licensed medical personnel for suspected health problems. A case also could be made for enacting massage laws to protect the massage professional from discrimination and provide the ability to practice a professional livelihood.

Therapeutic massage is not consistently regulated by law. Each state in the United States, each province in Canada, and each country in Europe have different ways of dealing with massage regulation. Because of this inconsistency, massage professionals must carefully research the governmental controls and the laws that apply in the areas where they plan to open their business.

Many old laws and local massage ordinances were written to control prostitution by preventing the practice of massage. This type of ordinance is easy to recognize because it specifies medical examinations for sexually transmitted disease and other degrading requirements. Although the situation is improving, local ordinances of this type are still found in states where the profession of massage has not yet been licensed.

Currently more than two thirds of the United States has some type of state licensing for the professional practice of therapeutic massage. The trend continues in this direction. Licensing requirements in the European and Asian countries, Canada, New Zealand, Australia, and other countries vary to such an extent that it is impossible to cover all of that information in this chapter. Overall, licensing requirements are changing quickly.

Educational requirements that allow a person to sit for a licensing examination are increasing, and the competencies reflected in the examinations are becoming more sophisticated, reflecting the evolving professionalism of therapeutic massage. Almost all licensed states require 500 to 1,000 contact hours of education (15 to 30 credits) from a state-approved school. To obtain the most current information on licensing requirements, massage therapists should contact licensed massage therapy schools or governmental licensing offices in their specific area.

In states where massage professionals must be licensed, the practitioner must still comply with local zoning ordinances and building requirements when setting up a professional practice. If the state licenses massage, the local government usually treats the massage professional like any other licensed health or service professional. The business is classified as a service, and it must be set up in the proper zoning location, usually an area of office or commercial zoning.

Local governments often discourage any type of business operation in residential areas but with special restrictions will designate what types of businesses can be operated from a home. These home occupations usually are service oriented rather than retail oriented (the sale of goods) and limit traffic to and from the home. To establish a home office, the massage therapist may need to have a special and separate area in the home, including a separate entrance. Another requirement might be that no employees other than the family in the home may be hired. Sometimes only those with a special need, such as a disability that prevents working outside the home, are eligible for a home office permit. Usually a special permit is required for a home office; each local government is different. Many massage practitioners choose to work from a home office. A massage practice is a business that fits well within these special requirements.

It is true that written tests and practical demonstrations cannot measure the massage professional's gentleness, care, nonjudgmental behavior, intuition, and touch. This does not mean that formal tests are not valid; they are. Local governments need to establish that the massage business is legitimate therapeutic massage and not a front for prostitution. State governments must protect the public's health, safety, and welfare from the unregulated practice of massage. Both units of government must protect the public from potentially dangerous acts by defining performance criteria based on education or the ability to pass a test.

Licensing, compliance with ordinances (Box 2-19), and passing any of the nationally recognized certification examinations are important in the professional practice of massage. The bottom line is, the massage professional must comply with the existing standards of practice, both required and voluntary. If a difficult state law or local ordinance is encountered, massage therapists must work together to change the regulation. The staff at a licensed massage school is the best resource on procedures for working with local governments to change a nonsupportive massage ordinance.

Reciprocity

Reciprocity is the right of exchange of privileges between governing bodies. Some states have similar licensing requirements for professionals. When this is the case, a state may accept a different state's license. This is not common for many professionals, and it is even less common for massage therapists. Individual state licensing or any type of certification does not secure the right to practice massage in any location other than that of the government issuing the license.

Regulations, standards of practice, codes of conduct, scopes of practice, and so forth are methods of setting the rules for cooperative professional relationships. All organized groups have rules that permit effective interaction between members. Respect is important, and working together as a team is essential in professional practice. Let us hope that the massage therapy profession is an example of cooperation, respect for other professions, and ethical standards of practice that provide for internal professional regulation and compliance with external governmental control.

DEALING WITH SUSPECTED UNETHICAL OR ILLEGAL BEHAVIOR OF FELLOW THERAPEUTIC MASSAGE PROFESSIONALS

SECTION OBJECTIVES

Using the information presented in this section, the student will be able to perform the following:

- List and explain the four steps involved in reporting unethical behavior

BOX 2-19

Steps for Complying with Licensing Requirements

1. Find out whether your state or province requires licensing. Contact the Department of Licensing and Regulation, Occupational Licensing Division, for this information. If state licensing is required, find out what educational requirements must be met to take the examination.

2. If your state does not have licensing, contact the local government where you intend to work to inquire about local ordinances. Obtain a copy of the ordinances and read them carefully. Look especially for the educational, zoning, and facility requirements. Whether you live in a city, township, or similar government unit, the clerk's office is the department that usually has this information.

   NOTE: Even if there is no state or local regulation, attending only a licensed school or an approved training program is a good idea. Other states or local governments may require this type of education, and without it you cannot practice in their areas.

3. Shop carefully for your school of massage training. Contact the state Department of Education and confirm that the school is licensed and in compliance with state regulations.

4. Before renting, buying, or setting up your massage practice, contact the local government concerning zoning requirements and building codes. If you are considering a home office, check the zoning ordinances to make sure you will be in compliance. Again, your city or township officials (usually the clerk) are your best sources of information.

   Zoning permits require a public hearing. Your neighbors are notified by mail, and the hearing is advertised in the newspaper. Contact the zoning department to find out what action is required. Whether you are establishing your business in a home office or a business zone, contact the neighbors to explain your business and find out their response. Without their approval, or at least lack of opposition, you are unlikely to obtain a permit. Attend the hearing at all costs. Remember: *no permit = no business.* Zoning permits may require 6 to 8 weeks to complete. If you start your business without proper permits, you could be shut down at any time by government authorities.

5. Before you rent space or begin your business, contact the local government and apply for any necessary permits or business licenses. Make sure you meet all regulations. Fees can run anywhere from $25 to $500.

The appropriate way to address unethical behavior and violations of standards of practice by colleagues can present a difficult dilemma. Everything covered in this chapter is an important consideration when dealing with inappropriate behavior by others (Proficiency Exercise 2-17). When concern develops about the conduct of a colleague, an approach that combines self-reflection, peer support, mentoring, supervision, and effective communication skills is the best way to deal with these situations.

 PROFICIENCY EXERCISE 2-17

Working in groups of three, make up and then develop a specific situation in which a colleague has acted in an unethical manner. Exchange responses with a different group and role play to resolve the situation. One student acts as the massage practitioner, one plays the colleague, and the other evaluates the way the situation was handled. Role play different situations until each student has had a chance to play each role. Use the problem-solving model and communication and conflict management skills during the role playing.

Self-Reflection

Carefully reflect on the personal motivation causing the concern. It is important that motives for confronting a fellow professional be based on a genuine concern for the person and his or her clients, as well as the higher good of the profession as a whole. It is necessary to make sure that the situation is purely one of professional ethical concern and not a reaction based on personal values or moral beliefs.

Mentoring and Peer Support

Discuss the situation with your mentor or a colleague in a peer support situation while maintaining the confidentiality of the suspected party. Explore the motives supporting your concern.

Talking with Those Involved

If others share your concern, speak directly to the colleague. Often the person is not aware of the breach of standards of practice or that the behavior appears to be unethical. Peer support and bringing the concern to the person's attention can help resolve the problem.

Formal Reporting

Depending on the seriousness of the infraction and the colleague's response, you may have to file a formal complaint through the professional organization or the legal system in your area.

Ignoring unethical behavior in colleagues is unprofessional. A willingness to be involved with profession-wide ethical concerns supports professional integrity as a whole.[3] Carefully document the concerns and the process of intervention. Follow all ethical principles in these types of situations.

■ ■ ■ SUMMARY

A tremendous amount of information has been covered in this chapter. Years of experience confirm that when a massage practitioner encounters difficulty in the professional setting, it is seldom a problem with a technical skill and almost always an ethical dilemma. Wise students will review this chapter time and again during the course of study and will find support in reviewing the information periodically as they mature in their professional practice after graduation.

Decision-making skills, achieved by using the problem-solving model and by developing effective communication and conflict management skills, will prove to be some of the most valuable information in this text. Both decision making and communication are skills to be learned, and massage professionals must practice these skills to gain proficiency. And as with any skill, when you first begin to use them, you will feel awkward and uncomfortable. That's okay. You probably will have the same feeling as you practice all the new skills in this text, such as body mechanics, draping procedures, and all the massage manipulations and techniques. It is not okay to avoid the practice needed to perfect the skills required of a massage professional.

evolve

2-1 Electronic flashcards for key terms in this chapter aid in information retention.

2-2 Complete an ethical behavior matching exercise.

Don't forget to study for your certification and licensure exams! Review questions for this chapter are located on Evolve.

Ethical behavior is professional behavior. It revolves around a high regard and respect for our clients; for other health, training, and service professionals; and for ourselves. Being a professional is a compassionate and caring responsibility that requires a commitment to continued learning, self-reflection, and the highest good for all concerned. For massage professionals, it is a privilege to serve others in such an important way and to watch as the respect we give our clients evolves into a respect for ourselves.

REFERENCES

1. *Hands On*: American Massage Therapy Association, accessed March 14, 1998.
2. Regulated Health Professions Act and the Massage Therapy Act, Ontario, Canada, 1992. https://www.cmto.com/regulations/mta.htm, accessed July 10, 2007
3. Corey G, Corey MS, Callanan P: *Issues and ethics in the helping professions,* ed 7, Pacific Grove, Calif., 2006, Wadsworth Publishing.
4. D'Arcy GG: The first and last word in privacy compliance, Phoenix Health Systems, 2003. http://www.phoenixhealth.com
5. American Dental Association. http://www.ada.org/prof/prac/issues/topics/hipaa/index.html accessed March 11, 2007.
6. *Webster's third new international unabridged dictionary deluxe,* ed 3, Springfield, Mass, 2002, Merriam-Webster.

Workbook Section

Answers for the Workbook Section for Chapter 2 are provided on p. 759.

■ ■ ■ SHORT ANSWER

1. Define ethics.

2. Why is it difficult to develop a definition for therapeutic massage?

3. Why does the massage professional need to understand the scope of practice for other professionals?

4. In what ways do massage practitioners avoid falling into a situation that could allow them to be accused of practicing medicine?

5. Why is it unethical to provide massage services to a client the practitioner does not like or with whom the practitioner is uncomfortable?

6. What is the importance of disclosure in the right of refusal?

7. Why is informed consent so important?

8. What are the implications of HIPAA and confidentiality?

9. In what way does the word *respect* relate to boundaries?

10. Determining the acts that constitute sexual misconduct is easy, but how do you decide whether more subtle activities and feelings are a breach of the trust between client and practitioner?

11. Why might a client interpret the experience of massage as a sexual one?

12. Why is it ethical to establish rules of conduct for the client and massage therapist and to maintain professional space in the client-practitioner relationship?

13. What are the important aspects of credentialing for the massage practitioner?

14. Why does the massage professional need to understand legislative issues, local ordinances, and zoning regulations?

15. What is the main purpose of a law?

16. What are the two types of massage therapy practice?

■ ■ ■ MATCHING

Match the term to the best definition.

1. Applied kinesiology
2. Bodywork
3. Boundary
4. Certification
5. Coalition
6. Craniosacral and myofascial
7. Credential
8. Disclosure
9. Energetic approaches
10. Essential touch
11. Ethics
12. Exemption
13. Informed consent
14. Integrated approaches
15. Intimacy
16. License
17. Manual lymph drainage
18. Medical rehabilitative massage
19. Neuromuscular approaches
20. Asian approaches
21. Right of refusal
22. Safe touch
23. Sexual misconduct
24. Scope of practice
25. Structural and postural integration approaches
26. Therapeutic massage
27. Wellness personal service massage
28. Conflict resolution

a. A term describing all the various forms of massage, movement, and touch therapy
b. Methods of bodywork that focus on subtle body responses
c. Vital, fundamental, primary touch that is crucial to well-being
d. A voluntary credentialing process that usually requires education and training, as well as testing administered privately or by governmental regulatory bodies
e. A tender, familiar, and understanding experience between human beings
f. A designation earned by completing a process that verifies a certain level of expertise in a given skill
g. Standards, ideals, morals, values, and principles of honorable, decent, fair, responsible, and proper conduct
h. Methods of massage that influence the movement of lymph
i. Methods of massage that evolved from the ancient Chinese systems
j. Methods of massage that influence the reflexive responses of the nervous system and its link to muscular function
k. Any sexually oriented behavior that occurs in the professional setting
l. The where, when, and how a professional may provide a service or function as a professional
m. Methods of massage derived from biomechanics, postural alignment, and the importance of the connective tissue structures
n. Personal space located within an arm's length perimeter; personal emotional space designated by morals, values, and experience
o. Combined methods of various forms of massage
p. A case in which a professional is not required to comply with an existing law because of educational or professional standing
q. Acknowledging any situation that interferes with or affects the professional relationship and informing the client of that situation
r. A scientific art and discipline involving assessment and the systematic, external application of touch to the superficial soft tissue of the skin, muscles, tendons, ligaments, and fascia and to the structures that lie in the superficial tissue; methods of touch include stroking (effleurage), friction, vibration, percussion, kneading (pétrissage), stretching, compression, passive and active joint movements within the normal physiologic range of motion, and adjunctive applications of water, heat, and cold
s. Methods of evaluation and adaptation that use an application of muscle testing, along with various forms of massage, for corrective procedures
t. Secure, respectful, considerate, sensitive, responsive, sympathetic, understanding, supportive, and empathetic contact
u. The level of professional responsibility, based on extensive education, that prepares the massage therapist to develop, maintain, rehabilitate, or augment physical function, to relieve or prevent physical dysfunction and pain, and to enhance the client's well-being; methods include assessment of the soft tissue and joints and treatment by soft tissue

manipulation, hydrotherapy, remedial exercise programs, actinotherapy (light therapy), and client self-care programs
v. A type of credential required by law as a means of regulating the practice of a profession to protect the public health, safety, and welfare
w. Client authorization for any service from a professional, based on the premise that the massage professional has provided adequate information to enable the client to make an educated choice
x. A nonspecific approach to massage that focuses on assessment for the purposes of detecting contraindications to massage or a need for referral to other health care professionals and also for developing a health-enhancing physical state for the client
y. A group formed for a particular purpose
z. Methods of therapeutic massage that work both reflexively and mechanically with the fascial network
aa. The right of both the client and the professional to stop the session
bb. The use of mediation, negotiation, and communication skills

■ ■ ■ STANDARDS OF PRACTICE ACTIVITY

Put an X on the line by the situations that indicate a person who is not able to provide informed consent.
____a. An elderly client living alone
____b. A 50-year-old man taking high blood pressure medication
____c. A freshman high school student
____d. A 30-year-old woman, the victim of a closed head injury, who communicates with a computer
____e. A 24-year-old developmentally disabled client
____f. A client who does not speak English, and no interpreter is present
____g. A client who seems to be under the influence of alcohol
____h. A 21-year-old woman in the third trimester of pregnancy
____i. A severely depressed client
____j. An elderly client with dementia
____k. A client who insists that you cure her sore knee
____l. A terminally ill hospice client

■ ■ ■ DETERMINING LICENSING NEEDS ACTIVITY

List five steps in determining licensing needs.

1.

2.

3.

4.

5.

■ ■ ■ ASSESS YOUR COMPETENCIES

Now that you have studied this chapter, you should be able to:

1. Define professionalism

2. Define therapeutic massage

3. Define a scope of practice for therapeutic massage

Workbook Section—cont'd

4. Develop and explain a code of ethics and the standards of practice for therapeutic massage

5. Complete an informed consent process

6. Take ethics into consideration in maintaining professional boundaries and the therapeutic relationship

7. Use basic communication skills to listen effectively and deliver an I-message

8. Identify and resolve conflict in the professional setting

9. Use a problem-solving approach to enhance ethical decision making

10. Identify legal and credentialing concerns of the massage professional

11. Identify and report unethical conduct of colleagues

12. Become familiar with HIPAA and its procedures

On a separate sheet of paper, write a short summary of the content of this chapter based on the competencies listed above. When writing this paper assume you are speaking to someone—a client, prospective employer, co-worker, or other interested person. Write the paper as if you were having a conversation and explaining the importance of the information and skills to professional massage development.

Next, in small student discussion groups, share the papers and compare and contrast how the information was presented. Discuss the content, looking for similarities, differences, potential misunderstanding of the information, and clear and concise methods of description.

■ ■ ■ PROBLEM-SOLVING EXERCISES

1. A new client tells you about the treatment he received during a massage in another community. Some of the information seems to conflict with the principles of the code of ethics presented in this text. The client tells you that the massage professional told him he needed to lose weight; she did not stop working on his feet when he asked her to do so; she did not explain that a trigger point area could be sore the next day; she gave him a hug at the end of the session without first asking permission; she told a joke that had some sexual innuendo; she let the drape slip while massaging his buttocks; she talked about difficulties with her children; she walked in to get a chart without knocking first while he was dressing after the session; she said that physical therapists were bad at dealing with neck pain and that she could fix his neck problem; and she did not give him a receipt when he paid for the massage.

Which of the 28 standards of practice presented in Box 2-5 did the massage professional breach, and in what way would you explain that you practice differently?

The following cases are situations in which intimacy issues must be explained. After reading each case, write three ways to deal with the issue. Use the clinical reasoning model to develop your answers.

2. Kathy has been a massage professional for 3 years. She has been seeing Mr. Adams for a monthly massage for 2 years. He is in the process of a divorce and begins to schedule a massage every week because of the stress. Last week he mentioned to Kathy how important the massage is for him and lightly touched her hand. Should Kathy be concerned?

3. Matt has been a massage therapist for 10 years. Recently he has been seeing a client, Jeff, who attended the same high school as Matt. Although they were only acquaintances during high school, Jeff speaks often of the good old school days. At the last appointment Jeff offered Matt an extra hockey ticket and asked if he would like to go to the game with him. How should Matt respond?

4. Mary is new to the massage therapy profession and has had only a few clients. She finds a new client very attractive and notices that she is spending extra time with that client each session. She recognizes that she is attracted to the client physically and emotionally. How should she handle the situation?

Medical Terminology for Professional Record Keeping

■ CHAPTER OBJECTIVES

After completing this chapter, the student will be able to perform the following:

- Identify the three word elements used in medical terms
- Combine word elements into medical terms
- Comprehend unfamiliar medical terms
- Identify pertinent abbreviations used in health care and their meanings
- Use relevant anatomic and physiologic terminology correctly
- Use the information in this chapter for effective professional record keeping

■ CHAPTER OUTLINE

■ KEY TERMS

Abbreviations
Care or treatment plan
Contraindication
Database
Goals
Indication
Motor tone
Muscle tone
Prefix
Qualified
Quantified
Root word
SOAP notes
Suffix

The study of medical terminology provides a key to understanding the accepted language of the sciences. As massage therapy again moves into the position of a medically valid service, the massage professional will find it increasingly important to be able to speak, write, and understand scientific language. In addition, the massage professional must be able to maintain client records accurately. The ability to record written information accurately and concisely depends on the correct use of terminology and an organized approach to charting procedures. This chapter provides an outline of the medical terminology most often encountered by the massage professional, particularly as it relates to charting and record-keeping procedures.

The chapter consolidates the vast array of medical terminology, focusing on the elements that are specifically useful to the massage professional. Success in mastering the information in this chapter depends on the use of a medical terminology textbook, a medical dictionary, and the Internet.

Developing skills in using medical dictionaries, medication reference books, and other reference materials is important. The expanding and changing knowledge base makes it almost impossible to remember all the details required for professional practice. The chapter includes a list of the terms most often encountered by the massage professional. Definitions for these words are available in a medical terminology text or medical dictionary, and learning involves looking them up. Exploring medical terminology automatically provides an overview of anatomy and physiology. This section is not meant to replace an anatomy and physiology text. The purpose of this information is to provide a quick reference as the student develops record-keeping and charting skills.

Used with a standard anatomy and physiology textbook and class instruction, this section can help the professional focus on information specific to the field of massage. The recommended anatomy and physiology text is *Mosby's essential sciences for therapeutic massage: anatomy, physiology, biomechanics, and pathology* by Sandy Fritz (Mosby, 2008), because it has been developed specifically for therapeutic massage students. However, the information in this chapter can be used with any comprehensive anatomy and physiology book.

The information presented here is especially pertinent to an understanding of massage as it relates to anatomy, physiology, pathophysiology, and client records. Because the basis for medical terminology is scientific language, understanding this information helps the massage student understand massage therapy research, as well as articles and books on subjects related to massage. Learning the names of muscles, bones, joints, and other anatomic structures lays a firm foundation for understanding and correctly using medical terminology.

It is important to have agreement across different medical fields regarding terminology. Without a common language, we cannot communicate. Massage professionals must be able to communicate with their clients in a common language that both can understand; it is just as important that they understand the communications of other health professionals.

Currently, the terminology used in massage therapy is inconsistent. Although similar words are used, the meanings of those words do not always coincide. The definitions for the massage therapy vocabulary in this textbook are based on traditional definitions, Canadian resources, available books, and common knowledge. This chapter offers a basis for agreement on terminology for the massage profession; this must occur before others in the health profession can communicate with us as a group. As mentioned in Chapter 1, Per Henrik Ling, the father of Swedish massage, had difficulty communicating with the established authorities of his time because he did not speak their language. To receive the respect and understanding of other health professionals, we as massage professionals must explain ourselves in terms other health professionals understand and patiently educate them in our language.

MEDICAL TERMINOLOGY

SECTION OBJECTIVES

Using the information presented in this section, the student will be able to perform the following:

- Define words by breaking them down into their word elements
- Use Appendix A to identify indications for and contraindications to massage
- List and define anatomic and physiologic terms by body system
- List and identify common abbreviations

evolve 3-1

Fundamental Word Elements

Medical terms are made up of a combination of word elements. A word can be interpreted easily by separating it into its elements. These word elements are called *prefixes, root words,* and *suffixes.*

Prefixes

A prefix is a word element placed at the beginning of a word to alter its meaning (Table 3-1). A prefix cannot stand alone; it must be combined with a root word.

TABLE 3-1

Common Prefixes

Prefix	Meaning	Prefix	Meaning
a-, an-	Without or not	intro-	Into, within
ab-	Away from	leuk-	White
ad-	Toward	macro-	Large
ante-	Before, forward	mal-	Bad, illness, disease
anti-	Against	mega-	Large
auto-	Self	micro-	Small
bi-	Double, two	mono-	One, single
circum-	Around	neo-	New
contra-	Against, opposite	non-	Not
de-	Down, from, away from, not	para-	Abnormal
dia-	Across, through, apart	per-	By, through
dis-	Separation, away from	peri-	Around
dys-	Bad, difficult, abnormal	poly-	Many, much
ecto-	Outer, outside	post-	After, behind
en-	In, into, within	pre-	Before, in front of, prior to
endo-	Inner, inside	pro-	Before, in front of
epi-	Over, on	re-	Again
eryth-	Red	retro-	Backward
ex-	Out, out of, from, away from	semi-	Half
hemi-	Half	sub-	Under
hyper-	Excessive, too much, high	super-	Above, over, excess
hypo-	Under, decreased, less than normal	supra-	Above, over
in-	In, into, within, not	trans-	Across
inter-	Between	uni-	One
intra-	Within		

Root Words

The **root word** provides the fundamental meaning of a term (Table 3-2). Combinations of root words, prefixes, and suffixes form medical and scientific terms. A vowel, called a *combining vowel*, often is added when two root words are combined or when a suffix is added to a root word; the combining vowel is usually *o* and occasionally *i*.

Suffixes

A **suffix** is a word element placed at the end of a root word to alter the meaning of the word (Table 3-3). Suffixes cannot stand alone; like prefixes, they must accompany a root word. The suffix should be the starting point when interpreting medical terms.

Root words that end in a consonant require a combining vowel. If the root word ends in a vowel and the suffix begins with a vowel, the vowel at the end of the root word is deleted.

Combining Word Elements

Word elements are the building blocks that are combined to create medical and scientific terminology. Prefixes always precede root words, and suffixes always follow root words (Proficiency Exercise 3-1).

Abbreviations

Abbreviations are shortened forms of words or phrases (Table 3-4). They are used primarily in written communication to save time and space. An extensive list of acceptable medical abbreviations can be found in most medical dictionaries.

When you use abbreviations in any type of record, including charting, provide an abbreviation key either on the forms or in a conspicuous place in the file. This is especially important if you generate a specialized list of abbreviations, such as *SWM* for Swedish massage or *CTM* for connective tissue method.

TABLE 3-2

Common Root Words

Root (Combining Vowel)	Meaning	Root (Combining Vowel)	Meaning
abdomin (o)	Abdomen	neur (o)	Nerve
aden (o)	Gland	ocul (o) Eye	Eye
adren (o)	Adrenal gland	orth (o)	Straight, normal, correct
angi (o)	Vessel	oste (o)	Bone
arterio (o)	Artery	ot (o)	Ear
arthr (o)	Joint	ped (o)	Child, foot
broncho (o)	Bronchus, bronchi	pharyng (o)	Pharynx
card, cardi (o)	Heart	phleb (o)	Vein
cephal (o)	Head	pnea	Breathing, respiration
chondr (o)	Cartilage	pneum (o)	Lung, air, gas
col (o)	Colon	proct (o)	Rectum
cost (o)	Rib	psych (o)	Mind
crani (o)	Skull	pulm (o)	Lung
cyan (o)	Blue	py (o)	Pus
cyst (o)	Bladder, cyst	rect (o)	Rectum
cyt (o)	Cell	rhin (o)	Nose
derma	Skin	sten (o)	Narrow, constriction
duoden (o)	Duodenum	stern (o)	Sternum
encephal (o)	Brain	stomat (o)	Mouth
enter (o)	Intestines	therm (o)	Heat
fibro (o)	Fiber, fibrous	thorac (o)	Chest
gastr (o)	Stomach	thromb (o)	Clot, thrombus
gyn, gyne, gyneco	Female	thyr (o)	Thyroid
hem, hema, hemo, hemat (o)	Blood	toxic(o)	Poison, poisonous
hepat (o)	Liver	trache (o)	Trachea
hydr (o)	Water	ur (o)	Urine, urinary tract, urination
hyster (o)	Uterus	urethr (o)	Urethra
ile (o), ili (o)	Ileum	urin (o)	Urine
laryng (o)	Larynx	uter (o)	Uterus
mamm (o)	Breast, mammary gland	vas (o)	Blood vessel, vas deferens
my (o)	Muscle	ven (o)	Vein
myel (o)	Spinal cord, bone marrow	vertebr (o)	Spine, vertebrae
nephr (o)	Kidney		

TABLE 3-3

Common Suffixes

Suffix	Meaning
-algia	Pain
-asis	Condition, usually abnormal
-cele	Hernia, herniation, pouching
-cyte	Cell
-ectasis	Dilation, stretching
-ectomy	Excision, removal of
-emia	Blood condition
-genesis	Development, production, creation
-genic	Producing, causing
-gram	Record
-graph	Diagram, recording instrument
-graphy	Making a recording
-iasis	Condition of
-ism	Condition
-itis	Inflammation
-logy	Study of
-lysis	Destruction of, decomposition
-megaly	Enlargement
-oma	Tumor
-osis	Condition
-pathy	Disease
-penia	Lack, deficiency
-phasia	Speaking
-phobia	Exaggerated fear
-plasty	Surgical repair or reshaping
-plegia	Paralysis
-rrhage, -rrhagia	Excessive flow
-rrhea	Profuse flow, discharge
-scope	Examination instrument
-scopy	Examination using a scope
-stasis	Maintenance, maintaining a constant level
-stomy, -ostomy	Creation of an opening
-tomy, -otomy	Incision, cutting into
-uria	Condition of the urine

Excessive use of abbreviations is discouraged. An overabundance of abbreviations results in a passage that is difficult to read and that requires interpretation. If you are unsure whether an abbreviation is acceptable, write the term out to communicate accurately.

Avoid using jargon. Jargon consists of word forms specially developed within a system or the use of existing words that have other definitions besides the dictionary meaning. For example, the word *mouse* is a computer jargon word. Many forms of jargon exist in the bodywork world, a situation that continues to confuse communication. In general, the words used in record keeping should be found in either a standard comprehensive dictionary or a medical dictionary and should represent the definition as listed.

On occasion jargon becomes understandable within the general community. Referring to the previous example of *mouse*, many readers would have thought immediately of the computer hand controller instead of a brown, furry creature.

 PROFICIENCY EXERCISE 3-1

Combine five words using the prefixes, root words, and suffixes listed in Tables 3-1 to 3-3. Define the words created. Look up each word in a medical dictionary to verify that it exists and that you have the correct meaning and spelling.

Example: Fibromyalgia
Divided into elements: Fibro- fiber; my- muscle; algia- pain
My definition: Pain in muscle fibers
Dictionary definition: Diffuse muscle pain

1.

2.

3.

4.

5.

TABLE 3-4

Common Abbreviations

Abbreviation	Meaning	Abbreviation	Meaning
abd	Abdomen	IBW	Ideal body weight
ADL	Activities of daily living	ICT	Inflammation of connective tissue
ad lib	As desired	id	The same
alt dieb	Every other day	L	Left, length, lumbar
alt hor	Alternate hours	lig	Ligament
alt noct	Alternate nights	M	Muscle, meter, myopia
AM (AM, am)	Morning	meds	Midline
ama	Against medical advice	ML	Medications
ANS	Autonomic nervous system	n	Normal
approx	Approximately	NA	Nonapplicable
as tol	As tolerated	OB	Obstetrics
BM	Bowel movement	OTC	Over the counter
BP	Blood pressure	P	Pulse
Ca	Cancer	PA	Postural analysis
CC	Chief complaint	PM (PM, pm)	Afternoon
c/o	Complains of	PT	Physical therapy
CPR	Cardiopulmonary resuscitation	Px	Prognosis
CSF	Cerebrospinal fluid	R	Respiration, right
CVA	Cerebrovascular accident, stroke	R/O	Rule out
DM	Diabetes mellitus	ROM	Range of motion
DJD	Degenerative joint disease	Rx	Prescription
Dx	Diagnosis	SOB	Shortness of breath
ext	Extract	SP, spir	Spirit
ft	Foot or feet	Sym	Symmetric
fx	Fracture	T	Temperature
GI	Gastrointestinal	TLC	Tender loving care
GU	Genitourinary	Tx	Treatment
h (hr)	Hour	URI	Upper respiratory infection
H_2O	Water	WD	Well developed
Hx	History	WN	Well nourished

This is an example of the way language can change. As massage becomes more generally accepted, much of our language will be standardized and lose its jargon quality. Until then, clarity and concise expression are crucial when choosing the words used for written records.

Terms Related to Diagnosis and Diseases

The massage practitioner must be able to understand medical terms related to diagnosis and various diseases. Two terms related to the diagnosis of a disease that massage professionals often encounter are *indication* and *contraindication*.

An **indication** is a condition for which an approach would be beneficial for health enhancement, treatment of a particular condition, or support of a treatment modality other than massage.

A **contraindication** is a condition or factor that may make an approach harmful (Proficiency Exercise 3-2). Contraindications may be further subdivided by severity:

- General avoidance of application—do not massage

- Regional avoidance of application—do massage but avoid a particular area
- Application with caution, usually requiring supervision from appropriate medical or supervising personnel—do massage but carefully select the type of methods to be used, the duration of application, the frequency, and the intensity of the massage.

Terminology of Location and Position

Directional Terms

Directional terms are used to describe the way one body part relates to another. The massage professional must be able to use directional terminology to describe the location of an area of the body accurately.

The directional terms in Figure 3-1 are used most often (Proficiency Exercise 3-3).

The abdomen is divided into four quadrants, and the locations of abdominal organs and the abdominal contents are

PROFICIENCY EXERCISE 3-2

1. *In a medical dictionary, look up and define each of the following terms related to the diagnosis of disease conditions of the body:*

acute

ambulatory

anomaly

atrophy

benign

chronic

clinic

clinical

diagnosis

malignant

metastatic

prognosis

sign

symptom

syndrome

systemic

2. *In a medical dictionary, look up and define each of the following terms related to diseases:*

bacterial

cancer

congenital

degenerative

epidemic

exacerbation

fungal

idiopathic

infectious

trauma

viral

3. *Write a descriptive statement about a fictional client. Use at least five terms listed in this section.*
Example: Mr. X reveals during the client history procedure that he is suffering from an <u>acute exacerbation</u> of a <u>chronic viral infectious process</u>.

Your Turn

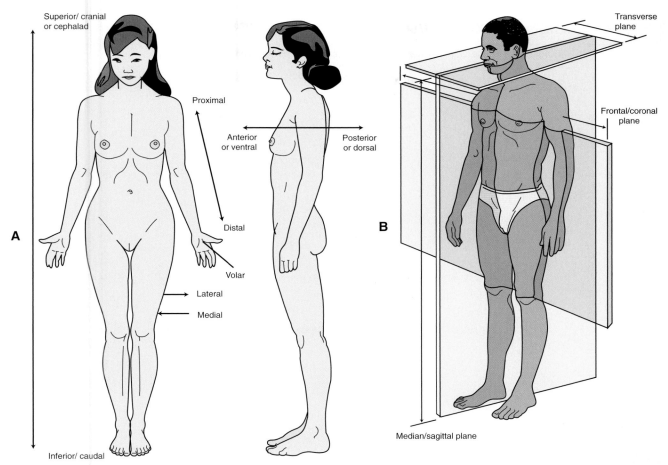

FIGURE 3-1 A, Directional terms. **B,** Anatomic planes. (From Fritz S: *Mosby's essential sciences for therapeutic massage: anatomy, physiology, biomechanics, and pathology,* ed 3, St Louis, 2009, Mosby.)

described in terms of the quadrants where they are found (Figure 3-2).

Positional Terms

Positional terms are used to describe the relationship of the body to the different planes (Proficiency Exercise 3-4):

1. *Anatomic position*—the stance of the body when it is erect, with the arms hanging at the sides, palms facing forward
2. *Erect position*—the body in a standing position
3. *Supine position*—the body lying in a horizontal position with the face up
4. *Prone position*—the body lying in a horizontal position with the face down
5. *Laterally recumbent position*—the body lying horizontally on either the right or left side

 3-2

The Structure of the Body

3-1

Tissues

The structure of the body is composed of tissues. A *tissue* is a collection of specialized cells that perform a special function. *Histo* is a root word meaning "tissue." *Histology* is the study

of tissue. The primary tissues of the body are the epithelial, connective, muscular, and nervous tissues (Proficiency Exercise 3-5).

Organs and Systems

An *organ* is a collection of specialized tissues. An organ has specific functions, but it does not act independenly of other organs.

Organs make up systems. The body as a whole is made up of several systems. Some of the systems are concentrated in a particular part of the body (e.g., the urinary system), whereas others reach out to all parts of the body, as the circulatory system does. The body has 10 general systems (Table 3-5). Each system is made up of organs that collectively perform specific functions. (A more extensive description of these systems can be found in any good anatomy and physiology textbook.)

Body Cavities

The body cavities, which contain the organs, are divided into ventral and dorsal regions (Figure 3-3). The two dorsal cavities are the cranial cavity and the vertebral cavity. The three ventral cavities are the thoracic, abdominal, and pelvic cavities. Sometimes the abdominal and pelvic cavities are considered as one (Proficiency Exercise 3-6).

PROFICIENCY EXERCISE 3-3

Consult your medical dictionary or medical terminology text to define the following terms:

anterior   medial

caudad   peripheral

cephalad   plantar

deep   posterior

distal   proximal

dorsal   superficial

external   superior

inferior   valgus

internal   varus

                                  volar

lateral

TABLE 3-5

Systems of the Body and Their Important Organs

System	Associated Organs
Musculoskeletal (can be classified separately as the skeletal, articular [joints], and muscular systems)	Bones, ligaments, skeletal muscles, tendons, joints
Nervous	Brain, spinal cord, nerves, special sense organs
Cardiovascular	Heart, arteries, veins, capillaries
Lymphatic	Lymphatic vessels, lymph nodes, spleen, tonsils, thymus gland
Digestive	Mouth, tongue, teeth, salivary glands, esophagus, stomach, small and large intestines, liver, gallbladder, pancreas
Respiratory	Nasal cavity, larynx, trachea, bronchi, lungs, diaphragm, pharynx
Urinary	Kidneys, ureters, urinary bladder, urethra
Endocrine	Endocrine glands: Hypothalamus, hypophysis (pituitary), thyroid, thymus, parathyroid, pineal, adrenal, pancreas, gonads (ovary or testis)
Reproductive	Female: Ovaries, uterine tubes (oviducts), uterus, vagina
	Male: Testes, penis, prostate gland, seminal vesicles, spermatic ducts
Integumentary	Skin, hair, nails, sebaceous glands, sweat glands, breasts

Right upper quadrant — Left upper quadrant

Right lower quadrant — Left lower quadrant

FIGURE 3-2 The quadrants of the abdomen. (From Fritz S: *Mosby's essential sciences for therapeutic massage: anatomy, physiology, biomechanics, and pathology,* ed 3, St Louis, 2009, Mosby.)

PROFICIENCY EXERCISE 3-4

1. *Act out each directional and positional term by creating a movement or a pantomime or by assuming the position.*
2. *With a partner, place each other in the positions listed above. Say each term as you position your partner.*

PROFICIENCY EXERCISE 3-5

Look up each of the following tissues in a medical terminology reference, anatomy and physiology textbook, or medical dictionary, and list the function of each tissue type.

Connective

Epithelial

Muscular

Nervous

Posterior Regions of the Trunk

The back, or posterior, surface of the trunk is also divided into regions. The terms used to describe these regions are related to the names of the vertebrae in the spinal column (Figure 3-4). In descending order they are:

■ The cervical region: The neck (seven cervical vertebrae)
■ The thoracic region: The chest (twelve thoracic vertebrae)

■ The lumbar region: The loin (five lumbar vertebrae)
■ The sacral region: The sacrum (five sacral vertebrae, which are fused into one bone)
■ The coccyx: The tailbone (four coccygeal vertebrae, which are fused into one bone)

The Skeletal System

3-2

The skeletal system consists of three types of tissue: bone, cartilage, and ligaments.

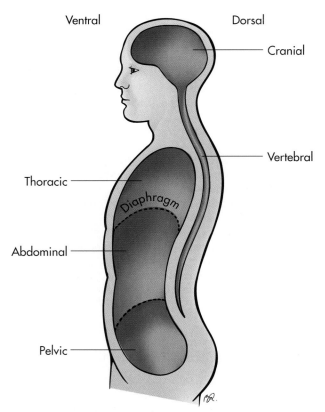

FIGURE 3-3 The body cavities.

   PROFICIENCY EXERCISE 3-6

Using clay or some other modeling compound, build the body cavities and the organs and structures they contain.

Bone

Bone is a dense connective tissue composed primarily of calcium and phosphate; *os-, ossa-, oste-,* and *osteo-* are all combining forms that mean "bone."

The human skeleton is composed of approximately 206 bones, and massage professionals must be familiar with most of them. Terms commonly used for some of these bones include *skull* or *cranium, cervical vertebrae, thoracic vertebrae, lumbar vertebrae, sacral vertebrae, coccygeal vertebrae, ribs, sternum, manubrium, body, xiphoid process, clavicle, scapula, humerus, ulna, radius, carpal bones, metacarpal bones, phalanges, pelvis, ilium, ischium, pubis, femur, patella, tibia, fibula, tarsal bones,* and *metatarsal bones* (see Figure 3-4; also Figure 3-5). Other terms related to bones and landmarks on bones are *malleolus, process, crest, insertion, joint, olecranon, origin, spine, trochanter,* and *tuberosity.*

Cartilage

The skeletal system includes two types of cartilage. *Hyaline cartilage,* which is very elastic, cushiony, and slippery, makes

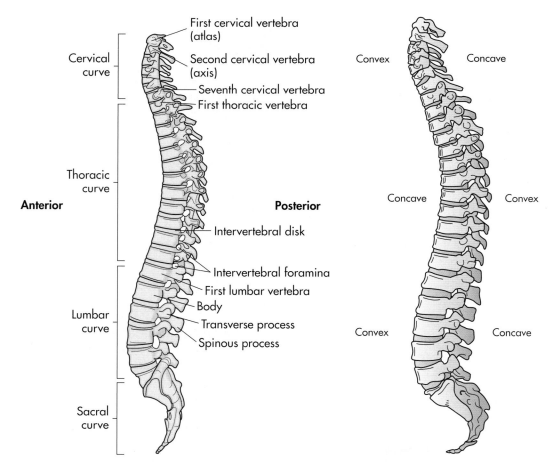

FIGURE 3-4 The vertebral column. (From Fritz S: *Mosby's essential sciences for therapeutic massage: anatomy, physiology, biomechanics, and pathology,* ed 3, St Louis, 2008, Mosby.)

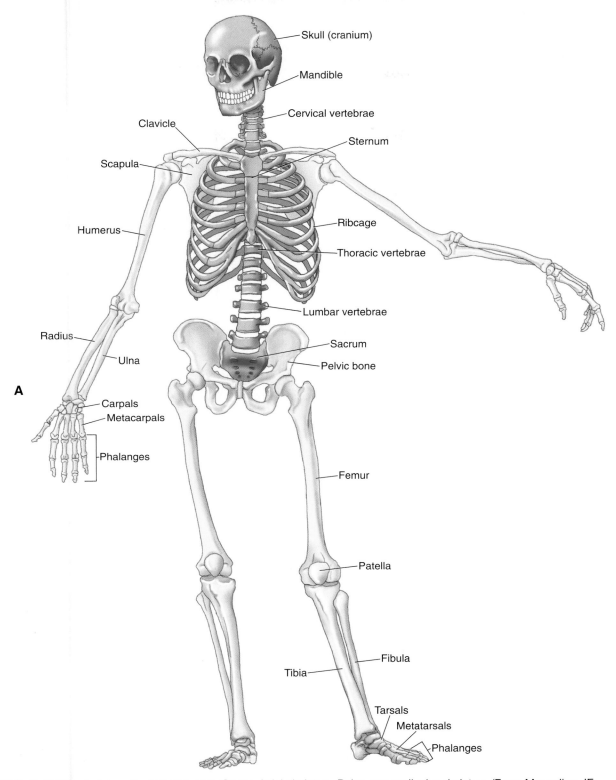

FIGURE 3-5 The skeleton. **A,** Anterior view. *Green*, Axial skeleton. *Beige*, appendicular skeleton. (From Muscolino JE: *Kinesiology: the skeletal system and muscle function,* enhanced edition, St Louis, 2007, Mosby.)

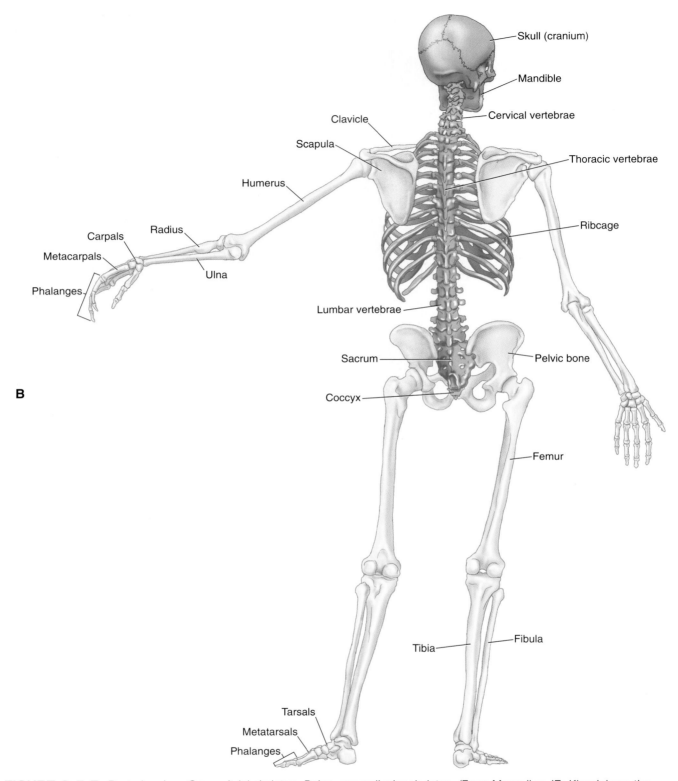

FIGURE 3-5 B, Posterior view. *Green*, Axial skeleton. *Beige*, appendicular skeleton. (From Muscolino JE: *Kinesiology: the skeletal system and muscle function,* enhanced edition, St Louis, 2007, Mosby.)

up the articular surfaces at the joints; the cartilage between the ribs and at the nose, larynx, and trachea; and the fetal skeleton. It has a pearly, bluish color. The term *hyaline* means glass. *White fibrocartilage,* which is elastic, flexible, and tough, is interarticular fibrocartilage found in joints such as the knee. The connecting fibrocartilage is cartilage that is only slightly mobile. It is found between the vertebrae (referred to as *disks*) and between the pubic bones (the symphysis pubis).

Ligaments

A *joint* or an *articulation* is a point where the bones of the skeleton meet. Movable joints are covered by cartilage and are held together by ligaments. Ligaments are made of white fibrous tissue. They are pliant, flexible, strong, and tough (Proficiency Exercise 3-7).

The Articular System

As mentioned, articulations are joints where two or more bones meet. The articular system concerns all of the anatomic and functional aspects of the joints.

Joints

Joints are places where bones come together, where limbs are attached, and where the motion of the skeletal system occurs. Some joints are rigid, and some allow a great degree of flexibility. The joints allow motion of the musculoskeletal system, bear weight, and hold the skeleton together.

Terms related to the articular system include *articulation, flexibility, synarthrodial, amphiarthrodial, diarthrodial, symphysis pubis, sacroiliac, symphysis, articular cartilage, articular disks, ligaments, synovial fluid,* and *tendon.*

Types of Movement Permitted by Diarthrodial Joints. The types of movement permitted by diarthrodial/synovial (freely movable) joints include the following (Figure 3-6):

- Flexion: Bending that reduces the angle of a joint
- Extension: Straightening or stretching that increases the angle of a joint
- Abduction: Movement away from (ab-) the midline
- Adduction: Movement toward (ad-) the midline
- Pronation: Turning of the palm downward
- Supination: Turning of the palm upward (you can hold a bowl of soup in a supinated hand)
- Eversion: Turning (-version) of the sole of the foot away from (e-) the midline (when you evert your foot, you move your little toe toward your ear)
- Inversion: Turning (-version) of the sole of the foot inward (in-)
- Plantar flexion: Bending of the plantar surface of the sole of the foot downward (plant your toes in the ground)
- Dorsiflexion: Bending of the top or dorsal surface of the foot toward the shin
- Rotation: Rolling to the side (internal rotation: rolling toward the midline, external rotation: rolling away from the midline)
- Circumduction: Making a cone; the ability to move the limb in a circular manner
- Protraction: Thrusting a part of the body forward (pro-)
- Retraction: Pulling a part of the body backward (re-)
- Elevation: Raising a part of the body
- Depression: Lowering a part of the body
- Opposition: The act of placing one part of the body opposite another, as in placing the tip of the thumb opposite the tips of the fingers

 PROFICIENCY EXERCISE 3-7

1. *Consult your medical dictionary or medical terminology text to define the following terms:*

Ankylosing spondylitis

Fracture

Osteoarthritis

Osteochondritis

Osteochondrosis

Osteoporosis

2. *Using Appendix A, choose one condition from the previous list and note any indications or contraindications involved.*

Condition:
Indications or contraindications:

3. *Palpate each bone listed in Figure 3-5 and say its name.*

4. *With a group of fellow students, assign each person to be a particular bone. By lying on the floor, build the skeleton by having each person assume the proper bone position. Be prepared to laugh and learn.*

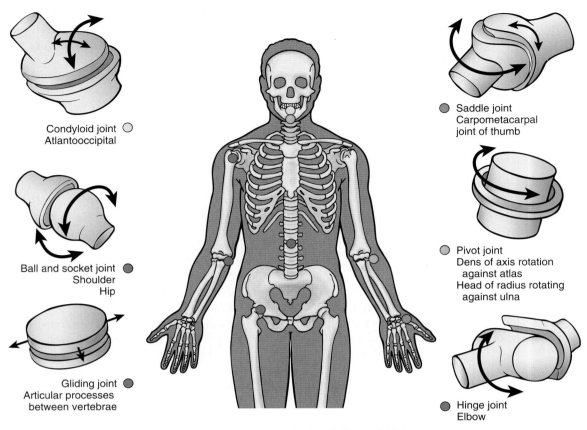

FIGURE 3-6 Types of diarthrodial/synovial joints.

Bursae. *Bursae* are closed sacs or saclike structures (bursa) that usually are found close to the joint cavities. The lining of bursae often is similar to the synovial membrane lining of a true joint. Some bursae are continuous with the lining of a joint. The function of a bursa is to lubricate an area between skin, tendons, ligaments, or other structures and bones where friction would otherwise develop (Proficiency Exercise 3-8).

The Muscular System

The muscular system is made up of contractile tissues. The three types of muscle tissue are cardiac muscle, smooth muscle, and skeletal muscle.

Many of the body's organs contain muscle tissue. Muscle tissue also makes up the muscles, which are themselves organs. These muscles give the body shape and produce movement. Muscle function is determined by the shape and location of the muscle and by the density and pliability of all the fluid, fibers, and connective tissue of the muscles; the term **muscle tone** is used to describe this aspect of muscle. The nervous system also controls how long or short a muscle is by regulating the degree of muscle fiber contraction; this is called **motor tone** (Figures 3-7 and 3-8).

Skeletal Muscle

Each skeletal muscle is made up of sections. Most muscles have two ends (proximal and distal), which are attached to other structures, and a belly. Muscles cause and permit motion by the actions of contraction and relaxation. Table 3-6 presents a list of terms used to describe the movements of different types of muscles.

Contraction refers to a reduction in size or shortening of a muscle. When one muscle contracts, another, opposite muscle is stretched and put in a state of tension. Relaxation occurs when tension is reduced, which allows the muscle to return to its resting length.

Muscles work in pairs of agonists and antagonists. *Agonists* are muscles responsible for the primary desired movement. The agonist is the prime mover, which shortens to produce movement. *Antagonists* are the muscles that oppose the action of the agonist and lengthen and control the movement produced by the agonist.

Synergists are muscles that assist the agonists by holding a part of the body steady, thereby providing leverage. In some cases synergists also produce the same action as the prime mover.

The agonist-antagonist-synergist relationship permits the skeletal muscles to work in a purposeful manner and gives fluidity to motion. This fluid movement is called *coordination*.

Terms related to the muscular system include *aponeurosis, asthenia, atrophy, belly, clonus, contracture, cramp, concentric, eccentric, fascia, fascicle, fasciculation, hyperkinesia, hypertrophy, insertion, isometric contraction, musculotendinous junction, myalgia, origin, proximal attachment, distal attachment, spasm, tendon,* and *tone.*

PROFICIENCY EXERCISE 3-8

1. *Consult your medical dictionary or medical terminology text to define the following terms:*

Ankylosis

Arthritis

Bursitis

Degenerative joint disease

Diastasis

Dislocation

Ganglion cyst

Genu valgum

Genu varum

Gout

Hallux malleus

Kyphosis

Lordosis

Rheumatoid arthritis

Scoliosis

Slipped disk

Spinal curvature

Spondylolisthesis

Sprain

Subluxation

Tendinitis

Tenosynovitis

2. *Using Appendix A, choose one condition from the previous list and note any indications or contraindications involved.*

Condition:
Indications or contraindications:

3. *Do a dance that incorporates each of the joint movements listed in this section. Call out the movement terms as the joint is moved.*

Length-tension relationship

A Actin — Myosin — Actin

Normal

Resting length

B Actin — Myosin — Actin

Short muscle contraction

C Actin — Myosin — Actin

Long muscle contraction

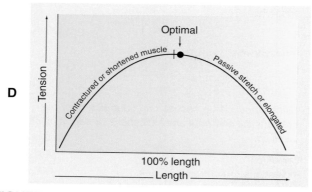

D

FIGURE 3-7 Length-tension relationship. **A,** Normal resting length. When a muscle is stimulated to contract, actin, in an appropriate position to attach to myosin, causes maximal contraction. **B,** Short muscle. Contraction ability is limited because actin has no space to "crawl" and cause contraction. **C,** Long muscle. Contraction ability is limited because actin is too far away to attach to myosin to begin contraction. **D,** Optimal length-tension relationship. (From Fritz S: *Sports and exercise massage: comprehensive care in athletics, fitness, and rehabilitation,* St Louis, 2006, Mosby.)

TABLE 3-6

Terms for Describing Muscle Movement

Term	Definition
Adductor	Muscle that moves a part toward the midline
Abductor	Muscle that moves a part away from the midline
Flexor	Muscle that bends a part
Extensor	Muscle that straightens a part
Levator	Muscle that raises a part
Depressor	Muscle that lowers a part
Tensor	Muscle that tightens a part

The names of muscles can be broken down into the word elements of medical terminology (Table 3-7). Muscles are named for a variety of reasons, including where they are located, what they do, and the way they are shaped. A basic understanding of medical terminology can assist the student in both remembering and understanding muscle names (Proficiency Exercise 3-9).

The Nervous System

The nervous system is the most complex system in the body. The information presented here on the workings of this system is very general but is expanded upon in the text where needed. Study of the nervous system is very important for the massage professional. Serious students of massage will challenge themselves to study the nervous system in depth.

For purposes of study, terms related to the nervous system are presented in the following three groups:

- The central nervous system (CNS)
- The peripheral nervous system (PNS)
- The autonomic nervous system (ANS)

Central Nervous System

The CNS is the center *(central)* of all nervous control. It consists of the brain and spinal cord, which are located in the dorsal cavity (cranial and vertebral).

Peripheral Nervous System

The PNS is composed of cranial and spinal nerves. The term *nerve* refers to a bundle of nerve fibers consisting of individual nerve cells outside the spinal cord or brain. The PNS consists of the nerves that carry impulses between the CNS and muscles, glands, skin, and other organs located outside (peripheral) the CNS. The ANS is the part of the peripheral nervous system that exerts nervous control over smooth muscle, heart muscle, and glands. Individual nerve cells are called *neurons.* The two types of nerve cells are the sensory neurons and the motor neurons.

Spinal Nerves. The 31 pairs of spinal nerves are attached to the spinal cord along almost its entire length. They are named for the region of the spinal column through which they exit.

FIGURE 3-8 The muscular system. **A,** Anterior view. **B,** Posterior view. (From LaFleur Brooks M: *Exploring medical language: a student-directed approach,* ed 5, St Louis, 2002, Mosby.)

TABLE 3-7

Muscle Descriptions Using Medical Word Elements

The muscles listed have been chosen because their names are made up of common word elements. After learning this list, the student should be able to figure out the meaning of muscles not listed.

Muscle	Description
Abductor digiti minimi pedis	Little *(minimi)* muscle that moves the little toe *(digit)* away from *(abductor)* the midline of the foot *(pedis)*
Adductor longus	Long muscle that moves the leg toward *(adductor)* the midline
Adductor magnus	Large *(magnus)* muscle that moves the leg toward *(adductor)* the midline
Biceps brachii	Muscle with two *(bi-)* heads *(ceps)* in the arm *(brachii)*
Deltoid	Triangular *(deltoid)* muscle of the shoulder
Dilatator naris posterior	Muscle of the nose *(naris)* that opens *(dilator)* the back *(posterior)* portion of the nostril
Extensor hallucis longus	Long *(longus)* muscle that extends *(extensor)* the great toe *(hallucis)*
Extensor pollicis brevis	Short *(brevis)* muscle that extends *(extensor)* the thumb *(pollicis)*
External oblique	Outermost *(external)* muscle that extends at an angle *(oblique)* from the ribs to the pelvis at the iliac crest
Flexor carpi radialis	Muscle that flexes *(flexor)* the wrist *(carpi)* toward the radius *(radialis)*
Flexor carpi ulnaris	Muscle attached to the ulna *(ulnaris)* that flexes *(flexor)* the wrist *(carpi)* and hand
Frontalis	Muscle over the frontal bone
Gastrocnemius	Muscle that makes up the belly *(gastroc)* of the lower leg *(nemius)*
Gluteus maximus	Largest *(maximus)* muscle of the buttocks *(gluteus)*
Gluteus medius	Muscle of the buttocks *(gluteus)* that lies in the middle *(medius)* between the other gluteal muscles
Gracilis	Slender *(gracilis)* muscle of the thigh
Iliopsoas	Muscle that is formed from the iliacus and psoas major muscles; the iliacus extends from the iliac bone *(iliacus),* and the psoas major is the large *(major)* muscle of the loin *(psoas)*
Latissimus dorsi	Broadest *(latissimus)* muscle of the back *(dorsi)*
Masseter	Muscle of chewing *(masseter)* or mastication
Orbicularis oculi and oris	Muscles circling *(orbicularis)* the eye *(oculi)* or mouth *(oris)*
Palmaris longus	Long *(longus)* muscle of the palm *(palmaris)*
Pectineus	Muscle of the pubic *(pectineus)* bone
Pectoralis major	Large *(major)* muscle of the chest *(pectoralis)*
Peroneus longus	Long *(longus)* muscle attached to the fibula *(peroneus)*
Plantaris	Muscle that flexes the foot *(plantaris)* and leg
Pronator teres	Long round *(teres)* muscle that turns the palm downward into a prone *(pronator)* position
Rectus abdominis	Muscle that extends in a straight *(rectus)* line upward across the abdomen *(abdominis);* the center border of the left and right rectus abdominis muscles in the linea alba or the white *(alba)* line *(linea)* at the midline of the abdomen
Rectus femoris	Part of the quadriceps muscle that is straight *(rectus)* and lies near the femur *(femoris)*
Sartorius	Muscle of the leg that enables a person to sit in a cross-legged tailor's *(sartorial)* position
Semimembranosus	Muscle made up partly *(semi-)* of membranous tissue; part of the hamstring group
Semitendinosus	Muscle made up partly *(semi-)* of tendinous tissue; this is one of the hamstring muscles
Serratus anterior	Sawtooth-shaped *(serratus)* muscle in front of *(anterior)* the shoulder and rib cage
Soleus	Muscle that resembles a flat fish *(sole)* located in the calf of the leg
Sternocleidomastoid	Muscle attached to the breastbone *(sterno),* the collarbone *(cleido),* and the mastoid *(mastoid)* process of the temporal bone
Temporalis	Muscle over the temporal *(temporalis)* bone
Tensor fascia lata	Muscle that tenses *(tensor)* the fascia of the thigh *(lata)*
Teres minor	Small *(minor)* round *(teres)* muscle that moves the arm
Tibialis anterior	Muscle in front *(anterior)* of the tibia *(tibialis)*
Trapezius	Four-sided, trapezoid-shaped *(trapezius)* muscle of the shoulder
Triceps brachii	Three- *(tri-)* headed *(ceps)* muscle of the arm *(brachii)*
Vastus lateralis, medialis, intermedialis	Large *(vastus)* lateral *(lateralis),* toward the midline *(medialis),* and middle *(intermedialis)* muscles of the quadriceps muscle group; the quadriceps has four *(quadri-)* heads *(ceps)*

PROFICIENCY EXERCISE 3-9

1. *Locate a more complete list of muscles in your anatomy and physiology textbook or medical dictionary. Break down five muscle names not listed in this section into their word elements. You will need a medical terminology book and/or medical dictionary to complete this exercise. Example: Auricularis superior: Aur- means ear; ar- means pertaining to; superior means above or upward.*

a.

b.

c.

d.

e.

2. *An excellent way to remember the names of muscles is to make up ridiculous sentences that explain listed muscle names. The crazier these sentences are, the better you will remember them. Use this memory aid as you study muscles in your anatomy and physiology classes.*

Examples:
Rectus femoris: Part of the quadriceps muscle that is straight (rectus) and lies near the femur (femoris)
Memory aid: Attention rectus! Straighten up and the other three of you in the quads head out to the femur.
Flexor carpi ulnaris: Muscle that flexes (flexor) the wrist (carpi) and hand and is attached to the ulna (ulnaris)
Memory aid: Help! There is a big carp pulling my wrist into flexion. It has my ulna in its mouth and my hand has it around the gills.

Many of the spinal nerves are located in groups called *somatic nerve plexuses.* The term *somatic* refers to the body wall; thus these nerve plexuses contain nerves that are involved with the wall of the body, as opposed to the organs within the body. A plexus is a network of intertwined (plexus) nerves. The major plexuses of spinal nerves are the cervical plexus, brachial plexus, lumbar plexus, and sacral plexus.

Autonomic Nervous System

The ANS is the part of the peripheral nervous system that is an automatic, or self-governing (self *[auto],* governing *[nomic]*), system. It is also called the *involuntary system* because the effects of this system are not usually under voluntary control. The ANS is divided in two parts: the sympathetic division and the parasympathetic division.

The sympathetic division controls the body's response to feelings *(sympath).* The nerves in this division come off the thoracic and lumbar segments of the spinal cord; thus this division is sometimes referred to as the *thoracolumbar division.* Actions resulting from these nerves include the fight-or-flight and fear responses. The reaction of some organs includes an increase in the heart rate, dilation of the pupils, and an increase in adrenaline secretion. A person may sometimes exhibit great strength as a result of a sympathetic response.

The nerves in the parasympathetic division come off the cranial and sacral segments of the spinal cord; thus this division is sometimes called the *craniosacral division.* The parasympathetic division generally causes effects opposite *(para-)* those caused by the sympathetic system. These effects include constriction of the pupils, the return of the heart rate to

normal, and stimulation of the lacrimal glands to produce tears.

Intertwined nerves *(plexus)* of the ANS are called the *autonomic plexuses.* Some examples of these plexuses are the cardiac plexus, or the intertwined nerves of the heart *(cardiac),* and the celiac plexus, or the intertwined nerves of the organs of the abdomen *(celiac).* The celiac plexus sometimes is called the *solar plexus* because of the sunray *(solar)* fashion in which the nerves exit the plexus.

Proprioception. Proprioception is the kinesthetic sense. Sensory receptors receive information about position, rate of movement, contraction, tension, and stretch of tissues through distortion of and pressure on the sensory receptor. After proprioceptive sensory information is processed in the CNS, motor impulses carry the response message back to the muscles. The muscles then contract or relax to restore or change posture, movement, or position. Proprioception maintains motor tone in muscle.

Terms related to proprioception include *mechanoreceptor, Golgi tendon organ, joint kinesthetic receptors, kinesthetic,* and *muscle spindle cells.*

Reflex

A *reflex* is an involuntary body response to a stimulus. Important reflexes stimulated by massage are crossed, extensor thrust, flexor withdrawal, gait, intersegmental, monosynaptic, nociceptive, optical righting, ocular pelvic, pilomotor, psychogalvanic, postural, proprioceptive, righting, startle, stretch, tendon, tonic neck, vasomotor, and visceromotor reflexes.

Function of the Nervous System

The function of the nervous system is to receive impressions from the external environment, organize the information, and provide appropriate responses. In other words, the nervous system allows the body to react to outside influences (environment). Outside information enters the nervous system through nerve endings in the skin and in special sense organs. These nerve endings are referred to as *receptors.*

Nerve endings in the skin are sensitive to pain, touch, pressure, vibration, and temperature. Special sense nerve endings are responsible for taste, smell, vision, hearing, and sense of position and movement. Sensations from the environment are picked up by these receptors and sent to the CNS by way of the PNS. The CNS sorts out the information and sends back a message, again by way of the PNS. Information is transferred from one nerve to another by chemicals called neurotransmitters.

The nervous system and neurotransmitters, along with the endocrine system, also maintain the internal environment, or the balance of the many activities within the body (homeostasis). Although the divisions of the nervous system may be treated independently, they do not function independently (Figure 3-9).

Terms Related to Nerves

Afferent nerves are nerves that carry *(ferent)* messages to *(af-* variation of *ad-)* the CNS; they are also known as *sensory nerves* because they pick up and transmit sensation *(sen)* (Proficiency Exercise 3-10).

FIGURE 3-9 A simplified view of the nervous system. (From LaFleur Brooks M: *Exploring medical language: a student-directed approach,* ed 5, St Louis, 2002, Mosby.)

PROFICIENCY EXERCISE 3-10

1. *List five of the disease conditions of the nervous system described in the indications and contraindications section in Appendix A.*

   a.

   b.

   c.

   d.

   e.

2. *Using Appendix A, choose one condition from your list and note any indications or contraindications involved.*

   Condition:
   Indications or contraindications:

3. *Choose one of the reflexes and look it up in a medical dictionary. Define the term and then write down how you think the reflex is implicated during massage.*

Example:

   Reflex: Psychogalvanic
   Definition: Psycho- **relates to the mind and** *galvanic* **pertains to electricity**
   Implication: *This reflex involves changes in electrical activity in the body connected with mind processes or thoughts. With the galvanic skin response, changes in electrical activity are related to activity of the sweat glands. Massage stimulates the skin as well as electrical activity in the body, which in turn may influence the mind.*

Your Turn
Reflex:
Definition:

Implication:

Efferent nerves are nerves that carry *(ferent)* messages away from *(ef-,* variation of *ex-)* the brain, resulting in motion *(motor)*. They are also known as *motor nerves*.

Cranial nerves are the 12 pairs of nerves that arise from the brainstem in the cranium or skull *(cranial)*.

Spinal nerves are the 31 pairs of nerves that branch off the spinal cord.

A *ganglion* is a mass of nerve cell bodies located outside the CNS; *ganglia* is the plural form. *Neuro* is the root word meaning "nerve."

The Cardiovascular System

The cardiovascular system consists of two parts, the heart and the blood vessels (Figure 3-10). The heart is a four-chambered pump. *Arteries* are tubes (vessels) that deliver oxygenated blood to the body. They carry blood under pressure and are located relatively deep within the body. *Veins* are vessels that return the blood to the heart. They are located in more superficial areas, therefore veins are easier to palpate. Veins have a valve system that prevents the backflow of blood. A breakdown of a valve may result in a varicose vein. *Capillaries* are very small, thin (usually one cell thick) vessels that allow for the exchange of blood gasses and nutrients. Blood vessels vasoconstrict, or become smaller inside, and vasodilate, or become larger inside.

Blood pressure is a measurement of the pressure exerted by the circulating volume of blood on the walls of the arteries, veins, and heart chambers. Blood pressure is maintained by the complex interaction of the homeostatic mechanisms of the body. Normal blood pressure varies according to age, size, and gender, but the average is approximately 120 mm Hg during systole and 70 mm Hg in diastole. High blood pressure is called *hypertension*, and low blood pressure is called *hypotension*.

Blood is composed of a clear, yellow fluid called *plasma*, blood cells, and platelets. The main function of blood is to transport oxygen and nutrients to the cells and remove carbon dioxide and other waste products. The amount of blood in muscle tissue influences the muscle tone. If muscle tissue contains too much blood, it is said to be congested and methods to encourage blood flow are used.

Terms and combining forms that relate to the cardiovascular system include *angio-, artery, arteriole, blood pressure, bruise, capillary, edema, phleb-, vasoconstriction, vasodilation, vein,* and *venule* (Proficiency Exercise 3-11).

The Lymphatic System

The lymphatic system is responsible for several functions and operates in the following ways:

1. It returns vital substances, such as plasma protein, to the bloodstream from the tissues of the body. The fluid around the cells in tissues is called *interstitial fluid*.
2. It assists in the maintenance of fluid balance by draining fluid from the body tissues.
3. It helps in the body's defense against disease-producing substances.

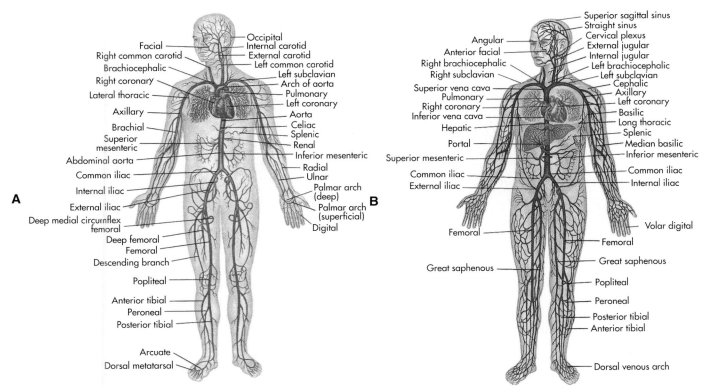

FIGURE 3-10 The systemic circulation. **A,** Arteries. **B,** Veins. (From Seidel HM et al: *Mosby's guide to physical examination,* ed 5, St Louis, 2003, Mosby.)

PROFICIENCY EXERCISE 3-11

1. *List five of the disease conditions of the cardiovascular system described in the indications and contraindications section in Appendix A.*

   a.

   b.

   c.

   d.

   e.

2. *Using your list, choose one condition and note any indications or contraindications involved.*

Condition:
Indications or contraindications:

3. *Look up the medication classification "anticoagulant" in Appendix C and in a pharmacology reference text. In the space provided, list contraindications and side effects of these medications. Also describe contraindications to massage that may exist if someone is taking anticoagulant medication.*

4. *Choose a partner and draw the major arteries and veins on the body with washable markers. Use red for arteries and blue for veins. Notice that you can almost trace the veins because they are located near the surface of the body.*

FIGURE 3-11 The principal lymph vessels and nodes.

4. It helps in the absorption of fats from the digestive system.

The lymphatic system is a network of channels and nodes in which a substance called *lymph* travels (Figure 3-11). Lymph is a clear, watery fluid similar to plasma. The system collects and drains fluid from around tissue cells from different areas of the body and carries it through the lymphatic channels back to the venous system. There it is deposited, mixed with venous blood, and recirculated.

Lymphatic capillaries are found near and parallel to the veins that carry blood to the heart. The ends of the lymphatic capillaries meet to form larger lymph vessels. The lymph vessels in the right chest, head, and right arm join the right lymphatic duct, which drains into the right subclavian vein. The lymph vessels from all other parts of the body join to meet the thoracic duct, which drains into the left subclavian vein.

Throughout the lymph system are *lymph nodes* (Table 3-8). Lymph nodes are small bodies present in the path of the lymph channels that act as filters for lymph before it returns to the bloodstream. The main locations of the more superficial lymph nodes are the cervical area, axillary region, and groin or inguinal area.

Plexuses of lymph channels are found throughout the body:

- Mammary plexus: Lymphatic vessels around the breasts
- Palmar plexus: Lymphatic vessels in the palm *(palmar)* of the hand
- Plantar plexus: Lymphatic vessels in the sole *(plantar)* of the foot

If soft tissue has too much interstitial fluid around the cells, or if the lymph vessels are full of fluid that is moving slowly or is stagnant, the tissue is said to be *infused* or *edematous*. Excess fluid in muscle tissue contributes to muscle tone problems.

The Immune System

The human body is able to resist organisms or toxins that tend to damage its tissues and organs. This ability is called *immunity* (Table 3-9). As a massage professional, you should explore the immune system in much greater depth. Use your anatomy and physiology textbook as a place to begin, but do not stop there. Exciting new research is being published in professional journals (Proficiency Exercise 3-12).

The Respiratory System

The respiratory system supplies oxygen to and removes carbon dioxide from the cells of the body (Figure 3-12). Respiration is divided into two phases, external and internal. *External respiration* involves the absorption of oxygen from the air by the lungs and the transport of carbon dioxide from the lungs back into the air. *Internal respiration* involves the exchange of oxygen and carbon dioxide in the cells of the body. The mechanisms of breathing and their relationship to massage are discussed in future chapters.

Terms and combining forms related to the respiratory system include *alveoli, lungs, nares, nostrils, olfactory cells, pneumo-, rhino-,* and *trachea* (Proficiency Exercise 3-13).

The Digestive System

The anatomy of the digestive system can be compared with a long muscular tube that travels a path through the body (Figure 3-13). The organs of the digestive system transport food through this muscular tube. The wavelike contraction of the smooth muscles of the digestive tube is called *peristalsis.* Accessory organs carry out functions directly related to digestion and are connected to the system by means of ducts. Understanding the flow of contents through the large intestine is important for the massage professional because methods of massage can be used to enhance this process. Investigate this process further by referring to your anatomy and physiology textbook (Proficiency Exercise 3-14).

TABLE 3-8

Types of Lymph Nodes

Nodes	Description
Parotid	Nodes around *(para-)* or in front of the ear *(otid)*
Occipital	Nodes over the occipital bone at the back of the head
Superficial cervical	Nodes close to the surface *(superficial)* of the neck *(cervic)*
Subclavicular	Nodes under *(sub-)* the collarbone *(clavicular)*
Hypogastric	Nodes in the area beneath *(hypo-)* the stomach *(gastric)*
Facial	Nodes draining the tissue in the face
Deep cervical	Deeply *(deep)* situated nodes in the neck *(cervic)*
Axillary (superficial)	Nodes in the armpit *(axilla)*
Mediastinal	Nodes in the mediastinal section of the thoracic cavity
Cubital	Nodes of the elbow *(cubit)*
Para-aortic	Nodes around *(para-)* the aorta *(aortic)*
Deep inguinal	Deeply *(deep)* situated nodes in the groin *(inguin)*
Superficial inguinal	Nodes in the groin *(inguin)* close to the surface *(superficial)*
Popliteal	Nodes in back of the knee *(popliteal)*

TABLE 3-9

Selected Terms Related to Immunology

Term	Meaning
Acquired immunity	Resistance *(immunity)* to a particular disease developed by people who have acquired the disease
Acquired immunodeficiency	A group of symptoms *(syndrome)* caused by the transmission *(acquired)* of a virus that causes a breakdown *(deficiency)* of the immune system (AIDS)
Active immunity	Resistance *(immunity)* in which the antibodies produced by the body currently exist
Allergy	A state of hypersensitivity to a particular substance; the immune system overreacts (over [hyper-], reacts [sensitive]) to foreign substances, and physical changes occur
Antigen	A substance that stimulates the immune response
Susceptible	An individual who is capable *(-ible)* of acquiring *(suscept)* a particular disease

PROFICIENCY EXERCISE 3-12

1. List five of the disease conditions of the lymphatic and immune system described in the indications and contraindications section in Appendix A.

a.

b.

c.

d.

e.

2. Using Appendix A, choose one condition from your list and note any indications or contraindications involved.

Condition:
Indications or contraindications:

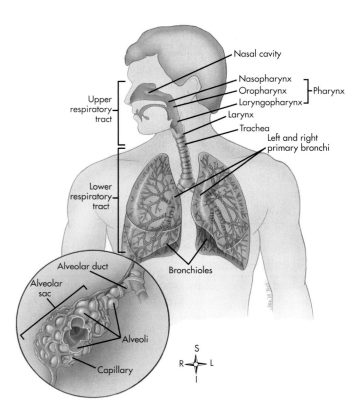

FIGURE 3-12 Structural plan of the respiratory system. The inset shows the alveolar sacs where the interchange of oxygen and carbon dioxide takes place through the walls of the grapelike alveoli. Capillaries surround the alveoli. (From Thibodeau GA, Patton KT: *Anatomy and physiology*, ed 6, St Louis, 2007, Mosby.)

BOX 3-1

SOAP

The SOAP note has four parts:

Subjective data: The patient's expression of his or her condition, pain, complaints, reactions, and so forth.

Objective data: The physical examination findings, results of tests, laboratory findings, observations, and the treatments used.

Assessment: (Think of this as an analysis). The healthcare professional's evaluation of the situation, which is based on both the subjective and objective information.

Plan: Details of the course of treatment chosen.

research on the mind/body phenomenon is being released too quickly to be current in any textbook. The massage professional must read medical and scientific research to remain current. The implications for massage are very important, because the effects of massage are connected with the nervous system and endocrine body control functions (Proficiency Exercise 3-15).

The Integumentary System

The integumentary system consists of the skin and its appendages, including the hair and nails.

The Skin

The skin is the largest organ of the body. It is composed of three layers of tissue: the epidermis, the dermis, and the subcutaneous tissue (Figure 3-15). The *epidermis* is the outer layer of skin, which contains many layers of tissue and melanocytes, the cells that give skin color. The *dermis,* or dermal layer, lies directly under the epidermis and is often called the *true skin.* It is made of connective tissue. Embedded in the dermis are the blood vessels, lymphatic vessels, hair follicles, and sweat glands. *Subcutaneous tissue* attaches the dermis to the underlying structures. This fatty tissue contains varying amounts of adipose tissue and acts as insulation for the body.

The functions of the fascial network of the skin are protection; control and maintenance of body temperature; detection of the sensations of touch, temperature, pain, and pressure; secretion of sweat and sebum; and production of vitamin D when the skin is exposed to the sun.

The Endocrine System

The endocrine system is composed of glands that produce hormones, which are secreted directly into the bloodstream to stimulate cells in a specific way or to set a body function into action (Figure 3-14). The endocrine system is complex and important because it serves as a control and regulation system for the body. As with the nervous system, the massage professional should commit to an in-depth study of the endocrine system, its relationship to the nervous system, and the connection to the mind/body processes. Information from

PROFICIENCY EXERCISE 3-13

1. *List five of the disease conditions of the respiratory system described in the indications and contraindications section in Appendix A.*

a.

b.

c.

d.

e.

2. *Using Appendix A, choose one condition from your list and note any indications or contraindications involved.*

Condition:

Indications or contraindications:

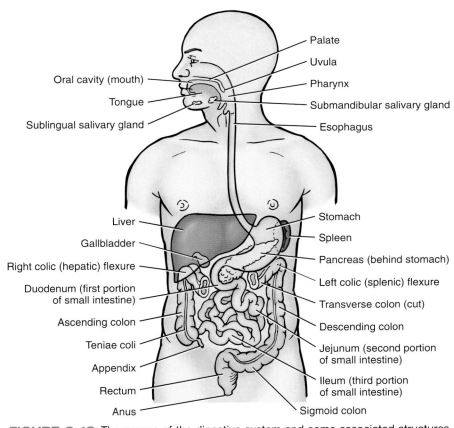

FIGURE 3-13 The organs of the digestive system and some associated structures.

Many disease signs (particularly color changes) may be first noticed in the skin. Terms relating to skin color changes include *cyanosis* (bluish), *erythema* (red), *jaundice* (yellow-orange), and *pallor* (a decrease in color).

Sebaceous Glands

Sebaceous glands are located in the skin. They secrete an oily substance, called *sebum,* that gives the skin and hair a glossy appearance. Most of these glands open into the walls of hair follicles. Other sebaceous glands are located at the corners of the mouth and around the external sex organs that open directly on the surface of the skin.

Sweat Glands

Sweat glands are found in most areas of the body. They function to cool the body. The most abundant type is the eccrine sweat gland. The palms of the hands and soles of the feet contain large numbers of these glands. Sweat from these glands is odorless. Another type of sweat gland is the apocrine sweat gland, which is connected to hair follicles in the armpits

PROFICIENCY EXERCISE 3-14

1. *List five of the disease conditions of the digestive system described in the indications and contraindications section in Appendix A.*

a.

b.

c.

d.

e.

2. *Using Appendix A, choose one condition from your list and note any indications or contraindications involved.*

Condition:
Indications or contraindications:

PROFICIENCY EXERCISE 3-15

1. *List three of the disease conditions of the endocrine system described in the indications and contraindications section in Appendix A.*

a.

b.

c.

2. *Using Appendix A, choose one condition from your list and note any indications or contraindications involved.*

Condition:
Indications or contraindications:

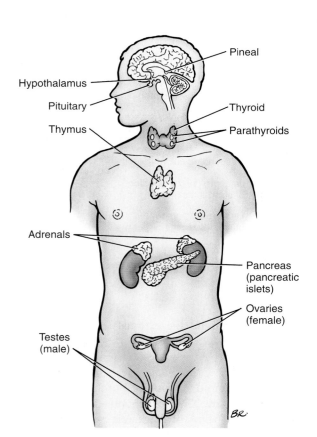

FIGURE 3-14 The locations of the major endocrine glands.

and the pubic area and is found at the navel and nipples. The secretions from these sweat glands increase in response to sexual stimulation. They function to lubricate the genital area, and they play a part in sexual arousal as a result of the mild odor (Proficiency Exercise 3-16).

Terminology as an Ongoing Study

The study of medical terminology, anatomy, physiology, and pathology must be an ongoing process for the massage professional, who needs this base to understand the research, books, and journal articles that relate to massage, record keeping, and charting. This base is also required if the massage professional is to communicate effectively with other health care professionals.

Many clients are not familiar with these terms, therefore it is important to use the language patterns of the people with whom you speak. Often the use of technical terms with a client is not appropriate; using big words and technical language is not necessary when presenting yourself to the general public. The massage professional must speak two languages and must be able to translate effectively back and forth between them.

When you speak with health care professionals and researchers who use this special language of the sciences, it is important that you ask questions about any term you do not understand. Acting as though you understand what is being said when you do not is unprofessional. The development of this language base has prepared the student to begin the process of maintaining records and charting.

▌▌▌ PROFICIENCY EXERCISE 3-16

1. *Using Appendix A, list at least three skin conditions that could be contagious.*

a.

b.

c.

2. *Using Appendix A, choose one condition from your list and note any indications or contraindications involved.*

Condition:

Indications or contraindications:

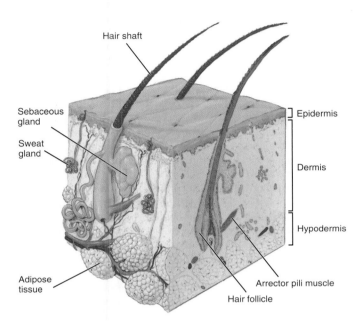

Hair shaft

Sebaceous gland

Sweat gland

Adipose tissue

Epidermis

Dermis

Hypodermis

Arrector pili muscle

Hair follicle

FIGURE 3-15 The structure of the skin. (From Jarvis C: *Physical examination and health assessment,* Philadelphia, 1992, WB Saunders.)

evolve 3-3

RECORD KEEPING

SECTION OBJECTIVES

Using the information presented in this section, the student will be able to perform the following:

- Complete a client intake process using sample forms
- Implement the clinical reasoning problem-solving/decision-making model for charting purposes
- Use a problem- or goal-oriented charting process
- Chart using a SOAP note format

The importance of maintaining professional documentation is becoming increasingly important for massage professionals. Massage has adopted and adapted documentation methods used by the medical profession (Box 3-1).

Dr. Lawrence Weed developed a method of record keeping that is organized around the patient's problems; this is known as the *problem-oriented medical record (POMR)* system. The total historical data are broken into clinical diagnoses, or problems. The first page in the patient's record is a list of all the problems—the medical, social, and psychological problems that can relate to physical findings, personal or social issues, and treatments.

The record then is organized around the various problems using a system known as the *SOAP format* (subjective, objective, assessment/analysis, and plan). The chief complaint and history portion of the record represents subjective information collected from the client or a significant other and from previous records. For each problem, the applicable parts of a traditional history (present illness, past medical history, personal/social history, family history, and review of systems) are summarized in a paragraph placed directly under the problem heading.

The objective data, which include the findings from the physical examination and the results of any tests, follow the list of problems. The physical examination usually is recorded in the traditional format; that is, the results are listed by the parts of the body. After the initial assessment, this section includes any changes in the physical findings and the results of any tests or treatment.

The next section, the assessment/analysis section, presents the conclusions reached based on the subjective and objective data.

The next section is the plan for that particular problem. A plan consists of three parts: diagnosis (Dx), treatment (Rx), and patient education. *Diagnosis* in this case means the diagnostic tests needed to identify the cause or follow the case. Treatment can include special therapy, drugs, radiation, chemotherapy, and other modalities such as massage. "Patient education" is the information the patient is given about the problem.

Organizing patient data in this way shows exactly what the medical caregiver is thinking. Each problem can easily be followed through the record. This saves valuable time for the caregiver and enables others to take over the care of the patient if necessary. The documentation process is based on a clinical reasoning pattern.

Progress Notes

Progress notes chart each patient visit. They should follow a systematic method of organizing the information for decision making. The SOAP method of organizing a progress note, taken from the problem-oriented medical record, is commonly used by massage professionals. This helps massage

BOX 3-2

Documentation Rules for Medical Records and Health Care Professionals

Medical records must be maintained in a specific way:

- Each page of the record should identify the patient by name and by hospital, clinic, or private physician clinical record number.
- Each entry in the record should include the date and time the entry was made and the signature and credential of the individual making the entry.
- No blank spaces should be left between entries.
- All entries should be written in ink or produced on a printer or typewriter or recorded appropriately in electronic format.
- The record must not be altered in any way. Erasures, use of correction fluid, and marked-out areas are not appropriate.
- Errors should be corrected in a manner that allows the reader to see and understand the error. Errors are corrected as follows:
  1. A single line is drawn through the error, and the legibility of the previous entry is checked.
  2. The correct information is inserted.
  3. The correction is dated and initialed by the person recording the data.
  4. If space is inadequate to allow the correction to be made legibly at the error, a note should be made indicating where the corrected entry can be found; this cross-reference should be dated and initialed. The correct information is entered in the proper chronologic order for the date the error was discovered and corrected.
- All information should be recorded as soon as possible. Memories can fade, and important facts can be omitted.

- Abbreviations should be used sparingly. Only those that have been approved by the organization are appropriate. The same abbreviation can have different meanings, which can be misleading. It is always better to write out the information than to use abbreviations that can be misinterpreted.
- Health care givers must write legibly. Because the patient record is used by so many other clinicians and practitioners in providing care, it is important to the quality of patient care that the record be legible. An electronic format helps in this area.
- All entries must be consistent with one another. The assessment must agree with the diagnostic testing, or an explanation must be given as to why it does not.
- Entries should be factual accounts.
- All information given to the patient before any procedures should be recorded. This ensures and verifies that the patient was properly informed of the benefits and risks before the person gave consent to the procedure.
- Telephone contacts with the patient should be entered into the record immediately.
- Some method of organizing entries, such as the SOAP format, must be used to ensure that the entries are comprehensive and reflect the thought processes involved when decisions were made about the patient's care.

These rules result in a record that is accurate, timely, specific, objective, concise, consistent, comprehensive, logical, legible, and reflective of the thought processes of the health care providers (including massage therapists). Not only will such a record be the best defense in a lawsuit, but it also will result in the best care for the patient.

---

therapists to externalize their reasoning and justify their actions. Also, the basic plan is easily modified to other charting styles. Computer record keeping is likely to be required in medical environments, therefore if you do not have basic computer skills, you need to take some classes.

Competent record-keeping skills provide the massage therapist with the information necessary to communicate with other personnel. They also allow the creation of an accurate record of specified treatment goals, the methods of massage, and the effectiveness of treatment.

Paper records are becoming a thing of the past, and are usually considered an impediment to effective delivery of high-quality health care. They are difficult to access, often lack information, and can be available only in a single location for a single use. The paper record has changed very little over the past 50 years, whereas the expectations for use of the data it contains have changed significantly.

Confidentiality of Medical Records

A patient's right to privacy has traditionally imposed an ethical responsibility on the people involved in the care of that patient. Many different people may see and treat a patient during the provision of health care, and each of them needs particular information. Protecting the patient's right to privacy while keeping all caregivers informed can present a dilemma. Passage of the Health Insurance Portability and Accountability Act (HIPAA) in 1996 substantially strengthened the patient's right to privacy.

HIPAA's privacy rules include standards that protect a patient's individually identifiable data; this type of data is considered protected health information (PHI). Generally speaking, PHI relates to information that identifies a patient and his or her health status. The privacy rules apply to health plans, health care clearinghouses, and other health care providers. The privacy rules cover a broad range of information. Protections apply to the information in many different formats, including electronic files (Internet, Intranet, private networks, and data moved from one location to another by disk, magnetic tape, or compact disk), paper records, and verbal information.

Most health care providers, and certainly hospitals, have policies and procedures governing the release of any information about a patient. Massage therapists must be aware of those policies. Policies on the release of information generally include provisions such as the following:

- A requirement for patient consent to release any information to any outside entity; any exceptions are outlined.
- Special considerations for release of information for sensitive conditions, such as alcohol, drug, or psychiatric diagnoses, and conditions related to infection with the human immunodeficiency virus (HIV).
- Required data elements for a proper consent form and how long the form is valid.
- Identification of those who can release information to outside parties.
- Appropriate fees or charges for copies that may be requested.

Other issues should be addressed in separate policies. For example, individuals by title who may release information to the media could be the subject of one such policy. Another policy could indicate what information hospital employees may disclose to telephone callers regarding the condition of the patient during hospitalization.

To be in compliance, health care providers have implemented policies and procedures in reaction to HIPAA. The massage therapist should be specifically trained in the HIPAA procedures in place in the medical environment. This needs to be in-house training. If it is not offered as part of the orientation training, massage therapists should request specific information on how they are expected to comply with these regulations.

All states have laws about which diseases, conditions, and events must be reported to appropriate agencies. Such incidents include births, deaths, gunshot wounds, communicable diseases, and evidence of child abuse. When reporting is required by law, confidentiality is no longer an issue. Reporting such incidents to anyone other than the responsible agency, however, is a breach of confidentiality.

Maintenance of a written record of the professional relationship with clients is essential. The informed consent procedure and the legal implications of documentation were presented in Chapter 2. Procedures for writing records and the ways to use various forms is sometimes called *documentation*.

The student also will continue to develop decision-making skills, as presented in Chapter 2. Ethical decisions are only one type of decision made in professional practice. Clinical decisions about what might be involved with a client's concerns and what methods to use to achieve clients' goals, as well as business decisions, are also necessary. This discussion focuses on clinical decision making and the records necessary for maintaining a written account of the professional interaction. Clinical decision making is discussed in further detail in future chapters. Chapter 14 more thoroughly discusses business records, and Chapter 15 provides examples of case studies.

Client record keeping involves creating a written or electronic record of intake procedures, including informed consent and needs assessments (including the history and physical assessment); obtaining release of information (if communication among health professionals is anticipated); and the ongoing process of recording each session, which is called *charting*.

NOTE: At this point, you, as students, would find it difficult to complete a needs assessment and devise an initial treatment plan because you are still developing the assessment skills and technical skills required to perform these procedures. The same is true of charting. Despite this, it is important to understand the mechanics of the record keeping and charting process so that as your technical skills improve, your ability to perform record-keeping procedures also develops.

Clinical Reasoning and Charting

As the volume of knowledge increases and as soft tissue modalities, such as massage, are integrated into health care systems, the ability to think or reason through an intervention process and justify the effectiveness of a therapeutic intervention is becoming increasingly important. Therapeutic massage practitioners must be able to gather information effectively, analyze that information to make decisions about the type and appropriateness of a therapeutic intervention, and evaluate and justify the benefits derived from the intervention. Charting is the process of keeping a written record of these professional interactions. Effective charting is more than writing down what happens during a session; it is a clinical reasoning methodology that emphasizes a problem-solving approach to client care.

As was noted at the beginning of this chapter, a practitioner needs a comprehensive knowledge base of medical terms, abbreviations, and anatomy and physiology in both normal and diseased states of functioning to be able to reason clinically and chart effectively.

Effective assessment, analysis, and decision making are essential to meeting the needs of each client. Routines or a recipe-type application of therapeutic massage often are limited and ineffective because each person's presenting circumstances and outcome goals are so varied. Effective clinical reasoning skills are the mark of an experienced professional. As with all skills, clinical reasoning can be learned.

Functionally Oriented Goals

Massage sessions are goal oriented. Goals describe desired outcomes. Decisions need to be made as to what goals are

---

 PROFICIENCY EXERCISE 3-17

Following the examples given in this section of the text, write three quantifiable and qualifiable functional goals that you might set for yourself using therapeutic massage.

1.

2.

3.

obtainable and the way the goals will be reached. Problems indicate limits in functions. Goals reclaim a support function. Consider the following example:

- Description of the problem: Client has disturbed sleep pattern due to multiple stressors.
- Goal set: Reduce physical stress symptoms to support more effective sleep.

Two primary reasons for developing treatment and care plans are to set achievable goals and to outline a general plan for the way the goals will be reached. Achievable goals often relate to day-to-day activities (functional goals), either personal or work related. It is important to develop measurable, activity-based goals that are meaningful to the client, such as improvement in the ability to perform activities of daily living.

Goals must be able to be **quantified;** that is, they must be measurable in terms of objective criteria, such as time, frequency, rating on a 1 to 10 scale, a measurable increase or decrease in the ability to perform an activity, or a measurable increase or decrease in a sensation, such as relaxation or pain.

Goals also need to be **qualified.** How will we know when the goal is achieved? What will the client be able to do after the goal has been reached that he or she is not able to do now? For example, how fast will the client be able to run, or how will the client behave when relaxed? Examples of functional goals include the following (Proficiency Exercise 3-17):

- Client will be able to manage independently (qualified) daily hygiene activities of bathing and dressing with a pain level of 5 on a scale of 1 to 10 (quantified), with 10 being unable to function without severe pain.
- Client will be able to work at the computer for 1 hour (quantified) without pain (qualified).
- Client will be able to incorporate a 30-minute walking program (quantified) without stiffness in left knee (qualified).
- Client will be able to fall asleep within 15 minutes (quantified) and sleep uninterrupted for 7 hours (qualified).
- Client will be able to increase duration of breath exhale to reduce sympathetic arousal (quantified), allowing her to drive car to and from market (qualified).
- Client will be able to meditate for 15 minutes (quantified) without racing thoughts (qualified).
- Client will be able to use massage to relax for 1 hour each week (quantified) to enjoy family more by being able to participate in a family outing after each massage (qualified).

Intake Procedures

Before massage therapists begin working with a client, it is important that they gather information on which to build the professional interaction, establish client goals, and develop a plan for achieving those goals. This is called a *database.*

Database. A **database** consists of all the information available that contributes to therapeutic interaction. It is created with information obtained from a history-taking interview with the client and other pertinent people, a physical assessment, prior records, and health care treatment orders. Information obtained during the history and assessment process becomes the needs assessment and provides the basis for the development of a treatment or care plan, identification of contraindications to therapy, and assessment of need for referral.

To gather the information, the professional must have effective communication skills. The same communication skills learned for ethical decision making in Chapter 2 are applied in this process. The I-message pattern can be altered slightly to develop effective, open-ended questions that support data collection.

The four basic questions are:

1. Will you please explain the situation or tell me what happened?
2. How did/do you feel about the situation?
3. What has been the result of the situation in terms of costs, limitations, and changes in activity or performance?
4. How would you prefer the situation to be or what would you like to occur?

NOTE: The answer to the last question can easily become the basis for the functionally oriented treatment goal.

History. The history interview provides information pertaining to the client's health history, the reason for contact, a descriptive profile of the person, a history of the current condition, a history of past illness and health, and a history of any family illnesses. It also contains an account of the client's current health practices (Figure 3-16).

Assessment. The physical assessment makes up the second part of the database. Assessment procedures identify both noneffective functioning and deviations from the norm. The extent and depth of this assessment vary from setting to setting, practitioner to practitioner, and the situation of the client. Practitioners of therapeutic massage generally use some sort of visual assessment process that looks for bilateral symmetry and deviations. Functional assessment looks for restricted, exaggerated, painful, or otherwise altered movement patterns. Palpation is used to identify changes in tissue texture and temperature, locate energy changes, and identify areas of tenderness. Various manual tests may be used to differentiate soft tissue problems from such other problems as joint dysfunction and muscle function (Figure 3-17).

Analysis of Data. After the information has been collected, it is analyzed. This is a very important process and follows the same model as that for decision making. Effective decision making depends on both thorough collection of data and effective analysis of those data.

The steps of the analysis process are as follows:

1. Review the facts and information collected.

   Questions that help with this process include the following:

   - What are the facts?
   - What is considered normal or balanced function?
   - What has happened? *(Spell out events.)*

CLIENT INTAKE INFORMATION FORM

Name: _____ Date: _____

Address: _____ City: _____ State: _____ Zip: _____

Phone: (day) _____ (eve) _____ Date of Birth: _____

Occupation: _____ Employer: _____

Referred by: _____ Physician: _____

Previous experience with massage:

_____

Primary reason for appointment / areas of pain or tension:

_____

Emergency contact—name and number: _____

**Please mark (X) for all conditions that apply now. Put a (P) for past conditions,
an (F) for family history of illness.**

Pain Scale: minor-1   2   3   4   5   6   7   8   9   severe-10

_____ headaches, migraines	_____ chronic pain	_____ fatigue
_____ vision problems, contact lenses	_____ muscle or joint pain	_____ tension, stress
_____ hearing problems, deafness	_____ muscle, bone injuries	_____ depression
_____ injuries to face or head	_____ numbness or tingling	_____ sleep difficulties
_____ sinus problems	_____ sprains, strains	_____ allergies, sensitivities
_____ dental bridges, braces	_____ arthritis, tendinitis	_____ rashes, athlete's foot
_____ jaw pain, TMJ problems	_____ cancer, tumors	_____ infectious diseases
_____ asthma or lung conditions	_____ spinal column disorders	_____ blood clots
_____ constipation, diarrhea	_____ diabetes	_____ varicose veins
_____ hernia	_____ pregnancy	_____ high/low blood pressure
_____ birth control, IUD	_____ heart, circulatory problems	
_____ abdominal or digestive problems	_____ other medical conditions not listed	

Explain any areas noted above:

_____

_____

Current medications, including aspirin, ibuprofen, herbs, supplements, etc.:

_____

_____

Surgeries: _____

Accidents: _____

Please list all forms and frequency of stress reduction activities, hobbies, exercise, or sports participation:

_____

_____

FIGURE 3-16 A sample history form. This information is provided by the client. The key to completing the form is: ask questions.

- What caused the imbalance? *(Can it be identified?)*
- What was done or is being done?
- What has worked or not worked?

2. Brainstorm the possibilities.

   Questions that help with this process include the following:

   - What are the possibilities? *(What could it all mean?)*

- What is my intuition suggesting?
- What are the possible patterns of dysfunction?
- What are the possible contributing factors?
- What are possible interventions?
- What might work?
- What are other ways to look at the situation?
- What do the data suggest?

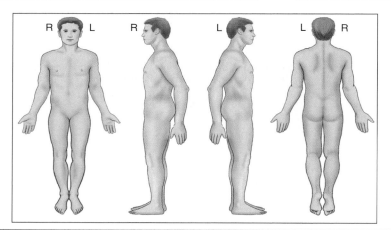

MASSAGE ASSESSMENT/PHYSICAL OBSERVATION/PALPATION AND GAIT   PRE   POST

Client Name: _____   Date: _____

OBSERVATION & PALPATION		
ALIGNMENT	**RIBS**	**SCAPULA**
Chin in line with nose, sternal notch, navel	Even	Even
Other:	Springy	Move freely
HEAD	Other:	Other:
Tilted (L)	**ABDOMEN**	**CLAVICLES**
Tilted (R)	Firm and pliable	Level
Rotated (L)	Hard areas	Other:
Rotated (R)	Other:	**ARMS**
EYES	**WAIST**	Hang evenly (internal) (external)
Level	Level	(L) rotated ☐ medial ☐ lateral
Equally set in socket	Other:	(R) rotated ☐ medial ☐ lateral
Other:	**SPINE CURVES**	**ELBOWS**
EARS	Normal	Even ☐
Level	Other:	Other:
Other:	**GLUTEAL MUSCLE MASS**	**WRISTS**
SHOULDERS	Even	Even
Level	Other:	Other:
(R) high / (L) low	**ILIAC CREST**	**FINGERTIPS**
(L) high / (R) low	Level	Even
(L) rounded forward	Other:	Other:
(R) rounded forward	**KNEES**	**PATELLA**
Muscle development even	Even/symmetrical	(L) ☐ movable ☐ rigid
Other:	Other:	(R) ☐ movable ☐ rigid

FIGURE 3-17 A sample physical assessment form. This information is obtained by observing (looking and feeling) and measuring. The key to completing the form is: identify what is the same on the two sides of the body and what is different.

ANKLES		TRUNK		LEGS	
Even		Remains vertical		Swing freely at hip	
Other:		Other:		Other:	
FEET		**SHOULDERS**		**KNEES**	
Mobile		Remain level		Flex and extend freely through stance and swing phase	
Other:		Rotate during walking		Other:	
ARCHES		Other:		**FEET**	
Even		**ARMS**		Heel strikes first at start of stance	
Other:		Motion is opposite leg swing		Plantar flexed at push-off	
TOES		Motion is even (L) and (R)		Foot clears floor during swing phase	
Straight		Other:		Other:	
Other:		(L) swings freely		**STEP**	
SKIN		(R) swings freely		Length is even	
Moves freely and resilient		Other:		Timing is even	
Pulls/restricted		**HIPS**		Other:	
Puffy/baggy		Remain level		**OVERALL**	
Other:		Other:		Rhythmic	
HEAD		Rotate during walking		Other:	
Remains steady/eyes forward		Other:			
Other:					

FIGURE 3-17, cont'd

3. Consider the logical outcome of each possibility.
   Questions that help with this process include the following:
   - What is the logical progression of the symptom pattern, contributing factors, and current behaviors?
   - What is the logical cause and effect of each intervention identified?
   - What are the pros and cons of each intervention suggested?
   - What are the consequences of not acting?
   - What are the consequences of acting?
4. Consider how people involved would be affected by each possibility.
   Questions that help identify these effects are the following:
   - In terms of each intervention being considered, what is the impact on the people involved: client, practitioner, and other professionals working with the client?
   - How does each person involved feel about the possible interventions?
   - Is the practitioner within his or her scope of practice to work with such situations?
   - Is the practitioner qualified to work with such situations?
   - Does the practitioner feel qualified to work with such situations?
   - Is there a feeling of cooperation and agreement among all parties involved?

Identification of Problems and Goals. Problems are then identified, based on a conclusion or decision resulting from examination, investigation, and analysis of the data collected. A problem is defined as anything that causes concern to the client or caregiver, including physical abnormalities, physiologic disturbances, and socioeconomic or spiritually based problems. Realistic and attainable functional outcome goals are established. A decision is then made about an intervention or care/treatment plan.

Not all therapeutic goals are related to problems. Clients commonly use massage for health maintenance, stress management, and fulfillment of pleasure needs. The same analysis process is used to best determine the methods and approach to meet the client's goals.

Care or Treatment Plan. After the analysis is complete and problems and goals have been identified, a decision needs to be made about the **care or treatment plan.** Anytime a decision must be made about the care plan, return to the problem-solving model, which includes consideration of the facts, possibilities, logical outcomes, and impact on others involved.

The care plan is not an exact protocol set in stone; rather, it is a guideline that has fluidity (the best professional educated guess). The care or treatment plan may evolve over the first three or four sessions and may be altered, with changes in the therapeutic goals. The development of the care or treatment plan is the end of the intake process (Figure 3-18).

As the plan is implemented, it is recorded sequentially,

TREATMENT PLAN

Client Name:_____

Choose One: ☐ Original plan   ☐ Reassessment date _____

Short-term client goals:

Quantitative:_____

Qualitative:_____

Long-term client goals:

_____

_____

Therapist objectives:

_____

_____

1) Frequency, 2) length, and 3) duration of visits:

1) _____   2) _____   3) _____

Progress measurements to be used: (Ex.— pain scale, range of motion, increased ability to perform function)

_____

_____

Dates of reassessment:

_____

Categories of massage methods to be used: (Ex.— general constitutional, stress reduction, circulatory, lymphatic, neuromuscular, connective tissue, neurochemical, etc.)

_____

_____

Additional notes:

_____

_____

_____

Client Signature: _____   Date:_____

Therapist Signature:_____   Date:_____

FIGURE 3-18 A sample form for a care/treatment plan.

session by session, in some form of charting process, such as **SOAP notes.** The plan is re-evaluated and adjusted as necessary.

SOAP Notes

Charting, or documentation, is the process of producing an ongoing record of each client session. As was mentioned earlier, commonly used methods of charting are based on the problem-oriented medical record system. The POMR system involves a problem-solving and clinical reasoning analysis process. Therefore after one method has been learned, adapting to any of the other charting methods is relatively easy. The

most important skill involved is the ability to reason logically and comprehensively through a therapeutic interaction. A charting process can provide the structure necessary to think through a process effectively and develop a written record of the process.

The charting process includes recording any therapeutic action taken, its effectiveness, and its outcome progressively from session to session. Effective charting requires an organized approach to recording the information that relates to the facts, possibilities, logical consequences of cause and effect, and impact on involved people, an approach similar to that used for the development of the initial care or treatment plan. This process again is a direct application of the decision-making model. While charting, a practitioner gathers and records subjective and objective information, records the methods used, and analyzes the effectiveness of the process. The plan for further sessions is then indicated and noted.

Although many different charting processes exist, massage professionals seem to be using the standardized SOAP model. This is a helpful choice in terms of learning because the four-part model correlates with the clinical-reasoning/decision-making model.

SOAP notes or similar charting methods are used to chart all massage sessions. After the initial intake and care/treatment plan development, subsequent visits require a modified and shortened subjective and objective assessment process to determine goals for each individual massage session. When a massage is given to the client after the intake session, specific treatment goals for the particular session are developed. Information from the history pertinent to the first session is transferred to *S* in SOAP notes. Physical assessment information pertinent to this session is transferred to *O* in SOAP notes.

When using SOAP note charting, the massage practitioner should use the following format[1]:

S stands for subjective data recorded from the client's point of view. Subjective information usually includes the following:
- Key symptoms that are quantified and qualified
- Activities that are affected by the situation; often stated as what can no longer be done or what increase in performance is desired
- The methods or activities currently used in treatment

O stands for objective data acquired from inspection and palpation. A list of assessment procedures and interventions used during the session is recorded. Objective information usually includes the following:
- Significant physical assessment findings
- Intervention modalities and locations used (limit specifics to interventions used to work toward treatment goals)
- General approach used, such as general massage focus, connective tissue focus, Swedish massage focus, neuromuscular focus, or circulatory focus
- If not recorded elsewhere, the duration of the session

A stands for analysis or assessment of the subjective and objective data. It includes an analysis of the effectiveness of the intervention and action taken, with a summary of the most pertinent data recorded.

(NOTE: Traditionally in SOAP charting, the *A* stands for assessment. However, observation of many students indicates that they confuse physical assessment information recorded in the objective data with assessment in the SOAP model, which is actually an analysis of the data and effectiveness of the interventions. Therefore this text uses the idea of analysis for the *A* section of SOAP charting.) Analysis information includes the following:

- Changes, whether *subjective* (i.e., related to the client's experience, such as "pain reduced" or "feel relaxed") or *objective* (i.e., measurable, such as "flexion of elbow increased by 15 degrees"). If no change occurs or if the condition worsens, record this also.
- Analysis of which methods were effective or not effective, such as "Trigger point methods most effective in increase of flexion of elbow," "Client indicated she responded best to rhythmic rocking for relaxation," "Tense-and-relax methods not effective in reducing pain in shoulder." Also indicate whether it is unclear which methods were effective: "Range of motion in neck increased 25%, but it is unclear which methods brought about the change."

The *A* (analysis/assessment) section of the SOAP charting process is very important. It is, in fact, the most important area in terms of determining future intervention procedures and communicating process information to other caregivers and insurance companies.

The *A* portion of the SOAP note is where the actual process of decision making is recorded. Decision making occurs during every step of the charting process; however, in the other areas of charting, only the decision is recorded, not the way the decision was made. Obviously a condensed version of the more detailed process is written down in the chart, but the components of the process (facts, possibilities, logical outcomes, impact on people) are evident in the *A* portion of the SOAP note.

P stands for plan, including the methodology for future intervention. The progress of the sessions is developed and recorded. Plan information usually includes the following:
- Frequency of appointments
- Continuation of a step-by-step process as it unfolds session by session to achieve treatment plan goals
- Client self-care
- Referrals

A sample SOAP charting form is presented in Figure 3-19; it has been modified for use by the beginning student. An example of SOAP charting is presented in Box 3-2.

Individual session goals need to be in line with the initial care/treatment plan agreed to in the informed consent process. If the goals are radically different, the client needs to sign an addendum to the informed consent form. Minor changes can be reflected in the SOAP notes or session charting procedure.

To maintain the integrity of client charts, make sure that any abbreviations used are universally understood, or write out the word. Use a black pen or type the notes. Make sure handwritten notes are readable. Never erase or white-out a correction. Draw a single line through any error and make the correction above or next to the error. It is important to share the charting notes with the client regularly and to explain them to him or her.

Computer-Based Patient Record (CPR) and Electronic Health Record (EHR)

Technology has improved over the past 10 years, allowing the design and implementation of electronic record-keeping

SESSION NOTES
SOAP CHARTING FORM

Client Name: _____ Date: _____
Practitioner Name: _____

Subjective

CLIENT STATUS
- **Information from client, referral source, or reference books:**
1) Current conditions/changes from last session: _____
_____
_____
_____

Objective

2) Information from <u>assessment</u> (physical, gait, palpation, muscle testing): _____
_____
_____

CONTENT OF SESSION
- **Generate goal (possibilities) from analysis of information in <u>client status</u>.**
1) Goals worked on this session. (Base information on client status this session and goals previously established in Treatment Plan): _____
_____
_____

What was <u>done</u> this session: _____
_____
_____

Analysis

RESULTS
- **Analyze results of session in relationship to what was done and how this relates to the session goals. (This is based on <u>cause</u> and <u>effect</u> of methods used and the effects on the persons involved).**
1) What worked/what didn't: (Based on measurable and objective Post Assessment) _____
_____

Plan

_____
_____

PLAN: Plans for next session, what client will work on, what next massage will reassess and continue to assess: _____
_____
_____

CLIENT COMMENTS: _____
_____

Time In: _____ Time Out: _____

Therapist signature: _____

FIGURE 3-19 A SOAP charting form modified for student learning. The key to completing the form is: answer the questions based on what happened during the massage.

systems. You will hear a variety of names for automated record-keeping systems, such as computer-based patient record (CPR), electronic patient record (EPR), computerized medical record, and electronic health record (EHR).

Whether the record-keeping system is electronic or paper, high-quality patient care depends on the practitioner's expertise in collecting information and his or her ability to interpret it. The clinical reasoning process is facilitated by electronic record keeping (see the Evolve Web site for practice using computer-based medical records).

Additional Information for the Client's File

Additional information found in a client's file includes the fee and payment record and, if applicable, signed release of information form(s); authorized communication with the client's health care provider(s); and massage therapy treatment orders.

Clients have the right to see their file, receive a copy of the file, and have any information contained in the file explained to them.

■ ■ ■ SUMMARY

Record-keeping and documentation skills, as well as the necessary language base for keeping records effectively, are important aspects of professional development. The ability to communicate clearly in both the written and spoken forms fosters understanding and the accurate exchange of information.

Paperwork usually is not the professional's favorite task. However, think of record keeping as writing the client's professional interaction story. Realize that reflection on the healing journey provided by reading this story allows both you and your client, as well as any other authorized individuals, to appreciate the process and to remember and replicate the steps toward achieving goals that honor the effort put forth by all concerned.

BOX 3-3

Example of SOAP Charting in Therapeutic Massage

The following is an example of the way SOAP charting would be done by a massage therapist for a new client who complains of frequent headaches. The SOAP format has been modified slightly to assist students in completing the documentation process

S (Subjective)

Client reports tension headache and indicates with hand placement that the major concentration of pain is at the occiput and upper cervical area with a secondary pain pattern at the temples. Client reports that on a pain scale of 1 to 10, the headache is a 7.

O (Objective)

Both shoulders are observed to be elevated, with increased elevation on the right. Range of motion of the neck appears to be generally limited to the left. Palpation of the upper back muscles elicited some pain behaviors, including pulling away, grimacing, and verbal indications of pain. The upper trapezius muscles seem to be warm but without indications of inflammation, suggesting tension in the muscles.

Approach Used (What I Did : General massage focus: Stress reduction with specific focus on shoulder and neck tension using positional release and lengthening. Basic methods used: Gliding, compression, rocking, and passive joint movement.

NOTE Postassessment: After the massage session, a postassessment is done. The client is asked how he or she feels and what is different from before the session. The client is asked what methods used seemed to be most beneficial. One or two of the methods identified are then modified for client self-care and are taught to the client.

After the massage and the postassessment, the **A** (analysis/assessment) part of the chart is recorded.

A (Analyze/Assessment)

Client indicates a reduction in headache by 50% (pain rating of 3), less tension in the shoulders, and increased range of motion of the neck to the left. Pain behaviors in the upper back are not observable, but the client still indicates tenderness in the area during palpation. Upper trapezius area is still warm, with exaggerated vasomotor response (reddening) and itching after massage, indicating possible connective tissue involvement in this area. Client now can look over his left shoulder, which he could not do without a catch before the massage. The shoulders are observed to be level within 1 inch, indicating a change in the right shoulder tension pattern. The methods that were most effective were compression and positional release. Rocking methods were ineffective, and the client reported an increase in head pain when rocking was used. *Note:* Make sure client's feet stay warm.

P (Plan)

Client selected self-help consisting of towel compression to the head and flexion/extension range of motion of the arms and shoulders. Client scheduled an appointment for 2 weeks and will monitor response to massage. Expect three to four sessions before beginning specific connective tissue work on the shoulder area. Client was advised to contact his personal physician and report that he has begun to receive massage.

NOTE: The interventions used and the plan recorded in SOAP charting need to reflect the original treatment plan developed during the intake procedure.

---

evolve

3-1   Categorize roots, prefixes, and suffixes to build your medical vocabulary.

3-2   Medical terminology flashcards are available for further study.

Don't forget to study for your certification and licensure exams! Review questions for this chapter are located on Evolve.

REFERENCE

1.   Thompson DL: *Hands heal: documentation for massage therapy: a guide for SOAP charting,* Philadelphia, 2005, Lippincott Williams & Wilkins.

Workbook Section

Answers for the Workbook Section for Chapter 3 are provided on p. 761.

■ ■ ■ SHORT ANSWER

1. What are the three word elements, and how are they used?

_____

_____

_____

_____

_____

_____

2. Define abbreviations and provide guidelines for their use.

_____

_____

_____

_____

_____

3. Explain what is meant by quantified and qualified functional goals.

_____

_____

_____

_____

_____

_____

4. What is the difference between an intake procedure and charting?

_____

_____

_____

_____

_____

_____

5. What are the four steps in the analysis of data acquired during the intake process, and how does analysis relate to the development of a care or treatment plan?

_____

_____

_____

_____

_____

_____

6. Explain the four parts of the SOAP charting process.

_____

_____

_____

_____

_____

_____

7. What is required to maintain the integrity of charts when writing in them?

_____

_____

_____

_____

_____

_____

■ ■ ■ MATCHING

Match the term to the best definition.

1. Abbreviation
2. Combining vowel
3. Prefix
4. Root
5. Suffix
6. Word element

a. A vowel added between two roots or a root and a suffix to facilitate pronunciation
b. A word element comprising the fundamental meaning of the word
c. A word element placed at the beginning of a word to alter the meaning of the word
d. A reduced form of a word or phrase
e. A part of a word
f. A word element placed at the end of a root to alter the meaning of the word

Match each of the following word elements to its proper meaning, then indicate whether it is a prefix (p), root word (r), or suffix (s). Remember that some of the root words may not have a vowel at the end because vowels are added only when combined with a suffix.

1. ab
2. ad
3. algia
4. arthro
5. chondr
6. circum
7. contra
8. cost
9. de
10. dia
11. dis
12. dys
13. epi
14. fibr
15. genesis
16. genic
17. gram
18. graph
19. graphy
20. hyper

21. inter
22. intra
23. intro
24. ism
25. itis
26. myo
27. myel
28. neuro
29. orth
30. osis
31. osteo
32. pathy
33. plegia
34. post
35. stasis
36. sterno
37. sub
38. supra
39. therm
40. thoraco

a. toward
b. over, on, upon
c. producing, causing
d. a diagram, a recording instrument
e. excessive, too much, high
f. around
g. against, opposite
h. joint
i. record
j. a condition
k. away from
l. nerve
m. condition
n. making a recording

o. paralysis
p. maintenance, maintaining a constant level
q. development, production, creation
r. pain
s. above, over
t. disease
u. chest
v. fiber, fibrous
w. cartilage
x. under
y. heat
z. rib
aa. bad, difficult, abnormal
bb. within
cc. down, from, away from, not
dd. across, through, apart
ee. inflammation
ff. spinal cord, bone marrow
gg. separation, away from
hh. between
ii. into, within
jj. straight, normal, correct
kk. bone
ll. after, behind
mm. sternum
nn. muscle

Match the lymph nodes and plexuses to their correct description.

1. Parotid
2. Occipital
3. Superficial cervical
4. Subclavicular
5. Hypogastric
6. Facial
7. Deep cervical
8. Axillary
9. Mediastinal
10. Cubital
11. Para-aortic
12. Deep inguinal
13. Superficial inguinal
14. Popliteal
15. Mammary plexus
16. Palmar plexus
17. Plantar plexus

a. deeply situated nodes in the groin
b. nodes in the groin close to the surface
c. nodes under the collarbone
d. nodes draining the tissue in the face
e. lymphatic vessels in the sole of the foot (plantar)
f. lymphatic vessels in the palm of the hand (palmar)
g. nodes around or in front of the ear
h. nodes over the bone at the back of the head
i. nodes in the area beneath the stomach
j. nodes around the aorta
k. deeply situated nodes in the neck
l. lymphatic vessels around the breasts
m. nodes in the armpit
n. nodes of the elbow
o. nodes close to the surface of the neck
p. nodes in back of the knee
q. nodes in the mediastinal section of the thoracic cavity

Workbook Section—cont'd

■ ■ ■ ASSESS YOUR COMPETENCIES

Now that you have studied this chapter, you should be able to:

1. Identify the three word elements used in medical terms
2. Combine word elements into medical terms
3. Comprehend unfamiliar medical terms
4. Identify pertinent abbreviations used in health care and their meanings
5. Use relevant anatomic and physiologic terminology correctly
6. Combine this information to be used for effective professional record keeping

On a separate sheet of paper, write a short summary of the content of this chapter based on the competencies listed above. When writing this paper assume you are speaking to someone—a client, prospective employer, co-worker, or other interested person. Write the paper as if you were having a conversation and explaining the importance of the information and skills to professional massage development.

Next, in small student discussion groups, share the papers and compare and contrast how the information was presented. Discuss the content, looking for similarities, differences, potential misunderstanding of the information, and clear and concise methods of description.

■ ■ ■ PROBLEM-SOLVING EXERCISE

This week, six new clients come to your office. Each of them has filled out a client history form ahead of time, providing you with the following information on medical conditions that have been diagnosed and treated by their physicians. Take each of the italicized medical terms and break it down into its word parts to define the various conditions.

Dermatitis of the hands
Neuropathy in the left leg
Hypothyroidism
Dyspnea
Hemangioma
Polyarthritis
Myocarditis
Hydronephrosis

■ ■ ■ RESEARCH FOR FURTHER STUDY

List three resource books or Internet sites you could use for further study of medical terminology. Include the title, publisher, and type of reference.

■ ■ ■ RECORD-KEEPING EXERCISE

Complete the forms in Figures 3-16 through 3-19, using the clinical reasoning process and yourself as the client. When you complete the SOAP form, make up a massage session that would be applicable to your personal situation as reflected on the intake forms.

Note: Before you do this exercise, you might want to make copies of the blank forms to use during practice sessions. Also, remember that these are sample forms, which are presented as a guide for learning and for the development of your own professional forms.

The Scientific Art of Therapeutic Massage

CHAPTER OBJECTIVES

After completing this chapter, the student will be able to perform the following:

- Describe the fundamentals of the Western scientific process
- Interpret a research paper
- Cite current research that validates the underlying physiologic mechanisms of therapeutic massage
- Classify massage methods into basic concepts
- Explain the effects of therapeutic massage in physiologic terms
- Use the Internet to do research

CHAPTER OUTLINE

KEY TERMS

Absolute risk
Art
Breathing pattern disorder
Centering
Circulation
Compression
Connective tissue
Conservation withdrawal
Cortisol
Counterirritation
Dopamine
Dynorphins
Endorphins
Enkephalins
Entrainment
Entrapment
Epinephrine/adrenaline
Ethics
Experiment
Gate control theory
General adaptation syndrome
Growth hormone
Hormone
Hyperstimulation analgesia
Hypothesis
Informed consent
Intuition
Joint kinesthetic receptors
Law
Mechanical methods

Continued.

STUDENT NOTE: Students will find it helpful to keep a medical dictionary and an anatomy and physiology textbook at hand to use as references while reading this chapter. ELECTRONIC REFERENCES ARE APPROPRIATE AS WELL AS PAPER REFERENCES. Many technical terms are used, and more in-depth reading may be needed to achieve the best understanding of the information presented. See the Evolve Web site for titles of recommended texts.

KEY TERMS

Muscle spindles	Scientific method
Neurotransmitter	Serotonin
Norepinephrine/noradrenaline	Stress
Oxytocin	Sympathetic
Parasympathetic patterns	Tendon organs
Placebo effect	Tensegrity
Reflexive methods	Toughening (hardening)
Relative risk	Trigger point
Science	

The *American Heritage Dictionary* defines science as "the intellectual process of using all mental and physical resources available to better understand, explain, and predict both normal and unusual natural phenomena." The scientific approach to understanding anything involves observation, measurement of things that can be tested, accumulation of data, and analysis of the findings. The scientific approach is different from an intuitive approach.

Intuition is knowing something without going through a conscious process of thinking. Other terms for intuition are *feelings, inspiration, instinct, revelation, impulse,* and *idea.* The term *intuition* is not used in this textbook to mean a psychic or extrasensory experience; rather, it means the ability to act purposefully on subconsciously perceived information. Intuition is the ability to bring subconscious information into conscious awareness. Biofeedback works on a similar principle. Using equipment that detects the heart rate, blood pressure, and skin temperature, a person can monitor and adjust involuntary, or subconscious, responses.

Centering is the ability to pay attention to a specific area of focus. Centering skills allow us to screen sensation and concentrate. Learning to pay attention to quiet, subtle information amid all the loud, exaggerated stimulation that blasts our sensory receptors every day takes practice. When we are centered, intuition is more apparent.

Art is craft, skill, technique, and talent. When massage professionals work with clients, they must trust their intuition. It is important to maintain the art of the profession by recognizing the validity of intuitional expression.

It is equally important to validate massage therapy on a scientific basis to separate that which is known scientifically from mere speculation about massage and related bodywork methods. In a taped lecture titled "Stress Without Distress: Evolution of the Concept,"[1] world-renowned researcher Hans Selye talked about the importance of both science and intuition. Unless there is first an idea (intuition), Dr. Selye said, there is nothing to research, and without research (science), an idea does not develop form and usefulness. One does not function without the other (Proficiency Exercise 4-1). The scientific art of therapeutic massage depends on the development of a concept or idea, the testing of the idea through research, and the use of skill and talent in applying the craft through its various techniques.

The beginning student of massage may find scientific justification intimidating. However, without this knowledge, the massage professional cannot make intelligent use of the simple methods of massage presented in this text. It is important to develop an understanding of this body of knowledge at the beginning of the educational process because it is the foundation of the profession. Therefore the purpose of this chapter is to help the student understand the strong physiologic basis for the effectiveness of therapeutic massage. Students must build a firm foundation in the anatomic and physiologic explanations of why massage works so that they can trust their intuition and design a massage based on the information they receive from the client during assessment procedures.

VALID RESEARCH

Effective outcomes are achieved when massage methods interact with physiologic processes. Because massage has demonstrable physiologic effects, those effects can be studied through the scientific method. The scientific method is a means of objectively researching a concept to determine whether it is valid. Research begins with a hypothesis (i.e., "if this happens, then that will happen"). The hypothesis must then be tested; this usually is accomplished through an experiment. Interpretation of the data collected during the experiment is expressed in statistical form, therefore it is necessary to be able to interpret terms used in statistical integration. The experiment must follow accepted design measures so that others can replicate

PROFICIENCY EXERCISE 4-1

Give your explanation of Dr. Selye's statement: "If there is not first an idea, there is nothing to research. Without research, an idea does not develop form and usefulness. One does not function without the other."

the experiment. The results of the experiment should either prove or disprove the hypothesis. Often the results of the research generate more questions, leading to more research.

The subjective (experiential) quality of massage complicates the research issue because of the complexity of human beings and the interactive psychological and energetic dynamics between the client and the practitioner, which affect the results of massage. Technologic advances have allowed researchers to see more deeply into the human experience than ever before. We are on the edge of being able to understand the more mysterious and hidden workings of the body. Only a growing body of research and data replication that establishes the positive biochemical and behavioral reaction to touch will convince the scientific community that massage is therapeutic. Fortunately, this type of research is now being done, and the health care professions and the public are responding by seeking massage therapy services. Validation through scientific research has opened these doors.

CURRENT RESEARCH

As a result of growing interest, and through funding provided by the National Institutes of Health (NIH) Research Centers, research on the benefits of massage is increasing in the United States. Similar research is underway in Canada, Europe, Australia, New Zealand, Japan, and China. These studies continue to validate therapeutic massage applications for various conditions. The data are beginning to identify patterns of the underlying physiologic mechanisms that massage addresses. In 2002, the Massage Therapy Foundation's comprehensive database for therapeutic massage research became available on the AMTA Web site (http://www.amtamassage.org). Medline is another excellent research Web site. (http://www.nlm.nih.gov/medlineplus). Research results are now within reach of all who desire to understand the underlying physiologic mechanisms of therapeutic massage benefits, and they continue to support the value of therapeutic massage. This chapter does not attempt to list individual research results, but rather consolidates the research into categories and physiologic processes. The student should become an avid research reader and can begin to explore the vast body of knowledge available.

Various types of research underway at the Touch Research Institute (TRI) of the University of Miami School of Medicine (www6.miami.edu/touch-research) and at other centers are helping to support the validity of the massage profession (Box 4-1). The TRI program is funded by Johnson & Johnson and other corporations and is directed by Tiffany Field, PhD. Dr. Field believes that the clinical health care system will come to incorporate touch therapy in the same way it incorporated relaxation therapy, exercise, and diet.[2] The studies that have been published by or are underway at the Touch Research Institute cover a broad range of subjects and conditions, and they show that massage affects many aspects of human physiology and experience.[3]

Dr. Field has noted the beneficial effects observed in these studies, as well as the need for further investigation:

> Across studies, decreases were noted in anxiety, depression, stress hormones (cortisol), and catecholamines. Increased para-

sympathetic activity may be the underlying mechanism for these changes. The pressure stimulation associated with touch increases vagal activity, which in turn lowers physiologic arousal and stress hormones such as cortisol. Appropriate application of pressure is critical because light stroking is generally aversive (much like a tickle stimulus) and does not produce these effects. Decreased cortisol levels in turn lead to enhanced immune function. Parasympathetic activity is also associated with increased alertness and better performance on cognitive tasks. Given that most diseases are exacerbated by stress and given that massage therapy alleviates stress, receiving massages should probably be high on the health priority list, along with diet and exercise.[2]

Further research is needed to replicate empiric findings on the benefits of massage and to investigate the underlying psychologic mechanisms. Until the underlying mechanisms are known, the medical community is unlikely to incorporate these therapies into general practice.

In addition to studies on mechanisms, treatment comparison studies are important for determining the best massage techniques for different conditions and the arousing versus the calming effects of different treatments. As these studies progress, the massage professional should evolve from method orientation (e.g., Swedish massage, deep tissue massage, Rolfing, shiatsu) to physiologic outcomes, using variations in pressure, speed, rhythm, direction, and duration to achieve the desired results.[2]

THE RESEARCH PROCESS

SECTION OBJECTIVES

Using the information presented in this section, the student will be able to perform the following:

- List the components of the scientific methods
- Describe three basic types of research
- Critically read a research paper

The focus of this section is to prepare the learner to become a consumer of research—not a researcher. Those interested in a more in-depth discussion of research methods or conducting research are directed to the textbook *Research methods for massage and holistic therapies,* by Glenn Hymel, in addition to other comprehensive works listed in the Suggested Readings at the end of the chapter. This section provides a brief survey of the way research is conducted, as well as how the reader can read research papers critically and decide two points:

- Whether the research is valid
- How the research influences massage application

Definition and Origin of Research

At its most basic level, research can be defined as a process in which researchers explore one or more areas of interest (called *factors* or *variables*) by analyzing numeric and/or verbal data (collected information) to advance the understanding of that subject. For example, a researcher might undertake the task

BOX 4-1

Research Findings on the Benefits of Massage

Studies done at the Touch Research Institute of the University of Miami School of Medicine have shown that massage provides the following benefits*:

- Facilitates growth
- Increases attentiveness and learning, which has positive implications for those with attention deficit disorder, hyperactivity, or learning disabilities
- Reduces stereotypical and off-task behavior in autistic individuals while normalizing social behaviors
- Alleviates pain
- Improves immune function (massage increases the number of natural killer cells, which has implications for those with acquired immunodeficiency syndrome [AIDS], cancer, and viral diseases)
- Reduces stress
- Promotes healing of psychiatric problems (child and adolescent psychiatric patients showed more open verbal communication, improved sleep, less depression, and lower anxiety levels, and clinical progress increased; similar results were achieved with depressed adolescent mothers and patients with eating disorders)
- Assists individuals in overcoming addictions, such as cigarette smoking
- Supports effective digestion and breathing through stimulation of the vagus nerve
- Diminishes premenstrual symptoms
- Encourages dietary compliance in people with diabetes, leading to more normal glucose levels

- Lowers blood pressure, anxiety, and hostility levels in individuals with hypertension
- Increases job performance (after a 15-minute chair massage, computation time with figures was cut in half and accuracy almost doubled)
- Reduces the number of headache days in migraine headaches
- Reduces pain and increases range of motion in individuals with low back pain
- Improves all clinical measures in pediatric eczema
- Improves grip strength, functional activities, positive mood, self-esteem, and body image in multiple sclerosis
- Improves caregiver-child relationships for abused and neglected children
- Has a therapeutic effect on the massage practitioner (i.e., reduces stress and improves sleep patterns)

Research is underway on the effects of massage for cystic fibrosis; childhood irritable bowel syndrome; arthritis in the elderly; sickle cell anemia (to mitigate pain); coma and spinal cord injuries (to improve circulation and retard muscle atrophy); mental depression and failure to thrive in the elderly; reduction of the formation of scar tissue from breast surgery, as well as reduction of anxiety, depression, and cortisol levels; Down syndrome (to improve muscle tone and cognitive skills); and cerebral palsy (to help infants gain more muscle flexibility).

*The Web site for the Touch Research Institute is www6.miami.edu/touch-research, accessed November 29, 2007.

of characterizing the percentage of adults surveyed nationwide who have used therapeutic massage as a form of complementary and alternative health care (Box 4-1). Researchers might also explore massage as an intervention for chronic low back pain. They might develop a detailed interview process to document a client's individual experience and perception of therapeutic massage over a designated period of time as an intervention for chronic low back pain. Research could explore the relationship, if any, between aquatic massage therapy and increased range of motion for clients recovering from bilateral hip replacement surgery, or a massage therapist could complete an exhaustive review and synthesis of what the professional literature has to say about therapeutic massage as a viable intervention for clients suffering from fibromyalgia. All of these examples describe different types of research processes.

Ethics in Research

Research involves several very important concerns related to **ethics** and the ethical conduct of research. **Informed consent, confidentiality,** the ability to exit the study at any time without prejudice, and debriefing are some of the ethical issues that researchers must face responsibly, for the obvious reason that the advancement of science must not occur at the expense of the safety and well-being of research participants.

Research in Plain Language

The **scientific method** is a model for conducting scientific research. The scientific method has eight primary steps, which include:

1. Defining the question
2. Locating resources and gathering information and materials
3. Forming a hypothesis (or hypotheses)
4. Planning data collection methods
5. Collecting data
6. Organizing and analyzing the data
7. Interpreting the data and drawing conclusions
8. Communicating the results

Defining the Question[4]

All research begins with the research question: What do I want to know? Examples of research questions might include the following:

1. Does using essential oils in combination with massage increase arterial circulation to the extremities?
2. What is the best position for the knee during massage to prevent joint strain?
3. Does bonding with a puppy occur differently when a specific pet massage routine is used, compared with general petting?

BOX 4-2

Research Vocabulary

absolute risk The chance of a specific occurrence happening over a specified time period.

adverse effect Any effect that produces functional impairment.

analytical study A type of epidemiologic study in which scientists observe certain behaviors (e.g., food choices) and track whether certain outcomes occur (e.g., the development of disease).

bias Problems in the design of a study that can lead to effects that are not related to the variables being studied. For example, *selection bias* occurs when study subjects are chosen in a way that can misleadingly increase or decrease the strength of an association.

blind (single or **double)** In a single-blind experiment, the subjects do not know whether they are receiving an experimental treatment or a placebo. In a double-blind experiment, neither the researchers nor the participants are aware of which subjects receive the treatment until after the study is completed.

clinical trial A type of experimental research in which people are used as subjects. The effectiveness and safety of a nutrient or medical treatment are evaluated through monitoring of its effect on the people participating in the clinical trial. Clinical trials may be small, involving a limited number of participants, or they may be large intervention trials that attempt to discover the outcome of treatments on entire populations. The more participants in a study, the greater the likelihood that the study results can be replicated in the general population.

cohort study An epidemiologic study in which scientists select the study population according to the participants' exposure, regardless of whether the group has the disease or of the health outcome being studied. The researchers then determine the outcomes and compare the results on the basis of the individuals' exposure. Cohort studies often are referred to as *prospective studies* because they follow the study population forward in time.

confounding variable (also **confounding factor** or **hidden variable**) A "hidden" variable that may cause an association that the researcher attributes to other variables. In some situations, a confounding factor may wrongly increase the effect of a substance.

control group The group of subjects in a study to whom a comparison is made to determine whether an observation or treatment has an effect. In an experimental study, it is the group that does not receive treatment.

correlation An association; when one phenomenon is found to be accompanied by another. A correlation does not prove cause and effect.

cross-sectional study A type of epidemiologic study that is basically the same as a survey. The epidemiologist defines the population to be studied and then collects information from members of the population about their disease and exposure status. Because the data represent a point in time, this type of study is somewhat like taking a snapshot of the population.

descriptive study A type of epidemiologic study in which scientists collect information to characterize and summarize a health event or problem.

epidemiologic study Considered the basic science of public health, this type of observational research usually focuses on the study of large groups, sometimes tens of thousands or hundreds of thousands of people. Epidemiologic studies attempt to identify possible factors that increase the risk or probability of a disease.

experimental group The group of subjects in an experimental study that receives treatment.

experimental research Research that generates data by investigating biochemical substances or biologic processes. Experimental research often is conducted in vitro, such as in test tubes. It also is conducted in vivo; that is, in both animals and humans.

generalizability The extent to which the results of a study can be applied to the general population.

mechanism of action The way in which a substance, such as a chemical, exerts its effects.

meta-analysis A quantitative technique in which the results of several individual studies are pooled to yield overall conclusions.

observational research This type of research may be used in the laboratory, but it is primarily conducted in a natural setting to study the relationship between a specific factor and some aspect of health or illness. For this reason, observational research may suggest an association but does not determine cause and effect.

outcomes research A type of research that provides information about the way a specific procedure or treatment regimen affects the subject (clinical safety and efficacy), the subject's physical functioning and lifestyle, and economic considerations, such as saving or prolonging life and avoiding costly complications.

phase I study (clinical trial) Researchers initially test a new treatment or intervention in a small group of people to evaluate its safety, determine a safe dosage range, and identify side effects.

phase II study The treatment is given to a larger group of people to see whether it is effective and to further evaluate its safety.

phase III study The treatment is given to large groups of people to allow researchers to confirm its effectiveness, monitor for side effects, compare it to commonly used treatments, and collect information that will allow the drug or treatment to be used safely.

phase IV study A study that is done after the treatment has been marketed to gather information about its effect in

Continued

BOX 4-2

Research Vocabulary—cont'd

various populations and about any side effects associated with long-term use.

placebo Sometimes casually referred to as a "sugar pill," a placebo is a "fake" treatment that seems to be identical to the real treatment. Placebo treatments are used to eliminate bias that may arise from the expectation that a treatment should produce an effect.

prevalence The number of existing cases of a disease in a defined population at a specified time.

prospective study Epidemiologic research that follows a group of people over a period of time to observe the potential effects of diet, behavior, and other factors on health and/or the incidence of disease.

random sampling A method of selecting subjects to participate in a study in which all individuals in a population have an equal chance of being chosen. This process helps to ensure the generalizability of a study's results.

randomization (or random assignment) The process of assigning subjects to experimental or control groups, with the subjects having an equal chance of being assigned to either group. Randomization is used to control for known variables, unknown variables, and variables for which it is difficult to control.

reliability Whether a test or an instrument used to collect data (e.g., a questionnaire) gives the same results if repeated with the same person several times. A reliable test gives reproducible results.

research design The way in which a study is set up to collect information or data. For valid results, the research design must be appropriate to answer the question or hypothesis being studied.

residual confounding The effect that remains after attempts have been made to statistically control for variables that cannot be perfectly measured. This is an important concept in epidemiologic studies, because researchers' knowledge of human biology is still developing. Unknown variables may

exist that could change conclusions based on epidemiologic research.

retrospective study Research that relies on recall of past data or on previously recorded information. This type of research often is considered to have limitations, because the number of variables cannot be controlled, and people's memories are fallible.

risk A term that encompasses a variety of measures of the probability of an outcome. It usually refers to unfavorable outcomes, such as illness or death.

risk factor Anything statistically shown to have a relationship with the incidence of a disease. It does not necessarily imply cause and effect.

statistical power A mathematical quantity that indicates the probability that a study will obtain a statistically significant effect. A high power of 80% (or 0.8) indicates that the study would produce a statistically significant effect 80% of the time if conducted repeatedly. A power of 0.1 means that a 90% chance exists that the research missed any effect or effects.

statistical significance The probability of obtaining an effect or association in a study sample that is as or more extreme than the effect or association observed if there was actually no effect.

validity The extent to which a study and/or study instrument or instruments measure that which the study is intended to measure. *Validity* refers to accuracy or truthfulness of a study's conclusion or conclusions.

variable Any characteristic that may vary in study subjects, including gender, age, body weight, diet, behavior, attitude, or other attribute. In an experiment, the treatment being investigated is called the *independent variable*. The variable that is influenced by the treatment is the ***dependent variable,*** which may change as a result of the effect of the independent variable.

Modified from Hymel GM: *Research methods for massage and holistic strategies,* St. Louis, 2006, Mosby and www.realmercuryfacts.com. Center for Food, Nutrition, and Agriculture Policy, University of Maryland, College Park, Maryland, 2006.

This first step of the scientific method involves narrowing down possible topics and then choosing the question that will be the focus of the research. The research question must be specific. For example, in the preceding sample question 1, the topics of essentials oils, massage, and arterial circulation are too broad. A better question would be: Does using lavender essential oil in combination with compression massage to the soles of the feet increase arterial circulation to the feet more than compression massage to the soles of the feet without lavender essential oil?

To develop a research question, the researchers must identify five specific goals: (1) what they want to know; (2)

the reason for asking the question; (3) what the answer will tell them; (4) how the information can be beneficial; and (5) whether the question can be answered through research.

Continuing with our previous example, the researchers want to know whether combining lavender oil with massage is better than massage alone for increasing circulation to the feet (goal 1). The reason for asking the question is to determine whether better results can be obtained in supporting circulation to the feet if lavender oil is used with massage (goal 2). The results (answer) will determine whether including lavender oil in compression massage of the feet is worth the expense and effort (goal 3). If using lavender oil with compression massage does increase arterial circulation more than massage alone, then clients with circulation problems in the feet would get better results (goal 4). An experiment could be conducted in which one group received massage with lavender oil and another group received massage without lavender oil; or, a group of people could be massaged one day without lavender oil and 2 days later with lavender oil. In both types of experiments, measurement tools are available for determining any changes in circulation, therefore research could answer the question (goal 5).

Locating Resources and Gathering Information and Materials

After defining the research question, the researchers must educate themselves on the topic to be studied by reading the existing literature and talking to experts. With regard to the lavender oil with massage question, the researchers would learn about essential oils in general and lavender oil specifically, as well as cardiovascular functioning specifically, arterial functioning in the extremities, massage in general, and compression methods specifically. They also would search through any existing, pertinent research. They would talk to an aromatherapist, a person who combines massage and essential oils, and other professionals who would be able to provide information.

Having learned as much as possible about the various aspects of the research question, the researchers then would develop a hypothesis.

Forming a Hypothesis

Based on the knowledge of the topic, the researcher should be able to make an educated guess as to what may happen at the end of the experiment. The hypothesis is important so that it can be compared to the factual information from the experiment and the conclusions, based on the experiment. The researcher can then determine if the hypothesis was correct. This does not affect the value of the research if the hypothesis is inaccurate at the conclusion of the research process.

For example, a hypothesis could be:

Using lavender essential oil during foot massage increases peripheral circulation.

The best position for massage of the knee would be the side lying position.

Planning Data Collection Methods

The fourth step of the scientific method involves making a specific, detailed plan for conducting the research. The procedure should be clear enough that other researchers could follow it exactly. During this planning phase, the following need to be determined:

- What steps are necessary to find the answer to the research question (i.e., to test the hypothesis)?
- What data need to be collected?
- How will the data be collected?
- What equipment, supplies, facilities, assistants, text subjects, support people, and so on will be required?

- What is the reference point (control) with which the data will be compared?
- How many samples, sites, tests, and so on are required?
- What variables will be manipulated and in what ways?
- What record-keeping techniques will be used (e.g., data sheet, journal)?
- How will data collection techniques be organized?
- What are the sequential steps to the research?
- What are the schedule, time line, and time expenditure?
- What are the financial obligations?

To complete this step, the researchers must determine the type of research design they intend to use.

Types of Scientific Research. Basically two types of research are used for scientific studies: observational research and experimental research. Researchers also use meta-analysis to reconcile differences among studies and to compile relevant findings.

Observational Research. Although observational research may be used in the laboratory, it is primarily conducted in a natural setting to study the relationship between a specific factor and some aspect of health or illness. For this reason, observational research may suggest an association, but it cannot be used to determine cause and effect.

- An example of observational research would be a study focusing on whether males or females receive massage more frequently.

Compared to experimental studies, observational research designs are very simple. Fundamentally, the research team simply observes the target groups or processes and uses statistical methods to determine whether an association exists. However, this approach gives rise to many problems. The results of the research may confuse the true effect of a variable and the possible effects of other factors in the environment. For example, an observational study may indicate that women received massage 50% more than men, but it cannot determine the reasons for this difference. This is why observational research often is followed by experimental studies that can validate cause and effect.

The most frequently used type of observational research is the *epidemiologic study,* which is considered the basic science of public health. Usually focused on the study of large groups (sometimes tens of thousands or hundreds of thousands of people), epidemiology attempts to identify possible factors that increase the risk or probability of a disease or behavior. Through one type of epidemiologic research, the *analytical study,* scientists observe certain behaviors (e.g., receiving massage) and track whether certain outcomes occur (e.g., the gender differences in massage frequency). Another type of epidemiologic research, the *descriptive study,* involves the collection of information to characterize and summarize a behavior, health event, or problem.

- For example, a descriptive study may examine the massage frequency associated with such factors as the time of day, the gender of the massage therapist, or the age of the client.

Scientists also use several other methods to conduct epidemiologic studies, and all of these methods have a number of significant limitations. One type of study design, the *cross-sectional study,* is basically the same as a survey. In this type of study, the researcher defines the population to be studied and then collects information from members of the group about their behavior. Because the data represent a point in time, this is like taking a snapshot of the population. Cross-sectional studies are good for examining the relationship between a variable and a behavior (e.g., receiving massage) or a disease (e.g., the flu), but not for determining cause and effect, which requires the collection of data over time.

In a *cohort study,* researchers select the study population according to the group members' exposure, regardless of the health outcome being studied or whether the group has the disease. The researchers then determine the outcomes of interest and compare the results on the basis of the individuals' exposures. Cohort studies often are referred to as *prospective studies* because they follow the study population forward in time, from suspected cause to effect.

- An example of a cohort study would be defining a group of people on the basis of massage received weekly and following them for 5 years to see whether they showed a reduced tendency for muscle tension headache.

Another option is the *case control study,* in which the research team works backward, from the effect to the suspected cause. For this reason, case control studies often are referred to as *retrospective studies.* Participants are selected on the basis of the presence or absence of the disease or outcome in question; the study therefore involves one group of people who have the behavior or problem (case subjects) and one group of people who do not (controls). These groups are then compared to determine the presence of specific exposures or risk factors.

- An example of a case control study would involve forming a group of people with tension headache and another group without it and then comparing the two groups for their history of receiving massage.

Regardless of the method used, the important thing to understand about the results of observational studies is that they are observations of associations and nothing more. They can tell us what, but not why. By conducting observational studies, researchers can add valuable information to the existing literature on a particular topic, which helps them design future research studies, including clinical trials.

Experimental Research. Basic research generates data by investigating biochemical substances or biologic processes. It often is conducted to confirm observations or to determine the way a particular process works.

- For example, an experiment might be conducted to examine how massage for 20 minutes on the head, hands, and feet helps promote falling asleep in less than 15 minutes after going to bed.

Basic research often is conducted in vitro (e.g., in test tubes) or with animals. Research with animals is an important tool for determining how humans may react when exposed to particular substances. However, it is important to note that, because of differences in physiology and the fact that animals are routinely exposed to levels of compounds far higher than those humans typically encounter, one cannot assume that results from animal studies can be generalized to humans. Therapeutic massage is extremely difficult to test in vitro, although various studies of blood samples or saliva samples might be possible.

For experimental research, study subjects, whether human or animal, are selected according to relevant characteristics and are then randomly assigned to an experimental group (i.e., the group that will receive the treatment or intervention) or a control group (i.e., the group that does not receive the treatment). Random assignment ensures that factors that may affect the outcome of the study, known as *variables,* are distributed equally among the groups and therefore cannot lead to differences in the effect of a treatment. As a result, any differences in results between the groups can be attributed to the treatment. However, controlled experimental research can be flawed, which is why it is important to know how the study was designed and conducted.

The most significant type of experimental research is the *clinical trial,* which uses human subjects to evaluate the effectiveness and safety of a nutrient treatment by monitoring its effect on large groups of people. Clinical trials generally are conducted by independent researchers or by researchers affiliated with a hospital or university medical program or private industry. These studies may be small, involving a limited number of participants, or they may be large intervention trials that attempt to discover the outcome of treatments on entire populations. The more participants in the study, the greater the likelihood that the results can be replicated in the general population.

Besides the size of the study, the other critical factor is how the research was designed. Scientists place the most value on the *double-blind, placebo-controlled study* that uses random assignment of subjects to experimental and control groups. Considered the "gold standard" of clinical research studies, the double-blind, placebo-controlled study provides dependable findings that are free of bias introduced by either the subject or the researcher. In this type of study, neither the subject nor the researcher conducting the study knows whether the test substance or a placebo has been administered. For the results to be valid and to ensure that the subject cannot violate the blinding, the placebo and the test substance must be virtually identical (i.e., look, smell, and taste similar). Blinding for massage is very difficult; what can be used as a placebo for massage? This is one of the hurdles researchers must overcome in conducting massage-based research.

To conduct a clinical trial, researchers must go through a series of steps, or phases, each of which is designed to answer a separate research question. The NIH defines the four phases of a clinical trial as follows:

- Phase I: Researchers test a new treatment or intervention in a small group of people for the first time to evaluate its safety, determine a safe dosage range, and identify side effects.
- Phase II: The treatment is given to a larger group of people to determine whether it is effective and to further evaluate its safety.

- Phase III: The treatment is given to large groups of people so that the researchers can confirm its effectiveness, monitor for side effects, compare it to commonly used treatments, and collect information that will allow the drug or treatment to be used safely.
- Phase IV: Studies are done after the treatment has been marketed to gather information about its effect in various populations and any side effects associated with long-term use.

Obviously, the findings of a phase III study are more significant for the public than those of a phase I or phase II study, which requires further investigation. Preliminary findings may make for interesting reading, but it is important for the public to recognize that the study represents only an initial step in the research process and needs to be confirmed through additional studies.

Meta-Analysis. Meta-analysis is conducted to reconcile differences among studies or to consolidate relevant findings across studies. It is a statistical method of combining results from separate studies to derive overall conclusions about a question or hypothesis. This method is most appropriate for examining studies that investigate the same question and use similar methods to measure relevant variables. For example, using one type of meta-analysis, researcher Chris Moyer examined the available massage literature to determine whether consistent, identifiable benefits for massage could be found.

This study is called "A meta-analysis of massage therapy research" and can be found in *Psychological Bulletin* 1:30(1), 2004.

"This meta-analysis supports the general conclusion that [massage therapy] is effective. Thirty-seven studies yielded a statistically significant overall effect as well as six specific effects out of nine that were examined," state the study's authors.

Although individual studies showed inconsistent results, pooling of data from similar studies showed benefits from massage for trait anxiety (an ongoing predisposition to anxiety over time) and depression.

The technique of meta-analysis is not without limitations. Data from flawed studies may be included, or the analysis may include data from studies that use different methods to measure variables, resulting in a comparison of apples and oranges.

Collecting Data

Researchers must collect all the information (data) that could affect the answer to the research question. The following criteria are useful in this process:

- All relevant data must be recorded.
- Researchers must keep track of the step-by-step process.
- Objectivity must be maintained in the data collection.

Organizing and Analyzing the Data

In the sixth step of the scientific method, the researchers pull together the data collected and examine them more closely.

The information is compared and contrasted. The data are:

- Organized and summarized
- Presented graphically (e.g., bar graphs, tables, pie charts, line graphs) so that others can see the results clearly
- Tested to determine whether the results are significant

Interpreting the Data and Drawing Conclusions

The researchers analyze the data and determine their conclusions, such as the following:

- What alternative hypotheses might explain these results?
- Were all relevant data, including extremes, or "oddball" data, analyzed?
- How might the sampling or data collection methods have affected these results?
- What answer do the results provide to the original question?
- How do the results compare to what was expected to happen (the hypothesis)?
- What can be concluded from the results? How do the conclusions affect the community or the "big picture" (implications)?

Communicating the Results

In the final step of the scientific method, the research and its findings are presented to the public. Important questions that must be considered in this process include the following:

- Who is the audience? (Who wants to read the research?)
- What is the best way to communicate the information (e.g., written report, oral or poster presentation, video)?
- What visual aids will help the audience clearly understand this research?

All of the following components of the research must be addressed:

- An introduction to the research question, the purpose of the research, and why it is interesting or matters
- A description of methods used to collect data
- The results
- The conclusions
- Questions raised by the research[4]

evolve

Reading and Interpreting a Research Paper*

The reader (consumer) of research needs to review the methodology of a study to ensure that the objective of the analysis is clearly stated and that the researchers explain the limitations of their findings so that the results can be put into context.

---

*The information in this section is modified with kind permission from Glenn Hymel's text, *Research methods for massage and holistic therapies.*

Besides knowing the limitations of the different types of studies, those who read research papers also must understand how the study was conducted. Important factors include the following:

- The setting of the study (e.g., a clinic, laboratory, or population)
- How variables were controlled (How did the researchers adjust for specific subject qualities or outside influences that could affect the results?)
- The sample size
- The number of study groups
- The treatment or variables observed (e.g., a vitamin supplement, a specific diet, massage)
- The length of the study
- How the data were collected
- How and by what statistical procedures the data were analyzed

One of the most significant factors in evaluating a study's findings is the study design, especially the randomness of the selection of the study's participants. If the subjects were selected randomly, the study results are more predictive of the population. If the only participants in the study were volunteers who belonged to an interest group or a media organization, greater potential exists for bias in the study.

Another important factor is the sample size. Although a small sample does not mean that the study is flawed, the conclusions that can be drawn clearly have limitations. For this reason, federal agencies, such as the Food and Drug Administration (FDA), require multiple studies involving large numbers of subjects before approving a new treatment or intervention.

In interpreting a study's findings, the reader also must understand the statistical significance. When conducting both observational and experimental research, scientists use statistical measures to convey the existence and strength of relationships. However, although statistics present the findings in an organized fashion, they do not provide information about cause and effect. Moreover, a statistically significant finding does not guarantee that the research is without bias or confounding factors that could make the statistical value irrelevant. Statistical significance is only part of the picture; to get the whole picture, the reader must consider the context of the study and the findings of other research on the subject.

A primary challenge in interpreting the findings of a research study for the public is communicating the potential risk. Those who use research must understand the difference between relative risk and absolute risk and must use these distinctions in explaining the findings of a study.

Absolute risk is the chance a person will develop a specific disease or potential injury over a specified time period. For example, a woman's lifetime absolute risk of breast cancer is 1 in 9; that is, one woman in every nine will develop breast cancer at some point in her life.

Relative risk puts the chance in comparative terms by describing the outcome rate for people exposed to the factor in question compared with the outcome rate for those not exposed to the factor. In most cases, the absolute risk is a far more relevant statistic for the public.

For example, suppose a study shows that people who get a massage once a week are 50% less likely to develop sacroiliac (SI) joint dysfunction in the next 3 years than people who get a massage only once a month. The relative risk is that a person who does not get a massage once a week will face a 50% greater likelihood of developing SI joint dysfunction. Yet the absolute risk for an individual who does not get a massage once a week may be only 1%. In this case, the relative risk makes the massage intervention seem more important than it really is. Therefore it is important to consider both the relative risk and the absolute risk when discussing study results.

As the research on massage increases and as current literature is interpreted, it is important for massage therapists to acquire adequate information on a study's original purpose, research design, and methods of data collection and analysis. Massage therapists also must have an understanding of the limitations of specific types of research and must recognize when a study is preliminary or when the findings differ from previous research.

Most important, proper interpretation of a new study's findings requires that the potential risk/benefit be put into perspective. It also requires clarification of cause and effect, which can be demonstrated only through rigorous experimental studies, not epidemiologic research.

A Framework for Reading a Research Article: Structure, Function, and Implied Criteria for Evaluation

Structure and Function (A Research Report's "Anatomy" and "Physiology")

The structure, or "anatomy," of an empirical research article is a rather standard feature of this form of scientific or technical writing. Because the intent is to enhance communication among professionals across various disciplines and professions, the composition of a research report is not left to the preferences or idiosyncrasies of individual researchers. The various sections and subsections that make up the structure of a research report are included specifically to accomplish certain functions, which are analogous to the "physiology" of the research report.

Examining the structure and function of a research article can help the reader identify several criteria or standards that might be used to determine whether the report provides appropriate information. The availability of appropriate information in the report allows the reader to evaluate the research effort with regard to its potential for advancing the knowledge base and, in turn, advancing the evidence-based practice that massage therapists provide for their clients.

The following is an overview of the six major sections, and their corresponding subsections, that constitute a research article.

The Preliminary Section (Title and Abstract)

The first section of a research article contains the title and an abstract of the study. Although fairly self-explanatory, the title of a study must be formulated so that a potential reader (e.g., a person scanning a list of studies by bibliographic citation only) can accurately determine the type of study, the major variables involved, and the participants who were the focal point of the researchers' efforts.

In the abstract, or summary, the author synthesizes as efficiently as possible the main body of the report (i.e., the introduction, method, results, and discussion sections). A well-written abstract gives the reader a precise idea of the actual functions the study accomplished, allowing the person to decide whether to read the report in its entirety.

The Introduction

The introduction provides the context for the rest of the report. It has five subsections: (1) a general review of the literature; (2) a specific review of the literature; (3) a purpose statement, which identifies the research question; (4) the rationale for the study's research hypothesis; and (5) a statement of the research hypothesis.

The general review of the literature identifies the broader context of the study's major research problem area. This addresses at a general level the earlier researchers and authors who have contributed to the research problem area. The specific review of the literature provides a more detailed treatment of related sources in the professional literature. This subsection allows the reader to become considerably more familiar with the earlier literature that informs the current study.

The two literature review subsections serve a dual purpose: (1) They establish in the reader's mind the study authors' familiarity with the existing sources of information in the research problem area; and (2) they inform the reader of the information and insight needed to better comprehend the current research report.

In the next subsection, the purpose statement, the research question at the very least must be implied, although an explicit formulation is considerably preferable. This subsection communicates to the reader what is truly the starting point in the study, because in any research endeavor, the many decisions are based precisely on the research question, which represents the reason the study was performed. The reader must always keep in mind that the research question is never formulated in a vacuum; this simply means that the researchers must have some familiarity with the relevant literature to identify the question. At the same time, the researchers must have at least the beginnings of a research question to know exactly where in the literature they must search.

The subsection on the rationale for the research hypothesis relies on and may even extend the preceding literature review subsections. The authors of a research report must rely on the available research literature in a given problem area to acknowledge the justification for what becomes their study's research hypothesis. The research hypothesis is basically the predicted answer to the study's research question; it is not a so-called educated guess. It is a predicted answer to the research question that is informed or justified primarily by concepts, theories, and/or existing empirical research contained in the professional literature. The rationale for the research hypothesis, then, should be presented immediately before the actual statement of the hypothesis. In this way, a context is already in place that clarifies the reasons the researchers predict a certain answer to the study's question. The rationale usually is only implied, but the preferred approach is to identify it explicitly for the reader's benefit.

The final subsection of the introduction is the statement of the research hypothesis. Unfortunately, far too many authors fail to provide an explicit statement of what they anticipate, with justification, will be the outcome of the study (i.e., the answer to the study's research question). Many authors tend to allow the research hypothesis simply to be implied. The major advantage of an explicit statement of the hypothesis is that it alerts the reader to several critical features of the study, including the research category, strategy, and method used; the variables investigated and their predicted relationship; the participants studied; and the context or setting of the study. Knowledge of a study's research hypothesis sets the stage for a more informed consideration of the study's methodology, which not coincidentally is the next major section in a research article.

The Method

Just as the name suggests, the method section of the research report provides a detailed account of the methodology used to carry out the study. It identifies the various research procedures used at different stages and explains them in such detail that the study can be replicated by others. This section also gives the reader as complete a basis as possible for determining whether the implementation of the study justifies (or in any way compromises) the results and conclusions reached.

To accomplish these tasks, the method section must describe how the participants were chosen, the instruments used to measure variables, and the procedures by which the study was actually implemented. Standard subsections that constitute the method section are (1) participants and sampling procedures; (2) research method and design; (3) variables investigated; and (4) instrumentation. These four subsections allow the authors to specify precisely what was done in carrying out the study. Readers should keep in mind that the labeling of these subsections can vary slightly across different studies; the important point is to make sure the method section addresses the issues of participants, measuring instruments, and procedures.

The first subsection, typically labeled participants and sampling procedures, describes the characteristics of the study participants and the activities used to select and assign them. The researchers identify and justify the inclusion and exclusion criteria used to determine who did and who did not qualify as study participants. Researchers also rely on this subsection to provide information about the power analysis used to determine the optimum sample size for a given study. In addition, the researchers must state the extent to which they used random selection of sample participants from an accessible population and random assignment of subjects to comparison groups. If the researchers used procedures other than random selection and random assignment, they must specify the alternatives chosen. These issues are critical when determining whether a study is valid. The participants and sampling procedures subsection also should specify the ethical provisions of the study that ensured the protection of participants, the overall integrity of the study, and prior approval from the appropriate Institutional Review Board.

The second subsection focuses on the research method and design. The third subsection addresses the variables investigated in the study. Although this is not the first time the variables are mentioned in the report, the important point is that here, the researchers describe the variables as specifically as possible. In this subsection the reader can learn all the details of how the researchers identified, defined, characterized, controlled, manipulated, and measured the study's variables.

The final subsection of the methods section is instrumentation. Although this refers primarily to measuring instruments used to generate numeric and/or verbal data, this subsection may also specify the type or model of equipment or apparatuses that played a role in the study. Technical factors, such as the validity and reliability of instruments, are crucial and therefore are prominent features of the information provided in this subsection.

The Results

The results section provides the reader with a full accounting of the outcomes or results of the data analysis performed in the study. This is accomplished mainly through disclosure of the descriptive and/or inferential statistical techniques used to analyze the data, the results of the analysis, and their interpretation.

The results section also provides the researchers the opportunity to specify other statistical findings beyond hypothesis testing if the study allowed this. For example, confidence intervals may be established and effect sizes may be cited in an attempt to augment traditional null hypothesis significance testing (NHST).

The Discussion

The fourth and final section of the report's main body is the discussion of the study's findings. This section provides the researchers with the opportunity to (1) reflect on the manner in which the study was conducted, including its limitations and delimitations (boundaries); (2) elaborate on the interpretation of the study's findings that was begun in the results section; (3) acknowledge the significance of the study's results, as well as their relationship to earlier research findings in the problem area investigated; (4) theorize as to the reason or reasons the results were obtained (i.e., which intervening variables may have come into play); and (5) suggest recommended areas of further research that would be logical sequelae to the current study.

The Conclusion (References and Other Material)

The concluding section of the research report begins with a list of the bibliographic citations for each of the sources cited in the research report. This list constitutes the references, and it is very important not only because it gives detailed credit to sources used in the study, but also because it provides the reader with the information necessary to access the sources cited. In addition to this list, research reports often include information in appendices, authors' notes, and footnotes.

Implied Criteria for Critiquing a Research Article

The structure and function of the sections and subsections of a research report provide the foundation for identifying certain criteria that can be used to evaluate the merits of a report. They also provide an organizational framework for systematically working through the process of reflecting on the contents of a report. Readers can use the following lists of specific questions to help them evaluate the designated sections and subsections of a research article.

- **Preliminary Section**
  1. Does the title of the study provide a basis for identifying the type of study, major variables, and participants?
  2. Does the abstract synthesize the main body of the report (i.e., the introduction, method, results, and discussion sections), with a particular focus on the research question, research hypothesis, participants, research method and design, major variables, instruments, statistical techniques, principal findings, and conclusions?

- **Introduction**
  1. Is the reader introduced to the professional literature that has bearing on the study being reported by means of a general overview of the research problem area and more specific coverage of individual studies?
  2. Is the purpose of the study identified by means of a detailed formulation of the research question?
  3. Is a rationale or justification, based on various features of the professional literature, presented as a context or framework for the study's research hypothesis?
  4. Do the authors state the study's research hypothesis in such a way that the predicted answer to the study's research question is clear and unambiguous?

- **Method**
  1. Are the study's participants clearly characterized, along with the inclusion and exclusion criteria used to choose them?
  2. Did the researchers justify the number of participants constituting the sample size by means of a power analysis?
  3. Was an accessible population of potential participants acknowledged, along with an indication of how the sample was derived from such a population, whether through random selection or some other procedure?
  4. Did the authors specify the manner in which the participants were assigned to the two or more comparison groups, whether through random assignment or some other means?
  5. Was any clarification provided as to how the ethical aspects of the study were governed, particularly with regard to protection of the participants, the overall

integrity of the research, and prior approval of the study by an Institutional Review Board?

6. Was the nature of the research effort adequately characterized in terms of its position in the research continuum (i.e., its position regarding research category, strategy, method, design, and defining procedures)?

7. Were the study's variables detailed in a comprehensive fashion so that their manipulation and measurement could be replicated?

8. Did the authors clearly specify the equipment and instruments used to manipulate and measure the variables, and did they provide documentation of the technical factors, including validity and reliability?

■ **Results**

1. Were the data analysis techniques used identified and justified?

2. Were the results of the study communicated by an appeal to descriptive and/or inferential statistics consistent with the nature of the research question, as well as the research method and measurement scales used?

3. Were the results of the data analysis related to an appropriate decision regarding the study's null or statistical hypothesis?

4. Was the decision regarding the null hypothesis acknowledged as a basis for inferring decisions concerning the alternative and research hypotheses?

5. If hypothesis testing was performed, were the analyses augmented with other statistical techniques, such as confidence interval estimation and/or effect size calculations?

6. Were tables and figures used appropriately to present the data analyses in a comprehensible manner?

■ **Discussion**

1. Did the researchers reflect on the manner in which the study was designed and conducted with regard to any limitations and/or delimitations (i.e., intentional or unintentional boundaries)?

2. Did the authors elaborate on the interpretation of the study's findings beyond the interpretation that was begun in the results section?

3. Did the researchers address the significance of the study and its findings, particularly as they relate to earlier studies in the problem area investigated?

4. Were possible intervening variables addressed that might explain the reason or reasons the results were obtained?

5. Were recommendations made regarding follow-up studies that might fully or partly replicate or at least augment the current study?

■ **Conclusion**

1. Does the list of references accurately reflect each of the sources cited in the research report, and is the list presented in a consistent bibliographic citation style?

2. Does the research report contain any appendices that provide more detailed information than that given earlier in the article?

3. Is any information provided, in the form of authors' notes, that gives insight into the funding support for the study, contact directives for communicating with the authors as a follow up, and/or collegial assistance in completing the study?

4. Are any footnotes provided, which elaborate on one or more aspects of the study, that would have been misplaced or distracting if embedded in the main body of the report?

WHY MASSAGE IS EFFECTIVE

SECTION OBJECTIVES

Using the information presented in this section, the student will be able to perform the following:

- Identify and categorize massage methods as reflexive or mechanical
- Explain the anatomic and physiologic influences of massage on the neuroendocrine system, connective tissue, body circulation, and energy systems

The manual techniques of massage are physiologically specific and well defined by (1) the mode of application (i.e., rubbing, pulling, pressing, touching); (2) the speed and depth of pressure (sustained or slow, rhythmic, staccato, or fast); (3) the intensity of touch (light touch, deep touch, or a combination of the two); and (4) the part of the therapist's body used to apply the techniques (fingers, hand, forearm, knee, or foot). The techniques of therapeutic massage and other types and styles of bodywork are merely variations of the fundamental application of manual manipulations. The benefits of the techniques are simply the result of basic physiologic effects.

Physiologic Effects

The fundamental concepts that explain the effects of therapeutic massage can be divided into two categories, mechanical methods and reflexive methods.

■ **Mechanical methods** apply various types of force (tension, bending, shear, torsion, and compression) directly to the body and directly affect the soft tissue through techniques that normalize the connective tissue or move body fluids and intestinal contents. Myofascial tissue (muscle and its associated connective tissues) and fluid content determine the density and pliability of a muscle structure (i.e., muscle tone). Mechanical methods primarily influence muscle tone.

■ **Reflexive methods** introduce various mechanical forces into body tissues to stimulate the nervous system, the endocrine system, and the chemicals of the body. A **reflex** is an involuntary response to a stimulus, and massage can be the source of the stimulus. Reflexes are specific and predictable. They also are purposeful and adaptive, and they explain most of the benefits of massage. The length of a muscle is determined primarily by the proprioceptive aspect of the nervous system; this is called *motor tone*. Reflexive massage methods influence motor tone.

The problem with this simple categorization is that the mechanism by which massage produces an effect cannot always be clearly identified. According to Dr. Philip E. Greenman, the effects of massage occur through the interrelationships of the peripheral and central nervous systems (and their reflex patterns and multiple pathways), the autonomic nervous system (ANS), and the neuroendocrine control.[3] Dr. John Yates has said, "It appears far more reasonable just to recognize that massage produces effects that are due to a combination of mechanical, neural, chemical, and psychological factors and to identify these wherever possible rather than to attempt to use them as a basis for classifying those effects."[5]

To understand the basis of research findings, it is necessary to understand the mechanisms by which massage applications achieve benefits. This understanding is grounded in the study of functional anatomy and physiology as they relate to therapeutic massage. The recommended text for this purpose is *Mosby's Essential Sciences for Therapeutic Massage: Anatomy, Physiology, Biomechanics, and Pathology*, by Sandy Fritz (Mosby, 2008). The anatomic and physiologic areas most affected by massage are:

- The nervous/neuroendocrine system (the central, autonomic, and somatic nervous systems, as well as neurochemicals and hormones)
- Circulation
- Connective tissue
- Energy systems

The Nervous/Neuroendocrine System

The Effects of Massage on the Nervous System

The responses to massage and its effects on the nervous system are primarily reflexive.

Briefly, the nervous system is divided into the central nervous system (CNS), which consists of the brain and the spinal cord and its coverings, and the peripheral nervous system (PNS), which consists of nerves and ganglions (Figure 4-1). The PNS is further divided into the autonomic and somatic divisions. The autonomic nervous system (ANS) division is subdivided into the sympathetic and parasympathetic systems. The sympathetic system is responsible for functions that expend energy in response to emergency or arousal situations. The parasympathetic system is more restorative and normalizing and returns the body to a nonalarm state. The somatic division of the PNS is made up of the peripheral nerve fiber innervation of the body wall (e.g., muscles, joints, and other structures).

The nervous system responds to therapeutic massage methods through stimulation of sensory receptors. Feedback loops are activated that intervene and adjust various homeostatic processes. The sensory stimulation from massage disrupts an existing pattern in the CNS control centers; this results in a shift of motor impulses, most often in the PNS, that re-establishes homeostasis. Usually both the somatic and autonomic divisions of the PNS are influenced as balance is restored.

FIGURE 4-1 The divisions of the nervous system. (From Thibodeau GA, Patton KT: *The human body in health and disease,* ed 3, St Louis, 2002, Mosby.)

Neuroendocrine Interactions

To understand the benefits of massage, as defined in current research, it is important to understand the functions of some of the neuroendocrine chemicals.

The endocrine system is regulated through the influence of the nervous system, and the endocrine system in turn influences the nervous system; this is a feedback loop, similar to the thermostat on a furnace. The feedback system and autoregulation (maintenance of internal homeostasis) are interlinked with all body functions. The controls for initiation of a reaction come through the nervous system and the endocrine system. Neuroendocrine chemicals are the communication transmitters of these control systems. A neuroendocrine chemical in the synapse of the nerve is called a **neurotransmitter.** A neuroendocrine chemical carried in the bloodstream is called a **hormone.** *Neuropeptide* is another term used to describe some of these substances.

The neuroendocrine substances carry messages that regulate physiologic functions. Neuroendocrine regulation is a continuous, ever-changing chemical mix that fluctuates with each external and internal demand on the body to respond, adapt, or maintain a functional degree of homeostasis. The immune system also produces and responds to these communication substances. The substances that make up this "chemical soup" remain the same, but the proportion and ratio change with each regulating function or message transmission. The "flavor" of the soup, which is determined by the ratio of the chemical mix, affects such factors as mood, attentiveness, arousal, passiveness, vigilance, calmness, ability to sleep, receptivity to touch, response to touch, anger, pessimism, optimism, connectedness, loneliness, depression, desire, hunger, love, and commitment. Food that contains additives, synthetic substances, and sometimes excessive sugar can affect mood and behavior; this is very often seen in children but also can occur in adults.

Research now indicates that most problems in behavior, mood, and perception of stress and pain, as well as other so-called mental and emotional disorders, are caused by dysregulation or failure of the biochemicals. Problematic behaviors, symptoms, and emotional and physical states often are normal chemical mixes that occur at inappropriate times.[6] For example, anxiety indicated by increased irresolvable stress is an appropriate chemical soup to have on the mental burner in a hostage situation, because the hypervigilance accompanying such a state may allow the hostage to see an opportunity for escape. However, this same chemical soup is not productive when it is bubbling away at the mall during holiday shopping.

Early Endorphin Research. In 1969 researchers observed that pain could be eliminated in rats without the use of anesthesia by stimulating the periaqueductal gray matter in the brainstem.[7] Other important discoveries soon confirmed this finding. The work of Dr. Candice Pert and others led to the discovery of the endogenous (made in the body) endorphin and nonendorphin pain-inhibiting systems of the CNS.[13] The body produces several endogenous, opiate-like compounds, including enkephalin and beta endorphins (beta endorphin is a fragment of the pituitary hormone beta lipotropin). These peptides attach to opiate receptors (as does morphine) and, in most cases, relieve pain, especially chronic pain, and produce euphoria. This finding supports the validity of acupuncture.

Acupuncture Studies and Implications for Massage. Acupuncture is an ancient healing art that involves much more than the insertion of needles into the body. Only the most fundamental concepts of acupuncture have been studied scientifically, but that research has revealed physiologic mechanisms affected by the method. Agreement has not been reached on what acupuncture points are, but the points used in acupuncture have anatomic components. The traditional acupuncture points correspond to nerves that are close to the surface of the body. Most of the points fall over neurovascular bundles (areas of nerves and vessels), motor points (places where nerves innervate muscles), the focal meeting of superficial nerves in the sagittal plane, superficial nerves or nerve plexuses, and muscle-tendon junctions at the Golgi tendons (Figure 4-2).[8]

Rather than needles, acupressure uses specific pinpoint compression over the same points. Some evidence indicates that acupuncture exerts its analgesic effect by causing the release of enkephalins, and this analgesia is said to be blocked by the morphine antagonist naloxone. In addition, a component of stress analgesia seems to arise from endogenous opiates, because in experimental animals some forms of stress analgesia are blocked by naloxone.

Acupuncture and acupressure seem to work by taking advantage of the body's natural inhibitory influences, which normally can block pain pathways. For example, it has been established that sensory pain fibers release a neurotransmitter called *substance P,* which increases the transmission of pain impulses. Enkephalin blocks the release of substance P, thereby inhibiting pain transmission to the brain. The effects of these and other neurotransmitters released during massage may explain and validate the use of sensory stimulation methods to treat chronic pain, anxiety, and depression.[9]

The effect of acupuncture or acupressure is delayed until the enkephalin level rises to inhibitory levels. It usually takes about 15 minutes for the blood level of enkephalin to begin to rise. The implication for massage is that the pain-inhibiting effects do not occur immediately. Massage practitioners should keep this in mind with regard to the intensity and duration of applications as they work. Similarly, the effect of acupuncture lingers after the twirling or vibration of the needles stops. The implication for massage is that the client should experience a prolonged effect from the massage, one that typically lasts about 48 hours.

The Influence of Massage on Neuroendocrine Substances

Much of the research on massage, especially that done at the Touch Research Institute, revolves around shifts brought about by massage in the proportion and ratio of the chemicals that make up the body's "chemical soup."[10]

Some of the main neuroendocrine chemicals influenced by massage are:
- Dopamine
- Serotonin
- Epinephrine/adrenaline
- Norepinephrine/noradrenaline
- Enkephalins/endorphins/dynorphins
- Oxytocin
- Cortisol
- Growth hormone

Dopamine. Dopamine influences motor activity that involves movement (especially learned, fine movement such as handwriting), conscious selection (the ability to focus attention), and mood in terms of inspiration, possibility intuition, joy, and enthusiasm. Dopamine is involved in pleasure states, seeking behavior to achieve pleasure states, and the internal record system. Low levels of dopamine result in the opposite effects, such as lack of motor control, clumsiness, inability to focus attention, and boredom. Massage increases the available level of dopamine in the body and can explain the pleasure and satisfaction experienced during massage.

Serotonin. Serotonin allows a person to maintain context-appropriate behavior; that is, to do the appropriate thing at the appropriate time. It regulates mood in terms of appropriate emotions, attention to thoughts, and calming, quieting,

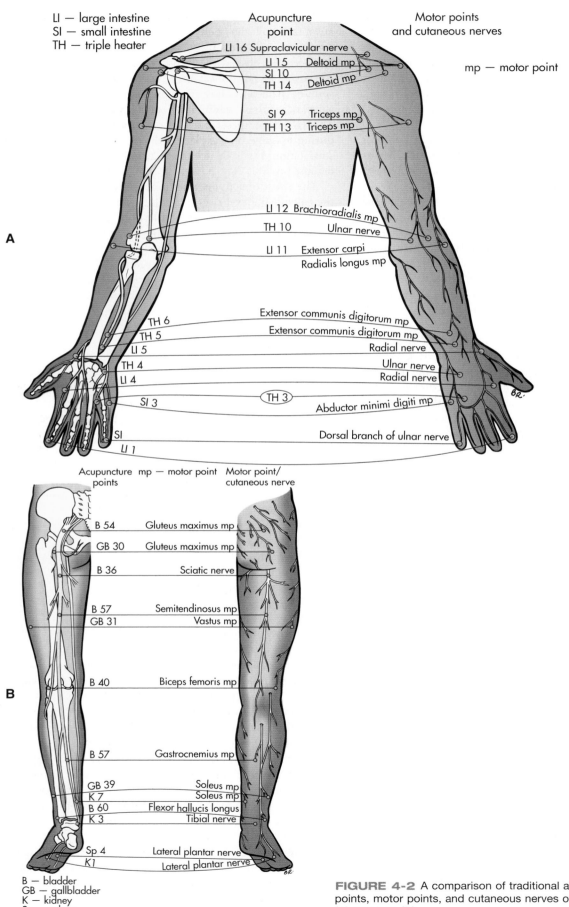

LI — large intestine
SI — small intestine
TH — triple heater

Acupuncture point

Motor points and cutaneous nerves

mp — motor point

LI 16 Supraclavicular nerve
LI 15 — Deltoid mp
SI 10
TH 14 — Deltoid mp

SI 9 — Triceps mp
TH 13 — Triceps mp

LI 12 Brachioradialis mp
TH 10 — Ulnar nerve
LI 11 — Extensor carpi
Radialis longus mp

TH 6 — Extensor communis digitorum mp
TH 5 — Extensor communis digitorum mp
LI 5 — Radial nerve
TH 4 — Ulnar nerve
LI 4 — Radial nerve
SI 3 — TH 3 — Abductor minimi digiti mp
SI — Dorsal branch of ulnar nerve
LI 1

A

Acupuncture points   mp — motor point   Motor point/cutaneous nerve

B 54 — Gluteus maximus mp
GB 30 — Gluteus maximus mp
B 36 — Sciatic nerve
B 57 — Semitendinosus mp
GB 31 — Vastus mp
B 40 — Biceps femoris mp
B 57 — Gastrocnemius mp
GB 39 — Soleus mp
K 7 — Soleus mp
B 60 — Flexor hallucis longus
K 3 — Tibial nerve
Sp 4 — Lateral plantar nerve
K 1 — Lateral plantar nerve

B

B — bladder
GB — gallbladder
K — kidney
Sp — spleen

FIGURE 4-2 A comparison of traditional acupuncture points, motor points, and cutaneous nerves of the arms (**A**) and legs (**B**).

comforting effects; it also subdues irritability and regulates drive states so that we can suppress the urge to talk, touch, and be involved in power struggles. For example, when someone tells you to "get a grip," they are saying that you could use a good boost in serotonin.

Serotonin also is involved in satiety; adequate levels reduce the sense of hunger and craving, such as for food or sex. In addition, it modulates the sleep/wake cycle. A low serotonin level has been implicated in depression, eating disorders, pain disorders, and obsessive-compulsive disorders. Massage seems to increase the available level of serotonin. A balancing effect occurs between dopamine and serotonin, much like agonist and antagonist muscles. Massage may support the optimum ratio of these chemicals.

Epinephrine/Adrenaline and Norepinephrine/Noradrenaline. The terms **epinephrine/adrenaline** and **norepinephrine/noradrenaline** are used interchangeably in scientific texts. Epinephrine activates arousal mechanisms in the body, whereas norepinephrine functions more in the brain. These are the activation, arousal, alertness, and alarm chemicals of the fight-or-flight response and of all sympathetic arousal functions and behaviors. If the levels of these chemicals are too high or if they are released at an inappropriate time, the person feels as though something very important is demanding attention or reacts with the basic survival drives of fight or flight (hypervigilance and hyperactivity). The person might have a disturbed sleep pattern, particularly a lack of rapid eye movement (REM) sleep, which is restorative sleep. With low levels of epinephrine and norepinephrine, a person is sluggish, drowsy, fatigued, and underaroused.

Massage seems to have a regulating effect on epinephrine and norepinephrine through stimulation or inhibition of the sympathetic nervous system or stimulation or inhibition of the parasympathetic nervous system. This generalized balancing function of massage seems to recalibrate the appropriate adrenaline and noradrenaline levels. Depending on the response of the ANS, massage can just as easily wake up a person and relieve fatigue as it can calm down a person who is angry and pacing the floor. It should be noted that initially, touch stimulates the sympathetic nervous system, whereas it seems to take 15 minutes or so of sustained stimulation to begin to engage the parasympathetic functions. Therefore it makes sense that a 15-minute chair massage tends to increase production of epinephrine and norepinephrine, which can help corporate workers become more attentive, whereas a 1-hour slow, rhythmic massage engages the parasympathetic functions, reducing epinephrine and norepinephrine levels and encouraging a good night's sleep.

Enkephalins, Endorphins, and Dynorphins. Enkephalins, **endorphins,** and **dynorphins** (endogenous opiates) are mood lifters that support satiety and modulate pain. Massage increases the available levels of these chemicals.

Oxytocin. Oxytocin is a hormone that has been implicated in pair or couple bonding, parental bonding, feelings of attachment, and care taking, along with its more clinical functions during pregnancy, delivery, and lactation. Massage tends to increase the available level of oxytocin, which could explain the connected and intimate feeling of massage.

Cortisol. Cortisol and other glucocorticoids are stress hormones produced by the adrenal glands during prolonged stress. Elevated levels of these hormones indicate increased sympathetic arousal. Cortisol and other glucocorticoids have been implicated in many stress-related symptoms and diseases, including suppressed immunity states, sleep disturbances, inappropriate inflammatory response, and increases in the level of substance P. Massage has been shown to reduce levels of cortisol and substance P.

Growth Hormone. Growth hormone promotes cell division and in adults has been implicated in the functions of tissue repair and regeneration. This hormone is necessary for healing and is most active during sleep. Massage increases the availability of growth hormone indirectly by encouraging sleep and reducing the level of cortisol.

Combined Neuroendocrine Influences. Massage balances the blood levels of serotonin, dopamine, and endorphins, which in turn facilitates the production of natural killer cells in the immune system and regulates mood. This response indicates that including massage in the treatment program for viral conditions, some forms of cancer, and mood disturbances would be beneficial. Oxytocin tends to increase supporting feelings of connectedness. At the same time, massage reduces cortisol and regulates epinephrine and norepinephrine, facilitating the action of growth hormone.

It is easy to see why massage is beneficial for so many conditions and indirectly influences many others. Consider the following examples:

- A lonely, depressed person feels more alive after a massage (increase in serotonin and oxytocin; decrease in cortisol).
- A child with attention deficit/hyperactivity disorder (ADHD) can do her homework after a 15-minute massage (increase in dopamine and noradrenaline).
- A person suffering from chronic pain functions better after a massage (increase in endorphin, serotonin, and oxytocin).
- A smoker trying to quit can forestall a craving for a cigarette after a massage (increase in noradrenaline, dopamine, serotonin, and endorphin).
- A person who has had surgery heals faster with massage (decrease in cortisol and adrenaline; increase in restorative sleep through pain reduction; increase in endorphin and serotonin, resulting in greater availability of growth hormone).
- An individual infected with the human immunodeficiency virus (HIV) may have a stronger immune response after massage (increase in serotonin, dopamine, and endorphin; decrease in cortisol).
- A couple may relate better to their newborn after learning to give the infant a massage (increase in serotonin and oxytocin; decrease in cortisol).

- People just feel better, cope more easily, and have more joy when massaged (neuroendocrine chemical processes give rise to higher levels of integrated thought, such as beliefs and values; interpreting context and meaning; forming intuition; making plans; and predicting, choosing, and carrying through with dreams).

Indications for massage are explored in greater depth in Chapter 5. This chapter is intended to help the student understand the current research findings that point toward neuroendocrine chemicals as a big piece of the "why massage works" puzzle.

The Autonomic Nervous System

Autonomic Influences

The effects of massage can be processed through the ANS. These effects, which are primarily reflexive, can influence the following:

- Sympathetic activation and stress
- Parasympathetic patterns and conservation withdrawal
- Entrainment
- Body/mind interaction
- Toughening/hardening
- Placebo effect

The ANS is best known for its regulation of the sympathetic "fight-flight-fear" and excitation response, and the parasympathetic "relaxation and restorative" response (Table 4-1). The sympathetic and parasympathetic systems work together to maintain homeostasis through a feedback loop system. These systems both affect and are affected by the endocrine glands. Specific muscle patterns are associated with both systems. Arm, leg, and jaw muscles may be tight during the sympathetic

response (the attack posture), whereas postural muscles often tighten with parasympathetic response (Figure 4-3).

Excessive sympathetic output causes most of the stress-related diseases physicians see, such as headaches, gastrointestinal difficulties, high blood pressure, anxiety, muscle tension and aches, and sexual dysfunction.

The ANS is regulated by several centers in the brain, particularly the cerebral cortex, hypothalamus, and medulla oblongata. The hypothalamus largely controls the ANS. It receives impulses from the visceral (organ) sensory fibers and from some somatic (muscle and joint) sensory fibers. The hypothalamus plays an important role in the body/mind connection.[11] It is one of the main components of the limbic system.

The *limbic system* is a group of brain structures, activated by emotional behavior and arousal, that influence the endocrine and autonomic systems. Limbic responses are reflected in a general alteration of mood and in feelings of well-being or distress. A property of limbic neural circuits is their prolonged afterdischarge following stimulation; this may explain why emotional responses generally are extended and outlast the stimuli that initiate them.

Research indicates that the cerebellum, the limbic pain and pleasure centers, and the various relay centers are all part of one circuit.[11] The cerebellum controls both conscious and subconscious movements of skeletal muscle, input from proprioceptors, feedback loops, posture, future positioning, and sensations of fear and pleasure.

Sympathetic Activation and Stress

Hans Selye called the body's response to stress the **general adaptation syndrome**, which he suggested can be divided into three stages:

TABLE 4-1

Functions of the Autonomic Nervous System

Component	Sympathetic Control	Parasympathetic Control
Viscera		
Heart	Accelerates heartbeat	Slows heartbeat
Smooth Muscle		
Most blood vessels	Constricts blood vessels	None
Blood vessels of skeletal muscle	None	Dilates blood vessels
Digestive tract	Decreases peristalsis; inhibits defecation	Increases peristalsis
Anal sphincter	Stimulates (closes sphincter)	Inhibits (opens sphincter for defecation)
Urinary bladder	Inhibits (relaxes bladder)	Stimulates (contracts bladder)
Urinary sphincters	Stimulates (closes sphincters)	Inhibits (opens sphincters for urination)
Iris	Stimulates radial fibers (dilation of pupil)	Stimulates circular fibers (constriction of pupil)
Ciliary muscles	Inhibits (accommodates for far vision; flattening of lens)	Stimulates (accommodates for near vision; bulging of lens)
Hair (pilomotor muscles)	Stimulates (goose bumps)	None
Glands		
Adrenal medulla	Increases secretion of epinephrine	None
Sweat glands	Increases secretion of sweat	None
Digestive glands	Decreases secretion of digestive juices	Increases secretion of digestive juices

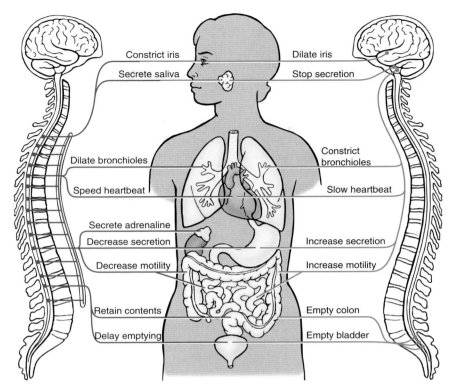

Constrict iris | Dilate iris
Secrete saliva | Stop secretion
Dilate bronchioles | Constrict bronchioles
Speed heartbeat | Slow heartbeat
Secrete adrenaline
Decrease secretion | Increase secretion
Decrease motility | Increase motility
Retain contents | Empty colon
Delay emptying | Empty bladder

FIGURE 4-3 Innervation of the major target organs by the autonomic nervous system.

1. The first stage is the *alarm reaction,* also called the *fight-or-flight response,* which is the body's initial reaction to the perceived stressor.
2. The second stage is the *resistance reaction,* which, through the secretion of regulating hormones, allows the body to continue fighting a stressor long after the effects of the alarm reaction have dissipated.
3. The third stage is the *exhaustion reaction,* which takes place if the stress response continues without relief.

Selye's general adaptation syndrome responses are commonly called sympathetic activation or sympathetic dominance. Activation of the sympathetic nervous system usually results in sensations that people call stress. Excessive stress can cause bodywide distress.[12]

So the question is, which comes first—the emotion or the release of the hormones? Science has discovered that it is rather like the chicken and the egg problem. Intense emotion, such as fear, rage, and anxiety, plays a part in activating the fight-or-flight response. The hormones epinephrine and norepinephrine are released in response to stimulation, and the alarm reaction begins. This is the stage of "do or die," "make it happen or get away." There is energy for action. The alarm reaction lasts 15 to 30 minutes. When this fight-or-flight response occurs, blood pressure increases, muscles tense, digestion and elimination shut down, circulation patterns shift, and glycogen is mobilized.

Long-term stress (i.e., stress that cannot be resolved by fleeing or fighting) may also trigger the release of cortisol, a cortisone manufactured by the body. Long-term high blood levels of cortisol cause side effects similar to those of the drug cortisone, including fluid retention, hypertension, muscle weakness, osteoporosis, breakdown of connective tissue, nonproductive inflammation, peptic ulcer, impaired wound healing, vertigo, headache, reduced ability to deal with stress, hypersensitivity, weight gain, nausea, fatigue, and psychic disturbances. This is the phase of enduring circumstances that are less than ideal and of constant vigilance in a world perceived as unsafe and hostile.

When the body can no longer tolerate the effects of stress, the exhaustion phase begins. In long-term sympathetic stress, tension builds until the body basically wears out. Cardiovascular, upper respiratory, and gastrointestinal problems tend to develop. The body begins to break down. This is the stage in which burnout occurs.

In our society most of us do not physically fight or flee from stressors, although the chemical reactions commanding these actions may be activated several times a day. So what happens to the chemicals? We each find our own way to dissipate them, such as yelling at our family or driving aggressively. Most of us would like to find more appropriate ways to release the chemicals. Moderate exercise is one of the best ways to burn up fight-or-flight chemicals (see Chapter 13).

Massage research studies have verified that the application of massage reduces sympathetic arousal.

Parasympathetic Patterns and Conservation Withdrawal

Because parasympathetic patterns are restorative, physical activity is curtailed and digestion and elimination increase. Peace and calmness are results of parasympathetic influence. When we become fatigued, parasympathetic functions signal the body to rest. Chronic fatigue syndrome is a good example of a parasympathetic reaction to stress. More drastically, depression can manifest with parasympathetic dysfunction.

Conservation withdrawal is another factor to be considered in a discussion of the parasympathetic patterns. In animals, conservation withdrawal is similar to "playing possum" or hibernation; in human beings it may arise as a result of intense negative experiences such as abuse, neglect, or starvation. To a lesser degree, conservation withdrawal patterns play a part in depression.

A massage that is more stimulating may help draw a client out of withdrawal patterns. All sensations, including touch, initially stimulate, whether they are received through visual, audio, or kinesthetic processes. Stimulation that is quick and unexpected arouses sympathetic functions. More commonly, massage encourages parasympathetic dominance and vagus nerve stimulation to counter the effects of sympathetic over-arousal.

Entrainment

Entrainment is an important reflexive effect that seems to be processed through the ANS. To entrain means "to drag with." Entrainment is the coordination or synchronization of rhythms. In the body, biologic oscillators, such as the heart and the thalamus, set the rhythm pattern. Research done at the Institute of HeartMath and other facilities indicates that the heart rhythm tends to be the guide for other body rhythms.[13] The heart rate/respiratory rate/thalamus synchronization supports the entrainment process, and the other, more subtle body rhythms follow. Synchronization of the rhythms of the heart, respiration, and digestion promotes balance, or *homeostasis,* which supports a healthy body. A balance between the sympathetic and parasympathetic divisions of the ANS influences the sinus node of the heart and the vascular systems, which in turn modulates the heart rate and blood pressure. Nasal reflexes, which are stimulated by the movement of air through the nose, rhythmically interact with the heart, lungs, and diaphragm.[14] Thus the entire body is affected because biologic rhythms are interconnected.

The body also entrains to external rhythms. Any activity that uses a repetitive motion or sound quiets or excites the nervous system (depending on the speed and pace of the rhythm) through entrainment and thereby alters the physiologic process of the body. Sometimes the body rhythms are disrupted. Music with disharmony and discord can be disruptive, as can multiple rhythms out of sync in the same environment, such as a shopping mall with flashing lights, many different types of music played at one time, and the humming of machinery. People often become fatigued or out of sorts in these disharmonic environments.

The body most easily entrains to natural rhythms, such as the sounds of a babbling brook, ocean waves, or the rustling of leaves in the breeze. Studies have shown that the rhythmic physiologic patterns of a dog's or cat's breathing or heart rate can be beneficial to the elderly. Music with a regular 4/4 beat at 60 beats per minute or slower tends to order rhythms and calm the body. A tempo faster than 60 beats per minute seems to excite physiologically, but if the rhythm is even, the body can achieve a focused, alert state. Many forms of classical music provide resourceful entrainment rhythms. Music therapy is one of the main sources of entrainment research. Music is a common addition to massage and provides an external entrainment rhythm for the practitioner and the client.

When a person experiences positive emotional states, the biologic rhythms naturally tend to begin to oscillate together, or entrain. Body entrainment processes also can be enhanced by techniques that shift the consciousness to the breathing patterns and heart rate. Most meditation processes or relaxation methods create an environment for entrainment by reducing external influences and focusing on internal rhythms, such as breathing. Many disciplines quiet the mind and body during meditation; yoga, for example, focuses attention on breathing, whereas Qigong focuses on the point below the navel. These systems center attention on body areas with known biologic oscillators. The location of the chakra system correlates with biologic oscillators. The rhythmic patterns of singing, chanting, and movement in our religious and social rituals interact with biologic patterns, resulting in a calming or exciting organization or disruption of body rhythms.

Many years of research will be required before we understand the magnitude of the influences that affect our body rhythms. Current research focuses on the possibility that disease processes might result from disruptions in body rhythms and on the effects of work environments that directly disturb or alter natural body rhythms.

The Influence of Massage on Entrainment. To encourage entrainment, massage is provided in a quiet, rhythmic manner. The rhythmic application of massage and the proximity of a centered, compassionate professional's breathing rate and heart rate can support restorative entrainment if body rhythms are out of sync. A focused, centered professional introduces his or her own ordered rhythms as part of the environment; these rhythms serve as an additional external influence that enables the client's body rhythms to synchronize. When synchronization occurs, homeostatic mechanisms seem to work more efficiently.

The Body/Mind Interaction

The ANS association is where the body/mind link is best understood. An *altered state of consciousness* is any state of awareness that differs from the normal awareness of a conscious person. Altered states of consciousness are a factor in body/mind interactions. Consciousness can be altered in many ways, such as by medications or foods that change chemical processes, by repetitive activities or sounds (entrainment), or by a trance state. For centuries many cultures and religions have explored altered states of consciousness and have used them readily in defensive actions, in healing, and in controlling pain. Meditation, tai chi, and yoga are examples of ancient methods used to achieve altered states of consciousness. We

THINK IT OVER

Rhythms tend to entrain to the rhythm that is strongest. What might happen if the practitioner is tired or a bit out of sorts while working with a client who is strongly out of sync? Who might entrain to whom? How might the professional and the client each feel? On the other hand, if the client is very focused and together, in what way might the entrainment be different?

can achieve a similar result by gardening, drawing, knitting, rocking in a rocking chair, or playing a musical instrument.

Both the practitioner and the client can achieve an altered state of consciousness during a massage session. After the altered state has been achieved, it must be maintained for at least 15 minutes to reap the most therapeutic benefit.

State-Dependent Memory. Another aspect of the body/mind connection that interacts with the ANS is state-dependent memory. The triggering of a pattern of movement or a particular pressure sensation related to pleasurable sensation or caused by trauma or learned habit sometimes is enough to enable the individual to achieve a particular altered state of consciousness, whether pleasurable or distressing. This results in a release of the chemical codes of the emotions involved in the initial memory encoding. Emotional input registers in the body through the ANS and the endocrine system. As described previously, a definite chemical factor is involved in the arousal of emotions based on the body's production of endorphins, enkephalins, epinephrine, norepinephrine, dopamine, serotonin, oxytocin, and other hormones and neurotransmitters. If these chemicals are released into the bloodstream during bodywork, the individual may once again feel the chemical arousal of an emotion, perhaps triggering a memory.

The adrenal hormones that interplay with the sympathetic responses are intimately involved with short-term memory. Norepinephrine depletion reduces memory storage, and elevation increases it. The "state" in state-dependent memory is either a sympathetic or a parasympathetic nervous system function coupled with a unique neuroendocrine chemical mix. If a person has an experience while in one of these states, the memory is encoded (stored in that state). Research shows that memory is accessible to an individual only when the particular body chemistry and function are similar to those of the experience as it first happened.[15]

Because of its effects on the ANS, massage can stimulate these state-dependent memory patterns. This can be useful in allowing the client to resolve a past experience that was irresolvable when it occurred. Often professional counseling is necessary to help the person sort out a memory pattern that is distressing and nonproductive and develop strategies for resolution, integration, and coping. These activities are outside the scope of practice for therapeutic massage; however, combined with effective counseling by trained professionals, massage can be a very beneficial part of an overall treatment plan. Exciting research currently is underway on state-dependent learning in sympathetic and parasympathetic patterns of function (see Chapter 12 for additional information) (Proficiency Exercise 4-2).

Toughening (Hardening)

The autonomic reaction to massage can be explained by a concept known as **toughening (hardening)**, which is the reaction to repeated exposure to stimuli that elicit arousal responses. The planned presentation of stimuli teaches the body to manage more efficiently with sympathetic stress responses. Forms of passive toughening, such as repeated exposure to cold shock, have been found to increase an individual's tolerance to stress. During exposure to the cold, two hormones of the adrenal medulla, epinephrine and norepinephrine, are released into the bloodstream.

Although massage is not as severe as cold shock, the increase in autonomic functioning and its passive nature may indeed be characterized as a form of passive toughening.[16] As with exercise, massage methods that require the client's active participation help dissipate sympathetic stress hormones (sympathoadrenal response), allowing the system to reestablish homeostasis (Proficiency Exercise 4-3).

PROFICIENCY EXERCISE 4-2

1. *In what way do you think the day-to-day activities listed below depend on the ANS?*
   - A person eats when tired but not hungry.

   - The driver of a car does not have to stop to use the restroom, although the children in the back seat do.

   - When the driver of the car tells the children that they are not going to stop to use the restroom and that they have to wait, the children start fighting.

   - A person's stomach starts growling half an hour after a boring lecture begins.

   - Watching a scary movie makes a person feel like doing something exciting and active.

2. *Give two other daily experiences that are influenced by the ANS.*

PROFICIENCY EXERCISE 4-3

In what way is exercise a form of "hardening"?

The Placebo Effect

Throughout history people have known that treatment in itself influences the course of a disease, even if the treatment is not specific. This placebo effect probably is caused by several mechanisms, most of which are not yet clearly understood. The environment, suggestions from and the attitude of the person giving the placebo, and the patient's confidence in its effectiveness act together to produce a placebo effect. Some studies have reported a success rate of 70% to 90% using placebos. The gentle, caring attention focused on the client during therapeutic massage may work with the powerful placebo effect.

The Influence of Massage on the Autonomic Nervous System

Because of its generalized effect on the ANS and associated functions, massage can cause changes in mood and excitement levels and can induce the relaxation and restorative response. Massage seems to be a gentle modulator, producing feelings of general well-being and comfort. However, this does not always mean that the client responds to the massage by becoming very relaxed. The most common response is a sense that "the edge is off," or there is a less urgent or intense emotional state.

The client may be better able to function in a self-regulating fashion, controlling the emotional state rather than being controlled by it. This ability to self-regulate is very important in the physiologic process. Another name for self-regulation is *internal control*. We tend to feel more at ease when we feel a sense of internal control.

Initially massage stimulates sympathetic functions. This really surprises students who think that they are giving a relaxation massage. The increase in autonomic sympathetic arousal is followed by a decrease if the massage is slowed and sustained with sufficient pleasurable pressure. To encourage more of a sympathetic response, participation in muscle energy techniques is helpful (see Chapter 9). Compression in a fast-paced massage style, similar to pre-event sports massage, stimulates sympathetic responses and may lift depression temporarily.

Slow, repetitive stroking, broad-based compression, or rhythmic movement initiates relaxation responses. It is the old "follow the watch" hypnosis induction approach. Rhythmic bodywork creates a trancelike effect. People are very open to suggestion at this time, and the therapist should be cautious of any type of leading discussion or suggestions. Sufficient pressure applied with a compressive force to the tissues supports serotonin functions.

Point holding, such as acupressure or reflexology (see Chapter 11), releases the body's own painkillers and mood-altering chemicals from the entire endorphin class. These chemicals stimulate the parasympathetic responses of relaxation, restoration, and contentment.

Acupressure causes sympathetic inhibition.[17] These methods of massage depend on the creation of a moderate, controlled pain to relieve pain. A greater pain or stress stimulus than the perception of the existing pain is required to generate the endorphin response. When the release of substance P triggers pain, enkephalins are released, suppressing the pain signal. A negative feedback system activates the release of serotonin and opiates, which inhibit pain.[7] Therapeutic massage methods can be used to create a controlled, noxious (pain) stimulation that triggers this cycle. Clients often refer to this noxious stimulation as *good pain*.

Breathing is a powerful way to interact with the ANS. Chest breathing and hyperventilation are common components of increased sympathetic stimulation. For the body to deal with stress, the muscular patterns of breathing must be normalized (see Chapter 13 for additional information on breathing). Most meditation breathing patterns, singing, and chanting are ways to normalize those patterns through entrainment.

Altering the muscles so that they are more or less tense or changing the consistency of the connective tissue affects the ANS through the feedback loop, which in turn affects the powerful body/mind phenomenon.

Somatic Influences

The effects of massage can be processed through the somatic division of the PNS; the somatic division controls movement and muscle contraction and relaxation patterns, as well as the motor tone of muscles. The length-tension relationship of a muscle is maintained through somatic influence. The *length-tension relationship* is how long or short the muscle fibers are and how this affects both the contraction ability and resting length of the muscle. A muscle that is either too short or too long cannot contract effectively. The effects of massage are primarily reflexive. Somatic effects are produced by means of the following:

- Neuromuscular mechanisms
- Hyperstimulation analgesia
- Counterirritation
- Reduction of impingement (entrapment and compression)

Neuromuscular Mechanisms

The prefix *neuro* refers to the nervous system; *muscular* refers to the muscles. The *neuromuscular effect* refers to the control of the muscles through signals from the nervous system and the response of the muscles to those signals.

Nerve cells stimulate muscles to contract or relax (release a contraction). Specialized nerve receptors called *proprioceptors* (or *mechanoreceptors*) provide a constant monitoring and protective function. Proprioceptors receive and transmit information about body position, muscle tension, static tone, degree of stretch, joint position and activity, and speed and direction of movement and equilibrium.

Dysfunction of soft tissue (muscle and connective tissue) without proprioceptive hyperactivity or hypoactivity is uncommon. Proprioceptive hyperactivity causes tense or spastic muscles and hypoactivity of opposing muscle groups. Put simply, a tight muscle area results in (or from) an inhibited (weakened) muscle area and vice versa.[18]

The three main types of proprioceptors are muscle spindles, tendon organs, and joint kinesthetic receptors.

- **Muscle spindles** are found primarily in the belly of the muscle; they respond to both sudden and prolonged stretches.
- **Tendon organs** are found in the tendon and musculotendinous junction; they respond to tension at the tendon. Articular (joint) ligaments, which have receptors similar to tendon organs, adjust reflex inhibition of the adjacent muscle when excessive strain is placed on the joints.
- **Joint kinesthetic receptors** are found in the capsules of joints; they respond to pressure and to acceleration and deceleration of joint movement. The two main types of joint kinesthetic receptors are type II cutaneous mechanoreceptors and pacinian (lamellated) corpuscles.

Somatic Reflexes. Stimulation of nervous system receptors is interpreted and processed through the somatic reflex arcs. Reflexes are fast, predictable, automatic responses to a change in the environment that help maintain homeostasis (Figure 4-4). The stimulation of therapeutic massage constitutes a change in the environment. When the body is called on to restore homeostasis, nonproductive nerve transmission pathways often are overridden.[18] The reflexes most often stimulated are the stretch reflex, tendon reflex, flexor reflex, and crossed extensor reflex.

The Stretch Reflex. The stretch reflex operates as a feedback mechanism to control muscle length by causing muscle contraction. It is activated by the muscle spindles, which sense muscle stretching. In response to massage methods that stretch muscles, a muscle spindle produces nerve impulses that stimulate a somatic sensory neuron in the posterior root of the spinal nerve. When the motor nerve impulse reaches the stretched muscle, a muscle action potential is generated, which causes the muscle to contract. Muscle contraction stops spindle cell discharge. The muscle stretch stimulates the stretch reflex, resulting in shortening of the muscle. The sensitivity of the muscle spindle in response to stretching influences the level of muscle tone throughout the body.

Therapeutic massage methods can make use of this reflex to stimulate inhibited muscle patterns by stretching the muscles and initiating the stretch reflex. An awareness of this reflex response is important in all stretches that are intended to lengthen and relax the muscles; in these instances the reflex must be avoided. Often this system of reflexes becomes hyperactive, resulting in an increase in muscle tension. Massage techniques that use isometric and isotonic muscle contraction to relax and lengthen muscles are helpful for normalizing short muscles and associated soft tissue.

The Tendon Reflex. The tendon reflex operates as a feedback mechanism to control muscle tension by causing muscle relaxation. This reflex is mediated by the tendon organs, which detect and respond to changes in muscle tension caused by the pull of muscular contraction.

The most common massage technique used to stimulate the tendon reflex is postisometric relaxation (see Chapter 9). This technique increases tension at the tendon. The tendon organ is stimulated, which sends a signal along a sensory neuron. In the spinal cord the sensory neuron synapses with an inhibitory association neuron, which inhibits motor neurons that innervate the muscle associated with the tendon organ. This inhibition causes the muscle to relax. The sensory neuron from the tendon organ also stimulates an association neuron in the spinal cord. The association neuron synapses with a motor neuron, controlling antagonistic muscles and causing them to contract. To simplify, when one muscle contracts, its antagonist, or opposing muscle group, inhibits. This is called *reciprocal innervation*. Massage practitioners can use reciprocal innervation to avoid the stretch reflex response and prepare a muscle for lengthening and stretching.

The Flexor and Crossed Extensor Reflexes. The flexor (withdrawal) and crossed extensor reflexes are polysynaptic reflex arcs. Stimulation of these reflexes affects both sides of the body through a series of intersegmental reflex arcs, which usually are linked in a pattern that includes postural muscles and muscle action in the limbs. A single sensory neuron can activate several motor neurons. The flexor reflex is involved in movement away from a stimulus, and the crossed extensor reflex is involved in maintaining balance. Synchronized control over the muscles that are contracting and those that are inhibited is achieved through contralateral reflex arcs, or

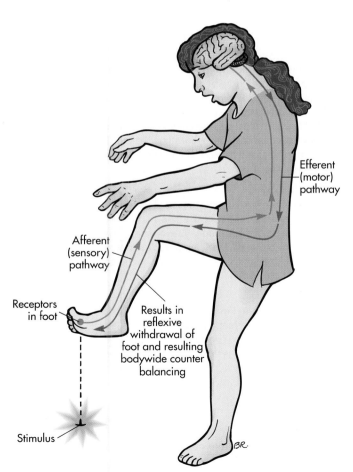

Efferent (motor) pathway

Afferent (sensory) pathway

Receptors in foot

Results in reflexive withdrawal of foot and resulting bodywide counter balancing

Stimulus

FIGURE 4-4 Reflex response. Localized stimulation of a few specific receptors leads to many outgoing impulses, which affect a large number of muscles.

reflex arcs on both sides of the body. Similar reflex patterns interact to coordinate movement; these are called *gait reflexes.* Others are involved with posture, such as the ocular pelvic reflex and righting reflexes.

By creating a noxious signal (i.e., pain or an unpleasant sensation), therapeutic massage can stimulate a withdrawal response to stimulate opposite-side patterns of tension or weakness. This is a powerful response, because withdrawal reflexes take priority over all other reflex activity occurring at the moment. If the massage application is so painful that the body tightens to guard against the noxious sensation, the effectiveness of the massage is lost. These reflex patterns also explain why tension patterns seldom occur only on one side of the body. The linked patterns of the reflex influence explain why dysfunctional patterns of groups of muscles often are identified.

The Influence of Massage on Neuromuscular Mechanisms. When working with the neuromuscular mechanism in massage, the massage therapist must keep in mind that the basic premises are (1) to substitute a different neurologic signal stimulation to support a normal muscle resting length through lengthening and stretching or strengthening of muscles and connective tissue and (2) to re-educate the muscles involved (e.g., take the joint through its increased range of motion).

Movement, stretch, and pressure methods of massage focus on the activities of the muscles, tendons, joints, and ligaments to stimulate the proprioceptors. Massage methods can stimulate the resetting of unproductive reflex actions.

The effects of therapeutic massage depend heavily on the reflex mechanism. The effectiveness of the techniques depends on how efficiently the receptors for these reflexes are stimulated. The targeted receptor must be accessed with the appropriate technique and intensity so that the stimulated reflex can function appropriately.

Various neurologic laws come into play to help explain the effects of therapeutic massage on the somatic nervous system (Box 4-3). A **law** is a scientific statement that is uniformly true for a whole class of natural occurrences.

Some controversy exists about the validity of some of these laws, primarily Pflüger's laws; however, it is valid to consider these neurologic laws in attempting to understand the physiologic effects of massage.

BOX 4-3

Laws of Neurology and Their Implications for Massage

Arndt-Schulz Law
Weak stimuli activate physiologic processes; very strong stimuli inhibit them.[20]
Implication for massage: To encourage a specific response, use gentler methods. To shut off a response, use deeper methods.

Bell's Law
Anterior spinal nerve roots are motor roots, and posterior spinal nerve roots are sensory roots.[21]
Implication for massage: Massage along the spine is a strong sensory stimulation.

Bowditch's (All or None) Law
The weakest stimulus capable of producing a response produces the maximum response contraction in cardiac and skeletal muscle and nerves.[19]
Implication for massage: Techniques need not be extremely intense to produce a response; all that is needed is enough sensory stimulation to begin the process.

Cannon's Law of Denervation
When autonomic effectors are partly or completely separated from their normal nerve connections, they become more sensitive to the action of chemical substances.[22]
This denervation supersensitivity involves injured nerves, which respond to all sensory stimulation regardless of whether the stimulation is specific to that nerve. Denervation supersensitivity is a universal phenomenon that affects muscles, nerves, salivary glands, sudorific glands, autonomic ganglion cells, spinal neurons, and even neurons in the cortex. Changes in muscle structure and biochemistry also occur, as does progressive destruction of the contractile elements of fibers.

Furthermore, unlike normal muscle fibers, which resist innervation from foreign nerves, degenerated muscle fibers accept contacts from other motor nerves, preganglionic autonomic fibers, and even sensory nerves.
Implication for massage: An injured area may hyperreact to all sensory stimulation, even after healing. If a person has a cold or is stressed at work or cannot sleep, previously injured areas may flare up.

Hilton's Law
A nerve trunk that supplies a joint also supplies the muscles of the joint and the skin over the insertions of such muscles.[21]
Implication for massage: Determining whether pain originates from the joint itself, the muscles around the joint, or the skin over the joint can be difficult; stimulation of each area affects all parts.

Hooke's Law
The stress used to stretch or compress a body is proportional to the strain experienced, as long as the elastic limits of the body have not been exceeded.[21]
Implication for massage: Methods that lengthen the tissue must be intense enough to match the existing shortening but must not exceed it.

Law of Facilitation
When an impulse has passed through a certain set of neurons to the exclusion of others one time, it will tend to take the same course on a future occasion, and each time it traverses this path, the resistance will be reduced.[20]
Implication for massage: The body likes sameness, which produces habitual patterns. After a pattern has been established, less stimulation is required to activate the response.

BOX 4-3

Laws of Neurology and Their Implications for Massage—cont'd

Law of Specificity of Nervous Energy

Excitation of a receptor always gives rise to the same sensation, regardless of the nature of the stimulus.[21]

Implication for massage: Whatever the method used, if a sensory receptor is activated, it will respond in a specific way.

Newton's Law

When two bodies interact, the force exerted by the first on the second is equal in magnitude and opposite in direction to the force exerted by the second on the first.

Implication for massage: This law explains various aspects of pressure delivery during massage. When two bodies interact (the massage therapist and the client), the force extended by the first (the massage therapist) on the second (the client) is equal in magnitude and opposite in direction (i.e., the client's body will push back). The point where they meet is a point of balance. This is especially important in body mechanics and with regard to the way tissue binds in response to pressure.

Pflüger's Laws

Law of Generalization

When an irritation becomes very intense, it is propagated in the medulla oblongata, which becomes a focus from which stimuli radiate to all parts of the cord, causing a general contraction of all muscles in the body.[20]

Implication for massage: This response must be avoided if possible. It is important to keep invasive massage measures (e.g., frictioning) below the intensity level that causes a general body response.

Law of Intensity

Reflex movements usually are more intense on the side of irritation; at times the movements of the opposite side equal the movements in intensity, but they usually are less pronounced.[20]

Implication for massage: See Law of Symmetry.

Law of Radiation

If excitation continues to increase, it is propagated upward, and reactions take place through centrifugal nerves coming from the higher cord segments.[20]

Implication for massage: See Law of Symmetry.

Law of Symmetry

If stimulation is increased sufficiently, a motor reaction is manifested not only on the irritated side but also in similar muscles on the opposite side of the body.[20]

Implication for massage: By using increasing levels of massage intensity, a bilateral effect can be created, even if only one side of the body is massaged. This is especially useful for massage applications to painful areas. By massaging the unaffected side, the painful areas can be addressed without receiving direct massage work.

Law of Unilaterality

If a mild irritation is applied to one or more sensory nerves, movement will take place usually on one side only and on the side that has been irritated.[20]

Implication for massage: Light stimulation remains fairly localized in response to massage.

Weber's Law

The increase in stimulus necessary to produce the smallest perceptible increase in sensation bears a constant ratio to the strength of the stimulus already acting.[21]

Implication for massage: To change a sensory perception, the intensity of a massage method must match and then just exceed the existing sensation.

Wolf's Law

Biologic systems (including soft and hard tissues) deform in relation to the lines of force imposed on them.

Implication for massage: Massage is the application of mechanical force. Massage therefore deforms tissue.

The Vestibular Apparatus and Cerebellum. The vestibular apparatus is a complex system composed of sensors in the inner ear (vestibular labyrinth), upper neck (cervical proprioception), eyes (visual motion and three-dimensional orientation), and body (somatic proprioception). These sensors send messages that are analyzed in several areas of the brain (brainstem, cerebellum, parietal and temporal cortices) and that affect the eyes (vestibulo-ocular reflexes), neck (vestibulocollic reflexes), and balance (vestibulospinal reflexes), while at the same time keeping us aware of where we are and how we are moving through the world (visuospatial orientation). A system this complex deserves to be called a sense, such as our sense of hearing, sense of sight, and so on.

The vestibular apparatus and the cerebellum are interrelated. The output from the cerebellum goes to the motor cortex and brainstem. Stimulating the cerebellum by altering muscle tone, position, and vestibular balance stimulates the hypothalamus to adjust ANS functions to restore homeostasis.

The Influence of Massage on the Vestibular Apparatus and Cerebellum. The techniques that most strongly affect the vestibular apparatus and therefore the cerebellum are those that incorporate rhythmic rocking into the application of massage. Rocking produces movement at the neck and head that influences the sense of equilibrium. Rocking stimulates the inner ear balance mechanisms, including the vestibular nuclear complex and the labyrinthine righting reflexes, to keep the head level. Pressure on the sides of the body may stimulate the body-righting reflex. Stimulation of these reflexes produces a bodywide effect involving stimulation of muscle contraction patterns, which pass throughout the body.

Massage alters body positional sense and the position of the eyes in response to postural change; it also initiates specific movement patterns that change sensory input from muscles, tendons, joints, and the skin and stimulates various vestibular reflexes. This feedback information, which adjusts and coordinates movement, is relayed directly to the motor cortex and the cerebellum, allowing the body to integrate the sensory data and adjust to a more efficient homeostatic balance.

Hyperstimulation Analgesia

In 1965 Melzack and Wall proposed the gate control theory. Although some aspects of the original theory have been modified over the past 40 years, the basic premise remains the same. According to this theory, a gating mechanism functions at the level of the spinal cord; that is, pain impulses pass through a "gate" to reach the lateral spinothalamic system. Painful impulses are transmitted by large-diameter and small-diameter nerve fibers. Stimulation of large-diameter fibers prevents the small-diameter fibers from transmitting signals. Stimulation (e.g., rubbing, massaging) of large-diameter fibers helps suppress the sensation of pain, especially sharp pain.

The skin over the entire body is supplied by spinal nerves that carry somatic sensory nerve impulses to the spinal cord. Each spinal nerve serves a specific segment of the skin, called a *dermatome*. Dermatomes, which can be affected by massage techniques that stimulate the skin, may account for hyperstimulation analgesia. The reduction of pain through stimulation (hyperstimulation analgesia) produced by massage and acupuncture has been used for many years.[8] In recent years transcutaneous electrical nerve stimulation (TENS) has become a popular method of producing hyperstimulation analgesia.

Massage and the Production of Hyperstimulation Analgesia. Stimulation of the PNS may produce analgesia by inducing neurophysiologic and neurohumoral inhibitory effects at the spinal gating mechanism (gate control theory). Evidence suggests that the development of analgesia depends on the stimulation of specific points in the muscle that correspond to certain types of muscle receptors. These same points correspond with many traditional acupuncture points (see Figure 4-2). If massage stimulates these points at a sufficient intensity, the large-diameter fibers can be stimulated and the gating mechanism and hyperstimulation analgesia may be activated.

Tactile stimulation produced by massage travels through the large-diameter fibers. These fibers also carry a faster signal. In essence, massage sensations win the race to the brain, and the pain sensations are blocked because the gate is closed. Many parents and small children seem to know this instinctively. They rub the injured spot, thus activating large-diameter fibers. Stimulating techniques, such as percussion or vibration of painful areas to activate stimulation-produced analgesia (hyperstimulation analgesia), also are effective.

Counterirritation

Taber's Cyclopedic Medical Dictionary defines counterirritation as superficial irritation that relieves some irritation of deeper structures.[21] Counterirritation may be explained by the gate control theory. Inhibition in central sensory pathways, produced by rubbing or shaking an area, may explain counterirritation. Noxious stimuli suppress nociceptive (pain) impulses. Changing the perception of pain by introducing a different pain signal is akin to stepping on a person's foot to relieve the pain in the thumb just hit by a hammer.

Inhibition in central sensory pathways may explain the effect of counterirritants. Stimulation of the skin over an area of pain or dysfunction produces some relief from the pain. The old-fashioned mustard plaster works on this principle, and various rubs and creams on the market also work in this manner.

Massage and the Production of Counterirritation. All methods of massage can be used to produce counterirritation. Many people have learned from practical experience that touching or shaking an injured area diminishes the pain of the injury. Any massage method that introduces a controlled sensory stimulation intense enough to be interpreted by the client as a "good pain" will work to create counterirritation. Massage therapy in many forms stimulates the skin over an area of discomfort. Techniques that result in reddening of the skin and underlying tissue (histamine response) are effective. Compression and movement methods require the body to attend to a different signal and temporarily ignore the original discomfort (Proficiency Exercise 4-4).

Trigger Points

No one is quite sure exactly what a trigger point is. A plethora of terms, including *myalgia, myositis, fibrositis, fibromyalgia, myofibrositis, fibromyositis, fasciitis, myofascitis, rheumatism, fibrositic nodule,* and *myogelosis* all seem to describe the myofascial trigger point.[18] For the purposes of this text, a trigger point is an area of local nerve facilitation in the muscle or associated connective tissue that creates small areas of shortening or microspasm. These points are sensitive to pressure and, when stimulated, can become the site of painful

---

 PROFICIENCY EXERCISE 4-4

Describe two more types of counterirritation.

sensation. Dr. Janet Travell spent much of her professional career researching and developing a treatment for myofascial trigger points.

Opinions differ as to whether trigger points are more a neuromuscular or a connective tissue phenomenon. Fortunately, the kinds of pathophysiologic mechanisms responsible for the development of trigger points are becoming clear, and the different mechanisms may explain why some therapeutic approaches are so effective and why others are of limited benefit for this condition.

Muscles with trigger points feel abnormal when palpated and have a reduced range of motion because of the increased tension of the palpable taut band that is associated with the trigger points. This palpable increase in muscle tension is commonly mistaken for muscle spasm. Muscle spasm is clearly identified by motor unit activity that is identified electromyographically, whereas taut bands show no motor unit activity at rest.

The increased tension of the palpable taut band is the result of regional shortening of the sarcomeres of involved muscle fibers in the taut band. In the region of a motor endplate, the sarcomeres in the area are hypercontracted; the remaining sarcomeres of an involved muscle fiber are noticeably stretched to compensate for the missing length of the shortened sarcomeres. Because of the nature of actin (the springlike molecule that holds the myosin molecules in place), the maximally contracted sarcomeres would tend to become stuck in this shortened position. The effect of these shortened sarcomeres is one likely source of increased resting tension in an involved muscle fiber.

The Effect of Massage on Trigger Points. Travell, Simons, and others suggest that the effects of massage on myofascial trigger points are a result of stimulation of proprioceptive nerve endings, changes in sarcomere length, release of enkephalin, stretching of musculotendinous structures that initiate reflex muscle relaxation through the Golgi tendon organ and spindle receptors, and increased circulation.[7,18,23,24]

Various massage methods, including pressure, positioning, and lengthening, provide this stimulation. (Trigger points are discussed in detail in Chapter 11.)

Nerve Impingement (Entrapment, Compression)

Soft tissue often impinges upon a nerve, a condition commonly called *pinched nerve.* Tissues that can bind include skin, fascia, muscles, ligaments, joint structures, and bones. Short muscles and stiff, dense connective tissue (fascia) often impinge upon major and minor nerves, causing discomfort.

Entrapment and compression are technically different dysfunctions. Entrapment results when soft tissue (e.g., muscles and ligaments) exerts inappropriate pressure on nerves. Compression occurs when hard tissue (e.g., bone) exerts inappropriate pressure on nerves.

Regardless of the source of impingement, the symptoms are similar; however, the therapeutic intervention is different. Soft tissue approaches are beneficial for entrapment but less so for compression.

The Effect of Massage on Nerve Impingement. Because of the structural arrangement of the body, impingement often occurs at major nerve plexuses (Figure 4-5). The specific nerve root, trunk, or division affected determines the condition, such as thoracic outlet syndrome, sciatica, or carpal tunnel syndrome. Therapeutic massage techniques work in many ways to reduce pressure on nerves. The main ways are to (1) reflexively change the motor tone pattern and lengthen the muscles, (2) mechanically stretch and soften connective tissue, and (3) interrupt the pain-spasm-pain cycle caused by protective muscle spasm that occurs in response to pain.

The Effect of Massage on the Somatic Nervous System. Massage methods directly stimulate the reflex mechanisms of the somatic functions. In fact, the bulk of the influence of massage is exerted through the somatic stimulation. Often the ANS and the endocrine system are influenced by secondary reflex activity in response to homeostatic changes caused by somatic

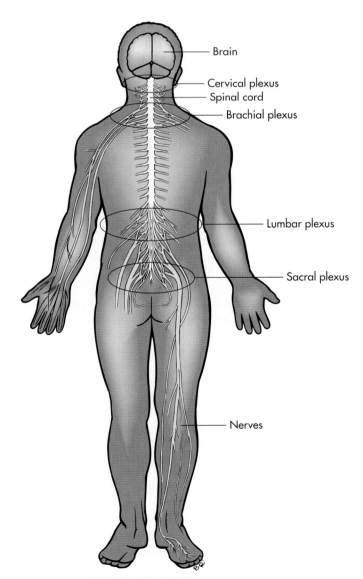

FIGURE 4-5 Major nerve plexuses.

Brain
Cervical plexus
Spinal cord
Brachial plexus
Lumbar plexus
Sacral plexus
Nerves

THINK IT OVER

Why might a combination of manipulations, such as chiropractic and massage, be a valid method of dealing with nerve impingement?

stimulation during massage. All massage methods are effective. The specific result depends on precise communication with the somatic sensory receptor. It is a language of pressure, pull, and movement.

Circulation

Three to five basic types of circulation have been recognized. All anatomy texts recognize arterial, venous, and lymphatic circulation. The other two types discussed in this text are respiratory and cerebrospinal fluid (CSF) circulation. These five systems depend on the pumping action of the skeletal muscles as they contract and relax. Arterial flow has the additional pumping action provided by the heart and muscle tissue in the arteries. Recent research indicates that the lymphatic system has its own rhythmic pumping action. The implication is that some of the benefits of massage may be a result of its influence on this rhythm.[25] These circulatory functions are both directly linked and interdependent. For example, the carbon dioxide level of the CSF affects the respiratory center in the medulla, helping to control breathing.

Increases in the blood and lymph circulations are the most widely recognized physiologic effects of massage therapy. According to Yates, many studies validate the increase in lymphatic movement caused by massage. Application of a mechanical device that produced a rhythmic massage in a proximal direction reduced edema, increased lymphatic movement from the tissues to the blood, and improved blood circulation.[5]

The Effect of Massage on Circulation. Increased blood flow on a local level is achieved by compression of tissues, which empties venous beds, lowers venous pressure, and increases capillary blood flow, which is quickly counteracted by autoregulation. Massage stimulates the release of vasodilators, especially histamine. Blood flow changes also may be induced through the autonomic vascular reflexes. This type of increase in blood flow has a bodywide effect. Compression against arteries mechanically influences the internal pressure receptors in the arteries. It seems that there is no way to avoid affecting the blood and lymph circulations in giving a massage. Massage and other forms of bodywork mimic and assist the pumping action of the muscle and respiratory pump.

The massage practitioner must know the anatomy and physiology of the blood and lymph circulations to understand the effect of massage on these systems. Circulation enhancement is fairly straightforward. Although it is true that more body fluids are moved by a 5-minute walk than by a 50-

minute massage, for those unable to walk or even get out of bed, manual facilitation of the movement of body fluids can be a viable and significant therapeutic option.

Arterial Flow. Arteries carry blood under pressure from the heart as a result of the pumping action of the heart muscle. The arteries themselves also have a muscular component that contracts rhythmically, facilitating arterial flow. Direct compression into the area of an artery effectively crimps the artery, much like crimping a hose, and allows some back pressure to build up. When the pressure is released, the blood rushes through like a waterfall. Arteries are accessible to compressive pressure on the soft medial areas of the arms and legs. Compressions should begin proximal to the heart and move in a distal direction. Heavy pressure or sustained compression is not necessary; rather, moderate pressure is used in the right location to pump rhythmically at the client's current heart rate as the practitioner moves distally toward the fingers or toes.

An increase in arterial flow is beneficial in any situation in which an increase in oxygenated blood is desirable. Such situations include sluggish circulation in a sedentary person or increased demand in an athlete (see Chapter 11).

Venous Return Flow. Venous return flow largely depends on contraction of the muscles against the veins. Back flow of blood is prevented by valves. Veins usually run more superficially than arteries. Because of the valve system in the veins and the fact that the blood is intended to flow back toward the heart, strokes to encourage venous flow move toward the heart. Short pumping, gliding, effleurage strokes are most effective in enhancing this flow.

Passive and active joint movements also encourage the muscles to contract against the deeper vessels, assisting venous blood flow. If this is not possible for the client, slow, meticulous mechanical work is required to drain the area. Placing the limb above the heart, allowing gravity to assist, is beneficial (see Chapter 11).

Lymphatic Drainage. The massage procedures for lymphatic drainage are similar to those for venous return. Because lymph vessels open into tissue space (interstitial space), surface work that pulls gently on the skin is performed over the entire affected body region instead of being focused over only the major veins. Pumping of jointed areas with passive joint movement seems to assist the movement of lymph through the areas of lymph node filtration. Deep breathing assists lymph movement in the thorax and abdomen. Unless the massage therapist is using manual lymphatic drainage as a specific therapeutic intervention in cases of a pathologic condition of the lymphatic system, it does not seem to be necessary to be precise about specific flow patterns. It is important to note that the lower abdomen (from the umbilicus down) drains into the inguinal area and eventually into the thoracic duct and that the right side (right arm and head) drains into the right lymphatic duct. Both major vessels dump into the vena cava (see Chapter 11).

Respiration

The muscular mechanism for the inhalation and exhalation of air is designed like a simple bellows system and depends on unrestricted movement of the musculoskeletal components of the thorax. The muscles of respiration include the scalenes, intercostals, serratus anterior diaphragm, abdominals, pelvic floor muscles, and lower leg muscles (which surprises many people). This can be demonstrated by contracting any of these muscle groups and attempting to take a deep breath; you will note that the ability to breathe is restricted. Disruption of function in any of these groups inhibits complete and easy breathing. Often subclinical overbreathing, called **breathing pattern disorder,** occurs, which causes many physical symptoms (Box 4-4).

Physiologists define *hyperventilation* as abnormally deep or rapid breathing in excess of physical demands. Dyspneic fear (no air) is a core factor in the cause of panic attacks, which result in rapid breathing.

The Effect of Massage on Respiration. All massage approaches that restore mobility to the thorax and the muscles of respiration affect the ability to breathe. Particularly with breathing pattern disorder, breathing retraining often is ineffective because the mobility of the respiratory mechanism is disrupted. Often massage can restore the normal function of the soft tissue involved with breathing, allowing breathing retraining to become effective.

Cerebrospinal Fluid Circulation

CSF cools, nourishes, and protects the brain and nerves and influences breathing through carbon dioxide levels. The movement of CSF has a pumping rhythm that some contend can be palpated. This rhythm seems to affect the phenomenon of fascial movement and is independent of the other body rhythms. Entrainment is implicated as a factor in fascial movement, as is lymphatic undulation.[25] More research must be done before the anatomic and physiologic mechanisms of the fascial movement phenomenon can be understood scientifically. Techniques of craniosacral therapy specifically target CSF circulation (Figure 4-6).[2] General massage also may influence this mechanism indirectly.

BOX 4-4

Breathing Pattern Disorder

Breathing pattern disorder is a complex set of behaviors that leads to overbreathing despite the absence of a pathologic condition. It is considered a functional syndrome because all the parts are working effectively, therefore a specific pathologic condition does not exist. Instead, the breathing pattern is inappropriate for the situation, producing confused signals to the central nervous system and resulting in a chain of events.

Increased ventilation is a common component of the fight-or-flight response. However, when the breathing rate increases but the body's actions and movements are restricted or do not increase accordingly, the person is breathing in excess of the metabolic need. Blood levels of carbon dioxide (CO_2) fall, and symptoms may occur. Because the person exhales too much CO_2 too quickly, the blood becomes more acidic. These biochemical changes can cause many of the following signs and symptoms:

- *Cardiovascular effects:* Palpitations, missed beats, tachycardia, sharp or dull atypical chest pain, "angina," vasomotor instability, cold extremities, Raynaud's phenomenon, blotchy flushing of the blush area, and capillary vasoconstriction (face, arms, hands)
- *Neurologic effects:* Dizziness; unsteadiness or instability; a sensation of faintness or giddiness (rarely actual fainting); visual disturbance (blurred or tunnel vision); headache (often migraine); paresthesia (numbness, uselessness, heaviness, pins and needles, burning, limbs feeling out of proportion or as if they "don't belong"), commonly of the hands, feet, or face but sometimes of the scalp or whole body; intolerance of light or noise; and enlarged pupils (needing to wear dark glasses on a dull day)
- *Respiratory effects:* Shortness of breath, typically after exertion; irritable cough; tightness or oppression of chest; difficulty breathing; "asthma"; air hunger; inability to take a satisfying breath; excessive sighing, yawning, and sniffing
- *Gastrointestinal effects:* Difficulty swallowing, dry mouth and throat, acid regurgitation, heartburn, hiatal hernia, nausea, flatulence, belching, air swallowing, abdominal discomfort, and bloating
- *Muscular effects:* Cramps, muscle pain (particularly in the occipital area, neck, shoulders, and between the scapulae; less commonly in the lower back and limbs), tremors, twitching, weakness, stiffness, or tetany (seizing up)
- *Psychological effects:* Tension, anxiety, "unreal" feelings, depersonalization, feeling "out of body," hallucinations, fear of insanity, panic, phobias, and agoraphobia
- *General effects:* Feelings of weakness; exhaustion; impaired concentration, memory, and performance; disturbed sleep, including nightmares; emotional sweating (axillae, palms, and sometimes the whole body); and woolly or thick head

Cerebrovascular constriction, a primary response to breathing pattern disorder, can reduce the oxygen available to the brain by about one half. Among the resulting symptoms are dizziness, blurring of consciousness, and, possibly, because of a decrease in cortical inhibition, tearfulness and emotional instability.

Other effects of breathing pattern disorder for which massage therapists should watch are generalized body tension and chronic inability to relax. In addition, individuals with a tendency for breathing pattern disorder are particularly prone to spasm (tetany) in muscles involved in the "attack posture"; they hunch their shoulders, thrust the head and neck forward, scowl, and clench their teeth.[23]

Connective Tissue

Connective tissue, the structural component of the body, is the most abundant body tissue. Its functions include support, structure, space, stabilization, and scar formation. It assumes many forms and shapes, from fluid blood to dense bone. The pliability of connective tissue, which is based on its water-binding components, is significant in effective connective tissue support and function. Connective tissue is adaptive and responsive to a variety of influences, such as injury, immobilization, overuse (increased demand), and underuse (decreased demand).

Connective tissue is made up of various fibers and cells in a gelatinous ground substance. In bone this ground substance is impregnated with minerals that harden the bone. The combination of the fibers and the cells that produce the fibers and the ground substance is called the *connective tissue matrix.*

During ANS sympathetic arousal, the ground substance thickens to provide protection from impact trauma. Enzyme action reverses this process during parasympathetic dominance. Healing of damage to body tissues requires the formation of connective tissue. The inflammatory response is one trigger that generates the healing process. Occasionally, more tissue than is needed forms, and adhesions develop. An adhesion is a binding of connective tissue to structures not directly involved with the area of injury. Fascia is a form of connective tissue that forms in sheets. Fascia is embedded with smooth muscle bundles that contribute to fascial tone (tautness).

In areas of *acute* (active) dysfunction, connective tissue initially may not play a role in the dysfunctional pattern. Connective tissue dysfunction usually is suspected as a factor in disorders older than 12 weeks.[26]

With overuse, additional connective tissue is formed to provide stabilization to the musculoskeletal areas involved. When the soft tissue problem is chronic, the connective tissue becomes fibrotic and involves areas surrounding the dysfunctional area.[26] After this has occurred, either of the following conditions may exist:

- The connective tissue may have thickened or thinned, or it may have dried out or become water-logged.
- Ligaments and tendons may fail to support joint stabilization, or the connective tissue may bind, restricting movement and function.

Piezoelectricity is an electrical current produced by applying pressure to certain crystals such as mica, quartz, or Rochelle salt. Collagen fibers of connective tissue have a piezoelectric property. The piezoelectric phenomenon in some way affects the connective tissue properties. With its piezoelectric properties, the collagen portion of connective tissue may be the link to energy-related forms of bodywork.

FIGURE 4-6 The flow of cerebrospinal fluid (CSF). Filtration of the blood by the choroid plexus of each ventricle produces the CSF, which flows inferiorly through the lateral ventricles, the interventricular foramen, the third ventricle, the cerebral aqueduct, the fourth ventricle, and the subarachnoid space into the blood. (From Thibodeau GA, Patton KT: *The human body in health and disease,* ed 3, St Louis, 2002, Mosby.)

The Effect of Connective Tissue Methods

Connective tissue massage was formalized in 1929 by Elizabeth Dicke, a German physiotherapist. Dr. James Cyriax also contributed extensively through his research on deep transverse friction massage. Fibrotic tissue responds well to the specific approaches of connective tissue massage (see Chapter 11). Studies indicate that massage may reduce the formation of adhesions and the scarring that often results from soft tissue injury. Similar approaches for the fascial or connective tissue component of muscles are called *myofascial techniques.* Connective tissue methods are primarily mechanical.

Connective tissue methods primarily affect the body structure. Methods that directly address the connective tissue do so by mechanically changing the consistency and pliability of the connective tissue, usually by softening it, and by creating physical space in the body. Mechanical dysfunctions call for more direct methods and depend on an actual physiologic change in the area. Cross-fiber frictioning (see Chapters 9 and 11) and inhibitory (direct) pressure approaches (see Chapter 9) are examples of mechanical massage methods. Mechanical force influences the smooth muscle bundles in fascia.

Massage methods most often affect the superficial and deep fascial sheaths, the ligaments, and the tendons. Three basic approaches are used:

- Methods that address the ground substance, which is *thixotropic,* meaning that the substance liquefies on agitation and reverts to gel when standing. Ground substance is also a colloid. A *colloid* is a system of solids in a liquid medium that resists abrupt pressure but yields to slow, sustained pressure.
- Methods that address the fibers within the ground substance; the fibers are collagenous (ropelike), elastic (rubber band–like), or reticular (meshlike).
- Methods that influence fascial tone through direct stimulus of muscle bundles and indirectly through influence of the nervous system.

Methods that primarily affect the ground substance have a quality of slow, sustained pressure and agitation. The shearing, bending, and torsion forces and tensile stretch applied during massage add energy to the matrix and soften it. Most massage methods can soften the ground substance as long as the application is not abrupt. Abrupt tapotement and compression (see Chapter 9) are less effective than slow, gliding methods that have a drag quality. Kneading and skin rolling (see Chapter 9) that incorporate a slow pulling action are effective as well. Parasympathetic activation helps create connective tissue pliability by effecting smooth muscle contraction and chemical response.

The fiber component is affected by methods that elongate the fibers past the elastic range (i.e., past the normal give) into the plastic range (i.e., past the bind or point of restriction). This creates either a freeing and unraveling of fibers or a small therapeutic (beneficial and controlled) inflammatory response that signals for change in the fibers. Transverse friction (see Chapter 11) also creates therapeutic inflammation.

Massage that provides for a gentle, sustained pull on the fascial component stimulates fascial smooth muscle bundles and cutaneovisceral (skin to organ) reflexes, and together with autonomic reflex pathways and endocrine responses produces the bodywide reactions to connective tissue massage. Connective tissue massage helps to harmonize the relationship between the sympathetic and parasympathetic divisions of the ANS. It also helps to normalize the circulation between organs and organ systems and other tissues. Locally, it improves the blood supply of the surface tissues in the area treated, especially in the particular connective tissue element. Connective tissue applications using massage methods are specifically addressed in Chapter 11.

Energy Systems (Biofields)

On the basis of the information presented thus far, we can begin to form a picture of the energy systems in the living body. Both styles of massage, mechanical and reflexive, influence the energy component of the body by stimulating electrochemical, electromagnetic, and piezoelectric effects.

Technology is just now enabling researchers to measure this subtle component of the body. Consequently, the validity of the effectiveness of any method based on the reaction of the electrochemical, electromagnetic, or piezoelectric component of the body is controversial. The terms *subtle energies* or *biofield therapies* cover a wide range of techniques that affect the subtle electrical fields of the body. These electrical fields exist. Animal behavior studies have shown that the platypus detects a living food source by sensing the weak electrical field around its prey.[27]

The connective tissues form a mechanical three-dimensional network continuum, extending throughout the body, even into the innermost parts of each cell. All movement, of the body as a whole or of its smallest parts, is created by tensions carried through the connective tissue structure.[28]

Each force introduced to or generated by the body causes the crystalline lattice of the connective tissues to generate piezobioelectronic signals that are precisely characteristic of those tensions, compressions, and movements. Stimulation of a piezomaterial causes either generation of electrical currents or a vibration. The connective tissue fabric is a semiconducting communication network that can carry the bioelectronic signals between every part of the body.

Tensegrity is an architectural principle developed in 1948 by R. Buckminster Fuller (Figures 4-7 to 4-9). The tensegrity principle is the foundation of the geodesic dome. A tensegrity system is characterized by a continuous tensional network (tendons, ligaments, and fascial structures) that is connected by a discontinuous set of compressive elements, or struts (bones). A tensegrity structure forms a stable yet dynamic system that interacts efficiently and resiliently with forces acting upon it. Attach tendons and muscles to the bones, and a three-dimensional tensegrity network emerges that supports and moves the body. Tensegrity of the body form explains how inflexibility or shortening in one tissue influences structure and movement in other parts.[28]

These concepts are useful for massage practitioners who work with athletes and other performers in whom flexible and well-organized fascia and myofascial relationships enhance

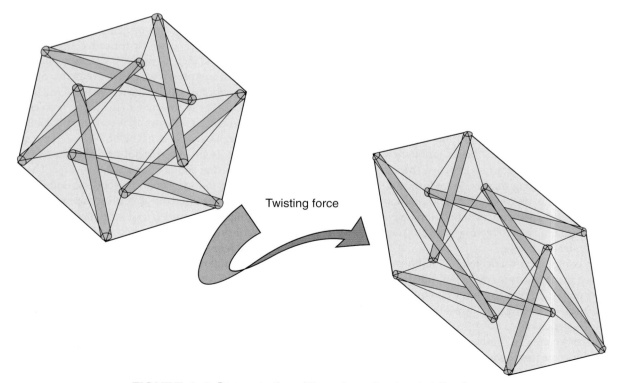

FIGURE 4-7 An abstract image of a cell that is kept together by tensegrity.

FIGURE 4-9 The head of the femur, a tensegrity structure, as it uses both compression and tension-resisting elements to support weight. (Modified from Oschman JL: *Energy medicine: the scientific basis,* London, 2000, Churchill Livingstone.)

Twisting force

FIGURE 4-8 Demonstration of the cell reacting to a twisting force.

performance and reduce the incidence of injuries. Because the living tensegrity network is both a mechanical and a vibratory network, restrictions in one part have both structural and energetic consequences for the entire organism.

Current research summarized here points to a remarkable model that may explain the unusual emissions of Qi, or "healing energy," and other phenomena observed in a wide variety of energy therapies. What these practices have in common seems to be periodic entrainments of brain waves and whole body biomagnetic emissions with the Schumann resonances in the earth's atmosphere. The Schumann resonance, in turn, is governed by terrestrial and extraterrestrial rhythms produced by cyclic astronomic activities. The result may be whole body collective oscillation, entrained with geophysical fields, involving virtually all of the billions of collagen cells, membrane phospholipid, and contractile protein molecules throughout the body, and possibly the associated water molecules. Brain electrical activity (measured by electroencephalography [EEG]) and the biomagnetic emissions from the body (measured with magnetometers) seem to be linked to the healing responses.

The thalamus maintains the rhythms, and "free-run" periods allow the brain waves to be entrained by rhythmic micropulsations that are tied to terrestrial and extraterrestrial rhythms. It is during these free-runs that we extract information on rhythms taking place in our environment.

Early in the twentieth century it was discovered that the various organs in the body produce electrical fields that can be detected on the skin. This led to important clinical tools, such as electrocardiography and electroencephalography. The laws of physics dictate that when electrical currents flow through tissues, magnetic fields must be created in the surrounding region. However, instruments to detect these fields were not developed until the 1950s. The superconducting quantum interference device (SQUID) magnetometer is being used in medical research laboratories around the world to map the biomagnetic fields produced by various organs. This has led to new clinical tools, such as magnetocardiography and magnetoencephalography.[15]

Medical researchers have explored the application of electric and magnetic fields to stimulate healing. Pulsing magnetic fields can also be emitted from the human hand under certain conditions. Sensitive photometers and thermographic imaging techniques have enabled scientists to map the patterns of light and heat emitted by cells, tissues, organs, and the whole body.

Spectroscopic methods reveal the roles of energy fields in molecular processes, including hormone-receptor, antibody-antigen, and allergic interactions. Spectroscopy provides the basis for pharmacology, homeopathy, aromatherapy, and herbal medicines.

Cell biologists are recognizing that nuclear, cytoplasmic, and extracellular matrices form a continuous and interconnected communication system that plays a key role in the integration of functions, including injury repair and defense against disease. Tensegrity concepts explain the various forms of energy that are absorbed and conducted throughout the framework of the body, affecting all cells. Movements, ten-

sions, and other energies conducted through this system interact with metabolism and the genetic material. Vibrations of living matrix molecules are affected by cellular activities, growth factors, carcinogenesis, and emotional states.

On the basis of what is now known about the roles of electrical, magnetic, elastic, acoustic, thermal, gravitational, and photonic energies in living systems, it is likely that there is no single "life force" or "healing energy." Rather, the living body seems to have many energy systems, and there seem to be many ways of influencing those systems. What we refer to as the "living state" and as "health" are all of these systems, both known and unknown, functioning collectively, cooperatively, and synergistically. The debate about whether there is such a thing as a healing energy or a life force is being replaced by study of the interactions between biologic energy fields, structures, and functions.

Complementing these scientific discoveries is a long history of experiential evidence and clinical technique developed by therapists of various kinds. The growing popularity of bodywork, energetic, and movement therapies is leading us to a synthesis of ideas that will be beneficial to all.

Of all the discoveries summarized, the most tenuous and yet the most exciting is the discovery of the biomagnetic fields emitted by the hands of therapists of various kinds. The phenomenon was originally described in the context of therapeutic touch and was confirmed for Qigong and other martial arts and meditation practices. A growing body of evidence indicates the effectiveness of these methods. However, the impact of even the most carefully controlled studies can be compromised if the findings cannot be connected logically to generally accepted biomedical paradigms.

Magnetic brain waves associated with the sensory and motor cortex become stronger when an action is practiced again and again, as occurs when a person rehearses with a musical instrument. Similar changes may occur with repeated practice of various "hands on" therapies. It would not be surprising if the various yogic, martial arts, and meditation practices also lead to amplification, the building of stronger and more coherent biomagnetic fields.

Although more research is needed, the most logical explanation for amplification is that the waves of electrical and magnetic activity from the brain are amplified as they pass through the peripheral tissues. Crystalline components of the living matrix, such as the collagen arrays in tendons, ligaments, and bones and the arrays of lipids in cell membranes, probably act as coherent, resonant molecular broadcasting systems. Vibrating molecules throughout the body may become cooperatively entrained with the brain rhythms. As more and more molecules within the crystalline living matrix become vibrationally entrained, the fields become stronger.

Bodywork, including massage and other repetitive practices such as yoga, Qigong, tai chi, meditation, and therapeutic touch, may gradually lead to more structural coherence (crystallinity) in the tissues, facilitating both the detection and radiation of energy fields.[29]

The nervous system is an energy system in the body. Its operation is studied by measuring electrical fields generated during the transmission of nerve impulses. Because electrical currents always give rise to magnetic fields, the nervous system is also a source of some of the biomagnetic fields present within and around an organism. Moreover, the nervous system regulates all muscular movements and therefore is one of the keys to the conversion of thoughts into energetic actions.

Neurophysiologists, who focus most of their attention on the "classic" nervous system (composed of the neurons that conduct information from place to place as electrical impulses), maintain that all functions of the nervous system result from the activities of the neurons. Hence integration of brain function, memory, and even consciousness has been assumed to arise from the massive interconnectivity of the neurons. This is a partial view because it neglects another energetic and informational system consisting of the perineural connective tissue system, which constitutes more than half of the cells in the brain (the prefix *peri* means *about, around, encircling,* or *enclosing*). Perineural cells surround each neuron in the brain and follow each peripheral nerve to its termination.

Robert O. Becker has been a pioneer in the exploration of the functions of the perineural system and its relationship with the semiconducting matrix that forms and surrounds it. To document the properties of this system, Becker refers to a "dual nervous system" consisting of the classic digital (all or none) nerve network and the perineural analog network, which regulates wound healing and tissue repair.

Pulses of electrical and magnetic energy begin in the brain before any movement occurs; these are called *anticipatory fields*. This "motor sequence" is the subject of much research around the world. It is an important phenomenon that is being investigated for its application in training for athletic events, dance, theater, music, and so on, because the benefit is derived from mental rehearsals or internal imaging, without the individual physically doing anything. Many athletes, performers, and therapists of various kinds have described the profound experience of being totally prepared, present, and focused. During such a period, sometimes referred to as "the zone," extraordinary accomplishments take place. Many therapeutic schools emphasize the importance of intention; that is, the practitioner deciding in advance the goals he or she wishes to attain for a particular client. This approach is based on the frequent experience that a vivid image of expectations facilitates change in that direction. Intention seems to be all the more effective when the client participates in it, as in directed movement therapies or image-based cancer treatments.

The effectiveness of various kinds of hands-on bodywork may derive from the entrainment of electrical and magnetic rhythms from therapist to client, and the anticipatory fields may be an important component of this entrainment.

If these speculations are correct, the next question is what function coherent biomagnetic emissions would serve in healing. The healing power of projected fields may arise from their ability to entrain similar coherent rhythms in the tissues of a client. Perhaps such entrainment enhances the regulatory systems involved in wound healing and defense. Various martial arts techniques appear to involve projecting fields at points in the body's energy system that are sensitive nodes in a solid-state informational and power distribution system.[29]

Scientific consensus has gone from a certainty that weak environmental energies can have no influence on living systems to agreement that such influences are extremely important and deserving of intense study to determine the precise mechanisms involved. Collectively, the discoveries of modern researchers tell a story of biologic sensitivity that coincides with the daily experiences of energy therapists ranging from medical doctors using imaging techniques to massage therapists, acupuncturists, polarity therapists, Reiki practitioners, herbalists, aromatherapists, and so on.

The new concepts do not require us to abandon our sophisticated understandings of physiology, biochemistry, or molecular biology. The definition of living matter is being expanded, not replaced, to incorporate the physics and chemistry of the solid state, including semiconduction, quantum mechanics, liquid crystals, and biologic coherence. Beneath the relatively slow-moving action potentials and billiard ball interactions of molecules lies a much faster and subtle realm of interactions. This dimension is subatomic, energetic, electromagnetic, and wavelike in character. Nerve impulses and chemical messengers are contained within the individual, whereas energy fields radiate indefinitely into space and therefore affect others who are nearby. For millennia, energy therapists have had a practical appreciation of these phenomena, which are finally open to scientific research.

The electromagnetic language has two aspects, frequency and intensity. After much confusion, extensive laboratory research is confirming what the homeopathic physician or aromatherapist has known for a long time: when it comes to triggering healing responses, "small is powerful," or "less is more."[29]

In her book, *Molecules of Emotion: Why You Feel the Way You Feel,* Dr. Candace Pert speculated on how energy healers may use their own energy fields to trigger receptors in the bodies of their patients. Receptors on the cell surface are the primary sites of action of low-frequency electromagnetic fields. It is at the receptor that cellular responses are triggered by hormones, growth factors, neurotransmitters, taste and smell molecules, pheromones, light, and a variety of other electromagnetic signals. Dr. Pert called for basic research into this promising area. Her careful research on neuropeptides can be integrated with the emerging understanding of electromagnetics in the living body to give us a much clearer picture of the human body in health and disease, as well as the biophysics of emotions.[13]

Certainly, for a culture that has become accustomed to having large numbers of tasks handled by invisible currents flowing through chips in computers and its television sets adjusted by invisible radiation from remote control devices, it is not too frightening to look at the ways our bodies are regulated and coordinated by invisible energies.

Massage and the Subtle Energy Approaches

Some methods of massage, especially the more subtle approaches, have not yet been researched enough to be scientifically validated. However, as previously explained, research is underway in these areas. These methods, based on the subtle electrical energy of the body, have been around for eons. Most ancient healing practices are based on the interaction with these subtle energy fields. The massage profession, as well as the health care and scientific professions, would be wise not to discount these methods just because current technology is not advanced enough to verify what the human being can perceive.

In time, many of the methods probably will show validity, or their use would not have stood the test of time. Entrainment is now being considered as a mechanism to explain the benefits of the more subtle approaches.[25] Currently the electrical energy generated by the body can be measured by electroencephalography, electrocardiography, magnetic resonance imaging, and other sophisticated scientific techniques.

The lack of sufficient Western scientific validation of the ancient energetic flows of chi, prana, meridians, chakras, auras, or whatever else they may be called causes us to represent this area of bodywork to the public carefully. Until our technology can prove the validity of energy techniques, it is important to remember the wisdom of Hippocrates, "Do no harm," and also Bernie Siegal's belief, "There is no false hope." It is important to represent subtle techniques simply, professionally, and without false expectations and mysticism. Additional training is required to learn to use the subtle energy approaches purposefully. It is also important not to discount the stimulation of the powerful placebo effect. If touch can activate it, why not use it? It will be exciting to watch science "discover" the validity of more and more of the ancient energy concepts.

The Effect of Massage on Body Energy

Physiologically, sufficient research exists to demonstrate that methods using "energy" have an effect through ANS activity and endocrine responses in regard to entrainment, motor nerve points, and the piezoelectric properties of connective tissue fibers. Acupuncture points and meridians can be correlated directly with the nerve tracts and motor nerve points; chakras are located over nerve plexuses and biologic oscillators.

The interrelationship among all the body's systems is sufficient to cause the body to respond to the stimulation of innate electrochemical energy by means of massage approaches. Therapeutic massage stimulates the nervous system and applies pressure on the connective tissues to produce a measurable electrical current via the piezoelectric properties of the connective tissue and the deformation of tensegrity structures. The generalized therapeutic approach of massage seems to have a normalizing effect on the body's energetic processes.

■ ■ ■   SUMMARY

Therapeutic massage methods are simple and effective in producing responses mediated through the nervous system, the interaction with the endocrine system, the connective tissue, and the circulatory systems. Massage techniques can replace pharmaceuticals as a treatment for mild symptoms in some illnesses. They also can be used as an adjunct to support medication therapy, possibly allowing the dosage and duration of treatment to be reduced, thereby reducing the risk of side effects. Massage is beneficial for anxiety, depression, and chronic pain as part of

an overall treatment protocol. Most forms of musculoskeletal pain and discomfort respond to massage at least temporarily. General daily stress responds well to massage.

Armed with an understanding of the physiologic effects of massage, massage professionals hopefully will be able to collaborate with medical, scientific, and trained personnel in the use of these very old and effective methods. When provided by trained professionals, therapeutic massage can be beneficial in conservative treatment plans for chronic pain and stress-induced disease before more invasive measures are attempted. Therapeutic massage can play an important role in prevention programs by providing a natural mechanism for stimulating the body to adjust to the stress of daily life and to restore the natural homeostatic balance.

Professional experience shows that most clients get a massage because it feels good and helps them feel better. Researching "good" and "better" scientifically is difficult. The massage professional can provide the services of this art and be confident that scientific explanations exist for why massage works and feels good. Let us not forget, as professionals, the importance of the "feel good" aspect of massage. Intuition and intent are necessary aspects of the professional application of massage. Clients do care about how much you know, but they care more about how much you care and about how good they feel after a massage.

The massage profession needs more research. Therefore the massage profession needs to cooperate with researchers and appreciate that research is tedious, painstaking work. The scientific community and the public need the research to strengthen their belief in massage so that they can justify receiving or recommending massage. The massage profession needs the public and the scientific community to support massage. We all need touch because it is so beneficial and, most of all, because it feels good. Whatever the massage or bodywork system used, the beneficial effects of therapeutic massage are elicited from the client's physiology as it adjusts to the external sensory information supplied by massage and responds to the compressive forces of massage.

As we said at the beginning of this chapter, massage is easy to validate. Additional information can be obtained by locating and studying the references in this chapter. Application of the techniques that bring about the physiologic effects is discussed in more detail in Chapters 9, 10, and 11.

THINK IT OVER

Can the various effects of massage really be separated from one another? Can you massage only connective tissue, or affect only circulation, or only the ANS?

4-1   PubMed research links for massage therapy are located on the Evolve Web site.

4-2   Identify the parts of a research paper.

4-3   Based on photographs, identify which type of reflex is occurring in each photo.

4-4   Label sympathetic and parasympathetic responses.

Don't forget to study for your certification and licensure exams! Review questions for this chapter are located on Evolve.

REFERENCES

1. Shealy NC: *The neurochemical substrate of behavior: the psychology of health, immunity and disease,* vol B, Mainsfield Center, Calif, 1992, National Institute for the Clinical Application of Behavioral Medicine.
2. Field T: *Touch therapy,* Edinburgh, 2000, Churchill Livingston.
3. Greenman PE: *Principles of manual medicine,* ed 3, Baltimore, 2003, Lippincott Williams & Wilkins.
4. Rural Girls in Science: Meeting the Challenge Through a Comprehensive Approach, a program funded by National Science Foundation Project HRD-94500053, Dr. Angela B. Ginorio, Principal Investigator. The program can be reached at: Rural Girls in Science Program Washington, Imogen Cunningham Hall, Box 351380, University of Washington, Seattle, WA 98195.
5. Yates J: *Physiological effects of therapeutic massage and their application to treatment,* Vancouver, BC, 1990, Massage Therapists Association of British Columbia.
6. Horacek HJ Jr: *Brainstorms: understanding and treating emotional storms of ADHD from childhood through adulthood,* Northvale, NJ, 2000, Jason Aronson.
7. Baldry PE: *Acupuncture, trigger points and musculoskeletal pain,* ed 3, New York, 2005, Churchill Livingstone.
8. Gunn CC: Reprints on pain, acupuncture and related subjects, Seattle, 1992, University of Washington.
9. Longworth JCD: Psychophysiological effects of slow-stroke back massage in normotensive females, *Adv Nurs Sci* 4:44, 1982.
10. Knaster M: Tiffany Field provides proof positive scientifically, *Massage Ther J* 37:84, 1998.
11. Hooper J, Teresi D: *The three pound universe,* Los Angeles, 1991, Tarcher.
12. Selye H: *The healing brain: understanding stress, stress without distress,* Institute for the Study of Human Knowledge, Los Altos, Calif, ISHK Paperbacks.
13. McCraty R, Tiller WA, Atkinson M: Head-heart entrainment: a preliminary survey, 1996, http://www.heartmath.org/research/research-papers/HeadHeart/index.html
14. Timmons BH, Ley R: *Behavioral and psychological approaches to breathing disorders,* New York, 1994, Plenum Press.
15. Pert CB: *Molecules of emotion: why you feel the way you feel,* New York, 1997, Scribner.
16. Levin SR: Acute effects of massage on the stress response, master's thesis, Greensboro, NC, 1990, University of North Carolina.
17. Ernst M, Lee MHM: Sympathetic effects of manual and electrical acupuncture of the Tsusanli knee point: comparison with the Hoku hand point sympathetic effects, *Exp Neurol* 94:101, 1986. Pressure on Acupoints Decreases Postoperative Pain.
18. Chaitow LND: *Muscle energy techniques,* ed 3, Edinburgh, 2006, Churchill Livingstone.
19. Anderson K, Anderson LE, Glanze WD, editors: *Mosby's medical, nursing, and allied health dictionary,* ed 6, St Louis, 2005, Mosby.
20. St John P: Workshop notes: seminar I, St John Neuromuscular Therapy Seminars, Largo, Fla, 1990, self-published.
21. Thomas CL, editor: *Taber's cyclopedic medical dictionary,* ed 20, Philadelphia, 2006, FA Davis.
22. DeGroot J, Chusid JG: *Correlative neuroanatomy,* ed 25, San Mateo, Calif, 2002, McGraw-Hill.
23. Simons D: Understanding effective treatments of myofascial trigger points, *J Bodywork Move Ther* 6(2), 2002.
24. Travell, Simons, Simons, Cummings: *Travell and Simons' myofascial pain and dysfunction: the trigger point manual,* ed 2, Baltimore, 1999, Lippincott Williams & Wilkins
25. Oschman JL: What is healing energy? III. Silent pulses, *J Bodywork Move Ther* 1:179, 1997.
26. Cailliet R: *Soft tissue pain and disability,* ed 3, Philadelphia, 1996, FA Davis.
27. Alcock J: *Animal behavior: an evaluatory approach,* Sunderland, Mass, 1989, Sinauer.
28. Oschman JL: Clinical aspects of biological fields: an introduction for health care professionals, *J Bodywork Move Ther* 6:117, 2002.
29. Oschman JL: *Energy medicine: the scientific basic,* Edinburgh, 2000, Churchill Livingstone.

Research at TRI: *Touch Therapy Times* 5(5), 1994. http://www6.miami.edu/touch-research/List%20of%20Studies.html

SUGGESTED READINGS

Gelbach SH: *Interpreting the medical literature* (Kindle edition), ed 4, 2002, McGraw-Hill/Appleton & Lange, 2002.

Hulley SB et al: *Designing clinical research; an epidemiologic approach,* ed 3, Baltimore, 2006, Lippincott, Williams and Wilkins.

Portney LG, Watkins MP: *Foundations of clinical research: applications of practice,* ed 3, 2008, Prentice Hall, 2008.

Stommel M, Wills CE: *Clinical research: concepts and principles for advanced practice nurses,* Baltimore, 2003, Lippincott, Williams, and Wilkins.

Workbook Section

Answers for the Workbook Section for Chapter 4 are provided on p. 761.

■ ■ ■ SHORT ANSWER

1. What are the five basic physiologic effects of massage?

2. In what way do chronic problems affect the connective tissue?

3. What are the five types of circulation?

4. What three words describe the sympathetic ANS functions?

5. What words describe the parasympathetic functions?

6. What is the importance of state-dependent memory to the massage therapist?

7. What is hyperstimulation analgesia?

8. How does massage promote the body's ability to maintain self-regulation and structural and functional balance?

9. Why is it easy to validate massage?

10. Why are research and its replication to verify the positive biochemical and behavioral responses to touch important?

11. Is it possible to separate the somatic, emotional, and cognitive elements in the response to massage? Is it possible to separate the mechanical, neural, chemical, and psychological effects?

12. How does the gate control theory explain hyperstimulation analgesia and counterirritation?

13. What role does massage play in relieving nerve impingement?

14. Why are reflexes important to the understanding of why massage works?

Workbook Section—cont'd

15. How does massage interact with the powerful body/mind phenomenon?

_____

_____

_____

16. How does massage stimulate the release of neurotransmitters, endorphins, and enkephalins?

_____

_____

_____

17. What seem to be the effects of massage on myofascial trigger points?

_____

_____

_____

18. In what ways does massage encourage circulation?

_____

_____

_____

19. What are the possible physiologic mechanisms that support energy methods?

_____

_____

_____

■ ■ ■ MATCHING

I. Match the term with the best definition.

1. Autoregulation	11. Hyperstimulation analgesia
2. Body/mind	12. Intuition
3. Centering	13. Law
4. Cognitive	14. Nerve impingement
5. Counterirritation	15. Noxious stimulation
6. Endogenous	16. Placebo
7. Endorphins	17. Reflex
8. Feedback	18. Science
9. Gate control theory	19. Somatic
10. Toughening/hardening	20. Subtle energies

a. the ability to focus on a specific circumstance by screening sensation

b. superficial stimulation that relieves deeper sensation by stimulating different sensory signals

c. weak electrical fields that are said to surround and run through the body

d. an involuntary response to a stimulus; the response is specific, predictable, adaptive, and purposeful

e. the interaction between thought and physiology connected to the limbic system, the hypothalamic influence of the ANS, and the endocrine system

f. a controlled pain sensation; "good pain"

g. a scientific statement found to be true for a whole class of natural occurrences

h. a method of teaching the body to deal with stress

i. a method of autoregulation to maintain internal homeostasis that interlinks body functions

j. made in the body

k. one of the endogenous opioid peptides that have morphinelike analgesic properties, behavioral effects, and neurotransmitter and neuromodulator functions

l. reduction of perception of a sensation by stimulation of large-diameter nerve fibers

m. awareness with perception, reasoning, judgment, intuition, and memory

n. knowing something by using subconscious information

o. the hypothesis that painful stimuli can be prevented from reaching higher levels of the CNS by stimulating larger sensory nerves

p. pressure against a nerve by skin, fascia, muscles, ligaments, and joints

q. a treatment for an illness that influences the course of the disease even if it is not specifically validated

r. pertaining to the body

s. the intellectual process of understanding through observation, measurement, accumulation of data, and analysis of the findings

t. control of homeostasis by alteration of tissue or function

II. Match the scientific laws affecting massage with their descriptions.

a. Hilton's law
b. Law of unilaterality
c. Law of facilitation
d. Hooke's law
e. Law of generalization
f. Arndt-Schulz law
g. Bowditch's (all or none) law
h. Bell's law
i. Law of specificity of nervous energy
j. Weber's law
k. Law of symmetry
l. Law of intensity
m. Law of radiation
n. Cannon's law of denervation

1. The weakest stimulus capable of producing a response produces the maximum response contraction in cardiac and skeletal muscle and nerves.

2. Anterior spinal nerve roots are motor roots, and posterior spinal nerve roots are sensory roots.

3. When an impulse has passed once through a certain set of neurons to the exclusion of others, it tends to take the same course on a future occasion, and each time it traverses this path, the resistance is smaller.

4. The stress used to stretch or compress a body is proportional to the strain experienced, as long as the elastic limits of the body have not been exceeded.

5. Excitation of a receptor always gives rise to the same sensation, regardless of the nature of the stimulus.

6. The increase in stimulus necessary to produce the smallest perceptible increase in sensation bears a constant ratio to the strength of the stimulus already acting.

7. A nerve trunk that supplies a joint also supplies the muscles of the joint and the skin over the insertions of such muscles.

8. If a mild irritation is applied to one or more sensory nerves, movement usually occurs only on one side, the side that is irritated.

9. If stimulation is increased sufficiently, a motor reaction is manifested not only on the side of irritation, but also in similar muscles on the opposite side of the body.

10. Reflex movements usually are more intense on the side of irritation; at times the movements of the opposite side equal them in intensity, but they usually are less pronounced.

11. If excitation continues to increase, it is propagated upward, and reactions take place through centrifugal nerves coming from the higher cord segments.

12. When an irritation becomes very intense, it is propagated in the medulla oblongata, which becomes a focus from which stimuli radiate to all parts of the cord, causing a general contraction of all muscles in the body.

13. Weak stimuli activate physiologic processes; very strong stimuli inhibit them.

14. When autonomic effectors are partly or completely separated from their normal nerve connections, they become more sensitive to the action of chemical substances.

Column 1	Column 2	Column 3	Control List
1. Heart muscle			a. increases the secretion of digestive juices
2. Digestive tract			b. increases the secretion of sweat
3. Skeletal muscle blood vessels			c. slows the heartbeat
4. Smooth muscle blood vessels			d. constricts blood vessels
5. Urinary bladder			e. relaxes the bladder
6. Iris			f. increases peristalsis
7. Pilomotor muscles			g. dilates blood vessels
8. Adrenal medulla			h. increases the secretion of epinephrine
9. Sweat glands			i. stimulates goose bumps
10. Digestive glands			j. constricts the pupil

Workbook Section—cont'd

III. Match the visceral functions with their sympathetic or parasympathetic controls. Column 1 lists visceral functions. Choose the best match from the Control List and place the corresponding letter in column 2. In column 3, write either "S" for sympathetic or "P" for parasympathetic, depending on the control response.

■ ■ ■ LABELING

Label the major nerve plexuses for Figure 4-10.
Brachial plexus
Brain
Cervical plexus
Lumbar plexus
Nerves
Sacral plexus
Spinal cord

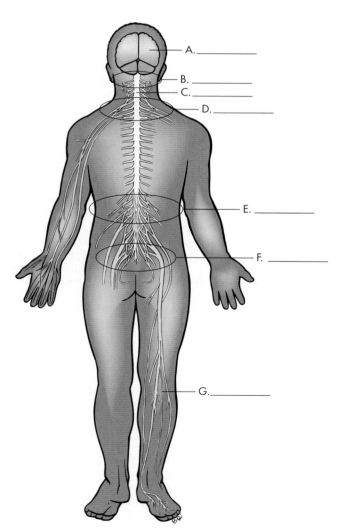

A. _____
B. _____
C. _____
D. _____
E. _____
F. _____
G. _____

FIGURE 4-10

■ ■ ■ ASSESS YOUR COMPETENCIES

Now that you have studied this chapter, you should be able to:

1. Describe the fundamentals of the Western scientific process.

2. Interpret a research paper.

3. Cite current research that validates the underlying physiologic mechanisms of therapeutic massage.

4. Classify massage methods into basic concepts.

5. Explain the effects of therapeutic massage in physiologic terms.

6. Use the Internet to do research.

On a separate sheet of paper, write a short summary of the content of this chapter based on the competencies listed above. When writing this paper assume you are speaking to someone—a client, prospective employer, co-worker, or other interested person. Write the paper as if you were having a conversation and explaining the importance of the information and skills to professional massage development.

Next, in small student discussion groups, share the papers and compare and contrast how the information was presented. Discuss the content, looking for similarities, differences, potential misunderstanding of the information, and clear and concise methods of description.

■ ■ ■ PROBLEM-SOLVING EXERCISES

1. A physician refers a client to you for basic relaxation massage to ease chronic pain of undetermined cause. Using the information presented in this chapter, list at least four principal reasons the massage could benefit the client.

2. After a series of massages, a client finds that her anxiety and impatience have diminished. How would you explain this?

3. A client brings in a research article about the use of massage for a specific condition, but he doesn't understand what it means. What steps would you take to explain it to him?

PROFESSIONAL APPLICATION
■ ■ ■ EXERCISE

1. Make a list of your daily experiences with ANS functions. Make a second list of ANS functions you encounter while performing massage.

2. Read through the various therapeutic massage journals. Find one or two articles on bodywork and classify the information presented according to the following effects:

   a. Mechanical or reflexive

   b. Nervous system primarily affected; benefits primarily somatic, visceral, peripheral, central or autonomic, connective tissue, or circulatory

   c. Stimulation of chemicals (i.e., hormones) and neurotransmitters

   d. Sensory receptor responsible for responding to the stimulation

■ ■ ■ RESEARCH FOR FURTHER STUDY

Design a possible research study. Develop an idea (a hypothesis), narrow the topic, then decide what measurements will be used. Identify possible outcomes. Identify other factors that may influence the outcome. Look at other research studies for examples of research design. Locate resources on ways to develop a research study.

CHAPTER 5

Indications and Contraindications for Therapeutic Massage

CHAPTER OBJECTIVES

After completing this chapter, the student will be able to perform the following:

- Define the terms *indication* and *contraindication*
- Define therapeutic change, condition management, and palliative care as a therapeutic approach
- Use a clinical reasoning model to determine the appropriate intervention process
- Develop a basic understanding of pathology and its connection to contraindications to massage
- Explain the stress response, inflammatory response, and pain response
- Identify indications for massage therapy and justify those indications
- Determine when to refer clients to licensed medical professionals

CHAPTER OUTLINE

KEY TERMS

Acute
Antagonistic
Benign tumors
Chronic
Communicable diseases
Compensation
Condition management
Contraindication
Dysfunction
Endangerment sites
General adaptation syndrome (GAS)
Health
Homeostasis
Impingement syndromes
Indication
Inflammatory response
Malignant tumors
Medications
Metastasis
Pain-spasm-pain cycle
Palliative care
Pathology
Referral
Referred pain
Signs
Suffering
Symptoms
Syndrome
Synergistic
Therapeutic change
Trauma

The massage professional must be able to identify indications and contraindications for therapeutic massage. An **indication** is a condition for which an approach would be beneficial for health enhancement, treatment of a particular disorder, or support of a treatment modality other than massage. A **contraindication** is a condition for which an approach could be harmful. The three types of contraindications are as follows:

- General avoidance of application—Do not perform any massage techniques.
- Regional avoidance of application—Do massage but avoid a particular area.
- Application with caution, usually requiring supervision from appropriate medical or supervising personnel—Do perform massage but carefully select the types of methods to be used, the duration of the massage, the depth and intensity of pressure, and the frequency of application.

INDICATIONS FOR MASSAGE

SECTION OBJECTIVES

Using the information presented in this section, the student will be able to perform the following:

- Identify and chart the benefits of massage
- Explain the difference between objective and subjective massage benefits
- Explain the benefits of massage to others

Indications for massage are based on the massage effect's *objective* and *subjective* health-enhancing benefits. Some results of massage can be measured (objective), whereas others are assumed effective based on experience (subjective). The effects of massage are both physical (objective, physically measured observation) and mental (subjective perception reporting) (Box 5-1 and Proficiency Exercise 5-1).

BOX 5-1

The General Benefits of Therapeutic Massage

Massage manipulations can be applied in a systematic approach or plan to influence conditions that affect physical function.

Skeletal muscles respond with direct biomechanical effects. Within this response, biomechanical effects encourage or produce reflex reactions that involve the nervous system and chemical responses. A variety of responses are reached at many levels. The nervous system can respond through the reflex arc, secretion of endorphins and other neural chemicals, and the release of histamine and other cellular secretions. The release of chemical substances affects a structure or system of the body directly or indirectly.

The foundation for understanding the benefits of massage therapy is an understanding of the nature of its effects on circulation, elimination, and nervous system control. Circulation is primarily improved by direct biomechanical responses to manipulations. A secondary benefit is obtained through reflex responses that encourage chemical secretion, which affects nervous system control.

Circulation improvement occurs as nutrients, oxygen, and arterial blood components are delivered to the local area being manipulated or are distributed to the general circulation. The benefit of circulatory improvement is the secondary effect of improved filtration and elimination of carbon dioxide, metabolites, and biochemical byproducts that are transported in the venous blood. Improved circulation, with its ability to affect elimination, generally enhances the abilities of the structures to benefit and support normal function. When nutrition is improved and elimination enhanced, the structures of localized areas, tissues, and systems are given the opportunity to maximize the potential for normal function.

Massage manipulations directly benefit restrictions to muscle tissue function. Mechanical benefits and reflex responses combine to help the muscular soft tissues respond through circulation improvement and elimination of byproducts. Mechanical effects on muscular tissues include influence on the stretch receptors and tendon apparatus, direct manual stretching of the muscle fibers, and changes in connective tissue structures. The reflex effects encourage relaxation of the tissues through change in the motor nerve output and chemical secretions.

Clients receiving massage therapy report a variety of sensations, emotions, feelings, and mental perceptions that are subjective, difficult to measure, and unique to the individual.

Therapeutic massage benefits conditions by encouraging the body through the phases involved in rehabilitation, restoration, and normalization of anatomic and physiologic function and ability. Psychological benefits occur subjectively, according to the individual, in response to therapy, with secondary effects that influence sensation and pain perception. Objective and subjective results of therapy combine to create individual responses that affect the desired health outcome.

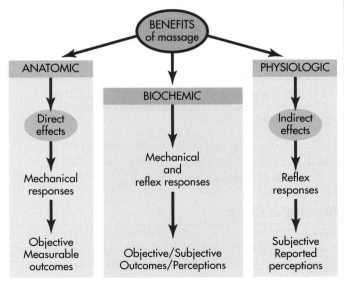

The benefits, effects, responses, and outcomes can occur separately, combined, or as a result of one another

Modified from Emily E.S. Cowall, Reg. MT, Ontario, Canada.

PROFICIENCY EXERCISE 5-1

In the spaces provided, write two dialogs that explain the benefits of massage. Direct one discussion to a group of health care professionals such as physicians, chiropractors, nurses, physical therapists, and psychologists; direct the other discussion to a group of business professionals, factory workers, construction workers, food service workers, and athletes.

Choose one: Physicians, chiropractors, nurses, physical therapists, psychologists

Type of health professional: _____

Choose one: Business professionals, factory workers, construction workers, food service workers, athletes

Type of group: _____

APPROACHES TO CARE

SECTION OBJECTIVES

Using the information presented in this section, the student will be able to perform the following:

- Define the term *therapeutic change*
- Explain the concepts of condition management and palliative care
- Implement a clinical reasoning process for making appropriate decisions as to the type of care most beneficial for the client

The benefits of massage occur as a result of therapeutic change, condition management, and palliative care. This section explains each of these approaches to care.

Therapeutic Change

Therapeutic change is a beneficial alteration produced by a therapeutic massage process that modifies a physical form or function, thereby affecting the client's physical, mental, and/or spiritual state.

Any change process, including beneficial change, requires energy and resource expenditure on the part of the client. The decision on whether to implement a therapeutic change process requires assessment of the client's ability to expend the energy required for active change and the availability of the support and resources often necessary during a change process. To facilitate a change process, the practitioner must have the appropriate knowledge and skills (current or acquired) and often a network of support from other professionals. The client must have the motivation and resources (information, finances, time, social support, and coping mechanisms) to complete a change process. Careful assessment helps identify whether a change process program holds a likely chance for success. If these components are not sufficient or in place or if the existing situation supports some sort of coping mechanism or has secondary gain for the client, the client will not be motivated to commit to the change process.

If the conditions are not suitable for active change, other intervention processes can be developed. Wise professionals understand and consider the complex dynamics of the lives of the people they serve. Although change often is indicated, it may not be realistically possible at a particular time or under a current set of circumstances. When the likelihood of a successful change outcome is not good, condition management and palliative care can be offered. These reduce suffering and allow clients to be more effective within their current set of circumstances.

Condition Management

Condition management is the use of massage methods to support clients who are not able to undergo a therapeutic change process but who want to be as effective as possible within an existing set of circumstances. Condition management is beneficial when a client is dealing with a chronic health condition or a set of life circumstances that creates chronic stress (e.g., caring for an ailing parent or child, stressful work environment, strain within a relationship, ongoing financial strain). Condition management also is beneficial when changing a situation is not a viable possibility (e.g., amputation, diabetes, job-related repetitive strain) or when the time frame for changing a situation needs to be postponed (e.g., pregnancy, chemotherapy, graduation from school, end of season for an athlete).

On a physical level, massage can offer benefits by managing the existing physical compensation patterns and sometimes by slowing the progression of chronic conditions or preventing a situation from becoming worse. On an emotional level, massage can assist in the management of physical stress symptoms, allowing the person to cope better with life stresses that cannot be altered.

Condition management accounts for the largest client base for therapeutic massage. Many people find themselves in undesirable or unchanging circumstances and search for ways to cope with—not change—the existing conditions while remaining productive. Most of us can relate to the importance of being able to remain resourceful and responsive to life events. Although the ideal is to make changes when life is not as we would like it to be, we all know that sometimes this is not possible for many reasons. Therapeutic massage offers support, acceptance, compassion, and a short-term respite.

Palliative Care

To *palliate* is to soothe or to relieve. Massage is soothing and provides comfort regardless of whether the client is seeking relaxation to meet pleasure needs, to cope with chronic pain of some type, or to make the transition from life to death.

In a health care context, palliative care attempts to relieve or reduce the intensity of uncomfortable symptoms, but it does not try to produce a cure. Palliative care is provided when the client's condition is most likely going to worsen and degenerative processes will continue (e.g., terminal illness, dementia). It often relates to approaches that reduce suffering.

Because the term *suffering* is inherently subjective and multifaceted, completely understanding this experience in the client often is difficult. Suffering can be defined as an overall impairment in quality of life. Some say that we may not have a choice about whether we experience pain (physical, emotional, or spiritual), but we can choose to suffer or not. Often, managing pain does not alleviate suffering. Dealing with only the physical aspects of pain may not address the mind and spirit of the client, because suffering often is a mental and spiritual issue. Many times suffering overshadows the client's ability to create or participate in meaningful experiences or to experience pleasure.

Palliative care is also appropriate when the condition should not be changed or the person does not desire a specific outcome other than pleasure and relaxation. Providing massage to a woman during labor, receiving a massage while on vacation, supporting an athlete during training for an event, providing massage at a public event such as a health fair, giving a massage to someone just before surgery, and providing massage to a wedding party the day before the event are all examples of the appropriate use of palliative care.

Massage approaches have great efficacy in palliative care. When presented through massage, the pleasurable experience of touch and human connection may be one of the greatest therapeutic gifts our profession offers.

All these facts give rise to some questions:

- When is change appropriate?
- When is change not desirable and condition management and palliative support more appropriate?
- How does the professional determine what type of care is appropriate: therapeutic change, condition management, or palliative care?
- How does the professional know when transitions in types of care occur (i.e., therapeutic change to condition management, or condition management to palliative care)?

Palliative care can progress to condition management and, with the gradual restoration of energy, the client may even progress to a therapeutic change process. Eventually, a therapeutic change process will end or transform, and condition management, such as stress management, becomes the professional focus once again (Proficiency Exercise 5-2).

Chapter 3 presented a detailed look at intake procedures, which include a client history, physical assessment, and methods to develop this information into a care or treatment plan. The clinical reasoning model provides a decision-making process for analyzing whether therapeutic changes or methods to maintain or support an existing state are the best approach. The ability to analyze data collected during assessment procedures is crucial in making decisions about what massage therapy intervention to use and whether the outcome is a therapeutic change process, condition management, or palliative care. The massage therapist must consider these factors to develop a plan that best serves the client (Proficiency Exercise 5-3).

PATHOLOGY, HEALTH, AND THERAPEUTIC MASSAGE

SECTION OBJECTIVES

Using the information presented in this section, the student will be able to perform the following:

- Define the terms *health, dysfunction,* and *pathology*
- Recognize when a client's condition should be evaluated by a primary health care provider
- List the mechanisms and risk factors that predispose people to disease processes
- Explain the general inflammatory response
- Explain the mechanisms of pain and evaluate pain for referral purposes

PROFICIENCY EXERCISE 5-2

Metaphor

Cleaning the house—Offer palliative and management care, reduce suffering, and encourage better coping in the existing situation

or

Remodeling the house—A process of active change

For both the professional and the client, list the differences between "cleaning the house" and "remodeling the house" in terms of skill levels, cost, time, materials, difficulties, disruption in daily living, and other factors.

Example:

Cleaning the house
    Professional—Ongoing service
    Client—Ongoing appointments

Remodeling the house
    Professional—Defined number of appointments with a specific outcome
    Client—Commitment to a specific set of appointments

Your Turn

List three differences in each area.
Cleaning the house
Professional

1.

2.

3.

Client

1.

2.

3.

Remodeling the house

Professional

1.

2.

3.

Client

1.

2.

3.

Pathology is the study of disease. To practice safely, massage practitioners need a basic understanding of pathologic processes. The diagnosis of disorders is not a function of a massage professional. However, to refer clients appropriately to a health care professional, the massage practitioner must be able to recognize when the client's condition represents an irregularity that should be evaluated by the person's primary health care provider. When working with a referral and under proper supervision, the massage professional also must be able to alter the application of massage in terms of any disease process present so that the client receives the benefits of massage without harm. Massage students should have both a general awareness of the types of disorders that occur in each major body system and more specific knowledge of the signs and symptoms of selected disorders that could endanger the health of either the client or the practitioner (see Appendix A for specific contraindications to massage). The massage professional also needs a basic understanding of pharmacology and the possible interactions between medications and massage (see Appendix C for specific information on these interactions).

It also is important to understand the way in which a disease process develops. The body is designed for health, and for disease to develop, a sequence of events must occur. Trauma is an abrupt shock or injury to the body or psyche, and like disease, trauma requires the body to use healing energy.

To understand disease, we first need to understand the definition of health. **Health** is optimal functioning with freedom from disease or abnormal processes. Health is influenced by many factors, including inherited (genetic) and constitutional conditions. Lifestyle, activity level, rest, loving relationships, exercise, a balanced diet, empowering beliefs and attitudes, self-esteem, authentic personality, and freedom from self-hindering patterns all support health. When a state of health no longer exists or is interrupted, dysfunction begins.

Dysfunction is the in-between state of "not healthy" but also "not sick" (i.e., experiencing disease). Unfortunately, many people experience dysfunctional states. Western medicine has a difficult time identifying and dealing with dysfunctions because these are prepathologic states and are often not apparent within current diagnostic methods. Actual pathology usually needs to exist before medical tests and diagnostic methods can detect a disease state.

Recent prevention methods, many modeled after more "Eastern" or "holistic" approaches, are beginning to address this area called *dysfunction.* Many ancient healing methods are more focused on the process of dysfunction, introducing restorative methods before a system breaks down into a disease process. When used in the prepathology state of dysfunction, these methods of mind/body medicine, stress management, and prevention are very effective. They are less effective when applied to an active pathologic

Text continued on p. 169

PROFICIENCY EXERCISE 5-3

Important Note to Students: These problem-solving activities can seem overwhelming, but it is important to understand how to do them. The only way to learn is to practice. Whenever you encounter these exercises in the book, attempt to do them. Don't worry whether you are correct or not; just practice the process.

After reading the following client case situations, decide whether you would introduce therapeutic change, condition management, or palliative care. Explain your reasons for the decision using the clinical reasoning model. An example is provided.

Example Case Study

A male client, age 47, is experiencing fatigue and neck and shoulder pain. He is a cross-country truck driver. He is married, has three children, and has the normal financial obligations of a house payment, car payment, and other responsibilities. One child just started college, and the client is somewhat concerned about the tuition expenses. He likes his job and is content with his family and social life. He can't seem to understand why he is tired or why his shoulder hurts. He can think of no reason for the pain other than the strain of the driving position and the long work hours. This pain never bothered him before. He went to the doctor for a physical examination, and nothing out of the ordinary was identified. The physician thinks that an old football injury, coupled with some age-related changes, is responsible. The doctor also thinks that the pain in the shoulder might be interfering with the client's sleep and might be a cause of fatigue. The doctor recommends an over-the-counter antiinflammatory agent and painkiller, such as aspirin, and suggests that massage might help. The doctor also recommends that the client cut back on his work hours and relax more. Aspirin helps the shoulder pain but upsets the client's stomach. He does not want to cut back on work hours. He is seeking help for shoulder pain and would like more physical energy.

Identify the Facts

Questions that can help with this process include the following:

What is considered normal or balanced function?
   The ability to work pain free with reasonable stamina at a job one enjoys.

What has happened? (Spell out events.)
   Nothing substantial has occurred to account for the changes other than age-related influences and a previous football injury.

What caused the imbalance? (Can it be identified?)
   A previous injury, long work hours, a static seated position with the arms elevated on the steering wheel and repetitive looking to the left during driving.

What was done or is being done?
   Treatment with aspirin

What has worked or not worked?
   Aspirin has benefits but upsets the client's stomach. The client has chosen to maintain his current work schedule.

Brainstorm the Possibilities

Questions that help with this process include the following:

What are the possibilities? (What could it all mean?)
   The fatigue and pain could be a result of age-related changes and the previous injury, coupled with repetitive use; this in turn could interfere with sleep, as suggested by the doctor.
   The condition could be related more to emotional stress caused by financial concerns.
   The client may have an undiagnosed health condition that is not sufficiently evident to allow a definitive diagnosis.

What is my intuition suggesting?
   I think we are likely dealing with a combination of the doctor's diagnosis and unexpressed emotional stress over financial concerns, particularly the tuition costs for the child in college.

What are the possible patterns of dysfunction?
   The static driving position may be aggravating the old football injury.

What are the possible contributing factors?
   Worry, postural distortion from the static position, and age-related tissue changes, because the body becomes somewhat less flexible with age and lack of exercise.

What are possible interventions?
   A job change
   A stretching program
   Massage therapy
   Short-term mental health support
   Treatment with a different medication that does not upset the client's stomach

What might work?
   Massage and a stretching program

What are other ways to look at the situation?
   The client does not seem to want to use medications, does not want to change his job, and does not seem to think that there is anything wrong with his emotional or social life. Maybe if the financial situation were different, the stress load would be low enough so that his energy levels would increase and he could ignore the pain. Maybe a financial advisor would be helpful, or maybe his wife could get a job.

What do the data suggest?
   Emotional stress seems to be a factor. The data seem to suggest that an age-related process and a previous injury are aggravated by repetitive job strain and a static seated position.

Consider the Logical Outcomes of Each Possibility

Questions that can help determine outcomes include the following:

What is the logical progression of the symptom pattern, contributing factors, and current behaviors?
   If the pain remains or worsens and sleep continues to be interrupted so that fatigue worsens, the immune system

Continued

PROFICIENCY EXERCISE 5-3—cont'd

can be compromised and other disease processes might occur. The client could become unable to work. His mood would be altered, which would affect family and social relationships.

What is the logical cause and effect of each intervention identified? What are the pros and cons of each intervention suggested?

Job change—Would remove repetitive strain on the shoulder and eliminate static seated position; drastic change in lifestyle, finances, and work environment

Stretching program—Would increase flexibility and counterbalance the static seated position; could make the situation worse if the stretching is too aggressive, not progressive, and intermittent instead of used daily; is self-initiated and once learned would not incur any ongoing costs; does not require a regular appointment schedule (helpful because client is frequently on the road); requires discipline to do the stretches

Massage therapy—Would help alleviate pain symptoms and support better sleep; does not require extensive self-discipline other than making regular appointments; would incur a financial obligation; would support a daily stretching program; would reduce the use of medication

Short-term mental health support—Would not require extensive self-discipline other than making regular appointments; would incur a financial obligation; does not address the physical condition but does address emotional strain

Treatment with a different medication that does not upset the client's stomach—Would help alleviate pain symptoms and support better sleep; does not require extensive self-discipline; would incur a small financial obligation; does not need regular appointment schedule because he is on the road; possible side effects and development of dependency on the medication

Consultation with a financial advisor—Would help client achieve better control of finances, eliminating the basis for worry and emotional stress; does not address physical conditions, long work hours, or job stress

Wife getting a job—Would eliminate financial burden; could create stress in the marriage; requires action on the part of a person other than the client; does not address physical conditions, long work hours, or job stress

What are the consequences of not acting?

The situation could stabilize and resolve itself, or the client's condition could become more problematic, requiring more drastic intervention measures in the future.

What are the consequences of acting?

The problem would remain stable or improve. The client would be better able to cope with the current situation.

Identify the Effect of Each Possibility on the People Involved

Questions that can help identify possible effects include the following:

In terms of each intervention being considered, what would be the impact on the people involved: client, practitioner, and other professionals working with the client?

Job change—Client is not supportive; wife may or may not like idea.

Stretching program—Client does not like to fuss with himself and avoids activities having to do with self-care.

Massage therapy—Client is open to idea but nervous; wife, doctor, and massage practitioner are supportive.

Short-term mental health support—Client and wife are not open to this possibility at this time; they do not think that this is an emotional problem. Massage practitioner is hesitant about the client being unwilling to seek mental health services and does think emotion is involved (worry over finances) and would like client to remain open to this possibility. Treatment with a different medication that does not upset the client's stomach—Client does not like to take medication, and the doctor is unwilling to prescribe at this time until other measures are explored. Consultation with a financial advisor—Client and wife think this is a good idea and will pursue this possibility. Wife getting a job—Not an option at this time.

How does each person involved feel about the possible interventions?

Job change—None are supportive.

Stretching program—Client is ambivalent; massage practitioner and wife are supportive.

Massage therapy—All are supportive.

Short-term mental health support—Massage therapist is supportive; client and wife are not supportive.

Treatment with a different medication that does not upset the client's stomach—Doctor and client are not supportive.

Consultation with a financial advisor—Client and wife are supportive.

Wife getting a job—Not an option.

Is the practitioner within his or her scope of practice to work with such situations?

Yes

Is the practitioner qualified to work with such situations?

Yes

Does the practitioner feel qualified to work with such situations?

The practitioner is concerned about the client's ambivalence toward a stretching program and his lack of interest in a mental health referral. These concerns raise questions for the practitioner about the ability to work effectively with the client's physical problems when other causal factors may exist.

Is there a feeling of cooperation and agreement among all parties involved?

There is a degree of cooperation, as well as some resistance. All agree on the benefit of massage therapy.

PROFICIENCY EXERCISE 5-3—cont'd

Based on this analysis of the information provided, the massage practitioner would recommend a condition management program rather than a therapeutic change process, for the following reasons:

Causal factors are involved that the client may not be able to address during a change process. Also he is resistant to the idea of an exercise or a stretching program that would interfere with his driving schedule.

Case Study 1

A 17-year-old volleyball player is in training for a playoff tournament in 4 weeks. She has been somewhat sore after practice and anxious about the playoffs. Her game is a bit "off," which is adding to her anxiety. Both her coach and her parents think that massage would be helpful to her. She is in good health and takes no medications, but she does have an erratic eating pattern and recently has been drinking soda with caffeine in it. She also has been working with visualization and progressive relaxation before sleeping. She thinks these methods help her sleep better.

Identify the Facts

Questions that can help with this process include the following:

What is considered normal or balanced function?

What has happened? (Spell out events.)

What caused the imbalance? (Can it be identified?)

What was done or is being done?

What has worked or not worked?

Brainstorm the Possibilities

Questions that can help with this process include the following:

What are the possibilities? (What could it all mean?)

What is my intuition suggesting?

What are the possible patterns of dysfunction?

What are the possible contributing factors?

What are possible interventions?

What might work?

What are other ways to look at the situation?

What do the data suggest?

Consider the Logical Outcomes of Each Possibility

Questions that can help determine outcomes include the following:

What is the logical progression of the symptom pattern, contributing factors, and current behaviors?

What are the logical cause and effect of each intervention identified? What are the pros and cons of each intervention suggested?

What are the consequences of not acting?

Continued

PROFICIENCY EXERCISE 5-3—cont'd

What are the consequences of acting?

Identify the Effect of Each Possibility on the People Involved

Questions that can help identify effects include the following:

In terms of each intervention being considered, what would be the impact on the people involved: client, practitioner, and other professionals working with the client?

How does each person involved feel about the possible interventions?

Is the practitioner within his or her scope of practice to work with such situations?

Is the practitioner qualified to work with such situations?

Does the practitioner feel qualified to work with such situations?

Is there a feeling of cooperation and agreement among all parties involved?

Based on this analysis of the information provided, the massage practitioner would recommend _____, for the following reasons:

Case Study 2

A 39-year-old woman is experiencing mood swings and headaches. She was in a car accident 3 years ago and suffered a whiplash injury, which was treated successfully with physical therapy. She still has some residual stiffness in her neck. She recently had visited her doctor because of the mood swings and headaches. She is premenopausal. No treatment other than stress management and moderate exercise has been recommended at this time. The woman's only child just graduated from high school and has joined the military. The woman was divorced 2 years ago. She has a supportive circle of friends and is financially stable and secure in her job. She says that she wants to feel more in control of her body and wants to be able to self-manage the mood swings and headaches. She is not opposed to hormone therapy for menopause but would like to see if she can manage without it. She is seeking massage as part of her lifestyle self-care program and is motivated.

Identify the Facts

Questions that help with this process are the following:

What is considered normal or balanced function?

What has happened? (Spell out events.)

What caused the imbalance? (Can it be identified?)

What was done or is being done?

What has worked or not worked?

Brainstorm the Possibilities

Questions that help with this process are the following:

What are the possibilities? (What could it all mean?)

PROFICIENCY EXERCISE 5-3—cont'd

What is my intuition suggesting?

What are the possible patterns of dysfunction?

What are the possible contributing factors?

What are possible interventions?

What might work?

What are other ways to look at the situation?

What do the data suggest?

Consider the Logical Outcomes of Each Possibility
Questions that can help determine outcomes include the following:

What is the logical progression of the symptom pattern, contributing factors, and current behaviors?

What are the logical cause and effect of each intervention identified? What are the pros and cons of each intervention suggested?

What are the consequences of not acting?

What are the consequences of acting?

Identify the Effect of Each Possibility on the People Involved
Questions that can help identify effects include the following:

In terms of each intervention being considered, what would be the impact on the people involved: client, practitioner, and other professionals working with the client?

How does each person involved feel about the possible interventions?

Is the practitioner within his or her scope of practice to work with such situations?

Is the practitioner qualified to work with such situations?

Does the practitioner feel qualified to work with such situations?

Is there a feeling of cooperation and agreement among all parties involved?

Based on this analysis of the information provided, the massage practitioner would recommend ____, for the following reasons:

Case Study 3
A 26-year-old man with asthma is experiencing an increase in symptoms. He was recently married and has just moved to a new city because of a job transfer. His wife is 3 months pregnant. He takes good care of himself and is careful with his diet. His exercise program was disrupted by the move, and he has not re-established a regular exercise program. Medication is effective in treating the asthma. His respiratory therapist recommends massage because she feels that the increased stress is a possible cause of the more severe asthma.

Continued

PROFICIENCY EXERCISE 5-3—cont'd

Identify the Facts

Questions that can help with this process include the following:

What is considered normal or balanced function?

What has happened? (Spell out events.)

What caused the imbalance? (Can it be identified?)

What was done or is being done?

What has worked or not worked?

Brainstorm the Possibilities

Questions that can help with this process include the following:

What are the possibilities? (What could it all mean?)

What is my intuition suggesting?

What are the possible patterns of dysfunction?

What are the possible contributing factors?

What are possible interventions?

What might work?

What are other ways to look at the situation?

What do the data suggest?

Consider the Logical Outcomes of Each Possibility

Questions that can help determine outcomes include the following:

What is the logical progression of the symptom pattern, contributing factors, and current behaviors?

What are the logical cause and effect of each intervention identified? What are the pros and cons of each intervention suggested?

What are the consequences of not acting?

What are the consequences of acting?

Identify the Effect of Each Possibility on the People Involved

Questions that can help identify effects include the following:

In terms of each intervention being considered, what would be the impact on the people involved: client, practitioner, and other professionals working with the client?

How does each person involved feel about the possible interventions?

Is the practitioner within his or her scope of practice to work with such situations?

PROFICIENCY EXERCISE 5-3—cont'd

Is the practitioner qualified to work with such situations?

Is there a feeling of cooperation and agreement among all parties involved?

Does the practitioner feel qualified to work with such situations?

Based on this analysis of the information provided, the massage practitioner would recommend ____, for the following reasons:

process, although they remain an important part of the total healing program. Often more aggressive approaches are required to reverse the pathologic condition and allow healing to begin.

Peak performance is defined as maximal conditioning and functioning in a particular action. Although most associated with athletes or entertainers such as dancers, peak performance can occur in more mental actions such as studying for school or dealing with a demanding workload or with family issues. Maximum use of body functions and resources becomes energy consuming and stressful to the body. During peak performance, the body does not hold back energy expenditure, and all available resources are used. If the person's lifestyle does not support recuperation time or if anatomic or physiologic limits are exceeded, injury or depletion commonly occurs, and illness results.

Disease

Disease, or pathology, occurs when homeostatic and restorative body mechanisms break down and can no longer adapt. It is seldom one thing that contributes to pathology, but rather a series of events.

For example, influenza (the flu) is caused by a virus, but not everyone exposed to the virus gets the flu. Consider the situations of one person who gets the flu and another who does not. The person who has the flu smokes, had a minor car accident 2 weeks ago, is experiencing a short-term financial setback, and got into an argument with a coworker 3 days before the onset of the flu. The person who does not have the flu has not experienced anything out of the ordinary for the past 3 months, exercises moderately, and follows a fairly supportive dietary plan with lots of fruits and vegetables. Stress and lifestyle habits are contributing factors for the breakdown of the body's healing mechanisms.

Functioning Limits

The body has anatomic and physiologic functioning limits. The heart can beat only so fast, the endocrine glands secrete

a maximum amount of hormones, the skeletal muscles can lift only so much weight or jump so high. Extraordinary events push the body's limits of functioning. Athletes and new parents, for example, often function at maximum body limits or peak performance.

Under normal conditions the body functions within a margin of safety. Normal physiologic mechanisms inhibit the tendency to function at the body's limits. We usually do not run as fast as we can, work as long as we could, or exert all of our energy to complete a task. Instead, the body signals fatigue, pain, or strain before the anatomic or physiologic limits are reached, and we back off. This very important protective mechanism allows us to live within a healthy range of energy expenditure while keeping functioning energy reserves in place in case of an emergency or extraordinary demand (Figure 5-1). Each time we tap into this reserve, the body tends to

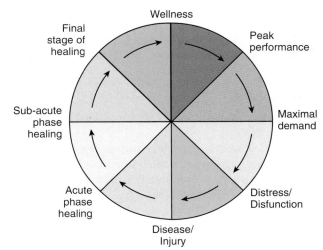

FIGURE 5-1 The health, wellness, injury, and illness continuum.

BOX 5-2

Dysfunction Related to Low Reserves

Example of Dysfunction Related to Functional Limits

A new mother with a fussy baby is unable to get restorative sleep; this continues for 6 months. The mother gets a cold that lingers. The infant is prone to recurring ear infections over the next 3 years, which continues to disturb the sleep pattern of the mother. In addition, the mother's diet becomes limited and begins to consist of mostly snack foods. The mother begins first to have headaches, then neck and shoulder pain, and then low back pain. Finally, 5 years after the birth, just as the child begins school, the mother develops chronic fatigue syndrome with fibromyalgia.

Massage intervention early in the process may help support restorative sleep, especially if help with the baby is provided. Massage and other similar stress-management systems could at least slow the progression of dysfunction. After the headaches appear, massage could be used to manage the pain and reduce the muscle tension patterns in an attempt to support innate body healing and restorative mechanisms. After chronic fatigue symptoms begin with fibromyalgia pain, a multidisciplinary team and lifestyle approach are necessary to reverse pathology.

Example of Dysfunction Related to Attempts to Maintain a Higher Energy Reserve

If a person plays tennis and overstretches the shoulder reaching for the serve, the body senses a danger of harm to the joint. Neurologic sensors may reset muscle patterns, limiting range of motion slightly to prevent this from happening again. Physiologically, protective space has been deposited in the body reserves even though range of motion has been sacrificed. If this continues, eventually the limited range of motion interferes with the ability to play tennis. Dysfunction occurs. If perpetuated and compensated for over a period of time, a pathologic condition usually develops. The person could end up with a "frozen" shoulder.

Massage intervention just after the first event, coupled with a more conservative playing style or improved playing form, might reverse the process, and dysfunction would not develop. Intervention applied at the point when range-of-motion limits were first observed would likely still be effective in reversing the dysfunctional process. However, the intervention plan would be more complex and time-consuming. Interventions introduced after a pathologic process has begun are complex, sometimes aggressive, and occasionally too late to support repair and restoration of function.

progress. Early intervention and referral to appropriate health care professionals are important for identifying potential problems; this allows appropriate measures to be taken to prevent these problems from actually developing. Massage also can support the restorative process to help maintain peak performance. The benefits of massage are most effectively focused on assisting people to stay within the healthy range of functioning.

Development of Pathology

Therapeutic massage has widespread effects on the physiologic functions of the body. Therefore the massage professional is responsible for acquiring a knowledge of pathology, contraindications, and endangerment sites. Obtaining a consensus on such information is difficult, however, because all sources do not agree.

Illness

Illness occurs when a body process breaks down. A person whose immune system did not effectively fight off a cold virus becomes ill with a cold. A person with diabetes is ill. Chronic fatigue syndrome, ulcers, cancer, and multiple sclerosis are all examples of illnesses.

Injury

Injury occurs when tissue is damaged. Cuts, bruises, burns, contusions, fractured bones, sprains, and strains are examples of injuries.

Illness tends to indicate general cautions and contraindications, whereas injury more often creates regional cautions and contraindications.

Therapeutic massage is indicated for both illness and injury. Massage techniques for illness involve very general application of massage to support the body's healing responses (e.g., stress management, pain control, restorative sleep). This approach to massage, sometimes called *general constitutional application,* is more reflexive in nature and is used to reduce the stress load so that the body can heal.

Massage for injury incorporates aspects of general constitutional massage, because healing is necessary for tissue repair. In addition, more mechanical application of lymphatic drainage is used to control edema. Gliding methods are used to approximate (bring close together) the ends of some types of tissue injuries, such as minor muscle tears and strains. Hyperstimulation analgesia and counterirritation reduce acute pain. Methods to increase circulation to the area support tissue formation. Connective tissue applications are used to manage scar tissue formation.

Healing an injury is taxing on the body and strains the restorative mechanism. If an injured person is not in a state of health to begin with, the stress of the injury frequently compromises the immune system, and the person then becomes susceptible to illness.

Inflammation is a factor in both illness and injury, because healing for both involves appropriate activation of the inflammatory response system.

work to restore what was used and, if possible, to add a little more to the reserve.

Dysfunction occurs when the reserve runs low because restorative mechanisms are unable to function effectively or when the body begins to limit function in an attempt to maintain higher energy reserves (Box 5-2).

Massage professionals serve many people at the beginning of dysfunctional patterns; that is, when the client does not feel his or her best but is not yet sick. It is important to monitor clients to make sure that the dysfunctional patterns do not

Because many diseases and injuries have similar symptoms, determining the specific underlying causes of pathology can be difficult. The massage professional must refer clients to qualified, licensed health care providers for a specific diagnosis.

Disease or injury conditions usually are diagnosed or identified by signs and symptoms. Signs are objective abnormalities that can be seen or measured by someone other than the patient. Symptoms are the subjective abnormalities felt only by the patient. A syndrome is a group of different signs and symptoms, usually arising from a common cause. A disease is classified as acute when signs and symptoms develop quickly, last a short time, and then disappear. Diseases that develop slowly and last for a long time (sometimes for life) are classified as chronic.

Communicable diseases can be transmitted from one person to another. The study of communicable diseases is an important process for the massage professional and is discussed in further detail in Chapter 6.

Homeostasis is the relative constancy of the body's internal environment. If homeostasis is disturbed, as occurs in a disease process, a variety of feedback mechanisms usually attempt to return the body to normal. A disease condition exists when homeostasis cannot be restored easily. In acute conditions, the body recovers its homeostatic balance quickly. In chronic diseases, a normal state of balance may never be restored, and compensation develops. Compensation is the process of counterbalancing a defect in body structure or function.

Risk Factors

Certain predisposing conditions may make the development of a disease or some types of injury more likely. Usually called *risk factors,* these conditions may put an individual at risk for developing a disease, but they do not actually cause the disease. Examples of risk factors include genetic factors, age, lifestyle, environmental factors, pre-existing conditions, and stress.

Genetic Factors. There are several types of genetic risk factors. An inherited trait may put a person at a greater than normal risk for developing a specific disease. A family history of disease processes and causes of death usually can reveal the possible genetic traits. Steps can be taken to support the body against the genetic tendency toward a disease process. Changes in diet and lifestyle may be beneficial.

Age. Biologic and behavioral factors increase the risk of developing certain diseases or injuries at certain ages. For example, musculoskeletal problems are common between the ages of 30 and 50 years.

Lifestyle. The way we live, work, and play can put us at risk for some diseases or injuries. Some researchers believe that the high-fat, low-fiber diet common among people in developed nations increases their risk of developing certain types of cancer and cardiovascular diseases. Playing hockey predisposes one to bruises, sprains, or broken bones.

Environmental Factors. Some environmental conditions put people at greater risk of contracting certain diseases. For example, living in an area with high concentrations of air pollution may increase a person's risk of developing respiratory problems. Snow and ice predispose people to injury from falls.

Pre-existing Conditions. A primary (pre-existing) condition can put a person at risk of developing a secondary condition. For example, a viral infection can compromise the immune system, rendering the individual more susceptible to bacterial infection.

Stress. *Stress* can be defined as any substantial change in routine or any activity that forces the body to adapt. Stress places demands on physical, mental, and emotional resources. Research has shown that as stresses accumulate, especially if the stress is long term, the individual becomes increasingly susceptible to physical illness, mental and emotional problems, and accidental injuries.

General Adaptation Syndrome. Dr. Hans Selye, a pioneer in stress research, labeled the body's response to stress the *general adaptation syndrome (GAS),* which involves three stages. The first stage is *alarm,* or the fight-or-flight response, which is the body's initial reaction to the perceived stressor. The second stage is known as the *resistance reaction.* This stage, through the secretion of regulating hormones, allows the body to continue fighting or to endure a stressor long after the effects of the alarm reaction have dissipated. The third stage is *exhaustion,* which occurs if the stress response continues without relief. *General adaptation* is a uniform, consistent, general response to the perceived stimuli.

The GAS describes the way the body mobilizes different defense mechanisms when threatened by harmful (actual or perceived) stimuli. In generalized stress conditions, the hypothalamus acts on the anterior pituitary gland to cause the release of adrenocorticotropic hormone, which stimulates the adrenal cortex to secrete glucocorticoid. In addition, the sympathetic subdivision of the autonomic nervous system (ANS) is stimulated by the adrenal medulla, resulting in the release of epinephrine and norepinephrine to assist the body in responding to the stressful stimulus. Unfortunately, during periods of prolonged stress, glucocorticosteroids (cortisol) may have harmful side effects, including a diminished immune response, altered blood glucose levels, altered protein and fat metabolism, and decreased resistance to stress.

Considering the variety and number of organs and glands innervated by the ANS, it is no wonder that autonomic disorders have varied and broad consequences. This is especially true of stress-induced diseases. A prolonged or excessive physiologic response to stress, the fight-or-flight response, can disrupt normal functioning throughout the body. Stress has been cited as an indirect cause or an important risk factor in many conditions.

Pathologic Conditions and Indications for Massage

Inflammatory Response

Inflammation may occur as a response to any tissue injury. Injury has components of inflammation and pain. The **inflammatory response** is a combination of processes that attempts to minimize injury to tissues and promote healing, thus maintaining homeostasis. Inflammation may also accompany specific immune system reactions. The inflammatory response is an active and important part of the healing process. Heat, redness, swelling, and pain are the four primary signs of inflammation.

Heat and Redness. As tissue cells are damaged, they release inflammatory mediators such as histamine, prostaglandins, and compounds called *kinins*. Some inflammatory mediators cause the blood vessels to dilate, increasing the blood volume available to the tissue. The increased blood volume produces the redness and heat of inflammation. This response is important, because it allows immune system cells (white blood cells) in the blood to travel quickly and easily to the site of injury.

Swelling and Pain. Some inflammatory mediators increase the permeability of blood vessel walls. When water (plasma fluid) leaks out of the vessel, tissue swelling, or edema, results. The pressure caused by edema triggers pain receptors. The fluid that accumulates in inflamed tissue, called *inflammatory exudate,* has the beneficial effect of diluting the irritant. Inflammatory exudate is removed slowly by the lymphatic system. Bacteria and damaged cells are held in the lymph nodes and are destroyed by white blood cells. Occasionally, lymph nodes enlarge when they process a large amount of infectious material.

Sometimes the inflammatory response is more intense or prolonged than desirable. Inflammation can be suppressed by antihistamines, which block the action of histamine, and by antiinflammatories such as aspirin, which disrupts the body's synthesis of prostaglandins.

Inflammatory Disease. Local inflammation occurs in a limited area, such as in a small cut that becomes infected. Systemic inflammation occurs when the irritant spreads throughout the body or when inflammatory mediators cause changes throughout the body. Conditions involving chronic inflammation are classified as *inflammatory diseases* (Table 5-1). Inflammatory conditions such as arthritis, inflammatory bowel disease, asthma, eczema, and chronic bronchitis are among the most common.

Indications for Massage. Therapeutic massage seems to be beneficial in cases of prolonged inflammation. Possible theories regarding this include the following:
- The stimulation from massage activates a release of the body's own antiinflammatory agents.
- Certain types of massage increase the inflammatory process (therapeutic inflammation) to a small degree, triggering the body to complete the process.

TABLE 5-1

Diseases Related to Chronic Inflammation

Seemingly unrelated diseases have a common link— inflammation. This is a partial list of common medical problems associated with chronic inflammation.

Disease or Disorder	Mechanism
Allergy	Mediators induce autoimmune reactions.
Alzheimer's disease	Chronic inflammation destroys brain cells.
Anemia	Mediators disrupt erythropoietin production.
Aortic valve stenosis	Chronic inflammation damages heart valves.
Arthritis	Inflammatory mediators destroy joint cartilage and synovial fluid.
Asthma	Mediators close the airways.
Cancer	Chronic inflammation causes most cancers.
Cardiovascular disease	Inflammation contributes to formation of plaque in the vessels.
Congestive heart failure	Chronic inflammation causes wasting of the heart muscle.
Fibromyalgia	Mediators are elevated in fibromyalgia.
Fibrosis	Mediators attack traumatized tissue.
Heart attack	Chronic inflammation contributes to coronary atherosclerosis.
Kidney failure	Mediators restrict circulation and damage nephrons.
Lupus	Mediators induce an autoimmune attack.
Pancreatitis	Mediators induce pancreatic cell injury.
Psoriasis	Mediators induce dermatitis.
Stroke	Chronic inflammation promotes thromboembolic events.
Surgical complications	Mediators prevent healing.

- Massage may facilitate dilution and removal of the irritant by increasing lymphatic flow.
- Massage supports parasympathetic function.

Tissue Repair. The processes of inflammation trigger tissue repair. Tissue repair is the replacement of dead cells with living cells. In a type of tissue repair called *regeneration,* the new cells are similar to those they replace. Another type of tissue repair is *replacement.* In replacement the new cells are formed from connective tissue and are different from those they replace, resulting in a scar. Often, fibrous connective tissue replaces the damaged tissue, resulting in a condition called *fibrosis.* Most tissue repairs are a combination of regeneration and replacement. A goal in the healing process is to promote regeneration and keep replacement to a minimum. Massage has been shown to slow the formation of scar tissue and to keep scar tissue pliable when it does form.

Therapeutic Inflammation. Because the inflammatory response is part of a healing process, the deliberate creation of inflammation can generate or "jump start" healing mechanisms. Certain methods of massage can be used to create a controlled, localized area of therapeutic inflammation. Deep frictioning techniques and connective tissue stretching methods are the most common approaches. In some healing practices the skin is burned to create inflammation. Acupuncture may also create very small localized areas of inflammation to generate healing mechanisms. These methods are most beneficial in resolving connective tissue dysfunction, particularly fibrotic changes of muscle tissue and areas of scar tissue adhesion.

The benefit derived from the use of therapeutic inflammation depends on the body's ability to generate healing processes. If healing mechanisms are suppressed, methods that create therapeutic inflammation should not be used. Therapeutic inflammation is not used in situations in which sleep disturbance, compromised immune function, a high stress load, or systemic or localized inflammation is already present. This method is also contraindicated if any condition that consists of impaired repair and restorative functions (e.g., fibromyalgia) is present, unless application is carefully supervised as part of a total treatment program.

Client use of antiinflammatory medications is another factor that must be considered. If a person is taking such medication, either the steroidal or nonsteroidal type, the effectiveness of therapeutic inflammation is negated or reduced and restorative mechanisms are inhibited. Any methods that create inflammation are to be avoided when these medications are used.

Pain

Massage professionals especially need to understand the mechanisms of pain. Chapter 4 presents reasons massage is beneficial for symptomatic reduction of pain perception. In this section, we consider the types of pain and the ways massage may be indicated or contraindicated for pain. Understanding the various types of pain helps the massage practitioner recognize when to refer the client to a physician.

Pain is a complex, private, abstract experience that is difficult to explain or describe. It is the main symptom or complaint that causes people to seek health care. Effective management of pain is a major challenge. Defining pain in descriptive and measurable terms is not easy, because pain has physiologic, psychological, and social aspects. Massage professionals need to recognize that pain is what the client says it is, and it exists when the client says it does. *Mosby's Medical, Nursing, and Allied Health Dictionary* defines *pain* as "an unpleasant sensation caused by noxious stimulation of the sensory nerve endings. It is a subjective feeling and an individual response to the cause."[1]

Four distinct processes are involved in pain sensation: transduction, transmission, modulation, and perception. *Pain transduction* is the process by which noxious stimuli lead to electrical activity in the pain receptors. *Pain transmission* involves the process of transmitting pain impulses from the site of transduction over peripheral sensory nerves to the spinal cord and the brain. *Pain modulation* involves neural activity through descending neural pathways from the brain that can influence pain transmission at the level of the spinal cord. Modulation also involves the chemical factors that produce or enhance activity in the primary afferent pain receptors. *Pain perception* is the subjective experience of pain by the person that is somehow produced by the neural activity of pain transmission.

Pain sensation is carried on two types of nerve fibers: large, myelinated A fibers and small, nonmyelinated C fibers. A and C nerve fibers can be distinguished by the two types of pain they elicit, fast pain and slow pain. Fast pain signals are transmitted to the spinal cord by the A nerve fibers and are felt within 0.1 second. Fast pain usually is local and specific and has a prickling, sharp, or electrical quality. Fast pain is elicited in response to mechanical or thermal stimuli on the skin surface but is not felt in deeper tissues of the body. Slow pain is transmitted by the C fibers and is felt 1 second after a noxious stimulus. Slow pain is less well localized and has a burning, throbbing, or aching quality. Slow pain may be elicited by mechanical, thermal, or chemical stimuli in the skin or most deep tissues or organs and is usually associated with tissue damage. Because of this double system of pain innervation, tissue injury often occurs as two distinct pain sensations: an early, sharp pain (transmitted by A nerve fibers), followed by a dull, burning, somewhat prolonged pain (transmitted by C nerve fibers).

Pain Sensations. Pain provides information about tissue-damaging stimuli and thus often enables us to protect ourselves from greater damage. Pain often initiates our search for medical assistance. The subjective description and indication of the location of the pain help pinpoint the underlying cause of disease.

The receptors for pain, called *nociceptors,* are simply the branching ends of the dendrites of certain sensory neurons. Pain receptors are found in almost every tissue of the body and may respond to any type of stimulus. When stimuli for other sensations, such as touch, pressure, heat, and cold, reach a certain intensity, they stimulate the sensation of pain as well. Injured tissue may release prostaglandins, making peripheral nociceptors more sensitive to the normal pain response (hyperalgesia). Aspirin and other nonsteroidal antiinflammatory drugs inhibit the action of prostaglandins and reduce pain.

Excessive stimulation of a sensory organ causes pain. Additional stimuli for pain receptors include excessive distention or dilation of a structure, prolonged muscular contractions, muscle spasms, inadequate blood flow to tissues, or the presence of certain chemical substances. Because of their sensitivity to all stimuli, pain receptors perform a protective function by identifying changes that may endanger the body.

Pain receptors adapt only slightly or not at all. *Adaptation* is the decrease or disappearance of the perception of a sensation even though the stimulus is still present. (An example is the way we get used to our clothes soon after dressing.) If adaptation to pain occurred, pain would cease to be sensed and irreparable damage could result.

Sensory impulses for pain are conducted by the central nervous system (CNS) along spinal and cranial nerves to the thalamus. From there the impulses may be relayed primarily to the parietal lobe of the brain. Recognition of the type and intensity of most pain ultimately is localized in the cerebral cortex of the brain. Pain is called a *thalamic sense* because it is probably brought to the consciousness in the thalamus. Neurons in the thalamus carry the pain impulses to the primary somatosensory cortex, where the sensory aspects of pain are identified by location, nature, and intensity.

This system of pain transmission influences the expression of pain in terms of tolerance, behavior, and sympathetic autonomic responses, especially in relation to chronic pain, because of the associated autonomic responses, emotional behavior, and lowered pain thresholds that often occur.

An understanding of the pain pathways is important because massage application can modulate pain transmission. Individuals perceive painful stimuli in different ways. Specific areas in the brain itself control or influence pain perception: the hypothalamus and limbic structures serve as the emotional center of pain perception, and the frontal cortex provides the rational interpretation and responses to pain. The CNS has a variety of mechanisms for modulating or suppressing nociceptive pain stimuli. Sensory input to the spinal cord may also be influenced by neurotransmitters or neuromodulators. *Neurotransmitters* are neurochemicals that inhibit or stimulate activity at postsynaptic membranes. Substance P, a neuropeptide, is a pain-specific neurotransmitter present in the dorsal horn of the spinal cord (at the "gate," as proposed by the gate control theory), among other sites. Other CNS neurotransmitters involved in pain transmission include acetylcholine, norepinephrine, epinephrine, dopamine, and serotonin.

Serotonin inhibits dorsal horn nociceptor neurons, thereby modulating pain transmission. In addition to serotonin other neurotransmitters such as norepinephrine, and endogenous opioid peptidesi (IE endorphins), are implicated in pain modulation. Opioid peptides, known as *neuromodulators* (pain reducers), are naturally occurring compounds that have morphinelike qualities. Massage influences these neurochemicals (see Chapter 4).

The point where a stimulus is perceived as painful is called the *pain threshold*, which varies somewhat from person to person. One factor that affects the pain threshold is perceptual dominance, in which the pain felt in one area of the body diminishes or obliterates the pain felt in another area. Not until the most severe pain is diminished does the person perceive or acknowledge the other pain. This mechanism is often activated with massage application that produces a "good hurt."

Pain tolerance refers to the duration or intensity of pain that the person endures before acknowledging it and seeking relief. Unlike the pain threshold, pain tolerance is more likely to vary from one individual to another. A person's tolerance to pain is influenced by a variety of factors, including personality type, psychological state at the onset of pain, previous experiences, sociocultural background, and the meaning of the pain to that person (e.g., the ways in which it affects the person's lifestyle). Factors that reduce pain tolerance include repeated exposure to pain, fatigue, sleep deprivation, and stress. Warmth, cold, distraction, alcohol consumption, hypnosis, and strong religious beliefs or faith act to increase pain tolerance.[2]

The origins of pain can be divided into two types, *somatic* and *visceral*. Somatic pain arises from stimulation of receptors in the skin (superficial somatic pain) or from stimulation of receptors in skeletal muscles, joints, tendons, and fascia (deep somatic pain). Visceral pain results from stimulation of receptors in the viscera (internal organs).

The ability of the cerebral cortex to locate the origin of pain is related to past experience. In most instances of somatic pain and in some instances of visceral pain, the cortex accurately projects the pain back to the stimulated area.

Pain usually is classified as acute, chronic, intractable, phantom, or referred.

Acute Pain. Acute pain is either a symptom of a disease condition or a temporary aspect of medical treatment. It acts as a warning signal because it can activate the sympathetic nervous system. *Acute pain* is usually temporary, of sudden onset, and easily localized. The client frequently can describe the pain, which often subsides with or without treatment. During acute pain, arousal of the sympathetic autonomic nervous system occurs.

Chronic Pain. Chronic pain is a major health problem for approximately 25% of the population. *Chronic pain* is pain that persists or recurs for indefinite periods, usually for longer than 6 months. It frequently has an obscure onset, and the character and quality of the pain change over time. Anxiety, sleep disturbances, and depression are common. Chronic pain usually is diffuse and poorly localized and often requires the efforts of a multidisciplinary health care team, which may include a massage therapist, for effective management.

Intractable Pain. Chronic pain that persists even when treatment is provided or that exists without demonstrable disease is called *intractable pain*. Intractable pain represents the greatest challenge to all health care providers. Massage may provide short, temporary, symptomatic relief of this type of pain. This is accomplished by flooding the sensory receptors with sensation, distracting the client temporarily from the perception of pain.

Phantom Pain. *Phantom pain* is a type of pain frequently experienced by clients who have had a limb amputated. These clients experience pain or other sensations in the area of the amputated extremity as if the limb were still there. This pain probably occurs because the remaining proximal portions of the sensory nerves that previously received impulses from the limb are being stimulated by the trauma of the amputation. Stimuli from these nerves are interpreted by the brain as coming from the nonexistent (phantom) limb.

Referred Pain. Pain may be felt in a surface area far from the stimulated organ; this is called **referred pain**. In general, the area or areas to which the pain is referred and the visceral organ involved receive their innervation from the same segment of the spinal cord. Figure 5-2 shows the cutaneous regions to which visceral pain may be referred. A client who has a recurring pain pattern that resembles the patterns on the chart should be referred to a physician for a more specific diagnosis.

As was already stated, irritation of the viscera frequently produces pain that is felt not in the viscera but in some somatic

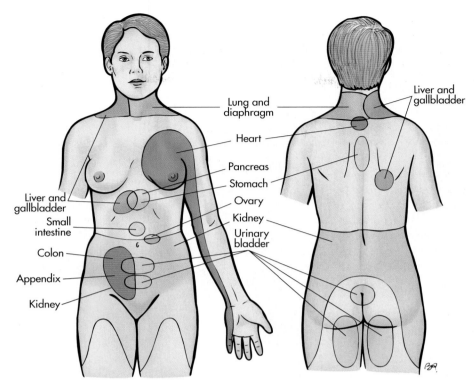

FIGURE 5-2 Referred pain. The diagram indicates cutaneous areas to which visceral pain may be referred. If pain is encountered in these areas during a massage, the massage practitioner needs to refer the client to a physician for diagnosis to rule out visceral dysfunction.

structure that may be located at a considerable distance. Such pain is said to be referred to the somatic structure. Deep somatic pain may also be referred, but superficial pain is not. When visceral pain is both local and referred, it sometimes seems to spread (radiate) from the local to the distant site. Visceral pain, like deep somatic pain, initiates reflex contraction of nearby skeletal muscle. Because somatic pain is much more common than visceral pain, the brain has "learned" to project the pain to the somatic area.

Obviously, a knowledge of referred pain and the common sites of pain referral from each of the visceral organs is very important to massage therapists and other health care professionals. However, sites of reference are not stereotyped, and unusual reference sites occur with considerable frequency. Heart pain, for instance, may be experienced as purely abdominal, may be referred to the right arm, and may even be referred to the neck. Any client with a referred or unexplained pain pattern should be referred to a physician, especially if the pattern is similar to visceral referred pain patterns (see Figure 5-2). When pain is referred, it usually is referred to a structure that developed from the same embryonic segment or dermatome as the structure in which the pain originates (Figure 5-3).

Evaluation of Pain. Because pain is a primary indicator in many disease processes, massage practitioners must have a basic evaluation protocol for pain so that they can determine when to refer their clients to the appropriate health care provider. The following guidelines for evaluating pain can help in this process.
- Location
  - Localized pain is pain confined to the site of origin.

- Projected pain is typically a result of proximal nerve compression. This pain is perceived in the tissue supplied by the nerve.
- Radiating pain is diffuse pain, which is not well localized, around the site of origin.
- Referred pain is felt in an area distant from the site of the painful stimulus.
- Types
  - *Pricking or bright pain:* This type of pain is experienced when the skin is cut or jabbed with a sharp object. It is short-lived but intense and easily localized.
  - *Burning pain:* This type is slower to develop, lasts longer, and is less accurately localized. It is experienced when the skin is burned. It often stimulates cardiac and respiratory activity.
  - *Aching pain:* Aching pain occurs when the visceral organs are stimulated. It is constant, not well localized, and often is referred to areas of the body far from where the damage is occurring. This type of pain is important because it may be a sign of a life-threatening disorder of a vital organ.
  - *Deep pain:* The main difference between superficial and deep sensibility is the different nature of the pain evoked by noxious stimuli. Unlike superficial pain, deep pain is poorly localized, nauseating, and frequently associated with sweating and changes in blood pressure. Deep pain can be elicited experimentally from the periosteum and ligaments by injecting them with hypertonic saline. Pain produced in this fashion initiates reflex contraction of nearby skeletal muscles. This reflex contraction is similar to the muscle spasm associated with injuries to bones,

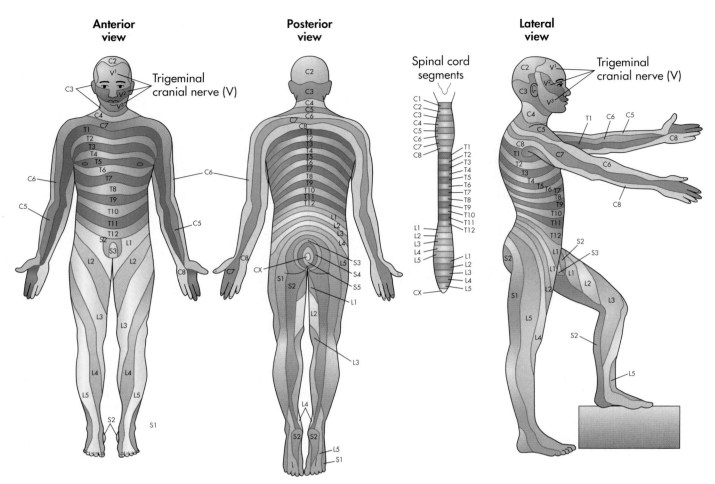

FIGURE 5-3 Dermatomes. Segmental dermatome distribution of spinal nerves to the front, back, and side of the body. *C,* Cervical segments; *T,* thoracic segments; *L,* lumbar segments; *S,* sacral segments; *CX,* coccygeal segment. (From Thibodeau GA, Patton KT: *The human body in health and disease,* ed 3, St Louis, 2002, Mosby.)

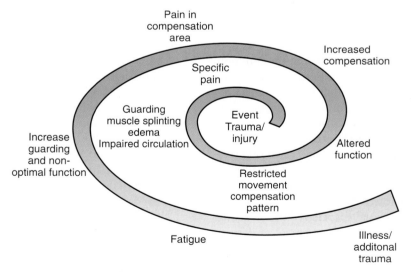

FIGURE 5-4 Pain-spasm-pain cycle.

tendons, and joints. The steadily contracting muscles become ischemic, and ischemia stimulates the pain receptors in the muscles. The pain, in turn, initiates more spasms, creating a vicious cycle called the **pain-spasm-pain cycle** (Figure 5-4).

■ *Muscle pain:* If a muscle with an adequate blood supply contracts rhythmically, pain does not usually result. However, if the blood supply to a muscle is occluded (cut off), contraction soon causes pain. The pain persists after the contraction until blood flow is re-established.

If a muscle with a normal blood supply is made to contract continuously without periods of relaxation, it also begins to ache because the maintained contraction compresses the blood vessels supplying the muscle.

Pain Assessment. Massage professionals gather subjective information by asking the client about symptoms associated with the pain. Practitioners should provide ample opportunity to discuss with the client what the pain means to that person by asking about its impact on the client's lifestyle. They also should document pain treatment methods (and their effectiveness) that the client has used in the past. Direct observation of nonverbal and verbal behavior may provide additional clues about the client's pain experience. Nonverbal behaviors such as facial grimacing, flinching, tearing, abnormal gait or posture, muscle tension, and guarding of the body are common indicators of pain. Verbal and emotional signals indicating pain may include crying, moaning, groaning, irritability, sadness, and changes in voice tone.

Gender and cultural differences exist in the types of displays people use to express pain. As described previously, acute pain often activates a sympathetic response, resulting in increases in the heart and respiratory rates and blood pressure, pallor, flushing, sweating, and pupil dilation. Very brief, intense pain may be followed by a rebound parasympathetic response.

The massage practitioner should inspect and palpate the painful area to test range of motion of involved joints, to determine whether muscle guarding is present, and to identify trigger points and other tender points of pain and areas of decreased sensation or increased sensitivity.

Indications for Massage. Pain is a complex problem with physical, psychological, social, and financial components. Subjective measurements of pain intensity are more reliable than observable ones. Pain scales, such as a 1 to 10 scale, are helpful for measuring necessary pain perception. Only the client can determine the degree of severity. Pain is rarely the same at all times. It is felt (perceived) differently over time and differs with various precipitating and aggravating factors. Pain can range from excruciating to mild and may be difficult for the client to verbalize. Pain can be alleviated in many ways. The massage professional, as part of a health care team, can contribute valuable manual therapy in various pain conditions, using direct tissue manipulation and reflex stimulation of the nervous system and the circulation. As a therapeutic intervention, massage may help reduce the need for pain medication, thus reducing the side effects of medication.

All medications, including over-the-counter (OTC) drugs (i.e., those available without a prescription), have some side effects. Obviously, with clients in extreme pain, the massage therapy must be monitored by a doctor or other appropriate health care professional. Most people experience pain in less severe forms occasionally throughout life. Massage may provide temporary symptomatic relief of moderate pain brought on by daily stress, replacing OTC pain medications or reducing their use.

Acute pain and chronic pain are managed somewhat differently, therefore distinguishing between the two is important. Intervention for acute pain is less invasive and focuses on supporting a current healing process. Chronic pain is managed either with symptomatic relief or with a more aggressive rehabilitation approach that incorporates a therapeutic change process. (See Chapter 12 for specific pain management strategies.)

Impingement Syndromes

The two types of nerve impingement syndromes are compression and entrapment. As was explained in Chapter 4, *compression* is pressure on a nerve by a bony structure, and *entrapment* is pressure on a nerve from soft tissue. Massage is beneficial for entrapment and can manage some symptoms of nerve compression, even though the direct causal factor is not addressed.

Cervical Plexus. If the impingement is on the cervical plexus, the person experiences headaches, neck pain, and breathing difficulties. The muscles most responsible for pressure on the cervical plexus are the suboccipital and sternocleidomastoid muscles. Shortened connective tissues at the cranial base also will press on these nerves.

The cervical plexus is formed by the ventral rami of the upper four cervical nerves. The phrenic nerve is part of this plexus. It innervates the diaphragm, and any disruption to this nerve affects breathing. Many cutaneous (skin) branches of the cervical plexus transmit sensory impulses from the skin of the neck, ear, and shoulder. The motor branches innervate muscles of the anterior neck.

Brachial Plexus. The brachial plexus, situated partly in the neck and partly in the axilla, provides virtually all the nerves that innervate the upper limb. Any imbalance that brings pressure on this complex of nerves results in shoulder pain, chest pain, arm pain, wrist pain, and hand pain.

The muscles most often responsible for impingement on the brachial plexus are the scalenes, pectoralis minor, and subclavius. Muscles of the arm occasionally impinge on branches of the brachial plexus. Brachial plexus impingement is responsible for thoracic outlet symptoms, which often are misdiagnosed as carpal tunnel syndrome. Whiplash injury involves the brachial plexus.

Lumbar Plexus. Impingement on the lumbar plexus nerve may give rise to low back discomfort with a belt distribution of pain, as well as pain in the lower abdomen, genitals, thigh, and medial lower leg. The main muscles that impinge on the lumbar plexus are the quadratus lumborum and the psoas. Shortening of the lumbar dorsal fascia exaggerates a lordosis and causes vertebral impingement on the lumbar plexus.

Sacral Plexus. The sacral plexus has approximately a dozen named branches. Almost half of these serve the buttock and lower limb; the others innervate pelvic structures. The main branch is the sciatic nerve. Impingement of this nerve by the piriformis muscle gives rise to sciatica.

Ligaments that stabilize the sacroiliac joint can affect the sacral plexus. Pressure on the sacral plexus can cause gluteal pain, leg pain, genital pain, and foot pain.

Indications for Massage. Massage methods can soften and stretch connective tissues that may impinge on nerves. They also can normalize muscle tension patterns, restoring a more normal resting length to shortened muscles and thereby reducing pressure on nerves.

Psychological Dysfunctions

Science has validated the body/mind link in terms of health and disease. Many risk factors for the development of physical (body) pathology are mentally (mind) influenced, such as stress levels and lifestyle choices. The same is true for mental health and pathology. The physical state of an individual has a strong influence on mental functioning. Usually when people feel well physically, they also feel well mentally; the reverse, too, is often the case; feeling bad mentally results in physical dysfunctions. Neurochemicals such as serotonin and dopamine exert a strong influence on a person's mental state.

The major mental health dysfunctions that affect Western society are trauma and post-traumatic stress disorder, pain and fatigue syndromes, anxiety and depressive disorders, and stress-related illness.

Trauma is defined as follows:

- Physical injury caused by violent or disruptive action or by a toxic substance
- Psychic injury resulting from a severe emotional shock, either short term or long term

Post-traumatic stress disorder, as defined by the *Diagnostic and Statistical Manual of Mental Disorders (DSM-IV),* includes flashback memory experiences, state-dependent memory, somatization, anxiety, irritability, sleep disturbance, concentration difficulties, times of melancholy or depression, grief, fear, worry, anger, and avoidance behavior. Post-traumatic stress disorder can have long-term effects.

Pain and fatigue syndromes are defined as multicausal and often chronic nonproductive patterns that interfere with well-being, activities of daily living, and productivity. Some current conditions in this category are fibromyalgia, chronic fatigue syndrome, Epstein-Barr viral infection, sympathetic reflex dystrophy, headache, arthritis, chronic cancer pain, neuropathy, low back syndrome, idiopathic pain, somatization disorder, and intractable pain syndrome. Acute pain can be a factor, as can acute "episodes" of chronic conditions.

Anxiety and depressive disorders are characterized by anxiety and depression. Anxiety is an uneasy feeling usually connected with increased sympathetic arousal responses. Depression is characterized by a decrease of vital functional activity and mood disturbances of exaggerated emptiness, hopelessness, and melancholy, or unbridled periods of high energy with no purpose or outcome.

Anxiety and depressive disorders are commonly seen with fatigue and pain syndromes. Panic behavior, phobias, and a sense of impending doom, along with the sense of being overwhelmed and hopeless, are common with these disorders. Mood swings, breathing pattern disorder, sleep disturbance, concentration difficulties, memory disturbances, outbursts of anger, fatigue, changes in habits of daily living, appetite, and activity levels are symptoms of these disorders.

Stress-related illness is defined as an increased stress load or reduced ability to adapt that depletes the reserve capacity of individuals, increasing their vulnerability to health problems. Stress-related illness can encompass the previously mentioned conditions as the primary cause of dysfunction or as the result of the stress of the dysfunction. Excessive stress sometimes manifests as cardiovascular problems, including hypertension; digestive difficulties, including heartburn, ulcer, and bowel syndromes; respiratory illness and susceptibility to bacterial and viral illness; endocrine dysfunction, particularly adrenal or thyroid dysfunction and delayed or reduced cellular repair; sleep disorders; and breathing pattern disorder, just to mention a few conditions (Proficiency Exercises 5-4 and 5-5).

Indications for Massage. Massage intervention has a strong physiologic effect through the comfort of compassionate touch, as well as a physical influence on mental state through the effect on the ANS and neurochemicals. Therefore people experiencing mental health problems may benefit from massage. Management of pain is an important factor. Because therapeutic massage often can offer symptomatic relief from chronic pain, the helplessness that accompanies these difficulties may dissipate as the person realizes that management methods exist. Soothing of any ANS hyperactivity or hypoactivity provides a sense of inner balance. Normalization of the breathing mechanism allows the client to breathe without restriction and can reduce the tendency for breathing pattern disorder, which feeds anxiety and panic.

Therapeutic massage can provide intervention on a physical level to restore a more normal function to the body, which supports appropriate interventions by qualified mental health professionals. Certainly strong and appropriate indications exist for the use of massage therapy in the restoration of mental health, but caution is indicated in terms of the establishment of dual roles and boundary difficulties. It is very important to work with mental health providers in these situations.

CONTRAINDICATIONS TO MASSAGE THERAPY

SECTION OBJECTIVES

Using the information presented in this section, the student will be able to perform the following:

- Evaluate a client's status to determine whether massage is contraindicated
- Effectively refer a client to a primary health care provider
- Interpret the reference list of indications and contraindications provided in Appendix A
- Recognize the warning signs of cancer
- List the endangerment sites for massage

As mentioned earlier in this chapter, a contraindication is any condition that renders a particular treatment improper or undesirable or that raises cautions concerning treatment, requiring supervision. Contraindications to massage are the

PROFICIENCY EXERCISE 5-4

Student Note: Give it a try and follow the example. The more you practice, the more you will understand the process.

Read the case study presented under Your Turn. Then use the clinical reasoning model (presented in the Example Case Study) to develop a statement validating the indication for the use of therapeutic massage.

Example Case Study

The client is a 45-year-old woman. She works 6 to 8 hours a day on the computer. She is experiencing mind fatigue and midback tension with pain. Her left arm tingles during sleep and wakes her up. She has a chronic compressed disk at L4. Currently she is involved in a large writing project and has a deadline to meet. Her exercise and stretching program has become sporadic. She also finds herself regularly driving for 3 and 4 hours at a time, which aggravates the nerve impingement in her low back. What are the indications for massage?

Identify the Facts

Questions that can help with this process include the following:

What is considered normal or balanced function?
   Regular movement without prolonged static positions

What has happened? (Spell out events.)
   Workload and a deadline are requiring more time at the computer. Long periods of time are required in the car. The exercise and stretching program has been interrupted.

What caused the imbalance? (Can it be identified?)
   Static seated position with the arm held in fixed position

What was done or is being done?
   Exercise and stretching, but this pattern has been interrupted.

What has worked or not worked?
   Exercise and stretching, but this pattern has been interrupted.

Brainstorm the Possibilities

Questions that can help with this process include the following:

What are the possibilities? (What could it all mean?)
   Muscles could be shortening in the front, changing the posture and straining the back muscles. Something may be interfering with circulation. Nerves could be impinged. Pain and increased tension could be contributing to mind fatigue.

What is my intuition suggesting?
   The client is tired, overworked, and sitting in one position too long.

What are the possible patterns of dysfunction?
   The existing back disk dysfunction could be causing compensation, which is being aggravated by the ongoing static seated position. A fixed position of the shoulder while driving or at the computer may cause muscle tension that is causing impingement upon a nerve. Stress from the deadline for the project is interfering with sleep.

What are the possible contributing factors?
   Pre-existing back injury, age, improper position at the computer, or an ergonomically incorrect chair

What are possible interventions?
   Massage, stretching, exercise, progressive relaxation, changing position of equipment

What might work?
   A combination of the possible interventions might be beneficial.

What are other ways to look at the situation?
   Excessive workload with equipment that is positioned to aggravate the problem

What do the data suggest?
   Multicausal factors

Consider the Logical Outcomes of Each Possibility

Questions that can help determine outcomes include the following:

What is the logical progression of the symptom pattern, contributing factors, and current behaviors?
   If the condition remains unchanged, the symptoms are likely to worsen. After the deadline is reached, the main causal factor will be eliminated and the condition could reverse itself.

What are the logical cause and effect of each intervention identified? What are the pros and cons of each intervention suggested?
   Massage: Pros—Reduces muscle tension, supports sleep
   Cons—Time away from work; effects may be short term
   Logical outcome—Massage may provide temporary relief until the condition changes.
   Stretching: Pros—Can be done throughout the day; would not require time away from job
   Cons—Effects short lived
   Logical outcome—Stretching would temporarily relieve the tension pattern and provide a counterbalancing activity to the static seated position.
   Exercise: Pros—Reduces muscle tension, supports sleep, clears mind fatigue
   Cons—Time away from work; effects may be short term
   Logical outcome—Exercise may provide temporary relief until the condition changes while supporting ongoing health maintenance.
   Progressive relaxation: Pros—Supports sleep and helps relieve muscle tension; can be done throughout the day; would not require time away from job
   Cons—Effects short lived
   Logical outcome—Progressive relaxation would provide some symptomatic relief.
   Changing position of equipment: Pros—Would address a possible causal factor; would not require any other energy expenditure
   Cons—Would not address emotional stress or physical symptoms
   Logical outcome—If equipment position is a causal factor, a change could eliminate a source of the problem.

Continued

PROFICIENCY EXERCISE 5-4—cont'd

What are the consequences of not acting?
   Situation may worsen or may resolve after project is completed.

What are the consequences of acting?
   Symptoms and further compensation patterns may be managed.

Identify the Effect of Each Possibility on the People Involved

Questions that can help identify effects include the following:

In terms of each intervention being considered identify potential impact on the people involved: client, practitioner, and other professionals working with the client.

How does each person involved feel about the possible interventions?
   Massage: Client is supportive, massage therapist is supportive.
   Stretching: Client is supportive.
   Exercise: Client is supportive.
   Progressive relaxation: Client does not feel that benefits are sufficient to justify time spent.
   Changing position of equipment: Client is supportive,

Is the practitioner within his or her scope of practice to work with such situations?
   Yes

Is the practitioner qualified to work with such situations?
   Yes, with cautions for disk compression

Does the practitioner feel qualified to work with such situations?
   Yes

Is there a feeling of cooperation and agreement among all parties involved?
   Yes

Based on this analysis of the information provided, the massage practitioner would recommend massage, stretching, exercise, and an equipment change, for the following reasons:
   The condition is short term until the project is completed. The client previously used stretching and exercise and needs encouragement to begin to use those methods again. Minor changes in the position of the computer may offer benefits. Massage is indicated to support sleep and address the general stress, the possible minor nerve impingement, the muscle tension from the static position, and management of muscle pain.

Your Turn

Case Study

The client is an 81-year-old man in good health for his age. He took a fall 6 months ago but recovered nicely. He is active in his church and works in his garden. His wife died 18 months ago after a long illness. Lately his age-related aches and pains are bothering him more, especially in his knees. This is interfering with his activities. He has mild hypertension and is taking medication for the condition. Currently the hypertension is under control. He takes aspirin for his arthritis as needed. No problems were detected during his last physical. What are the indications for massage?

Identify the Facts

Questions that can help with this process include the following:

What is considered normal or balanced function?

What has happened? (Spell out events.)

What caused the imbalance? (Can it be identified?)

What was done or is being done?

What has worked or has not worked?

Brainstorm the Possibilities

Questions that can help with this process include the following:

What are the possibilities? (What could it all mean?)

PROFICIENCY EXERCISE 5-4—cont'd

What is my intuition suggesting?

What are other ways to look at the situation?

What are the possible patterns of dysfunction?

What do the data suggest?

Consider the Logical Outcomes of Each Possibility
Questions that can help determine outcomes include the following:

What are the possible contributing factors?

What is the logical progression of the symptom pattern, contributing factors, and current behaviors?

What are possible interventions?

What are the logical cause and effect of each intervention identified? What are the pros and cons of each intervention suggested?

What might work?

Continued

PROFICIENCY EXERCISE 5-4—cont'd

What are the consequences of not acting?

What are the consequences of acting?

Identify the Effect of Each Possibility on the People Involved
Questions that can help identify effects include the following:

In terms of each intervention being considered, what would be the impact on the people involved: client, practitioner, and other professionals working with the client?

How does each person involved feel about the possible interventions?

Is the practitioner within his or her scope of practice to work with such situations?

Is the practitioner qualified to work with such situations?

Does the practitioner feel qualified to work with such situations?

Is there a feeling of cooperation and agreement among all parties involved?

Based on this analysis of the information provided, the massage practitioner would recommend _____

_____

for the following reasons:

PROFICIENCY EXERCISE 5-5

1. *Do a self-evaluation and list all your predisposing risk factors for disease in the space provided.*

2. *Pick one risk factor. Research a wellness plan to provide support for your body to prevent or reduce the likelihood of your developing the pathologic condition. Summarize the condition.*

BOX 5-3

Warning Signs of Cancer

- Sores that do not heal
- Unusual bleeding
- A change in the appearance or size of a wart or mole
- A lump or thickening in any tissue
- Persistent hoarseness or cough
- Chronic indigestion
- A change in bowel or bladder function

responsibility of both physicians and massage practitioners. The massage professional is not expected to diagnose any condition but should learn the client's particular condition by taking a thorough history and completing a physical assessment. The massage professional must be able to recognize indications and contraindications for therapeutic massage based on this information.

The massage practitioner also should have a current medical dictionary and comprehensive pathology reference available to research unfamiliar terms and pathologic conditions. Internet search programs are helpful as well. A massage practitioner is not a physician nor a mental health professional and is not expected to know the symptoms of all diseases, but resources must be available to locate specific information as needed.

Massage practitioners should not rely on lists of specific contraindications, but rather should use a set of medical and therapeutic guidelines pertinent to clinical applications and recent research developments. Unfortunately, such guidelines are not consistent in current literature. Contraindications are unique to each client and to each region of the body. The ability to reason clinically is essential to making appropriate decisions about the advisability of, modifications to, or avoidance of massage interventions. It is important to understand when to refer a client for diagnosis and when to obtain assistance in modifying the approach to the massage session so that it will best serve the client. A medical professional (including mental health and athletic training) must always be consulted if any doubt exists concerning the advisability of therapy. When in doubt, refer!

Contraindications can be divided into regional and general types.

- *Regional contraindications* relate to a specific area of the body. For our purposes, a regional contraindication means that massage may be provided but not to the problematic area. However, the client should be referred to a physician, who can make a diagnosis and rule out underlying conditions.
- *General contraindications* require a physician's evaluation to rule out serious underlying conditions before any

massage is indicated. If the physician recommends massage, he or she will need to help the massage therapist develop a comprehensive treatment plan with appropriate cautions. Mental health dysfunctions fall into the general contraindication category.

Therapeutic massage often is beneficial for clients who are receiving treatment for a specific medical or mental health condition or who are involved in a training program, such as a dancer or gymnast; however, caution is indicated.

In general, massage is indicated for musculoskeletal discomfort, circulation enhancement, relaxation, stress reduction, and pain control, as well as in situations in which analgesics, antiinflammatory drugs, muscle relaxants, and blood pressure, antianxiety, and antidepressant medications may be prescribed. Therapeutic massage, appropriately provided, can support the use of these medications, manage some side effects, and in mild cases may be able to replace them.

The general effects of stress and pain reduction and increased circulation, as well as the physical comfort derived from therapeutic massage, complement most other medical and mental health treatment modalities. However, when other therapies, including medication, are used, the physician must be able to accurately evaluate the effectiveness of each treatment the client is receiving. If the physician is unaware that the client is receiving massage, the effects of other therapies may be misinterpreted.

Clients with any vague or unexplainable symptoms of fatigue, muscle weakness, and general aches and pains should be immediately referred to a physician. Many disease processes share these symptoms. This recommendation may seem overly cautious, but in the early stages of some very serious illnesses, the symptoms are not well defined. If the physician is able to detect a disease process early in its development, often a more successful outcome is possible. A specific diagnosis is essential for effective treatment. Massage should be avoided in all infectious diseases suggested by fever, nausea, and lethargy until a diagnosis has been made and recommendations from a physician can be followed.

Tumors and Cancer

Benign tumors remain localized within the tissue from which they arise and usually grow very slowly. **Malignant tumors** (cancer) tend to spread to other regions of the body. The cells migrate by way of lymphatic or blood vessels; this manner of spread is called **metastasis.** Cells that do not metastasize can also spread by growing rapidly and extending the tumor into nearby tissues. Malignant tumors may replace part of a vital organ with abnormal tissues, which is a life-threatening situation.

Early detection of cancer is important, because cancer is most treatable in the early stages of primary tumor development, before metastasis and the development of secondary tumors. Box 5-3 presents the warning signs of cancer, as summarized by oncologists (cancer specialists). The massage practitioner may be the first to recognize these early warning signs in a client.

Although it is important to refer the client for proper evaluation to determine whether cancer is developing, the massage practitioner must *never* suggest to the client that cancer is evident. Instead, the practitioner should simply point out the changes and explain that it is important that they be evaluated by a qualified professional.

Massage is not necessarily contraindicated for people with cancer. Current research indicates that massage can support the immune system's battle with cancer cells and manage the side effects of treatment. However, massage must be used as part of the entire treatment program and supervised by qualified medical personnel. As with any stressful condition, the massage practitioner must not overtax the system of a client with cancer; instead, massage must be used as a general support to the body's healing mechanisms.

Medications

The massage professional needs to be aware of any medications the client is taking. Massage therapists should have a current edition of *Mosby's Drug Consult, Physicians' Desk Reference, Medical Economics,* or a similar drug reference book so that all medications listed on the client information form can be researched. Internet search programs for researching medications also are available. In addition, the client may be able to provide information about each medication he or she takes.

In general, a medication is prescribed to do one of the following:

- Stimulate a body process
- Inhibit a body process
- Replace a chemical in the body

Therapeutic massage can also stimulate, inhibit, and replace body functions. When the medication and massage stimulate the same process, the effects are synergistic, and the result can be too much stimulation. If the medication and massage inhibit the same process, the result is again synergistic, but this time with too much inhibition. If the medication stimulates an effect and massage inhibits the same effect, massage can be antagonistic to the medication. Although massage seldom interacts substantially with a medication that replaces a body chemical, it is important to be aware of possible synergistic or inhibitory effects.

Massage often can be used to manage undesirable side effects of medications. In particular, medications that stimulate sympathetic ANS function can cause uncomfortable side effects such as digestive upset, anxiety or restlessness, and sleep disruption. The mild inhibitory effects of massage resulting from stimulation of parasympathetic activity can sometimes provide short-term relief of the undesirable effects of the medication without interfering with its desired action. Especially in these instances, caution is required, and close monitoring by the primary care physician is necessary.

For example, a side effect of some medications is anxiety. Massage may help the client by reducing anxiety, or it may be the cause of an adverse reaction. If the doctor is using the level of anxiety to monitor the correct medication dosage and if anxiety levels are lowered through massage, the medication dosage may appear to be too high.

Massage professionals should be able to assess the effects of medications and should be aware of the ways massage may influence these effects. Massage practitioners need to be specifically knowledgeable about antiinflammatory drugs, muscle relaxants, anticoagulants (blood thinners), analgesics (pain modulators), and other medications that alter sensation, muscle tone, standard reflex reactions, cardiovascular function, kidney or liver function, or personality. They also should be aware of the effects of over-the-counter medications, herbs, and vitamins. If a client is taking medication, it is important to have the physician confirm the advisability of therapeutic massage. (See Appendix C for information on basic pharmacology and a list of common medications and possible interactions with massage.)

Endangerment Sites

Endangerment sites are areas in which nerves and blood vessels surface close to the skin and are not well protected by muscle or connective tissue. Deep, sustained pressure in these areas can damage the vessels and nerves. Areas containing fragile bony projections that could be broken off are also considered endangerment sites. The kidney area is considered an endangerment site because the kidneys are loosely suspended in fat and connective tissue. Heavy pounding is contraindicated in that area. When the massage therapist is working over an endangerment site, avoidance or light pressure is indicated to prevent damage. The areas shown in Figure 5-5 are commonly considered endangerment sites for the massage therapist (Proficiency Exercise 5-6).

Other endangerment sites and activities include the following:

- Eyes
- Area inferior to the ear (fascial nerve, styloid process, external carotid artery)
- Posterior cervical area (spinous processes, cervical plexus)
- Lymph nodes
- Medial brachium (between the biceps and triceps)
- Musculocutaneous, median, and ulnar nerves

PROFICIENCY EXERCISE 5-6

Locate all endangerment sites on a fellow student.

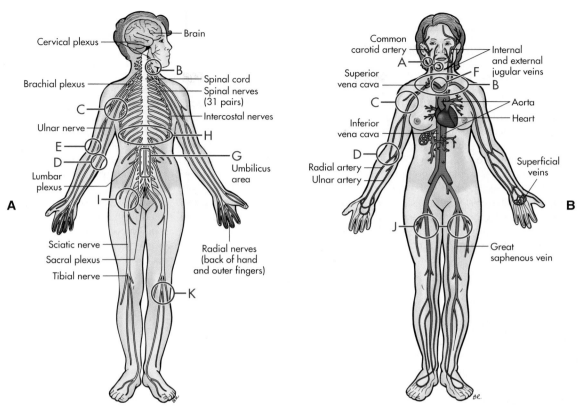

FIGURE 5-5 Endangerment sites of the nervous system and the cardiovascular system. **A,** Anterior triangle of the neck—Carotid artery, jugular vein, and vagus nerve, which are located deep to the sternocleidomastoid muscle. **B,** Posterior triangle of the neck—Specifically the nerves of the brachial plexus, the brachiocephalic artery and vein superior to the clavicle, and the subclavian arteries and vein. **C,** Axillary area—The brachial artery, axillary vein and artery, cephalic vein, and nerves of the brachial plexus. **D,** Medial epicondyle of the humerus—The ulnar nerve; also the radial and ulnar arteries. **E,** Lateral epicondyle—The radial nerve. **F,** Area of the sternal notch and anterior throat—Nerves and vessels to the thyroid gland and the vagus nerve. **G,** Umbilicus area—To either side; descending aorta and abdominal aorta. **H,** Twelfth rib, dorsal body—Location of the kidney. **I,** Sciatic notch—Sciatic nerve (the sciatic nerve passes out of the pelvis through the greater sciatic foramen, under cover of the piriformis muscle). **J,** Inguinal triangle located lateral and inferior to the pubis—Medial to the sartorius, external iliac artery, femoral artery, great saphenous vein, femoral vein, and femoral nerve. **K,** Popliteal fossa—Popliteal artery and vein and tibial nerve.

- Brachial artery
- Basilic vein
- Cubital (anterior) area of the median nerve, radial and ulnar arteries, and median cubital vein
- Deep stripping over a vein in a direction away from the heart (contraindicated because of possible damage to the valve system)
- Application of lateral pressure to the knees

Some acupuncture authorities consider the ankle area on pregnant women to be an endangerment site.

Referral

Referral is a method by which a client is sent to a health care professional for diagnosis and treatment of a disease. When a client is ill, he or she is aware of it. If the client is very sick, it shows. Common sense should be the guide. Although massage cannot cure anything, it can assist in the client's healing process. Massage professionals may pick up subtle changes in the tissue before the client consciously recognizes that some-

thing is out of balance. When this happens, the client should be referred to a qualified professional for specific diagnosis.

Massage practitioners should become familiar with the health professionals in their area, including medical doctors, osteopathic doctors, podiatrists, chiropractors, physical therapists, occupational therapists, psychologists, licensed counselors, athletic trainers, exercise physiologists, and dentists. Some health care providers offer alternative therapies, such as acupuncture and homeopathy. Because clients trust the massage practitioner, before referring a client to a specific health care professional, the massage practitioner should take the time to get to know that health professional. This can be done by calling the professional's office and making an appointment for a short visit, during which the professional's feelings about massage could be discussed. Information about massage should be left for reference.

Clients must always be referred to their personal health care professionals. The massage therapist should make no attempt to direct them to different health care professionals. If the client does not have a doctor, chiropractor, or coun-

BOX 5-4

Example of a Referral by a Massage Therapist

Sandy, a veteran massage practitioner, has been seeing a client, Ms. Jones, every other week for massage for about 1 year. Ms. Jones has a mole on her left shoulder. At the last two visits, Sandy noticed that the mole had started to change shape and looked different. Sandy feels that these signs should be evaluated by a health care professional with more specific training. She says to Ms. Jones, "The mole you have on your left shoulder looks a little different to me. Have you noticed any change? It is important to have your doctor look at any changes in a mole. Will you please make an appointment with your personal physician to have the mole examined? Have your doctor give you a written statement that you were seen and that massage may be continued, along with any special instructions. It is important for you to do this

before we schedule the next massage. After I determine it is a good idea to refer a client, and I put that on your record, I need written verification from the doctor to see you again."

If the client does not have a personal physician, Sandy could say, "I have talked with various health care professionals in our area and have developed a referral list. I am sure one of the doctors listed will be able to help you, or you can ask a family member or friend for a recommendation."

Ms. Jones says, "What do you think the change in the mole is?" Sandy replies, "I am trained to notice changes in the body and when to refer a client, but I am not trained to be able to diagnose what any specific condition is. That is the role of a physician. It is best for you to go and have it checked by someone who has much more training in this area."

---

selor, a list of professionals who have been contacted and educated about therapeutic massage should be provided.

When referral is indicated, the massage practitioner should simply tell the client why a referral to a health care professional is being recommended, explaining that the observed set of signs or symptoms should be evaluated by someone who has more specialized training (Box 5-4). No specific condition should be named. The client should be given the massage professional's business card or brochure to give to the health care professional to facilitate contact. The client must sign a release of information before information can be exchanged between professionals.

If the massage therapist feels that it is necessary to refer a client for diagnosis, some sort of written permission from the doctor is needed for the therapist to continue to see the client. The client should obtain the written documentation and bring it to the next massage session. This information is kept in the client's file. If the doctor or other health care professional has given any specific directions or recommendations, they must be followed exactly. Massage therapy must never interfere with or contradict the care plan of the physician, nor should the massage therapist assume the role of counselor. If it is necessary to contact the health care professional directly, the massage professional should always work through the receptionist. Leave whatever information is needed with the front desk, and if the doctor feels it is necessary to speak with the massage therapist directly, he or she will call.

The reason for referral and the date of referral must be noted on the client's record, along with the signs and symptoms. If the client responds in any unusual way, such as by panicking or refusing to go to the doctor, this must be indicated on the client record as well. The written permission for continuation of massage from the health professional must also be placed in the client's file.

Most disease processes present a few basic symptoms (see Appendix A for more comprehensive information). A client should always be referred for diagnosis if the symptoms listed in Box 5-5 do not have a logical explanation (e.g., if the client

BOX 5-5

Indications for Referral

If any of the following conditions are present and cannot be explained logically, the client should be referred to a health care professional.

- Pain (local, sharp, dull, achy, deep, superficial)
- Fatigue
- Inflammation
- Lumps and tissue changes
- Rashes and changes in the skin
- Edema
- Mood alterations (e.g., depression or anxiety)
- Infection (local or general)
- Changes in habits (e.g., appetite, elimination, or sleep)
- Bleeding and bruising
- Nausea, vomiting, and diarrhea
- Temperature (hot [fever] or cold)

---

has been up late or working long hours, naturally he or she will show the symptom of fatigue). Massage practitioners should use common sense tempered with accurate information and caution (Proficiency Exercises 5-7 and 5-8)

■ ■ ■ SUMMARY

Indications for massage are based on the physiologic effects that provide the benefits of massage. Massage is beneficial for most people, yet contraindications do exist. Responsible massage professionals always refer a client for diagnosis and treatment by a qualified health professional, without delay, as soon as they notice any condition that may suggest an underlying physical or mental health problem. After the condition has been diagnosed and appropriate treatment has been established, the massage professional may provide massage under the supervision of a medical professional. Massage may prove beneficial and supportive to the interventions of the health care professional and may enhance the healing process by temporarily reducing pain,

PROFICIENCY EXERCISE 5-7

1. Using the reference section in Appendix A, list five regional contraindications to massage that you have encountered (or that you think you may encounter) with clients.

a.

b.

c.

d.

e.

2. List the five general contraindications you think you will encounter most often.

a.

b.

c.

d.

e.

3. Using the Oregon Model in Appendix A, list two specific disease conditions that correspond to the seven basic symptoms listed in Box 5-3.

a.

b.

c.

4. Choose a condition from each of the categories in the Oregon Model in Appendix A. Pretend that clients display symptoms of that condition or actually role play in the classroom, having a fellow student act out the signs and symptoms of the condition. Write down what you would notice about each condition that would make you want to refer the patient to a health professional. Also write down or act out a referral process with the pretend client.

5. Choose two medications from Appendix C and describe the possible interactions with massage.

a.

b.

6. On a separate piece of paper, write down the names of health care providers in your area whom you would like to place on a referral list. Because they need to support your work, set up a plan to meet and interview each one. Write down a list of questions you should ask and information that you must provide about your skills. Have at least three professionals from each category so that the client has a choice. If time permits, contact these people while you are still a student.

PROFICIENCY EXERCISE 5-8

Important Note to Student: Keep practicing the clinical reasoning process. Keep working at answering the questions. It's okay to be frustrated; just keep practicing. Remember, there's no correct answer—just (in your opinion) an effective decision.

After reading the case study, use the clinical reasoning model to identify whether contraindications exist for the use of therapeutic massage and whether referral is necessary. If you determine that referral is necessary, list the reasons for it.

Case Study

A 32-year-old female client is seeking massage for stress management and pain management for headaches. A coworker recommended massage therapy. Over the past 3 months, she has been increasingly unable to maintain her work schedule, and work time missed is increasing to the point where her job is in jeopardy. She is a production line worker in a small plastics factory. The work environment has adequate ventilation but requires repetitive movement of the arms. She is getting afternoon headaches almost daily. She has been moody and temperamental, which is unusual for her. Her weight has increased by 15 pounds over the past year. She sporadically exercises and crash diets. She is single and has no children, but she has close family ties in a nearby town. Her last physical examination was 5 years ago, and at that point no problems were identified. Her menstrual cycle is somewhat erratic, and she had episodes of heavy bleeding during her last two periods. She is prone to hay fever and is currently self-medicating with an over-the-counter antihistamine. She takes aspirin for the headaches and also takes a multiple vitamin tablet. She takes no other medications. She thinks the cause of her problems is job stress, but she does not feel that a job change is possible at this time.

Continued

PROFICIENCY EXERCISE 5-8—cont'd

Identify the Facts

Questions that can help with this process include the following:

What is considered normal or balanced function?

What has happened? (Spell out events.)

What caused the imbalance? (Can it be identified?)

What was done or is being done?

What has worked or not worked?

Brainstorm the Possibilities

Questions that can help with this process include the following:

What are the possibilities? (What could it all mean?)

What is my intuition suggesting?

What are the possible patterns of dysfunction?

What are the possible contributing factors?

What are possible interventions?

What might work?

What are other ways to look at the situation?

What do the data suggest?

Consider the Logical Outcomes of Each Possibility

Questions that can help determine outcomes include the following:

What is the logical progression of the symptom pattern, contributing factors, and current behaviors?

What are the logical cause and effect of each intervention identified? What are the pros and cons of each intervention suggested?

PROFICIENCY EXERCISE 5-8—cont'd

What are the consequences of not acting?

What are the consequences of acting?

Identify the Effect of Each Possibility on the People Involved

Questions that can help identify effects include the following:

In terms of each intervention being considered, what would be the impact on the people involved: client, practitioner, and other professionals working with the client?

How does each person involved feel about the possible interventions?

Is the practitioner within his or her scope of practice to work with such situations?

Is the practitioner qualified to work with such situations?

Does the practitioner feel qualified to work with such situations?

Is there a feeling of cooperation and agreement among all parties involved?

Based on this analysis of the information provided, the massage practitioner would identify the following contraindications for the following reasons:

Is referral indicated? What are the reasons for referral?

evolve

5-1 Categorize several pathologies into "indicated" or "contraindicated" columns.

5-2 Read two pathology-related case studies—one on shingles and one on eczema—and answer true/false questions at the end.

Don't forget to study for your certification and licensure exams! Review questions for this chapter are located on Evolve.

relaxing the client, reducing stress responses, increasing circulation, and much more. In addition, the one-on-one contact given by the massage professional may provide support and compassionate touch during a difficult time, thereby reducing the feelings of frustration, isolation, anxiety, and depression that often accompany illness or periods of stress.

REFERENCES

1. Anderson K, Anderson LE, Glanze WD, editors: *Mosby's medical, nursing, and allied health dictionary,* ed 6, St Louis, 2005, Mosby.
2. Price SA, Wilson LM: *Pathophysiology: clinical concepts of disease processes,* ed 6, St Louis, 2002, Mosby.

Workbook Section

Answers for the Workbook Section for Chapter 5 are provided on p. 762.

■■■■ SHORT ANSWER

1. What is an indication for a massage?

2. What is a contraindication to a massage?

3. What are three approaches to care? Define them.

4. Define health.

5. What is dysfunction as defined in this text, and how is massage beneficial in dysfunctional situations?

6. How do acute and chronic conditions affect homeostasis?

7. Why would a massage practitioner need to be aware of risk factors?

8. Why does the massage practitioner need to understand tumor pathology?

9. Why does the massage therapist need to understand the inflammatory response?

10. Define therapeutic inflammation.

11. Under what conditions should therapeutic inflammation not be used?

12. Why is pain difficult to describe?

13. What would the benefits of massage be for acute pain, chronic pain, and intractable pain?

14. What is the difference between localized pain, radiating pain, referred pain, and projected pain?

15. What is the difference between somatic and visceral pain?

16. Why is a knowledge of referred pain patterns important?

17. What role do dermatomes play in the pain pattern?

Workbook Section—cont'd

18. What is phantom pain?

_____

_____

_____

19. What is the difference between entrapment and compression impingement, and when is massage most indicated?

_____

_____

_____

20. What are endangerment sites?

_____

_____

_____

21. What are some important warning signs that indicate that the client should be referred to a physician for specific diagnosis?

_____

_____

_____

22. What resource materials should massage practitioners have available to help them understand medications and terminology?

_____

_____

_____

23. Why should the massage therapist understand the actions of medications?

_____

_____

_____

24. How do you refer a client to a health care professional?

_____

_____

_____

25. How can the student best make use of Appendix C, which provides information on massage interactions with medications?

_____

_____

_____

■■■ MATCHING I

Match the term to the best definition.

1. Acute pain
2. Arterial circulation
3. Autonomic nervous system
4. Cerebrospinal fluid
5. Chronic diseases
6. Chronic pain
7. Connective tissue
8. Contraindication
9. Dermatome
10. Disease
11. Endangerment site
12. General contraindications
13. Health
14. Homeostasis
15. Indication
16. Inflammatory response
17. Intractable pain
18. Lymphatic drainage
19. Metastasis
20. Pain
21. Pain-spasm-pain cycle
22. Pathology
23. Phantom pain
24. Referral
25. Referred pain
26. Regeneration
27. Regional contraindications
28. Respiration
29. Risk factors
30. Signs
31. Somatic pain
32. State-dependent memory
33. Stress
34. Symptoms
35. Syndrome
36. Venous circulation
37. Visceral pain

a. cutaneous (skin) distribution of spinal nerve sensations
b. tumor cell migration by way of lymphatic or blood vessels
c. an unpleasant sensory and emotional experience associated with actual or perceived tissue damage or described in terms of such damage
d. the most abundant tissue in the body; its functions include support, structure, space, stabilization, and scar formation
e. a warning signal that activates the sympathetic nervous system; it can be a symptom of a disease or a temporary aspect of medical treatment; it usually is temporary, of sudden onset, and easily localized
f. dynamic equilibrium of the internal environment of the body through the processes of feedback and regulation
g. diseases that develop slowly and last for a long time
h. pain arising from stimulation of receptors in the skin or skeletal muscles, joints, tendons, and fascia
i. encoding and storage of a memory based on the ANS and the resulting chemical balance of the body; only retrievable during a similar situation in the body
j. any substantial change in routine or any activity that causes the body to have to adapt, including changes for the better and for the worse
k. a diffuse, poorly localized discomfort that persists or recurs for indefinite periods, usually for more than 6 months
l. regulates energy by using sympathetic fight-or-flight and fear responses and the restorative parasympathetic relaxation response; sympathetic and parasympathetic systems work together to maintain homeostasis through a feedback loop system
m. subjective abnormalities felt only by the patient
n. a collection of different signs and symptoms, usually having a common cause, that present a clear picture of a pathologic condition
o. the return of deoxygenated blood to the heart by way of the veinsp. pain that results from stimulation of receptors in the internal organs

q. an abnormality in a body function that threatens well-being
r. a liquid that nourishes and protects the brain and nerves
s. movement of oxygenated blood under pressure from the heart to the body through the arteries
t. a healing process in which new cells are similar to those they replace
u. a method for sending a client to a health care professional for specific diagnosis and treatment of a disease
v. a therapeutic application that promotes health or assists in a healing process
w. any condition than renders a particular treatment improper or undesirable
x. a normal mechanism that usually speeds recovery from an infection or injury characterized by pain, heat, redness, and swelling
y. physical, mental, and social well-being, not merely the absence of disease
z. the study of disease
aa. a kind of pain frequently experienced by patients who have had a limb amputated
bb. a steady contraction of muscles that causes them to become ischemic, which stimulates the pain receptors in the muscles; the pain, in turn, initiates more spasms, setting up a vicious cycle
cc. a specific type of massage that enhances lymphatic flow
dd. chronic pain that persists even when treatment is provided or that exists without demonstrable disease
ee. an area of the body where nerves and blood vessels surface close to the skin and are not well protected by muscle or connective tissue; deep, sustained pressure into these areas could damage these vessels and nerves
ff. findings that require a physician's evaluation to rule out serious underlying conditions before any massage is indicated
gg. contraindications that relate to a specific area of the body
hh. the movement of oxygen in the body during breathing
ii. predisposing conditions that may make a person more likely to develop a disease than some other person
jj. objective abnormalities that can be seen or measured by someone other than the client
kk. pain felt in an area different from the source of the pain

■■■ MATCHING II

Match the correct terms with the primary responses.

1. Heat and redness
2. Swelling and pain
a. release of histamine, prostaglandins, and kinins
b. increased permeability of vessel walls
c. enlargement of lymph nodes
d. dilation of blood vessels
e. triggering of pain receptors by pressure from edema
f. irritant diluted through excess fluid
g. destruction of bacteria by white blood cells
h. increase in blood volume

Workbook Section—cont'd

■ ■ ■ LABELING I

Use the following list of terms to label the areas of referred pain in Figure 5-6 with the corresponding letter or letters. Terms may be used more than once.

A. Urinary bladder

B. Colon

C. Appendix

D. Heart

E. Lung and diaphragm

F. Liver and gallbladder

G. Ovary

H. Pancreas

I. Small Intestine

J. Kidney

K. Stomach

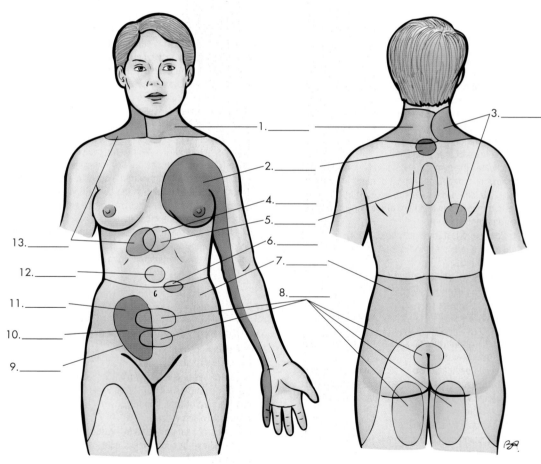

FIGURE 5-6

■■■ LABELING II

Using the following list of terms, label the endangerment sites in Figure 5-7 with the corresponding letter or letters. Terms may be used more than once.

A. Anterior triangle of neck

B. Posterior triangle of neck

C. Axillary nerve

D. Ulnar nerve

E. Radial nerve

F. Vagus nerve, nerves and vessels to thyroid gland

G. Abdominal and descending aorta

H. Kidney

I. Sciatic nerve

J. Inguinal triangle

K. Tibial nerve, popliteal artery and nerve

L. Kidney

FIGURE 5-7

Workbook Section—cont'd

■ ■ ■ RISK FACTORS EXERCISE

1. List all the risk factors for developing disease. Make separate columns for your personal risk factors and the risk factors of two friends.

2. When interviewing a client or doing a massage, how would you find out if the person has any of the possible warning signs of cancer? A list of the signs is found below; state how or when you would find out the information if the client did not reveal it.

The warning signs of cancer are as follows:
    Sores that do not heal
    Unusual bleeding
    A change in a wart or mole
    A lump or thickening in any tissue
    Persistent hoarseness or cough
    Chronic indigestion
    A change in bowel or bladder function
    Example:
    Sores that do not heal:
    Noticed during proper draping techniques—skin on body has open wounds

■ ■ ■ ASSESS YOUR COMPETENCIES

Now that you have studied this chapter, you should be able to:

1. Define the terms indication and contraindication.

2. Define therapeutic change, condition management, and palliative care as a therapeutic approach.

3. Use a clinical reasoning model to determine the appropriate intervention process.

4. Develop a basic understanding of pathology and its connection to contraindications to massage.

5. Explain the stress response, inflammatory response, and pain response.

6. Identify indications for massage therapy and justify those indications.

7. Understand when to refer clients to licensed medical professionals.

On a separate sheet of paper, write a short summary of the content of this chapter based on the competencies listed above. When writing this paper assume you are speaking to someone—a client, prospective employer, co-worker, or other interested person. Write the paper as if you were having a conversation and explaining the importance of the information and skills to professional massage development.

Next, in small student discussion groups, share the papers and compare and contrast how the information was presented. Discuss the content, looking for similarities, differences, potential misunderstanding of the information, and clear and concise methods of description.

■ ■ ■ PROBLEM-SOLVING EXERCISE

You just ran into a friend you have not seen in 5 years. That friend is now a college professor, teaching anatomy and physiology. When you mention that you are studying massage, your friend says, "It sounds interesting, but I don't think I'd ever need one." Take 5 minutes to list all the reasons you think your friend might need a massage.

Hygiene, Sanitation, and Safety

 CHAPTER OBJECTIVES

After completing this chapter, the student will be able to perform the following:

- Identify good health and personal hygiene practices
- Explain the major disease-causing agents
- Describe methods for preventing and controlling disease
- Give specific recommendations for sanitary practices for massage businesses
- Implement standard precautions
- Provide information about human immunodeficiency virus infection, acquired immunodeficiency syndrome, and hepatitis
- Establish a hazard-free massage environment

 CHAPTER OUTLINE

PERSONAL HEALTH, HYGIENE, AND APPEARANCE
  Smoking
  Alcohol and Drugs
  Hygiene

SANITATION
  Pathogenic Organisms
  Disease Prevention and Control
  Indications for the Use of Standard Precautions by the
    Massage Professional

**PREVENTING THE TRANSMISSION OF HIV INFECTION,
  HEPATITIS, TUBERCULOSIS, AND OTHER
  CONTAGIOUS CONDITIONS**
  The Mechanics of Transmission
  Hepatitis
  Tuberculosis
  Severe Acute Respiratory Syndrome (SARS)

PREMISE AND FIRE SAFETY

SUMMARY

 KEY TERMS

Acquired immunodeficiency syndrome (AIDS)
Aseptic technique
Bacteria
Environmental contact
Fungi
Hepatitis
Human immunodeficiency virus (HIV)
Opportunistic invasion
Pathogenic animals
Person-to-person contact
Protozoa
Sanitation
Severe acute respiratory syndrome (SARS)
Standard precautions
Tuberculosis (TB)
Viruses

This chapter discusses hygiene and sanitation practices in a professional setting. The information may seem to be mere common sense, but specific skills are needed to practice massage in a way that protects the safety of both the client and the massage professional. Many local and state laws governing massage deal extensively with sanitary procedures. The Oregon health code requirements,[1] which have been used as a model for part of this chapter, are both typical and well defined.

The primary importance of **sanitation** is to prevent the spread of contagious disease. Diseases caused by "germs," or viruses, bacteria, fungi, and parasites, are considered contagious. Some contagious diseases are rare, and others are becoming more common. Until recently, tuberculosis, a bacterial disease, was considered to be under control; however, the incidence of the disease has begun to rise, and strains resistant to current medications have emerged. Various streptococcal bacteria also are becoming resistant to the antibiotics currently available. The common cold and influenza (the "flu") are caused by viruses that constantly mutate, thwarting scientific development of any sort of consistent vaccine. The key, then, is prevention; contagious diseases are best controlled before infection occurs, by the use of sanitary practices.

Considerable concern, misinformation, and misunderstanding have arisen about the spread of hepatitis, the human immunodeficiency virus (HIV), and acquired immunodeficiency syndrome (AIDS). Intense education of the public through the media about HIV and AIDS has dispelled some of the misunderstanding about these conditions. Better care and research developments are beginning to move the prognosis of HIV infection to that of a chronic disease. The infection rate for hepatitis is increasing alarmingly, which poses a significant health danger. Currently, concern is rising about the global spread of infectious diseases caused by several viruses, including the various forms of the influenza virus. An extensive section of this chapter is devoted to these topics in order to provide accurate information about hepatitis, HIV, AIDS, and other contagious diseases and also to explain in detail the massage practitioner's responsibilities.

Because new information about the spread and control of contagious diseases becomes available almost daily, it is important that massage practitioners keep up-to-date. As information develops, the federal Centers for Disease Control and Prevention (CDC) adjusts its standards and guidelines for communicable diseases. Massage practitioners are responsible for updating themselves semiannually on changes in the CDC's recommendations and for following the most recent standards and guidelines.

In addition to a sanitary environment, the massage professional must provide a safe environment. It is important to consider fire and accident prevention for both the client and the professional. The massage professional is well served by becoming certified in first aid and cardiopulmonary resuscitation (CPR) through the Red Cross or a similar organization.

Let's begin with the personal care of the massage practitioner. It is important that we take care of ourselves, not only so that we function at our best, but also because, as wellness and health professionals, we set an example for our clients. Clients notice the way we look and act, as well as our energy and vitality levels. Clients respect professionals who care for themselves, because the professional thus teaches clients to care for themselves. The ethical principle of respect, discussed in Chapter 2, is reflected in the way we care for ourselves and for our clients.

PERSONAL HEALTH, HYGIENE, AND APPEARANCE

SECTION OBJECTIVE

Using the information presented in this section, the student will be able to perform the following:

- Identify the basic hygiene procedures important to a professional environment

One of the best ways to control disease is to stay healthy. If our bodies are strong and our immune systems are functioning properly, we do not become sick easily. If injured, we heal better if we are healthy. Diet, sleep, rest, body mechanics (the way we use our bodies), exercise, and lifestyle all must be considered in the overall health picture. It also is important to keep to a schedule of regular physical checkups, because early detection of disease leads to more successful treatment.

Smoking

Smoking is considered one of the leading causes of disease. It is directly linked to cardiovascular disease and is the leading cause of lung cancer.[2] Exposure to secondhand smoke has been found to cause cancer and other health problems in nonsmokers. Besides its dangerous health effects, smoking is offensive to many people. Smoke odors linger in the air and on the hands, hair, and clothing. Many nonsmokers find this smell obnoxious, and the smell of smoke can cause reactions in sensitive individuals. Because the massage professional works physically close to the client, any smoke odors from the professional are reason for concern.

Massage professionals should never smoke in the massage therapy room, even when clients are not present, because the smell of smoke lingers in carpets, draperies, and furniture. If the practitioner must smoke during business hours, it should be done outside, away from any access doors or windows. The practitioner who smokes should wash his or her hands carefully before touching a client; he or she also should inform clients when they make appointments that the practitioner smokes. If the client is bothered by smoke odors, referral to a different massage professional is appropriate.

Alcohol and Drugs

Alcohol and drugs interfere with the ability to function as a massage professional. Because these substances affect thinking, feeling, behavior, and functioning, the practitioner must never be under the influence of alcohol or illegal drugs when working with a client. Any prescription or over-the-counter medications that affect mental or physical abilities must be considered carefully, because use of these substances by the massage professional can place the client at risk. A massage professional should wait at least 12 hours after the last alcoholic drink before working with a client, because it takes this long for the direct effects of alcohol to wear off. The indirect effects last for the next 24 hours. In this condition, often called a *hangover,* the body is exhausted and toxic; it is not a good condition to be in while giving a massage. Clients should be referred or rescheduled if the professional's ability to function is affected.

Hygiene

The massage professional must pay careful attention to personal hygiene. Preventing breath and body odor without using chemical cover-ups is essential. Massage professionals should not wear perfume, aftershave, or perfumed hair products because many clients are sensitive to these odors.

Massage professionals should bathe or shower at the start of each workday. The armpits, genitals, and feet should be washed carefully with soap or a similar cleaning agent. Female professionals must be especially mindful of odor during menstruation.

Because breath odor is offensive, careful brushing and flossing of the teeth and scraping of the tongue after each meal are important. Any food that may cause breath odor should be avoided during work hours. Gum chewing is unprofessional and irritating to many people and is ineffective in combating breath odors. Breath mints, however, may help.

Hair should be kept clean. Chemicals such as hair spray or gel must be avoided because they may cause an allergic reaction in sensitive people. The hair must not fall onto the professional's face or drag on the client. If it is long, it should be kept pulled back.

Proper care of the hands is especially important. Nails should be kept short and well manicured and should not extend past the tips of the fingers. Fingernails can harbor bacteria and other pathogens. Care must be taken to keep the space under the nails clean, a task that is best accomplished with a nailbrush. Any hangnails, breaks, or cracks in the skin of the hands must be kept clean and covered during a massage. An intact, strong skin is the professional's first line of defense against infection. Nail polish and synthetic nails promote the growth of bacteria, and hand jewelry can harbor pathogens; these should not be worn while the practitioner gives a massage.

Massage uniforms should be loose and made of cotton or a cotton blend. Because body temperature increases while the professional gives a massage, clothing must "breathe" and absorb and evaporate perspiration. Sleeves should be above the elbow, but the uniform should not be sleeveless. All clothing should be opaque and modest. T-shirts and shorts usually are inappropriate. If skirts or shorts are worn, they should be knee length or longer; loose pants are preferable.

White clothing is not necessary or even desirable because lubricant stains are less evident on colored clothing. Clothing should be laundered in a disinfectant, usually bleach, and the uniform chosen must be able to withstand this type of laundering. If perspiration is heavy or if the clothing becomes stained, the practitioner may need to change clothes. A spare uniform should be kept available. Underclothing must be changed daily, more often if perspiration is heavy. Many professionals use uniforms called *scrubs*. Scrubs meet all the previously mentioned criteria, are inexpensive, and are easy to obtain.

The practitioner should wear clean, comfortable shoes while giving a massage. Going barefoot or wearing only stockings is neither sanitary nor professional. Changing socks daily helps prevent foot odor.

Makeup should be modest to avoid a painted, severe appearance; heavy makeup is never appropriate. Male practitioners must keep facial hair shaved or neatly trimmed.

Jewelry of all types creates sanitation and safety hazards and should not be worn while giving a massage. Necklaces, bracelets, and hair jewelry can become tangled or can drag on the client, and jewelry of all types, including piercings, can harbor pathogens and collect debris, creating a sanitation hazard (Figure 6-1).

If the client or professional is ill and if there is any concern that the condition might be contagious, the massage professional should refer or reschedule the client until the condition changes (Proficiency Exercise 6-1).[3]

FIGURE 6-1 Properly groomed massage professionals.

PROFICIENCY EXERCISE 6-1

1. *Design your ideal uniform and ask three massage professionals their opinion of your idea.*
2. *Develop a class project in which fellow students' personal hygiene and professional appearance are evaluated anonymously.*
3. *Ask honest, trusted family members or friends if you have breath or body odor.*

SANITATION

SECTION OBJECTIVES

Using the information presented in this section, the student will be able to perform the following:

- Identify the transmission routes for disease-causing pathogens
- Implement sanitation practices, including standard precautions, to prevent and control the spread of disease

Sanitary massage methods promote conditions that are conducive to health. This means that pathogenic organisms must be eliminated or controlled. Pathogens are spread by direct contact, through blood or other body fluids, or by airborne transmission.

Pathogenic Organisms

Pathogenic organisms include viruses, bacteria, fungi, protozoa, and pathogenic animals. These organisms cause many diseases.

Viruses

Viruses invade cells and insert their own genetic code into the host cell's genetic code. They use the host cell's nutrients and organelles to produce more virus particles. By bursting the cell membrane, the new virus particles may escape to infect other cells.

Bacteria

Bacteria are primitive cells that have no nuclei. They cause disease in one of three ways: (1) by secreting toxic substances that damage human tissues; (2) by becoming parasites inside human cells; or (3) by forming colonies in the body that disrupt normal function. Because bacteria can produce resistant forms, called *spores,* under adverse conditions, pathogenic bacteria are difficult for the human body to destroy.

Fungi

Fungi are a group of simple parasitic organisms that are similar to plants but have no chlorophyll (green pigment). Most pathogenic fungi live on the skin or mucous membranes (e.g., athlete's foot, vaginal yeast infections). Yeasts are small, single-celled fungi, and molds are large, multicellular fungi. Because fungal, or mycotic, infections can be resistant to treatment, they can become quite serious.

Protozoa and Pathogenic Animals

Protozoa are one-celled organisms that are larger than bacteria. They can infest human fluids and cause disease by parasitizing (living off) or directly destroying cells.

Pathogenic animals, sometimes called *metazoa,* are large, multicellular organisms. Most are worms that feed off human tissue or cause other diseases.

Many of these pathogens cause skin diseases when the pathogen commonly is spread through direct contact. Because massage professionals spend much time working directly with skin, they would be wise to learn to recognize these various skin conditions. Most anatomy, physiology, and pathology textbooks have color plates showing different skin diseases (see Appendix B for color illustrations showing examples of skin disorders).

An intact skin (skin integrity) prevents infection and various skin diseases, whereas abrasions and cuts breach the protective layer of the skin. Therefore it is important that the massage professional obtain additional information about pathologic skin conditions. (See Works Consulted for the list of recommended texts for this chapter.)

Disease Prevention and Control

The key to preventing many diseases caused by pathogenic organisms is to prevent the organisms from entering the body. This sounds simple enough, but often it is difficult to accomplish. Three primary means by which pathogens can spread are as follows:

- **Environmental contact.** Many pathogens are found in the environment; that is, in food, water, and soil and on various surfaces. Diseases caused by environmental pathogens often can be prevented by avoiding contact with certain materials and by following safe sanitation practices.
- **Opportunistic invasion.** Some potentially pathogenic organisms are found on the skin and mucous membranes of nearly everyone. These organisms do not cause disease until they have the opportunity to do so. Preventing opportunistic infection involves avoiding conditions that promote infection. Changes in pH (acidity), moisture, temperature, or other characteristics of the skin and mucous membranes often promote these infections. Aseptic treatment and cleansing of wounds can prevent them.
- **Person-to-person contact.** Small pathogens often can be transmitted in the air from one person to another. Direct contact with an infected person or with materials handled by the infected person is a familiar mode of transmission. The rhinovirus that causes the common cold often is transmitted in these ways. Some viruses, such as the hepatitis B virus (HBV), are transmitted when infected blood, semen, or other body fluids enter the bloodstream.

Aseptic Technique

Aseptic technique kills or disables pathogens on surfaces before they can be transmitted (Table 6-1).

Most sanitation conditions for massage require disinfection. Occasionally protective apparel is necessary. In rare instances use of a mask, gown, and gloves may be appropriate

TABLE 6-1

Common Aseptic Techniques for Preventing the Spread of Pathogens

Method	Action	Example
Sterilization	Destroys all organisms by means of heat	Pressurized steam bath, extreme temperature, irradiation
Disinfection	Destroys most or all pathogens (but not necessarily all microbes) on inanimate objects	Chemicals (e.g., iodine, chlorine, alcohol, soap)
Isolation	Separates potentially infectious people or materials from uninfected individuals	Quarantining infected patients; wearing protective apparel while giving treatments; and sanitary transport, storage, and disposal of body fluids, tissues, and other materials

FIGURE 6-2 Hand-washing technique. **A,** Create a lather with the soap. Interlace your fingers to wash between them, keeping your hands pointed down. **B,** Rinse the hands well, keeping your fingers pointed down. **C,** Use the blunt edge of an orangewood stick to clean under your fingernails. **D,** After drying your hands, use a dry paper towel to turn off the water. (From Zakus SM: *Mosby's clinical skills for medical assistants,* ed 4, St Louis, 2001, Mosby.)

to protect the massage professional or the client. These cases are discussed later in the chapter.

evolve **6-1** **Hand Washing.** Proper hand washing is the single most effective deterrent to the spread of disease (Figure 6-2). The hands must be washed before and after each massage, after blowing the nose or coughing into the hands, and after using the toilet. The hands and forearms must be washed in hot, running water to remove any infectious organisms. Soap or another antiseptic hand-washing product must be used, and a clean towel is used to dry the hands and forearms. Faucets and door handles are contaminated and should

not be touched after washing the hands. The towel should be used to turn off the water and open the door. Because frequent hand washing may dry and chap the skin, using a lotion after washing helps replace natural oils. Using the clean towel to hold the lotion bottle helps prevent contamination of the hands.

Suggested Sanitation Requirements

Box 6-1 provides a summary of sanitation procedures all massage professionals should observe. State and local laws may mandate additional procedures, and the professional should be aware of these (Proficiency Exercise 6-2).

BOX 6-1

Sanitation Practices for Massage Professionals

The following sanitation requirements for practicing massage professionals have been developed from the Oregon model.

- The massage professional must clean and wash the hands and forearms or feet thoroughly with an antibacterial/antiviral agent before touching each client. Any professional known to be infected with any communicable disease or to be a carrier of such disease or who has an infected wound or open lesion on any exposed portions of the body is excluded from practicing massage until the communicable condition is alleviated.
- The professional must wear clean clothing. If at all possible, lockers or closets for personnel should be maintained apart from the massage room for the storage of personal clothing and effects.
- All doors and windows opening to the outside must be tight fitting and must ensure the exclusion of flies, insects, rodents, or other vermin. All floors, walks, and furniture must be kept clean, well maintained, and in good repair.
- All rooms in which massage is practiced must meet the following requirements: (1) heating must be adequate to maintain a room air temperature of 75° F; (2) ventilation must be sufficient to remove objectionable odors; and (3) lighting fixtures must be capable of producing a minimum of 5 foot-candles of light at floor level; this level of lighting should be used during cleaning.
- All sewage and liquid waste must be disposed of in a municipal sewage system or approved septic system. All interior water distribution piping should be installed and maintained in conformity with the state plumbing code. The water supply must be adequate, deemed safe by the health department, and sanitary. Drinking fountains of an approved type or individual paper drinking cups should be provided for the convenience of employees and patrons.
- Every massage business must have a sanitary toilet facility with an adequate supply of hot and cold water under pressure, and it must be conveniently located for use by employees and patrons. Bathroom doors must be tight fitting, and the rooms must be kept clean, in good repair, and free of flies, insects, and vermin. A supply of soap in a covered dispenser and single-use sanitary towels in a dispenser must be provided at each lavatory installation, as well as a covered waste receptacle for proper disposal; a supply of toilet paper on a dispenser must be available for each toilet.
- Lavatory and toilet rooms must be equipped with fly-tight containers for garbage and refuse. These containers should be easily cleanable, well maintained, and in good repair. Any refuse must be disposed of in a sanitary manner.
- Massage lubricants, including but not limited to oil, alcohol, powders, and lotions, should be dispensed from suitable containers, to be used and stored in such a manner as to prevent contamination. The bulk lubricant must not come in contact with the massage professional. It should be poured, squeezed, or shaken into a separate container or the massage professional's hand. Any unused lubricant that comes into contact with the client or massage professional must be discarded.
- The use of unclean linen is prohibited. Only freshly laundered sheets and linens should be used for massage. All single-service materials and clean linens should be stored at least 4 inches off the floor in shelves, compartments, or cabinets used for that purpose only. All soiled linens must be placed in a covered receptacle immediately and kept there until washed in detergent and an antiviral cleaning agent (e.g., a 10% bleach solution, or one part bleach to nine parts water) in a washing machine that provides a hot water temperature of at least 140° F.
- Massage tables must be covered with impervious material that is cleanable and must be kept clean and in good repair. Equipment that comes in contact with the client must be cleaned thoroughly with soap or other suitable detergent and water, followed by adequate sanitation procedures before use with each individual client (a 10% bleach solution, made up daily, is recommended). All equipment must be clean, well maintained, and in good repair.
- When cleaning the massage area, observe the following rules:
  - Do not shake linen, and dust with a damp cloth to minimize the movement of dust.
  - Clean from the cleanest area to the dirtiest. This prevents soiling of a clean area.
  - Clean away from your body and uniform. If you dust, brush, or wipe toward yourself, microorganisms will be transmitted to your skin, hair, and uniform.
  - Store used linens in a closed bag or container while in the massage room or during transport.
- Floors are dirty; any object that falls on the floor should not be used on or for a client.

Modified from Oregon Board of Massage Technicians: Sanitation requirements for the state of Oregon, Oregon Administrative Rules, November, 2006.

PROFICIENCY EXERCISE 6-2

1. *Contact your local health department for information on disease control, health practices, and sanitation requirements.*
2. *Review your local and state laws concerning sanitation requirements.*

evolve 6-2

Indications for Use of Standard Precautions by the Massage Professional

Under normal circumstances the massage professional does not come in contact with a client's blood, body fluids, or body substances (e.g., urine, feces, and vomit). However, in rare

BOX 6-2

Standard Precautions

Standard precautions synthesize the major features of universal precautions (blood and body fluids), which are designed to reduce the risk of transmission of blood-borne pathogens, and body substance isolation, which is designed to reduce the risk of transmission of pathogens from moist body substances. Standard precautions apply to (1) blood; (2) all body fluids, secretions, and excretions, except sweat, regardless of whether they contain visible blood; (3) nonintact skin; and (4) mucous membranes. Standard precautions are designed to reduce the risk of transmission of microorganisms from both recognized and unrecognized sources of infection in hospitals.

Hand Washing and Gloving

Hand washing is considered by many to be the single most important measure for reducing the risk of transmitting organisms from one person to another or from one site to another on the same patient. Washing your hands as promptly and thoroughly as possible between clients is very important. In addition to hand washing, gloves play an important role in reducing the risk of transmission of microorganisms.

Gloves are worn for two important reasons: (1) to provide a protective barrier and (2) to reduce the likelihood that microorganisms on the massage practitioner's hands will be transmitted to clients. Wearing gloves does not replace the need for hand washing, because gloves may have small, unapparent defects or may be torn during use, and hands can become contaminated during the removal of gloves. Gloves must be changed and the old ones discarded after each use.

A mask provides protection against the spread of infectious, large-particle droplets that are transmitted by close contact and that generally travel only short distances (up to 3 feet) from infected patients who are coughing or sneezing. Massage professionals occasionally use masks.

Gowns and Protective Apparel

Various types of gowns and protective apparel are worn to provide barrier protection and to reduce the opportunity for transmission of microorganisms in medical settings.

Immunocompromised Clients

Standard precautions, or the equivalent, are used for the care of all clients.

Hand Washing

1. Wash the hands after touching blood, body fluids, secretions, excretions, and contaminated items, regardless of whether gloves are worn. Wash the hands immediately after removing gloves, between client contacts, and when otherwise indicated to avoid transfer of microorganisms to other clients or environments. It may be necessary to wash the hands between tasks and procedures on the same client to prevent cross-contamination of different body sites.
2. Use a plain (nonantimicrobial) soap for routine hand washing.
3. Use an antimicrobial agent or a waterless antiseptic agent if hand washing is not possible.

Gloves

1. Wear gloves (clean, nonsterile gloves are adequate) when touching blood, body fluids, secretions, excretions, and contaminated items. Put on clean gloves just before touching mucous membranes and nonintact skin.
2. Change gloves between tasks and procedures on the same client after contact with material that may contain a high concentration of microorganisms.
3. Remove gloves promptly after use, before touching uncontaminated items and environmental surfaces, and before going to another client, and wash hands immediately to avoid transferring microorganisms to other clients or environments.

Mask, Eye Protection, and Face Shield

Wear a mask and eye protection or a face shield to protect the mucous membranes of the eyes, nose, and mouth during procedures and client care activities that are likely to generate splashes or sprays of blood, body fluids, secretions, and excretions.

Gown

Wear a gown (a clean, nonsterile gown is adequate) to protect skin and to prevent soiling of clothing during procedures and client care activities that are likely to generate splashes or sprays of blood, body fluids, secretions, or excretions. Select a gown that is appropriate for the activity and the amount of fluid likely to be encountered. Remove a soiled gown as promptly as possible, and wash hands to avoid transfer of microorganisms to other clients or environments.

Modified from the Division of Healthcare Quality Promotion, National Center for Infectious Diseases, Centers for Disease Control and Prevention. http://www.cdc.gov/ncidod/dhqp/guidelines.html Accessed July 20, 2007.

cases an accident may occur in which such contact is possible. The best recommendation is always to make **standard precautions** part of the professional practice (Box 6-2). Gloves are not necessary for most massage sessions unless the skin of the massage practitioner's hands or any skin area of the client has a rash, cut, abrasion, infection, or any other condition that would allow the transmission of fluids. A mask may be appropriate if transmission of an airborne pathogen, such as the flu virus, is a concern. In most cases use of a mask protects the client from the massage professional's pathogens; therefore a

mask is used with clients who have any form of immune suppression, including excessive stress, which makes the client more susceptible to infection.

Required Use of Standard Precautions

With additional training and under medical supervision, massage professionals may work with clients who have a contagious condition. In these cases, knowledge of standard precautions is essential. However, it is wise to remember the importance of the massage professional's gentle, nurturing touch. The human connection becomes difficult through layers of protective coverings. We must remember that our normal germs can be very dangerous for any immune-suppressed client, and standard precautions must be used to protect the client from viruses and bacteria. Extra effort is required to follow standard precautions, but this extra effort should not hinder the safety of either client or practitioner.

Clients considered contagious may feel isolated and "unclean." We do not want to make such clients feel ashamed and guilty for having a contagious disease. Many of them desperately need to be touched in a supportive, nonjudgmental way. It is the pathogen that is undesirable, not the client, and all clients must be treated with respect, dignity, and kindness. The professional must remember to touch the person and not the disease, to see and listen to the person rather than the disease. These are *people* who are sick—not sick people.

The massage professional may need to wear gloves if a client is infected with a contagious, transmittable disease or if a client is in an immunosuppressed state, such as might occur with chemotherapy, and must be protected from germs. In these situations the massage therapist would be working under the supervision of a medical professional. It is important to follow all of his or her directions carefully.

If massage professionals work in the health care setting (e.g., hospitals, extended care facilities, rehabilitation centers), it is essential that they follow standard precautions. Each setting has approved procedures posted. Most often special training is provided. If this is not the case and the massage professional is concerned in any way about the application of required sanitation procedures, he or she should speak directly to the supervisor.

Possible Exposure to Contaminants and Body Fluids. Any person who touches a spill of blood or other body substances, such as vomit, urine, or feces, should wear single-use, disposable gloves (Figure 6-3). Such contact conceivably could

FIGURE 6-3 Procedure for removing gloves. **A,** Grasp the glove below the cuff. **B,** Pull the glove down over the hand, turning the glove inside out. **C,** Insert the fingers of the ungloved hand into the other glove. **D,** Pull the glove down and over the hand, turning the glove inside out. (Modified from Sorrentino SA: *Mosby's textbook for nursing assistants,* ed 5, St Louis, 2000, Mosby.)

happen during a massage. The most common blood exposure is to menstrual blood, an incidence that can occur if the client's protective product is inadequate. In rare cases men who have a history of premature ejaculation could be stimulated indirectly by the general massage and ejaculate or leak fluid. An incontinent client could leak urine or feces, or a client could suddenly become sick and vomit. Standard precautions should be followed during any cleanup.

Cleanup Procedures Using Standard Precautions

A 10% bleach solution (one part bleach to nine parts water) should be used to clean up spills of body fluids. The spill should be surrounded with solution and then mopped or wiped up, with the professional working slowly and carefully inward to avoid splashes or aerosols (airborne particles). Stronger bleach solutions should be used if excessive amounts of blood or other substances are present. Afterward, the mop head or cloth should be soaked in the bleach solution. The mop head should be agitated carefully to ensure that all its surfaces are exposed to the cleaning fluid. All linens should be rolled away and double-bagged in plastic, separate from other soiled linens. The outside bag should be marked "contaminated with body fluids." The table should be washed with a strong disinfectant solution and allowed to air dry. Latex gloves should be worn during the cleanup process.

If a contaminated substance comes in contact with a person's skin, the skin should be washed immediately with soap and water and an antiviral agent, such as 10% bleach solution. If an open wound is exposed to a contaminated substance, it should be flushed immediately with large amounts of hydrogen peroxide or a 10% bleach solution. Hydrogen peroxide should not be used on mucous membranes or in any body orifice (e.g., mouth, vagina, anus, eyes, or urethra).

Bleach is the preferred cleaning agent. A bleach and water solution should be prepared daily, and any leftover solution should be discarded at the end of the day. If blood or body fluid seepage is excessive, a stronger mixture of bleach should be used.

Although hot, soapy water kills HIV, dishes that are visibly soiled with blood or other body substances should be soaked in 10% bleach solution before they are washed in hot, soapy water.

Bathroom surfaces are hazardous only if they are visibly soiled with tainted bodily waste or substances. Any contaminated surface must encounter a mucous membrane surface or an open wound to transmit pathogens. Bathrooms should always be cleaned as if they were contaminated.

Approved Cleaning Solutions. The CDC has recognized the following three levels of solutions and products that destroy HIV, HBV, and other viral organisms. These recommendations should be followed in every practice.

- *High-level sanitation:* Products labeled "sterilant/disinfectant glutaraldehyde—air dry"; massage professionals do not need to practice high-level sanitation techniques under normal conditions.

PROFICIENCY EXERCISE 6-3

1. Call the National AIDS Hotline, which is open 24 hours, at (Spanish: [800] (800) CDC-INFO and TTY: [800] 243-7889) and ask a representative to send you information, or check the Internet Web site at http://www.ashastd.org.
2. Contact the information center at the Centers for Disease Control and Prevention (CDC) in Atlanta, Georgia (800-232-4636 CDC-INFO). Request information about communicable diseases or check the Internet Web site at http://www.cdc.gov.

- *Medium-level sanitation:* Bleach solution—one part bleach to nine parts water, made up daily (10% solution) or a hospital disinfectant labeled "tuberculocidal."
- *Low-level sanitation:* Hot, soapy water (with air drying) or a hospital disinfectant effective against viruses and bacteria. Hands are to be washed in hot, soapy water or with surgical soap.

Medium- and low-level sanitation are adequate for most therapeutic massage procedures. Cleanup of a body fluid spill might require high-level procedures. Massage professionals should update their information on recommended sanitary practices at least every 6 months (Proficiency Exercise 6-3). The CDC can provide current information. The Internet Web site for the CDC is http://www.cdc.gov.[4]

PREVENTING THE TRANSMISSION OF HIV INFECTION, HEPATITIS, TUBERCULOSIS, AND OTHER CONTAGIOUS CONDITIONS

SECTION OBJECTIVES

Using the information presented in this section, the student will be able to perform the following:

- Define AIDS in detail
- Identify behavior that could result in the transmission of HIV or HBV infection and other contagious conditions

A *syndrome* is a group of clinical symptoms that constitute a disease or abnormal condition. (*Clinical* means reported or observed symptoms not discovered by laboratory tests.) With syndromes, an individual need not have all the symptoms. Syndromes may be caused by many different things, but with AIDS, the cause is a dysfunction in the body's immune system, one of the body's primary defenses against disease.

The diseases of AIDS are caused by germs we encounter every day. In fact, some of these germs live permanently in small numbers inside the human body. When the immune system weakens, these germs are able to multiply freely, therefore the diseases they cause are called *opportunistic diseases*.

HIV, which seems to be responsible for AIDS, is a retrovirus. As a group, retroviruses can live in the host for a long time without causing any sign of illness. In most animals, retrovirus infections last for life. These viruses die when exposed to heat, they can be killed by many common disinfectants, and they usually do not survive well if the tissue or blood they are in dries up. However, retroviruses have a high mutation rate and consequently tend to evolve very quickly into new strains. HIV shares this and other traits with other known retroviruses.

HIV replicates (lives) in the group of white blood cells called *lymphocytes,* or *T cells.* Among the T cells, HIV's favorite target is the T4 cell. The T4 cell, also called the *helper/inducer T cell,* performs a vital job in the immune system. HIV infection of the T4 cells creates a defect in the body's immune system, which may eventually result in AIDS. Long-term infection with HIV without the development of AIDS is becoming more common. Improved treatment, a better understanding of the disease on the part of health care professionals, increased public education, and less stress from public stigma support this process.

The Mechanics of Transmission

For transmission, HIV must travel from inside one person to the inside of another person. Because viruses are unable to enter the body through intact skin, they must enter through an open wound or one of a number of possible body openings (most of which contain mucous membranes). *Mucous membranes* are thin tissues that protect most openings and passages in the human body. These membranes secrete mucus, which contains antigerm chemicals and keeps the surrounding tissues moist. Mucous membranes can be found in the mouth, inside the eyelids, in the nose and air passages leading to the lungs, in the stomach, along the digestive tract, in the vagina, in the anus, and inside the eye and the opening of the penis. From the surface of a mucous membrane, many viruses can travel through the membrane and enter the tiny blood vessels inside. The mucous membranes of the eyes and mouth often are doorways for highly infectious viruses, such as the flu virus. The danger with HIV is very different. The major infection sites for this virus are the bloodstream and the central nervous system. HIV can be found in any body fluid or substance that contains lymphocytes.

The presence of HIV in a substance does not necessarily indicate that the substance is capable of transmitting the infection. In theory, all body fluids are capable of transmitting disease; in reality, however, the most dangerous substances seem to be blood, semen, and pre-ejaculate fluid; cervical and vaginal secretions; and perhaps feces. Despite much research, a clear-cut case of saliva causing transmission has not been found, although kissing theoretically could transmit the virus. The concentration of HIV (i.e., the number of viral particles per unit of volume) is very important in infectivity. If a substance has a high concentration of HIV, it is more likely to transmit the virus. A pregnant woman can transmit the virus to her unborn child. The concentration of HIV in mother's milk and in saliva, urine, and tears is low, but theoretically these are infectious substances that could transmit HIV infection. However, no cases have been reported to be caused by contact with these secretions. Sweat cannot transmit HIV.

HIV Survival Outside the Host

If HIV is present in a substance that leaves the body, the viral particles are capable of remaining infectious until the substance dries up. Depending on the circumstances, this could be a matter of minutes or hours. If the substance stays moist, the viral particles can survive much longer. For example, in water and blood solutions (10% blood, 90% saline), HIV can survive at room temperature for 2 weeks. In refrigerated blood, such as that used for transfusions, HIV can survive indefinitely.

The public has a widespread fear that AIDS can be contracted through casual contact, such as shaking hands, being in the same room with an individual infected with HIV, touching doorknobs, or sharing bathroom facilities. The fear is far, far greater than the risk. Diseases spread by casual contact invariably are spread through saliva or sputum, and they exist in the saliva or sputum in very high concentrations. The concentration of HIV in saliva and sputum is very low, if it exists in these substances at all. After 10 years of documentation of the AIDS epidemic, there are no known cases of AIDS or HIV infection being transmitted by casual social contact, not even among people living in the same household. In some cases household members have even shared toothbrushes with infected housemates without contracting the virus.

To date no medical or health care workers have contracted HIV from casual contact. The contact between the massage professional and the client falls under this classification. We touch only the skin, which is not a transmission route.

Hepatitis

Hepatitis is an inflammatory process, an infection of the liver caused by a virus. It is classified as type A, B, C, D, E, or G. Hepatitis A, caused by the hepatitis A virus (HAV), is a less serious form and is usually transmitted by fecal contamination of food and water. Hepatitis B is a potentially fatal disease caused by the hepatitis B virus (HBV), which is transmitted through routes similar to those for HIV. HBV is 100 times more contagious than HIV, and it is estimated that more than 1 million people in the United States are carriers of HBV. Two types of vaccine are available for preventing the transmission of HBV. Hepatitis C accounts for 86% of new cases of hepatitis each year. The hepatitis D virus (HDV) infects only those who have hepatitis B, and its symptoms are more severe than other forms of hepatitis. Vaccines do not appear to be effective for HDV. Hepatitis E is transmitted through food and water contaminated by fecal material. Hepatitis G is a sexually transmitted virus.[5]

Standard precautions prevent the spread of hepatitis. It is important to be cautious of all behaviors in which body fluids are contacted or unsanitary conditions may be present that may allow the transmission of HIV and the hepatitis viruses (Proficiency Exercise 6-4).

PROFICIENCY EXERCISE 6-4

1. *Contact a local hospital, the police, the fire department, and an emergency rescue team and investigate their procedures for standard precautions.*
2. *Practice putting on and taking off gloves.*

Tuberculosis

Tuberculosis (TB) is an infection caused by a bacterium that usually affects the lungs but may invade other body systems. It is estimated that approximately 1.86 billion people—more than one third of the world's population—are infected with TB. Transmission occurs via airborne droplets that are produced when an infected person coughs, sneezes, or talks. TB can also be spread through contaminated food.

In many infected individuals, tuberculosis is asymptomatic. In others, symptoms develop so gradually that they are not noticed until the disease is advanced. However, symptoms can appear in immunosuppressed individuals within weeks of exposure to the bacillus. Symptoms include fatigue, weight loss, lethargy, anorexia (loss of appetite), and a low-grade fever that usually occurs in the afternoon. A cough that produces purulent sputum develops slowly and becomes more frequent over several weeks or months. Night sweats and general anxiety often are present. Because these are common signs and symptoms of all chronic infections, referral is necessary for diagnosis. Dyspnea, chest pain, and hemoptysis may also occur as the disease progresses.

Tuberculosis is diagnosed by a positive tuberculin skin test (PPD), sputum culture, and chest x-ray. A positive tuberculin skin test indicates that an individual has been infected and has produced antibodies against the bacillus. By itself the positive skin test does not indicate the presence of an active disease. Treatment consists of antibiotic therapy to control active or dormant tuberculosis and to prevent transmission. Massage professionals should be tested yearly because of their contact with the public.

Severe Acute Respiratory Syndrome (SARS)

Severe acute respiratory syndrome (SARS) is a respiratory illness that has been reported in Asia, North America, and Europe. In general, SARS begins with a fever over 100.4° F (38° C). Other symptoms may include headache, an overall feeling of discomfort, and body aches. Some people also experience mild respiratory symptoms. After 2 to 7 days, SARS patients may develop a dry cough and have trouble breathing. SARS appears to spread primarily through close person-to-person contact. Most cases of SARS have involved people who cared for or lived with someone with SARS or who had direct contact with infectious material (e.g., respiratory secretions) from a person with SARS.

Potential ways SARS can be spread include touching the skin of other people or touching objects that are contaminated with infectious droplets and then touching the eyes, nose, or mouth. Droplet contamination occurs when someone who is sick with SARS coughs or sneezes droplets onto themselves, other people, or nearby surfaces. SARS may possibly be spread more broadly through the air or in other currently unknown ways. Most U.S. cases of SARS have occurred among travelers returning from other parts of the world that were experiencing a SARS outbreak. A small number of cases resulted from spread of the disease to close contacts, such as family members and health care workers.[4]

The transmission of SARS to health care workers has resulted from close contact with sick people before recommended infection control precautions were put into use. The CDC has issued interim infection control recommendations for health care settings as well as for the management of exposure to SARS in health care and other institutional settings.

Although SARS is not commonly contracted by health care workers, it is essential that massage professionals strictly follow standard precautions (see Box 6-2) to reduce the spread of diseases such as SARS. The practitioner also is responsible for consistently checking the CDC Web site for updates on all diseases.

PREMISE AND FIRE SAFETY

SECTION OBJECTIVES

Using the information presented in this section, the student will be able to perform the following:

- Recognize and avoid fire and safety hazards
- Complete an accident report

The massage professional's facility must be kept free of hazards. Some clients will need additional assistance to prevent falls or other injury. The following safety rules are guidelines for creating a hazard-free massage environment.

- Infants and young children should not be left unattended. Parents or guardians should always be present during massage for minors.
- Women in the last trimester of a pregnancy should not be left in the massage room alone and may need assistance getting on and off the massage table.
- Elderly individuals may be less steady on their feet and should not be left in the massage room unattended.
- Any client whose mobility is impaired, including those with visual impairments, may need assistance getting on and off the massage table. People with disabilities should be asked what assistance they need, and their instructions should be followed carefully.

Preventing falls is very important. The massage professional should observe the following rules to prevent falls.

- Provide barrier-free access.
- Provide good lighting; never perform a massage in a dark room.
- Do not use throw rugs, because they may slip or tangle in the feet.
- Avoid slippery tile floors.
- Keep floors and walkways uncluttered.
- Keep electrical and phone cords out of traffic areas.

6-1 The Evolve Web site has a video demonstrations of proper hand-washing procedures.

6-2 Electronic flashcards review key terms from this chapter.

6-3 Complete a matching exercise by corresponding the levels of sanitation to the products used by a massage therapist.

Don't forget to study for your certification and licensure exams! Review questions for this chapter are located on Evolve.

- Regularly check all massage equipment to make sure it is sturdy and in good repair.
- Make sure all outside entrances are free of clutter and hazards caused by ice, snow, or rain.

If an accident occurs, all information about the accident must be written down. An insurance company will need the following information:

- Where and when the accident occurred
- Detailed information about the accident
- Names and addresses of the person or people involved in the accident
- Names of any witnesses to the accident
- Names of manufacturers, if equipment is involved

Most accidents can be prevented. Knowing the common safety hazards, recognizing which clients need extra assistance, and using common sense are all necessary to promote safety.

Fire prevention also is essential (Proficiency Exercise 6-5). The massage professional should observe the following rules to prevent fires:

- Provide a nonsmoking environment. In places where smoking is allowed, make sure proper ashtrays are used. Empty ashtrays only into a metal container that is partly filled with sand or water.
- Regularly check all electrical cords and equipment to make sure they are in good condition. Do not plug more than two cords into an electrical outlet.
- Never use candles, incense, or any open flame.

PROFICIENCY EXERCISE 6-5

1. *Contact your local fire marshal and learn more about fire prevention.*
2. *Draw up a fire escape route and emergency plan for your massage business.*
3. *Contact the local building and safety inspector and find out more about accident prevention.*
4. *Contact a local insurance agent and find out about the requirements for reporting accidents to the insurance company, as well as the insurance plan recommended for this type of protection.*
5. *Take basic and advanced first aid classes and learn cardiopulmonary resuscitation (CPR).*

- Make sure the massage area is equipped with a smoke detector and fire extinguisher. Check them regularly to make sure they are functional.

SUMMARY

The information in this chapter supports a safe, professional practice. Massage professionals should review these procedures regularly to maintain the attention to detail that ensures a safe, sanitary massage environment for our clients. It is our responsibility to act reliably in emergencies. As massage professionals, we must understand the use of standard precautions and fire and premise safety measures to serve our clients in a health-promoting and hazard-free manner.

REFERENCES

1. Oregon Board of Massage Technicians: *Sanitation requirements for the state of Oregon, Oregon Administrative Rules,* July 1991, The Board.
2. Thibodeau GA, Patton K: *Anatomy and physiology,* ed 6, St Louis, 2007, Mosby.
3. Board of Directors of Masseurs, Province of Ontario: *Ontario, Canada, therapeutic massage curriculum guidelines,* Toronto, 1992, The Board.
4. http://www.cdc.gov/ncidod/sars/factsheet.htm
5. McCance K, Huether S: *Pathophysiology: the biologic basis for disease in adults and children,* ed 5, St Louis, 2005, Mosby.

Workbook Section

Answers for the Workbook Section for Chapter 6 are provided on p. 763.

■ ■ ■ SHORT ANSWER

1. Why is the massage professional's hygiene so important?

_____

_____

_____

2. What odors may be offensive or a health risk to clients?

_____

_____

_____

3. Why does the use of alcohol and certain drugs interfere with the ability to function as an effective massage professional?

_____

_____

_____

4. Why should the massage professional study pathogenic organisms?

_____

_____

_____

5. Why is the integrity of the skin so important?

_____

_____

_____

6. What are the main ways diseases caused by pathogenic organisms are spread?

_____

_____

_____

7. What are the aseptic methods?

_____

_____

_____

8. What are the main concepts presented in the section on sanitation requirements?

_____

_____

_____

9. What is the main goal of standard precautions?

_____

_____

_____

10. Why should the massage professional understand hepatitis, HIV, AIDS, and SARS?

_____

_____

_____

11. What one sanitation method is most effective in controlling the spread of disease?

_____

_____

_____

12. What are the main precautions necessary for preventing falls and accidents?

_____

_____

_____

13. What are the main ways to prevent a fire?

_____

_____

_____

14. Why should the massage professional study emergency care and CPR?

_____

_____

_____

Workbook Section—cont'd

■■■ MATCHING I

Match the term to the best definition. You may need to use your anatomy and physiology text or a medical dictionary to complete this exercise.

1. AIDS
2. Asepsis
3. Centers for Disease Control and Prevention
4. Communicable disease
5. Contamination
6. Dermatosis
7. Dermatitis
8. Disinfection
9. First aid
10. Hazard
11. Hemorrhage
12. Host
13. Hygiene
14. HIV
15. Infection
16. Microorganism
17. Pathogen
18. Sanitation
19. Shock
20. Sterilization
21. Transmission
22. Standard precautions

a. the absence of pathogens
b. excessive loss of blood from a blood vessel
c. the human immunodeficiency virus
d. the formulation and application of measures to promote and establish conditions favorable to health, especially public health
e. the process by which an object becomes unclean
f. procedures developed by the CDC to prevent the spread of contagious disease
g. a disease caused by pathogens that are easily spread; a contagious disease
h. skin inflammation
i. a condition that results from inadequate blood supply to body organs and tissues
j. the process by which all microorganisms are destroyed
k. a disease state that results from the invasion and growth of microorganisms in the body
l. the person, animal, or environment in which microorganisms live and grow
m. acquired immunodeficiency syndrome
n. a small living plant or animal that cannot be seen without the aid of a microscope
o. a microorganism that is harmful and capable of causing an infection; a virus, bacterium, fungus, protozoan, or pathogenic animal
p. emergency care given to an ill or injured person before medical help arrives
q. the spread or transfer of pathogens
r. the process by which pathogens are destroyed
s. a division of the U.S. Public Health Service that investigates and controls diseases with epidemic potential
t. any skin condition
u. anything that poses a safety threat
v. practices and conditions intended to promote health and prevent disease

■■■ MATCHING II

Match the ways pathogens can be spread or controlled with the proper description.

1. Pressurized steam bath, extreme temperature, or irradiation
2. Chemicals such as iodine, chlorine, alcohol, and soap
3. Quarantine of affected individuals; protective apparel worn while giving treatments
4. Pathogens found in the environment, such as in food, water, and soil and on assorted surfaces
5. Disease that does not develop until the pathogens have the opportunity
6. Transferal of pathogens from one person to another
7. Killing or disabling of pathogens on surfaces before they can spread to other people

a. aseptic technique
b. person-to-person contact
c. opportunistic invasion
d. environmental contact
e. isolation
f. disinfection
g. sterilization

■■■ ASSESS YOUR COMPETENCIES

Now that you have studied this chapter, you should be able to:

1. Identify good health and personal hygiene practices.
2. Explain the major disease-causing agents.
3. Describe methods for preventing and controlling disease.
4. Give specific recommendations for sanitary practices for massage businesses.
5. Implement standard precautions.
6. Provide information about HIV, AIDS, and hepatitis.
7. Establish a hazard-free massage environment.

On a separate paper, write a short summary of the content of this chapter based on the competencies listed above. When writing this paper assume you are speaking to someone—a client, prospective employer, co-worker, or other interested person. Write the paper as if you were having a conversation and explaining the importance of the information and skills to professional massage development.

Next, in small student discussion groups, share the papers and compare and contrast how the information was presented. Discuss the content, looking for similarities, differences, potential misunderstanding of the information, and clear and concise methods of description.

▪ ▪ ▪ PROFESSIONAL ACTIVITY

List 20 suggested sanitation requirements developed from the Oregon model.

1.
2.
3.
4.
5.
6.
7.
8.
9.
10.
11.
12.
13.
14.
15.
16.
17.
18.
19.
20.

▪ ▪ ▪ PROFESSIONAL APPLICATION EXERCISE

Completing an accident report

It is a fact of life that accidents happen daily. When they involve personal injury or property damage, information is needed so that the involved parties and any insurance companies can recognize and repair the damage. A massage practitioner, like any other business person, may be called on to fill out an insurance report.

This exercise presents a practice story about an accident. The story is followed by some standard questions, and the correct answers are supplied so that you can see how the information should be presented. (Please note that the following scenario is intended to be humorous.)

This afternoon you had a new client. He was the contortionist from the traveling circus, which is in town for the next week. He brought along his wife, who works with him, to observe your techniques so that she can help him as they travel. Unfortunately, some interesting things happened. You sit for a few minutes to recollect the events, and this is what you remember:

You had completed the massage with Mr. Gummy and had just asked him to roll over when you noticed that the table had started swaying. Ms. Gummy, who is an acrobat, was doing a handstand on Mr. Gummy's shoulders. Your table was sturdy enough, but because of the lubricant on your client's shoulders, his wife slid off and out the window. She was able to catch herself on the awning of the store below your office, but in doing so she bent the frame and tore the canvas. No one was injured, but the other tenant called emergency services, so reports had to be filed.

Because your immediate supervisor was not available, you had to complete the accident report yourself. Using your narrative, fill out the following information for the police and insurance companies.

1. State where and when the accident occurred.

2. Provide detailed information about the accident.

3. Give the names and addresses of the person or people involved in the accident.

4. Give the names of any witnesses to the accident.

5. Give the names of manufacturers, if equipment was involved.

6. Describe all property damage.

7. Detail any injuries to the people involved.

Answers to questions

1. The accident occurred at The Massage Center, 38 Falls Drive, Anytown, ML 48999, on Thursday, June 12, 2003, at approximately 11:15 AM.

2. The incident occurred during a massage therapy session at the above location, in room #4 on the second floor. As I was working with my client, Mr. Victor Gummy, his wife, Ms. Viola Gummy, began doing a handstand on Mr. Gummy's shoulders. Because of the lubrication on his shoulders, Ms. Gummy slid off of Mr. Gummy's shoulders and out the window. To prevent herself from hitting the sidewalk, Ms. Gummy caught the outer aluminum trim of the front door awning. The awning frame bent, and the canvas covering was torn.

3. The people involved in the accident included myself, Cathie Balevit, 38 Falls Drive, Anytown, ML 48999; my client, Victor Gummy; and his wife, Viola Gummy, of Fred's Traveling Funshows, 826 Cartwheel Drive, Caravan, FN 81234.

4. Mr. Victor Gummy and I both witnessed Viola Gummy fall out the window. Mr. William Bill of Bill's Locksmith Company, 41 Falls Drive, Anytown, ML 48999, actually saw Viola catch herself on the awning, which then gave way.

5. No one was injured.

Now, read the following incident narrative and provide the information requested.

Today's date is Thursday, May 1, 2——. Your client, Mr. James Jackson, arrived for his weekly 4 PM massage appointment. Twenty minutes into the session, you asked him to roll over from his stomach to his side. As he did so, the table cracked and started to collapse. It did not collapse completely because the cable supports held it up. Other than being a little scared, Mr. Jackson was not injured, and you

Workbook Section—cont'd

were able to help him off the table. Every Friday you check the tables for safety and perform any maintenance. This table had been checked the previous Friday, and no problems were found.

You immediately contacted the table distributor to tell him of the problem with the table. He works for Buy-Low Products, at 12 Buy-Low Drive in Anytown, VN 84848. He contacted the manufacturer, Fred's Cut Rate Tables, 480 W. Shady Lane, Market Town, ML 29341 The table is model #83, called "The Basic," and retails for $99.95.

1. State where and when the accident occurred.

2. Provide detailed information about the accident.

3. Give the names and addresses of the person or people involved in the accident.

4. Give the names of any witnesses to the accident.

5. Give the names of manufacturers, if equipment was involved.

6. Describe all property damage.

7. Detail any injuries to the people involved.

Body Mechanics

CHAPTER OBJECTIVES

After completing this chapter, the student will be able to perform the following:

- Use the body, especially the hands and forearms, in an efficient and biomechanically correct manner when giving a massage
- Alter the position of both the client and the practitioner to maximize body mechanics

CHAPTER OUTLINE

KEY TERMS

Asymmetric standing
Balance point
Compressive force
Leverage
Physical ergonomics

Body mechanics allow the massage practitioner's body to be used in a careful, efficient, and deliberate way. They involve good posture, balance, leverage, and use of the strongest and largest muscles to perform the work. Fatigue, muscle strain, and injury, including overuse syndromes, can result from improper use and positioning of the massage practitioner's body while giving a massage. In this chapter the student will learn methods of working more efficiently so that providing 8 hours of massage in a day does not cause any dysfunction or pain. The ability to work for 8 full hours a day is important, because to make a living doing massage full time, the practitioner must be able to give 15 to 30 sessions per week. Efficient use of the body helps prevent burnout. (The DVD has more information on this subject.)

The information in this chapter has been taken from standard ergonomics recommendations for service professions, personal observation, and the author's professional and teaching experience. The principles of body mechanics presented

STUDENT NOTE: Most models in this chapter are pictured in sportswear to enhance and clarify the various body positions. The properly groomed massage professional would wear a uniform as shown in Figure 6-1 (p. 199). Draping materials are not used in the examples in this chapter so that positions may be seen more clearly.

in this text rely on leverage, balance, and biomechanics. Static and dynamic postures assumed at work and during recreational activities may have adverse effects on the body. These effects usually manifest in the musculoskeletal system. Also, safe professional practice is a consideration.

The delivery of therapeutic massage makes unique postural and physical demands. For most professionals, body mechanics focus on lifting or exerting a force in an upward direction, such as when a nurse lifts a patient from the bed to a chair. Other aspects of body mechanics apply to dynamic movement, such as for dancing and participating in athletics or the martial arts. By contrast, most of the effort exerted to give a massage is a sustained, restrained, and somewhat static movement, with pressure focused downward and forward to deliver compressive and tension force. The massage practitioner makes extensive use of the forearms, wrists, hands, fingers, thumbs, knees, and foot to deliver compressive force. Because of this difference, the standard recommendations provided to most professionals for safe use of the body are of little help to massage practitioners. In fact, attempting to modify these forms of body mechanics may actually result in injury to the massage professional.

Massage professionals need to consider their body types and musculoskeletal limitations. The suggestions in this chapter will help most students develop the best personal body mechanics style for them as individuals.

Physical ergonomics deals with the human body's responses to physical and physiologic loads. Relevant topics include manual materials handling, workstation layout, job demands, and risk factors such as repetition, vibration, force, and awkward or static posture as they relate to musculoskeletal disorders and repetitive strain injury. Work activities should allow the worker to adopt several different postures, all equally healthy and safe. When muscular force must be exerted, it should be done by the largest appropriate muscle groups available. Awkward posture is associated with an increased risk for injury, and the more a joint deviates from the neutral (natural) position, the greater the risk of injury. Every joint in the body has a neutral position where joint spaces are even and symmetric. The muscles around a joint in neutral position are neither short nor long, but at their neutral physiologic resting lengths. Joint stability is provided with the least amount of muscle activity and maximizing stability provided by joint shape, joint capsule, ligaments, and normal co-contraction of the muscles around the joint.

Four basic concepts of body mechanics are common to all techniques used to apply compressive force to the body tissues during massage:

- Weight transfer
- Perpendicularity
- Stacking the joints
- Keeping the back straight and maintaining core stability

With weight transfer, massage practitioners transfer their body weight by shifting the center of gravity forward to achieve a pressure that is comfortable to the client. To transfer weight, the practitioner stands (or kneels) with one foot forward and the other foot (or knee) back in an asymmetric stance. In the standing position, the front leg is in a relaxed knee flexion with the foot forward enough to be in front of the knee. The back leg is straight, and the hips and shoulders are aligned so that the back is straight. The transfer is made by taking the weight off the front leg and moving it to the heels of the hands, thumbs, or whichever part of the arm is used to apply pressure. Pressure is increased or decreased by moving the back leg farther away from or closer to the client. The weight of the body is distributed to the heel of the weight-bearing leg, not the toes.

Perpendicularity is an important concept that ensures that the pressure is sinking straight into the tissues. The line from the shoulders to the point of contact (e.g., the forearm or heel of the hand) must be 90 degrees to the plane of the contact point on the client's body.

Stacking the joints one on top of another is essential to the concepts of perpendicularity and weight transfer. The practitioner's body must be a straight line from the feet and then through the shoulder to the forearm, or through the elbow acting as an extension of the shoulder, to the heels of the hands. The ankle, knee, hip of the back leg, and spine are stacked. The shoulder is stacked over the elbow, which in turn is stacked over the wrist. Stacking the joints in this way allows the pressure to go straight into the client's body effortlessly as the center of gravity moves forward.

A straight back and a pressure-bearing leg are essential components of body mechanics. If the back is not straight, the practitioner often ends up pushing with the upper body instead of using the more effortless feeling of transferred weight. The practitioner's weight should be held on the back leg and on the heel of the foot. At first this may feel uncomfortable; however, some of the biggest muscles in the body are in the legs. If you carry the weight on your back, fatigue sets in more quickly, and eventually the pain can become debilitating. The muscles of the torso, especially the abdomen, make up the body's core. *Core stability is necessary for back stability* (Figures 7-1 to 7-4).

Practical Application

The following exercise puts all these components together to demonstrate the concept of transferring weight by shifting the center of gravity to apply compressive force.

1. Stand facing a wall and put both hands on the wall, shoulder-width apart and at shoulder height.

2. Step back with both feet so that your body is at a 45-degree angle and you're leaning into the wall. Your feet should be shoulder width apart. Bring your hips forward and under you so that your shoulders, back, and feet are aligned. Hold your abdomen in while exhaling to stabilize the core. Hold the abdomen in, but continue to breathe. Do not suck in your belly; pull it in by contracting the muscles. Notice that all your weight is on your feet and your hands.

3. Now, bring one leg forward and bend it. Make sure your foot is forward enough so that your toes are in front of your knee. The other leg stays back and straight. Keep your hips aligned with your shoulders and your back foot. Maintain core stability.

FIGURE 7-1 Draw-in maneuver.

A

B

FIGURE 7-2 Prone core exercises.

4. Drop the arm on the same side as your back foot. Keep the arm that remains on the wall straight and relax your shoulders. If you have range-of-motion limitations in your wrist, adjust the hand that is on the wall so that you're comfortable. Sometimes slightly curling your fingers is enough. Another option is using your fist with a straight wrist.

5. Now, try to hold your weight in your front leg so that your hand is not supporting you at all. Begin by slowly transferring the weight of your body from your front leg (slowly lift it from the floor) to the heel of your hand on the wall. Keep the arm that is against the wall straight and your hips aligned. Your hips don't need to move at all. Maintain core stability. As you feel the weight transfer to the heel of your hand, you'll notice that weight is also moving to the heel of your back foot.

DYSFUNCTIONS CAUSED BY IMPROPER BODY MECHANICS

Massage professionals who are not attentive to body mechanics commonly feel the effects in the neck and shoulder, wrist and thumb, lower back, knee, ankle, and foot. The following recommendations are methods for protecting the practitioner's body.

Neck and Shoulder (Figure 7-5)

Neck and shoulder problems most often develop when the massage practitioner uses upper body strength to push and exert the pressure for massage. These problems can be avoided

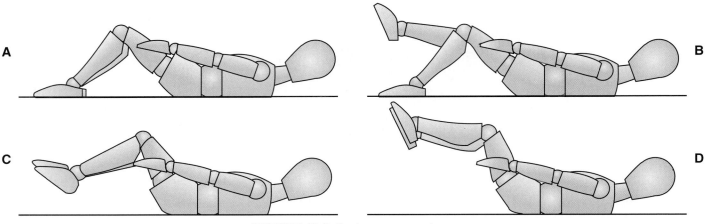

FIGURE 7-3 Supine core exercises.

FIGURE 7-4 Ball curl exercises.

if the student learns to use leverage and leans with the body weight to provide pressure. The practitioner's arms and hands should be relaxed while giving a massage, because tension in the arms and hands translates to the shoulders and neck. Remember, the joints need to be stacked and stable so that the force is easily distributed from the body weight through the joint structure to create compressive force. If the core is not stable, the scapula will be unstable, making it difficult to maintain shoulder stability.

Forearm, Wrist, and Hand (Figure 7-6)

Massage professionals need to protect their wrists by preventing the development of excessive compressive forces from the delivery of massage methods. Using a proper wrist angle and staying behind the massage stroke protect the wrist. Tense wrists and hands also contribute to shoulder problems. It is important always to maintain a relaxed hand and wrist while giving a massage. Whenever possible, use the forearm to apply massage to spare the hands and wrists.

Low Back (Figure 7-7)

Some reasons for low back problems include core instability, inappropriate bending, bent static positions, twisting, improper knee position, improper foot position, bending of the elbows, and reaching for an area with the arm while giving a massage instead of moving the feet to the area. Massage professionals must learn to keep the lower back straight and avoid bending or curling at the waist while working. Maintaining a stable spinal line and a strong core helps prevent this problem. Frequent posture shifting of the massage practitioner's body also helps protect the lower back, as does learning to lift by leaning back during stretching. Using an asymmetric stance, normal knee-lock position in the weight-bearing leg, and variations using a short or tall stool provide protection for the back. The lower back is further supported by avoiding twisting and reaching while working and by keeping the point of contact with the client below the practitioner's waist (Figure 7-8).[1] The joints of the arm must be kept effectively stacked,

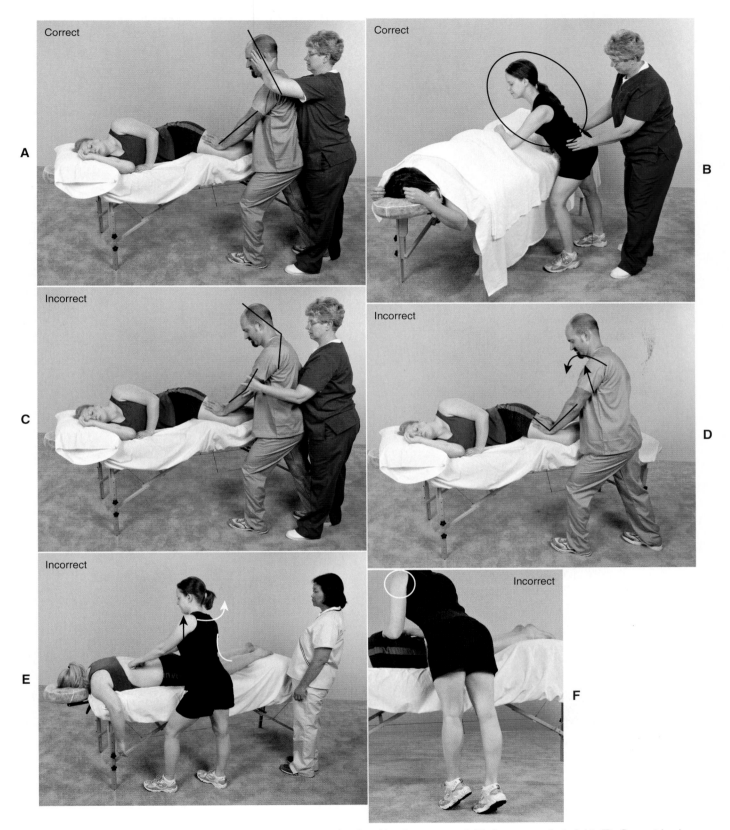

FIGURE 7-5 The neck and shoulder. **A,** Correct body mechanics: Head up, arms at 45 degrees and straight. **B,** Correct body mechanics. **C,** Incorrect body mechanics: Elbows bent, head forward. **D,** Incorrect body mechanics: Shoulders up, rotated, and forward. **E,** Incorrect body mechanics: Shoulders up and rotated with low back sway. **F,** Incorrect body mechanics.

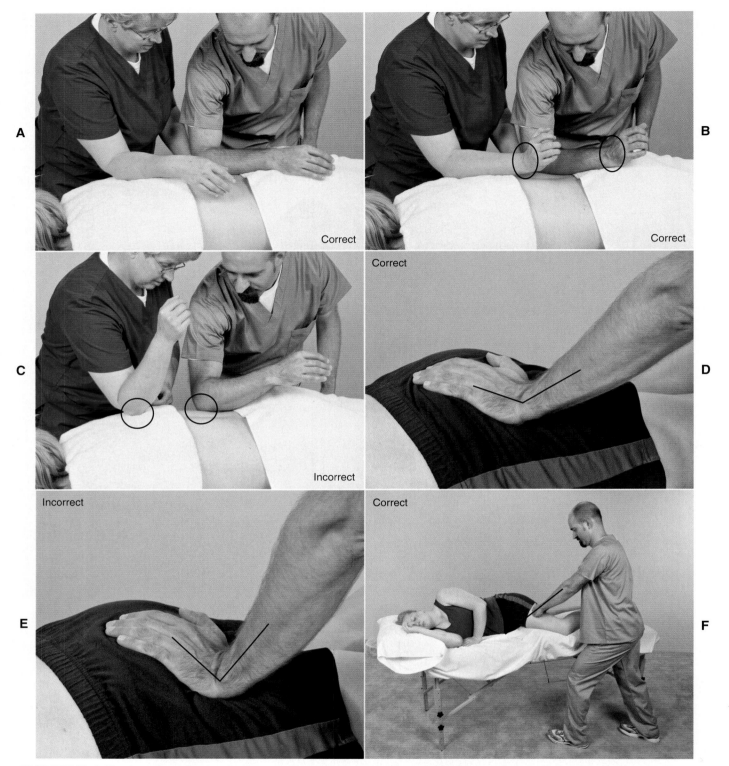

FIGURE 7-6 The forearm and wrist. **A,** Forearm. Incorrect body mechanics. Stiff wrist. **B,** Forearm. Correct body mechanics. Relaxed and flat. **C,** Forearm. Incorrect body mechanics. Using wrong point of elbow. **D,** Wrist. Correct body mechanics. **E,** Wrist. Incorrect body mechanics. **F,** Wrist. Correct body mechanics.

FIGURE 7-6, cont'd **G,** Wrist. Incorrect body mechanics. Hand stiff. **H,** Wrist. Correct body mechanics. Hand relaxed.

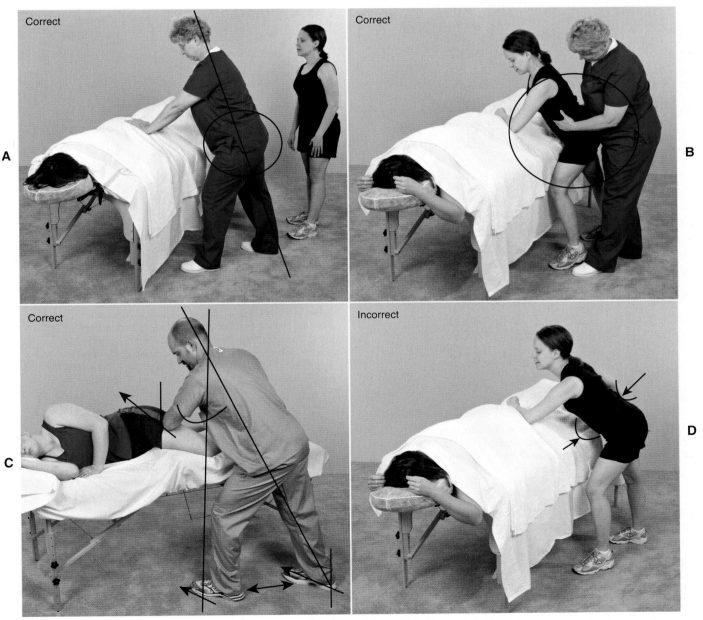

FIGURE 7-7 The low back and hips. **A,** Correct body mechanics: Back straight, core stability. **B,** Correct body mechanics: Maintaining core stability. **C,** Correct body mechanics: Back straight; feet wide enough apart and pointed in the same direction as the arm; center of gravity correct. **D,** Incorrect body mechanics: Loss of core stability.

Continued

Incorrect

E

Incorrect

F

FIGURE 7-7, cont'd E, Incorrect body mechanics: Torsion. **F,** Incorrect body mechanics: Lower body sticks out because knee is extended; sway back; no core stability.

with the elbow straight. If the elbow is bent, there is a tendency to curl at the waist and slouch in the lower back.

Knee (Figure 7-9)

Knee problems can be avoided by respecting the basic stability design of the knee and frequently shifting the weight from foot to foot. The most efficient standing position involves the normal screw-home, or knee-lock, position in the last 15 degrees of extension on the back weight-bearing leg. This

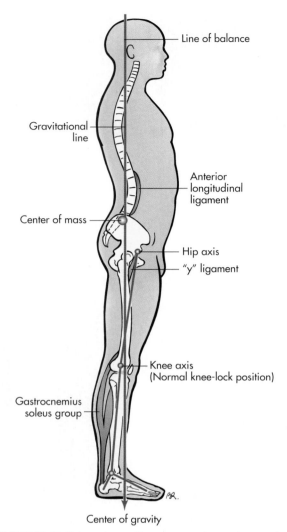

FIGURE 7-8 Relaxed standing posture that supports the gravitational line with normal knee-lock position in the last 15 degrees of extension. The gravitational force line falls behind the hip joint, in front of the knee joint, and in front of the ankle joint. The only muscle group used for balance is the gastrocnemius-soleus group. The relaxed stance involves leaning on the "y," or iliofemoral, ligament, the anterior longitudinal ligament, and the posterior knee ligaments.

position provides the least compressive force on the knee capsule and the least muscular action for stability. As the knee is flexed, compressive forces increase in the joint capsule, and muscular action for stability increases (Figure 7-10). Full hyperextension should be avoided.

Confusion and disagreement exist about the proper position of the knee while giving a massage. Some recommend a slightly flexed knee, opposing this text's recommendation of a locked knee. Others express some concern with the locked-knee position, opposing the blocking of body energy flow and interference with concepts of grounding and being centered. These concerns tend to arise from information founded on movement principles such as tai chi, forms of dance, and martial arts. Although a flexed knee is appropriate for these systems, massage requires the application of sustained pres-

FIGURE 7-9 The knees. **A,** Correct body mechanics: Normal knee extension and flexion in asymmetric stance. **B,** Incorrect body mechanics: Bilateral flexion. **C,** Incorrect body mechanics: Bilateral hyperextension. **D,** Incorrect body mechanics: Bilateral flexion.

sure from a stable position with the least amount of effort, muscular activity, and compressive force to the joint.

The knee needs to be in a slightly flexed position as the massage practitioner changes position and moves around the table. However, when pressure is applied, the anatomic design of the knee provides stability in the knee-lock position in the last 15 degrees of extension. Practitioners must honor their own bodies in terms of the individualized approach to body position. The body mechanics presented in this chapter have been developed to support the knee.[2,3]

Ankle and Foot (Figure 7-11)

Asymmetric standing (i.e., standing with one foot in front of the other) is the most efficient standing position. The weight is shifted from one foot to the other in an energy conservation mechanism. Symmetric standing, in which the weight is equally distributed on the two feet, is fatiguing, interferes with circulation, and should be avoided.[3] The ankle and foot are

protected by the asymmetric stance, frequent position changes, and sitting, when possible, to do massage. The body mechanics presented in this chapter are based on the asymmetric stance so as to best use the massage professional's energy and avoid fatigue.

APPLICATION OF COMPRESSIVE FORCES

The human body is designed for movement and range of motion, not the applied compressive forces required when giving a massage. Therefore it is vital to use body weight and leverage and not muscle strength to provide the pressure required during a massage.[4] This is accomplished by shifting the body weight center of gravity (as described previously) so that the balance point shifts (remember Newton's Law in Chapter 4) to the contact point between the massage professional's hand or forearm and the client's body. It is important to redistribute the body mass and to move the body's center

FIGURE 7-10 Improper leg position, which puts excessive strain on joints and requires muscle activity to maintain balance. The gravitational line improperly falls behind the knees.

FIGURE 7-11 The ankle and foot. **A,** Correct body mechanics: Feet pointed in the direction of the stroke, asymmetric stance, feet shoulder width apart. **B,** Correct body mechanics: Feet pointed in the direction of the stroke, asymmetric stance, feet shoulder width apart.

of gravity forward. Increasing the amount of pressure applied is accomplished by widening the stance, which is done by moving the back leg farther away from the point of contact and making sure the weight bearing is originating from the heel.

Massage uses primarily a force generated forward and downward with a 90-degree contact against the body. The combination of a 45-degree slant from the contours of the client's body plus the 45-degree angle of force used during appropriate body mechanics results in the 90-degree contact (Figure 7-12). Therefore the center of gravity and the weight force must be redistributed by keeping the weight on the back foot, the knee and back straight, the weight distribution coming from the abdomen, and the balance point at the object-contact point. The joints of the wrist, arm, shoulder, back, hip, weight-bearing knee, and ankle are stacked for effective delivery of force. As the body's stance widens, the base of support enlarges. The arm generating the pressure is

opposite the weight-bearing leg, which allows proper counterbalance and prevents twisting of the body at the shoulder and pelvic girdle.[4] The shoulder girdle must stay in line with the pelvic girdle, with the head held up and the eyes forward (Figures 7-13 and 7-14).

FIGURE 7-11, cont'd C, Correct body mechanics. **D,** Incorrect body mechanics: Weight on wrong foot. **E,** Incorrect body mechanics: Feet too far apart and not properly aligned, resulting in torsion strain. **F,** Incorrect body mechanics: Tightrope effect.

Continued

Although there is no one correct way to use the human body efficiently, these recommendations are effective. The important thing is that the massage practitioner must learn to remain relaxed, to stay comfortable, and to avoid straining when doing massage. If the practitioner looks and feels as if he or she is working hard while giving a massage, something is wrong with the body mechanics. If proper body mechanics are used, the practitioner will look and feel relaxed and graceful while giving a massage. Shifts in balance, not harder pushes, are used to apply the various degrees of pressure. In fact, using body mechanics effectively eliminates the need for pushing to create compressive pressure. As compressive force is applied during massage, a gradual increase in pressure accesses the various layers of body tissues from the skin to the bone. This requires changes in body mechanics throughout the massage.

Text continued on p. 231.

FIGURE 7-11, cont'd **G,** Incorrect body mechanics: Feet too close together. **H,** Incorrect body mechanics: Feet in symmetric stance.

FIGURE 7-12 Correct body mechanics for compressive force required for massage.

FIGURE 7-13 Basic principles of body mechanics: Correct positioning. **A,** Weight on back foot. **B,** Lean uphill.
C, Weight transfer balance point. **D,** Proper alignment for body mechanics.

Continued

FIGURE 7-13, cont'd E, Maintain normal knee-lock position (feet shoulder width apart) and weight on back of foot. **F,** Feet shoulder width apart, asymmetric stance. **G,** Correct center of gravity. Straight back, solid core. **H,** Center of gravity between contact on body and back, weight-bearing foot.

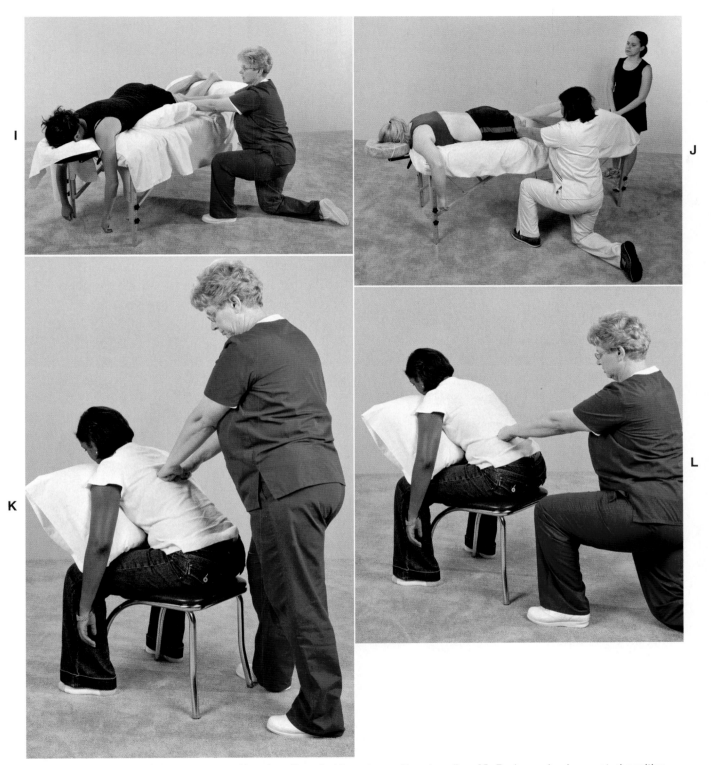

FIGURE 7-13, cont'd I, Alternate position, kneeling. **J,** Alternate position, kneeling. **K,** Body mechanics, seated position. **L,** Seated position, kneeling.

FIGURE 7-14 Basic principles of body mechanics: Incorrect positioning. **A,** Incorrect posture. Feet are too close together and not aligned with direction of stroke. Both knees are straight, and bottom sticks out. Shoulders and head twisted. **B,** Incorrect posture. Feet are improperly aligned to the direction of stroke and too far apart. Practitioner should not be bent at the hips. **C,** Incorrect posture. Feet should not have a "tightrope effect." Back leg knee is hyperextended and torso is twisted. **D,** Head tipped back. Sway back. Shoulder up and scapula winged. No core stability.

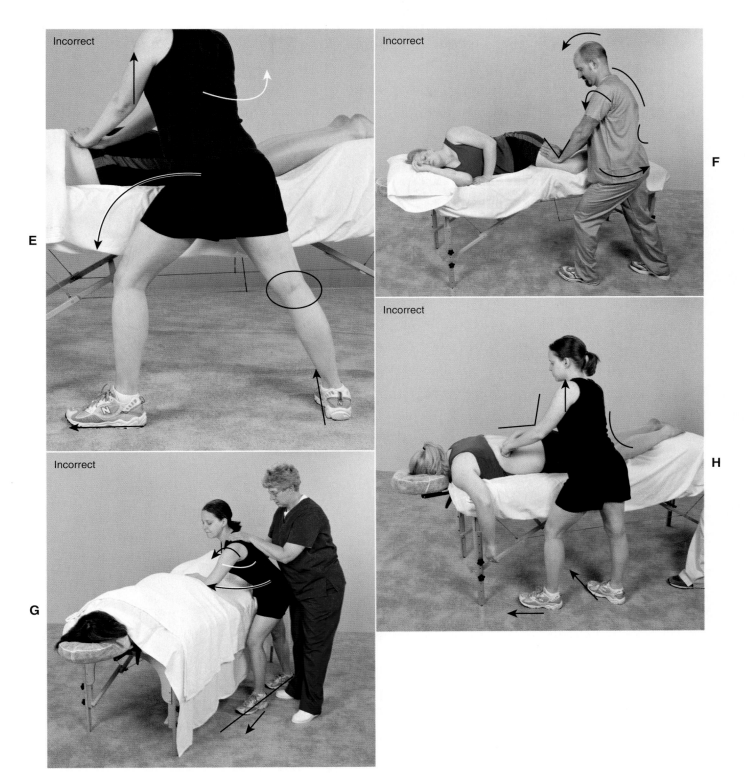

FIGURE 7-14, cont'd E, Stance too wide. Misalignment of feet. Hyperextended knee. Torso torsion. High shoulder. **F,** Wrist angle incorrect, rounded shoulders. Sway back. Twisted torso. Head down. **G,** Tightrope foot placement. Twisted torso. Rounded shoulders. Arm too far in front. **H,** Bent elbow. Elevated shoulder. Sway back. Misaligned feet.

Proper

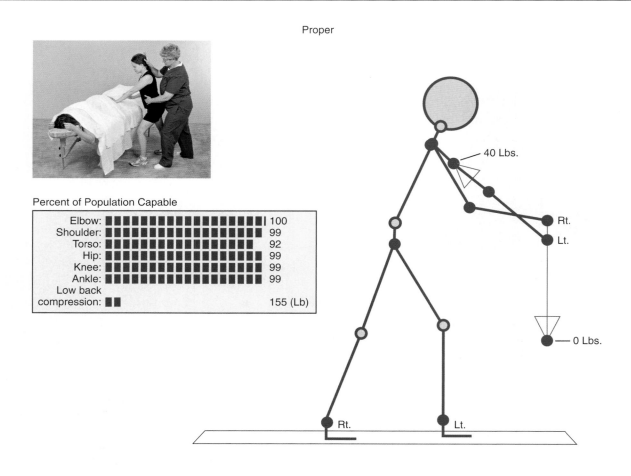

Percent of Population Capable

Elbow:	████████████████████	100
Shoulder:	████████████████████	99
Torso:	████████████████	92
Hip:	████████████████	99
Knee:	████████████████	99
Ankle:	████████████████	99
Low back compression:	██	155 (Lb)

Improper

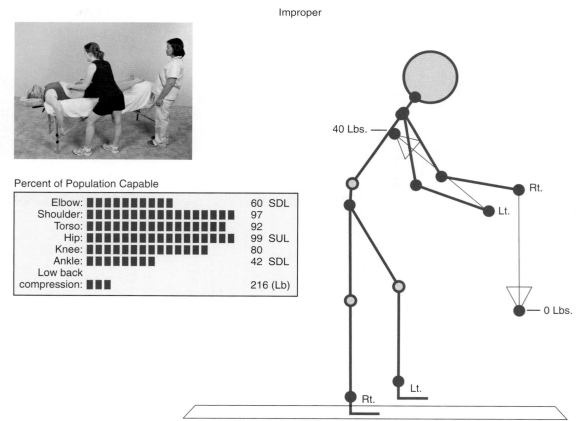

Percent of Population Capable

Elbow:	██████████	60	SDL
Shoulder:	████████████████	97	
Torso:	████████████████	92	
Hip:	████████████████	99	SUL
Knee:	████████████	80	
Ankle:	███████	42	SDL
Low back compression:	███	216 (Lb)	

BASIC PRINCIPLES OF BODY MECHANICS

7-1

Leverage and Leaning and Moving

The basic concept of this style of body mechanics is the use of leverage by "leaning" on the client, just as someone would comfortably lean against a wall or on a table. The practitioner seldom "pushes" against the client. Pushing requires a tense body, using muscle contraction to exert pressure. By leaning to transfer weight, the practitioner can substantially reduce muscle tension in the shoulders, neck, wrists, thumbs, elbows, and lower back.

Leaning pressure can also be used to evaluate the client. *Evaluation* means gathering information but making no changes. If a change in soft tissue is desired, the signal to the tissues must be carefully overridden and intensified slightly to substitute a different pattern. For the client's body to accept this change, the new signal must be presented in a nonthreatening manner and applied slowly. As soon as clients feel trapped, pressed, or pushed on, they tense up to protect themselves. The existing muscle pattern is reinforced, and little or no change occurs.

If the pressure levels are too intense, if the pressure feels "bony" or "pokey," or if a sensitive area is touched, the client's body automatically responds with a protective movement by flinching, tensing, pushing, or moving away. These subtle evaluation cues are easily missed if the massage practitioner is pushing on the client and stabilizing the movement. The style of body mechanics presented in this text provides the essential component for enabling the practitioner to receive feedback through body signals. While leaning, the practitioner becomes extremely sensitive to subtle body changes in the client, which supports the ongoing assessment process during massage (see Chapter 10). Moving and gliding involves leaning forward as body weight is transferred to the front foot (Figures 7-15 and 7-16).

Balance Point

While giving a massage, the practitioner's body is relaxed, which allows body weight to do the work. The point of contact between the practitioner and the client is the balance point. The practitioner would fall forward if the hand was moved off the client. The practitioner's center of gravity has moved forward, not dropped between the feet as in martial arts or similar systems. With the balance point located at the point of contact with the client's body, the practitioner can be moved or swayed by the subtle movements of the client's body. This prevents the use of too much pressure and allows the client to direct the movement and pressure intensity of the massage without feeling pressed and pinned against the table. The client should never feel trapped or constrained by the massage practitioner.

Firm Pressure Distributed over a Wide Area

Clients appreciate a firm, even pressure that is distributed over a wide area. For example, firm pressure on the back using the forearm is pleasant. However, the same pressure using the point of the elbow or the thumb would be painful, because the pressure is concentrated in a small area instead of dispersed over a broad area. The tissue feels poked, and the potential for tissue damage arises. When the practitioner's weight is maintained on the back foot, the pressure levels are more even; however, when the weight shifts to the front foot, the pressure becomes more concentrated and uneven and may be uncomfortable to the client.

FIGURE 7-15 Examples of how to glide. **A,** Start. **B,** Leaning forward with weight shift. *Continued*

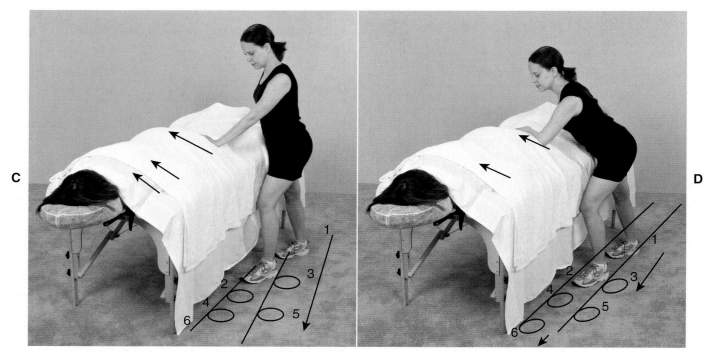

FIGURE 7-15, cont'd C, Move parallel to table by changing the position of back foot on *1, 3,* and *5.* Front foot should be on *2, 4,* and *6.*

FIGURE 7-16 Examples of how to knead. **A,** Position of hands. **B,** One hand compresses forward as the other hand moves back.

Pressure, Drag, and Duration

The task of describing various pressures and drag intensity is difficult because a number of factors influence these elements, including client factors, massage practitioner factors, the location of the pressure, and the desired outcome of the massage. The perception of the application depends extensively on the client. Pressure that one client perceives as deep may be perceived as lighter pressure by another client. Various authors and teachers (including myself) have presented a number of approaches to teaching massage students how to gauge the most beneficial and safe pressure and drag intensity (Figure 7-17).

Pressure

Pressure has been defined in numerous ways: compressive force; force application depth; light, medium, and deep pressure; and so forth. For the purposes of this text, *pressure* means compressive force down into the tissue at a 90-degree contact.

Drag is the resistance to glide. Glide moves horizontal to the tissues. Drag applies tension force to tissues to stretch them. The angle of force can be anything greater than 180 degrees to just less than 90 degrees and away from the point of contact. Therefore, pressure combined with drag can produce a multitude of intensities. For example, light pressure

FIGURE 7-17 Pressure levels. **A,** Level 1, light. The therapist's fingertips do not blanch. **B,** Level 2. **C,** Level 3. **D,** Level 4, **E,** Level 5. **F,** Level 6.

Continued

G

H

I

FIGURE 7-17, cont'd G, Level 7. **H,** Minimal drag. **I,** Maximal drag.

with extensive drag significantly stretches the skin. If the pressure is increased slightly and significant drag is maintained, the superficial fascia is stretched (tension force is applied).

Duration can modify intensity. In general, long duration is more intense and short duration is less intense.

Another factor that influences the application of pressure is the size of the point of contact. Pressure over a large contact area is less intense than that applied through a small contact point. More pressure can be applied safely with a broad base of contact, such as the forearm or full hand, than through a small point of contact, such as when thumb pressure is used.

As we have seen, the factors that determine the intensity of a massage application are compressive force, drag, duration, and the size of the contact point. In addition, a fast rhythmic application is more intense than a slow rhythmic application. Obviously, determining the right pressure is more difficult than it appears.

With compressive force, increasing force is needed to affect various layers of soft tissue. Hypothetically speaking, the tissues in the fleshy areas of the body (i.e., between the joints) can be divided into seven layers, which require seven levels of compressive force. The seven tissue layers, surface to deep, are as follows:

1. Skin surface
2. Skin
3. Superficial fascia
4. First muscle layer
5. Second muscle layer
6. Third muscle layer
7. Bone

The corresponding levels of pressure required to reach each layer are as follows:

- Level 1 pressure just touches the skin but does not dent it. It slides on the skin and cannot produce drag or tension of the skin. The therapist's fingertips do not blanch (change color). A bathroom scale or other scale does not move at this pressure (Figure 7-17, *A*).
- Level 2 pressure slightly dents the skin. It moves (drags) the skin to bind but cannot apply a tension force to stretch the skin past bind. The therapist's fingertips blanch, but the nail bed does not change color. A scale would move just 0 to 5 pounds, depending on the density of the person's skin (Figure 7-17, *B*).
- Level 3 pressure is compressive force that penetrates through the skin but not to the muscle; palpation of muscle structure indicates that the force is too intense. The therapist's fingertips and nail beds blanch. A scale would move 3 to 10 pounds. Body mechanics involve slight leaning into the tissue (Figure 7-17, *C*).
- Level 4 pressure is compressive force that penetrates through the skin and superficial fascia. The skin layer is displaced (pressed away), and the therapist should be able to palpate muscle tissue. Body mechanics require moderate leaning into the tissue. A scale would move 7 to 16 pounds, depending on the tissue density of the recipient (Figure 7-17, *D*).
- Level 5 pressure displaces the surface tissues (i.e., skin, fascia, and first muscle layer), and the compressive force penetrates to the middle muscle layer. Point or narrow base contact would feel "pokey." Broad-based contact with leaning body mechanics typically is used. A scale would move 12 to 35 pounds, depending on the recipient's tissue density and the bulk of the first layer of muscle (Figure 7-17, *E*).

- Level 6 pressure displaces surface tissues (skin, fascia, and first and second muscle layers), and the compressive force penetrates to the third muscle layer. This layer of muscle is smaller than the first and second layers and lies next to the bone. Applying force compresses the muscle against the bone; however, if bone is felt, the force is too intense. Full leaning body mechanics with simultaneous counterpressure may be required to reach this layer. Counterpressure involves pulling up against the table or the client's body while compressive force is applied (see p. 245). Broad-based contact must be used, or pain and protective guarding will occur in the first and second muscle layers. A scale would move 25 to 60 pounds (sometimes higher), depending on the recipient's muscle bulk and tissue density (Figure 7-17, *F*).
- Level 7 pressure is slightly more intense than level 6. The therapist would feel bone pressing against the tissue, except around the joints when the muscle layers are not prominent and the bone is beneath the skin and superficial fascia (Figure 7-17, *G*).

Drag

An arbitrary scale can be applied to drag:

    0—Minimal drag (Figure 7-17, *H*)
    1—Moves tissue but not to bind
    2—Moves tissue to bind
    3—Moves tissue past bind (Figure 7-17, *I*)

Duration

As mentioned previously, duration can modify intensity. Some guidelines for duration are as follows:

- For a specific application, a short duration is 10 seconds, a moderate duration is 30 seconds, and a long duration is 60 seconds.
- For a whole massage session, a short duration is 5 to 15 minutes, a moderate duration is 15 to 30 minutes, and a long duration is 45 to 60 minutes

Speed

Speed of the massage application can also influence the intensity of the massage and influence outcomes. Typically, the slower the speed, the more relaxing. The faster the speed, the more stimulating.

    Speed can be considered to be:

- Slow—from beginning to end of stroke: 10 seconds
- Moderate—from beginning to end of stroke: 5 seconds
- Fast—from beginning to end of stroke: 2 seconds

If the elements of pressure level, drag intensity, and duration are combined, the following general guidelines can be used.

Fragile patient outcomes: Comforting and soothing
    Pressure level—1 or 2
    Drag—0
Palliative, pleasure-based massage (nonfragile)
    Pressure level—2 or 3
    Drag—1-2
    Speed—Slow

    Duration (full session)—Short to moderate or moderate to long
Lymphatic drainage, surface tissues
    Pressure level—2 or 3
    Drag—2
    Speed—Slow
    Duration—Varies; moderate to long
Lymphatic drainage, deep tissues
    Pressure level—4 or 5
    Drag—2
    Speed—Slow
    Duration—Short
Myofascial release, superficial fascia
    Pressure level—3
    Drag—3
    Speed—Slow
    Duration (specific application)—Moderate to long
General relaxation (inhibition of sympathetic arousal)
    Pressure level—4 or 5
    Drag—2
    Speed—Slow
    Duration—Long
Trigger point therapy
    Pressure level—4 to 6, depending on location
    Drag—0
    Speed—Not a factor
    Duration (specific application)—Moderate
Scar tissue surface (mature scar)
    Pressure level—2 or 3
    Drag—2 or 3
    Speed—Slow
    Duration (specific application)—Moderate
Adhesion of muscle layers
    Pressure level—4 to 6
    Drag—3
    Speed—Slow
    Duration (specific application)—Short to moderate
Arterial support
    Pressure level—4 or 5
    Drag—0
    Speed—Moderate to fast over arteries
    Duration (specific application)—Short to moderate
    Duration (entire session)—Short to moderate
Support for venous return
    Pressure level—3 or 4
    Drag—1
    Speed—Slow
    Duration (specific application)—Moderate
    Duration (entire session)—Short to moderate
Client who takes anticoagulants
    Pressure level—1 or 2
    Drag—0 to start; monitor results
Fragile bone (osteoporosis)
    Pressure level—1 to 3
    Drag—0 to 3
Stimulation of sympathetic autonomic nervous system tone
    Pressure level—2 to 5

Drag—0 to 1
Speed—Moderate to fast
Duration—Short to moderate

ADDITIONAL CONSIDERATIONS IN BODY MECHANICS

Care of the Practitioner

Attention to body mechanics begins before the massage even takes place. The practitioner's body should be warmed up with general aerobic activity and stretching. Massage professionals need to be comfortable and should dress in loose, unrestrictive clothing that does not interfere with movement.

They should take a short break after each massage, using the time to stretch all the muscles involved in giving a massage. Besides getting a professional massage weekly, the practitioner should massage his or her own hands, arms, and shoulders during the day. The Evolve Web site includes a PowerPoint presentation on how to perform self-massage.

Massage Table

The massage table must be kept at a comfortable height, which depends on the practitioner's body size, the size of the client (thick or thin), and style of massage applied. An individual with long arms may need a shorter table than a person with short arms. A person with a short torso, short arms, and long legs often needs a taller table (Figure 7-18).

FIGURE 7-18 Table height. **A,** Measure height of practitioner with a cord. **B,** Fold cord in half to identify table height. **C,** Measure table. **D,** Table is too short.

FIGURE 7-18, cont'd E, Raise the table for better body mechanics. **F,** Efficient body mechanics with table at appropriate height. **G,** Table too tall. **H,** Lower table to proper height—much better. **I,** Correct table height supports efficient body mechanics.

As a general rule, the table height should be one half the practitioner's height. Therefore, if the practitioner is 5 feet, 6 inches tall (66 inches), the table should be approximately 33 inches high. Then, depending on torso, arm, and leg ratios, the correct height for the table will be 2 to 3 inches higher or lower. The best thing a practitioner can do is experiment to find what feels best. For example, if the practitioner has a tendency to bend and curl at the waist when giving a massage, the table may be too short, and raising the table will help. Each practitioner must experiment to find the most comfortable table height.

A table 24 to 28 inches wide provides adequate space for the client to lie down comfortably, but it is not so wide that the practitioner must reach for the client in the middle of the table.

Massage professionals who carry a portable table must pay attention to the body mechanics used to lift and move the table. The table should be lifted using the knees and hips, not the waist. A table that is 28 inches wide is easier to transport than one that is 30 inches wide. The extra 2 inches of lift needed to clear the ground requires additional effort, espe-

cially if the practitioner is short. Some massage table manufacturers have developed shoulder straps, wheel bases, and other devices to aid the transport of tables. These aids help redistribute the weight load. If a table is carried into a location with the left arm, it should be carried out with the right arm, because consistently carrying the table on only one side of the body may be harmful.

Floor Mats

If the massage professional chooses to work on a mat on the floor, the same body mechanics principles apply. The weight-bearing balance points on the floor are then from the knees instead of the feet (Figure 7-19).

Seated Massage

Massage provided with the client in a seated position uses similar principles of body mechanics. Compression is the primary method. It is important to remember that compressive force is applied 90 degrees to client tissues.

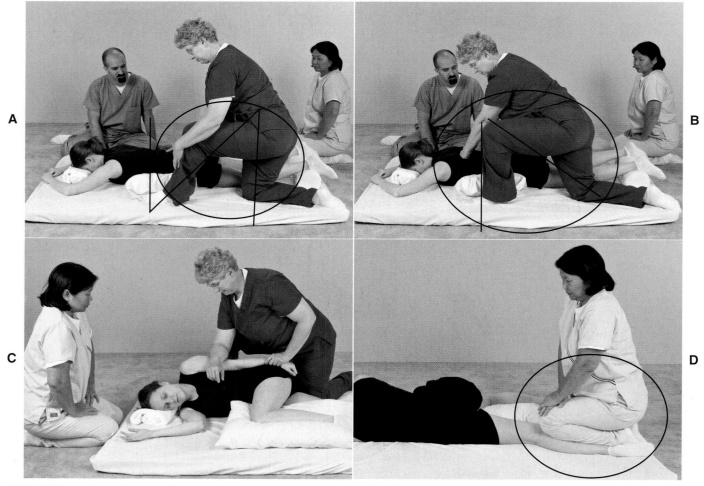

FIGURE 7-19 Body mechanics on the mat. **A,** Basic position. **B,** Correct weight transfer. **C,** Arm massage using correct body motions. **D,** Apply pressure using leg.

Specially designed massage chairs help with positioning the client so that compression can be correctly applied. Variations are necessary to access the arms, legs, and feet, including grasping tissue. Figure 7-20 provides body mechanics suggestions for complete chair-based massage.

BODY MECHANICS WHILE GIVING A MASSAGE

The following general rules apply to body mechanics.

1. The practitioner's body must be in good alignment, with the feet placed apart for support. The arm generating the downward pressure is opposite the back, weight-bearing leg.

2. The practitioner's body weight is kept on the back leg and foot, concentrated at the heel, with the client's body in front of the practitioner. This position provides adequate leverage. Putting weight on the front leg and placing the client's body directly under the pressure results in no leverage; therefore all pressure results from pushing with the upper body muscles instead of using body weight. The front, non-weight-bearing leg is used to modulate pressure levels and provide some stability. The massage practitioner should be able to lift the front leg off the floor and still

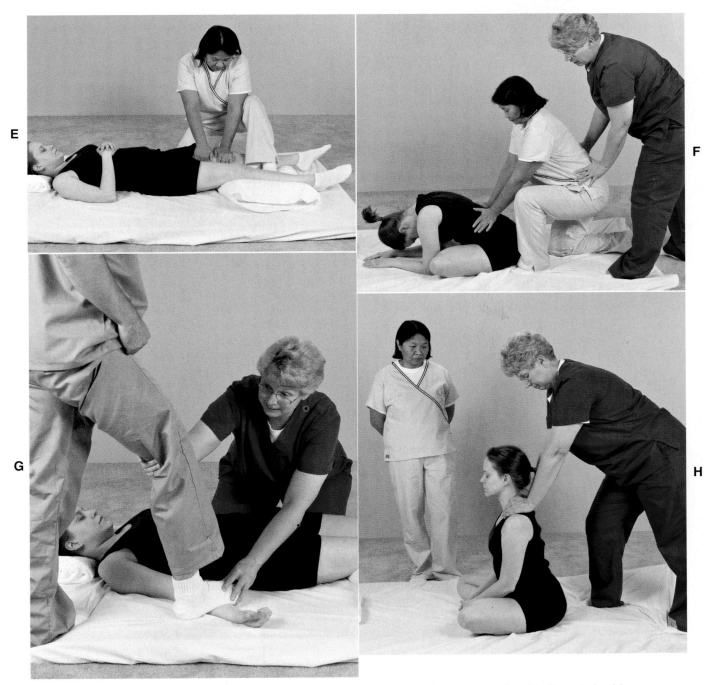

FIGURE 7-19, cont'd E, Kneading. **F,** Maintain straight back. **G,** Correct foot compression. **H,** Correct shoulder compression.

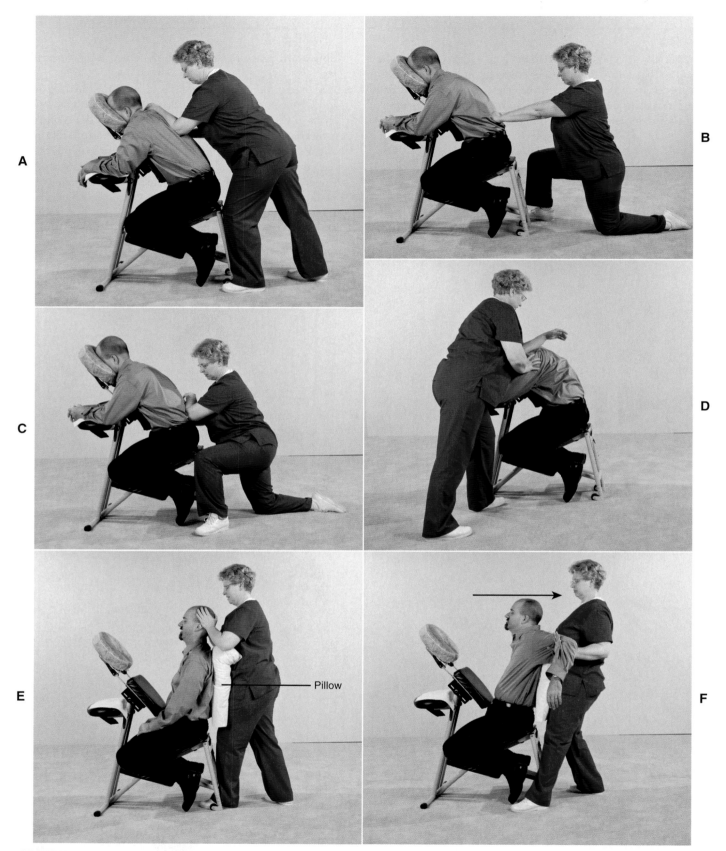

FIGURE 7-20 Body mechanics for chair massage. **A,** Forearm compression, standing. **B,** Fist compression, kneeling. **C,** Forearm position, kneeling. **D,** Forearm compression, shoulder. **E,** Position client against pillow. **F,** Stretch, lean back.

Pillow

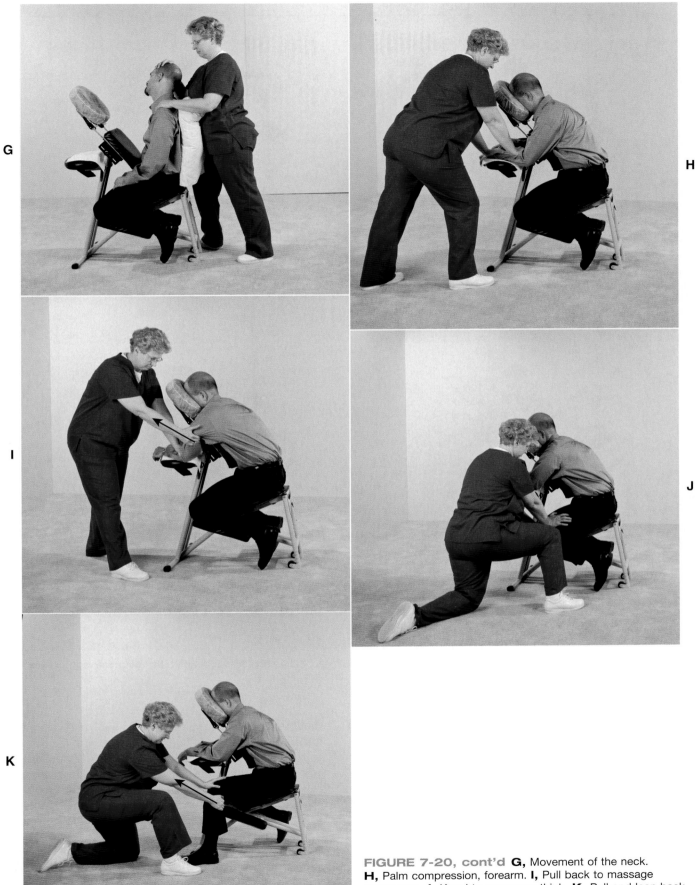

FIGURE 7-20, cont'd G, Movement of the neck.
H, Palm compression, forearm. **I,** Pull back to massage
upper arm. **J,** Kneel to compress thigh. **K,** Pull and lean back
to massage calf.

FIGURE 7-21 Body mechanics for chair/seated massage. **A,** Feet should be shoulder width apart. **B,** Bring one foot forward halfway between client and the other foot. **C,** Lean. **D,** Put weight on back foot/heel.

maintain a stable balance point at the client-practitioner contact point. It is important that the practitioner use body weight. Although muscle strength is not a big factor, leverage is essential.

3. It is important to stay behind the stroke. The practitioner should be able to look down the arm at a 45- to 60-degree angle and see the hand at the point of contact with the client. If the angle is 90 degrees, the practitioner is on top of the stroke, muscle tension in the arm will result, and the massage practitioner has a tendency to push to apply pressure.

4. The wrists and hands must always be relaxed. Tension in this area transfers to the shoulder and may develop into

shoulder and neck problems. When applying a massage manipulation, the practitioner should be sure the deltoid and shoulder muscles remain soft and the wrists and hands stay relaxed. When the practitioner is working with the hands, the elbow must remain straight. If the elbow is allowed to bend, pressure is unevenly distributed to the wrist and there is a tendency to curl or bend at the waist, straining the low back.

5. Use of the fingers and thumbs should be avoided. These joints are not built for compressive forces, and the saddle joint of the thumb cannot be easily stabilized.

Most massage methods are performed using the whole hand or forearm. Creative use of the forearm and palm is

FIGURE 7-21, cont'd **E,** Front foot is non-weight bearing. **F,** Kneel; use knee pads if necessary. **G,** Maintain core stability. **H,** Incorrect stance.

Continued

important. Grasping manipulations, such as kneading, are stressful on the hands. Massage should not be applied with the individual fingers. Instead, the fingers are used as a unit and closed against the pad of the thumb. The position is similar to that of a lobster claw. Massage is provided with the palms. Direct pressure is best applied with the forearm, except in small areas where using the forearm is not feasible. In these areas the stacked finger with hinge joints is preferable to the thumb with a saddle joint. When the forearm is used, the other hand is placed near the contact point to assess the tissue and the client's response. The ulnar nerve can be damaged by use of the triceps portion of the arm. Do not use the point of the elbow; the fleshy portion of the forearm

nearest the ulna below the elbow is the best part to use for massage.

The practitioner follows the natural contours (hills and valleys) of the body and uses various methods of positioning of the client's body. This allows the practitioner to lean "uphill" to provide pressure.

The stroke should be kept at a 45- to 60-degree angle in front of the practitioner and at a 90-degree contact with the client's body. An equilateral triangle is formed by the hip, shoulder, and client contact point. Reaching farther may cause low back strain and shifting of the weight to the front foot; this requires the use of upper body strength to apply pressure, which pins the client to the table. The shoulder angle should

FIGURE 7-21, cont'd I, Incorrect stance. **J,** Improved body mechanics, but there is still a problem with shoulder position. **K,** Kneel to apply compression at lower back and maintain elbow stability.

be fixed in the 45- to 60-degree range and not moved. Forward movement is accomplished by shifting the entire body forward in a smooth forward lean of the body. As soon as the angle increases beyond 60 degrees, the weight tends to shift from the back foot to the front foot and the pressure begins to poke the client. If this happens, the practitioner should step forward without moving closer to the table and then redistribute weight bearing to the back leg.

Hyperextension of the wrists or knees can cause damage. The weight-bearing knee moves into the normal knee-lock position; this is not hyperextension. The wrist angle must never be less than 110 degrees to avoid compression of the nerves in the wrist.

The practitioner should face the area being worked on, with his or her navel and back weight-bearing foot pointed at the area being massaged and toward the "slope of the hill" of the body contours that are being leaned against. The shoulder and pelvic girdle should be in alignment, and the head should be up. When the direction of movement is changed, the body must be turned, including both feet, and the weight shifted to the back foot.

If kneading, the practitioner should grasp and rock back to lift the tissue. A rhythm of rocking should be developed by moving forward as the tissue is grasped and back as the tissue is kneaded and pulled as previously explained.

Counterpressure

The practitioner should not push, even if intense pressure is required. Instead, the practitioner should lean on the area of the client's body that requires the intense pressure and then, using the nonworking hand, lift the body area back into the practitioner's compressive force. By shifting the weight on the feet as the practitioner grasps the client's body, the client is automatically lifted into the practitioner (Figure 7-22). No set pattern or particular point to grasp has been established; anything available and comfortable for the client can be used. The original contact arm pressure increases as the body area is pulled into it, squeezing the pressure forces together. As the pulling arm leans back, the contact arm moves forward into the client. This technique must be monitored by the client for pressure levels. The practitioner can use the table as a source of counterpressure by pulling up on the table edge and leaning into the client's body, squeezing the forces together to increase the intensity of the pressure delivered. Contact must remain broad and must not narrow and poke the client.

Client Rhythm

It is important that massage practitioners allow their bodies to rock and sway with the massage movements. Slow rocking keeps the massage manipulations slow; this is crucial for efficient adaptation or change in the client's muscle tissue or in the consistency of the connective tissue. The resulting rhythmic movement keeps the practitioner's body relaxed and is comforting to the client. Practitioners should remember to work with smooth, even movements, shifting position often.

FIGURE 7-22 Examples of counterpressure.

Body Mechanics During Range-of-Motion, Lengthening, and Stretching Methods

The same principles apply to stretching methods used during massage. Range of motion is more often restricted by faulty physiologic signals than by an anatomic barrier. The protective proprioceptive mechanism sets up this physiologic barrier. Pushing or pulling the stretches or range-of-motion movements can bypass this physiologic barrier, thereby fully activating the protective neuromuscular mechanism, and spasms may result. Slowly leaning while performing the lengthening and stretching movements automatically accesses the physiologic barrier. The practitioner then can feel the subtle push back as the stretch reflex response signals that the muscles have been lengthened or stretched enough.

■ ■ ■   SUMMARY

The massage professional's body is a vital, irreplaceable tool. It is crucial that massage professionals use caution while giving a massage. If the practitioner is uncomfortable, the client will become uncomfortable. If the practitioner can give a massage in a relaxed, efficient, and energy-conserving manner, the client will be able to relax and more easily accept the touch. Students should practice over and over until they develop graceful, efficient body mechanics.

PROFICIENCY EXERCISE 7-1

1. Practice leaning on a wall the correct way and the incorrect way. Feel the difference.
2. Videotape yourself giving a massage. Do you look graceful and relaxed, or are you working too hard?
3. Experiment with different positions with the client so that you can effectively "lean."
4. Tie one end of a short rope around your waist and the other end around your wrist. The length of the rope should allow you to reach out at a 45- to 60-degree angle. Perform a massage. The rope will prevent you from reaching too far with the stroke and will tug at the waist when it is time to shift the body by taking a step forward.
5. Practice with a standing partner. Lean on your partner as you would lean on a wall. Pay attention to how you feel as your "wall" slightly changes position by moving forward, backward, or twisting. If your partner cannot easily move you with subtle body shifts, you are stabilizing your body and pushing.
6. Have your partner lie on the table and repeat the exercise in no. 5.
7. Practice using your hand as a unit and grasping objects with the palm of your hand. Make sure not to pinch during the grasping movement.
8. Practice a massage using all the positions illustrated and explained in this chapter.

evolve

7-1 Take a true/false quiz on proper and improper body mechanics.

7-2 Learning exercise: Identify correct and incorrect body mechanics by viewing several more photos.

Don't forget to study for your certification and licensure exams! Review questions for this chapter are located on Evolve.

REFERENCES

1. Birnbaum JS: *The musculoskeletal manual,* ed 3, Philadelphia, 1982, Academic Press.
2. Norkin CC, Levangie PK: *Joint structure and function: a comprehensive analysis,* ed 2, Philadelphia, 2005, FA Davis.
3. Smith LK, Weiss E, Lemkuhl LD: *Brunnstrom's clinical kinesiology,* ed 5, Philadelphia, 1996, FA Davis.
4. Kreighbaum E, Barthels KM: *Biomechanics: a qualitative approach for studying human movement,* ed 4, New York, 1995, Macmillan.

Workbook Section

Answers for the Workbook Section for Chapter 7 are provided on p. 765.

■ ■ ■ SHORT ANSWER

1. How do practitioners maintain good body mechanics?

_____

_____

_____

2. How can massage professionals protect their necks and shoulders?

_____

_____

_____

3. How can massage professionals protect their wrists?

_____

_____

_____

4. How can massage professionals protect their thumbs and fingers?

_____

_____

_____

5. How can massage professionals protect their lower backs?

_____

_____

_____

6. How can massage professionals protect their knees?

_____

_____

_____

7. How can massage professionals protect their ankles and feet while giving a massage?

_____

_____

_____

8. What is asymmetric standing, and why should it be used instead of symmetric standing?

_____

_____

_____

9. What are the basic principles of body mechanics?

_____

_____

_____

10. Where is the balance point during a massage?

_____

_____

_____

11. What premassage preparations are important to support good body mechanics?

_____

_____

_____

12. What are the general rules for body mechanics?

_____

_____

_____

13. How do the general principles of body mechanics apply to stretching?

_____

_____

_____

Workbook Section—cont'd

■ ■ ■ ASSESS YOUR COMPETENCIES

Now that you have studied this chapter, you should be able to:

1. Use the body, especially the hands and forearms, in an efficient and biomechanically correct manner when giving a massage.

2. Alter the position of both the client and the practitioner to maximize body mechanics.

On a separate sheet of paper, write a short summary of the content of this chapter based on the competencies listed above. When writing this paper assume you are speaking to someone—a client, prospective employer, co-worker, or other interested person. Write the paper as if you were having a conversation and explaining the importance of the information and skills to professional massage development.

Next, in small student discussion groups, share the papers and compare and contrast how the information was presented. Discuss the content, looking for similarities, differences, potential misunderstanding of the information, and clear and concise methods of description.

■ ■ ■ PROBLEM-SOLVING ACTIVITIES

1. A female massage practitioner has been doing massage for 4 years. She tends to provide deep pressure with her forearms and the point of her elbow and works very hard to sustain the pressure throughout the massage. In the past 6 months she has developed shoulder pain with numbness and tingling. What might be problematic about her body mechanics and what corrective action could be taken?

_____

_____

_____

_____

2. A male massage professional is experiencing tenderness in his wrist on the ulnar side. He has long arms and prefers a tall table. He tends to use the palms of his hands for most of his work because of concern about applying too much pressure with his forearm. What might be problematic about his body mechanics, and what corrective action could be taken?

_____

_____

_____

_____

3. A female massage practitioner with 10 years of experience has been aware of right knee pain over the past 2 years. She learned to keep her knees flexed as part of her initial training. She tends to rotate her right leg externally, so she often does not line up her body so that her right foot is directed toward her application of pressure. What might be problematic about her body mechanics, and what corrective action could be taken?

_____

_____

_____

_____

4. A female massage professional has recently developed low back pain. She tends to keep her weight on the front foot or evenly distributed between both feet in a symmetric stance. She has long legs, a short torso, and very short arms. A year ago she was advised to work at a taller table, but she never made this adjustment. What might be problematic about her body mechanics, and what corrective action could be taken?

_____

_____

_____

_____

5. A male massage practitioner with 2 years of experience is exhausted after giving five 1-hour massage sessions. He needs to be able to increase his client base by one massage per day but does not know whether his energy can hold out. He feels that he has good body mechanics. He usually stands and provides a variety of massages, but his specialty is a vigorous massage with a lot of pétrissage and frictioning methods. He tends to adjust his position instead of altering the client's position to his advantage. What might be problematic about his body mechanics, and what corrective action could be taken?

_____

_____

_____

_____

Preparation for Massage:
Equipment, Supplies, Professional Environment, Positioning, and Draping

CHAPTER OBJECTIVES

After completing this chapter, the student will be able to perform the following:

- Construct a massage setting in different types of environments
- List the equipment, supplies, and setup procedures required to prepare for a massage session
- Explain massage procedures to a client
- Effectively drape and position a client

CHAPTER OUTLINE

EQUIPMENT
    Care of the Massage Practitioner's Hands and Body
    The Massage Table
    The Massage Chair
    The Massage Mat
    Body Supports
    Draping Materials
    Lubricants
    Additional Equipment
THE MASSAGE ENVIRONMENT
    General Conditions
    A Typical Massage Room, Home Office, or Clinical Setting
DETERMINING A NEW CLIENT'S EXPECTATIONS
FEEDBACK
    Client Feedback
    Practitioner Feedback
    Client Conversation
GENDER CONCERNS
PREMASSAGE PROCEDURES
    Orientation Process
    Focus/Centering
POSITIONING AND DRAPING THE CLIENT
    Positioning
    Draping

AFTER THE MASSAGE
    Helping the Client off the Massage Table
    Closing the Session, Collecting the Fee, and Making the Next Appointment
SUMMARY

KEY TERMS

Body supports
Draping
Draping material
Feedback
Focus/centering
Lubricants
Massage chair
Massage mat
Massage table
Positioning

The massage practitioner must make certain preparations before beginning the massage. The room must be set up, and all necessary supplies must be gathered. The type of lubricant used and how it is dispensed, the temperature of the massage room, and the warmth of the practitioner's hands are all considerations. Massage professionals benefit from developing a method, referred to as *centering*, to help them focus on the client and the session to come. Client positioning and modest, appropriate draping procedures also must be considered. The practitioner then uses history taking and assessment procedures to identify client outcomes and to formulate the approach for the massage. The plan is discussed with the client, and informed consent is obtained. All this is done before the massage begins. This chapter is designed to help the student develop these important premassage

249

procedures, which support the massage relationship and professional environment first discussed in Chapter 2.

EQUIPMENT

SECTION OBJECTIVES

Using the information presented in this section, the student will be able to perform the following:

- Care for and protect his or her hands, arms, and general health
- Make informed decisions about the purchase of a massage table, chair, mat, body supports, draping materials, and lubricants
- Make the most effective use of massage equipment

Care of the Massage Practitioner's Hands and Body

For massage professionals, their most important pieces of equipment are their hands, arms, and body. They should make sure to protect their hands from abrasion and damage by wearing gloves when doing outdoor chores or other work in which the hands may be injured. Using the forearms during a massage protects and limits use of the hands. In some circumstances the knees and feet are used for certain massage techniques. The massage practitioner has a professional responsibility always to be attentive to efficient and proper body mechanics (as presented in Chapter 7) and the maintenance of personal health.

The Massage Table

The next piece of equipment to consider is a surface on which the client may sit or lie while receiving the massage. The first choice of most practitioners for this purpose is a **massage table**. The table must be sturdy and properly assembled so that there is no chance of it collapsing while a client is lying on it. The two primary types of massage tables are the portable table, which folds into a smaller unit and can be carried easily from place to place (Box 8-1), and the stationary table, which remains in one location.

Most manufacturers offer a basic model, and many have tables with all sorts of features, such as automatic height and tilt adjustments, arm supports, and face cradles. The more features, the more expensive the table.

Almost all portable tables are built with a hinge in the middle that allows them to fold in half for ease of carrying (Figure 8-1). This hinged area is a weak spot in the table, and cable supports on the legs counterbalance this weakness. Most tables are strong and can hold about 300 pounds if the weight is distributed evenly over the entire surface of the table. Problems occur when the client sits in the middle of the table when lying down or sitting up, which focuses all the weight in one spot. With cumulative use the hinge weakens. It is important to check the cable tension consistently to ensure that no sag develops. Otherwise, the table may buckle, injuring the client and damaging the table. Adjustable legs allow the massage table to be lowered or raised to accommodate the various body builds of clients while allowing the practitioner to use proper body mechanics.

BOX 8-1

Features of a Portable Massage Table

A portable massage table is the most versatile type of massage table. At minimum, it should have the following features:

- Sturdy construction, including cable support on the legs
- Manual height adjustment
- A face cradle
- A washable covering (usually vinyl) that also can be cleaned with disinfectant
- Adequate padding to ensure comfort and firm support
- A width of 24 to 28 inches (most tables are about 6 feet long); tables narrower than 24 inches are too narrow for the client's comfort. 28 inches appears to be most suitable for a majority of situations. Tables wider than 30 inches are difficult to carry and ergonomically inefficient.

FIGURE 8-1 A generic portable massage table with center hinge, support cables, and face cradle.

Stationary tables do not have the instability problem because the table is heavier; cross-bracing and leg supports make the table even safer. However, the lack of portability is a major drawback if the massage practice involves any on site work (Figure 8-2).

Ideally a massage professional should have both a stationary table and a portable one. A stationary table can easily be built at home by an average carpenter at a reasonable cost. A portable table, however, should be purchased from an experienced manufacturer. Buying a product that has been tested for safety is worth the investment. All massage tables must be checked daily for structural stability. It is important to perform a complete maintenance check on all connectors, bolts, cables, and hinges every week and to repair any defects immediately.

Many clients may be concerned about the sturdiness of the table. The lightweight, portable tables may look weak, but a quality table is well built and strong. Before the massage, demonstrate the stability of the table to the client or offer alternatives, such as a chair or massage mat.

FIGURE 8-2 A generic stationary massage table.

Support bar

Face cradle

Chest support

Arm rest

Seat

Leg supports

FIGURE 8-3 A generic massage chair.

The Massage Chair

Instead of a massage table, equipment designed for a seated massage can be used. A special massage chair can be purchased for this purpose, and these chairs are a worthwhile investment (Figure 8-3). The sit-down massage, often referred to as an on site or corporate massage, usually takes place in a public setting (e.g., business location) and is done over clothing. Massage chairs also are excellent for working with clients who are more comfortable sitting upright, such as a woman in the last trimester of pregnancy or a person who has difficulty getting on and off a massage table (Box 8-2).

A straight-backed chair with no arms also can be used. The client sits facing the back of the chair and leans on the chair back, supported by pillows. A stool or chair pushed up to a table or desk is another option. The client leans forward on a

BOX 8-2

Advantages and Disadvantages of a Massage Chair

Advantages
1. Massage chairs, which are specially designed for that purpose, usually are very comfortable and easy to use.
2. Professionally manufactured equipment adds to the professional atmosphere of the massage setting and ensures safety through quality workmanship in construction and design.
3. Professionally manufactured massage chairs are lightweight and portable.
4. Clients with certain respiratory, vascular, and cardiac conditions are best given a massage in a seated position.

Disadvantages
1. Some people have difficulty getting into and out of the semikneeling position required to use the massage chair.
2. Access to certain body areas is limited.

supporting pillow placed on the table. Special triangular or block-shaped foam forms can be purchased to provide support. A professionally manufactured desktop support, which could replace the pillows, also is available (Figure 8-4).

The Massage Mat

A mat on the floor is used for some methods of massage (Box 8-3). The massage mat can be a futon or an exercise mat, but it must be protected by a sanitary covering (Figure 8-5).

Body Supports

Body supports are used to bolster the body during the massage and give contour to the flat working surface (Figure 8-6).

Commercial body support products are available that consist of various shapes and sizes of pillows and foam forms. As an alternative, the practitioner can buy assorted shapes and densities of hypoallergenic foam and make covers for them. A wedge, a round tube, and two or three square or oblong pieces will be needed, each with a different depth and density. Additional supports are needed for working with pregnant women (Proficiency Exercise 8-1).

Draping Materials

Opaque draping material is used to provide the client with privacy and warmth. Standard bed linens are the coverings most commonly used because they are large enough to cover the entire body and are easily used for most draping procedures. Both full and twin-size sheets fit nicely on most massage tables. The practitioner can either buy these linens and launder them in a sanitary fashion or use a linen service. Sheets made of cotton or cotton blends are the best choice because they do not slip on the client. Cotton flannel sheets are nice because

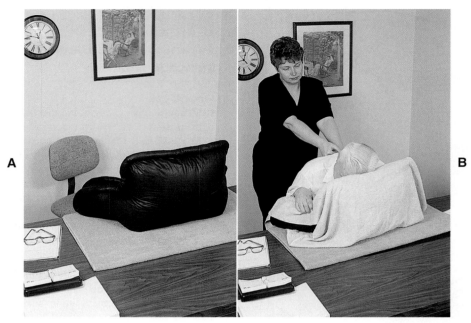

FIGURE 8-4 A, Use of a support pillow to provide massage in an office chair and at a desk. **B,** Positioning of the client for massage.

BOX 8-3

Key Features, Advantages, and Disadvantages of a Massage Mat

Key Features
1. The mat should be soft enough and provide sufficient support to ensure the client's comfort.
2. It should be large enough to allow the massage practitioner to move around the client's body while staying on the cushioned surface, thereby protecting his or her own knees and body.
3. The mat should be made so that it can be covered with a sanitary covering.

Advantages
1. A mat often is less expensive than a massage table.
2. A mat may be lighter and therefore easier to carry than a massage table.
3. Mats are particularly safe (i.e., there is little chance of a client falling off).
4. A mat is a popular choice when working with infants and children.

5. Mats are portable.
6. Because a mat is so safe and comfortable, it may be the best choice for working with clients who have certain physical disabilities; a transfer from a wheelchair to a mat may be accomplished more easily.

Disadvantages
1. Proper training is needed to work effectively on the floor; many massage practitioners are not familiar with this kind of work.
2. The floor may be drafty or colder for the client.
3. Physically challenged or elderly clients may have difficulty getting down on or up from the floor.
4. Mats do not have face cradles to maintain alignment of the neck in the prone position.

---

they feel warm to the skin. Whatever linen is used, it must be able to withstand being washed in bleach or other disinfecting solution (Figure 8-7).

Large towels may be used for draping because they are both warm and opaque. They must be at least the size of a beach towel and have a soft texture. Be sensitive to the client's comfort and provide a choice of towels or sheets. Because towels are smaller, a client may feel more exposed and may prefer the security offered by a sheet. As an alternative, both sheets and towels can be used, with a bath-size towel used as a chest covering.

Disposable linen also is available. Some higher-quality disposable products may look and feel like a cotton fabric, but they do not provide the same warmth. Disposable linens are convenient and sanitary, but they cannot be washed or recycled.

Draping Material Recommendations

Either a twin fitted sheet or a flat sheet should be put over the vinyl table top to protect the table. Laundering this additional sheet is much less expensive than replacing the covering on the table. A full or twin flat sheet then is placed over the

FIGURE 8-5 A generic massage mat covered with a sheet.

FIGURE 8-6 Various sizes and shapes of body supports.

protective covering. The top sheet can be either a full or a twin sheet. Twin sheets fit a bit better on the table but can be somewhat skimpy for draping. Full sheets provide more material, which facilitates draping, but can be cumbersome. Also, for sanitary purposes, care must be taken that sheets do not drag on the floor. Face cradles should be draped with a hand towel, a pillowcase, or an additional piece of fabric sewn just to fit the face cradle. All body supports and pillows are covered with pillowcases.

In addition to the sheets and pillowcases, a bath-size towel is used for various draping procedures. A large beach-size towel, a flannel sheet, or a light blanket should be available in case the client becomes chilled.

It is helpful to have different colors of sheets and towels for each set of drapery material, because if all are the same color, distinguishing between the top and bottom sheets can be difficult. For example, the protective fitted sheet may be white; the bottom flat sheet, blue; the top flat sheet, green; and the towel and pillowcase, yellow. The blanket or flannel sheet for additional warmth could be a printed material.

PROFICIENCY EXERCISE 8-1

1. *Collect information from at least three manufacturers of massage tables and massage chairs. Compare the cost, quality, and construction of the equipment.*
2. *Research a variety of styles of body supports for clients with specific needs.*
3. *Locate a source for foam (an upholstery or a mattress company is a good start). See how many different body supports you can build from foam scraps.*

FIGURE 8-7 A, Bolsters and draping material. *1,* Sanitizing wipes. *2,* Disposable face cover. *3,* Bolsters and pillows—various sizes and shapes. *4,* Sheets, pillowcases, blankets. *5,* Rolling carry bag. **B,** Additional material. *1,* Disposable face cover. *2,* Bottom sheet. *3,* Fitted sheet. *4,* Top sheet. *5,* Neck roll (rolled towel). *6,* Pillow for placement underneath abdomen or knees. *7,* Mat sheet. *8,* Ankle support. *9,* Bolster (knee or abdomen). *10,* Ankle bolster. *11,* Blanket. *12,* Various lubricants and hand sanitizers. *13,* Top sheet.

The draping material required for one client includes the following:

1 twin fitted sheet (table protector)
2 full or twin flat sheets (bottom and top drapes)
1 pillowcase or hand towel (face cradle)
Additional pillowcases (body supports)
1 bath-size towel
1 flannel sheet, light blanket, or beach-size towel (which is easiest to launder) for warmth

When possible, soft pastel colors should be chosen for draping materials because they withstand bleaching, are more opaque than white linens, and tend not to show lubricant stains. Some people are allergic to cotton blends, which may irritate their skin. If the client has sensitive skin, the practitioner should use white, pure cotton sheets to reduce the risk of a reaction.

At least 10 full sets of draping material are needed; this is sufficient for 2 standard business days, with laundry done every other day. If you use a laundry service, order enough linen for 10 days to make sure you do not run out of linens if delivery is late. Whenever linens come in contact with the client, they must be laundered in an approved fashion before they are reused. Most linens must be replaced every 1 to 2 years if used often. Lubricants build up, and bleach wears out the fabric (Proficiency Exercise 8-2).

Lubricants

Lubricants serve only one purpose for the massage practitioner: they reduce drag on the skin during gliding-type massage strokes. Medicinal and cosmetic use of lubricants is out of the scope of practice for therapeutic massage.

Scented Lubricants

Because headaches and other allergic responses to lubricants often are caused by the volatile oils in scented products, scented lubricants should not be used. This recommendation does not discount the therapeutic benefit of aromatherapy; the sense of smell is a very powerful sensory mechanism, and many emotional and physiologic processes can be triggered by deliberate use of aroma. However, this textbook does not cover all these applications, and additional education is required to use aromas specifically, purposefully, and therapeutically. Until you receive this training, do not use them. (A short discussion of the use of essential oils is included in Chapter 11.)

FIGURE 8-8 Massage lubricants.

Lubricant Types

Oils and creams can be vegetable, mineral, or petroleum based, and powders can be talc or cornstarch based (Figure 8-8). If possible, use the most natural products available and avoid using petrochemicals and talc, because many people are allergic to these substances. All lubricants must be dispensed from a contamination-free container.

The lubricant traditionally used for massage is oil. It is easy to dispense from a squeeze bottle and can be kept free of contamination. However, natural vegetable oils can become rancid quickly, and some commercial products use additives that may cause allergic reactions in clients. In addition, oils are messy, they can spill and drip, and they stain linens (although specialized laundry products are available for removing oil stains).

Massage creams must be dispensed in a contamination-proof manner. Some creams are thin enough to be kept in a squeeze bottle. Others are thick, and the amount to be used must be removed in a sanitary fashion before the massage. Various processing methods have produced many natural vegetable oil–based massage creams and lotions that do not feel greasy. Some products are water based, and these wash out of linens without leaving stains.

Powders are used when creams and oils are undesirable, usually because of skin conditions (e.g., acne) or excessive body hair. Do not inhale the dust from powders, because this could cause respiratory problems. Powders with a cornstarch base are preferable because they pose less of a risk of respiratory irritation. If the client and practitioner are in agreement, disposable masks can be used to reduce the risk of respiratory irritation even further.

Using Massage Lubricants

Only a small amount of lubricant is needed for a massage. Remember that the reason for using lubricant is to reduce drag on the skin from the massage movements. More lubricant is required to work over body hair. In some cases powder

▥ PROFICIENCY EXERCISE 8-2

1. *Obtain a set of sheets, some towels, and some disposable linen. Practice draping methods with them. Which type of material did you prefer to use?*
2. *Have another student or a massage practitioner give you a massage using the different draping materials. Which type did you prefer to have used on you?*

may be a better choice. Sometimes the use of any type of lubricant is contraindicated, therefore it is important to be able to perform massage without a lubricant.

In Chapter 9 you will learn about different massage manipulations. The long, gliding methods are best for applying lubricant. Keep the application even and very thin. It is easy to apply more but difficult to remove excess. Keep a clean towel available in case removal is necessary.

Do not pour the lubricant directly onto the client. It first is warmed in the practitioner's palms by rubbing the hands together. Apply the lubricant to one area at a time rather than to the entire body. Do not use lubricant on the face or hair, because it disturbs makeup and hairstyles. For sanitary reasons the practitioner's hands must be washed and dried before working in the area of the face. Some practitioners begin the massage with the face and head, before using any lubricant.

Some clients may appreciate having the lubricant removed after the massage. An alcohol-based product can do this, but alcohol is drying to the skin. Rubbing the skin with an absorbent towel removes most of the lubricant.

Additional Equipment

Other aids to a massage, besides a massage table, draping material, supports, and lubricants, might include disposable tissues, a clock, and music.

Music

Music often is used to distract the client from or to block out surrounding noise. A less recognized use is to achieve interaction and modulation of the autonomic nervous system through entrainment. Simple, soft music with a base beat under 60 beats per minute tends to activate a parasympathetic response, which produces a soothing, relaxing effect. Music faster than 60 beats per minute encourages sympathetic responses, producing a stimulating, invigorating effect.

When using music, the practitioner must consider the effect to be created and whether both the client and the massage practitioner enjoy the music. The best recommendation is that the massage practitioner have available a variety of music from which the client is allowed to choose. An assortment of styles, rhythms, and instruments, as well as equipment to play music, should be available. The volume should be kept low but loud enough so that the music can be heard without straining.

The music itself can be very helpful in pacing the massage, because the massage practitioner can gain a sense of the passage of time without having to look at the clock (Proficiency Exercise 8-3).

THE MASSAGE ENVIRONMENT

SECTION OBJECTIVES

Using the information presented in this section, the student will be able to perform the following:

- Design an efficient therapeutic massage environment
- Organize an office and massage room

PROFICIENCY EXERCISE 8-3

1. *Obtain the three basic types of lubricant: oil, cream, and powder. Give a massage with each type. Which do you prefer to use?*
2. *Find a practice client with a hairy body and practice using the different types of lubricant. Which one was the easiest to use? Which one did the client prefer?*
3. *Have a fellow student give you a massage using all three types of lubricant on different parts of the body. While receiving the massage, compare and decide which type you preferred.*
4. *Practice giving a massage with as little lubricant as possible.*
5. *Assemble a music library consisting of different types of music. Mark each 15-minute segment to assist with timing of the massage.*

Clients return for another massage because they appreciate the quality of the service and a professional personality and environment. Thoroughly plan the image that your massage environment is to convey to the public. To maintain the integrity of the professional relationship, the environment created for the massage setting, including decorations and the reading material provided for clients, should reflect the scope of practice of massage.

When most people think of massage, they picture a quiet, private room with low lighting and soft music. However, therapeutic massage can be provided almost anywhere and under almost any conditions. Successful massage practices have been developed in noisy public locations, such as airports, in a client's home, in the workplace, and outdoors at sporting events or retreats. Whatever the physical location of the massage environment, the most important aspect is to present and deliver the highest standard of professional care to the public.

GENERAL CONDITIONS

General conditions for massage areas that must be considered are the room temperature, the fresh air supply, privacy, and accessibility.

Room Temperature

The air temperature in the massage room should be kept at 72° to 75° F. Massage produces a vasodilative effect, which brings the blood closer to the surface of the body and allows internal heat to escape, cooling the client. It is impossible for clients to relax if they are cold. The massage practitioner is active and fully dressed and can become warm while doing the massage. Some practitioners put an electric blanket on the table to keep clients warm. A piece of lamb's wool may be used because it traps and retains body heat. Placing a hot water bottle or other form of heating device at the client's feet and another at the neck or wherever comfortable may increase body temperature.

The most comfortable massage practitioner's uniform is cotton or a cotton blend to wick away moisture and perspiration from the skin. It should have short sleeves and be loose fitting to help prevent the practitioner from becoming too warm.

Fresh Air and Ventilation

The room should have access to fresh air, but a window that opens to the outside is not always available. Ventilation of some sort is important. A small fan in the room pointed at the ceiling or the wall keeps the air moving without causing a draft on the client.

Privacy

Clients need privacy for removing their clothes in preparation for the massage treatment. If the massage room is separate from other public areas, the client can be left alone to get ready for the massage. Sometimes a screen or curtained area can be used to divide one large room into two distinct areas.

Accessibility

It is important to locate the massage practice so that it is easily accessible to clients with mobility impairments. Barrier-free access and restrooms are required.

Lighting

The massage area must be lit well enough to meet the standards for proper cleaning and safety (see Chapter 6). Bright overhead lighting often is too harsh and glaring for the client. Indirect or natural light from a window is much better. If the massage area has overhead lights, turn them off and use a lamp in the corner of the room instead. A dimmer switch is excellent because it allows adjustment of the lighting. Never work in a dark room, to prevent accidents caused by tripping, and never work by candlelight, because an open flame is a safety hazard.

Scents, Incense, Flowers, and Plants

Massage practitioners work with a variety of people during a day, each one with different ideas about what is pleasant and what is offensive. Many clients are also environmentally sensitive and react to scents, incense, and flowers. The best recommendation is to avoid using such items because the fragrance lingers and can cause problems for a client.

Nonflowering (foliage) plants usually are less of a problem. However, if the practitioner serves an allergic population, the best course may be not to use them. If their use is not a problem, foliage plants are a wonderful natural air purifier that can supply oxygen to the massage areas.

Hygiene, Chemicals, Perfume, and Warm Hands

It is important for the massage professional to attend to personal hygiene and to prevent body odors because people are sensitive to these smells. Avoid heavy use of aftershave, perfume, scented cosmetics, hair spray, or other scented products. Clients usually do not comment on offensive breath or body odors; they simply do not return for further sessions. Because recognizing odors on ourselves can be difficult, ask a family member or friend who will answer truthfully if you have such a problem.

If the massage practitioner is a smoker, the smell of smoke can linger in fabric, carpeting, and furniture and on the practitioner. This can be very distasteful to a nonsmoking client. Because it is difficult to remove the odor, the massage environment should be located in a nonsmoking area. Refraining from smoking during professional hours may help prevent the smell from clinging to the hands, clothes, hair, and breath.

Cold hands are a real problem for many massage practitioners. The hands should be heated with warm water, on a hot water bottle or other warming device, or by rubbing them together before touching the client.

A Typical Massage Room, Home Office, or Clinical Setting

Business and Massage Areas

It is desirable for the massage area to be separate from the business area in the massage setting. People associate behavior with locations and expect certain activities at those locations. It is important that these two activities remain separate in the client's mind. The interaction that takes place when appointments are made and money is taken is very different from the one that takes place during a massage.

The business or reception area should be near the entrance. An appointment book, calendar, forms, receipts, pencils, and telephone, as well as a chair and a small table, should be set up in the business area. Appropriate reading material should be available for clients. The massage area should be located farther from the door or in an adjacent room (Figure 8-9).

Make sure clients have a place to sit and to hang their clothes. Use an enclosed cabinet to store linens and lubricants, and designate a place to keep the body supports. A covered hamper, located away from the massage table, is needed for used linens.

Hand-washing and restroom facilities must be easily accessible. If the massage room has no sink, a liquid hand cleanser must be available. If there is no direct access between the massage room and the restroom, make sure the client uses the facilities before the massage session begins. It also is important to have a plan for getting the client to the restroom during the massage session if necessary. This can get tricky if the only way to the facilities is down a public hall, past offices that share the restroom facilities.

Room Size

The reception and business area can be small, about 8 feet by 8 feet (64 square feet). A room for massage should be at least 10 feet by 10 feet (100 square feet). If the two areas are in the same room, a space at least 12 feet by 12 feet (144 square feet) is needed to provide the necessary working area (Figure 8-10).

The Office at the Practitioner's Home

Designating a professional area in your home is a business option if zoning regulations allow home office businesses (see

Chapter 14). Establishing a professional office in the home involves special considerations. If at all possible, the massage area should have a private entrance (zoning regulations usually require this). Barrier-free access and restrooms are a major consideration in planning a home office. Most homes are not designed with these accommodations.

If pets are in the home, potential clients must be informed in case of allergy or fear of animals. Pets should not be allowed in the business or massage areas. Family members must understand the privacy issue of the massage environment, and massage clients must understand the boundaries of the private home area. This more personal environment requires very careful attention to professional boundaries.

The Public Environment: Event Sports Massage, Demonstration Massage, On Site or Corporate Massage

In the public setting, the massage practitioner goes to the location rather than having the client come to the practitioner's office. These public massage sessions normally last less than 30 minutes and the client remains fully clothed. As the practitioner, you usually have little control over noise, lighting, and other conditions. Clear enough space to set up the massage table or chair. If indoors, try to locate this area in a corner, which gives two walls to provide some privacy.

Regardless of the massage location, it is always important to create both a business area and a massage area. Find a flat surface and use it to set up a portable office from a briefcase or similar carrying case that contains receipts, an appointment book, and handouts such as cards and brochures. Set up the massage area a few steps away.

Although the use of linens and lubricants usually is limited in these circumstances, it is still important to have them available. They should be carried in a closed bag to maintain sanitation. Make provision for hand-washing or hand-cleaning products to maintain hygiene and sanitation.

The Client's Residence (On Site Massage)

On site massage can be provided in the home for many reasons, including service and convenience for the client, especially if the person is housebound. A 60- or 90-minute massage usually is given in these situations. Because the

FIGURE 8-9 An example of the layout of a massage office with separate business office and massage area.

FIGURE 8-10 An example of the layout of a massage office with the business office and massage area in one room.

massage takes place in the client's residence, this is the most difficult environment in which to maintain professionalism and professional boundaries. A professional uniform is especially important in this environment. A portable table most often is used, but a massage chair or mat also is acceptable.

Find a private location for the massage, but avoid the bedroom; opt for a family room or den. If the only room available is a bedroom, try to use the guest room or a child's room rather than the client's bedroom. Make sure it is near an area where hands can be washed. Set up a business area using a briefcase as the office and maintain the professional atmosphere. Do not sit at the kitchen table or in the living room, because the professional role of the massage practitioner may be obscured in these traditional conversation locations.

Linens, body supports, and lubricants are needed. It also may be wise to carry a small fan to keep the air moving and to drown out noise from other areas. Never lock the door, because a locked door invites secrecy and creates an environment in which maintaining professionalism is difficult. Under rare circumstances it could constitute entrapment, or the client could perceive it as a violation of the boundaries of the therapeutic relationship. Carry a sign to hang on the door that says, "Massage in session." If you are going to use music, bring portable equipment. (More information about on site massage practice is provided in Chapter 12.)

Outdoors

Outdoor massage usually is provided at a sports massage event or promotional activity. Some massage professionals also work on ships, on the beach, and at poolside at spas and resorts. Although these are very casual settings, the massage practitioner's behavior must reflect professional and ethical standards. Again, a professional uniform is especially important in these more casual and public environments.

Wind, sun, rain, and insects create special conditions. The wind blows the drapes, but picnic table clips can be used to prevent this. Instructing clients to wear a swimsuit or loose clothing for an over-the-clothing massage also helps. A firm, level location is needed for the table because tables that sink into the sand are dangerous. This can be avoided by putting sample carpet squares and coffee cans under the legs of the massage table. It is important to do massage in the shade to avoid sunburn.

A roof or canopy is helpful in case of rain. If the area is screened in, technically it is not outdoors. True outdoor massage has insects; just blend the brushing away of insects into the massage as best you can. If an area for washing hands is not available, use a special disinfectant hand cleanser. Set up the portable office in an area away from the massage setting (Figure 8-11) (Proficiency Exercise 8-4).

DETERMINING A NEW CLIENT'S EXPECTATIONS

SECTION OBJECTIVE

Using the information presented in this section, the student will be able to perform the following:

- Interview a new client to gain a better understanding of the client's expectations of massage in general and of the outcome for a particular massage session

It is important that massage practitioners carefully explain the limitations of massage to clients, put expectations into perspective, and help define the outcome for the massage. This must be done in the beginning as part of the informed consent procedures, before the massage is started.

An important consideration is how the new client thinks a massage is given. If the client has never had a massage, his expectations will be determined by what he has heard, read, or

---

PROFICIENCY EXERCISE 8-4

1. *Arrange to give a massage in each of the four basic environments. What was different about each experience?*
2. *Put together a briefcase office.*
3. *On separate pieces of paper, design three different setups for a clinical massage environment. Indicate the business and massage areas.*

FIGURE 8-11 A, On site massage in an office setting. **B,** Outdoor sports massage setting involving use of a massage chair.

observed. Because methods and applications of massage vary so much, the client may not expect the style of massage that is offered. The difference between what is expected and what is received may be confusing. The client's answer to a simple question such as, "What do you think a massage is like?" or "Describe for me how a massage is done" gives the massage practitioner an idea of the client's expectations for the session. The massage practitioner should explain the different approaches used so that the client is not on the table wondering why this massage is so different from what he expected.

If a new client has had a massage before from someone else, it is natural to compare the different styles. The massage practitioner must explain the procedures and methods used so that the client understands that massage can be done in many ways. Never discount another massage professional's methods or approach and say that your way is better; this is unethical behavior. The only exception is if the previous massage violated professional ethics, scope of practice, and standards of practice. Explain to the client that massage practitioners do not conduct themselves in a manner that violates professional codes of ethics. The code of ethics example in this textbook or one from a professional organization can be used as a framework for the discussion (see Chapter 2).

The outcome for massage is what the client can anticipate in response to the benefits of the proposed massage plan. Each massage manipulation has an anticipated response (discussed in Chapters 4 and 9). A client can be made aware of these responses and any risks inherent in the proposed massage interventions (see Chapter 5).

Do not confuse expectations with outcome. Consider this example: A new client has never had a massage, but a friend of hers in another city regularly receives therapeutic massage. The client explains that the massage her friend receives is for a chronic headache problem that seems to be related to daily stress and that the massage helps a lot (expectation). When you ask your client why she came for a massage (the outcome), she says that she has no real problems, although sometimes she has headaches just as her friend does. Your client thinks a massage would feel good, and her outcome is a general massage that feels good, not the more specific approach to address headaches.

The client's expectations were based on information from her friend. A first-time client naturally considers this type of information, but the outcome may be very different. If the massage practitioner is not careful to differentiate the two, the massage provided for the client may not meet the client's expectations.

The practitioner can ask a number of questions to help determine a new client's expectations, such as the following:

- How do you want to feel after the massage?
- What do you think massage will do for you?
- What results do you want from the massage?

After determining the client's expectations and the outcome, the practitioner should carefully go over all the client policies and procedures discussed in Chapter 2. Never assume that a client understands the complexities of massage practice. Explain everything in detail in terms the client can understand.

FEEDBACK

SECTION OBJECTIVES

Using the information presented in this section, the student will be able to perform the following:

- Elicit feedback from the client
- Provide the client with appropriate feedback

Feedback is a noninvasive, continual exchange of information between the client and the professional. Feedback is not social conversation. It is common for a client to talk during the massage and appropriate for a massage professional to listen to the client while remaining focused on the massage. Note: It is inappropriate for the professional to engage in social conversation with clients, particularly about their personal lives.

Client Feedback

Whether working with a new client or providing regular massage services to an existing client, encouraging feedback from the client is important. Explain the importance of feedback concerning comfort levels (e.g., warmth, positioning, restroom needs) and the quality of any pain sensations (i.e., "good pain," such as is often experienced with deeper massage methods, and "undesirable pain," which the client may feel if the methods are too aggressive). DVD 1 at the back of this book shows video case studies with pre-massage interviews.

The practitioner benefits from feedback about the effectiveness or ineffectiveness of the various massage methods. Session-to-session reports of progress, postmassage sensations and experiences, and the duration of effects help the practitioner adjust the application of the massage. Feedback from the client about professionalism and the quality of the professional relationship also is valuable.

Some clients may find giving feedback difficult. They may not have enough body awareness to give an accurate report on sensations during the massage or the effectiveness of the methods used. With education from the practitioner, this communication can improve.

It is far more common for clients to have difficulty providing feedback about what they did not enjoy about the massage, methods that were uncomfortable or ineffective, and inappropriate behavior by the practitioner. People generally tend to avoid confrontational situations, or they try not to hurt another's feelings. Both of these behaviors interfere with the client's ability to provide effective feedback to the practitioner. The massage professional is responsible for developing a professional trust relationship that allows the client to feel safe in giving both positive and constructive feedback.

Clients should be told during premassage procedures about the importance of feedback. Explain to the client that all feedback is taken as constructive, that it is not personalized, and that it enhances the service of massage therapy. It is important to ease the client's concerns about the practitioner's possible reaction to "negative feedback." Gentle, open-ended questions before, during, and after the massage encourage feedback. Reminder statements also are helpful.

Questions and reminder statements that could be used before the massage include the following:

- Is there a position in which you are most comfortable?
- Does the temperature of the room feel comfortable?
- I am going to place my forearm on the massage table, and you apply pressure to it at a level you think you would like, and explain how you want the massage to feel.
- Remember to tell me if a method is too deep or painful.
- I would appreciate it if you would indicate when a method seems particularly beneficial or enjoyable.

Questions and reminder statements that might be used during the massage include the following:

- I'll use three different pressure levels on your back; please tell me which you prefer.
- Might there be a more comfortable position for you?
- Are you comfortable with massage in this area?
- Remember that it's OK to tell me if you are uncomfortable.
- Remember to turn over slowly.

Questions and reminder statements to use after the massage include the following:

- What methods were most effective for you today?
- What might I improve on during the next session?
- Remember to evaluate the aftereffects of the massage, and we'll discuss them at the next session.

Instilling the idea of "client as a teacher" is one way to encourage feedback from the client. The client teaches the massage professional about himself or herself and guides the practitioner in providing the best massage for them both. This knowledge and experience accumulate, adding depth to the knowledge base of the massage professional.

Practitioner Feedback

Massage practitioners also provide feedback to their clients. Practitioners must develop communication skills (see Chapter 2) to ensure that the feedback they give is not personalized by the client but rather taken as valuable information to be used.

Forms of feedback that the practitioner can give the client include the following:

- Do you notice that your breathing is beginning to slow a bit as you relax?
- Are you aware that you have a bruise on the back of your calf?
- The muscle tension in your shoulder appears greater than before. Can you think of a logical reason?
- You seem to tense up when I apply pressure to this area.
- I noticed that your skin color improved after the massage.

Client Conversation

New clients often talk quite a bit during the first massage. This usually is the result of nervousness, and in future sessions,

particularly those for relaxation and stress reduction outcomes, the talking diminishes.

Clients commonly talk more during the first 15 minutes of massage as they acclimate to the environment and begin to relax. Some talk during the entire massage; this is appropriate and should be accepted. Many people seek massage not only for the therapeutic physical benefit but also, unconsciously, for the social interaction. The professional respectfully listens to the client and limits conversation to appropriate feedback and necessary verbal exchanges to indicate understanding of what the client is saying.

The following is an example of an appropriate dialog:

Client: "My, it has been a very busy week. My son was in two band competitions. I was only able to attend one. It disturbs me when I miss these events. He placed second and third. I'm very proud of him. Do you remember that last week I told you he might get a scholarship to college for music?"

Practitioner: "Yes, I do remember you speaking of that possibility. If I remember correctly, it was to Mott College, right?"

Client: "Yes. You know, it's hard being a single parent. My work interferes with my ability to be with my son as much as I think is important."

Practitioner (replying with feedback): "Were you aware that your shoulders became more tense just now?"

Client: "Yes, it felt as if you were applying more pressure all of a sudden. Were you?"

Practitioner: "No, I didn't increase the pressure, but your muscles did tense while you were speaking about your lack of time with your son."

Client: "What would you do about this if you were me?"

Practitioner: "I don't have the professional skills to help you with your feelings about your time availability with your son, but I can use some methods to relax your shoulders and teach you some methods to keep them relaxed throughout the week."

Here is the same dialog presented in an inappropriate way (Proficiency Exercise 8-5):

Client: "My, it has been a very busy week. My son was in two band competitions. I was only able to attend one. It disturbs me when I miss these events. He placed second and third. I am very proud of him. Do you remember that last week I told you he might get a scholarship to college for music?"

Practitioner: "Yes, I do remember you speaking of that possibility. If I remember correctly, it was to Mott College, right? My daughter went to Mott College. She had difficulty with the registration procedure, and it took forever to work out the snag. Make sure your son doesn't work with Mrs. Jones. She was very rude."

Client: "Yes, Mott College is correct, but now I wonder if he'll be OK. You know, it's hard being a single parent. My work interferes with my ability to be with my son as much as I think is important."

Practitioner: "I sure do understand, because my sister is a single parent, and she just read a real good book about it. I told her she needs a day away once a month, and so do you. By the way, were you aware that your shoulders became more tense just now?"

Client: "Yes, it felt as if you were applying more pressure all of a sudden. Were you?"

Practitioner: "No, I didn't increase the pressure, but your muscles did tense while you were speaking about the guilt feelings about your lack of time with your son."

Client: "What would you do about this if you were me?"

Practitioner: "Well, a social group or even a support group might help. I think I would talk with my son and see if the situation really bothers him, but you know teenage boys, he probably won't tell you anything. My daughter was so hard to get any information from when she was that age. I can use some methods to relax your shoulders and teach you some methods to keep them relaxed throughout the week, since you seem to get more upset when you think about these issues, and I am sure that this entire situation is a big reason for this muscle tension."

GENDER AND AGE CONCERNS

SECTION OBJECTIVE

Using the information presented in this section, the student will be able to perform the following:

- Recognize differences based on gender in clients' expectations and interpretation of touch

Male and female practitioners may experience some difference in a client's expectations and interpretation of touch. It is important to establish clear boundaries concerning the inappropriateness of sexual interaction and to create a safe, nonsexual professional environment with first-time clients. These boundaries may need to be reinforced as the professional relationship evolves.

Without passing judgment on the correctness of the behavior, both men and women frequently seem, at least initially, to be more comfortable with a middle-aged (30 or over) female practitioner. This appears to be based on several factors:

- Body image on the part of female clients (they are more comfortable having another woman see their bodies)
- Women's male partners (e.g., husbands) are not comfortable having a male massage professional interact with their wives or significant others

- Women's concern about safe touch from men
- Men's discomfort with being touched in a pleasurable way by another man
- Men's social conditioning to accept comfort and touch in a caring manner from women
- Cultural influences

Male massage professionals must be aware of the possibility of encountering these preconceived ideas. They must present themselves in such a way as to alleviate concerns (with education when possible) and to respect the feelings of the individual client through referral to a female professional if necessary. As public awareness of massage increases, this gender difference probably will begin to dissipate.

Age is also a concern. Both male and female massage practitioners under 25 years of age can experience bias based on the relative perception of lack of experience from older clients and peer stress from clients their own age.

In both situations, it is essential for young massage professionals and male massage professionals to present themselves as neutral, competent, and ethical. Acknowledging the situation also can be effective. For example, a male therapist greets a new client as follows: "Hello, my name is _____. I'm aware that it may be unusual to have a male massage therapist, since currently the profession is female dominant. However, as with the nursing profession, more and more males are entering the field of massage. I function as a health care professional, and you can be assured of competent care."

A young (male or female) massage practitioner might greet a client as follows: "Hello. My name is _____. I know I'm young, but I assure you that I assume my professional responsibilities with a mature focus."

PREMASSAGE PROCEDURES

SECTION OBJECTIVES

Using the information presented in this section, the student will be able to perform the following:

- Set up an orientation process for a new client
- Develop a personal method of focus/centering

 PROFICIENCY EXERCISE 8-5

Compare the two dialogs presented in the chapter and list three differences between them.

Example
In the first dialog, the client did most of the talking.

Your Turn
1.

2.

3.

Orientation Process

After the intake process, a new client is ready to learn about the massage process. The orientation proceeds as in the following manner.

1. Take the client to the massage area.
2. Show her where she may hang her clothes, and explain that she needs to remove only the amount of clothing necessary and only what she is comfortable with. Instruct her to leave her underclothing on. Most clients, especially new clients, are more comfortable with the underclothes left on to cover the genital area. If you have any other special requirements about clothing, now is the time to explain them.
3. Demonstrate the massage table, how it is draped, and how the draping works. Explain the requested starting position on the table (prone, supine, or side-lying).
4. If you are using a massage chair or mat, show the client how to use the chair or mat for proper positioning.
5. Ask about the use of music and offer a few selections.
6. Show the client where the restroom is and how to get there if it is not next to the massage area.
7. Briefly explain any charts you may have on the walls.
8. Ask about a lubricant. Show the client what you have and offer a choice. It is important for clients to choose the type of lubricant or to have the option of no lubricant to avoid any misrepresentation by the massage practitioner of diagnosing or prescribing.
9. Explain that you will leave the room to allow the client privacy while she undresses. The exception to this is if a client is a very elderly person or a woman in an advanced stage of pregnancy who requests assistance, or any other special situation in which the client requires the practitioner's assistance. If you will be staying in the room, explain how you will help the client and maintain modesty. This usually is done by holding up a sheet in front of the client or by using a screen. If direct assistance is necessary for disrobing, present yourself in a professional and matter-of-fact way while providing the help needed.
10. Explain all sanitary precautions.
11. Show the client the sign on the door stating that a massage is in session and explain why the door is not locked.
12. Give a general idea of the massage flow. For example, that the massage will start on the back and take about 10 minutes, and then the legs and feet will be done for 15 minutes. Explain the effect of any change in a basic pattern; for example, that spending more time on the neck means that less time will be available for the back.
13. Instruct the client to get on the table by sitting between the end of the table and the hinged area (if the table is a portable one) or in the middle of the table (if it is a free-standing table). Next, the client should lean on one side to position herself side-lying or roll to the supine or prone position. To get off the table, the client reverses the procedure; she rolls to one side, pushes up to a seated position, and sits for a minute to prevent dizziness. She then gets off the table. If any chance exists that the client may fall or may need assistance getting on or off the table, stay in the room to help. Demonstrate the procedures, if nec-

essary, but do not use any draping materials on the table. It is unsanitary for anything or anyone to touch the drapes before the client uses them.

14. Ask the client if she has any questions.
15. Explain that you will be washing your hands and forearms and preparing for the massage while the client gets ready.
16. Tell the client how long you will be gone and that you will knock and announce yourself before entering the room.

Any modifications that need to be made because of the location and environment of the massage should be taken into consideration. People can become anxious if they do not know how to do what they are supposed to do. Do not assume that a client remembers the instructions or knows what is expected. Explain all steps in detail.

It is important to remind repeat clients of the previously mentioned procedures. Just as the information gathered during the intake procedure is updated each week and reassessment continues as the massage sessions progress, clients must be kept updated on any changes in procedures, new equipment, and so forth.

Focus/Centering

While waiting for the client to prepare for the massage, the practitioner should do the same through focus/centering. This can be done in many ways. Slow, deep breathing combined with stretching slows the mind and focuses the attention into the body. Looking at a nature scene or a painting is another way. Listening to music or performing some sort of repetitive behavior, such as washing your hands under warm water while visualizing the water carrying away all concerns for the next hour, can become a trigger for focus. The goal is to be present in the moment for the client and not focused on lists of things that need to be done. Developing a routine sequence for focusing enables the practitioner to become calm and centered much faster (Proficiency Exercise 8-6). During the focusing moments, the massage professional solidifies a clear intention for the massage based on the client outcomes. A very important aspect of professional behavior is to be clearly focused on the client and delivering the massage with intentionally based outcomes.

PROFICIENCY EXERCISE 8-6

1. Develop a checklist of everything the client needs to know before preparing for the massage.
2. Role play with two other students. One student is the first-time client, another is the massage practitioner, and the third evaluates the performance. Practice using the checklist and explaining procedures to the client. Switch roles so that each student plays all three parts.
3. Develop three different ways to focus your attention before beginning a massage. Make note of your ideas for future reference.
4. Work with three students and teach each other ways to focus. Discuss what works and what does not work in focusing.

POSITIONING AND DRAPING THE CLIENT

SECTION OBJECTIVES

Using the information presented in this section, the student will be able to perform the following:

- Position and drape a client and perform a massage using the four basic positions
- Drape effectively with two basic styles

Positioning

Positioning is placing a client into the position that best enhances the benefits of the massage. The four basic massage positions are supine (face up), prone (face down), side-lying, and seated (Figure 8-12). This section explains the use of body supports and proper draping for these basic positions.

A client may be placed in all four positions during a massage session, because remaining in one position longer than 15

FIGURE 8-12 Positioning the client, seated, prone, side-lying, and supine. **A,** Prone. *1,* Rolled towel. *2,* Face cover. *3,* Bottom sheet. *4,* Rolled towel at forehead. *5,* Top sheet. *6,* Support for abdomen or chest. *7,* Ankle support. *8,* Support for abdomen or chest. *9,* Ankle support. *10,* Blanket. *11,* Bottom sheet. *12,* Top sheet. *13,* Shoulder support. *14,* Fitted sheet. **B,** Side-lying. *1,* Towel roll or pillow. *2,* Pillow. *3,* Knee support (under sheet). *4,* Fitted sheet. *5,* Blanket. *6,* Bottom sheet. *7,* Knee/leg bolster. *8,* Top sheet. *9,* Pillow for arm and shoulder. *10,* Pillow. *Continued*

FIGURE 8-12, cont'd C, Supine. *1,* Pillow. *2,* Knee support. *3,* Knee support. *4,* Chest towel.

minutes may become uncomfortable. The exception is a painful situation that limits the client's ability to be comfortable in a certain position.

Pillows or other supports, such as folded towels, blankets, or specially designed pieces of foam, are used to make the client comfortable. The supports fill any gaps in contour when the client is positioned and provide soft areas against which the client can lean. Supports generally are used under the knees, ankles, and neck.

After the first trimester, a pregnant woman probably will be most comfortable in a side-lying position. If a client has a large abdomen, supports should be used to lift the chest and support the abdomen. This can be done by using a foam form with an area cut out for the abdomen. Women with large breasts may need a chest pillow.

Side-lying positions require pillows or supports for the arms and a small support between the knees. Clients with lower back pain may be more comfortable with a support under the abdomen when lying prone.

Changing the client's position requires shifting of the body supports. All supports must be under the sanitary drape or protected with sanitary coverings that are changed after each client. If the supports are located under the sheets, simply fold the bottom sheet over the top to expose the supports and move them.

Draping

Draping has two purposes:

- *To maintain the client's privacy and sense of security.* The drape becomes the boundary between the practitioner and the client. It is a way to establish touch as professional. Skillfully undraping an area to be massaged and

purposefully redraping the area is much more professional and less invasive than sliding the hands under the draping materials. Respect for the client's personal privacy and boundaries fosters an environment in which the client's welfare is safeguarded.
- *To provide warmth.*

Principles of Draping

Draping can be done in many ways, although certain primary principles apply.

- All reusable (multiple use) draping material must have been freshly laundered with bleach or other approved solution for each client (see Chapter 6). Disposable (single use) linens if used must be fresh for each client and then disposed of properly.
- Only the area being massaged is undraped.
- The genital area is never undraped. The breast area of women is not undraped during routine wellness massage. Specific massage targeting the breast under the supervision of a licensed medical professional may require special draping procedures for the breast area of women. In Canada, breast massage for medical purposes has a specific methodology and a consent process. These methods are out of the scope of practice for the wellness massage practitioner. (Specific recommendations for therapeutic breast massage are provided in Chapter 12.)
- Draping methods should keep the client covered in all positions, including the seated position.

Draping materials can be a bit clumsy to use at first. To ensure the modesty of the first few practice clients, have them leave their clothing on. If the client uses a dressing area away from the massage table, a robe, top sheet, or wrap large enough to cover the body will be needed for the walk to the massage area. If a wrap or top sheet is used, it can become the top drape once the client is on the table.

The two basic types of draping are flat draping and contoured draping.

Flat Draping Methods

With flat draping, the top sheet is placed over the client in the same manner that a bed is made, with a bottom sheet and a top sheet. Instruct the client to lie supine, prone, or side-lying between the drapes on the massage table. The entire body is then covered. The top drape, and sometimes the bottom drape, is moved in various ways to cover and uncover the area to be massaged.

NOTE: To ensure the privacy of men, the massage practitioner should avoid smooth, flat draping over the genitals while the client is supine. The penis may become partly erect as a result of parasympathetic activation or a reflexive response to the massage. This response is purely physiologic and does not necessarily suggest sexual arousal. Loose draping that does not lie flat against the body provides for a visual shield and reduces the client's embarrassment.

Contoured Draping

Contoured draping can be done with two towels or with a sheet and a towel. The drapes are wrapped and shaped around the client. This type of draping is very effective for securely covering and shielding the genital and buttock areas. Positioning of the drape may feel invasive to the client, but having the client assist in placement of the drapes preserves a sense of modesty. For women, a separate chest towel can be used to drape the breast area.

Alternative to Draping

As an alternative to draping, the client can wear a swimsuit or shorts and a loose shirt. The table or mat must have a sanitary covering, such as a bottom drape, and a top drape must be available because the client may become chilled even if partly clothed. When working with a client wearing clothing or a swimsuit, the practitioner must still observe all the precautions for sanitation, privacy, and respect.

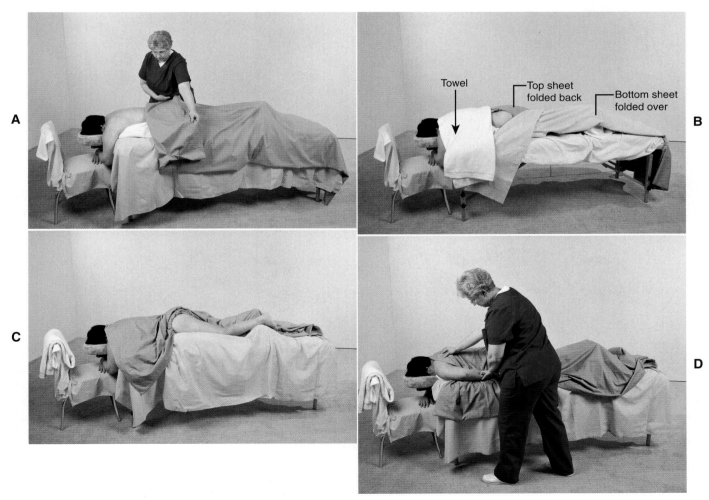

FIGURE 8-13 Draping. **A,** Prone: Undraped back. **B,** Draping for the gluteal area. **C,** Prone: Draping for leg. **D,** Prone: Draping for arm.

Continued

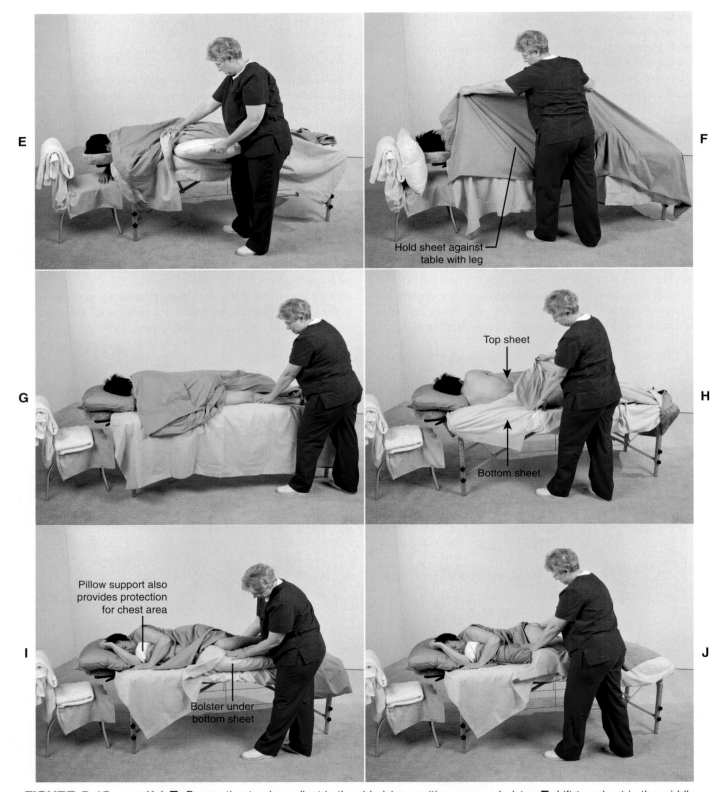

FIGURE 8-13, cont'd E, Preparation to place client in the side-lying position: remove bolster. **F,** Lift top sheet in the middle to allow client to roll. **G,** Side-lying: Draping for leg. **H,** Side-lying: Draping for back. Use bottom sheet to fold over leg and glutes. **I,** Side-lying: Draping for leg. **J,** Move drape to provide access to upper thigh and gluteal area.

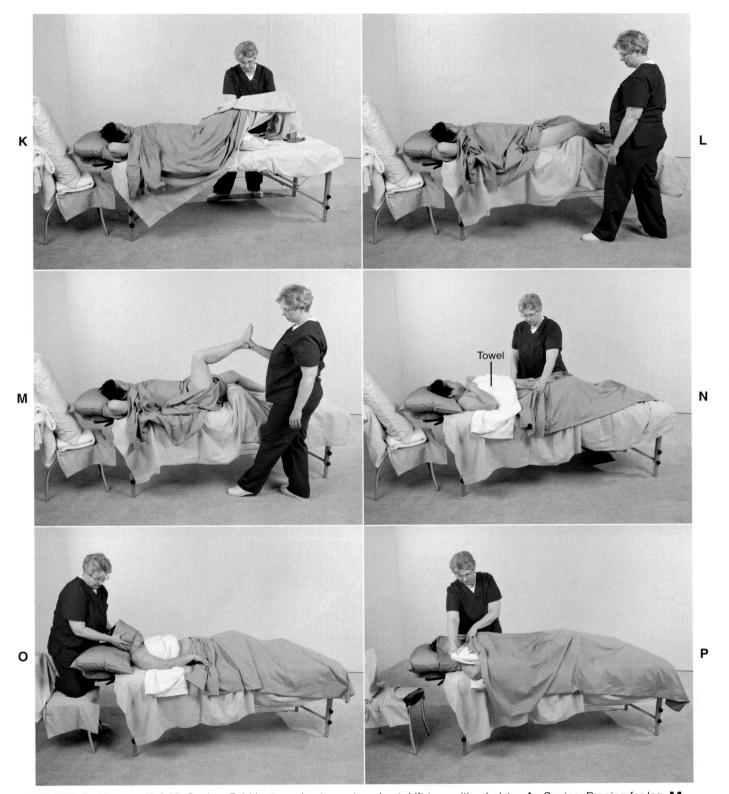

FIGURE 8-13, cont'd K, Supine: Fold bottom sheet over top sheet. Lift to position bolster. **L,** Supine: Draping for leg. **M,** Contour drape to prevent exposure of the groin area. **N,** Towel over top sheet: Client holds towel while sheet is moved. **O,** Draping for abdomen. Optional use of a pillowcase to cover the eyes. **P,** Redrape and remove towel.

Continued

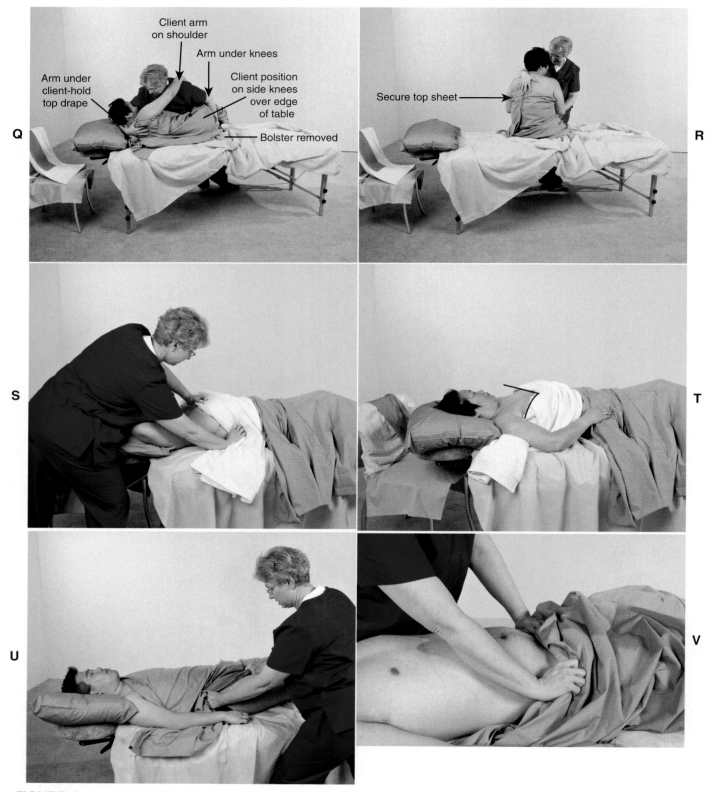

FIGURE 8-13, cont'd Q, Help client from the table. **R,** Lift by standing; secure drape. **S,** Working around the female breast. Use towel to move breast tissue. **T,** Contour drape around the breast. **U,** Working in the groin area, use a top sheet to slide drape tightly into area. For males, this will move the genitals out of the massage area. **V,** Use drape to slide to the top of the pubic bone. For males, this will move the genitals away from the massage area.

FIGURE 8-13, cont'd W, Avoid flat draping on males in the supine position. **X,** Bunched sheets disguise the genital area.

Suggested Draping Procedures

The photograph sequence for draping procedures is presented in Figure 8-13. Practice them and then combine the methods to fit the particular needs of the client. The DVD provides additional examples.

Notice how the draping material is placed so that the practitioner's clothing does not come in contact with the client. This maintains sanitation.

These draping procedures are a starting point for modest, secure use of towels and sheets for proper and appropriate draping. Modification is encouraged. Many other methods are available and can be used instead or combined with the procedures presented here (Proficiency Exercise 8-7).

AFTER THE MASSAGE

When the massage is finished, the client should be left alone for 5 to 10 minutes to rest. If necessary, re-enter the massage area to help the client off the table.

Helping the Client off the Massage Table

Use the following procedure when helping a client off the table.
1. Reach under the client's neck and knees.
2. Support the sheet loosely around the client's neck and hold it so that it does not slip when the client is lifted.

PROFICIENCY EXERCISE 8-7

1. *Receive three different professional massages and observe how the massage practitioner drapes and uses body supports.*
2. *With a fellow student or practice client, practice each draping method shown in Figure 8-13.*

3. Lift the client's torso off the table while swinging the knees around to the edge of the table. Make sure the client's arm is over your shoulder and not around your neck.
4. In case of dizziness, stabilize the client for a moment after he is in the seated position.
5. Still holding the sheet, help the client to a standing position.
6. Shift the position of the sheet so that the client can hold it securely.

In rare instances the client may need help dressing. Let the client do as much as possible. Be matter-of-fact and deliberate with any assistance.

If a client will be left to get off the table alone, remind him of the following:
1. Roll to one side.
2. Use your arms to push up to a seated position.
3. Sit for a minute before getting up.
4. Leave the sheets on the table.
5. Get dressed and return to the business area.

Closing the Session, Collecting the Fee, and Making the Next Appointment

When the client is dressed and ready to leave, make the next appointment or provide a written reminder if it already has been made. If the fee was not collected in advance, the client should pay at this time.

Saying Good-Bye

After the massage is finished, do not linger in conversation. The attitude in the business area is one of courteous completion. Often, getting a client to leave can be difficult. After spending time in a comfortable, caring environment, many people want to talk. Breaking this pattern when business picks up can be a problem, so the best course is to establish a short, consistent departure routine in the beginning. People respond well to sameness. A client will get used to leaving and making

PROFICIENCY EXERCISE 8-8

1. *Practice helping people off the massage table. Find 10 different body shapes and sizes to work with and note the difference in leverage needed for each client.*
2. *Write down your departure routine and practice it with other students. What will you do to end a massage session successfully with a client who does not want to leave? Have one of the students in your practice group role play this situation and see how successful your procedure is.*

the break from the massage practitioner in a reasonable period more easily if the sequence is always the same.

For example, the client approaches the desk, and the massage practitioner takes the money, writes a receipt, and confirms the next appointment. The massage practitioner gets up from the desk and says, "I really enjoyed working with you today. I am glad that you continue to feel that the massage is beneficial. It will be nice to see you again in 2 weeks. I hope the stretches we talked about are helpful. Keep track of any changes, and we'll discuss them next time I see you."

The massage practitioner then extends a hand for a warm handshake. (In some situations, a quick, friendly hug is appropriate, but only if it is initiated by the client and the practitioner is comfortable with the interaction. Professionally and respectfully accept hugs or physical contact initiated by the client.) Then say good-bye while gesturing or looking toward the door. At this point it is important for the massage practitioner to make a move to leave the area, or the client may initiate additional conversation.

evolve

8-1   Watch video clips on proper draping technique in addition to the content on the DVD.

8-2   Categorize items as appropriate or inappropriate for a massage office.

Don't forget to study for your certification and licensure exams! Review questions for this chapter are located on Evolve.

After the Session

After the client has left, the practitioner should update all records, prepare the room for the next client, and attend to personal hygiene and self-care (Proficiency Exercise 8-8).

■■■ SUMMARY

The information discussed in this chapter is just as important as any other aspect of professional therapeutic massage. The different locations and environments for massage set the mood and reflect the personality of the massage practitioner.

Careful consideration of equipment (e.g., massage tables, body supports), supplies (e.g., oils, linens), music, and other amenities results in a professional yet personalized approach.

Taking time to explain massage procedures to a client, taking a basic history, and learning and understanding the expectations and outcome for each massage help create an approach that meets the client's needs. Providing safe, respectful touch by using careful, modest draping and positioning is very important.

This chapter has described professional skills that create the confidence, respect, and trust important to successful application of therapeutic massage. Professional massage practice requires attention to these details.

Workbook Section

Answers for the Workbook Section for Chapter 8 are provided on p. 766.

■ ■ ■ SHORT ANSWER

1. What factors must be considered before the massage actually begins?

2. What is the most important piece of massage equipment?

3. How do massage practitioners protect their hands?

4. What types of massage equipment provide a surface that supports the client while the massage is given?

5. What features should be considered when looking for a massage table?

6. What must be checked on the massage table to ensure the client's safety?

7. What are body supports?

8. What are drapes?

9. What types of draping materials are available?

10. What accommodation should be made for clients with sensitive skin?

11. What sanitary measures must be taken with draping materials?

12. What is the purpose of lubricants?

13. What types of lubricants are used?

14. What are some important things to remember about lubricants?

15. What are some general considerations for creating a professional massage environment?

16. What are the main types of massage environments?

17. What special considerations are important for the use of music?

18. What considerations are important for lighting in the massage room?

Workbook Section—cont'd

19. Why is a scentless environment so important?

_____

_____

_____

20. What other considerations are necessary to ensure the client's comfort?

_____

_____

_____

21. Why must the massage practitioner educate the client about appropriate expectations for the massage session?

_____

_____

_____

22. Why should the massage practitioner carefully explain all procedures to the client before the massage?

_____

_____

_____

23. What are the basic massage positions for a client, and how are body supports used in these positions?

_____

_____

_____

24. What are the specific guidelines for draping?

_____

_____

_____

25. In what way is the drape a type of boundary?

_____

_____

_____

26. What are the two basic types of draping procedures?

_____

_____

_____

27. How is a chest towel used?

_____

_____

_____

28. How do you assist a client into a seated position?

_____

_____

_____

29. What is the massage practitioner's attitude at the conclusion of the session?

_____

_____

_____

30. After the client leaves, the massage practitioner should attend to what activities?

_____

_____

_____

▪▪▪ PROBLEM-SOLVING EXERCISES

1. A client indicates on the client information form that he does not wish to have an oil-based lubricant used on his back, face, or chest. What are your options? List them on a separate piece of paper.

2. You are scheduled to travel to a client's home to do a massage. When you arrive, you realize that there is no private location large enough to accommodate the massage table. What are some of your options? List them on a separate piece of paper.

▪▪▪ ASSESS YOUR COMPETENCIES

Now that you have studied this chapter, you should be able to:

1. Construct a massage setting in different types of environments.

2. List the equipment, supplies, and setup procedures required to prepare for a massage session.

3. Explain massage procedures to a client.

4. Effectively drape and position a client.

On a separate sheet of paper, write a short summary of the content of this chapter based on the competencies listed above. When writing this paper, assume you are speaking to someone—a client, prospective employer, co-worker, or other interested person. Write the paper as if you were having a conversation and explaining the importance of the information and skills to professional massage development.

Next, in small student discussion groups, share the papers and compare and contrast how the information was presented. Discuss the content, looking for similarities, differences, potential misunderstanding of the information, and clear and concise methods of description.

▪▪▪ PROFESSIONAL APPLICATION EXERCISE

You have been contracted to provide on site massage in an office setting using a chair. Before you begin, you will have a chance to visit the location. On a separate piece of paper, list the specifics you will look for in locating the massage area, what supplies you need to include in the traveling office, and what materials you will need.

▪▪▪ RESEARCH FOR FURTHER STUDY

Check nursing texts and study the positioning and draping procedures; record any procedures that are applicable to massage.

CHAPTER 9

Massage Manipulations and Techniques

CHAPTER OBJECTIVES

After completing this chapter, the student will be able to perform the following:

- Explain the basic theories for the physiologic effects of massage methods and techniques
- Organize massage methods and techniques for application in four positions
- Perform a full-body massage using the methods and techniques presented in the chapter

CHAPTER OUTLINE

KEY TERMS

STUDENT NOTE: Most models in this chapter are pictured in sportswear to enhance and clarify the various body positions. A properly groomed massage professional, of course, wears a uniform (see Figure 6-1). For draping procedures, see Chapter 8.

KEY TERMS—cont'd

Frequency	Percussion (tapotement)
Friction	Physiologic barriers
Gliding (effleurage)	Positional release technique (PRT)
Isometric contraction	Postisometric relaxation (PIR)
Isotonic contraction	Proprioceptive neuromuscular facilitation (PNF)
Joint end-feel	Pulsed muscle energy procedures
Joint movement	Reciprocal inhibition (RI)
Joint play	Resting position
Kneading (pétrissage)	Rhythm
Lengthening	Rocking
Multiple isotonic contractions	Shaking
Muscle energy techniques	Skin rolling
Oscillation	Speed
Osteokinematic movements	Strain/counterstrain
Passive joint movement	Stretching
Passive range of motion	Target muscle
Pathologic barrier	Vibration

The massage professional is in the process of clarifying terminology. In addition, there are ongoing changes in anatomical terminology. To address this issue, varying terms are presented together so the reader can identify multiple terms for the same concept. Although the author is aware that this can be confusing, there does not seem to be a more logical solution to the issue until there is a regarding terminology.

Chapter 9 is a core technical chapter. It includes definitions, descriptions, and directions for the application and use of the most common massage methods and techniques. As a student of therapeutic massage, you must learn to problem solve by using clinical reasoning to devise variations of the applications of massage methods. Massage routines offer limited benefits. Each session needs to be designed specifically for the individual client (see Chapter 10).

Examine each of the individual massage manipulations and techniques and learn to use them well. It is important to understand both why and where massage methods and techniques are used and how to organize a process that uses the various therapeutic approaches efficiently. In the practice of therapeutic massage, practitioners use their fingers, thumbs, hands, forearms, and, for some applications, their knees and feet. This chapter focuses on methods that use the fingers, thumbs, hands, and forearms, but be open to how application can be provided using your legs and feet to spare the arms and hands. You should always stay mindful of how to best use your body when applying massage manipulations and techniques (see Chapter 7).

The massage professional uses a structured, purposeful application of various forms of touch for specific reasons.

Since the late 1800s, these massage manipulations have been called *effleurage, pétrissage, compression, vibration, friction,* and *tapotement.* However, the terminology is changing, and the current trend is to use descriptions that are more relevant to the application of mechanical forces created by the method.

Mosby's Medical, Nursing, and Allied Health Dictionary defines *manipulation* as "the skillful use of the hands in therapeutic or diagnostic procedures . . . see also *massage*."[1] This dictionary also defines *massage* as "the manipulation of the soft tissue of the body through stroking, rubbing, kneading, or tapping." The word *manipulation* is used in this chapter to indicate each of these methods.

It is important to distinguish between the soft tissue manipulations of the massage professional and the joint manipulations of the chiropractor, osteopath, or physical therapist. The massage professional does not perform specific, direct joint manipulations. The massage techniques presented in this text incorporate passive and active joint movement, as well as lengthening and stretching methods, within the comfortable limits of the joint. These methods may indirectly affect the range of motion of a joint through changes in the soft tissue. The particular focus of the massage professional is the soft tissue, not the osseous structure of the joint.

Often a combination of soft tissue work and specific joint manipulation is required to achieve the functional goals of the client. In these instances the massage practitioner, with appropriate training, becomes part of the multidisciplinary team under the supervision of the health care professional. This team approach provides the skills and expertise of multiple professionals to best serve the client.

THE PHYSIOLOGIC EFFECTS OF MASSAGE

SECTION OBJECTIVES

Using the information presented in this section, the student will be able to perform the following:

- Categorize the effects of massage methods and techniques as stimulating or inhibiting physiologic responses
- Classify massage manipulations and techniques as reflexive, mechanical, or chemical, according to their effects

All massage methods apply forms of external mechanical force processed as sensory information that can stimulate or inhibit body processes, depending on their use. Some methods are better at stimulation, and others are better at inhibition. In general, a fast, specific application of methods tends to stimulate, whereas a slow, general application tends to inhibit. Some methods work better for producing mechanical effects, through the application of forces such as tension, compression, shearing, bending, and torsion. Others are better at initiating chemical responses.

Assigning a wholly mechanical, reflexive, or chemical effect to massage manipulations and techniques is not always possible. Often the combination of the effects of massage, coupled with the client's physiologic state and receptivity to the massage, produces the response.

In general, reflexive massage manipulations and techniques either stimulate or inhibit a response. Simply stated, imbalances fall into two categories: conditions of the body that are "too much" or "not enough." Massage methods help the body restore balance by inhibiting "too much" conditions and by stimulating "not enough" conditions. In terms of muscle responses, think of contraction or lengthening (reducing the neural stimulation causing contraction) of the muscle, with imbalance reflected as a muscle that is either too short or too strong, or too long or too weak. Connective tissue methods deal with tissue that is too hard, too soft, too thick, or too thin. Circulation may be marked by a rushing fluid flow or a sluggish fluid flow. With nervous system activity, think of overactivity or underactivity.

Consider these general guidelines:
- Methods that move through the skin to the underlying tissue tend to be more mechanical and stimulate localized chemical responses and arterial circulation. Painless, deep, broad-based compression encourages parasympathetic dominance.
- Massage manipulations and techniques that stay within the skin and superficial fascial layer tend to have a more direct reflexive effect on the nervous system because many sensory nerves are located in the skin. These methods also tend to stimulate the release of hormonal and other body chemicals that provide for a general systemic (whole body) effect. The venous and lymphatic circulations are influenced. These approaches, especially if delivered briskly, stimulate sympathetic dominance.
- Methods that move the body, cause muscles to contract and relax and joint positions to change, and deliver sensory input to the proprioceptors are more reflexive in nature.
- Methods that exert force on soft tissues are reflexive, mechanical, and chemical.

QUALITY OF TOUCH

SECTION OBJECTIVES

Using the information presented in this section, the student will be able to perform the following:

- Evaluate massage manipulations based on seven criteria
- Effectively establish and adjust the physical contact with the client

Gertrude Beard (1887-1971), a highly respected educator in massage therapy as an integral part of physical therapy, described the components of massage as follows:

> The factors that must be considered as components in the application of massage techniques are: the direction of the movement, the amount of pressure, the rate and rhythm of the movements, the medium used, the frequency and duration of the treatment, the position of the patient and of the physical massage practitioner.[2]

Beard's definition of *medium* referred to the application of lubricants or other instruments used. The definition of *frequency* reflected how often per day or week the massage was given. Individual massage methods vary with regard to depth of pressure, drag, direction, speed, rhythm, frequency, and duration. From Beard's information and other sources, the following components of the quality of touch have been compiled and are discussed in this textbook.

9-1

- Depth of pressure (compressive force) can be light, moderate, deep, or variable. Depth of pressure is extremely important. Most soft tissue areas of the body consist of three to five layers of tissue, including the skin; the superficial fascia; the superficial, middle, and deep layers of muscle; and the various fascial sheaths and connective tissue structures. Pressure must be delivered through each successive layer, displacing the tissue to reach the deeper layers without damage and discomfort to the tissues. The deeper the pressure, the broader the base of contact with the surface of the body. More pressure is required to address thick, dense tissue than delicate tissue. Pressure delivers compressive force to the tissue (Figure 9-1).
- Drag is the amount of pull (stretch) on the tissue (tensile force). In this context, the term drag refers to the effort of overcoming resistance. When skin is dry, it has a high resistance to slip. Lubricant is used during massage to increase slip and therefore reduce drag. When a tensile force is used during assessment or to bring about a physiologic change during the massage application, the amount of drag on the tissue increases or decreases in relationship to the degree of slipperiness of the skin.
- Direction means that the massage can proceed from the center of the body outward (centrifugal) or inward from the extremities to the center of the body (centripetal). It can proceed from proximal to distal attachments of the muscle (or vice versa) following the muscle fibers, transverse to the tissue fibers, or in circular motions.
- Speed of manipulations can be fast, slow, or variable.

FIGURE 9-1 **A,** Massage applications systematically generate force through each tissue layer. This figure provides a graphic representation of the application of force. It begins with light, superficial application and progresses with increased pressure to the deepest layer. The varying degrees of pressure are: **B,** Light. **C,** Light. **D,** Medium. **E,** Medium.

Continued

FIGURE 9-1, cont'd **F,** Deep. **G,** Deep.

- Rhythm refers to the regularity of application of the technique. A method that is applied at regular intervals is considered even, or rhythmic. A method that is disjointed, or irregular, is considered uneven, or nonrhythmic.
- Frequency is the rate at which the method repeats itself within a given time frame. In general, each method is repeated about three times before the practitioner moves or switches to a different approach.
- Duration is the length of time the method is applied or that the manipulation remains in the one location.

Through these variations in touch, simple massage methods are adapted to produce the outcomes desired by the client. These qualities of touch provide the therapeutic benefit. The *mode of application* (e.g., gliding, kneading) provides the most efficient application. Each method can be varied, depending on the desired outcome, by adjusting depth, drag, direction, speed, rhythm, frequency, and duration. As you strive to perfect your practice of massage application, remember that the quality of touch is more important than the method. Quality of touch is altered when a contraindication or caution for massage exists. For example, when a person is fatigued, the duration of the application often is shortened; if a client has a fragile bone structure, the depth of pressure is altered.

Establishing and Adjusting Physical Contact

The massage professional must make contact with the client's body in a secure and confident way. Be sure to inform the client verbally that you are about to touch him or her; then, make sure the approach of the touch is steady, not abrupt, and that your hands are warm.

After touch contact has been made with the client and the massage has begun, the intention of the contact should not be broken. This means that the massage practitioner remains focused on the client for the entire session. Maintaining contact does not mean that the practitioner never removes his or her hands from the client. It is nearly impossible to drape effectively, or have the client change position, or apply lubri-

cant to a different area without removing the hands from the client's body. When removing your hands, simply establish verbal contact by telling the client that you will be removing your hands for a moment, shifting the draping, or altering position. Before re-establishing touch, again tell the client that you will be touching him or her, and where, so that the person does not startle. Centering facilitates this process of remaining focused on the client (see Chapter 8).

ORGANIZING THE MASSAGE AND POSITIONING THE CLIENT

SECTION OBJECTIVE

Using the information presented in this section, the student will be able to perform the following:

- Organize a massage sequence using the four basic positions

Organization of the various massage manipulations and techniques follows a cohesive pattern. During a full-body massage, all the soft tissues are addressed, and the joints are moved within the limits of the client's comfortable range of motion.

The illustrations in the protocol and the DVD included with this text show body placement. Any methods can be used in any combination in a particular body area. Some students will find these simple guidelines helpful, whereas others will find it easier to develop a structure themselves. For learning purposes, beginning with the suggestions provided and then modifying them as needed is a good course of action. Remember, the examples in the book and on the DVD are only a place to begin as you work to understand the organization of massage application. (A sample protocol is presented on p. 335.)

The four positions for client positioning are prone, supine, side-lying, and seated. All four are commonly used in combination during a massage. As was discussed in Chapter 8, client comfort is important when positioning and supports are used. The client may appreciate a positional shift during the massage to maintain general comfort. About every 15 minutes, ask the client whether he or she is comfortable

The different approaches can be combined in many different ways to create different massage patterns. You may find it helpful to study the illustrations and incorporate the suggestions into your practice massage sessions. Use the illustrations while generating your own ideas, and be open to experimentation, creation, and modification of massage applications based on individual clients according to body shape, style of massage, and equipment available.

TYPES OF MECHANICAL FORCE AND MASSAGE MANIPULATIONS

SECTION OBJECTIVES

Using the information presented in this section, the student will be able to perform the following:

- Perform six basic massage manipulations: gliding, kneading, compression, oscillation (vibration, shaking, rocking), tapotement (percussion), and friction
- Combine the six massage manipulations into a basic full-body massage

In *Massage in Athletics,* author Albert Baumgartner quotes Plato as saying, "Massage must be simple."[3] Baumgartner also says, "Many endeavor to introduce improvements into the science of massage but fail to gain adherents to their preventive methods. It would be well to advise these witty inventors of the new sub-methods to keep their improvements to themselves."

The massage manipulations and techniques in this textbook are explained and organized in a manner that consolidates, condenses, and simplifies therapeutic massage methods based on what seems to be the consensus from the historical material and currently accepted terminology and theory. The infinite variations of massage application do not come from many different methods but from skilled use of the fundamental application and variation of the quality of touch in terms of depth of pressure, drag, direction, speed, rhythm, frequency, and duration.

Terminology

Ling called the massage methods passive movements. In 1879 the terms *effleurage, pétrissage, friction,* and *tapotement* first appeared in the *VonMosegeil* (Proceedings of the German Society for Surgery) to describe Mezger's methods (see Chapter 1). Since then, almost every textbook on massage has included these terms. Kellogg described the resting position in terms of passive touch.[4] Most historical textbooks did not distinguish between superficial stroking and effleurage, and many described compression by classifying it as part of pétrissage or pressure. Current trends divide the methods of compression into distinct categories. Most references agree that *tapotement* and *percussion* are synonymous, yet resources seem evenly split between classifying "vibration" and "shaking" separately or together. *Friction* is classified many different ways, but the definitions usually are similar. This textbook refers to passive movements by the names developed through Ling's and Mezger's works in combination with current usage, which is moving away from the historical terminology. The current trend is to describe something based on how the method is applied (i.e., gliding, effleurage): these are listed in the massage manipulations section. Active movements or gymnastics, as defined by Ling, Taylor, and others, are listed in the massage techniques section using current terminology. Although the approach presented in this text is comparable to the method currently called *Swedish or classical massage,* it is much more expansive and should not be limited by a label. The more appropriate term is *therapeutic massage.*

All massage manipulations introduce mechanical forces into the soft tissues, stimulating various physiologic responses.

Types of Force

9-2

Force may be perceived as mechanical (discussed in this chapter) or as field forces, such as gravity or magnetism. Actions that involve pushing, pulling, friction, or sudden loading (e.g., a direct blow) are examples of mechanical forces. Mechanical forces can act on the body in a variety of ways. Learning the different types of mechanical forces and understanding the ways in which mechanical forces applied during massage act therapeutically on the body are important aspects of massage.

The five kinds of force that can affect the tissues of the body are *compression, tension, bending, shear,* and *torsion.* Not all tissue is affected the same way by each type of force. We will look at each of the five types of force, the different ways they can produce tissue injuries, and more important, the ways in which they produce therapeutic benefits when applied by a skilled massage practitioner.

Compression (Figures 9-2 and 9-3)

Compressive forces occur when two structures are pressed together. Compressive force is a component of massage application and is described as depth of pressure. This kind of force may be sudden and strong, as with a direct blow (percussion), or it may be slow and gradual, as with gliding strokes. The magnitude and duration of the force are important in determining the outcome of the application of compression.

Some tissues are quite resilient to compressive forces, whereas others are more susceptible. Nerve tissue is an interesting example. Nerve tissue can withstand moderately strong compressive forces if they do not last long (e.g., a sudden blow to the back of your elbow that hits your "funny bone"). However, even slight force applied for a long time (as occurs with carpal tunnel syndrome) can cause severe nerve damage. The practitioner needs to take this into account when

FIGURE 9-2 Illustration of compression.

FIGURE 9-3 Examples of compression.

FIGURE 9-4 Illustration of tension.

FIGURE 9-5 Examples of tension.

determining the duration of a massage application using compression.

Ligaments and tendons are quite sturdy and resistant to strong compressive loads. Muscle tissue, on the other hand, with its extensive vascular structure, is not as resistant to compressive forces. Excess compressive force can rupture or tear muscle tissue, causing bruising and connective tissue damage. This is a concern when pressure is applied to deeper layers of tissue. To prevent tissue damage, the practitioner must distribute the compressive force of massage over a broad contact area on the body; the more compressive force used, the broader the base of contact with the tissue.

Compressive force is used therapeutically to affect circulation, sensory and autonomic nerve stimulation, nerve chemicals, and connective tissue pliability.

Tension (Figures 9-4 and 9-5)

Tension forces (also called *tensile force*) occur when two ends of a structure are pulled in opposite directions. This is different from muscle tension. Muscle tension is created by excess muscular contraction, which results from an increase in motor tone or an increase in tissue density caused by fluid accumulation and connective tissue changes (muscle tone). Muscles that are long as a result of being pulled apart are affected by tensile force. Certain tissues, such as bone, are highly resistant to tensile forces. An extreme amount of force would be required to break or damage a bone by pulling its two ends apart. Soft tissues, on the other hand, are very susceptible to tension injuries. In fact, tensile stress injuries are the most

common soft tissues injuries. Such injuries include muscle strains, ligament sprains, tendinitis, fascial pulling or tearing, and nerve traction injuries (i.e., sudden stretching of nerves, such as occurs in whiplash).

Tension force is used during massage with applications that drag, glide, lengthen, and stretch tissue to elongate connective tissues and lengthen short muscles.

Bending (Figures 9-6 and 9-7)

Bending forces are a combination of compression and tension. One side of a structure is exposed to compressive forces while the other side is exposed to tensile forces. Bending occurs during many massage applications. Force is applied across the fiber or across the direction of the muscles, tendons or liga-ments, and fascial sheaths. Bending forces rarely damage soft tissues; however, they are a common cause of bone fractures. Bending force is very effective in increasing connective tissue pliability and affecting proprioceptors in the tendons and belly of the muscles.

Shear (Figures 9-8 and 9-9)

Shear is a sliding force, and significant friction often is created between the structures that slide against each other. The massage method of friction uses shear forces to generate

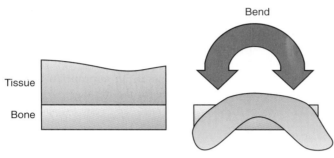

FIGURE 9-6 Illustration of bending.

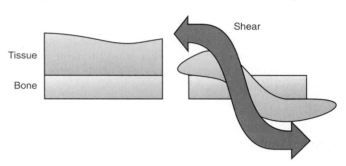

FIGURE 9-8 Illustration of shear.

FIGURE 9-7 Examples of bending.

FIGURE 9-9 Examples of shear.

physiologic change by increasing connective tissue pliability and creating therapeutic inflammation. However, excess friction (shearing force) may produce an inflammatory irritation that causes many soft tissue problems.

Torsion (Figures 9-10 and 9-11)

Torsion forces are best understood as twisting forces. Massage methods that use kneading introduce torsion forces and target connective tissue changes and fluid movement.

The application of torsion force to a single soft tissue structure is not very common and is rarely the cause of significant tissue injury. Torsion force applied to a group of structures (e.g., a joint) is much more likely to be the cause of significant injury. For example, when the foot is on the floor and the individual turns the body, the knee as a whole is exposed to significant torsion force.

Massage Manipulations (Mode of Application)

The methods of massage described in the following sections introduce one or a combination of the five types of mechanical force into the body to achieve a therapeutic benefit (Figure 9-12). This process is influenced by the quality of touch, depth of pressure, drag, duration, speed, rhythm, and frequency. Appropriate use of mechanical force is necessary. If insufficient force or the wrong type of mechanical force is used, the application will not be effective; conversely, excessive or inappropriate use of force can damage tissues.

FIGURE 9-10 Illustration of torsion.

The variety of massage and bodywork modalities in the profession (see Chapter 2) can be clarified by describing what is done during the application, using qualities of touch, mechanical forces, and mode of application. For example, the modality called *deep tissue massage* is not a unique form of massage but appears to be a compressive force application at a "deeper" tissue level.

Those studying this textbook should be able to modify the massage application from surface to deep, fast to slow, long to short, as appropriate based on the individual needs of the client and to appropriately influence the fluid movement, nervous system function, musculoskeletal function, and connective tissue pliability in a focused and compassionate manner (see Chapters 4 and 5). The following massage manipulations, which are modes of application, are used to apply mechanical force during massage in an appropriate way to achieve the determined outcome for the massage.

Resting Position

The act of placing your hands on another person seems so simple; yet this initial contact must be made with respect and a client-centered focus with the intention of meeting the client's goals. With the resting position, we enter the client's personal boundary space, as defined by sensitivity to changes in air movement and heat picked up by the sensory receptors in the skin. The root hair plexus is one of the most sensitive receptors to the movement of air. Activation of the heat sensors indicates that something is close enough to cause physical harm. Because of these sensors, the fight-or-flight responses of the sympathetic autonomic nervous system often are activated with the initial contact.

The instinctive survival and protective mechanisms designed to protect human beings from hand-to-hand combat dictate that the physiologic safety zone generally is an arm's length. If another person is at this distance, the sensory mechanisms of sympathetic arousal are less sensitive than if the person is close enough to touch. For this reason, the first

FIGURE 9-11 Examples of torsion.

FIGURE 9-12 Combined loading. **A,** Bend and tension. **B,** Compression and tension.

approach to touch by the massage professional is very important.

The resting position provides time for the client to become acclimated to the proximity of another human being. It gives the client time to evaluate, on a subconscious level, whether this touch is safe. This first application of touch sets the stage for the first 15 to 30 minutes of the massage, because it takes that long for the sympathetic arousal fight-or-flight response, which causes the release of adrenaline into the blood, to reverse itself.

The resting position also allows stillness when intermixed with the other movements of massage. The body needs time to process all the sensory information it receives during massage. Stopping the motions and simply resting the hands on the body provides for this moment of stillness.

The resting position is an excellent way to call attention to an area through stimulation of the cutaneous (skin) sensory receptors. Simple, sustained touch over an area of imbalance often is enough stimulation to cause a reflexive response. This position also adds body heat from the massage practitioner's hand to an area of the client's body. In addition, it is an excellent way to re-establish contact with the client if the flow of the massage is interrupted or if physical contact is broken.

Applying the Resting Position. An open, soft, relaxed, warm, dry hand is best for application of the resting position (Figure 9-13). It is a signal to the physiologic survival mechanism that no weapon is nearby nor is there any intent to strike. A cool, clammy hand suggests sympathetic activation in the practitioner. Subconscious survival mechanisms in the client can recognize this and will respond to perceived danger by tensing for protection.

Practice extending an open, relaxed hand. Rub your hands together to warm them and then towel-dry them before touching the client.

In most circumstances a slow, steady approach by the practitioner, with deliberate hesitation at the arm's length boundary, accompanied by a verbal announcement that you will

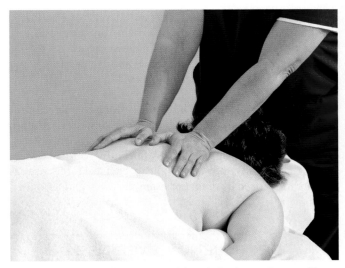

FIGURE 9-13 Open, relaxed hands in the resting position.

begin touching, is the best way to avoid excessive sympathetic arousal. Most of the time, the massage practitioner seeks to activate the restorative parasympathetic state for the client. Yet even when the massage is designed to stimulate sympathetic activation, the first touch should be slow, gradual, and deliberate, using pressure level 1 or 2 (see Chapter 7).

Apply the resting position slowly and gradually, in a confident, secure manner. As part of the survival mechanism, the body innately responds to a hesitant touch by withdrawing. An unsure touch is difficult to interpret and unsettling to the client. Mastering the application of the resting position makes flowing into the other methods easy (Proficiency Exercise 9-1).

Gliding (Effleurage)

The historical term for gliding strokes is *effleurage*. The term *effleurage* originates from the French verb meaning "to skim" and "to touch lightly on." The most superficial applications of gliding (effleurage) do this, but the full spectrum is determined by pressure, drag, speed, direction, and rhythm, making this one of the most versatile massage manipulations. The most common forces introduced by gliding are tension force, bending force, and compression force.

After application of the initial touch, or resting position, gliding often is next in the sequence, especially if a lubricant is used. The long, broad movements of this method are excellent for spreading the lubricant on the skin surface. The ease of application makes this an effective manipulation to use repetitively while gradually increasing the depth of pressure. This is one of the preferred manipulations to warm or prepare the tissue for more specific bodywork. Because of the horizontal nature of the manipulation, the flow pattern of the massage can progress smoothly from one body area to another. Gliding also is a good method to use to evaluate for hard and soft tissue, hot and cold areas, or areas that seem stuck. It is the preferred method for abdominal massage and for massage to facilitate circulation.

The more superficial the stroke, the more reflexive the effect. Slow superficial strokes (pressure level 2 or 3) are very soothing, whereas fast superficial strokes (pressure level 1 or 2) are stimulating. If a deeper stroke pressure (levels 3 to 5) is applied at a slower rate, the effect is more mechanical and stimulates parasympathetic dominance.

Applying Gliding Strokes. The distinguishing characteristic of gliding strokes is that they are applied horizontally in relation to the tissue fibers, generating a tensile force (Figure 9-14). Gliding also can be applied across fibers to create a bending force. The intensity and result of the mechanical force application are influenced by drag. For example, when gliding is used

to influence superficial fascia, there is significant drag on the tissue. During a palliative (relaxation) massage approach, lubricant is typically used to reduce the drag.

During gliding, light pressure remains on the skin, and moderate pressure extends through the subcutaneous layer of the skin to reach muscle tissue; however, it is not so deep as to compress the tissue against the underlying bony structure. Moderate to heavy pressure that exerts sufficient drag on the tissue mechanically affects the connective tissue and the proprioceptors in the muscle (i.e., spindle cells and Golgi tendon organs). Heavy pressure produces a distinctive compressive force on the soft tissue, pressing it against the bone.

Depth of pressure is a result of leverage and of leaning on the body. Pressure increases as the angle of the lean increases. Increases in pressure are *not* achieved by pushing with muscle strength.

Increasing pressure adds a compressive force and drag to the stroke. Light stroking is done with the fingertips or palm. Small body areas, such as the fingers, can be grasped and surrounded as gliding is applied to the entire area. The surface contact increases with full hand and forearm application of the manipulations.

Gliding that proceeds from the trunk of the body outward, using superficial pressure, usually follows the dermatome distribution and is more reflexive in its effects (Proficiency Exercise 9-2).

Strokes that use moderate pressure from the fingers and toes toward the heart, following the direction of the muscle fibers, are excellent for mechanical and reflexive stimulation of blood flow, particularly as it affects venous return and the lymphatics. Light to moderate pressure with short, repetitive gliding that follows the patterns for the lymph vessels is the basis for manual lymphatic drainage (see Chapter 11) (Figure 9-15).

Kneading (Pétrissage)

The historical term for kneading is *pétrissage*, which comes from the French verb petrir, meaning "to knead." In kneading (pétrissage), the soft tissue is lifted, rolled, and squeezed (Figure 9-16).

Just as gliding is focused horizontally on the body, kneading is focused vertically and involves twisting. The main purpose of this manipulation is to lift tissue, applying bend, shear, and torsion forces. After the tissues have been lifted, the full hand is used to squeeze the tissue as it rolls out of the hand, while the other hand prepares to lift additional tissue and repeat the process (Figure 9-17).

Because skin and the underlying muscles cannot be lifted without first pressing into them, compression is a component of kneading and is done first. Kneading is very good for reducing motor tone. The lifting, rolling, and squeezing action affects the spindle cell proprioceptors in the muscle belly. As the belly of the muscle is squeezed (which squeezes the spindle cells), the muscle feels less tense. When lifted, the tendons are stretched, thus increasing tension in both the tendons and the Golgi tendon receptors, which have a protective function. The result of this sensory input is reflexive relaxation of the muscle to protect it from harm, restoring a more normal resting

PROFICIENCY EXERCISE 9-1

1. *Purposeful touch may be simple, but it is not easy. Diligent practice is required. If you enjoy animals, practice your approach with them. They do not hide responses as people do. Practice using the resting position to touch a dog, cat, or other animal while the animal is asleep, and see if you can do it without waking the animal.*
2. *Babies and young children are good for practice as well. Practice the resting position with a baby or child. Acceptance of the touch is indicated if the child does not startle or move away.*

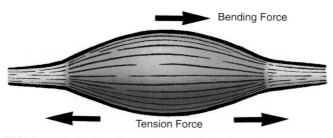

FIGURE 9-14 The focus of gliding is horizontal strokes.

PROFICIENCY EXERCISE 9-2

Do five massages and experiment with the following suggestions, plus any other application of gliding stroke you can create.

1. Use finger stroking of the face, first following the direction of the muscle fiber and then moving across the muscle fibers. Have a chart of the facial muscles available.

2. Use the forearm on the back, first following the muscle fiber directions from proximal to distal attachment and then moving across the muscle fiber direction. Keep a muscle chart nearby.

3. Use the palm or the pads of the fingers to lightly stroke the dermatome pattern from the spine to the fingers and toes. This method is sometimes called nerve stroking. Have a chart of dermatome distribution available.

4. Use the palm to glide from the toes and fingers toward the heart along the main pathways of the superficial veins. Use an anatomy chart as needed.

5. Grasp the fingers and toes and "milk" the tissue with gliding.

6. Use the forearm to glide on the quadriceps, hamstrings, abductors, fasciae latae, and iliotibial band of the thigh. Use a muscle chart to follow the fiber direction. Then glide across the fibers.

7. Grasp the foot at the toes with both hands and glide to the ankle.

8. Use the knuckles to glide on the bottom of the foot from the toes to the base of the heel.

9. Use the thumbs to glide in a very specific pattern to gently separate the muscles in the hamstring and quadriceps groups.

10. Use the four basic flow patterns and design an entire massage with only gliding strokes using variations of depth, drag, direction, speed, rhythm, frequency, and duration.

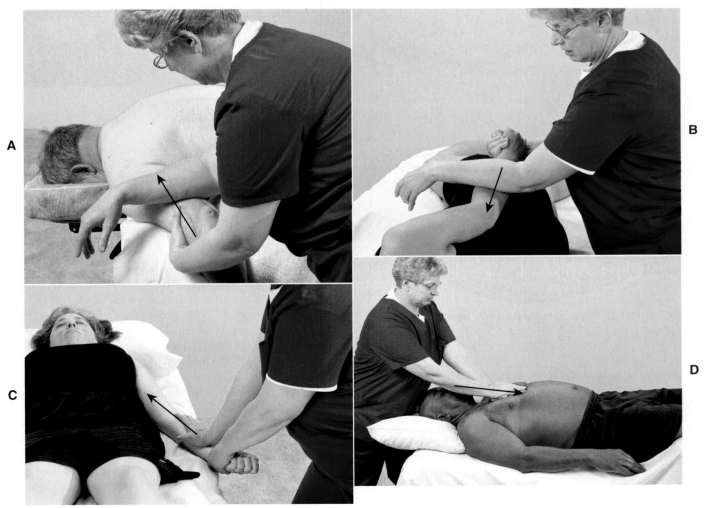

FIGURE 9-15 Examples of gliding applications.   *Continued*

FIGURE 9-15, cont'd

FIGURE 9-16 The focus of kneading is vertical lifting and twisting.

length of the muscle. Kneading is very good for mechanically softening the superficial fascia. This type of connective tissue, located under the skin, is similar to gelatin. It is made up of a glycol (sugar) protein that binds with water. If gelatin is mixed with water and allowed to sit, it becomes thick and solidifies, resulting in reduced pliability and increased density. If the gelatin is pressed into smaller pieces and stirred, it softens (i.e., decreased density and increased pliability). This is similar to the effect of kneading on connective tissue with the bend, shear, and tension forces exerted on the tissue. The difference

in feeling in the muscles after kneading is the same as comparing the stiffness of a brand new pair of shoes or jeans with the comfort of an old pair of jeans or a broken-in pair of shoes.

The fascia forms a major part of each muscle. Kneading has the mechanical effect of softening and creating space around the muscle fibers, making the tendons more pliable. The tension on the tendon as it is pulled during kneading deforms the connective tissue and mechanically warms it in a manner similar to that by which a piece of metal bent back and forth becomes warm. Instead of metal fibers, collagen fibers are bent and warmed. When something is warm, its molecules are moving faster and are farther apart. The space, which is created at the molecular level, translates into a softer, more pliable structure.

Kneading may incorporate a wringing or twisting component (torsion) after the tissue is lifted. Changes in depth of pressure and drag determine whether the client perceives the manipulation as superficial or deep. By the nature of the manipulation, the pressure and pull peak when the tissue is lifted to its maximum and are less at the beginning and the end of the manipulation.

FIGURE 9-17 Examples of kneading applications.

Continued

FIGURE 9-17, cont'd

Kneading methods are effective for supporting circulation because they squeeze the capillary beds in the tissues and support fluid exchange.

Skin Rolling. Skin rolling is a variation of the lifting manipulation. Deep kneading attempts to lift the muscular component away from the bone; skin rolling, however, only lifts the skin from the underlying muscle layer. It has a warming and softening effect on the superficial fascia, causes reflexive stimulation of the spinal nerves, and is an excellent assessment method. Areas of "stuck" skin (bind) often suggest underlying problems. Skin rolling is one of the very few massage methods that can safely be used directly over the spine. Only the skin is accessed and the direction of pull on the skin is up and away from the underlying bones; thus no risk of injury is posed to the spine, unlike with methods that involve any type of downward pressure (Figure 9-18).

Sometimes the tissue will not lift. This may be a result of excessive edema (swollen tissue), a heavy fat layer, scarring that extends into the deeper body layers, or thickened areas of connective tissue, especially over aponeuroses (flat sheets of superficial connective tissue). If these conditions are present, applications of kneading or skin rolling are uncomfortable for the client. Shifting to gliding and compression may soften the tissue enough that kneading can be used more effectively later in the massage session.

Excessive body hair may hamper the use of kneading or skin rolling. The massage practitioner must be careful not to pull the client's hair when using these massage manipulations.

Applying Kneading. Kneading must be rhythmic to feel correct. The speed of the manipulation is limited. The speed and frequency of the application are determined by how much tissue can be lifted and how long it takes to roll and squeeze the tissue through the hand. Lifting the tissue quickly or squeezing it too fast is uncomfortable for the client. Although

FIGURE 9-18 Skin rolling.

the concept is difficult to explain, it is much like milking a cow or kneading bread dough; the consistency of the material determines how it is to be kneaded.

Kneading begins with palmar compression on a 45-degree angle to move the tissue forward and up. The massage practitioner produces the compression pressure by leaning into the body—not by using muscle strength to push downward. As the tissue bunches in front of the hand, the fingers, used as a unit with the palm, close over the mound of tissue. The tissue is then lifted, rolled, and squeezed through the hand as the practitioner rocks his or her entire body away from the direction used to produce the compressive force and initiates the lifting action. As the practitioner's body sways back, the tissues lift and roll through the grasping hands. The massage practitioner again rocks forward and leans into the body to apply compression, and the movements are repeated to create a rhythmic pattern of kneading.

Except in very delicate areas, such as the face, the fingers and thumbs should not be used to lift the tissue because of a tendency to pinch and cause discomfort to the client.

To get a feel for the method, practice with some clay. Keep your fingers pressed together, using use them as a single unit pressed against the thenar eminence (the pad at the base of the thumb). Do not use the thumb itself. It is important to use as large a part of the palmar surface as possible. Slowly extend the upward pull until you feel the end of the elastic give of the tissue; this is where a sense of resistance (bind) is felt. This type of kneading works on both the skin and the tendons. In most cases only one hand at a time is used to lift, squeeze, and twist the tissue. Kneading becomes continuous when a hand-over-hand rhythm is established. Two hands can also be used against each other on larger areas, such as the hamstring muscle.

In skin rolling, the entire hand is used to lift the skin, and the thumbs then are used to feed the skin to the fingers in a rolling motion (Proficiency Exercise 9-3).

NOTE: Although kneading is very effective for softening and relaxing tissue, it is energy-consuming for the massage practitioner. As mentioned earlier, the fingers should be used as a unit with the thenar eminence of the thumb. The massage practitioner should take care not to use this manipulation excessively. A better practice is to use kneading intermittently with gliding and compression, which do not require such labor-intensive use of the hands. Constant attention must be paid to body mechanics.

Compression

Compression uses a lift-press method that is applied at a 90-degree angle to the tissue. Compressive force is an aspect of gliding and kneading. Compression is particularly suited for use when a lubricant is undesirable. It also is a very good method to use on hairy bodies, because the manipulations do not glide on the skin, pull the tissue, or require lubricant. As with gliding, the deeper the pressure, the more mechanical the effect. Likewise, the more superficial the pressure, the more reflexive the effect.

Compression directs pressure downward into the tissues (Figure 9-19), with varying depths of pressure adding bending and compressive forces. The superficial application of compression resembles the resting position but uses more pressure. The manipulations of compression usually penetrate the subcutaneous layer, whereas in the resting position, they remain on the skin surface. Much of the effect of compression results from pressing tissue against the underlying bone, causing it to spread and be squeezed from two sides, similar to flattening out a tortilla or a ball of clay or pressing pizza dough into a pan.

Compression can disconnect from the body with each lift and reconnect with each press in a pistonlike fashion. Pressing rhythmically into connective tissue softens it mechanically. Pressing tissue against the underlying hard bone spreads the tissue mechanically, enhancing the softening effect on the connective tissue component of the muscle. Compression at 90 degrees takes all the slack out of the tissue (the barrier) to produce bind (sense of resistance) and then pushes or pulls at a 45-degree angle without slipping produces a drag (tension force) on the tissue that affects the connective tissue.

Compression applied to the belly of a muscle spreads the spindle cells, causing the muscle to sense that it is stretching. To protect the muscle from overstretching, the spindle cells signal the muscle to contract. The lift-press application stimulates the muscle and nerve tissues. The combination of these two effects makes compression a good method for stimulating muscles and the nervous system. Because of this stimulation, compression is a little less desirable for a relaxation or soothing massage. It is important to remember that not all people want to feel like a relaxed rag doll after a massage. If the client wants to be alert and energized, a stimulating massage should be done.

A muscle needs to contract or at least have the nerve "fire" (as occurs in a contraction) before it can relax. This is due to the threshold stimulation pattern of the nerve and its effects on muscle tone. Nerves build up the energy needed to spark the nerve impulse. The automatic response of muscle fibers to contraction is a period of relaxation called the *refractory period*. Sometimes the signals are enough to get everything ready to fire, but they are not strong enough to actually cause the contraction or discharge of the nerve. As a result, the muscle tenses but cannot quite contract, and the tension

PROFICIENCY EXERCISE 9-3

1. *Knead a variety of sizes of bread dough. Small pieces can be used to practice the delicate applications used on the face and anterior neck; larger pieces can mimic big muscles, such as the gluteals. Bread dough is good for practice because it is resilient (like body tissue) and will not allow you to pétrissage too fast.*

2. *Pétrissage an inflated balloon. If it slips out of your grasp, you just pinched your "client." Using a balloon helps develop the use of the palm in place of the fingers.*

3. *For learning purposes only, practice using pétrissage or kneading for an entire body massage using all four basic flow patterns. Make sure to practice different depths of pressure, drag, direction, speed, rhythm, frequency, and duration of the application. Notice that some parts of the body are more easily kneaded. Because of the repetitive use of the hand for pétrissage, avoid extensive long-term use.*

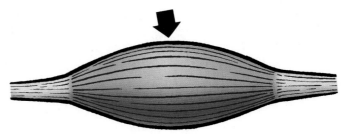

FIGURE 9-19 The focus of compression is a vertical downward pressure.

remains. If stimulation of the nerves can be increased just enough to prompt the nerve to discharge, the muscle contracts and can reset to a normal resting length. Applying compression to the belly of the muscle, and the resultant effect on the spindle cells, elicits this response. Any sustained, repetitive use of a stimulation method that causes muscle fibers to maintain a contraction or to contract repeatedly eventually fatigues the muscle fibers. Compression used in this manner initiates a relaxation response in muscles.

Compression is an excellent method for enhancing circulation. The pressure against the capillary beds changes the pressure inside the vessels and encourages fluid exchange. Compression appropriately applied to arteries allows back pressure to build, and release of the compression encourages increased arterial flow. This manipulation can be done over the clothing or without lubricant.

Very specific, pinpoint compression is called *direct pressure* or *ischemic compression* and is used on acupressure points and trigger points.

Applying Compression. Compression can be applied with the point of the thumb or with a stabilized finger, the palm and heel of the hand, the fist, the knuckles, the forearm and, in some systems, the knee and heel of the foot (Figure 9-20). It is applied perpendicular to the tissue (i.e., 90 degrees). Usually it is applied against the contours (hills) of the body that are oriented at around 45 degrees.

When using your palm to apply compression, avoid hyperextending or hyperflexing your wrist by keeping the application hand in front of rather than directly under your shoulder. Even though the compressive pressure is perpendicular to the tissue, the position of the forearm in relation to the wrist is about 120 to 130 degrees. Application against a 45-degree angle of the body (hill) plus the 45-degree angle of the practitioner's hand and forearm results in the 90-degree contact on the tissue. If you are using your knuckles or fist, make sure the forearm is in a direct line with the wrist. Use of the thumb should be avoided, if possible, because the thumb can be damaged by extensive use, especially on large muscle masses.

The tip and the radioulnar side of the elbow should not be used to apply compression. Because the ulnar nerve passes just under the skin and damage can result from extensive compression, use the forearm near the elbow for compression. The massage professional's arm and hand must be relaxed, or neck

FIGURE 9-20 Examples of compression applications.

FIGURE 9-20, cont'd

Continued

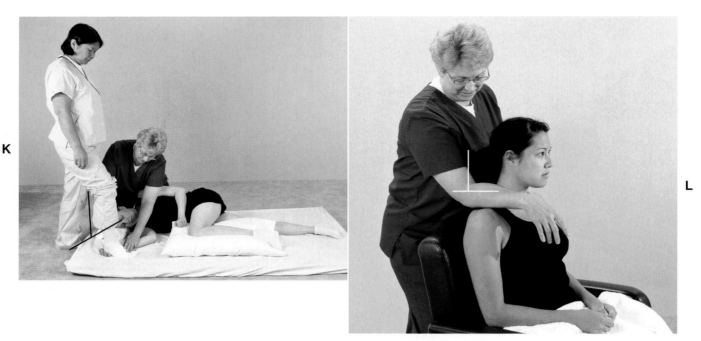

FIGURE 9-20, cont'd Examples of compression applications.

and shoulder tension will develop. Leverage applied through appropriate body mechanics does the work, not muscle strength. Compression also can be applied with the practitioner's leg and foot.

The depth of compression is determined by what is to be accomplished, where compression is to be applied, and how broad or specific the contact is with the client's body. Deep compression presses tissue against the underlying bone. Because of the diagonal pattern of the muscles, the massage practitioner should stay perpendicular to the bone, with actual compression somewhere between a 60- and 90-degree angle to the body. Beyond those angles, the stroke may slip and turn into a glide.

Compression can replace gliding if gliding strokes cannot or should not be used, such as in areas of excessive body hair, areas where a person is ticklish, and areas where the skin is sensitive to lubricant. Compression bypasses the tickle response by activating deep touch receptors. Also, compression does not slip or roll on the tissue (Proficiency Exercise 9-4).

Oscillation

Attempts to clarify massage terminology cluster vibration, shaking, rocking, and percussion under the umbrella term of *oscillation*. Oscillation is any effect that varies in a back-and-forth, or reciprocating, manner. The term *vibration* sometimes is used more narrowly to mean a mechanical oscillation.

Very simply, oscillation involves action in the form of springs and swings. In terms of springs, it is logical to include massage methods that bounce off the tissue (later called *percussion*), just as beating a drum creates oscillation. The concept of swings can be related to any massage method that moves

PROFICIENCY EXERCISE 9-4

1. *Inflate a series of balloons with different internal pressures. Fill some with water and others with gelatin and use these to represent the density and pliability of different tissue types. The use of balloons is great for practicing the angle and pressure of the manipulation. The best angle allows good, firm compression into the balloon without it slipping out from under you.*
2. *Use pieces of foam of various densities and place them over objects of different sizes and shapes. Determine how much pressure it takes to feel each object. Pay attention to the difference with the low-density foam compared with the high-density foam.*
3. *Design a complete massage for each of the basic flow patterns using only compression. Pay very close attention to ways in which you can use compression manipulations in all of the variations to access the client's body successfully. Adjust depth of pressure, speed, rhythm, frequency, and duration and observe the different physiologic effects. Experiment with using your leg and foot to apply compression while the client is on a mat.*

the body. Vibration is an action of moving back and forth really fast; shaking is moving back and forth but is much bigger than vibration; and rocking is a rhythmic, swinging motion.

Vibration. Edgar Cyriax, one of the foremost authorities on massage and manual techniques, describes vibration as follows:

Almost every author who attempts to describe the modus operandi for generating these vibrations prefaces his remarks by stating that they are extremely tiring to produce. Vibration is generated by means of the operator tensing all the muscles of his or her arm (some even include the muscles of the shoulder) into a state of powerful complete tetanus. This method is very fatiguing; no one can sustain such a contraction evenly for more than a minute or so. The correct technique for production of manual vibrations is to set up a small amount of alternating contraction and relaxation in some of the muscles of the forearm, those of the upper arm and the shoulder being kept quite passive (unless required for fixation purposes).[5]

Vibration is very powerful if it can be done long enough and at an intensity sufficient to produce reflexive physiologic effects. The massage practitioner can use manual vibration to stimulate muscles by applying the technique at the muscle tendons for up to 30 seconds. When this is complete, the antagonist muscle pattern relaxes through neurologic reciprocal inhibition.

Vibration also can be used to break up the monotony of the massage. If the same methods are used repeatedly, the body adapts and does not respond as well to the sensation or stimulation. Because vibration is used to "wake up" nerves, it is a good method for stimulating nerve activity. The nerves of the muscles around a joint also innervate the joint itself. Muscle pain often is interpreted by the client as joint pain and vice versa. Used specifically and purposefully, vibration is a great massage manipulation to confuse and shift the muscle-joint pain perception.

Applying Vibration. All vibration begins with compression. After the depth of pressure has been achieved, the hand needs to tremble and transmit the action to the surrounding tissues. As described by Cyriax, the muscles above the elbow should be relaxed; the action comes only from the alternating contraction and relaxation of the forearm muscles (Figure 9-21).[5] Of all the massage methods, vibration may be the most difficult to master.

To start with coarse vibration, place one hand on the client and compress lightly. Begin moving the hand back and forth using only the forearm muscles and limiting the motion to about 2 inches of space. Gradually quicken the back-and-forth movement, checking to make sure your upper arm stays relaxed. Next, make the back-and-forth movement smaller until the hand does not move at all on the tissue but is trembling at a high intensity. This is vibration.

Because considerable energy is needed to perform this manipulation, it should be used sparingly and only for short periods. A forearm gliding method should be used after vibration, because the gliding action essentially massages and relaxes the practitioner's arm, protecting it from repetitive use problems (Figure 9-22).

Some professionals use mechanical vibrators to replace manual vibration. This is acceptable as long as the practice is allowed by licensing regulations, the equipment is safe, and the client approves its use (Proficiency Exercise 9-5).

Shaking. Shaking is effective for relaxing muscle groups or an entire limb. Shaking manipulations confuse the positional proprioceptors because the sensory input is too disorganized for the brain's integrating systems to interpret; muscle relaxation is the natural response in such situations.

Shaking warms and prepares the body for deeper bodywork and addresses the joints in a nonspecific manner. It is effective when the muscles seem extremely tight. Shaking has a reflexive effect, but a small mechanical influence also may

FIGURE 9-21 The focus of vibration is downward and back and forth in a fast, oscillating manner.

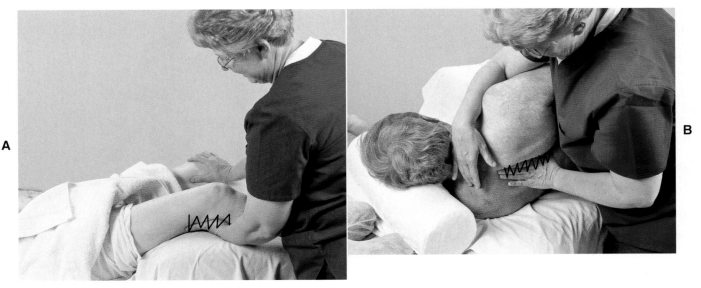

FIGURE 9-22 Examples of vibration.

be exerted on the connective tissue because of the lift-and-pull component of the method.

Shaking sometimes is classified as a form of vibration; however, the application is very different, because vibration begins with compression and shaking begins with lifting.

Applying Shaking. Shaking begins with a lift-and-pull technique. Either a muscle group or a limb is grasped, lifted, and shaken. To begin to understand shaking, think of a dog shaking water from its coat, a person shaking out a rug or blanket, a dog or cat tugging on a toy, or a horse swishing its tail.

For massage purposes, the focus of shaking is more specific and less intense than shaking a rug, but the idea is the same. There is a lift and then a fairly abrupt downward or side-to-side movement that ends suddenly, as if something is being thrown off. Even the most subtle shaking movements deliberately move the joint or muscle tissue with the intention of a "snap" at the end of the movement.

Shaking should not be used on the skin or superficial fascia, nor is it effective for use on the entire body. Rather, it is best applied to any large muscle groups that can be grasped and to the synovial joints of the limbs. Good areas for shaking are the upper trapezius and shoulder area, biceps and triceps groups, hamstrings, quadriceps, gastrocnemius and, in some instances, the abdominals and the pectoralis muscles close to the axilla. The joints of the shoulders, hips, and extremities also respond well to shaking.

The larger the muscle or joint, the more intense the method. If the movements are performed with all the slack out of the tissue, the focal point of the shaking is very small and the technique is extremely effective. The more purposeful the approach, the smaller the focus of the shaking. The practitioner should always stay within the limits of both joint range of motion and the elastic give of the tissue. The goal is to see how small the shaking action can be and still achieve the desired physiologic effect. To accomplish this, first lift the tissue or limb, grasp it, and then lean back gently until the tissue becomes taut. Begin the shaking movement from this position (Figure 9-23).

PROFICIENCY EXERCISE 9-5

The first two exercises to teach vibration were developed by a professional magician who is also a massage practitioner and instructor. Many sleight-of-hand movements required for his illusions use the same movements as vibration. Perfecting these two balloon exercises will enhance your vibration skills.

1. *Use a clear, 5-inch balloon. Put a penny inside it and then inflate and tie the balloon. Grasp the tied end of the balloon, cupping it in the palm of the hand. Using wrist action only, circle the balloon until the penny begins to roll inside. Once you can do this, make the wrist circles smaller and smaller while continuing to roll the penny in the balloon. Eventually the action will be the movement required for vibration.*

2. *Use the same balloon and put the fattest part in the palm of your hand. Place your other hand on top of the balloon. Using just the bottom hand, use a coarse vibration to get the penny to jump and dance in the balloon. Once you can do this, make the movements smaller and smaller until you can make the penny dance with fine vibration movements.*

3. *Combine all the methods presented so far into a massage. Incorporate vibration at each tendon, paying attention to the results as the muscles contract or tense slightly in response to the stimulation.*

A   B

FIGURE 9-23 Examples of shaking.

FIGURE 9-24 Examples of rocking.

Rocking. Rocking is a soothing, rhythmic method used to calm people. It has both reflexive and chemical effects (Figure 9-24).

Rocking also works through the vestibular system of the inner ear and feeds sensory input directly into the cerebellum. Other reflex mechanisms probably are affected as well. For these reasons, rocking is one of the most productive massage methods for achieving entrainment. For rocking to be most effective, the client's body must move so that the fluid in the semicircular canals of the inner ear is affected, initiating parasympathetic mechanisms.

Applying Rocking. Rocking is rhythmic and should be applied with a deliberate, full-body movement. Rocking involves the up-and-down and side-to-side movement of shaking, but no flick or throw-off snap occurs at the end of the movement. The action moves the body as far as it will go, then allows it to return to the original position.

After two or three rocks, the practitioner will be able to sense the client's rhythm. This attunement to the client's rhythm is a powerful interface point to synchronize entrainment. The massage practitioner works within the rhythm to maintain and amplify it by attempting to gently extend the limits of movement or by slowing the rhythm. Incorporation of a rocking movement that supports this entrainment process into all massage applications effectively individualizes the application and speed of the method. The client seems to relax more easily when a subtle rocking movement, matching his or her innate rhythm pattern, is incorporated as part of the generalized massage approach, along with such techniques as gliding, kneading, compression, and joint movement, especially passive movements. The body mechanics described in this text tend to produce a rocking motion.

With a tense, anxious client who initially may resist rocking, begin the process with slightly bigger and more abrupt shaking manipulations. As the muscles begin to relax, switch to rocking methods.

During rocking, nothing is abrupt; the methods have an even ebb and flow. All movement is flowing, like a wind chime in a gentle breeze or a porch swing on a hot summer night. Rocking is one of the most effective relaxation techniques the massage practitioner can use. Many parasympathetic responses are elicited by the rocking of the body during gliding, kneading, and compression (Proficiency Exercise 9-6).

Percussion (Tapotement)

Percussion (tapotement) moves up and down on the tissue. The term *tapotement* comes from the French verb *tapoter*, which means "to rap, smack, drum, or pat." In percussion techniques, the hands or parts of the hand administer springy blows to the body at a fast rate. The blows are directed downward, creating rhythmic compression of the tissue (Figure 9-25).

Percussion is characterized as light or heavy. In light percussion, the compressive force of the blows penetrates only to the superficial tissue of the skin and subcutaneous layers; in heavy percussion, the force penetrates deeper into the muscles, tendons, and visceral (organ) structures, such as the pleura in the chest cavity.

Percussion is a stimulating manipulation that operates through the response of the nerves. Because of its intense stimulating effect on the nervous system, it initiates or enhances sympathetic activity of the autonomic nervous system. The effects of the manipulations are reflexive except for the mechanical results of percussion, which are loosening and moving mucus in the chest. Children with cystic fibrosis are treated with percussion, but massage therapy of this type is beyond the beginning skill levels of the massage technician.

The most noticeable effect of percussion results from the response of the tendon reflexes. A quick blow to the tendon stretches it. In response, protective muscle contraction occurs. To obtain the best result, stretch the tendon first. The most common example of this reflexive mechanism is the knee-jerk

PROFICIENCY EXERCISE 9-6

1. *Lay a sheet on your massage table or other flat surface. Lift one end and practice shaking the sheet to achieve a wavelike motion from one end of the sheet to the other. Practice directing the ripple to various locations on the table.*
2. *Swing in a playground swing, using your legs to pump yourself. This exercise will give the full-body effect of the shake. Pay close attention to the feeling as you reach the top of the swing and begin to head back.*
3. *Using your own body for practice, systematically shake each joint, lying down to do the legs. See how small you can make the movement and still feel the effects. Grab the muscles of your arm and leg. Lift and shake the tissue, paying attention to the sensations.*

4. *Sit in an old-fashioned rocking chair and let the chair rock you. See what happens when you rock the chair. Vary the speed to go faster and slower than the chair's movement. Put the chair on different surfaces, such as carpet, hard floor, sand, and grass. Again, let the chair rock you and notice the difference. Remember, each person has an individual rhythm that needs to be identified, supported, and respected.*
5. *Put on music with a 4/4 beat at less than 60 beats per minute. Pick up the sway of the music and rock with it. Repeat the exercise with different beats of music.*
6. *Design an entire massage for all four basic flow patterns using a combination of shaking and rocking. Be aware of all the qualities of touch during the application.*

FIGURE 9-25 The focus of percussion (tapotement) is a vertical, abrupt downward snapping.

(or patellar) reflex, but this response happens in all tendons to some degree. This is very helpful when the massage practitioner is preparing the muscles for lengthening, such as when a client indicates that the hamstrings are tight and need to be lengthened. With the client supine, the hip flexed to 90 degrees, and the knee flexed to 90 degrees, percussion on the stretched quadriceps tendon causes the quadriceps to contract. As a result, the hamstrings are inhibited, making them easier to lengthen to a more normal resting length.

When applied to the joints, percussion affects the joint kinesthetic receptors responsible for determining the position and movement of the body. The quick blows confuse the system, similar to the effect of joint-focused rocking and shaking, but the body muscles are stimulated rather than inhibited. This method is useful for stimulating weak muscles. The force used must move the joint but should not be strong enough to damage the joint. For example, a single finger may be used to administer percussion over the carpal joints, whereas the fist may be used over the sacroiliac joint.

Percussion is very effective when used at motor points that usually are located in the same area as the traditional acupuncture points. The repetitive stimulation causes the nerve to fire repeatedly, stimulating the nerve tract.

Tapotement focused primarily on the skin affects the superficial blood vessels of the skin, initially causing them to contract. Heavy tapotement or prolonged lighter application dilates the vessels by causing the release of histamine, a vasodilator. Although prolonged tapotement seems to increase blood flow, surface tapotement enhances the effect of cold application used in hydrotherapy.

Applying Percussion. Two hands usually are used alternately to do percussion. One or two fingers can be used to tap a motor point (sometimes called *neurotapping*). The forearm muscles contract and relax in rapid succession to move the elbow joint into flexion and then allow it to release quickly. This action travels down to the relaxed wrist, extending it; the wrist then moves back and forth to provide the action of the percussion. Percussion is a controlled flailing of the arms as the wrists snap back and forth. Remember that the wrist must always stay relaxed. Beginning students usually want to use the wrists to provide the snap action. This is especially tempting when using small movements of the fingers; however, it should not be done because it will damage the wrist (Figure 9-26).

Heavy percussion should not be done in the kidney area or anywhere pain or discomfort is present (Proficiency Exercise 9-7).

The following are methods of percussion.

- *Hacking.* Hacking is applied with both wrists relaxed and the fingers spread, with only the little finger or the ulnar side of the hand striking the skin surface. The other fingers hit each other with a springy touch. Point hacking can be done by using the fingertips in the same way. Hacking is done with the whole hand on the larger soft tissue areas, such as the upper back and shoulders. Point hacking is used on smaller areas, such as the individual tendons of the toes, or over motor points (Figure 9-26, *A*).
- *Cupping.* To perform cupping, the fingers and thumbs are positioned as if making a cup. The hands are turned over, and the same action used in hacking is performed. When done on the anterior and posterior thorax, cupping is good for stimulating the respiratory system and for loosening mucus. If the client exhales and makes a monotone noise during cupping, enough pressure is used so that the tone begins to break up, changing from "AAAAAAAAAAAAH-HHHHH" to "AH AH AH AH AH AH" (Figure 9-26, *B*).
- *Beating and pounding.* These moves are performed using a soft fist with the knuckles down or vertically with the ulnar side of the palm. This technique is used over large muscles, such as the buttocks and heavy leg muscles (Figure 9-26, *C* and *D*).

FIGURE 9-26 Examples of percussion. **A,** Hacking. **B,** Cupping. **C,** Fist beating.

PROFICIENCY EXERCISE 9-7

1. Play a drum or watch a drummer, paying attention to the action of the arms and wrists and the grasp of the drumsticks. Notice that the drummer holds the drumstick loosely.

2. Get a paddleball or yo-yo and see what actions it takes to make these toys work. Play with a rattle or tambourine.

3. Use the foam from the compression exercises and practice the different methods and intensity of percussion (light to deep, slow to fast).

4. While shaking your hands very quickly, use hacking to strike the foam or a practice client. Without stopping, change hand positions so that all the methods are used.

5. Design a stimulating massage with various applications of percussion. Notice which qualities of touch are most reflected with these methods.

FIGURE 9-26, cont'd D, Beating over the palm. **E,** Slapping. **F,** Finger tapping.

■ *Slapping (splatting).* For this technique, the whole palm of a flattened hand makes contact with the body. This is a good method for causing the release of histamine, thereby increasing vasodilation and its effects on the skin. It also is a good method to use on the bottoms of the feet. The broad contact of the whole hand disperses the force laterally instead of downward, and the effects remain in the superficial tissue. Kellogg called this movement *splatting* (Figure 9-26, *E*).[4]

■ *Tapping.* In tapping, the palmar surface of the fingers alternately taps the body area with light to medium pressure. This is a good method to use around the joints, on the tendons, on the face and head, and along the spine (Figure 9-27, *F* and Proficiency Exercise 9-7).

Friction

One method of friction, formalized by James Cyriax, consists of small, deep movements performed on a local area; this

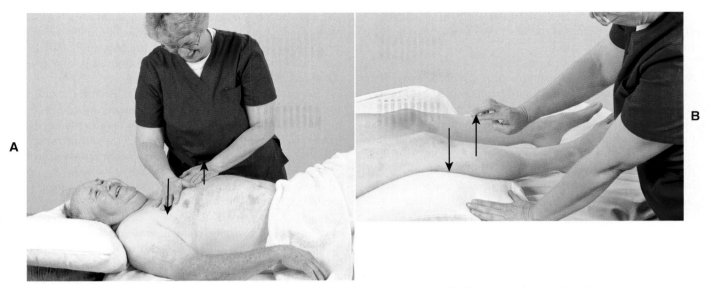

FIGURE 9-27 More examples of percussion. **A,** Rocking to assess for mobility. **B,** Finger tapping to stimulate acupuncture point.

FIGURE 9-28 The focus of friction is a vertical downward pressure that is applied with a back-and-forth movement to underlying tissues.

provides shear force to the tissue. This method uses deep transverse friction massage without the application of lubricant. The skin moves with the fingers (Figure 9-28). Friction burns may result if the fingers are allowed to slide back and forth over the skin. Friction creates therapeutic inflammation.

Friction manipulation prevents and breaks up local adhesions in connective tissue, especially over tendons, ligaments, and scars, by creating therapeutic inflammation. This method is not used over an acute injury or fresh scars. Modified use of friction, after the scar has stabilized or the acute phase has passed, may prevent adhesions and can promote a more normal healing process.

The Cyriax application also provides for pain reduction through the mechanisms of counterirritation and hyperstimulation analgesia. In many older textbooks, friction is explained as a back-and-forth, brisk movement focused on the skin and subcutaneous tissue to promote dilation of the vessels in the skin. Excessive use causes a friction burn on the skin similar to a rug burn. Historical literature on massage indicates that friction burns were created on purpose to produce long-term stimulation of the nerve. This method of counterirritation is seldom used today.

Connective tissue has a high water content. To remain pliable, it must remain hydrated. Friction increases the water-binding capacity of the connective tissue ground substance.

The movement in friction is usually transverse to the fiber direction. Friction generally is performed for 30 seconds to 10 minutes (although some authorities have suggested a duration of 20 minutes). This type of friction initiates a small, controlled inflammatory response. The chemicals released during inflammation result in activation of tissue repair mechanisms, with reorganization of the connective tissue. This type of work, coupled with proper rehabilitation, is very valuable. Because of its specific nature and direct focus on rehabilitation, deep transverse friction is not suitable for the beginning level massage technician. The method is discussed in more depth in Chapter 11.

A modified application of friction that is used to keep high-concentration areas of connective tissue soft and pliable is appropriate for the beginner. The modified application is essentially the same as deep transverse friction in that the focus is transverse to the muscle fiber direction and moves the tissue beneath the skin; however, the duration and specificity are reduced. The direction can be transverse or circular, pinpointed or more generalized, but the tissue under the skin is still affected.

Friction is a mechanical approach best applied to areas of high concentrations of connective tissue, such as the musculotendinous junction. Microtrauma from repetitive movement and overstretching are common in this area. Microtrauma predisposes the musculotendinous junction to inflammatory problems, connective tissue changes, and adhesions. Friction is a good way to keep this tissue healthy. Experts disagree over the need to stretch an area that is to receive friction. Because both the stretching and not stretching approaches have merit, both should be included when frictioning.

Friction also can be combined with compression, a combination that adds a small stretch component. The movement includes no slide. This application has mechanical, chemical, and reflexive effects and is the most common approach used today for applying friction.

Applying Friction. When using friction, the main focus is to move tissue under the skin. No lubricant is used because the tissues must not slide. The area to be frictioned should be placed in a soft or slack position. The movement is produced by beginning with a specific and moderate to deep compression using the fingers, palm, or flat part of the forearm near the elbow. After the pressure required to contact the tissue has been reached, the upper tissue is moved back and forth across the grain or fiber of the undertissue for transverse or cross-fiber friction or around in a circle for circular friction (Figure 9-29).

As the tissue responds to the friction, gradually begin to stretch the area and increase the pressure. The feeling may be intense for the client; if it is painful, the application should be modified to a tolerable level so that the client reports the sensation as a "good hurt." The recommended way to work within the client's comfort zone is to use sufficient pressure

such that the person feels the specific area but does not complain of pain. Friction should be continued until the sensation diminishes. Gradually increase the pressure until the client again feels the specific area. Begin friction again and repeat the sequence for up to 10 minutes.

The area being frictioned may be tender to the touch for 48 hours after use of the technique. The sensation should be similar to a mild after-exercise soreness. Because the focus of friction is the controlled application of a small inflammatory response, heat and redness are caused by the release of histamine. Also, increased circulation results in a small amount of puffiness as more water binds with the connective tissue. The area should not bruise.

Another effective way to produce friction is a combination of compression and passive joint movement, with the bone under the compression used to perform the friction (Figure 9-30). The process begins with compression as just described, but instead of moving the tissue back and forth or in a circle, the massage practitioner moves the client's body under the compression. This automatically adds the slack and stretch positions for the friction methods. The result is the same. This

FIGURE 9-29 Examples of friction.

FIGURE 9-30 Compression + movement = friction.

method is much easier for the massage professional to perform and may be more comfortable for the client as well. The movement of the joint provides a distraction from the specific application of the pressure and generalizes the sensation. Broad general methods can be used with a higher degree of intensity than a pinpointed specific focus (Box 9-1) (Proficiency Exercise 9-8).

MASSAGE TECHNIQUES

SECTION OBJECTIVES

Using the information presented in this section, the student will be able to perform the following:

- Use movement in a purposeful way to create a specific physiologic response
- Explain the proprioceptive mechanisms and their importance in the physiologic effects of massage techniques
- Move the synovial joints through the client's physiologic range of motion using both active and passive joint movement

Incorporate muscle energy techniques to enhance lengthening and stretching procedure

In his book, *An Illustrated Sketch of the Movement Cure*, which was published in 1866, George H. Taylor wrote:

The purpose of an active movement is to convey to, and concentrate upon a selected point, the nutrition and energies of the system. Such a movement may accomplish a twofold purpose, that of supplying a part, and of relieving another part more or less distant.

The mode of effecting this purpose is as follows: the person to receive the application is placed in an easy, unconstrained position, sitting, lying, half lying, kneeling, or in a convenient position that will suitably adjust all parts of the body to the purpose. The body is fixed either by the hands of an assistant, or by means of an apparatus so as to prevent as much as possible any motion of all parts of the body, except the acting part. The patient is in

some cases directed to move the free part in a particular direction, the effort to do so is resisted by the operator, with a force proportionate to the exertion made very nicely graduated to the particular condition of the part and of the system at large. The resistance is not uniform, but varies according to the varying action of muscles, as perceived by the operator. In other cases the operator acts while the patient resists. The action is the same, but in one case the patient's acting muscles are shortened and in the other lengthened. The operator is a wrestle, in which a very limited portion of the organism is engaged. The motion must be much slower than the natural movement of the part engaged, which fact strongly fixes the attention and concentrates the will. The act is repeated two or three times with all the care and precision the operator can command, being cautious not to induce fatigue.[6]

The use of movement as described in the next section follows Taylor's guidelines and recommendations, which were his interpretations of Ling's gymnastics or active movements (Box 9-2). The principles of massage today are built on the same principles described in the historic literature. The names may be different and the physiologic explanations more precise, but the methods are the same.

The efficient use of massage techniques reduces the need for repetitive massage manipulations. If these techniques are used well, the neuromuscular mechanism can be activated and influenced quickly, with less physical effort by the massage professional.

Physiologic Influences of Massage Techniques

The passive and active joint movement and muscle energy techniques presented in this chapter work with the neuromuscular reflex system to *lengthen* short muscles. In contrast, *stretching* has both a reflexive and a mechanical aspect. The reflexive component of stretching is an initial neuromuscular lengthening phase used to prepare the area for the more mechanical stretching effect of elongating connective tissue. (Stretching is discussed in greater detail on p. 424.)

BOX 9-1

Sequence for Basic Massage

Four initial methods are used on each part of the body:
1. Gliding
2. Kneading
3. Compression
4. Oscillation or percussion, depending on the body area

These four methods form the basis of therapeutic massage. Once mastered, they become the foundation for palpation assessment. Each method, whether used alone or in combination with therapeutic intervention methods, can be adjusted to create reflexive or mechanical change in the body.

Basic Sequence

The following basic sequence is performed on each body area.
1. Gliding: Use four strokes to cover the area. The first stroke is light and superficial. The second stroke is slower and deeper and moves the skin. The third stroke is progressively slower and deeper to access muscle layers. The fourth stroke is superficial again.
2. Kneading: Cover the area three times, with each application becoming slower and lifting more tissue. Make sure to use a broad base and do not pinch. Identify areas where compression plus movement is better than kneading.
3. Compression: Cover the area three times, with each application becoming slower and deeper. Use a broad base of the whole hand, double hand, forearm, or leg. To replace kneading, compress tissue away from bone and have the client move the joint below (distal to) the pressure. Move the joint back and forth or in small circles.
4. Oscillation or percussion: Apply the appropriate method to the area for about 30 to 60 seconds.
5. Repeat gliding (step 1).

Appropriate sanitation, draping, and body mechanics are used consistently.

The following example protocol is one way to approach a massage sequence. The protocol is a combination of the positioning and applications described in the chapter text. Address each area using the glide—knead—compression—oscillation or percussion—glide sequence, unless an alteration is noted. Use this written protocol in combination with the photo example and the example on the DVD that accompanies this book. There are additional examples of massage application on the Evolve site as well as the written protocol so that it can be printed and used during practice.

Example Protocol

Client lies on the stomach (prone).
Use bolster under ankles (possibly under abdomen as well).
Right side back from top of gluteus to top of shoulder blade
Left side back from top of gluteus to top of shoulder blade
Left and right side glutes with the applications

Turn client on left side.
Use bolster as needed.
Right upper arm
Right lower arm
Hand
Left upper arm
Left lower arm
Hand
Right upper shoulder
Right side of the neck
Right side of the head

Move to legs.
Left inner thigh
Left calf
Left foot
Right outer thigh
Right calf
Right foot

Turn client on right side.
Use bolster as needed.
Left upper arm
Left lower arm
Hand
Right upper arm
Right lower arm
Hand
Left upper shoulder
Left side of the neck
Left side of the head

Move to legs.
Right inner thigh
Right calf
Right foot
Left outer thigh
Left calf
Left foot

Turn client on back (supine).
Use bolster under knees and head.
Left upper thigh
Right upper thigh
Abdomen
Left chest
Right chest

Wash or sanitize hands.
Face
Have client move to a seated position (you may have to assist some clients).
Bilateral upper shoulders

Also see the General Protocol on p. 335.

PROFICIENCY EXERCISE 9-8

1. *Put a towel over toothpicks laid in a haphazard fashion. Use fingertip friction to line up all the toothpicks.*
2. *Get a piece of rope ½ inch in diameter. Use friction to separate the fibers of the rope.*
3. *Access as many surface areas of the musculotendinous junction as possible. Gently friction across the grain of the fibers using the fingers, palm, and ulnar side of the elbow.*
4. *Using palmar, forearm, leg, or foot compression on larger muscle groups, combine passive and active joint movement (see the following section) to design a massage session.*

BOX 9-2

Taylor's Principles for the Application of Massage Techniques

1. Be specific.
2. Be mindful of patterns of "too much" and "not enough."
3. Position the client purposefully.
4. Stabilize the body so that only the focused target area is affected.
5. You may move the area (client passive) or may cooperate in the effort with the client (client active).
6. Be sure the force and exertion are gradual and vary with the demand.
7. Remember that the purpose is to lengthen shortened tissue and stimulate weakened muscles.
8. You are a facilitator in the process.
9. Make sure the application is slow and purposeful.
10. Repeat the movement two or three times but not to fatigue.

A working knowledge of the proprioceptive interaction between the prime mover (muscle shortening) and the antagonist (muscle elongating), as well as bodywide reflex patterns, is necessary to understand and implement massage techniques. With this knowledge, the massage practitioner can choose methods that provide specific information to the neuromuscular mechanism about current function, encouraging a reset to the more normal neutral state, which allows the optimal range of functioning. The neuromuscular mechanism makes adjustments based on the information it receives. If the information is clear and accurate, the muscles operate as designed; if the information is unclear, incorrect, or inconsistent, imbalances can occur.

For example, if a client spends the day talking on the phone, holding the phone with the shoulder, the lateral neck flexors and shoulder elevators are in constant contraction (tight, short, concentric contraction), whereas the other side of the neck is in constant extension (taut, long, eccentric). An adaptation takes place, and when the neck muscles are used, painful resistance occurs to any use other than that allowed by the

new reset position. This type of interaction is responsible for most muscle discomfort or reduced functioning.

Muscle imbalances result because the body adapts to a different muscle spindle set point and a new muscle resting length (usually shortened). Massage techniques can provide clearer neurologic information so that the body can restore optimal or as close to optimal function as possible. This allows the body's homeostatic mechanism to restore a neutral mode.

All the massage manipulations described previously affect proprioception reflexively but usually have a general, nonspecific effect. In this section you will learn ways to deliver accurate, specific information to the neuromuscular system that supports normal functioning. The difference is similar to providing a general announcement to a group of people (massage manipulations) and calling out individuals' names and delivering a message (massage techniques).

Joint Movement

To understand joint movement, you must first understand the joint. A simplified review is included here. Students are encouraged to consult anatomy and physiology resources for further clarification and descriptions of individual joints (Figure 9-31).

How Joints Work

Joints allow us to move. Joint position and velocity receptors inform the central nervous system where and how the body is positioned in gravity and how fast it is moving. These sensory data are the major determining factors for muscle motor tone patterns.

Joint movement techniques focus on the *synovial*, or freely movable, joints in the body (see Chapter 3). To a lesser extent, the joints of the vertebral column, hand, and foot are also considered, as are other joints, such as the facet joints of the ribs, the sacroiliac joint, and the sternoclavicular joint. These joints are not directly influenced by muscles, but rather move through indirect muscle action.

We can control some joint movements voluntarily; we can move our limbs through various motions, such as flexion, extension, abduction, adduction, and rotation. These are referred to as *physiologic movements,* or osteokinematic movements. For normal physiologic movement, other types of movements (*accessory movements,* or arthrokinematic movements) must occur as a result of the inherent laxity, or joint play, that exists in each joint. This laxity allows the ends of the bones to slide, roll, or spin smoothly on each other inside the joint capsule. These essential movements occur during movement of the joint and are not under voluntary control.

Comparing a Joint to a Door Hinge. A good example of joint motion is found on a door. The hinge holds the door both to the casing and away from the casing. For the door to open and close efficiently *(osteokinematic movement),* the space between the door and the door casing must be maintained and the fit must be correct. If the fit of the door in the door casing is incorrect or if the space is not maintained, the door will not

Text continued on p. 308.

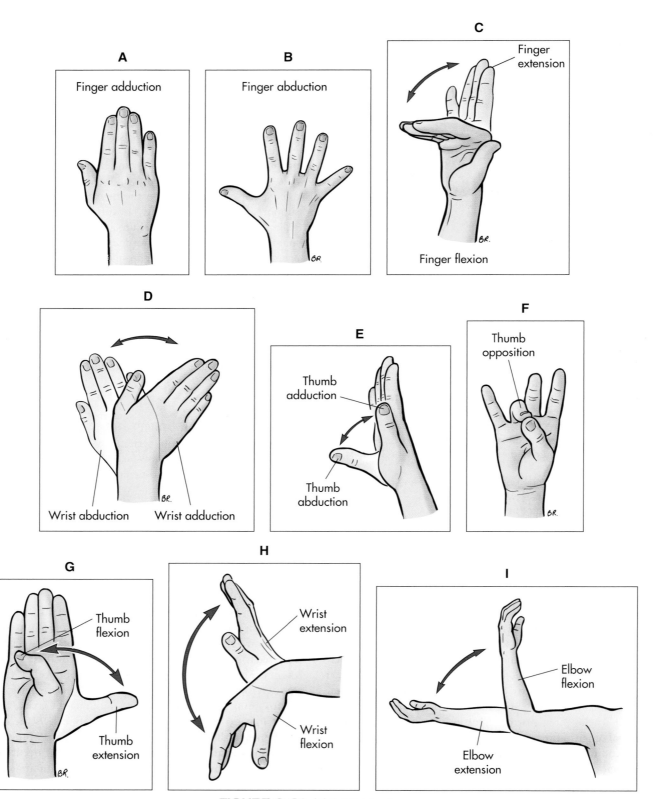

FIGURE 9-31 Joint movements.

J

Forearm pronation

K

Forearm supination

L

Shoulder elevation

M

Shoulder depression

N

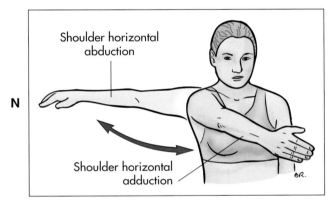

Shoulder horizontal abduction

Shoulder horizontal adduction

O

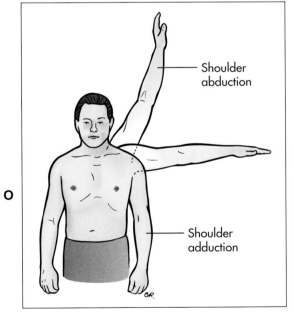

Shoulder abduction

Shoulder adduction

P

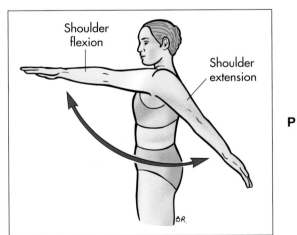

Shoulder flexion

Shoulder extension

FIGURE 9-31, cont'd

Continued

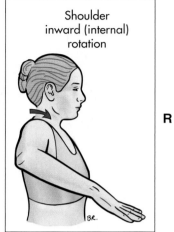

Q — Shoulder outward (external) rotation

R — Shoulder inward (internal) rotation

S — Toe extension / Toe flexion

Toe adduction / Toe abduction

T, U — Ankle inversion / Ankle eversion

V — Ankle dorsiflexion

W — Ankle plantar flexion

FIGURE 9-31, cont'd

X

Knee
flexion

Knee
extension

Y

Hip
abduction

Hip
adduction

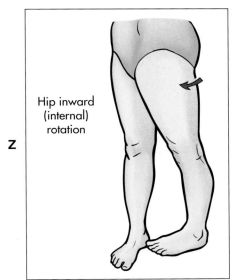

Z

Hip inward
(internal)
rotation

AA

Hip outward
(external)
rotation

BB

Hip
flexion

Hip
extension

Hip
hyperextension

CC

Trunk
hyperextension

Trunk
extension

Trunk
flexion

FIGURE 9-31, cont'd

Continued

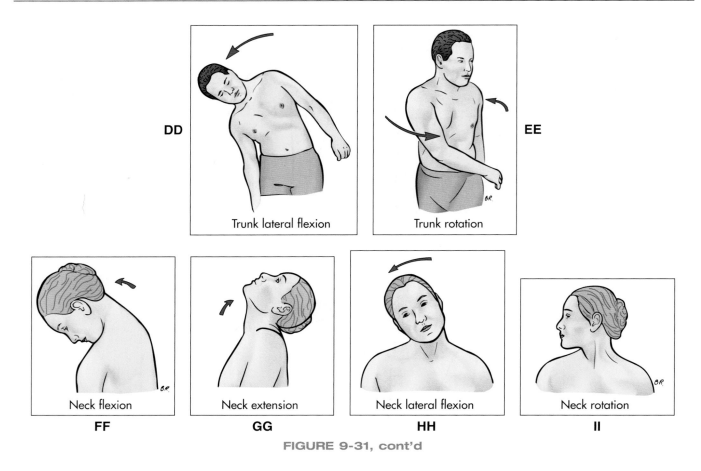

FIGURE 9-31, cont'd

open and close correctly. In the body, ligaments act as the hinges.

The door hinge must be oiled. In the joint, the synovial membrane secretes synovial fluid, produced on demand by joint movement. If a joint does not move or is not moved, it will lock up like a rusty door hinge, and movement will be restricted or lost.

If you look closely at a door hinge, you will notice the space around the pin in the hinge. If you move the hinge back and forth (not swing the door), the hinge and pin mechanism moves a little (arthrokinematic movement). This little movement can be likened to joint play. If the ligaments and connective tissue that make up the joint capsule are not firm enough to maintain joint space, the joint play is lost. If the capsule is too tight, joint play is lost as well. Muscles around a joint can shorten, pulling the bone ends together and affecting joint play.

If the ligaments and joint capsule are not pliable, flexibility is lost. If the ligaments and joint capsule do not support the joint, the fit is disrupted. Muscle contraction may pull the joint out of alignment. Muscle groups that flex and adduct the joints are about 30% stronger and have more mass than the extensors and abductors. If the body uses muscle contraction to stabilize a joint, the uneven pull between flexors and extensors and adductors and abductors disturbs the fit of the bones at the joint.

Limitations on Joint Movement. Joints have various degrees of range of motion. Anatomic, physiologic, and pathologic barriers to motion exist. A barrier is a point of resistance and can feel hard, such as when bone contacts bone or during binding, when soft tissue is short.

Anatomic barriers are determined by the shape and fit of the bones at the joint. The anatomic barrier is seldom reached because the possibility of injury is greatest in this position. Instead, the body protects the joint by establishing physiologic barriers.

Physiologic barriers are the result of the limits in range of motion imposed by protective nerve and sensory function to support optimal function. The sensation at the barrier is soft and pliable.

An adaptation in a physiologic barrier that causes the protective function to limit instead of support optimal functioning is called a pathologic barrier. Pathologic barriers often are manifested as stiffness, pain, or a "catch."

When massage therapists use joint movement techniques, they must remain within the physiologic barriers. If a pathologic barrier exists that limits motion, massage techniques are used to gently and slowly encourage the joint to increase the limits of the range of motion to the physiologic barrier.

Joint End-Feel. When a normal joint is taken to its physiologic limit, usually still a bit more movement is possible, a sort of springiness in the joint. This type of joint end-feel is called a *soft end-feel.* When a joint is restricted or a muscle shortened by a pathologic barrier, resulting in reduction of the range of motion, movement is always limited in some direction. As the limit is reached and exceeded, comfortable movement is no longer possible. In the case of abnormal restriction, the limit does not have any spring, as is found at a physiologic barrier. Rather, similar to a jammed door or drawer, the joint is fixed at the barrier, and any attempt to take it farther causes discomfort and is a distinctly "binding" or leathery feel. A distinct jamming rather than springy sensation is called a *hard end-feel.*

Effects of Joint Movement Methods

Joint movement is effective because it provides a means of controlled stimulation to the joint mechanoreceptors. Movement initiates muscle tension readjustment through the reflex center of the spinal cord and lower brain centers. As positions change, the supported movement gives the nervous system an entirely different set of signals to process. The joint sensory receptors can learn not to be so hypersensitive. As a result, the protective spasm and movement restriction may lessen.

Joint movement also encourages lubrication of the enhanced joint and contributes an important addition to the lymphatic and venous circulations. Much of the pumping action that moves these fluids in the vessels results from compression against the lymph and blood vessels during joint movement and muscle contraction. The tendons, ligaments, and joint capsule are warmed from the movement. This mechanical effect helps keep these tissues pliable.

Figure 9-31 shows the direction and range of motion for each joint. Normal joint movements are often indicated by the degree of movement available, with the anatomic, or neutral, position labeled 0 degrees. For example, the elbow is said to be able to flex 106 degrees and extend 180 degrees from neutral. Wrist flexion is 90 degrees and wrist extension 70 degrees from neutral. The degrees of movement have been left off the figure to avoid creating an expectation of what normal should be. Instead, the "normal" range of motion for each joint should be identified for each individual. For additional study, consult a comprehensive anatomy and physiology book for the degrees of movement for joints.

Remember that each person is unique, and many factors influence available range of motion. Just because a joint does not have the textbook range of motion does not mean that what is displayed is abnormal. Abnormality is indicated by nonoptimal function. This can be either a limit or an exaggeration in the "textbook normal" range of motion. Study Figure 9-31 carefully. When working with clients, use it as a guide for moving each joint through its full range of motion, always being mindful to go slowly and stay within the client's comfort limits. (A video of a joint movement sequence is presented on the DVD.)

Types of Joint Movement Methods

9-4

Joint movement involves moving the jointed areas within the client's physiologic limits of range of motion.

The two types of joint movement are active joint movement and passive joint movement. In **active joint movement,** the client moves the joint by active contraction of muscle groups. The two variations of active joint movement are **active assisted movement,** which occurs when both the client and the massage practitioner move the area, and **active resistive movement,** which occurs when the client actively moves the joint against resistance provided by the massage practitioner.

In **passive joint movement,** the client's muscles remain relaxed and the massage practitioner moves the joint with no assistance from the client. When doing passive joint movement, the massage practitioner should feel for the soft or hard end-feel of the joint range of motion. This is an important evaluation.

Whether active or passive, joint movements are always done within the comfortable limits of the client's range of motion.

The client's body must always be stabilized; only the joint being addressed should be allowed to move. Occasionally the entire limb is moved to allow for coordinated interaction among all the joints of the area, but the rest of the body is stabilized. It is essential to move slowly, because quick changes or abrupt moves may cause the muscles to initiate protective contractions.

Nerves stimulate muscles to contract, moving the joints. Nerves respond to sensory stimulation. If the signal is not quite strong enough, the muscle may tense but not contract; this is called *facilitation.* A facilitated area responds to a lower intensity sensory stimulation. Sensory stimulation must reach a certain intensity before activation occurs; this is called the *threshold.* If a threshold sensory signal does not occur, the nerve stays activated, waiting to contract the muscle and discharge the tension.

All massage professionals have had to deal with a leg or an arm that is extremely stiff, even though the client thinks it is relaxed. Most practitioners instruct the client to relax the muscles, or they use some other ineffective statement, such as, "Now, just let me do it." It is important to recognize that the client cannot let go of the tension in the muscles because of the facilitation of the nerves and lack of threshold stimulus.

Systems that incorporate progressive relaxation recognize that a muscle relaxes best if it contracts first. Active resistive range of motion provides a mechanism to contract muscles, discharge the nervous system, and then allow the normal relaxation phase to take over. A good approach is to have the client use active joint movement, pressing the area to be moved against stabilizing pressure provided by the massage practitioner. The practitioner then shakes or rocks the area to relax it.

Caution in Working with Joints

Joint-specific work, including any type of high-velocity thrust manipulation, is beyond the scope of practice of the beginning massage professional. Because of the interplay among the joint proprioceptors, muscle tone, innervation of the joint, and surrounding muscles by the same nerve pattern, any damage to a joint can cause long-term problems. Working within the physiologic ranges of motion for the particular client is within the scope of practice of the massage professional. Specific corrective procedures for pathologic range of motion are best applied in a supervised health care setting.

Relationship of Joint Movement to Lengthening and Stretching Methods

Joint movement becomes part of the application of muscle energy techniques to lengthen muscles and of stretching methods to elongate connective tissues. For this reason, the massage professional should concentrate on developing the ability to use joint movement efficiently and effectively.

Applying Joint Movement Methods

Hand placement with joint movement is very important. Make sure the area is not squeezed, pinched, or restricted in its movement pattern. One hand should be placed close to the joint to act as a stabilizer and allow evaluation. The other hand is placed at the distal end of the bone; this is the hand that actually provides the movement. Proper use of body mechanics is essential when using joint movement. The stabilizing hand must remain in contact with the client and must be placed near the affected joint.

As an alternative method of positioning the stabilizing hand, the jointed area can be moved without stabilization while the massage practitioner observes where the client's body moves most in response to the range of motion action. The stabilizing hand then is placed at this point.

Avoid working cross-body. Usually, the hand closest to the joint is the stabilizing hand. The actual movement comes from the massage practitioner's whole body, not from the shoulder, elbow, or wrist. The movements are rhythmic, smooth, slow, and controlled.

Before joint movement begins, the moving hand lifts and leans back to produce the slight traction necessary to put a small stretch on the joint capsule. If this is not done, the technique is much less effective. When tractioning has been mastered and the joint is moved simultaneously, the size of the movement becomes smaller and the effectiveness increases. It is neither necessary nor desirable to have the client's limbs flailing about in the air (Figure 9-32).

Active Range of Motion. In active range of motion, the client moves the area without any type of interaction by the massage practitioner. This is a good assessment method and should be used before and after any type of joint work, because it pro-

FIGURE 9-32 Examples of joint movement. **A,** Neck. **B,** Shoulder joint. One hand stabilizes at the shoulder joint. **C,** The other hand produces a slight traction to the shoulder joint and moves the shoulder through circumduction range of motion. (*Circumduction* is a circular movement of a jointed area.) **D,** Elbow joints. The stabilizing hand holds above elbow while the moving hand produces a slight traction and moves the joint through flexion and extension. Supination and pronation can also be achieved. **E,** Wrist joints. the stabilizing hand holds below the wrist while the moving hand produces a slight traction and moves the joint through circumduction. **F,** Hip joint. The stabilizing hand holds above the hip while the moving hand and arm produce a slight traction and move the joint through circumduction.

FIGURE 9-32 cont'd G, Hip joint (alternate position). The stabilizing hand holds at the opposite anterosuperior iliac spine while the moving hand moves the hip through flexion and extension. No traction is produced in this position. **H,** Pelvis. The stabilizing hand and arm hold the legs at the calf. **I,** The moving arm and hand move the pelvis to a side-lying figure-eight pattern. **J,** Knee. The stabilizing hand holds above the knee while the moving hand produces a slight traction and moves the joint through flexion and extension. **K,** Ankle. The stabilizing hand holds above the ankle. **L,** The moving hand produces a slight traction and moves the joint through circumduction.

vides information about the limits of range of motion and the improvement after the work is complete. Active range of motion is also great to teach as a self-help tool. As mentioned previously, the two variations of active range of motion methods are active assisted range of motion and active resistive range of motion.

Active Assisted Range of Motion. In active assisted range of motion, the client moves the joint through the range of motion and the massage practitioner helps or assists the movement. This approach is very useful in cases of weakness or pain with movement. The action remains within the comfortable limits of movement for the client. The focus is to create movement within the joint capsule, encouraging synovial fluid lubrication to warm and soften connective tissue and support muscle function.

Active Resistive Range of Motion. In active resistive range of motion, the massage practitioner firmly grasps and holds the end of the bone just distal to the affected joint. The massage practitioner leans back slightly to place a small traction on the limb to take up the slack in the tissue. Then the practitioner instructs the client to push slowly against a stabilizing hand or arm while moving the joint through its entire range. A tap or light slap against the limb to begin the movement works well to focus the client's attention.

Another method is to stabilize the entire circumference of the limb and instruct the client to pull gently or move the area. The massage practitioner's job is to maintain a gentle traction to prevent slack in the tissue, keep the movement slow, and give the client something to push or pull against, discharging the nervous system so that the area can relax.

The counterforce applied by the massage practitioner does not exceed the pushing or pulling action of the client, but rather matches it and then allows movement.

After a form of active range of motion has been completed, the client's body is more apt to accept passive range of motion.

Passive Range of Motion. If a client is paralyzed or very ill, only passive range of motion or joint movement may be possible. Some clients do not wish to participate in active joint movement and prefer to take a very passive role during the massage. Client participation is not necessary.

PROFICIENCY EXERCISE 9-9

Using the Basic Massage Sequence on p. 330, incorporate joint movement into the general sequence. At each body area use joint movement to assess for range of motion before using glide, knead, compress, oscillate, and rhythmic movement. Then use active and passive joint movement as each area is finished to assess for changes.

PROFICIENCY EXERCISE 9-10

1. *Using Figure 9-31 for reference, move each of your joints, using a variety of speeds, one at a time, through the normal range of motion. Notice the difference when you move slowly.*
2. *Pretend that a piece of plastic wrap is a joint. Hold one end tightly in your "stabilizing" hand. Now move the plastic wrap around, but do not stretch it or put drag on the "tissue." Use your "moving hand" to traction the plastic wrap. Pull on it as far as it will go without stretching the tissue. Pretend to assess range of motion from this point and feel the difference. Last, pull the plastic wrap just a little more. Feel the pliability and do the joint movement from this position. Feel for the difference in effect.*
3. *Design and perform a massage incorporating joint movement using each of the basic flow patterns. As always, remain aware of the variation in depth of pressure, drag, direction, speed, rhythm, frequency, and duration.*

Because the protective system of the joints does not like to be out of control, it takes time to prepare the body for passive range of motion. Shaking, rocking, and the active joint movement sequence previously described work well for this purpose.

To perform passive range of motion, instruct the client to relax the area by letting it lie heavy in your hands. Slowly and rhythmically move the joint through a comfortable range of motion for the jointed area. Repeat the action three or more times, increasing the limits of the range of motion as the muscles relax (Proficiency Exercise 9-9).

Suggested Sequence for Joint Movement Methods

When incorporating joint movement into the massage, follow these basic suggestions:

- If possible, perform active joint movement first. Assess range of motion by having the client move the area without participation by the practitioner.
- Have the client move the area against a stabilizing force supplied by the practitioner to increase the intensity of the signals from the contracting muscles, which discharges the nervous system.
- Incorporate any or all of the previously discussed massage methods.
- After the tissue is warm and the nervous system relaxed, do the passive range of motion/joint movement.
- During a massage session, strive to move every joint approximately three times. Each time, take up any slack in the tissues and gently encourage an increase in the range of motion.
- Joint movement should be incorporated into every massage when possible (Proficiency Exercise 9-10).

Muscle Energy Methods and Proprioceptive Neuromuscular Facilitation: Techniques to Lengthen Neurologically Shortened Muscles

Muscle energy methods emerged from the osteopathic profession. Dr. T. J. Ruddy developed a technique he called *resistive induction.* Dr. Fred K. Mitchell is the acknowledged father of the system now known as muscle energy technique. He built on Dr. Ruddy's method, turning it into a whole body approach.[7] Dr. Karel Lewit, author of *Manipulative Therapy in Rehabilitation of the Locomotor System,* described the importance of methods that use postisometric relaxation.[8] Dr. Leon

Chaitow, author of many textbooks on manual techniques, synthesized these gentle methods, which fall within the scope of practice of therapeutic massage when used for general body normalization.

Proprioceptive neuromuscular facilitation techniques grew out of physical therapy approaches during the 1950s. The first book on the subject, written by Margaret Knott and Dorothy Voss, was *Proprioceptive Neuromuscular Facilitation.*[9] This system, which was formalized as a rehabilitation method for spinal cord injury and stroke, involved the use of maximal contraction and rotary diagonal movement patterns to re-educate the nervous system. In recent years, massage professionals have begun to use pieces of the system to enhance muscle lengthening and stretching.

The diagonal movement patterns of **proprioceptive neuromuscular facilitation (PNF)** incorporate cross-body movement, which is used in repatterning for children born with various types of damage to the motor areas of the brain. Popularized as *cross crawl,* the technique causes the left and right brain hemispheres to function simultaneously by moving one leg and the opposite arm into flexion and adduction to cross the midline of the body. This stimulates the contralateral reflexes. The same movement is repeated with the other leg and arm. These types of movements reflexively stimulate the gait or walking pattern and are a valuable addition to any massage system. Other names for approaches based on muscle energy techniques include *manual resistance techniques, contract-relax-antagonist-contract (CRAC),* and *active isolated stretching.* There are certainly other names for methods that involve contraction of the muscles in various patterns followed by lengthening of the muscles.

The main differences among common methods are the origin of the approach, the intensity of the muscle contraction, and the specificity of the approach. Massage techniques as described in this text are incorporated as nonspecific aspects of a general massage. However, adaptive methods are used if massage outcomes are based on condition management or therapeutic change (Chapter 5). Friction is an adaptive method used only if changes in the tissue are desired. Muscle energy methods are also adaptive and are used specifically to address shortened muscles and support optimal muscle/soft tissue and joint function. Only the methods applicable to general massage are presented here, but the system of muscle energy methods has much more to offer. A diligent student of therapeutic massage should pursue additional training at more advanced levels. Most of the information in the following section has been adapted from Dr. Chaitow's books and workshop notes. A good text to study is *Muscle Energy Techniques* (third edition) by Leon Chaitow (Churchill Livingstone, 2006).

Muscle Energy Techniques

9-5

Muscle energy techniques involve a voluntary contraction of the client's muscles in a specific and controlled direction, at varying levels of intensity, against a specific counterforce applied by the massage practitioner. Muscle energy procedures have a variety of applications and are considered active techniques in which the client contributes the corrective force. The amount of effort may vary from a small muscle twitch to a maximal muscle contraction. The duration may be a fraction of a second to several seconds. All contractions begin and end slowly, gradually building to the desired intensity. No jerking is done in the movement.

The focus of muscle energy techniques is to stimulate the nervous system to allow a more normal muscle resting length. The term lengthening is used to describe this process, because lengthening is more of a neurologic response that allows the muscles to stop contracting and to relax. Stretching is more correctly defined as a mechanical force applied to elongate connective tissue. However, the terms are used interchangeably, which can create confusion.

Muscle energy techniques focus on specific muscles or muscle groups. It is important to be able to position muscles so that the proximal muscle attachment (origin) and the distal attachment (insertion) are either close together or in a lengthening phase with the attachments separated. Study muscle charts until you understand the configuration of the muscle structures and practice isolating as many muscles as possible, keeping in mind that proper positioning is very important. When practicing, make sure the muscles can be isolated whether the client is supine, prone, or in a side-lying or seated position (Figure 9-33).

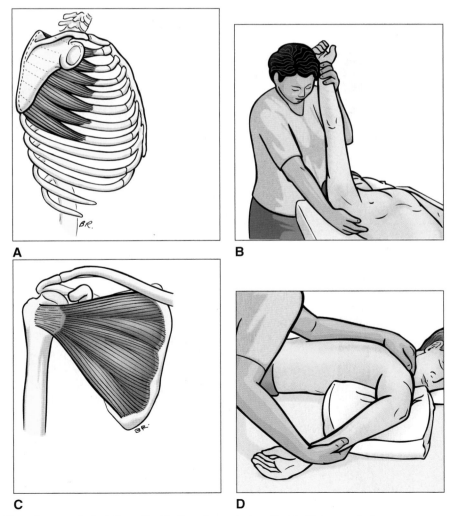

A **B** **C** **D**

FIGURE 9-33 Positions for muscle isolation. **A, B,** Serratus anterior. **C, D,** Subscapularis.

Continued

FIGURE 9-33, cont'd E, F, Latissimus dorsi. **G, H,** Deltoid. **I, J,** Biceps and brachialis.

FIGURE 9-33, cont'd K, L, Triceps. **M, N,** Gluteus medius. **O, P,** Gluteus maximus and hamstrings.

FIGURE 9-33, cont'd **Q, R,** Gastrocnemius and soleus. **S, T,** Peroneus.

Counterpressure is the force applied to an area that is designed to match the effort or force exactly (isometric contraction) or partially (isotonic contraction). The person providing the resistance (the massage practitioner) can apply this holding force with one or both hands, or it can be applied against an immovable object or against gravity where appropriate. The response to the method is specific to a certain muscle or muscle group, referred to as the target muscle (or muscles).

Types of Muscle Contractions. The massage practitioner uses three types of muscle contraction to activate muscle energy

techniques: *isometric contraction, isotonic contraction,* and *multiple isotonic contractions.*

In an isometric contraction, the distance between the proximal and distal attachments (origin and insertion) of the target muscle is maintained at a constant length. A fixed tension develops in the target muscle as the client contracts the muscle against an equal counterforce applied by the massage practitioner; this prevents shortening of the muscle. In this contraction the effort of the muscle or group of muscles is exactly matched by a counterpressure so that no movement occurs, only effort.

In an isotonic contraction, the effort of the target muscle or muscles is not quite matched by the counterpressure, which allows a degree of resisted movement. With a concentric isotonic contraction, the massage practitioner applies a counterforce but allows the client to move the proximal and distal attachments of the target muscle together against the pressure. In an eccentric isotonic contraction (more accurately, an "action," since contraction specifically describes a shortening, and eccentric action results in lengthening), the massage practitioner applies a counterforce but allows the client to move the jointed area so that the proximal and distal attachments of the target muscle separate as the muscle lengthens against the pressure.

Multiple isotonic contractions require the client to move the joint through a full range of motion against partial resistance applied by the massage practitioner.

Strength of Contraction. Muscle energy techniques usually do not use the client's full contraction strength. With most isometric work, the contraction should start at about 25% of the strength of the muscle. Subsequent contractions can involve progressively greater degrees of effort but never more than 50% of the available strength.

Many experts use only about 10% of the available strength in muscles treated in this way, and they find that they can increase effectiveness by using longer periods of contraction. Pulsed contractions (a rapid series of repetitions) using minimal strength are also effective.

Using coordinated breathing to enhance particular directions of muscular effort is helpful. During muscle energy applications, all muscular effort is enhanced by inhaling as the effort is made and exhaling during the lengthening phase.

Eye positions can be used as well (Figure 9-34). Looking down activates flexors, looking up activates extensors, when looking left all muscles used to turn left are activated, looking right all muscles used to turn right are activated.

Neurophysiologic Principles. Two neurophysiologic principles explain the effect of the techniques as a result of physiologic laws, not of mechanical force, as in stretching. These principles are postisometric relaxation (PIR) and reciprocal inhibition (RI). Recent research indicates that the physiologic mechanism for benefit may not be directly related to PIR or RI. Rather, any type of muscle activation seems to increase tolerance to stretching by alternating perceived pain sensation. In addition, some evidence indicates that the connective tissue component of the muscle is influenced, allowing for changes in tissue length.[10]

Even though the scientific rationale for benefit is changing, the process of performing muscle energy applications remains basically the same; these are described in the following pages. At the end of the sections, recommendations for applications based on research are provided.

Postisometric Relaxation. PIR, which occurs after isometric contraction of a muscle, results from the activity of the Golgi tendon bodies. This response is an aspect of methods called contract/relax (CR), hold/relax (HR). In the brief latent period of 10 seconds or so after such a contraction the muscle can be lengthened painlessly, farther than it could before the contraction. After an isometric contraction (which loads the Golgi tendon organs and the musculotendinous junction and reflexively inhibits the extrafusal fibers of the muscle spindles), a brief period ensues during which nerve impulses to the target muscle are inhibited. This period is called the *refractory state;* it allows the target muscle to be lengthened passively to its comfort barrier. The comfort barrier is the first point

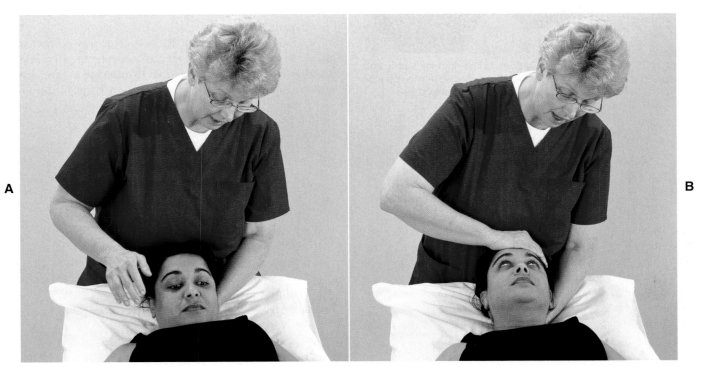

A   **B**

FIGURE 9-34 Eye positions. **A,** Eyes down facilitates flexors. **B,** Eyes up facilitates extension and inhibits flexors.

Continued

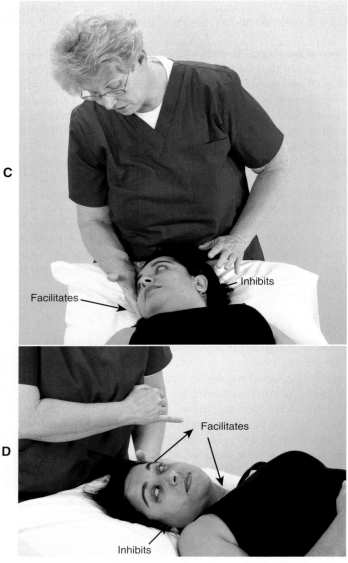

C

Inhibits

Facilitates

D

Facilitates

Inhibits

FIGURE 9-34, cont'd C, Eyes to the right facilitates and opposing muscles are inhibited. **D,** Eyes moved left to the side inhibits previously facilitated muscle and facilitates those previously inhibited.

of resistance short of the client perceiving any discomfort at either the physiologic or pathologic barrier. The isometric contraction involves minimal effort lasting 7 to 10 seconds. Repetitions continue until no further gain is noted. The procedure for PIR is as follows (Figure 9-35):

1. Lengthen the target muscle to the comfort barrier. Then back off slightly.
2. Tense the target muscle for 7 to 10 seconds.
3. Stop the contraction and lengthen the target muscle.
4. Repeat steps 1 through 3 until the normal full resting length is obtained.

Reciprocal Inhibition. RI takes place when a muscle contracts, causing its antagonist to relax to allow for more normal movement. Generally, isometric contraction of the antagonist of a shortened target muscle allows the muscle to relax and to be taken to a new resting length. Such contractions usually begin in the midrange rather than near the barrier of resistance and last 7 to 10 seconds. Reciprocal inhibition relaxes a target muscle as the tension increases in its antagonist. This response works through the central nervous system, which cannot allow the prime movers and the antagonists to tighten at the same time in this reflex arc pattern. The procedure for RI is as follows (Figure 9-36):

1. Isolate the target muscles by putting them in passive contraction (massage practitioner moves the proximal and distal attachments of the muscles together using joint positioning).
2. Contract the antagonist muscle group (the muscle in extension).
3. Stop the contraction and slowly bring the target muscle into a lengthened state, stopping at resistance.
4. Place the target muscle slightly into passive contraction again.
5. Repeat steps 2 through 4 until the normal full resting length is obtained.

Activating muscles using RI is a great way to soften a muscle so that it can be massaged at deeper levels. All massage practitioners know what it is like to massage a hard, tense muscle, especially when trying to get to tissue under that

A

B

FIGURE 9-35 Procedure for postisometric relaxation (PIR)/contract-and-relax techniques targeting hamstring. **A,** Hamstring contracts. **B,** Relax and lengthen hamstring.

FIGURE 9-35, cont'd **C,** Latissimus dorsi contracts target muscle. **D,** Relax and lengthen latissimus dorsi.

FIGURE 9-36 Procedure for initiating reciprocal inhibition (RI)/antagonist contraction. **A,** RI/antagonist contraction (hamstrings)—target quadriceps. **B,** Lengthen quadricep. **C,** Identify antagonist muscles (lateral neck flexors) and contract antagonist. **D,** Lengthen target muscles.

FIGURE 9-37 Procedure for contract-relax-antagonist-contract (CRAC). **A,** Contract target muscles, and then relax. **B,** Contract-antagonist quadriceps. **C,** Lengthen hamstring.

muscle. The following procedure reflexively creates a soft muscle, which in turn makes massage much easier:

1. Isolate the target muscle or muscle group into passive contraction.
2. Place the hand that will massage the "soft muscle" on the target muscle. Place the other hand or some other stabilizing object on the antagonist muscle group (the one that is stretched out at this point).
3. Have the client actively contract the antagonist muscles against the stabilization. The target muscle will be inhibited reciprocally and will become a soft muscle, which will be easier to massage, and the massage practitioner will be able to reach the deeper areas.

Combined Methods: Contract-Relax-Antagonist-Contract.
CRAC, or contract and relax and antagonist contract, can be used to enhance the lengthening effects. The procedure for CRAC is as follows (Figure 9-37):

1. Position the target muscles as in contract and relax procedures.
2. Lengthen the target muscle to the barrier. Then back off slightly.
3. Contract the target muscle for 7 to 10 seconds and then relax.
4. Contract the antagonist (reciprocal inhibition).
5. Stop the contraction of the antagonist.

6. Lengthen the target muscle to a more normal resting length.

Pulsed Muscle Energy. Pulsed muscle energy procedures involve engaging the comfort barrier and using small, resisted contractions (usually 20 in 10 seconds); this introduces mechanical pumping as well as PIR or RI, depending on the muscles used. The procedure for pulsed muscle energy is as follows (Figure 9-38):

1. Isolate the target muscle by putting it into a passive contraction.
2. Apply counterpressure for the contraction.
3. Instruct the client to contract the target muscle rapidly in very small movements for about 20 repetitions. Go to step 4 or use this variation: maintain the position, but switch the counterpressure location to the opposite side and have the client contract the antagonist muscles for 20 repetitions.
4. Slowly lengthen the target muscle.
5. Repeat steps 2 to 4 until the normal full resting length is obtained.

NOTE: All contracting and resisting efforts should start and finish gently.

Direct Applications. In some circumstances the client does not wish to or cannot participate actively in the massage. The

A

B

FIGURE 9-38 Pulsed muscle energy method targeting the hamstring.

principles of muscle energy techniques can still be used through direct manipulation of the spindle cells or Golgi tendons. Pushing muscle fibers together in the direction of the fibers in the belly of a muscle weakens the muscle by working with the spindle cells. As the fibers of the muscle are pushed together, the spindle cells (which sense muscle length) determine that the muscle is too short. The proprioceptive response is to relax the muscle fibers so that the muscle can be comfortable in its chosen position. Pushing muscle fibers together in the belly of the muscle is a way to relieve a muscle cramp. This is sometimes called **approximation.**

Separating the muscle fibers in the belly of the muscle in the direction of the fibers strengthens the muscle. When this occurs, the spindle cells determine that the muscle is too long; they signal the brain's proprioceptive intelligence to shorten the muscle so that the muscle can do the job it is supposed to do.

The same responses can be obtained by using the Golgi tendon organs, except that the manipulation of the proprioception signal cells is reversed. Manipulation of the Golgi tendon organs occurs at the ends of the muscle where it joins the tendons. To weaken the muscle, pull apart on the tendon attachments of the target muscle; this tells the body's proprioception center that tension on the tendon is excessive and the muscle should loosen to remain in balance. To strengthen the muscle, push the tendon attachments together; this signals the body that there is too little tension on the tendon (in relation to the tension within the muscle belly). The muscle, in turn, contracts.

The pressure levels used to elicit the response must be sufficient to contact the muscle fibers. Pressure that is too light does not access the proprioceptors, and excessive pressure negates the response by activating protective reflexes. Moderate pressure where the muscle itself can be palpated is most effective.

The procedure for direct manipulation of the spindle cells to initiate the relaxation and lengthening response is as follows (Figure 9-39):

1. Place the target muscle in comfortable passive extension.
2. Press the spindle cells together on the target muscle.

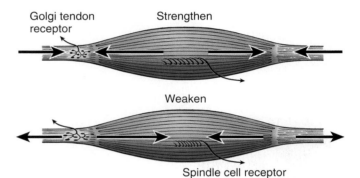

FIGURE 9-39 Proprioceptive manipulation of muscles. (Modified from Chaitow L: *Modern neuromuscular techniques,* Edinburgh, 1996, Churchill Livingstone.)

3. Pull the spindle cells apart on the antagonist muscle.
4. Lengthen the target muscle.
5. Repeat steps 2 through 4 until the normal full resting length is obtained.

Direct Manipulation of the Golgi Tendon Organs to Initiate the PIR Response. The procedure for direct manipulation of the Golgi tendon organs to initiate the PIR response is as follows (Figure 9-40):

1. Place the target muscle in comfortable passive extension.
2. Pull apart on the tendon attachments of the target muscle.
3. Push the tendon attachments together on the antagonist muscle.
4. Lengthen the target muscle.
5. Repeat steps 2 through 4 until normal full resting length is obtained.

Positional   Release/Strain-Counterstrain. Strain/counterstrain, a technique formalized by Dr. Lawrence Jones, involves the use of tender points to guide the positioning of the body into a space where the muscle tension can release on its own. The Orthobiotomy method, which grew from the foundation of strain-counterstrain, encompasses similar concepts.

FIGURE 9-40 Direct manipulation used to stimulate muscle lengthening at muscle belly. **A,** Target quadriceps—push together. **B,** Pull apart antagonist at muscle belly. **C,** Push muscle ends toward middle of antagonist muscle. **D,** Pull muscle ends apart on target muscle. **E,** Position target muscle in lengthened position. **F,** Stabilize and lengthen target muscle.

According to Dr. Chaitow, during a **positional release technique (PRT),** a muscle's spindles are influenced by methods that take them into an ease state and that theoretically allow them an opportunity to reset and reduce hypertonic status. Strain-counterstrain and other positional release methods use the slow, controlled return of distressed tissues to the position of strain as a means of offering spindles a chance to reset and thus normalize function. This is particularly effective if the spindles have inappropriately held an area in just such protective splinting.

Positional release is a more generic term used to describe these methods. Positional release methods are used on painful areas, especially recent strains, before, after, or instead of muscle energy methods. The tender points often are located in the antagonist of the tight muscle because of the diagonal balancing process the body uses to maintain an upright posture in gravity.

Repositioning of the body into the original strain (often the position of a prior injury) allows proprioceptors to reset and stop firing protective signals. By moving the body into the direc-

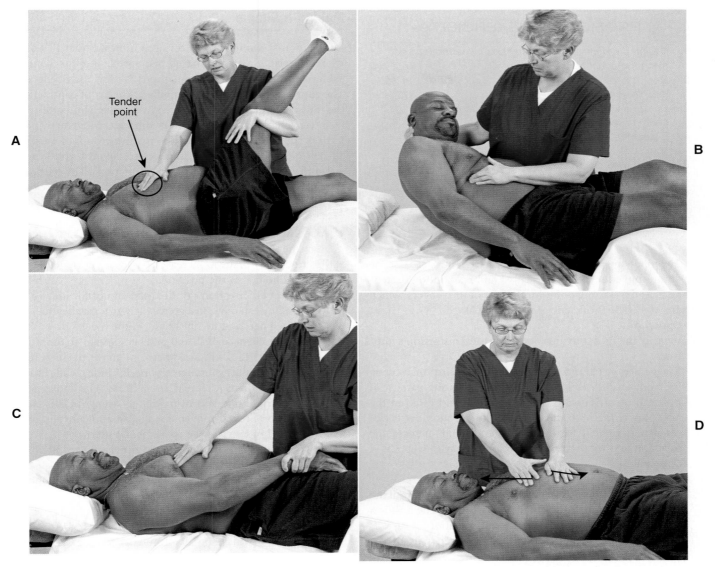

FIGURE 9-41 Procedure for generalized positional release. **A,** Identify tender points in **B** and **C** and begin to move the client into pain-relieving positions. **D,** Direct lengthening of tender area.

tion of ease (i.e., the way the body wants to go and out of the position that causes the pain), the proprioception is taken into a state of safety. Remaining in this state for a time allows the neuromuscular mechanism to reset itself. The massage practitioner then gently and slowly repositions the area into neutral.

The positioning used during positional release is a full-body process. Remember, an injury or loss of balance is a full-body experience. For this reason, areas distant to the tender point must be considered during the positioning process. The position of the feet very likely will have an effect on a tender point in the neck.

The procedure for positional release is as follows (Figure 9-41):

1. Locate the tender point.
2. Gently initiate the pain response with direct pressure. Remember, the sensation of pain is a guide.
3. Slowly position the body until the pain subsides.
4. Wait at least 30 seconds or longer until the client feels the release, lightly monitoring the tender point.
5. Slowly lengthen the muscle.

6. Repeat steps 1 through 5 until the normal full resting length is obtained.

Positional release techniques are important because they gently allow the body to reposition and restore balance. They also are highly effective ways of dealing with tender areas regardless of the pathology. Sometimes it is impossible to know why the point is tender to the touch. However, if tenderness is present, a protective muscle spasm surrounds it. Positional release is an excellent way to release these small areas of muscle spasm without causing additional pain.

Integrated Approach. Muscle energy methods can be used together or in sequence to enhance their effects. Muscle tension in one area of the body often indicates imbalance and compensation patterns in other areas of the body. Tension patterns can be self-perpetuating. Often, using an integrated approach introduces the type of information the nervous system needs to self-correct. The procedure outlined here relies on the body's innate knowledge of what is out of balance and how to restore a more normal functioning pattern.

PROFICIENCY EXERCISE 9-11

1. *Design a progressive relaxation sequence for yourself using the concept of PIR.*
2. *Design a lengthening sequence for yourself using pulsed muscle contraction.*
3. *Design a complete massage using kneading and compression on "soft muscles."*
4. *Experiment with positional release concepts to relax sore spots on your body.*
5. *Design a complete massage incorporating all of the muscle energy methods presented.*
6. *Repeat the massage sequence from step 5 using the Making It Simple pattern. Compare the results.*

The following procedure is an integrated approach. Use the position from either option A, steps 1 and 2, or option B, steps 1 and 2, as the starting point for the rest of the process, which begins at step 3 (Proficiency Exercise 9-11).

Option A
1. Identify the most obvious of the postural distortion symptoms.
2. Exaggerate the pattern by increasing the distortion, moving the body into ease. This position becomes the pattern of isolation of various muscles that will be addressed in the next part of the procedure (e.g., if the left shoulder is elevated and rotated forward, exaggerate and increase the elevation and rotation pattern). Continue with step 3.

Option B
1. Identify a painful point.
2. Use positional release to move the body into ease until the point is substantially less tender to pressure. The position of ease found becomes the pattern of isolation of various muscles that will be addressed in the next part of the procedure. Continue with step 3.

After choosing from option A or option B, continue the procedure as follows:

3. Stabilize the client in as many different directions as possible.
4. Instruct the client to move out of the pattern. Be as vague as possible and do not guide the client, because it is important for the client to identify the resistance pattern.
5. Provide resistance for the client to push or pull against.
6. Modify the resistance angle as necessary to achieve the most solid resistance pattern for the client.
7. Spend a few moments noticing when the client's breathing changes; then, while still providing modified resistance, allow the client to move through the pattern slowly.
8. When the client has achieved as much extension as he can on his own, recognize that what he has achieved is the lengthening pattern.
9. Gently increase the lengthening. If additional elongation in this position is desired, connective tissue stretching can be achieved.
10. Pay attention to what body areas become involved besides the one addressed. This is your guide to the next position.

Making It Simple

As mentioned, some current research indicates that PIR and RI mechanisms may not be as responsible for the benefit achieved using muscle energy methods as previously believed. The approaches thus can be simplified. The act of contracting the muscles appears to be involved in a movement pattern to facilitate lengthening of the short muscles. Movement patterns occur at each jointed area and involve groups of muscles all neurologically linked—prime mover, agonist and synergist, and antagonist (eccentric control function). The eye position also influences the neurologic signaling to the muscles.

The following is a combined simplified approach (Figure 9-42):
1. Assess movement patterns with passive and active joint movement and identify short tissue (the target).
2. Position short tissue in increased passively shortened position and hold it in the position.
3. Stabilize in all directions at the distal end of the area (e.g., for the elbow, stabilize just above the wrist; for the hip, just above the knee; and for the ankle, at the toes).
4. Instruct the client to push and pull back and forth for hinge joints (fingers/toes, elbows, knees) or move the area in a circle (wrist, ankle, shoulder/hip, neck, spine) while at the same time moving the eyes in a circle. The movement should be rhythmic and of moderate strength. This back and forth or circular movement against applied resistance activates all muscles in the movement pattern.
5. Slowly lengthen the target area (short tissue) to the bind (resistance barrier) and hold for a few seconds.
6. Repeat steps 3 to 5 of this sequence two or three more times.
7. Massage the target tissue, primarily using gliding, compression, and kneading, both with and against the muscle fiber direction; this manually stimulates receptors, connective tissue, and fluid. Then shake or rock the area and lengthen again.

This sequence basically uses all the muscle energy methods described.

Stretching

Stretching is a mechanical method of introducing various forces into connective tissue to elongate areas of shortening. Again, ongoing research is shifting the understanding of connective tissue structure and function in the body. How-ever, for practical application purposes, the description that follows is sufficient. Stretching affects the fiber component of connective tissue by elongating the fibers past their normal give so that they can enter the plastic range, past the existing bind. This creates either a freeing and unraveling of fibers or a small therapeutic inflammatory response that signals for change in the fibers. Stretching also affects the ground substance, warming and softening it and thereby increasing pliability.

Because fascial sheaths provide structural support, it is important to work with a sense of three-dimensional awareness, realizing that shifts in structure have more than a localized effect. Because the body supports stability before mobility

FIGURE 9-42 Making it simple. **A,** Identify short tissue. **B,** Increase passive shortening of tissue. **C, D,** Move distal joints in circle.

and compensation patterns are bodywide, changes in structure need to be balanced with either lengthening or strengthening activities that allow the body to maintain a sense of perpendicular orientation in gravity.

If the stability/mobility factor is not considered, the body's method of reacting to changes in structure is to increase muscle spasm and acute pain. This results in a decreased ability to adapt effectively to the changes introduced; it reduces the effectiveness of the methods. Stretching introduces forces of bend, torsion, and tension that mechanically affect connective tissue.

Applying Stretching

As explained previously, stretching and lengthening are different. Before stretching, the muscles usually must be lengthened or those in the area may develop protective spasms; this occurs because stretching often moves into pathologic barriers formed by connective tissue changes. The connective tissue component cannot be accessed until the muscle has been lengthened. Without stretching, any neuromuscular lengthening may be restricted by shortened connective tissue. Although lengthening without stretching is possible and often desirable, lengthening must always be done before stretching. During stretching the two methods work in conjunction. Muscle energy techniques are used to prepare muscles to stretch by activating lengthening responses.

Longitudinal stretching pulls connective tissue in the direction of the fiber configuration. Cross-directional stretching pulls the connective tissue against the fiber direction. The two approaches accomplish the same thing, but longitudinal stretching is done in conjunction with movement at the joint and gliding manipulations applied with drag in the direction of the force. If longitudinal stretching is not advisable, if it is ineffective in situations of hypermobility of a joint, or if the area to be stretched is not effectively stretched longitudinally, cross-directional stretching is a better choice. Cross-directional stretching focuses on the tissue itself and does not depend on joint movement (Figure 9-43).

The **direction of ease** is the way the body allows for postural changes and muscle shortening or weakening compensation patterns, depending on its balance in gravity. Although compensation patterns may be inefficient, the patterns developed serve a purpose and need to be respected. It may seem logical to locate a shortened muscle group or a rotated movement pattern and use direct methods to reverse the pattern. However, this may not be the best approach. Protective sensory receptors prevent any forced stretch out of a compensation pattern. Instead, the pattern of compensation is respected, and the body position is exaggerated and coaxed into a more efficient position.

Take the example of a client who has shortened pectoralis muscles that pull the shoulders forward, giving the person a gorilla-like appearance. Instead of pulling the pectoralis muscles into a stretch by forcing the arms back, curl the shoulders and arms more into adduction, providing slack and space to the receptors in the pectoralis muscles. Begin corrective action from this point.

The procedure for longitudinal stretching is as follows:

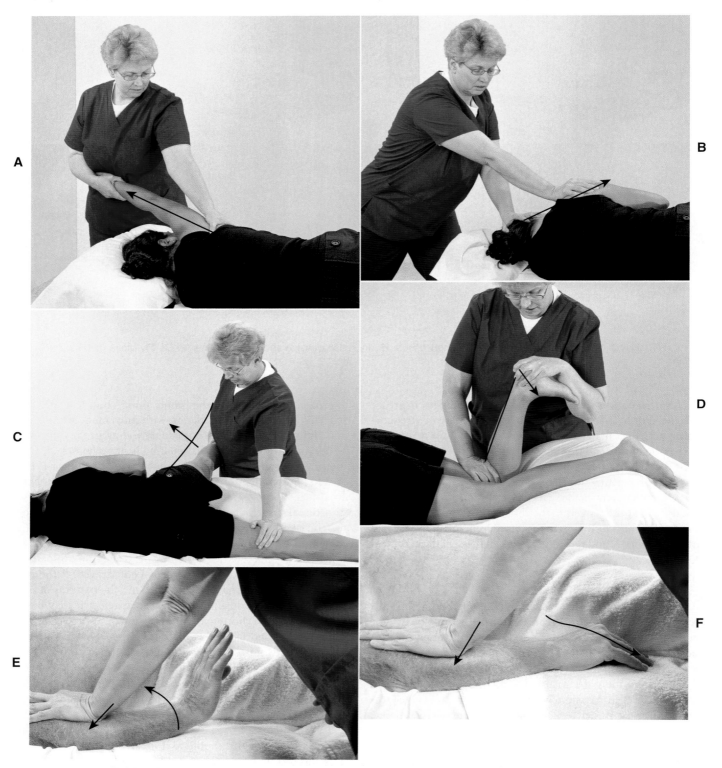

FIGURE 9-43 Examples of stretching. **A** to **D,** Longitudinal stretching. **E, F,** Active release.

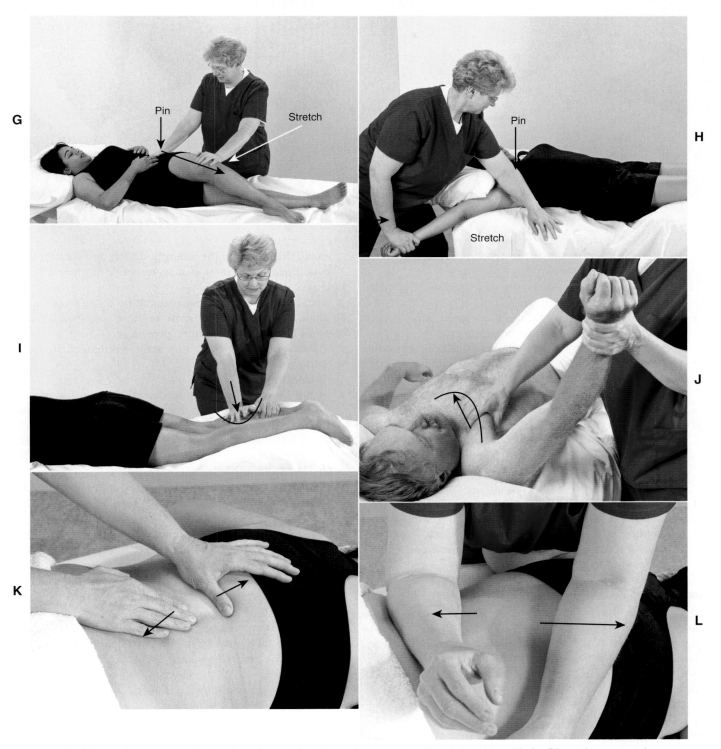

FIGURE 9-43, cont'd G, H, Pin and stretch. **I, J,** Cross-directional stretching. **K, L,** Direct tissue stretch.

Continued

FIGURE 9-43, cont'd M, Direct tissue stretching. **N,** Combined cross-directional and longitudinal stretch.

1. Position the target muscle in the direction of ease. Stabilize and isolate a muscle group.
2. Choose a method to prepare the target muscle to stretch (e.g., gliding, compression, kneading).
3. After the target muscle has been prepared, stretch the muscle to its physiologic or pathologic barrier or to wherever protective contraction is engaged; this is the point of bind. Back off slightly to avoid muscle spasm. Stay in line with the muscle fibers. Exert effort or movement as the client inhales. Stretch as the client exhales.

The following two approaches are used for the actual stretch phase:

1. Hold the position just off the physiologic or pathologic barrier for at least 10 seconds to allow for the neurologic reset; this is the lengthening phase. Feel for secondary response (a small give in the muscle).
2. Take up slack by further lengthening the muscle for up to 20 seconds to create longitudinal pull (tension force) on the connective tissue. You must hold the muscle stretch as instructed to allow for changes in the connective tissue component of the muscle.

Alternate Procedures for Longitudinal Stretching. If only a small section of muscle needs to be stretched, if the muscle does not lend itself to stretching with joint movement, or if the joints are so flexible that not enough pull is put on the muscles to achieve an effective stretch to the tissues, the following alternate procedure for longitudinal stretching should be used:

Alternative A

1. Locate the fibers or muscle to be stretched.
2. Place the hands, fingers, or forearms in the belly of the muscle or directly over the area to be stretched.
3. Contact the muscle with sufficient pressure to reset the neuromuscular mechanism.
4. Separate the fingers, hands, or forearms (tension force) or lift the tissue with pressure sufficient to stretch the muscle (bending or torsion force). Take up all slack from length-

ening, then increase the intensity slightly and wait for the connective tissue component to respond (this may take as long as 30 seconds).

NOTE: All requirements for preparation of the muscle and direction of stretch are the same as those described for the previous longitudinal stretching procedure.

The following procedure is for active assisted longitudinal stretching.

Alternative B

1. Identify and isolate the muscle, making sure it is not working against gravity in this position. Remind the client to exhale during the stretching phase of this technique.
2. Lengthen the muscle to its physiologic or pathologic barrier, move slightly beyond this point, and stretch gently for 1 to 2 seconds.
3. Return the muscle to its starting position. Repeat this action in a rhythmic, pulselike fashion for 5 to 20 repetitions.
4. The client can benefit from contracting the antagonist while the target muscle is lengthened and stretched. As in all proper lengthening and stretching movements, attention must be paid to the stretch reflex; bouncing is never done because it initiates this reflex.

Alternative C

Other effective methods involve the application of compression into the short binding tissue to hold it, followed by either active or passive movement:

1. Locate the area to be stretched.
2. Apply compression into the short tissue and hold it in a fixed position.
3. The client moves the adjacent joints and lengthens the tissue (sometimes called *active release*), or the massage practitioner uses the other hand to move the tissue or joint into a stretched position (sometimes called *pin and stretch*).

Cross-directional tissue stretching uses a pull and twist component, introducing torsion and bend forces. The procedure for cross-directional stretching is as follows:

1. Access the area to be stretched by moving against the fiber direction using compression.
2. Lift or deform the area slightly and hold for 30 to 60 seconds until the area gets warm or seems to soften.

Use the following procedure for skin and superficial connective tissue:

1. Locate the area of restriction.
2. Lift and pull (like taffy), first moving into the restriction and then pulling and twisting out of it, keeping a constant tension on the tissue (remember the plastic wrap exercise). Go slowly. Take up slack until the area warms and softens.

Use of Cold Applications and Stretching. Dr. Janet Travell popularized the cold spray and stretch technique.[11] The cold spray stimulates cold receptors, blocking other sensory signals; the proprioceptors thus are inhibited momentarily, allowing the muscle to relax.

An ice pop (made by freezing water in a paper cup with a wooden stick inserted) can be used to create the same effect as cold spray. Move the ice pop on the skin from the proximal to the distal attachment along the path of the target muscle. Move at a speed of about 1 inch per second while stretching the muscle.

Use of Percussion with Stretching. Using forms of percussion on the skin over the muscle along the same pathway as the ice pop massage facilitates stretching. The skin is snapped quickly with a move like shooting marbles. If a tendon is tapped quickly, the muscle will contract. To assist stretching, apply the tap to the antagonist muscles so that they contract reflexively. The target muscle thus is inhibited reciprocally, allowing for a relaxation response and the ability to stretch with reduced protective muscle spasm.

Stretching Deep Fascial Planes. Accessing deep fascial planes requires an understanding of the deep structures involved. Specific soft tissue systems, such as myofascial release and soft tissue manipulation, provide instruction in these very valuable methods. Chapter 11 expands on this information.

It is important to realize that the human body is made up of interconnecting parts. Therefore all stretching affects deep connective tissue structures. The body cannot be divided into separate layers; the only difference is the access point. A house may have three or four doors, each of which will let you inside. Where you enter may be different, but once you are inside, you are able to have an effect on all the areas. Therefore effective stretching of the more superficial connective tissues, as presented in this chapter, indirectly affects the deeper connective tissue structures as well (Proficiency Exercise 9-12).

SEQUENCE AND FLOW

SECTION OBJECTIVE

Using the information presented in this section, the student will be able to perform the following:

- Design a basic full-body massage

PROFICIENCY EXERCISE 9-12

1. *Knead extra flour into bread dough so that the consistency is quite firm. Practice stretching the dough. Feel for the give of the tissue as opposed to the tissue breaking.*
2. *Design a lengthening and stretching sequence for yourself that accesses the major muscle groups and connective tissue areas. Pay attention to the difference in the feel of neuromuscular lengthening, with its quick release, and connective tissue stretching, with its softer, slower give.*
3. *Have a fellow student assume various stretch positions. Tell him or her to stretch as far as is comfortable and hold. Take the area and stretch it 1/8-inch farther and hold it. Pay attention to the feeling and talk with the student to get feedback.*
4. *Practice tapping antagonist tendons and using ice massage on a client as you position the body for various stretches.*
5. *Working with a partner, see how many massage manipulations and techniques you can combine and do at once (e.g., joint movement combined with compression, gliding combined with a stretch, percussion combined with a stretch, kneading combined with muscle energy methods—especially the "make a soft muscle" concept).*
6. *Design a massage incorporating each of the basic positions that combines at least two methods or techniques for every body area.*

The previous section presented massage manipulations and techniques. The next concern is how to combine the methods into a focused massage session. There are a million ways to give a massage, and the choices massage therapists make each time they give a massage develop from an understanding of the principles and practice of therapeutic massage. Each massage is different, because the client is different each time, even if that client has been seen for many massage sessions.

The focus of the session depends on the stated outcomes for the client. To understand what those outcomes are, the massage practitioner must be able to take a general history and do a basic assessment of the client. These procedures were presented in Chapter 3. Based on the information gathered in the history and assessment process, the therapeutic massage professional designs the best massage for the individual client by choosing the appropriate methods, pressure, rhythm, pacing, intensity, duration, and amenities (e.g., music). (Refinement of the assessment process and the criteria for decision making are addressed in Chapter 10 and in the case studies in Chapter 15.)

When doing a massage, the massage practitioner uses a variety of methods and techniques in a manner that allows easy transition from one method into another as a particular part of the body is addressed. Once students learn the technical aspects of performing methods, they learn to perfect the massage sequence; that is, to combine the methods in a logical way so as to address specific body areas and eventually to generate specific outcomes, such as relaxation, pain control, mobility, and improved circulation.

General sequencing principles guide the massage application. These principles describe the direction and progression of manipulations. They are:

- General→Specific→General
- Superficial→Deep→Superficial

General to specific to general and *superficial to deep to superficial* refer to the ways in which methods are applied to an area of the body. The first application of a method is done generally and superficially; this is followed by applications that are more specific and deeper. The methods then return to more general and superficial techniques before the practitioner moves to another area.

This sequencing has many effects. It accustoms the client to the touch, and it allows the practitioner to palpate through layers of tissue in a systematic manner for assessment, as well as for application for therapeutic change. Without this approach, especially after deep work, the client may experience postmassage soreness for hours or days after the session.

The Basic Full-Body Massage

9-1

The basic full-body massage is a common approach in massage. The full-body general massage stimulates all the sensory nerve receptors, contacts all the layers and types of tissues, and moves all the major joints of the body. The General Protocol is shown on pp. 335–352 and also on the DVD that accompanies this textbook.

The session lasts about 1 hour. The purpose of the massage is to affect the whole body using primarily gliding, compression, oscillation, and range of motion to the joints, along with limited use of kneading, shaking, and general friction methods. The other manipulations and techniques are chosen as needed to address specific problem areas.

Regardless of the type of massage approach, the first and perhaps most important massage manipulation is the resting position, or the first touch. The next massage manipulations are used for general, broad applications and to connect all the other methods during the massage session. Methods most commonly used for general broad applications are gliding strokes, compression, rhythmic rocking and shaking, and joint range of motion.

Gliding strokes are effective in the following situations:
- A lubricant is to be used.
- A large surface area must be covered efficiently.
- Changes are made between manipulations.
- The practitioner moves from one area to another.
- The client prefers a soothing massage with generalized body responses.

Compression is effective in the following situations:
- Lubricant will not be used.
- The client is hairy or ticklish.
- The client prefers a more stimulating massage.

Rhythmic rocking and *shaking* are effective in the following situations:
- Lubricant will not be used.

- Excessive rubbing or pressing on the skin or underlying tissue is not desirable.
- The client desires a soothing massage with generalized body responses.

Joint range of motion is effective for the following situations:
- Lubricant will not be used.
- The client is hairy or ticklish.
- Excessive rubbing or pressing on the skin or underlying tissue is not desirable.
- The client desires a general increase in mobility.

It is beneficial to blend these four methods to provide the general base of the massage. The other massage manipulations and techniques provide uniqueness to the massage.

The full-body general massage has a sense of wholeness, with a beginning point and an ending point. The basic flow patterns explained earlier in the chapter provide the basis for this sense of organized and integrated structure. The massage should have a general sense of continuity. In simple words, the massage needs to flow, to feel connected, like one continuous experience made up of all the applications of the massage methods chosen to achieve the individual client's outcomes.

The general sequence of contact is gliding, kneading, compression, oscillation (rocking, shaking), and movement (usually passive joint movement). Each body area is addressed. Each method usually is applied three or four times (frequency), becoming slower and deeper with each application. The rhythm, duration, and direction vary, depending on the goal of the massage. A basic sequence can be developed (e.g., glide, glide, glide—knead, knead, knead—compress, compress, compress—rock or shake or move a joint as appropriate). The practitioner then can move to a different body area and repeat the sequence.

GENERAL MASSAGE SUGGESTIONS

SECTION OBJECTIVES

Using the information presented in this section, the student will be able to perform the following:

- Understand how to deal with difficult or unusual situations regarding body hair, skin problems, and avoidance of tickling
- Make thoughtful decisions regarding the application of massage techniques by body region

Body Hair

Excessive body hair requires an alteration in the massage procedure. Gliding and kneading methods can pull the hair. A lubricant may feel uncomfortable. Compression and oscillation (vibration, rocking, and shaking), coupled with lengthening and stretching procedures, can be an effective alternative.

Skin Problems

People who have rashes, acne, psoriasis, and other skin problems require an alteration of massage procedures. The integrity of healthy skin prevents the transmission of pathogens. Physician referral and approval may be required. Massage can usually be provided by placing a clean, white bath towel or triple-folded sheet over the affected area and using compression methods over the fabric. Be very careful to avoid contact with any body fluids.

Working over a clean towel or sheet can be helpful for clients who have sensitive skin and find the movement of massage irritating. Any method that does not glide on the skin can be used over a towel, sheet, or loose, nonrestrictive clothing. Using a towel to lift tissue, especially the tissue of the abdomen, is helpful for gaining an effective grip and is more comfortable.

Avoidance of Tickling

Tickling usually can be avoided by reducing the speed and increasing the pressure of the stroke. Also, because tickling oneself is difficult, the problem often can be solved by placing the client's hand on the area you want to massage and massaging with it. Tickling frequently can be avoided by working over a towel or sheet.

Considerations and Suggestions for Massage Applications by Body Region

Head and Face Massage

- To avoid disturbing the client's hairstyle and makeup, always ask before massaging the head and face.
- Use lubricants carefully, keeping in mind the sensitivity of the facial skin. Avoid using lubricant on the face if possible.
- Remember that the delicate nature of the facial skin and muscles requires a confident yet moderate approach.

Because of the extensive motor/sensory sensitivity of the face, massage can stimulate considerable nervous system activity, which may be beneficial for relaxation and pain control. Also, the facial muscles create the expressions that reflect our moods and emotions. Changes in expression are processed in the emotional centers of the brain. Careful attention to massage of the face may gently interact with the way the client feels emotionally.

Always clean your hands before massaging the face. Pathogens can easily be spread through the mucous membranes of the eyes, nose, and mouth. Avoid direct contact with these areas.

Neck Massage

- Keep in mind that side-lying is the most effective position for massage of the neck. The head is stabilized against the table, and the neck area is opened up for easy access.
- Always provide lengthening and stretching for the neck from the shoulder with the head stabilized. Injury may result if the neck is lengthened or stretched by moving the head.
- Avoid deep pressure into the anterior triangle of the neck (the general area between the sternocleidomastoid muscle and the trachea). Damage to blood vessels and nerves in this area can result.

- Use broad, generalized methods of massage applied with the forearm or the whole hand; this feels less invasive than using the fingers and thumbs when massaging the neck.

The neck is a crowded, complex area. It can be affected by responses to stress and by chest and shoulder breathing, which can cause the neck muscles to become rigid and hypertonic. Effective massage of the neck is necessary to provide for relaxed breathing and reduced stress perception.

Careful study of the anatomy of the neck shows that the direct soft tissue influence extends from the forehead to the second and third ribs, the middle thoracic vertebrae, and the middle of the humerus. Because the neck area balances the head against gravity, postural distortion anywhere in the body is reflected in the neck. Massage to this area, in conjunction with an entire body approach, is most beneficial.

The brachial nerve plexus exits from the neck. It is helpful to think of most arm, wrist, and hand problems as beginning at the neck. Problems result from either a direct dysfunction of the neck or difficulties in the arm and hand, which often indirectly cause a neck problem.

Shoulder Massage

- Keep in mind that the side-lying position is most effective for massage, range of motion, and lengthening and stretching of the shoulder.

The shoulder complex (scapula, clavicle, humerus, and associated muscles, ligaments, and tendons) floats on the trunk. It is constructed with a loose fit at the shoulder (glenohumeral) joint to provide for a wide range of motion. Soft tissue (muscles, tendons, ligaments, and fascia) connects the shoulder to the trunk, with multidirectional forces coming from the back, chest, and neck. The practitioner should consider all these areas when massaging the shoulder.

The shoulder is stabilized at the iliac crest and sacrum by the latissimus dorsi muscle and the lumbar dorsal fascia. With any shoulder massage, the practitioner needs to consider massage of the low back area.

The joint design reflects the fact that flexor muscles (which narrow a joint angle) and adductor muscles (which pull toward the midline of the body) exert more pull and are stronger than the extensors (which increase the joint angle) and abductors (which pull away from the midline). Joint fit may be compromised by an imbalance in the tone pattern of these muscles. The practitioner should keep this in mind when working with the shoulder.

The brachial nerve plexus, which supplies the arm, may be affected by soft tissue dysfunction in the shoulder area. This is a very important consideration for clients who have arm pain and discomfort, often resulting from repetitive use injury. Massaging the shoulder may help reduce muscle tension and soften connective tissue in the area, which may alleviate discomfort in the shoulder and arm.

Arm Massage

- Positioning and stabilizing of the arm for massage can be aided by massaging the arm in all the basic positions: supine, prone, and side-lying. Each offers advantages.

- Massage only the areas of the arm that are easily accessible in each position. Return to the arm as the client changes position.
- Massage the arm with the forearm stabilized against the massage table in the prone or supine position or against the body in the side-lying position.
- The arm is often small enough in circumference to grasp with the hands, surrounding a bulk of the tissue.

This approach provides a compressive effleurage to facilitate fluid movement. When massaging the arm, it is useful to remember that the fingers actually begin at the elbow, and the shoulder mechanism extends to the elbow.

The elbow joint area is more complex than a hinge joint because of the pronation (palm down)/supination (palm up) action at the elbow. Flexion, extension, pronation, and supination movement patterns need to be considered when the practitioner massages the arm.

The nerves of the brachial nerve plexus run the entire length of the arm. Nerve impingement from soft tissue at the neck, shoulder, and elsewhere in the entire length of the arm needs to be considered if pain exists in the arm.

Hand and Wrist Massage

- Because the hand is usually in a flexed position, opening and spreading the tissue of the palm is very beneficial.
- The use of compression to provide a pumping action on the palm of the hand stimulates the lymphatic plexus in the palm, which in turn encourages lymphatic flow. This can be very helpful for those whose hands swell.

The hand and wrist have an intricate, complex joint and soft tissue structure. Thorough attention to massage of these structures and range of motion of the hand and wrist requires time and a focus on detail.

Slow circumduction (moving in a circle) of the wrists, both passive and active against resistance, accesses the joint movement patterns of the wrist. The carpal and metacarpal (palm) joints of the hand can be addressed with a scissoring action. The phalangeal (finger) joints are hinge joints that respond well to active movement against resistance and passive range of motion.

The extensive motor/sensory sensitivity of the hand provides for intense neurologic stimulation through massage methods. The hand is an effective area for massage to initiate relaxation and pain control.

Massage of the hand can be a time of increased connection between the client and the massage practitioner. This is a result of the hand-in-hand position. The sense of intimacy created by the act of holding hands may shift the therapeutic focus from the client to the massage practitioner. Extra care is suggested to avoid transference/countertransference and professional boundary issues while not disturbing the closeness created at this time.

Chest Massage

- The breast area of the female can pose difficulties in accessing the chest area. The side-lying position is effective because the breast tissue falls toward the table, allowing access to the side of the chest and axilla (armpit) area.

Using the person's hand as a "buffer" between the practitioner's hand and the client, as when avoiding tickling, can be helpful when working around the clavicles and ribs.

- Broad compressive methods to the rib area in the side-lying position are effective in providing general range of motion to the ribs.
- Avoid the breast tissue and nipple area on both males and females. During general massage there is no reason to massage this area, and the tissue often is very sensitive to touch and can be easily irritated.
- Be extra attentive to changes in the tissue in the chest area. Without any alarm reaction, refer clients to their physician if you notice any lumps or tissue changes.

The intercostal muscles (those between the ribs) are very important in respiratory function. Slow, deliberate work between the ribs with the client in the side-lying position can be valuable in restoring mobility and breathing function.

The pectoralis muscles and associated connective tissue are involved in arm and shoulder movement. This large soft tissue area is often shortened, not only affecting arm action but causing breathing difficulties as well. Effective massage, lengthening, and stretching are beneficial.

Abdominal Massage

The Abdominal Sequence. Not all researchers agree that massage has a substantial effect on peristalsis or even that mechanical emptying of the colon is possible. Nonetheless, with abdominal massage it seems prudent to approach the area as though massage does have an effect. Theoretically, to support peristalsis and mechanical emptying of the colon, all massage manipulations are directed in a clockwise fashion. To avoid any chance of impaction of fecal material, the manipulations begin in the lower left quadrant at the sigmoid colon. The methods progressively contact the large intestine and eventually end up encompassing the entire colon area (Figure 9-44).

Standing on the left side of the body when the client is in the supine position facilitates the body mechanics of the practitioner (see Figure 9-44). The body mechanics for the massage practitioner and elimination patterns are most efficient when the client is lying on his or her left side.

The direction of flow for emptying of the large intestine and colon is as follows:

1. Massage down the left side of the descending colon, using short strokes directed to the sigmoid colon.
2. Massage across the transverse colon to the left side, using short strokes directed to the sigmoid colon.
3. Massage up the ascending colon on the right side of the body, using short strokes directed to the sigmoid colon.
4. End at the right ileocecal valve, located in the lower right quadrant of the abdomen.
5. Massage the entire flow pattern, using long, light to moderate strokes, from the ileocecal valve to the sigmoid colon. Repeat the sequence.

- The abdomen can be massaged with the client in the supine or side-lying position. Side-lying on the left is the most

FIGURE 9-44 A, Colon (the arrows indicate the flow pattern). All massage manipulations are directed in a clockwise fashion. The manipulations begin in the lower left quadrant (on the right side as you view the illustration) at the sigmoid colon. The methods progressively contact all of the large intestine and eventually end up covering the entire colon area. **B,** Abdominal sequence. The direction of flow for emptying of the large intestine and colon. Make the change as suggested. Massage down the left side of the descending colon using short strokes directed toward the sigmoid colon. **C,** Massage across the transverse colon to the left side using short strokes directed toward the sigmoid colon. **D,** Massage up the ascending colon on the right side of the body using short strokes directed toward the sigmoid colon. End at the right-side ileocecal valve, which is located in the lower right quadrant of the abdomen. **E,** Massage the entire flow pattern of the abdominal sequence, using long, light to moderate strokes, from the ileocecal valve to the sigmoid colon. Then repeat the sequence.

effective position. During abdominal massage the knees usually are bent about 90 degrees to the trunk to tilt the pelvis and allow for more relaxed abdominal muscles.

- Because the abdomen contains no bony structure against which to apply pressure, much abdominal work is done with lateral pressure. The tissue is pushed against pressure from the massage practitioner's opposing hand or with kneading that lifts the tissue.

The abdomen has an expansive fascial system. Lifting methods to stretch this connective tissue can be beneficial. Using a towel to lift the abdominal tissue provides grip and protects against pinching.

The abdomen often is ticklish; this is a protective mechanism. Follow the instructions given earlier for avoiding tickling.

Be careful of pressure down into the abdomen. Always move slowly, allowing the tissue to soften under the touch. If you feel a pulse or throbbing, immediately reduce the pressure.

Many times the abdomen is given only superficial attention during the massage. Avoid this tendency. This is an important area that deserves effective massage application.

Back Massage

- Avoid spending excessive time on massage of the back. Often the reason for back pain or stiffness is shortening and weakness of muscles in the chest and abdomen. The resulting change in posture is responsible for the back tension.
- The back is effectively massaged in the prone, side-lying, and seated positions.
- Use of the forearm is very effective for back massage. The lumbar dorsal fascia responds well to skin rolling (tissue lifting) and connective tissue stretching methods. Pressure directly over the spine is not appropriate. However, skin rolling techniques that lift the skin over the spine are effective.

The low back, including the deep quadratus lumborum muscle, is easily massaged in the side-lying position with the client's arm raised over the head to lift the ribcage away from the iliac crest. Deep, even pressure with the forearm often feels best to the client.

Gentle range of motion to provide for rotation of the spinal column is most effectively done in the side-lying position.

Nerve roots are located all along the spine. Massage close to but not on the spine is beneficial.

Gluteal and Hip Massage

- Massage of the gluteals and hips is most effective when the client is in the side-lying or prone position. Lengthening and stretching methods are most easily done in the side-lying or supine position.
- This area is heavily muscled and reinforced with extensive ligament and tendon structures. The bones and joints in this area are large compared with other body areas. Deeper pressure, with increased duration, is often required to relax these tissues. Methods need to work slowly into the tissue. Avoid work with the hands and make extensive use of the forearm, knee, or foot; these are less intimate, which may be an important consideration when working with the gluteals and hips.

The sacroiliac joints are large joints that are not directly moved by muscular action. Range-of-motion actions are indirectly achieved through movement of the leg through a range-of-motion sequence.

The coxal articulations (hip joints) are massive joints with an extensive ligament structure. The joint provides considerable range of motion, second only to the shoulder joint. When doing range-of-motion methods, include as many variations of flexion, extension, abduction, adduction, and internal and external rotation as possible to involve all the soft tissue elements.

The lumbar and sacral plexuses both innervate this region. Nerve distribution patterns include the entire lower body, and the largest nerve is the sciatic nerve. When using heavy pressure to address the soft tissue, avoid sustained deep pressure on the nerve tracts.

Leg Massage

- Supine, prone, and side-lying are all effective positions for massage of the leg and are best used in combination to access all parts of the leg easily. For the most efficient use of time in the massage session, make sure each area of the leg is massaged only once. For instance, if you massage the back of the leg in the prone position, it is not necessary to repeat the back of the leg again in the supine position unless a specific reason exists for doing so.
- The side-lying position offers the easiest access in the medial and lateral aspect of the leg. The supine position provides access to all aspects of the leg, whereas the prone position is the most limited.
- The soft tissue mass of the leg lends itself to massage with the forearm, leg, and foot. Kneading is often uncomfortable on the leg because of body hair and the tight adherence of the skin and superficial fascia to the underlying tissue. Gliding and compression are effective methods to use instead.
- Varicose veins most often occur in the leg, particularly in the saphenous veins. Thromboembolism and thrombophlebitis are serious conditions involving a blood clot in a vein. If the clot moves, it can lodge in the heart, lung, kidney, or brain and cause severe problems. Symptoms of

deep vein thrombophlebitis in the legs are aching and cramping that can be mistaken for muscle pain. Massage of any type is contraindicated, and immediate referral is indicated for varicose veins, thromboembolism, and thrombophlebitis. Diagnosis is beyond the scope of practice for massage practitioners, therefore remain cautious of any leg pain and refer the client to the appropriate health care professional.

- Range of motion for the leg above the knee is hip range of motion. Make sure to effectively stabilize at the pelvis. Stabilizing pressure in this area can be uncomfortable. The use of a small pillow or folded towel over the stabilizing point provides comfort.

The knee is a complex joint influenced by muscles from above and below the joint. Knee instability is often compensated for by increased motor tone in the leg muscles and thickening and shortening of the iliotibial tract (a large connective tissue structure on the outside of the leg). This is resourceful compensation, and the protective nature of the muscle and connective tissue tension must be considered. The gluteus maximus and tensor fascia lata muscle exert a pull at the iliotibial crest. Relax these muscle structures to reduce tension on the iliotibial tract and knee. When massaging the leg of a person with a hypermobile knee, you can use the proper methods to reduce excessive motor tone and connective tissue shortening, but you should not try to remove the splinting action entirely. To do so may result in increased knee pain.

The lumbosacral plexus nerves supply the leg, with the sciatic nerve running the entire length of the leg. Impingement can occur anywhere along the nerve pathways. The distribution of leg pain can indicate the nerve portion affected. When located, the entire nerve tract needs to be searched above and below the impingement site for soft tissue restriction to provide soft tissue normalization around the nerves. Light stroking along the nerve tracts is very soothing.

Foot and Ankle Massage

- The feet often are a safe place to begin a massage for a client who is nervous or in pain.
- Because of the number of joints in the foot and ankle, careful and deliberate range-of-motion work is beneficial in this area. Slow circumduction (circular movements), both passive and active against resistance, accesses the ankle movement patterns. The tarsal and metatarsal (main foot) joints can be accessed with a scissoring or bending movement of the foot. Phalangeal (toe) joints are hinge joints and benefit from both active range of motion against resistance and passive range of motion.

The foot and ankle mechanism is a highly complex structure. It has many joints, muscles, and nerves that provide stability and neurologic positional information during walking and standing. An extensive connective tissue network provides stability. Any disruption of normal foot and ankle action often results in a compensatory pattern through the entire musculoskeletal system.

Massage of the foot is one of the best ways to provide a high degree of nervous system input for relaxation and pain control. Many beneficial effects are obtained with foot massage because of the stimulation of parasympathetic activity, which results in the relaxation or quieting response.

The sole of the foot contains a vast lymphatic plexus that acts as a pump to move lymphatic fluid in the foot and legs. Compression used in a rhythmic pumping action is effective in stimulating the lymphatic system.

The tibial nerve, off the sciatic nerve, branches into the medial and lateral plantar nerve, which in turn branches to provide extensive nerve distribution in the foot. Sciatic nerve impingement can be felt into the foot. Nerve pain in the foot can indicate impingement anywhere along the nerve tract from the lumbosacral plexus to the foot. Nerve pain in the foot needs to be addressed with massage of the entire leg, with the practitioner noticing which areas of restriction refer pain to the foot (Proficiency Exercise 9-13).

PROFICIENCY EXERCISE 9-13

Design a 1-hour massage sequence on paper using a variety of methods and techniques from this chapter. Trade papers with another student and perform the other person's massage sequence on him or her. When you are finished, list what you learned from the experience and share the list with your partner in this exercise. Have your partner critique his or her massage design.

GENERAL MASSAGE PROTOCOL

The following series of photographs provides one example of how a massage can be designed. Examples of massage applications are provided, incorporating the various methods described in this chapter. It is assumed that the student would perform the methods on both sides of the body where appropriate. Variations also are shown, providing options for massage of a particular area. This series of photographs is complemented by the demonstration provided on the DVD. By studying these examples, you should be able to modify and adapt applications to make each massage unique.

The series of photographs that follow is organized as an example of a full-body massage in three positions: prone, side-lying, and supine. Draping is shown, but not in such a way as to obstruct the view of the application. Ideally, the massage is applied using all of the best positioning. Most areas of the body can be massaged in the three positions; however, some positions related to body areas support the optimal body mechanics, and circumstances may require that variations be used. (See the DVD for a complete demonstration of the General Protocol.)

1. Review intention focus for massage. Center. Then apply resting stroke.

2. Palpation. Wet/dry skin drag, ease/bind, hot/cold, rough/smooth.

Continued

GENERAL MASSAGE PROTOCOL—cont'd

3. Glide on back. Vary speed, drag, and depth of pressure.

4. Shift position. Glide/compress.

5. Knead.

6. Move underwear.

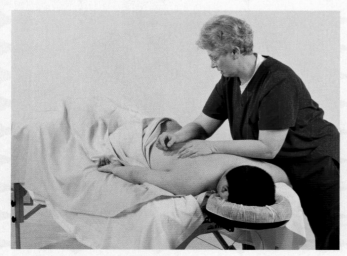

7. Glide lumbar and gluteal region.

8. Compression to gluteal area.

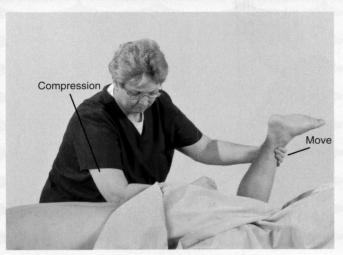

9. Combined loading. Compression and move.

10. Knead.

11. Percussion. Repeat opposite side.

12. Shift position. Glide/compress upper back/shoulder.

13. Compression.

14. Compression/kneading.

Continued

GENERAL MASSAGE PROTOCOL—cont'd

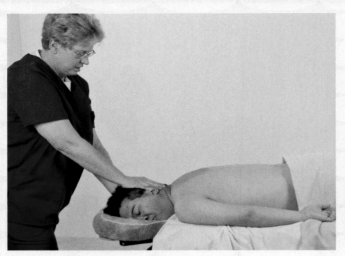

15. Turn head, massage scalp.

16. Reposition head. Compress muscles of the head.

17. Knead neck.

18. Glide/compression on shoulder.

19. Oscillation. Shaking and move scapula.

20. Bolster shoulder.

21. Knead and glide around scapula.

22. Position arm, then rock and shake, assessment.

23. Glide arm.

24. Glide using palm.

25. Knead arm and forearm.

26. Compression forearm and hand. Repeat opposite side.

Continued

GENERAL MASSAGE PROTOCOL—cont'd

27. Move to hip and thigh. Glide/compression. Begin glide.

28. Compression.

29. Repeat gliding—slower and deeper.

30. Knead on thigh.

31. Glide on calf.

32. Knead calf.

33. Reposition leg, knee straight, glide and knead/compression.

34. Joint movement knee, ankle, foot.

35. Stretch and move. Position leg for foot massage.

36. Compression of lateral foot using palm. Reposition leg.

37. Compression of sole of foot using forearm.

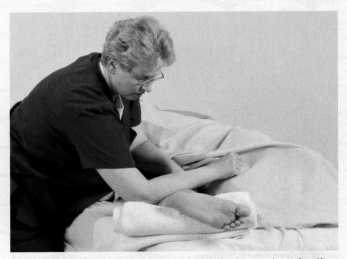

38. Reposition client sidelying with glide/compression of calf and foot.

Continued

GENERAL MASSAGE PROTOCOL—cont'd

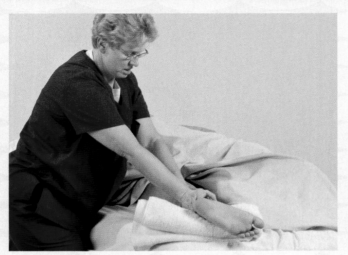

39. Compression/glide of ankle and heel, medial side.

40. Knead calf.

41. Muscle energy techniques.

42. Stretch.

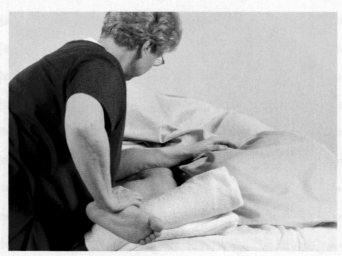

43. Glide of the inner (medial) thigh.

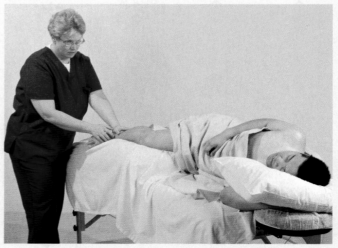

44. Client remains side-lying. Switch to opposite leg.

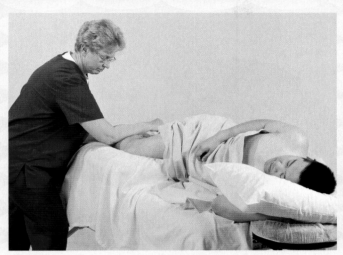

45. Glide/compression on calf, lateral side.

46. Knead calf.

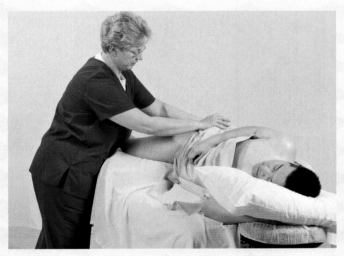

47. Move drape to provide access to thigh and hip.

48. Glide, thigh.

49. Knead.

50. Knead while kneeling.

Continued

GENERAL MASSAGE PROTOCOL—cont'd

51. Joint movement.

52. Arm. Glide/compression using forearm.

53. Glide using palm.

54. Knead.

55. Move to opposite arm. Glide/compression.

56. Change position. Glide using forearm.

57. Knead arm.

58. Joint movement and compression combined with glide.

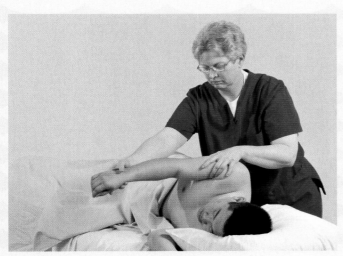

59. Joint movement and position arm.

60. Knead lateral chest and back.

61. Compression of neck.

62. Compression of shoulder.

Continued

GENERAL MASSAGE PROTOCOL—cont'd

63. Knead neck.

64. Massage the head. Repeat opposite side.

65. Turn client supine—Begin with leg. Assess and palpate.

66. Massage abdomen.

67. Knead.

68. Glide on chest. Drape appropriately for women.

69. Knead anterior thigh.

70. Position leg. Glide anterior thigh combined with muscle energy technique and lengthen and stretch.

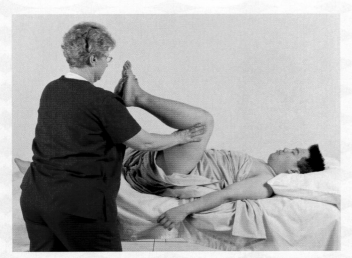

71. Joint movement of hip.

72. Joint movement/assessment.

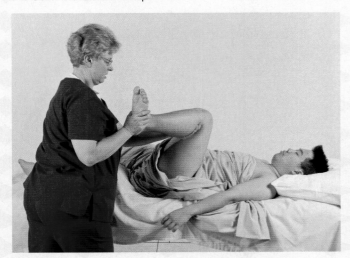

73. Joint movement/muscle energy technique, stretch.

74. Assessment/joint movement, stretch (hip and knee).

Continued

GENERAL MASSAGE PROTOCOL—cont'd

75. Position leg to massage foot, medial leg and foot.

76. Compression of foot.

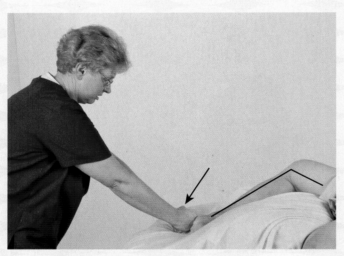

77. Compression of foot. Note: leg position.

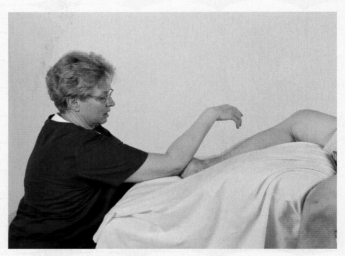

78. Compression of foot, therapist kneeling.

79. Stretch toes. Repeat other side.

80. Change position and massage anterior thorax.

81. Move arm. Glide/compression on pectoralis muscle.

82. Position arm. Compression and kneading.

83. Compression of hand.

84. Massage fingers.

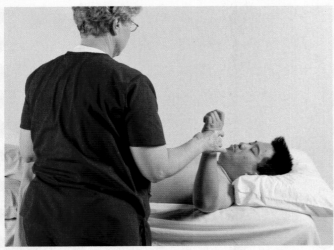

85. Joint movement of shoulder and elbow.

86. Position arm. Glide/compress.

Continued

GENERAL MASSAGE PROTOCOL—cont'd

87. Kneading of arm, therapist kneeling.

88. Hand compression and glide. Repeat other side.

89. Bring arms up. Joint movement and muscle energy techniques.

90. Lengthen and stretch.

91. Compression of upper anterior thorax.

92. Joint movement of neck. Stretch is applied at shoulder.

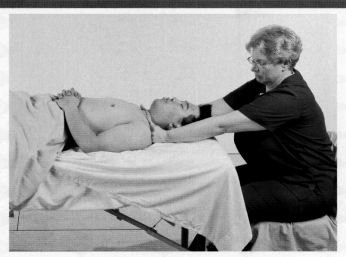

93. Compression of shoulder and neck massage, therapist seated.

94. Compression.

95. Compression/glide.

96. Ears.

97. Face/compression of sinus points.

98. Face.

Continued

GENERAL MASSAGE PROTOCOL—cont'd

99. Percussion. Tapping.

100. Finish.

SEATED MASSAGE PROTOCOL

Massage methods can be adapted to the seated position. The accompanying photographs demonstrate how to apply massage to the various body regions using primarily compression and movement, because clothing typically is left on during a seated massage. (See the DVD for a complete demonstration of the Seated Massage Protocol.)

1. A regular chair with a pillow placed against the chair back—appropriate body mechanics.

2. A pillow placed between the chair and the massage practitioner for comfort.

3. Range of motion and stretching.

4. Use of a pillow to provide a boundary and a comfortable place for the client's head as it rests against the massage therapist's chest.

5. Kneeling position for kneading the arm. A towel is used to protect clothing if lubricant is used.

6. Compression applied to the leg.

7. A sanitary drape.

8. Foot position and a sanitary drape.

9. An example of positioning in a massage chair.

9-3 MAT MASSAGE PROTOCOL

The following series of photographs provides an example of massage application using a mat. An entire sequence is not provided, but the photographs show positioning, bolstering, sequencing, and body mechanics, along with examples of gliding, kneading, and compression, the three basic components of general massage. It is impossible to show all the massage variations, but the examples given should provide enough structure to allow the student to begin to perfect techniques for massage on a mat. (See the DVD for a complete demonstration of the Mat Protocol.)

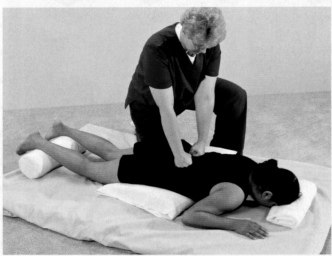

1. Kneeling body mechanics, roll bolster, bed pillow, and rolled towel.

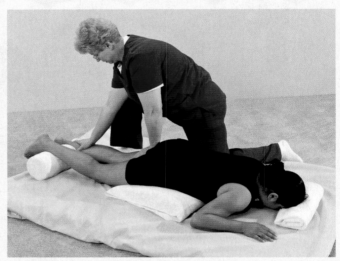

2. Altered body mechanics for application of gliding strokes.

3. Kneading.

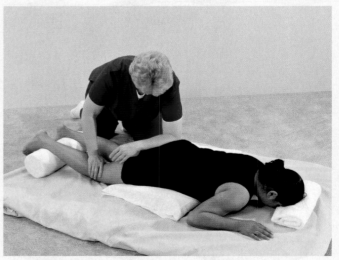

4. Kneeling position, weight bearing, stabilization, and producing force.

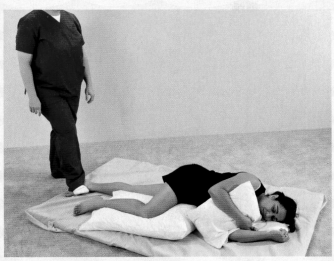

5. Side-lying with bolstering; compression of foot using the arch of the foot.

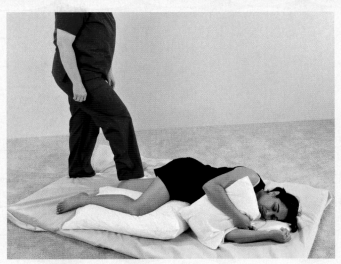

6. Compression on the calf using the foot.

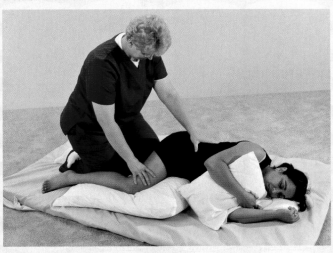

7. Compression on inner thigh using leg.

8. Position for applying massage to the arm.

9. Example of massage for neck and head.

10. Supine; compression using arch of the foot on arms.

MAT MASSAGE PROTOCOL—cont'd

11. Position for chest compression.

12. Gentle and focused end.

■■■ SUMMARY

Now that you have all the individual skills to give a great massage, your job is to practice using them in combination. It is common to be clumsy with massage applications at first. Skills evolve with experience and practice. Very few people, if any, do something perfectly on their first attempt. Expertise is a never-ending process of learning, modification, and change. If you work with a client-centered focus, allow the client's needs to direct the massage, and do not try to force a particular response, the client should experience beneficial results.

Massage manipulations and techniques can be combined to produce an infinite number of therapeutic massage applications. Give yourself permission to practice and improvise. As you practice, ask the client for feedback on how a particular application of a technique or massage manipulation feels and what its effects are. Always be open to innovation, and do not be afraid to experiment with new techniques.

𝘦𝘷𝘰𝘭𝘷𝘦

9-1 See the Evolve Web site for additional examples of client positioning.

9-2 An additional General Protocol sequence is presented on the Evolve Web site.

Don't forget to study for your certification and licensure exams! Review questions for this chapter are located on Evolve.

REFERENCES

1. Anderson KE, Anderson LE, Glanze D, editors: *Mosby's medical, nursing, and allied health dictionary,* ed 4, St Louis, 1990, Mosby.
2. Beard G: A history of massage technique, ed 5, St. Louis, 2007, Saunders.
3. Baumgartner AJ: *Massage in athletics,* Minneapolis, 1947, Brugess Publishing.
4. Kellogg JH: *The art of massage: a practical manual for the nurse, the student and the practitioner,* Kila, Mont, 2004, Kessinger Publishing.
5. Cyriax E: Some misconceptions concerning mechano-therapy, *Br J Physical Med* October 1938.
6. Taylor GH: *An illustrated sketch of the movement cure: its principal methods and effects,* New York, 1866, The Institute.
7. Greenman PE: *Principles of manual medicine,* Baltimore, 2003, Lippincott Williams & Wilkins.
8. Lewit K: *Manipulative therapy in rehabilitation of the locomotor system,* ed 3, Oxford, 1998, Butterworth-Heinemann.
9. Knott M, Voss D: *Proprioceptive neuromuscular facilitation: patterns and techniques,* Baltimore, 1985, Lippincott Williams & Wilkins.
10. Chaitow L: *Muscle energy techniques,* Edinburgh, 2006, Churchill Livingstone.
11. Travell JG, Simons DG: *Myofascial pain and dysfunction: the trigger point manual,* vol 2, Baltimore, 1999, Lippincott Williams & Wilkins.

Workbook Section

Answers for the Workbook Section for Chapter 9 are provided on p. 767.

■ ■ ■ SHORT ANSWER

1. What are the three effects that massage methods and techniques have on the body? Explain each one.

2. Which massage methods seem more mechanical?

3. Which methods seem more reflexive?

4. What are the seven aspects of quality of touch?

5. What is the importance of varying the quality of touch with regard to speed, rate, rhythm, and duration?

6. Why do you think that similar trends, applications, and methods continue to make up the body of knowledge of therapeutic massage?

7. What are the major differences between massage manipulations and massage techniques?

8. What are the main uses for the resting position?

9. How does the massage practitioner first approach the client?

10. What is the distinguishing characteristic of gliding?

11. Why should deeper applications of gliding always move slowly?

12. What are some specific uses of the gliding massage manipulation?

13. What are the distinguishing qualities of kneading?

14. Why should the massage professional use kneading sparingly?

15. What conditions interfere with the use of kneading?

16. What are the physiologic effects of compression?

17. What are some things massage practitioners should remember to protect their hands and arms while doing compression?

18. Where are the best anatomic locations to do vibration? Why?

Workbook Section—cont'd

19. How is rocking different from shaking?

_____

_____

_____

20. What is the strongest physiologic effect of percussion (tapotement)?

_____

_____

_____

21. From where does the movement for percussion come?

_____

_____

_____

22. What are the distinguishing characteristics of friction?

_____

_____

_____

23. How long does friction need to be done to accomplish the desired results?

_____

_____

_____

24. Describe two methods for applying friction.

_____

_____

_____

25. Why does the use of joint movement and muscle energy techniques make massage manipulations more effective?

_____

_____

_____

26. What are the three types of proprioceptors affected by movement techniques? What do they detect?

_____

_____

_____

27. What are the two different types of joint movement described in this text?

_____

_____

_____

28. What is the pathologic range-of-motion barrier?

_____

_____

_____

29. Explain hand placement for joint movement.

_____

_____

_____

30. What are the major uses of muscle energy techniques?

_____

_____

_____

31. Describe the concept of lengthening.

_____

_____

_____

32. What is the importance of positioning?

_____

_____

_____

33. What types of muscle contraction are used for muscle energy techniques? Explain each one.

_____

_____

_____

34. What is postisometric relaxation (PIR)?

_____

_____

_____

35. What is reciprocal inhibition (RI)?

_____

_____

_____

36. How do pulsed muscle energy methods differ from the other methods described?

_____

_____

_____

37. What is the target muscle?

_____

_____

_____

38. How much strength is required during the contraction for the muscle energy method to work?

_____

_____

_____

39. When is direct manipulation of spindle cells and Golgi tendons used?

_____

_____

_____

40. When is positional release/strain-counterstrain used?

_____

_____

_____

41. Define stretching.

_____

_____

_____

42. Why must lengthening methods be used before stretching?

_____

_____

_____

43. When might stretching be an inappropriate method to use?

_____

_____

_____

44. What are the two basic types of stretch?

_____

_____

_____

45. What is direction of ease and why is it important?

_____

_____

_____

46. Explain the concept of the massage as being a mixture of techniques.

_____

_____

_____

47. What is the goal of the general massage?

_____

_____

_____

48. Why are there a million ways to do a massage?

_____

_____

_____

Workbook Section—cont'd

■ ■ ■ MATCHING I

Match the massage manipulation or technique with its description.

1. Active joint movement
2. Beating
3. Compression
4. Cross-directional stretching
5. Cupping
6. Gliding stroke
7. Friction
8. Hacking
9. Joint movement
10. Lengthening
11. Longitudinal stretching
12. Manipulation
13. Muscle energy techniques
14. Passive joint movement
15. Kneading
16. Positional release
17. Postisometric relaxation (PIR)
18. Proprioceptive neuromuscular facilitation (PNF)
19. Pulsed muscle energy
20. Reciprocal inhibition (RI)
21. Resting stroke
22. Rocking
23. Shaking
24. Skin rolling
25. Slapping
26. Stretching
27. Stroke
28. Tapotement
29. Tapping
30. Techniques
31. Traction
32. Vibration

a. a type of alternating tapotement in which the massage therapist strikes the surface of the body with quick snapping movements
b. the movement of the joint through its normal range of motion
c. the assuming of a normal resting length by a muscle through the neuromuscular mechanism
d. a stretch applied along the fiber direction of the connective tissues and muscles
e. tissue stretching that pulls and twists connective tissue against its fiber direction
f. moving the body out of a position causing discomfort and into the direction it wants to go, thereby taking the proprioception into a state of safety, which may allow it to stop signaling for protective spasm
g. occurs after isometric contraction of a muscle, resulting from the activity of minute neural reporting stations called the *Golgi tendon bodies*
h. application of muscle energy techniques that combine muscle contractions with stretching and muscular pattern retraining
i. rhythmic movement of the body
j. grasping and shaking a body area in a quick, loose movement; sometimes classified as rhythmic mobilization
k. a form of pétrissage that lifts skin
l. movement of a joint through its range of motion by the client
m. methods of therapeutic massage that provide sensory stimulation or mechanical alteration of the soft tissue of the body
n. pressure exerted into the body to spread tissue against underlying structures; a massage manipulation sometimes classified with pétrissage
o. a gentle pull on the joint capsule to increase the joint space
p. a fine or coarse tremulous movement that creates reflexive responses
q. a type of tapotement that uses a cupped hand; often used over the thorax
r. horizontal strokes, applied with the fingers, hand, or forearm, that follow the fiber direction of the underlying muscle or fascial planes or a dermatome pattern
s. circular or transverse movements that are focused on the underlying tissue and do not glide on the skin
t. procedures that involve engaging the barrier and using minute, resisted contractions (usually 20 in 10 seconds), which introduces mechanical pumping and PIR or RI (depending on the muscles used)
u. takes place when a muscle contracts, obliging its antagonist to relax to allow normal movement
v. the first stroke of the massage; the simple laying on of hands
w. a form of tapotement that uses a flat hand
x. mechanical tension applied to lengthen the myofascial unit (muscles and fascia); the two types are longitudinal and cross-directional
y. a form of heavy tapotement that uses the fist
z. a technique of therapeutic massage applied on the surface of the body, whether superficial or deep
aa. springy, fast blows to the body to create rhythmic compression to the tissue; also called *percussion*
bb. a type of tapotement done with the fingertips
cc. skillful use of the hands in a therapeutic manner; massage manipulations focus on the soft tissues of the body and are not to be confused with joint manipulation using a high-velocity thrust
dd. specific use of active contraction in individual muscles or groups of muscles to initiate a relaxation response; activation of the proprioceptors to facilitate muscle tone, relaxation, and stretching
ee. movement of the jointed areas by the massage practitioner, without the assistance of the client
ff. rhythmic rolling, lifting, squeezing, and wringing of soft tissue

■ ■ ■ MATCHING II

Match the movement activity with its proper description.

1. Arthrokinematic movement
2. Concentric isotonic contraction
3. Counterpressure
4. Eccentric isotonic contraction
5. Isokinetic contraction
6. Isometric contraction
7. Osteokinematic movements

a. accessory movements that occur because of inherent laxity or joint play that exists in each joint; these essential movements occur passively with movement of the joint and are not under voluntary control
b. during the contraction of a muscle, the massage practitioner applies a counterforce but allows the client to move, bringing the origin and insertion of the target muscle together against the pressure
c. flexion, extension, abduction, adduction, and rotation; also referred to as *physiologic movements*
d. contraction in which the effort of the muscle, or group of muscles, is exactly matched by a counterpressure so that no movement occurs, only effort
e. the client moves the joint through a full range of motion, using full muscle strength, against partial resistance supplied by the massage practitioner; a multiple isotonic movement
f. during the extension of a muscle, the massage practitioner applies a counterforce but allows the client to move the muscle, enabling the origin and insertion to separate
g. the force produced by the muscles of a specific area, designed to match the effort exactly (isometric contraction) or partially (isotonic contraction)

▪▪▪ MATCHING III

Match the term with the proper definition.

1. Antagonists
2. Barrier
3. Compressive force
4. Depth of pressure
5. Direction
6. Direction of ease
7. Drag
8. Facilitation
9. Golgi tendon receptors
10. Heavy pressure
11. Distal attachment
12. Insertion
13. Joint kinesthetic receptors
14. Moderate pressure
15. Motor point
16. Neuromuscular mechanism
17. Proximal attachment
18. Positioning
19. Pressure
20. Prime movers
21. Proprioceptors
22. Range of motion
23. Refractory period
24. Reflex
25. Soft tissue
26. Spindle cells
27. Stabilization
28. Stimulation
29. Superficial fascia
30. Target muscles
31. Tone
32. Tonic vibration reflex
33. Touch

a. a limitation in movement; anatomic barriers are caused by the fit of the bones at the joint; physiologic barriers arise from the limits of range of motion from protective nerve and sensory function
b. contact with no movement
c. some sort of excitation that activates the sensory nerves
d. the connective tissue layer just under the skin
e. a compressive pressure that can be light, moderate, deep, and variable
f. the muscle or groups of muscles on which the response to the methods is specifically focused
g. the state of causing the muscle to contract or strengthen
h. the reflex that tones a muscle with stimulation through vibration methods at the tendon
i. the amount of pull on the tissue
j. the muscles that oppose the movement of the prime movers
k. the state of a nerve when it is stimulated but not to the point of the threshold at which it will transmit a nerve signal
l. postural changes assumed by the body and muscle shortening or weakening, depending on the way in which it has balanced against gravity
m. the flow of massage strokes can be from the center of the body out (centrifugal), or from the extremities in toward the center of the body (centripetal); it can be from the origin to the insertion of the muscle following the muscle fibers, transverse to the tissue fibers, or in a circular motion
n. compressive pressure that extends to the muscle layer but does not press the tissue against the underlying bone
o. placing the body in such a way that specific joints are isolated
p. compressive force
q. the amount of pressure against the surface of the body needed to apply pressure to the deeper body structures
r. the muscles responsible for a movement
s. one of three types of sensory nerves in the joint that detect position and speed of movement
t. the point at which a motor nerve enters the muscle it innervates and will cause a muscle twitch if stimulated
u. the movement of joints
v. a response that depends on nervous system function; reflexive methods work by causing a stimulation of the nervous system (sensory neurons) and the tissue changes in response to the body's adaptation to the neural stimulation
w. holding the body in a fixed position during joint movement, lengthening, and stretching
x. sensory receptors in the belly of the muscle that detect stretch
y. the skin, fascia, muscles, tendons, joint capsules, and ligaments of the body
z. the length of time a muscle is unable to contract after it has contracted
aa. sensory receptors that detect joint and muscle activity
bb. the attachment point of a muscle at the fixed point during movement
cc. the interplay and reflex connection between sensory and motor neurons and muscle function
dd. receptors in the tendons that sense tension
ee. a compressive force that extends to the bone under the tissue
ff. to diminish or stop a response or function
gg. the muscle attachment point that is closest to the moving joint

▪▪▪ PROBLEM-SOLVING EXERCISES

1. A client has achy legs. She also has a history of varicose veins. This contraindicates direct massage of the area. What methods can be used to relax the legs?

2. A client has very sensitive skin that cannot tolerate any type of lubricant. What massage methods can you use that do not involve lubricant?

3. A client's nose becomes stuffy and he gets a sinus headache when he lies on his stomach. How will you give him a massage?

▪▪▪ ASSESS YOUR COMPETENCIES

Now that you have studied this chapter, you should be able to:

1. Explain the basic theories for the physiologic effects of massage methods and techniques.

2. Organize massage methods and techniques for applications in four positions.

3. Perform a full-body massage using the methods and techniques presented.

4. Divide into groups of three. One student gives massage to another student while the third student evaluates the competency of the massage. Rotate among all three students until each has given a massage and received feedback.

▪▪▪ PROFESSIONAL APPLICATION EXERCISE

A massage professional finds that he becomes fatigued with the style of massage he tends to provide, which consists mostly of gliding, kneading, and percussion. He would like to be able to perform massage more effectively. What recommendations would you make?

CHAPTER 10

Assessment Procedures for Developing a Care/Treatment Plan

CHAPTER OBJECTIVES

After completing this chapter, the student will be able to perform the following:

- Conduct an effective client interview
- Perform a basic physical assessment
- Interpret assessment information and develop a care/ treatment plan

CHAPTER OUTLINE

ASSESSMENT
    Establishing Rapport
    How to Observe
    Interviewing and Listening: The Subjective Aspect of Assessment
    Physical Assessment: the Objective Aspect of Assessment
    Outcome Documentation Instruments
    Posture Assessment: Standing Position
    Gait Assessment
    Assessment by Range of Motion
    Overpressure and End-Feel
    Assessment by Palpation
    Assessment Procedures for Muscle Testing
    Functional Biomechanical Assessment
INTERPRETATION AND ANALYSIS OF ASSESSMENT INFORMATION
    General Presence
    Gesturing
    Posture Assessment
    Gait Assessment
    Range of Motion Assessment
    Palpation Assessment
    Muscle and Joint Imbalance, Muscle Testing, Functional Assessment, and Range of Motion
    Compensation Patterns
    Dysfunction as a Solution

CLINICAL REASONING AND PROBLEM SOLVING TO CREATE MASSAGE CARE/TREATMENT PLANS
    Care or Treatment Plan
SUMMARY

KEY TERMS

Applied kinesiology
Assessment
End-feel
Neurologic muscle testing
Palpation
Phasic muscles
Postural muscles
Rapport
Resourceful compensation
Strength testing

As the learning process begins, it is important that the student understand the value of the sequence and general flow of the massage application. Although modeling precise massage routines is a valuable learning exercise, after the student grasps the concepts, the routine must evolve to meet the unique needs of the individual client. If the student knows how to perform a certain massage routine but does not understand how to modify and alter the application of therapeutic massage, his or her ability to serve the client will be limited. People do not fit neatly into a routine sequence of massage techniques. To achieve the best results, the massage practitioner must use the concepts learned from performing the routines to design an application that fits the client's individual needs, based on physiologic outcomes, rather than trying to make the client fit the routine. Instead of providing the structure of a precise, step-by-step routine, this chapter teaches the student to perform an assessment to evaluate current function and then to determine short- and long-term outcomes for the client. Then, based on the assessment information and the client's goals, an individual care or treatment plan is developed.

The assessment process can be as simple as ruling out contraindications to a one-time session in a personal service environment (e.g., day spa, cruise ship, resort) or as comprehensive as determining a client's needs for therapeutic massage provided as a health care component (e.g., as part of a rehabilitation or pain management program or in the development of coping strategies for anxiety disorder).

Care and treatment plans can be as simple as providing a 1-hour vacation from daily stress, a present for Mother's Day or Father's Day, or a session of pleasure and pampering for a client. They also can be complex, such as using massage to aid in the management of asthma, depression, stroke rehabilitation, side effects caused by chemotherapy, and sports training protocols.

This chapter presents the assessment skills a practitioner needs to function effectively with supervision in a health care setting, providing massage as part of a comprehensive treatment plan developed by health care professionals. The massage professional should be able to participate in this process by providing reliable information to be considered in the development of the treatment plan. These skills exceed those usually required in the personal service setting; however, as more employment opportunities open in the health care setting, it is important to be able to function as part of a multidisciplinary health care team. The ability to reason clinically at this level supports the effectiveness of all massage interactions, be it for relaxation and pleasure outcomes or for the management of complex health conditions.

For the professional, it is better to have the skill and not use it than to need a skill and not have it. Because most of the physiologic changes and benefits of massage result from the most basic technical skills, expertise comes from the decisions made in applying those skills. The practitioner's ability to make those decisions depends on his or her ability to gather the client's history data, perform assessment and analysis, and interpret the information collected during assessment. Then, with the information gathered and the client outcomes determined, the massage methods and variations (depth of pressure, drag, frequency, direction, speed, and rhythm) are identified to develop the treatment plan.

Finally, competency in assessment and intelligent development and implementation of treatment plans based on outcome goals differentiates the massage technician, who applies a method, from the massage therapist, who can support client outcomes with layered therapeutic intervention. What is your career goal: technician or therapist? If your choice is to be a technician, you may find it difficult to proceed; however, if your goal is to be a therapist, then the information in this chapter will excite and challenge you.

ASSESSMENT

SECTION OBJECTIVES

Using the information presented in this section, the student will be able to perform the following:

- Interview a client effectively
- Complete a basic physical assessment, a gait assessment, a 14-level palpation assessment, and a muscle testing assessment

Assessment is a learned skill. The ability to incorporate this skill into massage sessions enhances the quality of treatment given by the massage professional. Assessment is the collection and interpretation of information provided by the client, the client's consent advocates (parent or guardian), and the referring medical professionals, as well as information gathered by the massage practitioner. In a growing number of clinical health care settings, the massage professional's assessment is considered in the treatment plan developed by the multidisciplinary health care team. Therefore the massage practitioner must understand and practice standard assessment and charting procedures. Chapter 3 introduced these concepts; this chapter refines and synthesizes them. Although the massage professional observes, interprets, and makes decisions based on information gathered during assessment procedures, it is important to remember that the massage professional is not equipped to diagnose any specific medical condition or to treat one except under the direct supervision of a licensed medical professional.

For the massage practitioner, interpreting the information gathered during a premassage assessment has three purposes:

- To determine whether the client should be referred to a medical professional and to discover any cautions that would modify the massage application
- To obtain input from the client that is used in developing the massage care/treatment plan
- To design the best massage for the client; specifically, the types of methods used and the mechanical forces generated by those methods, as well as the proper application of depth of pressure, drag, direction, speed, rhythm, frequency, and duration of each method, to achieve the desired physiologic outcome (Figure 10-1)

In reality, the assessment and the application of massage techniques are almost the same thing. Not uncommonly, massage manipulations and techniques are used during a massage to evaluate the tissue and then use the same manipulations and techniques, altered slightly in intensity, to normalize the situation (adaptation).

For teaching purposes, the two approaches have been separated. One of the truly difficult concepts to teach and to learn is pure assessment. Students typically rush into localized adaptation techniques without taking the time to discover the larger pattern of dysfunction that the client presents. *Assessment does not change a condition; rather it is an attempt to understand it.* Interventions cause change. To understand the results of the massage session, the student must learn to separate assessment information obtained before, during, and after the massage from methods of intervention. To support

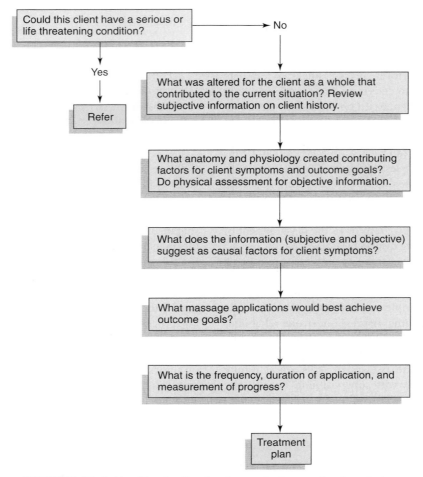

FIGURE 10-1 Algorithm for the development of a care/treatment plan.

the learning process, this chapter is divided into two distinct areas: (1) pure assessment and (2) interpretation of assessment information with general suggestions for massage intervention.

Establishing Rapport

The client is the most important resource involved in the assessment process. The skills a massage professional requires for the process of gathering information from the client are (1) an ability to establish rapport, (2) keen observation, (3) successful interviewing methods, and (4) active listening.

Rapport is the development of a relationship based on mutual trust and harmony. It is the massage professional's responsibility to establish a sense of rapport with clients.

The best way to begin establishing rapport is to learn and use the client's name. The massage practitioner needs to show a genuine interest in the person that goes beyond the problems and goals the person presents. What happens to a person affects the whole being.

Many people need time to sort out their thoughts and feelings and develop their statements. The conversation should proceed slowly, and the client should never be rushed. By giving the person full attention and by observing what makes

the client most comfortable, the practitioner will find it easier to resist the urge to treat everyone in the same manner. Rapport is enhanced if the massage professional uses words, a tone of voice, and body language similar to those of the client. The process of rapport has actual neurons in the brain called *mirror neurons* that coordinate the process of looking and acting like the person we are communicating with. This process is a very instinctual survival mechanism. If the body language and the voice tone are similar—like a dance—then the client and massage therapist connect. If for some reason the mirroring is not established, the communicating persons will feel odd and may avoid contact. This is an overlooked issue in client retention. Unless the client feels rapport, they will not be able to relax during the massage and will likely avoid further contact. Some people have mannerisms or voice tone that is out of sync and may have difficulty establishing rapport with a potential client . The may be from social conditioning or some sort of physical cause. For example, if a person has experienced a closed head injury, he may not be able to modulate eye contact or body language. If the reason for the disconnect is not evident, the potential client will not understand why he is uncomfortable. Medication can sometimes interfere with rapport mechanisms as do almost all substances of abuse. If the massage professional has a physical condition, making it difficult to "mirror," they need to briefly explain the situation. If massage professionals find that they have clients with whom they are out of sync, they need to learn more effective rapport skills. This may require taking communication classes or seeking help to understand the nature of their behavior as well as that of their client.

How to Observe

Attention to detail and the needs of the client provide a sensitive, well-trained massage therapist with essential information. Clients notice the difference between a massage professional who takes the time to honor the client's space and adjust to it and one who tries to make the client fit into a routine method of massage application. During the initial conversation, it is important to pay very close attention to the client visually. If the practitioner has a visual impairment, information gathered from the interview and physical assessment replaces visual assessment. An effective therapist uses all the senses—hearing, sight, smell, touch, and intuition—in the assessment of the client.

At this point, information is only gathered, not interpreted; resist the urge to try to understand what all the information means. Interpretation comes after all the information has been gathered. This may take several sessions. Any massage provided at this stage is a form of assessment. Although the client experiences generalized benefits from the assessment-focused massage, only when sufficient information has been gathered can the client's expected outcomes be specifically addressed.

At the beginning of each session, the practitioner gets a sense of the client's general presence. How well does the client move and breathe? Does the client's presence suggest sympathetic or parasympathetic dominance? Sympathetic dominance is the display of restlessness, anxiety, fear, anger, agitation, elation, or exuberance. Parasympathetic dominance is indicated by a generally relaxed appearance, contentment, slowness, or depression. Because therapeutic massage can either stimulate or relax, this needs to be considered in the massage design.

If a client is active and exuberant (sympathetic dominance), the initial massage approach and the massage practitioner's energy level need to match the client's energy level. If the focus of the session is to calm the client, the therapist begins to slow down as the massage progresses and may introduce appropriate rhythmic entrainment approaches to provide a calming effect.

If the client is tired or moderately depressed, the therapist should proceed slowly in the initial pace of the massage. During the session, the energy and activity level of the massage practitioner and the methods used can be increased as the client's energy increases.

The practitioner pays attention to where and how a client indicates a problem on his or her body. These gestures often reveal whether a client has a muscle, joint, or visceral problem. It also is important for the therapist to observe the client's body language and nonverbal responses while discussing various topics. Everything the person does is important. Everyone's behavior has a pattern, and all the bits of information combine to reveal that pattern (Proficiency Exercise 10-1).

PROFICIENCY EXERCISE 10-1

1. *Watch people in a public place, such as a mall or an airport. Is the general presence of each person you observe sympathetic or parasympathetic in nature?*
2. *Ask 10 people to explain a physical ache or pain to you. Watch their gestures carefully. What similarities do you notice in their explanations?*

Interviewing and Listening: the Subjective Aspect of Assessment

Communication skills first were presented in Chapter 2. These skills are used during interviewing sessions and throughout client-practitioner interactions.

Open-ended questions encourage conversation. It is important to avoid questions that can be answered with only one word. The point of the interview is to help the client communicate his or her health history and to reveal the reason for the massage. For example, the question, "Have you ever had a professional massage before?" requires the client to answer only "Yes" or "No." A better question would be, "What is your experience with therapeutic massage?" This question requires the client to give more detail when answering. When the client provides information, it is important for the practitioner to restate what the client has said. The client then has the opportunity to correct any information and is reassured that the therapist was listening.

When speaking to a client, it is important that the massage professional use words the client can understand. Although professionalism is important, medical terminology need not be used. If the client uses a word that is unclear, the therapist should ask what the person means. Asking for clarification enhances knowledge and understanding of the information obtained from the client.

Certain specific information must be obtained from the client. When encouraging conversation, the massage professional can easily forget to ask the important questions. A client information form (see Chapter 3) provides a framework for obtaining necessary and important information during the interview.

When listening, the massage practitioner must do nothing but listen. You cannot listen while thinking about what is going to be said, writing, or interpreting information. An active listener nods or shows other signs of interest to encourage the person to continue speaking.

The client must be allowed to finish a sentence and must not be rushed or interrupted. Some people rehearse what they say internally before speaking. They speak with pauses between statements, and the practitioner must wait for the client to complete her thoughts. If interrupted, the client often forgets what she was going to tell you. Other clients talk nonstop. They may need to sort through their information by saying it aloud.

When the client has completed a thought and verbalized it, it is important for the massage therapist to summarize and restate the information to make sure that she understood it.

PROFICIENCY EXERCISE 10-2

1. *With a partner, practice asking three open-ended questions that you might use during an interview.*
2. *Hold conversations with 10 different people. Practice restating information given to you in response to a question you asked.*

It is amazing how often information is misinterpreted. A competent professional is very careful of any preconceived ideas and keeps an open mind while the assessment is in progress (Proficiency Exercise 10-2).

Physical Assessment: The Objective Aspect of Assessment

After the subjective assessment has been completed, the massage practitioner may choose to do a physical assessment before beginning the massage. For a single-session general massage, the physical assessment usually is limited to having the client show the massage technician any movements that feel restricted or may be causing pain. It is important to ask the client to point out any bruises, varicose veins, or areas of inflammation to avoid working over these areas. The massage technician should ask, "Are there any areas you feel I should avoid?" Be sure the information is indicated on the client information form and then take care to avoid those areas.

The assessment for basic therapeutic massage, including the development of a treatment plan and agreed-on outcomes over a series of massage sessions, includes a general evaluation of the client's posture (Figure 20-2), gait (walking pattern), and biomechanical function.

Components of the Physical Assessment

For the physical assessment, the main considerations are body balance, efficient function, and basic symmetry. Functional assessment considers posture, gait, and range of motion.

People are not perfectly symmetric, but the right and left halves of the body should be similar in shape, range of motion,

FIGURE 10-2 Learning posture assessment.

and ability to function. For example, the ear, shoulder, hip, and ankle should be in a vertical line. The greater the discrepancy in symmetry, the greater the potential for soft tissue dysfunction.

Disruption of the gait reflexes creates the potential for many problems. Common gait problems include a functional short leg caused by muscle shortening, tight neck and shoulder muscles, aching feet, and fatigue. The massage therapist must understand basic biomechanics, including posture, interaction of joint functions, and gait.

Outcome Documentation Instruments

Because health care intervention is based on evidence of benefit, the massage therapist must be able to show that beneficial changes in the client's status derive from massage. Both the value and quality of evidence-based interventions can be assessed using standardized assessment tools called *instruments.*

Two important aspects of treatment plan development and effective documentation (charting) are preassessment and postassessment. As the preassessment and postassessment data are compared, the benefits of massage can be identified, as can parts of the care/treatment plan that may need to be adjusted in future massage sessions. To assess outcomes accurately, massage therapists must use the same instruments for follow-up evaluations that they used for the baseline (beginning) evaluation.

Instruments for evaluating outcomes can be divided into two categories: subjective measurements, which focus on data provided by the client, and objective measurements, which focus on data provide by the practitioner's assessment.

The evaluation of pain has classically been a subjective measurement. Examples of assessment instruments that focus on subjective outcomes include the following:

- Visual analog scale (measures the intensity of pain)
- Pain Drawing (measures the location and quality of pain)
- McGill Pain Questionnaire (measures the sensory and cognitive experience of pain)

The Evolve Web site presents examples of these types of subjective outcome assessment instruments.

The McGill Pain Questionnaire (MPQ) is used to specify the subjective pain experience using sensory, affective, and evaluative word descriptors. The three primary measures are (1) the pain rating index, which is based on two types of numeric values that can be assigned to each word descriptor; (2) the number of words chosen; and (3) the present pain intensity, which is rated on a 1 to 5 intensity scale.[1]

The short form of the McGill Pain Questionnaire (SF-MPQ) has 11 questions related to the sensory dimension of the pain experience and four related to the affective dimension.[2] Each descriptor is ranked on a four-point intensity scale (0 = none, 1 = mild, 2 = moderate, 3 = severe). The pain rating index of the standard MPQ is included, as is a visual analog scale.

Physical assessment procedures typically are classified as objective and cover isolated function of muscles and/or joints, range of motion, strength, and endurance. These functions are measured and compared to what is considered normal function, and the differences (deviations from the norm) are recorded.

Functional capacity, or whole body movement capabilities, can also be measured. Examples of functional capacity tests include lifting, carrying, walking, sitting, standing, balancing, and hand function. These types of assessment procedures are especially helpful for measuring qualitative goals, such as improvement in performing activities of daily living and occupation-related rehabilitation.

A number of questionnaires can help identify the client's perception of his or her own well-being, distress, or activity intolerance. These include the Oswestry Low Back Pain Disability Questionnaire, Roland-Morris Questionnaire, and Functional Assessment Screening Questionnaire (FASQ).

Examples of Pain Measurement Instruments

The Pain Drawing is a very popular tool for assessing pain in terms of quality (e.g., sharp, aching, numbness, burning) and location.

Pain assessment tools help patients describe their pain. For example, a pain scale commonly is used to describe the intensity of the pain or how much pain the patient is feeling. Pain scales include the numerical rating scale, the visual analog scale, the categorical scale, and the pain faces scale.

On the numerical rating scale, the person is asked to identify how much pain they are having by choosing a number from 0 (no pain) to 10 (the worst pain imaginable).

The visual analog scale is a straight line, on which the left end represents no pain and the right end represents the worst pain. Individuals are asked to mark on the line where they think their pain is.

The categorical pain scale has four categories: none, mild, moderate, and severe. Individuals are asked to select the category that best describes their pain. The pain faces scale uses six faces with different expressions on each face. Each face is a person who feels happy because he or she has no pain or feels sad because he or she has some or a lot of pain. The person is asked to choose the face that best describes how he or she is feeling. This rating scale can be used by people age 3 years and older (Figure 10-3).

Physical/Objective Measurements

Assessment data can be quantified in a number of ways.

Standardized Palpation of Tenderness. The American College of Rheumatology has developed a quantifiable method of assessing tissue tenderness.[3] The examiner observes the response to palpatory stimulus by noting pain behaviors, such as facial grimacing and signs of withdrawal. By comparing the painful sites to uninvolved body areas, the examiner can determine whether the response is due to increased physiologic activity or his same assessment process can be used to detect a change in pain perception at the same pressure. Instruments for gauging pressure, called *algometers,* can further objectify the assessment.

Using a baseline of 4 kg of pressure (enough to blanch the tip of a thumbnail pressed on a table), results are rated as follows:

Grade 0 = No tenderness

Grade I = Tenderness with no physical or verbal response

Grade II = Tenderness with grimacing and/or flinching

Grade III = Tenderness with withdrawal (positive jump sign)

Grade IV = Withdrawal from non-noxious stimuli

Physical Capacity (Impairment) Assessment. Physical capacity tests measure functions such as joint mobility and muscle strength and endurance, such as cervical rotation mobility, hip range of motion, and trunk extensor endurance.

1. Walking 1 mile
2. Climbing two flights of stairs (16 steps)
3. Squatting
4. Kneeling
5. Sitting for prolonged periods with the knees bent in one position
6. Climbing four flights of stairs (32 steps)
7. Running a short distance (100 yards, the length of a football field)
8. Walking a short distance (1 block)

Muscle Testing Assessment. Various instruments have been developed to measure muscle and joint function (Figure 10-4).

10-1

Posture Assessment: Standing Position

Three major factors influence posture: heredity, disease, and habit. These factors must be considered in the evaluation of posture. The easiest factor to adjust is habit. By normalizing the soft tissue and teaching balancing exercises, the massage practitioner can play a beneficial role in helping clients over-

0	1	2	3	4	5
No hurt	Hurts little bit	Hurts little more	Hurts even more	Hurts whole lot	Hurts worst

FIGURE 10-3 Categorical/numeric pain scale. (Modified from Whaley L, Wong, D. *Nursing care of infants and children,* ed 3, St Louis, 1987, Mosby.)

Muscle Strength Grading Scale (Oxford Scale)
Medical Research Council [MRC] grading scale

Grade	Value	Muscle Strength
5	Normal	Complete range of motion (ROM) against gravity with full resistance
4	Good	• Complete ROM against gravity with some resistance: Full range of motion with decreased strength • (sometimes this category is subdivided further into $4^-/5$, 4/5, and $4^+/5$)
3	Fair	Complete ROM against gravity with no resistance; active ROM
2	Poor	Complete ROM with some assistance and gravity eliminated
1	Trace	Evidence of slight muscular contraction, no joint motion evident
0	Zero	No evidence of muscle contraction NT: Not testable

FIGURE 10-4 Muscle strength grading scale (Oxford Scale). Aids to the examination of the peripheral nervous system. London: Medical Research Council, The Stationary Office, 1976 (Memorandum No. 45, ISBN 0-11450-033-9).

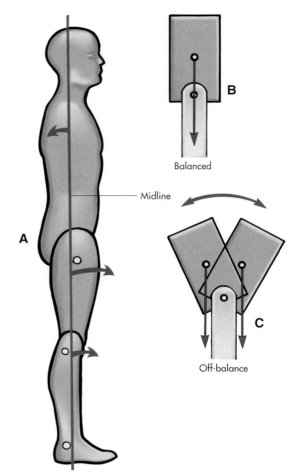

FIGURE 10-5 A, In a normal, relaxed stance, the leg and trunk tend to rotate slightly off the midline of the body but maintain a counterbalance force. Balance is achieved in **B** but not in **C.** Anytime the trunk moves off this midline balance point, the body must compensate.

come habitual postural distortion. Effects may arise from occupational habits (e.g., a shoulder raised from talking on the phone) and recreational habits (e.g., a forward-shoulder position in a bike rider), or they may be sleep related (long-term use of high pillows).

Clothing, shoes, and furniture affect the way a person uses the body. Tight collars or ties restrict breathing and contribute to neck and shoulder problems. Restrictive belts, control-top undergarments, and tight pants also limit breathing and affect the neck, shoulders, and midback. Shoes with high heels or those that do not fit the feet comfortably interfere with postural muscles. Shoes with worn soles imprint the old postural pattern, and the client's body assumes the dysfunctional pattern if she puts them back on after the massage. If postural changes are to be maintained, the client must change to shoes that do not have a worn sole. Sleep positions can contribute to a wide range of problems. Furniture that does not support the back or that is too high or too low perpetuates muscular dysfunction.

When assessing posture, the massage practitioner must take care to notice the complete postural pattern, head to toe. Every action has a reaction, and the reaction can be compensation. Most compensatory patterns (reactions) occur in response to external forces imposed on the body. The body makes countless compensatory changes daily. This is normal, and if other pathologic conditions are not present, they seldom become problematic. However, if the client has had an injury, maintains a certain position for a prolonged period, or over-

uses a body area, the body may not be able to return to a normal dynamic balance efficiently. The balance of the body against the force of gravity is the fundamental determining factor in a person's posture, or upright position. Even subtle shifts in posture demand a whole body compensatory pattern (Figure 10-5).

The cervical, thoracic, lumbar, and sacral curves (Figure 10-6) develop because of the body's need to maintain an upright position against gravity. In adults, the cervical vertebrae, when viewed laterally, form a symmetric anterior convex curve. The thoracic vertebrae curve posteriorly, and the lumbar vertebrae reverse and curve in the anterior direction, with a posterior curve of the sacrum. The sharp angulation above C1, the atlas that allows the head to maintain a level, horizontal plane, has also been considered a curve. Changes in the normal spinal curves result in scoliosis, lordosis, and kyphosis.

Mechanical Balance

A mechanically balanced, weight-bearing joint must be in the gravitational line of the mass it supports and is located exactly through the axis of rotation. Placement of the feet influences the stability of the standing position by providing a base of

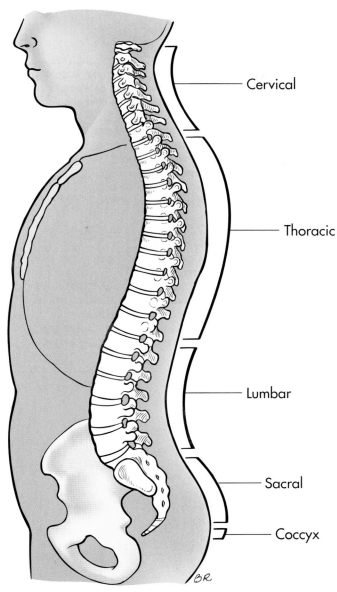

FIGURE 10-6 Normal spinal curves.

Cervical

Thoracic

Lumbar

Sacral

Coccyx

support. The most common position is one leg in front of the other, with mild external rotation of the forward leg. People commonly have a functionally long and short leg. When a person is standing, the long leg often is the front one. When the person is seated with the legs crossed, the long leg often is on top.

The standing posture requires various segments of the body to cooperate mechanically as a whole. Passive tension of ligaments, fascia, and the connective tissue elements of the muscles supports the skeleton. Muscle activity plays a small but important role. Postural muscles maintain small amounts of contraction that stabilize the body upright in gravity by continually repositioning the body weight over the mechanical balance point.

In relaxed symmetric standing, both the hip and the knee joints assume a position of full extension to provide for the most efficient weight-bearing position. The knee joint has an additional stabilizing element in its *screw home mechanism.* The femur rides backward on the medial condyle and rotates medially about its vertical axis to lock the joint for weight bearing; this happens only in the final phase of extension. The normal screw home extension pattern of the knee is not hyperextension, which puts a strain on the knee. The hamstrings are the major muscles that resist the force of gravity at the knee.[4,5]

At the ankle joint, bones and ligaments do little to limit motion. Passive tension of the two-joint gastrocnemius muscle (i.e., the muscle crosses two joints) becomes an important factor. This stabilizing force is diminished if high-heeled shoes are worn. The heel of the shoe puts the gastrocnemius on a slack. If these heels are worn constantly, the muscle and the Achilles tendon shorten.

Body sway is limited by the intermittent action of appropriate antigravitational postural muscles. During prolonged standing, the average person shifts position frequently. The two basic positions used are the symmetric stance, with the weight distributed equally on both feet, and the asymmetric stance, in which nearly all the weight rests on one foot (Figure 10-7). The asymmetric stance is the most common, with the

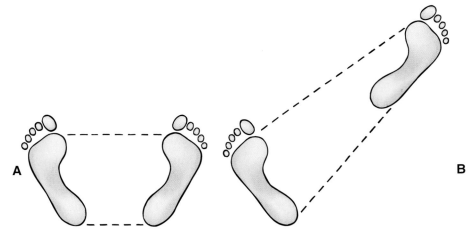

A

B

FIGURE 10-7 A, Symmetric stance. **B,** Asymmetric stance. The asymmetric stance, with the weight shifted from foot to foot, is the most efficient standing position.

BOX 10-1

Landmarks That Help Identify Lack of Symmetry

The following landmarks can be used to compare the symmetry of the body in different aspects. Be sure to observe the client from the back, the front, and the left and right sides.

- The middle of the chin should sit directly under the tip of the nose. Check the chin alignment with the sternal notch. These two landmarks should be in a direct line.
- The shoulders and clavicles should be level with each other. The shoulders should not roll forward or backward or be rotated with one forward and one backward.
- The arms should hang freely and at the same rotation out of the glenohumeral (shoulder) joint.
- The elbows, wrists, and fingertips should be in the same plane.
- The skin of the thorax (chest and back) should be even and should not look as if it pulls or is puffy.
- The navel, located on the same line as the nose, chin, and sternal notch, should not look pulled.
- The ribs should be even and springy.
- The abdomen should be firm but relaxed and slightly rounded.
- The curves at the waist should be even on both sides.

- The spine should be in a direct line from the base of the skull and on the same plane as the line connecting the nose and the navel. The curves of the spine should not be exaggerated.
- The scapulae should appear even and should move freely. You should be able to draw an imaginary straight line between the tips of the scapulae.
- The gluteal muscle mass should be even.
- The tops of the iliac crests should be even.
- The greater trochanter, knees, and ankles should be level.
- The circumferences of the thigh and calf should be similar on the left and right sides.
- The legs should rotate out of the acetabulum (hip joint) evenly in a slight external rotation.
- The knees should be locked in the standing position but should not be hyperextended. The patellae (kneecaps) should be level and pointed slightly laterally.
- A line dropped from the nose should fall through the sternum and the navel and should be spaced evenly between.

A   **B**

FIGURE 10-8 Proper (A) and improper (B) foot position in walking.

weight shifted back and forth between the two feet. This allows for rest periods and shifting of the gravitational forces.

Assessment Procedures for the Standing Position

When the massage practitioner assesses the posture of a client in the standing position, it is important that the client use the symmetric stance. The feet are about shoulder-width apart, and the eyes are closed. With the eyes closed, most of the client's postural patterns are exaggerated, because the client is unable to orient the body visually. Often the client will tip the head or rotate it slightly to feel balanced; this indicates muscular imbalance and internal postural imbalance information relayed by positional receptors.

Box 10-1 presents a list of indicators of lack of symmetry. The physical assessment form in Chapter 3 is a helpful tool for performing the physical assessment.

Gait Assessment

Understanding the basic body movements of walking can help the massage practitioner recognize dysfunctional and inefficient gait patterns. It is important to observe the client from the front, the back, and both sides. First, the massage practitioner should watch the client walk, noting the heel-to-toe foot placement. The toes should point directly forward with each step (Figure 10-8).

FIGURE 10-9 Efficient gait position.

Observe the upper body. It should be relaxed and fairly symmetric. The head should face forward with the eyes level with the horizontal plane. A natural arm swing occurs opposite the leg swing. The arm swing begins at the shoulder joint. On each step, the left arm moves forward as the right leg moves forward and vice versa. This pattern provides balance. The rhythm and pace of the arm and leg swing should be similar. Increasing the walking speed increases the speed of the arm swing. The length of the stride determines the arc of the arm swing (Figure 10-9).

Observe the client walking, and notice the person's general appearance. The optimal walking pattern is as follows:

1. The head and trunk are vertical, with the eyes easily maintaining forward position and level with the horizontal plane; the shoulders are level and perpendicular to the vertical line.
2. The arms swing freely opposite the leg swing, allowing the shoulder girdle to rotate opposite the pelvic girdle.
3. The step length and timing are even.
4. The body oscillates vertically with each step.
5. The entire body moves rhythmically with each step.
6. At the heel strike, the foot is approximately at a right angle to the leg.
7. The knee is extended, not locked, in slight flexion.
8. The body weight is shifted forward into the stance phase.
9. At push-off, the foot is strongly plantar flexed, with defined hyperextension of the metatarsophalangeal joints of the toes.
10. During the leg swing, the foot easily clears the floor with good alignment, and the rhythm of movement remains unchanged.
11. The heel contacts the floor first.
12. The weight then rolls to the outside of the arch.
13. The arch flattens slightly in response to the weight load.
14. The weight then is shifted to the ball of the foot in preparation for the spring-off from the toes and the shifting of the weight to the other foot.

During walking the pelvis moves slightly in a side-lying, figure-eight pattern. The movements that make up this sequence are transverse, medial, and lateral rotation. The stability and mobility of the sacroiliac (SI) joints play very important roles in this alternating side, figure-eight movement. If these joints are not functioning properly, the entire gait is disrupted. The SI joint is one of the few joints in the body that is not directly affected by muscles that cross the joint. It is a large joint, and the bony contact between the sacrum and the ilium is broad. The rocking of this joint often is disrupted (Figure 10-10).

The hips rotate in a slightly oval pattern beginning with a medial rotation during the leg swing and heel strike, followed by a lateral rotation through the push-off. The knees move in a flexion and extension pattern opposite each other. The extension phase never reaches enough extension to initiate the normal knee-lock pattern that is used in standing. The ankles rotate in an arc around the heel at heel strike and around a center in the forefoot at push-off. Maximal dorsiflexion at the end of the stance phase and maximal plantar flexion at the end of push-off are necessary.

Procedures for Assessing Gait

Observing areas of the body that do not move efficiently during walking is a good means of detecting dysfunctional areas. Pain causes the body to tighten and alters the normal relaxed flow of walking. Muscle weakness and shortening interfere with the neurologic control of the agonist (prime mover) and antagonist muscle action. Limitation of joint movement and hypermobility result in protective muscle contraction. If the situation becomes chronic, both muscle shortening and muscle weakness result. Changes in the soft tissue, including all the connective tissue elements of the tendons, ligaments, and fascial sheaths, restrict the normal action of muscles. Connective tissue usually shortens and becomes less pliable.

Amputation disrupts the body's normal diagonal counterbalance function. Obviously, any amputation of the leg disturbs the walking pattern; what is not so obvious is that amputation of any part of the arm affects the counterbalance movement of the arm swing during walking. The rest of the body must compensate for the loss. Loss of any of the toes greatly affects the postural information sent to the brain from the feet. So often these details are overlooked, when in fact

FIGURE 10-10 The mechanism of the slight rocking movement of the sacroiliac joint.

they may be major contributing factors in posture and gait problems.

Soft tissue dysfunction can exist without joint involvement. Any change in the tissue around a joint has a direct effect on the joint function. Changes in joint function eventually cause problems with the joint. Any dysfunction with the joint immediately involves the surrounding muscles and other soft tissue.

Any disruption of the gait demands that the body compensate by shifting movement patterns and posture. Because of this, all dysfunctional patterns are whole body phenomena. Working only on the symptomatic area is ineffective and offers limited relief. Therapeutic massage with a whole body focus is extremely valuable in dealing with gait dysfunction (Proficiency Exercise 10-3). (For further information on gait, see Chapter 10 of *Mosby's Essential Sciences for Therapeutic Massage,* Mosby, 2009.)

Assessment by Range of Motion

Active range of motion is performed when the client moves the joint through the planes of motion that are normal for that joint. Any pain, crepitus, or limitation that manifests during the action is reported. This assessment identifies what the client is willing or able to do.

Passive range of motion is performed when the massage therapist moves the joint passively through the planes of motion that are normal for the joint. The assessment identifies

PROFICIENCY EXERCISE 10-3

1. *Watch people walk.*
2. *Pay attention to yourself when walking. Put on two different shoes and notice what happens when you walk. Tie one arm to your leg and pay attention to what happens when you walk.*
3. *Place your thumbs on a person's sacroiliac joints and walk behind as the person walks. Feel for the movement. Notice whether the figure-eight pattern is even or lopsided.*
4. *Using the information just presented and the form provided in Figure 3-16, do a physical assessment of 10 people.*

limitation (hypomobility) or excess movement (hypermobility) of the joint. Passive movement is performed carefully and gently to allow the client to fully relax the muscles during the assessment. The client reports the point at which pain or bind, if present, occurs. The massage therapist stops the motion at the point of pain or bind. Passive range of motion provides information about the joint capsule and ligaments and other restricting mechanisms, such as muscles (Figure 10-11).

The range of motion of joints is measured in degrees, starting at the neutral line of anatomic position, which is considered 0. Movement of a joint in the sagittal, frontal, or transverse plane is described as the number of degrees of flexion,

A

B

FIGURE 10-11 Assessment using range of motion. **A,** Assessment of the internal shoulder rotators. **B,** Assessment of the extensor hip rotators.

extension, adduction, abduction, and internal and external rotation (Figure 10-12). For example, the elbow has approximately 150 degrees of flexion at the end range. Anything less than this is hypomobility, and anything more is considered hypermobility. The normal range of motion of joints is found in anatomy texts, such as *Mosby's Essential Sciences for Therapeutic Massage.*

Overpressure and End-Feel

The stretch on the soft tissues, such as muscles, tendons, fascia, and ligaments, and the arrangement of the joint surfaces determine the range of motion of the joint and therefore the joint's normal end-feel. In using overpressure, the massage therapist gradually applies more pressure when the end of the available passive range of joint motion has been reached. The sensation transmitted to the therapist's hands by the tissue resistance at the end of the available range is the end-feel of a joint.

Types of End-Feel

Normal End-Feel. *Soft tissue approximation end-feel* occurs when the full range of the joint is restricted by the normal muscle bulk; it is painless and has a feeling of soft compression. *Muscular,* or *tissue stretch, end-feel* occurs at the extremes of muscle stretch, such as in the hamstrings during a straight leg raise; it has a feeling of increasing tension, springiness, or elasticity. *Capsular stretch,* or *leathery, end-feel* occurs when the joint capsule is stretched at the end of its normal range, such as with external rotation of the glenohumeral joint; it is painless and has the sensation of stretching a piece of leather. *Bony,* or *hard, end-feel* occurs when bone contacts bone at the end of normal range, as in extension of the elbow; it is abrupt and hard.

Abnormal End-Feel. *Empty end-feel* occurs when no physical restriction to movement exists except the pain expressed by the client. *Muscle spasm end-feel* occurs when passive movement stops abruptly because of pain; a springy rebound may occur as a result of reflexive muscle spasm. *Boggy end-feel* occurs when edema is present; it has a mushy, soft quality. *Springy block,* or *internal derangement, end-feel* is a springy or rebounding sensation in a noncapsular pattern; this indicates loose cartilage or meniscal tissue within the joint. *Capsular stretch (leathery) end-feel that occurs before normal range* indicates capsular fibrosis with no inflammation. *Bony (hard) end-feel that occurs before normal range* indicates bony changes or degenerative joint disease or malunion of a joint after a fracture.

Assessment by Palpation

10-5

Palpation is the use of touch to examine the body. Our hands are our most versatile and exquisite assessment tool. Technology does not come close to the sensitivity and accuracy of a trained assessing hand. Our hands need to be trained to interpret what they perceive accurately. Palpation is more than touching and information gathered by sensory receptors in the hands and joints of the upper limb. Sometimes the foot and leg are used during massage and can be effective for palpation assessment. For the therapeutic massage professional, palpation is an essential and continuous process, and the hands become skilled with experience.

With palpation assessment, the main considerations for basic massage are the ability to differentiate between different types of tissue, the ability to distinguish differences of tissue texture in the same tissue types, and the ability to palpate through the various tissue layers from superficial to deep. Palpation includes assessment for hot and cold and observation of skin color and general skin condition. Palpation also assesses various body rhythms, including breathing patterns and pulses.

The tissues the massage therapist should be able to distinguish are the skin, superficial fascia, fascial sheaths, tendons, ligaments, blood vessels, muscle layers, and bone.

FIGURE 10-12 Examples of visual assessment of movements and degrees of range of motion. **A,** 170 degrees. **B,** 180 degrees. **C,** 30 degrees, lateral trunk flexion. **D,** 25 degrees, leg extension. **E,** 30 degrees, hip adductor. **F,** 90 degrees, hip flexion. **G,** 10 degrees, dorsiflexion. **H,** 40 to 45 degrees, internal hip rotation.

Mechanisms of Palpation

Before launching into any discussion of actual palpation skills, the student must understand the mechanism that makes palpation an effective assessment tool. The proprioceptors and mechanoreceptors of the shoulder, arm, and hand (or hip, leg, and foot) receive stimulation from the tissue being palpated. This is the reception phase. These impulses are transmitted through the peripheral and central nervous systems to the brain, where they are interpreted.

The somatosensory region of the brain that interprets this sensory information devotes a massive area to the hand. The refined discriminatory sense of the hand can perceive very subtle shifts and changes. The ability to interpret usually is a sense of comparison; that is, this tissue is softer than that tissue, or this feels rougher than that. Because comparison is a necessity, the practitioner must be careful to compare apples with apples; for example, the skin on the back cannot be compared with the skin on the feet.

This same mechanism makes self-massage less effective. The brain has difficulty deciding which signals to pay attention to when the hand is doing the massage and trying to send sensory information, and the body area being massaged is also trying to decide what is happening. Because the hand sensory and motor areas in the brain are so large, the information from the hand may supersede the information from the part of the body being self-massaged. The body seems to respond to the strongest set of signals. Consequently, the brain pays attention to the hand and does not focus enough motor response to the area being massaged. If the same area is massaged by another person, the area can respond without conflicting sensory input.

It is essential that the massage therapist's entire self become sensitive to subtle differences in the client's body. This is especially true with palpation skills. With palpation, what is going on must be felt and not thought about. Too much thinking shifts awareness away from kinesthetic input.

How to Palpate

Palpation can begin in many different ways. After you have learned the skills, you need not follow the particular protocol presented in this text. The best course is to begin with the lightest palpation and move to the deepest levels, because after the hands have been used for deep compression, the sensitivity of the light touch sensors is momentarily diminished.

During palpation, varying depths of pressure must be used to reach all the tissue types and layers. Do not stay in one area too long or concentrate on a particular spot. The receptors in the practitioner's hands, forearms, or other body areas adapt quickly, and what is subsequently felt or perceived is then lost. The practitioner's first impression should be trusted; if the area feels hot, it probably is. The differences often are small. For practice, put your thumb and first finger together. Close your eyes and then just move the finger on the thumb only enough so that you feel the movement. Open your eyes and notice that the observable difference is tiny. Palpation assessment occurs at this level of awareness.

Near-Touch Palpation. The first application of palpation does not involve touching the body; rather, the intent is to detect hot and cold areas. This is best done just off the skin using the back of the hand, which is very sensitive to heat. The general temperature of the area and any variations should be noted. It is important to move fairly quickly in a sweeping motion over the areas being assessed because heat receptors adapt quickly.

Very sensitive cutaneous (skin) sensory receptors also detect changes in air pressure and currents and the movement of the air. This is one reason we can feel someone come up behind us when we cannot see the person. The movement and change in the surrounding air pressure alert us; this is a protective survival mechanism. Being able to consciously detect subtle sensations is an invaluable assessment tool. It is important to realize where the information comes from and why it can be sensed, to dispel the notion that this is an extrasensory ability. We are subconsciously aware of all the sensory stimulation that we have receptor mechanisms to detect. With practice, we can become consciously aware of these more subtle sensory experiences. Sensitivity, or intuition, is the ability to work with this information on a conscious level.

Near-touch assessment just above the skin feels somewhat similar to putting two poles of a magnet together; a very subtle resistance occurs. Areas that seem thick, dense, or bumpy or that tend to push the therapist away are hyperactive. Deeper palpation often reveals muscular hyperactivity or hot spots. Areas that seem thin or feel as though holes are present usually are underactive. Impaired circulation, fibrotic tissue, and inhibited muscle activity often develop in underactive areas.

Palpation of the Skin. The second application of palpation is very light surface stroking of the skin. First, determine whether the skin is dry or damp. Damp areas feel a little sticky, or the fingers drag. This light stroking also causes the root hair plexus that senses light touch to respond. It is important to notice whether a particular area gets more goose bumps (i.e., the pilomotor reflex) than other areas. This is a good time to observe for color, especially blue or yellow coloration. In addition, the practitioner should note and keep track of all moles and surface skin growths, pay attention to the quality and texture of the hair, and observe the shape and condition of the nails.

In palpation, the examiner uses gentle, small stretching of the skin in all directions and compares the elasticity of these areas (Figure 10-13). The skin also can be palpated for surface texture. Roughness or smoothness can be felt by applying light pressure to the skin surface.

The skin should move evenly and glide on the underlying superficial fascia tissues. Areas that are stuck, restricted, or too loose should be noted, as should any areas of the skin that become redder than surrounding areas.

Palpation of the Superficial Connective Tissue. The third application of palpation is the superficial connective tissue, which separates and connects the skin and muscle tissue. It allows the skin to glide over the muscles during movement.

FIGURE 10-13 Skin stretching can be used to assess elasticity. Skin that seems tight compared with the surrounding skin may indicate dysfunctional areas.

FIGURE 10-14 The use of skin rolling (i.e., lifting of the tissues) to assess the superficial connective tissues.

This layer of tissue is found by using compression until the fibers of the underlying muscle are felt. The pressure then should be lightened so that the muscle cannot be felt, but if the hand is moved, the skin also moves. This area feels a little like a sponge. The tissue should feel resilient and springy, like gelatin. The superficial fascia holds fluid and fat. If surface edema is present, it is in the superficial fascia. This water-binding quality gives this area the feel of a water balloon, but it should not feel boggy or soggy or show pitting edema (i.e., the dent from the pressure stays in the skin). Fat is stored in the superficial fascia; the method known as skin rolling should really be called superficial fascia rolling. By lifting and rolling the tissue folds, the massage practitioner can compare binding and density (Figure 10-14).

Palpation of Vessels and Lymph Nodes. The fourth application of palpation involves the circulatory vessels and lymph nodes. The more superficial blood vessels lie just above the muscle and still in the superficial connective tissue. The vessels are distinct and feel like soft tubes. Pulses can be palpated, but the feel of the pulse is lost if the pressure is too intense (Figure 10-15). Feeling for pulses helps detect this layer of tissue.

In this same area are the more superficial lymph vessels and lymph nodes. Lymph nodes usually are located in joint areas and feel like small, soft gel caps. The compression of the joint action assists in lymphatic flow. A client with enlarged lymph nodes should be referred to a medical professional for diagnosis. Very light, gentle palpation of lymph nodes and vessels is indicated in this circumstance.

Palpation of Muscles. The fifth application of palpation is skeletal muscle. Muscle has a distinct fiber direction that can be felt. This texture feels somewhat like corded fabric or fine rope. Muscle is made up of contractile fibers embedded in connective tissue. Individual muscles are contained in layers of deep fascia. The area of the muscle that becomes the largest when the muscle is concentrically contracted is in the belly of

the muscle. The tendon develops where the muscle fibers end and the connective tissue continues; this is called the *musculotendinous junction*. A good practice activity involves locating both of these areas for all surface muscles and as many underlying ones as possible. Almost all muscular dysfunctions, such as trigger points or microscarring from minute muscle tears, are found at the musculotendinous junction or in the belly of the muscle. Most acupressure points and motor points are also located in these areas.

Often three or more layers of muscle are present in an area. These layers are separated by deep fascia, and each muscle layer should slide over the one beneath it. Compressing systematically through each layer until the bone is felt is important. Pressure used to reach and palpate the deeper layers of muscle must travel from the superficial layers down to the deeper layers. To accomplish this, the compressive force must be even, broad based, and slow. There should be no "poking" quality to the touch nor abrupt pressure pushing through muscle layers, because the surface layers of muscle will tense up and guard, preventing access to the deeper layers.

Muscle tends to push up against palpating pressure when it is concentrically contracting. Having the client slowly move the joint that is affected can aid the identification of the proper location of muscles being assessed.

Make sure to slide each layer of muscle back and forth over the underlying layer to detect any adherence between the muscle layers. The layers usually run cross-grain to each other. The best example of this is the abdominal muscle group. Even in the arm and leg, where all the muscles seem to run in the same direction, a diagonal crossing and spiraling of the muscle

FIGURE 10-15 Palpation of arterial pulses. **A,** Carotid. **B,** Brachial. **C,** Radial. **D,** Femoral. **E,** Popliteal. **F,** Dorsalis. **G,** Posterior tibial. (From Seidel HM et al: *Mosby's guide to physical examination,* ed 5, St Louis, 2003, Mosby.)

groups is evident. Muscles can feel tense and ropy in both concentric (short) and eccentric (long) patterns. Therefore, think of muscle functioning as short and tight and long and taut.

Palpation of Tendons. The sixth application of palpation is the tendons. Tendons have a higher concentration of collagen fibers and feel more pliable and less ribbed than muscle. Tendons feel like duct tape. Tendons attach muscles to bones. These attachments can be directly on the bone, but just as often tendons attach to ligaments, other tendons, and deep fascia for indirect attachment to the bone. The important

point to remember is that these attachment areas are made up of various types of connective tissue. The difference in the connective tissue is the ratio of collagen, elastin, and water. Beneath many tendons is a fluid-filled bursa cushion that assists the movement of the bone under the tendon. Bursae feel like small water balloons or bubbles.

Palpation of Deep Fascia. The seventh application of palpation is the deep fasciae. The deep fasciae feel like sheets of plastic wrap and duct tape. Unlike the superficial fascia, which is thick and spongy, the deep fasciae are thin but very fibrous. Deep fasciae separate muscles and expand the connective tissue area of bone for muscular attachment. Some deep fasciae, such as the lumbodorsal fascia, the abdominal fascia, and the iliotibial band, run on the surface of the body and are thick, like a tarp. Other types of deep fasciae, such as the linea alba and the nuchal ligament, run perpendicular to the surface of the body and the bone, like a rope. Still others run horizontally through the body. The horizontal pattern occurs at joints, the diaphragm muscle (which is mostly connective tissue), and the pelvic floor. Deep fasciae separate muscle groups and provide a continuous, interconnected framework for the body that follows the principles of tensegrity (see Chapter 4). The shapes and sheets of deep fasciae are kept taut by the design of the cross-pattern and the action of muscles that lie between sheaths, such as the gluteus maximus, which lies between the iliotibial band and the lumbodorsal fascia.

The larger nerves and blood vessels lie in grooves created by the fascial separations. Careful comparison reveals that the location of the traditional acupuncture meridians corresponds to these nerve and blood vessel tracts. The fascial separations can be felt by palpating with the fingers. With sufficient pressure, the fingers tend to fall into these grooves, which can then be followed. These areas need to be resilient but distinct, because they serve as both stabilizers and separators (Figure 10-16).

Palpation of Ligaments. The eighth application of palpation is the ligaments. Ligaments are found around joints. They are high in elastin and somewhat stretchy; they feel much like

bungee cords, although some ligaments are flat. The ligaments hold joints together and maintain joint space in the synovial joints by keeping the joint apart. Ligaments should be flexible enough to allow the joint to move, yet stable enough to restrain movement for joint stability. It is important to be able to recognize a ligament and not mistake it for a tendon. With the joint in a neutral position, if the muscles are isometrically contracted, the tendon moves but the ligament does not.

Palpation of Joints. The ninth application of palpation is the joints (Box 10-2). Joints are found where two bones come together. Careful palpation should reveal the space between the synovial joint ends. Joints often feel like hinges. Most assessment, at the basic massage level, is done with active and passive joint movements. An added source of information is palpation of the joint while it is in motion. The sense should be that of a stable, supported, resilient, and unrestricted range of motion.

With joint movements, it is important to assess for end-feel, as previously described. Simply, *end-feel* is the perception of the joint at the limit of its range of motion, and it feels either soft or hard. In most joints it should feel soft; this means that the body is unable to move any more through muscular contraction, but a small additional move by the therapist still produces some give. A hard end-feel is what the bony stabilization of the elbow feels like on extension. No more active movement is possible, and passive movement is restricted by bone.

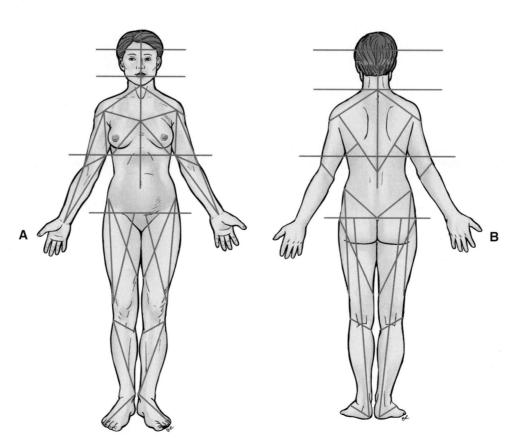

FIGURE 10-16 Fascial sheaths. **A,** Anterior view. **B,** Posterior view.

BOX 10-2

Joint Function

For the most part, massage practitioners work with synovial (freely movable) joints. These joints are the focus of this text. However, all joints are basically the same. The amount of joint movement depends on the bone structure, supportive elements of the ligaments, and arrangement of the muscles. Almost all joint movement is based on the basic flexion-extension concept. Flexion reduces the angle of a joint, and extension increases it. Circumduction is a combination of flexion-extension and adduction-abduction movements.

For a joint to move, the muscular elements must function properly, and the joint structure, including the cartilage, must also be functional. Joints are designed to fit together in a specific way. For a joint to move, there must be a space between the bone ends. The bone ends must be smooth and lubricated to prevent friction. Anything that interferes with these key elements interferes with joint function.

Balance is another key element in joint function. If the positional receptors in a joint relay information to the central nervous system indicating that damage to the joint may occur, motor activity (i.e., muscular action) is affected.

Joints are characterized as one-joint muscles or two-joint muscles, depending on the basic configuration of the muscles around the joint. One-joint muscles cross a single joint and consist of short levers and long levers. Short levers initiate and stabilize movement. They often have the best mechanical advantage in joint movement, and they usually are located deep to the long levers. Long levers have the strength and pulling range to carry out the full range of motion of the joint pattern. They are superficial to the short levers and deep to the two-joint muscles. Two-joint muscles cross two joints and coordinate movement patterns. They usually are the most superficial of the muscles. A noted exception to this is the psoas muscle.

When evaluating joint function, the massage professional is most concerned with pain-free, symmetric range of motion. Determining whether pain on movement is a muscle or tendon problem or a ligament or joint problem can be difficult. Therapeutic massage can deal with nonspecific soft tissue dysfunction. Joint dysfunction is out of the scope of practice for massage professionals unless they are specifically supervised by a chiropractor, physician, or physical therapist.

It is important to be able to distinguish between the muscle and tendon components and the ligament and joint components in a restricted movement pattern. When in doubt, always refer suspected joint problems to a medical professional.

Muscle and tendon problems can be differentiated from ligament and joint problems in two ways:

- Pain on gentle traction usually indicates a soft tissue such as a muscle or tendon problem; pain with gentle

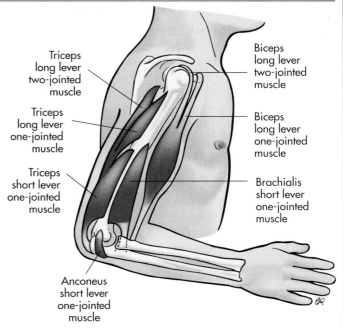

One- and two-joint muscles. functional short- and long-lever muscles.

compression usually indicates a ligament or joint problem.
- If active range of motion produces pain and passive range of motion does not, the cause usually is a muscle or tendon problem. If both passive and active range of motion produce pain, the cause usually is a ligament or joint problem.

When massage practitioners work with joints, it is important that they distinguish between the anatomic barrier and the physiologic barrier. The *anatomic barrier* is the bone contour and the soft tissue (especially the ligaments) that serve as the final limit to motion in a joint. Beyond this motion limit, tissue damage occurs. The *physiologic barrier* is more of a nervous system protective barrier that prevents access to the anatomic barrier when damage to the joint could occur. A pathologic barrier exists when the movement is limited by some sort of injury, dysfunction, or inappropriate compensation pattern. The massage therapist must stay within the limits of the physiologic barrier to avoid possible hypermovement of a joint. Therapeutic massage may increase the range of motion of a jointed area by resetting the confines of the pathologic barrier.

Palpation of Bones. The tenth application of palpation is the bones. Those who have developed their palpation skills find a firm but detectable pliability to bone. Bones feel like young sapling tree trunks and branches.

For the massage practitioner, it is important to be able to palpate the bony landmarks that indicate the tendinous attachment points for the muscles and to trace the bone's shape.

Palpation of Abdominal Viscera. The eleventh application of palpation is the viscera, which are the internal organs of the body. The abdomen contains the viscera. It is important for the massage professional to be able to locate and to know the positioning of the organs in the abdominal cavity. A good anatomy atlas can help with this information. The massage therapist should be able to palpate the distinct firmness of the liver and the large intestine. Although deep massage to the abdomen is not suggested for those trained in basic massage, light to moderate stroking of the abdomen is beneficial for the large intestine. The massage therapist should be able to locate and palpate this organ.

Palpation of Body Rhythms. The twelfth application of palpation is the body rhythms. Body rhythms are felt as even pulsations. Body rhythms, those mentioned and not mentioned, are designed to operate in a coordinated, balanced, and synchronized manner. In the body the rhythms all entrain (synchronize). When palpating body rhythms, the practitioner should get a sense of this harmony. Although the trained hand can pick out some of the individual rhythms, just as one can hear individual notes in a song, it is the whole connected effect that is important. When a person feels "off" or "out of sync," he or she often is speaking of disruption in the entrainment process of body rhythms.

The three basic rhythms are the respiration, circulation and lymph, and craniosacral rhythms. There may also be more subtle energetic rhythms in the body that can be identified with increased palpation sensitivity. However, the rhythms discussed next are the three with the most scientific understanding.

Respiration. The breath is easy to feel. It should be even and should follow good principles of inhalation and exhalation (see Chapter 13). Palpation of the breath is done by placing the hands over the ribs and allowing the body to go through three or more cycles as the practitioner evaluates the evenness and fullness of the breath. Relaxed breathing should result in a slight rounding of the upper abdomen and lateral movement of the lower ribs during inhalation. Movement in the shoulders or upper chest indicates potential difficulties with the breathing mechanism.

Circulation. The movement of the blood is felt at the major pulse points. The pulses should be balanced on both sides of the body. Basic palpation of the movement of the blood is done by placing the fingertips over pulse points on both sides of the body and comparing for evenness.

The vascular refill rate is another means of assessing the efficiency and rhythm of the circulation. To assess this rate, press the nail beds until they blanch (push blood out), then let go and count the seconds until color returns. Lymph vessels have an undulating peristalsis type of rhythm.

Craniosacral Rhythm. The craniosacral rhythm is a subtle but detectable widening and narrowing movement of the cranial bones. A to-and-fro (back-and-forth) oscillation of the sacrum should be noted.[6] Specific training for craniosacral therapy focuses on this mechanism. Basic palpation of the craniosacral rhythm is done by lightly placing the hands on either side of the head and sensing for the widening and narrowing of the skull. The same undulation can be sensed in any symmetrically placed hand position on the body, such as on both shoulders, the two sides of the back, the two sides of the rib cage, the iliac crests, the knees, and the feet. Also, place a hand over the sacrum and feel for the to-and-fro movement. These sensations normally occur at a rate of 10 to 14 times per minute.[6] The movement should feel coordinated and even. This sensation may be the rhythmic lymphatic undulation instead of a specific focus on the craniosacral system (Proficiency Exercise 10-4) (Figure 10-17).

PROFICIENCY EXERCISE 10-4

1. *Palpate several objects with different textures. Then palpate the same objects through a sheet, towel, blanket, and foam. See how many you can recognize.*
2. *Have people walk up to you while you are blindfolded. Pay attention to when you sense the person's presence.*
3. *Feel heat radiating off various objects. How far away can you get from the object before you cannot feel the heat?*
4. *Feel appliances or machinery as the motor runs. Pay attention to the vibrations. How far away can you get and still feel the vibrations?*
5. *Put a dime in a phone book under two pages. Locate the dime. Keep increasing the number of pages over the dime until you cannot feel it.*
6. *Get two magnets and play with them. Feel for the "force field."*
7. *Using the list below, palpate and observe all of the following on five clients. Compare with related areas.*
   - Heat and cold
   - Air pressure and current shifts
   - Damp or dry skin
   - Goose bumps
   - Color
   - Hair
   - Nails

- Skin texture
- Skin roughness or smoothness
- Superficial connective tissue/superficial fascia
- Blood vessels
- Pulses
- Lymph nodes
- Direction of skeletal muscle fiber
- Musculotendinous junction
- Motor points
- Muscle layers
- Tendons
- Fascial sheaths
- Ligaments
- Bursae
- Joints
- Joint space
- Joint movement
- Joint movement end-feel
- Bone
- Bony landmarks
- Bone shape
- Viscera
- Craniosacral rhythms or lymphatic undulation
- Breathing

FIGURE 10-17 Palpation. **A,** Near touch. **B,** Skin stroking. **C,** Skin elasticity. **D,** Compare skin fold. **E,** Palpation of superficial connective tissue. **F,** Vessels and lymph nodes.

Continued

FIGURE 10-17 cont'd G, Palpation of muscle layer sliding. **H,** Palpation of tendons. **I,** Palpation of fascial sheaths. **J,** Palpation of ligaments. **K,** Palpation of joints. **L,** Palpation of bone.

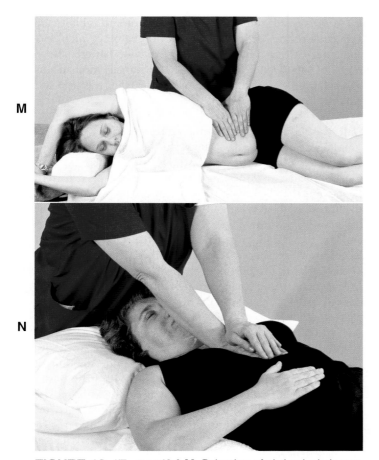

FIGURE 10-17, cont'd M, Palpation of abdominal viscera. **N,** Palpation rhythms.

Assessment Procedures for Muscle Testing

Muscle testing procedures are used for different purposes. The purpose of **strength testing** is to discover whether the muscle responds with sufficient strength to perform the required body functions. The purpose of **neurologic muscle testing** is to discover whether the neurologic interaction of the muscles is working smoothly. The third type of muscle testing, which is used in **applied kinesiology**, relies on muscle strength or weakness as an indicator of body function. It is somewhat like a body biofeedback mechanism. The system itself is too complex to cover in this book, but it is important to identify applied kinesiologic muscle testing procedures as a method of assessment and evaluation.

Strength Testing

In general, the purpose of strength testing is to determine whether the muscle or muscle groups are able to respond with adequate force to a demand without excessive recruitment of other muscles and whether the muscle strength patterns are similar on both sides of the body.

Strength testing determines a muscle's force of concentric contraction. The preferred method is to isolate the muscle or muscle group by positioning the muscle with its attachment points as close together as possible. The muscle or muscle

BOX 10-3

Muscle Assessment Grades

Grade 5	Normal strength
Grade 4	Movement against gravity and resistance
Grade 3	Movement against gravity (resistance eliminated)
Grade 2	Movement with gravity eliminated
Grade 1	Only a flicker of movement

group being tested should be isolated as specifically as possible. Many good kinesiology manuals are available that provide instruction on ways to isolate a specific muscle or muscle group. The client holds or maintains the contracted position of the muscle isolation while the therapist slowly and evenly applies a counterpressure to pull or press the muscle out of its isolated position. The massage therapist must use sufficient force to recruit a full response by the muscles being tested but not enough to recruit other muscles in the body. If strength testing is done this way, there is little chance the therapist will injure the client. As with palpation, it is necessary to compare the muscle test with a similar area, usually the same muscle group on the opposite side (see Chapter 10 of *Mosby's Essential Sciences for Therapeutic Massage*). Various assessment scales are used to describe the result of the findings from strength testing. The most common is the numerical scale. The muscles assessed should be able to hold against the applied resistance without any pain or recruitment of other muscles. The assessment findings are graded as shown in Box 10-3 (Figure 10-18).

A tested muscle or muscle group may be unable to hold against applied force for many reasons, including atrophy, joint dysfunction, and neurologic inhibition.

Testing the Coordination of the Agonist-Antagonist Interaction. Another testing method is to compare a muscle group's strength with its antagonist pattern. The body is designed so that the flexor, internal rotator, and adductor muscles are about 25% to 30% larger and therefore stronger than the extensor, external rotator, and abductor muscles. It is also designed so that flexors and adductors usually work against gravity to move a joint. The main purposes of extensors and abductors are to restrain and control the flexor and adductor movement and to return the joint to a neutral position. Less strength is required because gravity is assisting the function.

Strength testing should reveal a difference in the pattern between the flexors, internal rotators, and adductors, and the extensors, external rotators, and abductors in an agonist/antagonist pattern. These groups should not be equally strong (i.e., able to hold against the same applied force). Flexors, internal rotators, and adductors should show more muscle strength than extensors, external rotators, and abductors.

Muscle Testing of Gait Patterns. It also is important to consider the pattern of muscle interactions that occurs with

FIGURE 10-18 A, Muscle test. **B,** Learning strength test.

walking. Remember that gait has a certain pattern for efficient movement. For example, if the left leg is extended for the heel strike, the right arm also is extended. This results in activation of the flexors of both the arm and leg and inhibition of the extensors. Strength imbalances are common in this gait pattern. One muscle out of sequence with the others can set up increased motor tone (too strong) or inhibited (unable to hold) muscle imbalances. Whenever a muscle contracts with too much force, it overpowers the antagonist group, resulting in inhibited muscle function. The imbalances can occur anywhere in the pattern (Proficiency Exercise 10-5).

Strength muscle testing should reveal that the flexor and adductor muscles of the right arm should activate, facilitate, and coordinate with the flexors and adductors of the left leg. The opposite is also true: left arm flexors and adductors activate and facilitate with the right leg flexors and adductors. Extensors and abductors in the limbs coordinate in a similar fashion.

If the flexors of the left leg are activated, as occurs during strength testing, the flexors and adductors of the right arm should be facilitated and strength test strong. The flexors and adductors of the right leg and left arm should be inhibited and strength test weak. Also, the extensors and abductors in the right arm and left leg should be inhibited. All associated patterns follow suit (i.e., activation of the right arm flexor pattern facilitates the left leg flexor pattern and inhibits left arm and right leg flexor muscles while facilitating extensors and abductors). In a similar way, activation of the adductors of the right

leg facilitates the adductors of the left arm and inhibits the abductors of the left leg and right arm. The other adductor/abductor patterns follow the same interaction pattern.

All of these patterns are associated with gait mechanisms and reflexes. If any pattern is out of sync, gait, posture, and efficient function are disrupted.

Gait Muscle Testing as an Interventional Tool. An understanding of gait provides a powerful intervention tool. For example, a person trips and strains the left leg extensor muscles. Gait muscle testing reveals the imbalanced pattern by showing that the left leg extensor muscles are weak, whereas the flexors in the left leg and right arm are overly tense. The leg is sore and cannot be used for work, but the arm muscles are fine. By activating the extensors in the right arm, the left leg extensor muscles can be facilitated. By activating the flexors of the left arm, the flexors of the left leg are inhibited. This process may restore balance in the gait pattern. Many combinations are possible based on the gait pattern and reflexes. Gait muscle testing provides the means of identifying these interactions.

Careful study of this interaction is important for work with individuals such as athletes or dancers. An understanding of this interaction also is helpful in working with people who have various forms of spastic paralysis and spastic muscle conditions. For example, a child with a head injury that causes flexor spasms in the right arm may be helped temporarily by a reduction in the spasm pattern through activation of left leg extensor patterns, especially if the child has more coordination in that area. All other possible interactions follow suit. If voluntary activation of the muscles is not possible, tapotement at the tendons of the muscle required to contract usually provides the appropriate neurologic signal. (See Chapter 10 of *Mosby's Essential Sciences for Therapeutic Massage.*)

Neurologic Muscle Testing

Neurologic muscle testing focuses more on the patterns of muscle communication. A small force is used for testing because only the nervous system is assessed. An efficient pattern is one in which the muscles contract evenly, without jerking and without a lot of synergistic (helper muscle) activity. The same isolation of muscle groups is used as in strength testing. The client holds the contraction, and the massage therapist provides moderately light pressure against the muscle.

As always, the goal is to locate the muscle interaction pattern, not only for the muscle directly tested but also for all other muscles linked through gait and postural reflexes. In tests of neuromuscular activity, it is important that the examiner notice what the rest of the body does when the isolated muscle group is tested. For example, if testing of the neck flexor muscles causes the left leg to roll in, a pattern of interaction has shown itself. These patterns may be natural, such as the gait reflexes, but they often are a mixed-up set of signals that cause the body to respond inappropriately. Inefficient patterns cause some muscles to contract more than is necessary. Muscles may not be able to stop contracting and thus maintain tension

Text continued on p. 396.

Protocol for Kinetic Chain Testing

To complete this exercise, you first must know two important definitions:

Control group: *For this particular purpose, the control group is the group of muscles that initiates the reflex response.*

Test group: *Again, in this case, the test group is the muscle group that responds to the stimulus from the control group.*

There are many gait-related kinetic chain patterns. This exercise concentrates on the main patterns involved in flexion, extension, abduction, and adduction at the shoulder and pelvic girdle. For testing of the arm flexors and extensors, the humerus should be stabilized superior to the elbow joint, and the femur should be stabilized above the knee.

The control group is activated first, the test group is next, and the contractions in the two groups are held simultaneously. Both groups should hold strong and steady during the test. You should chart the data to show any inhibitions.

The antagonist pattern should be inhibited during the test; that is, the antagonists should let go. If they do not let go, the contraction maintained is concentric rather than eccentric. Be sure to chart the data.

I. Contralateral Flexors

A. Left Arm Flexor Test (Figures A1 to A4)

1. Isolate and stabilize the left arm and the right leg in supine flexion.

2. Control group: Use the right leg as the control and have the client hold the right leg position against inferior/caudal pressure provided by you.

3. Test group: Test the left arm flexors by having the client hold the left arm position against inferior/caudal pressure provided by you.

4. The two groups should be equally strong and steady. If the test group is inhibited (i.e., lets go), chart the data.

Antagonist test: Test the left arm extensors by having the client hold against superior/cranial pressure provided by you. These muscles should inhibit (let go). If the test group remains concentrically contracted and holds, chart the data.

B. Right Arm Flexor Test

1. Isolate and stabilize the left leg and the right arm in supine flexion.

2. Control group: Use the left leg as the control and have the client hold the left leg position against inferior/caudal pressure provided by you.

3. Test group: Test the right arm flexors by having the client hold the right arm position against inferior/caudal pressure provided by you.

4. The two groups should be equally strong and steady. If the test group is inhibited, chart the data.

Antagonist test: Test the right arm extensors by having the client hold the right arm position against superior/cranial pressure provided by you. These muscles should inhibit. If the test group remains concentrically contracted and holds, chart the data.

Left arm flexor test
Reverse arm and leg for right arm flexor test

Continued

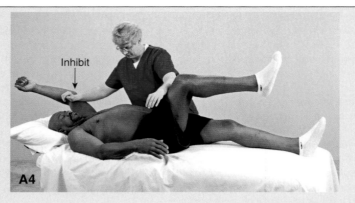

A4

Inhibit

C. Left Leg Flexor Test

1. Isolate and stabilize the left leg and the right arm in supine flexion.
2. Control group: Use the right arm as the control and have the client hold the right arm position against inferior/caudal pressure provided by you.
3. Test group: Test the left leg flexors by having the client hold the left leg position against inferior/caudal pressure provided by you.
4. The two groups should be equally strong and steady. If the test group is inhibited, chart the data.

Antagonist test: Test the left leg extensors by having the client hold against superior/cranial pressure provided by you. These muscles should inhibit. If the test group remains concentrically contracted and holds, chart the data.

D. Right Leg Flexor Test (Figures B1 to B4)

1. Isolate and stabilize the left arm and the right leg in supine flexion.
2. Control group: Use the left arm as the control and have the client hold the left arm position against inferior/caudal pressure provided by you.
3. Test group: Test the right leg flexors by having the client hold the right leg position against inferior/caudal pressure provided by you.
4. The two groups should be equally strong and steady. If the test group is inhibited, chart the data.

Antagonist test: Test the right leg extensors by having the client hold the right leg position against superior/cranial pressure provided by you. These muscles should inhibit. If the test group remains concentrically contracted and holds, chart the data.

Control

Should remain strong

Should inhibit

B1

Right leg flexor test
Reverse arm and leg position for left leg flexor test

B2

Control

B3

Control

Strong

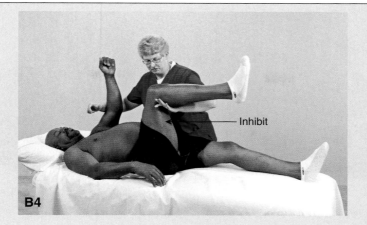

B4 — Inhibit

II. Contralateral Extensors

A. Left Arm Extensor Test (Figures C1 to C6)

1. Isolate and stabilize the left arm and the right leg in supine flexion.
2. Control group: Use the right leg as the control and have the client hold the leg position against superior/cephalad pressure provided by you.
3. Test group: Test the left arm extensors by having the client hold the arm position against superior/cephalad pressure provided by you.
4. The two groups should be equally strong and steady. If the test group is inhibited, chart the data.

Antagonist test: Test the left arm flexors by having the client hold the left arm position against inferior/caudal pressure provided by you. These muscles should inhibit. If the test group remains concentrically contracted and holds, chart the data.

B. Right Arm Extensor Test

1. Isolate and stabilize the left leg and the right arm in supine flexion.
2. Control group: Use the left leg as the control and have the client hold the leg position against superior/cephalad pressure provided by you.
3. Test group: Test the right arm extensors by having the client hold the arm position against superior/cephalad pressure provided by you.
4. The two groups should be equally strong and steady. If the test group is inhibited, chart the data.

Antagonist test: Test the right arm flexors by having the client hold the right arm position against inferior/caudal pressure provided by you. These muscles should inhibit. If the test group remains concentrically contracted and holds, chart the data.

Should inhibit

Should remain strong

Control

C1

Left arm extensor test
Reverse arm and leg for right arm extensor test

Continued

C2

C3

C4

C5

C6

C. Left Leg Extensor Test

1. Isolate and stabilize the left leg and the right arm in supine flexion.
2. Control group: Use the right arm as the control and have the client hold the arm position against superior/cephalad pressure provided by you.
3. Test group: Test the left leg extensors by having the client hold the leg position against superior/cephalad pressure provided by you.

4. The two groups should be equally strong and steady. If the test group is inhibited, chart the data.

Antagonist test: Test the left leg flexors by having the client hold the left leg position against inferior/caudal pressure provided by you. These muscles should inhibit. If the test group remains concentrically contracted and holds, chart the data.

D. Right Leg Extensor Test (Figures D1 to D4)

1. Isolate and stabilize the left arm and the right leg in supine flexion.
2. Control group: Use the left arm as the control and have the client hold the arm position against superior/cephalad pressure provided by you.
3. Test group: Test the right leg extensors by having the client hold the leg position against superior/cephalad pressure provided by you.
4. The two groups should be equally strong and steady. If the test group is inhibited, chart the data.

D1

Right leg extensor test
Reverse arm and leg position for left leg extensor test

D2

D3

D4

Continued

Antagonist test: Test the right leg flexors by having the client hold the right leg position against inferior/caudal pressure provided by you. These muscles should inhibit. If the test group remains in a concentrically contracted pattern and holds, chart the data (Figure E).

A + A = Strong
B + B = Strong
A + B = Inhibit

Composite of contralateral tests

III. Unilateral Flexors

A. Left Arm Flexor Test (Figures F1 to F4)

1. Isolate and stabilize the left arm and the left leg in supine flexion.
2. Control group: Use the left leg as the control and have the client hold the leg position against superior/cephalad pressure (contracting extensors) provided by you.
3. Test group: Test the left arm flexors by having the client hold the arm position against inferior/caudal pressure (testing flexors) provided by you.
4. The two groups should be equally strong and steady. If the test group is inhibited, chart the data.

Antagonist test: Test the left arm extensors by having the client hold the left arm position against superior/cranial pressure provided by you. These muscles should inhibit. If the test group remains concentrically contracted and holds, chart the data.

B. Right Arm Flexor Test

1. Isolate and stabilize the right arm and the right leg in supine flexion.
2. Control group: Use the right leg as the control and have the client hold the leg position against superior/cephalad pressure (contracting extensors) provided by you.
3. Test group: Test the right arm flexors by having the client hold the arm position against inferior/caudal pressure (testing flexors) provided by you.
4. The two groups should be equally strong and steady. If the test group is inhibited, chart the data.

Antagonist test: Test the right arm extensors by having the client hold the right arm position against superior/cranial pressure provided by you. These muscles should inhibit. If the test group remains concentrically contracted and holds, chart the data.

Should inhibit

Should remain strong

Control

F1

Left arm flexor test
Reverse arm and leg position for right arm flexor test

C. Left Leg Flexor Test

1. Isolate and stabilize the left arm and the left leg in supine flexion.
2. Control group: Use the left arm as the control and have the client hold the arm position against superior/cephalad pressure (contracting extensors) provided by you.
3. Test group: Test the left leg flexors by having the client hold the leg position against inferior/caudal pressure (testing flexors) provided by you.
4. The two groups should be equally strong and steady. If the test group is inhibited, chart the data.

Antagonist test: Test the left leg flexors by having the client hold the left leg position against inferior/caudal pressure provided by you. These muscles should inhibit. If the test group remains concentrically contracted and holds, chart the data.

D. Right Leg Flexor Test (Figures G1 to G4)

1. Isolate and stabilize the right arm and the right leg in supine flexion.
2. Control group: Use the right arm as the control and have the client hold the arm position against superior/cephalad pressure (contracting extensors) provided by you.
3. Test group: Test the right leg flexors by having the client hold the leg position against inferior/caudal pressure (testing flexors) provided by you.
4. The two groups should be equally strong and steady. If the test group is inhibited, chart the data.

Antagonist test: Test the right leg extensors by having the client hold the leg position against superior/cranial pressure provided by you. These muscles should inhibit. If the test group remains concentrically contracted and holds, chart the data.

Right leg flexor test
Reverse arm and leg position for left leg flexor test

G1

Continued

IV. Unilateral Extensors

A. Left Arm Extensor Test

1. Isolate and stabilize the left arm and the left leg in supine flexion.
2. Control group: Use the left leg as the control and have the client hold the leg position against inferior/caudal pressure (contracting flexors) provided by you.
3. Test group: Test the left arm extensors by having the client hold the arm position against superior/cephalad pressure (testing extensors) provided by you.
4. The two groups should be equally strong and steady. If the test group is inhibited, chart the data.

Antagonist test: Test the left arm flexors by applying inferior/caudal pressure. These muscles should inhibit. If the test group remains concentrically contracted and holds, chart the data.

B. Right Arm Extensor Test (Figures H1 to H4)

1. Isolate and stabilize the right arm and the right leg in supine flexion.
2. Control group: Use the right leg as the control and have the client hold the leg position against inferior/caudal pressure (contracting flexors) provided by you.
3. Test group: Test the right arm extensors by having the client hold the arm position against superior/cephalad pressure (testing extensors) provided by you.
4. The two groups should be equally strong and steady. If the test group is inhibited, chart the data.

Antagonist test: Test the right arm flexors by applying inferior/caudal pressure. These muscles should inhibit. If the test group remains concentrically contractor and holds, chart the data.

H1

Right arm extensor test
Reverse arm and leg position for left arm extensor test

H2 — Control

H3 — Strong

H4 — Inhibit

C. Left Leg Extensor Test

1. Isolate and stabilize the left arm and the left leg in supine flexion.
2. Control group: Use the left arm as the control and have the client hold the arm position against inferior/caudal pressure (contracting flexors) provided by you.
3. Test group: Test the left leg extensors by having the client hold the leg position against superior/cephalad pressure (testing extensors) provided by you.
4. The two groups should be equally strong and steady. If the test group is inhibited, chart the data.

Antagonist test: Test the left leg flexors by applying inferior/caudal pressure. These muscles should inhibit. If the test group remains in concentric contraction and holds, chart the data.

D. Right Leg Extensor Test (Figures I1 to I4)

1. Isolate and stabilize the right arm and the right leg in supine flexion.
2. Control group: Use the right arm as the control and have the client hold the arm position against inferior/caudal pressure (contracting flexors) provided by you.
3. Test group: Test the right leg extensors by having the client hold the leg position against superior/cephalad pressure (testing extensors) provided by you.

Should remain strong · Should inhibit · Control

I1

Right leg extensor test
Reverse arm and leg position for left leg extensor test

Continued

4. The two groups should be equally strong and steady. If the test group is inhibited, chart the data (Figure J).

A + A = Strong
B + B = Strong
A + B = Inhibit

Composite of unilateral patterns

Antagonist test: Test the right leg flexors by applying inferior/caudal pressure. These muscles should inhibit. If the test group remains concentrically contracted, chart the data.

V. Medial/Lateral Symmetry

A. Bilateral Arm Adductor Test (Figures K1 to K5)

1. Isolate and stabilize the arms bilaterally in supine 90% flexion and the legs bilaterally in flexion.
2. Control group: Use the bilateral legs as the control and have the client either hold position against lateral pressure provided by you or squeeze a ball (contracting adductors).
3. Test group: Test the bilateral arm adductors by having the client hold the arm position against lateral pressure (testing adductors) provided by you.

4. The two groups should be equally strong and steady. If the test group is inhibited, chart the data.

Antagonist test: Test bilateral arm abduction by having the client hold position against medial pressure provided by you. These muscles should inhibit. If the test group remains concentrically contracted, chart the data.

B. Bilateral Leg Adductor Test

1. Isolate and stabilize the arms bilaterally in supine 90% flexion and the legs bilaterally in flexion.
2. Control group: Use the bilateral arms as the control and have the client hold position against lateral pressure provided by you, or have the client press the palms together (contracting adductors).

3. Test group: Test the bilateral leg adductors by having the client hold position against pressure provided by you (testing adductors).
4. The two groups should be equally strong and steady. If the test group is inhibited, chart the data.

Antagonist test: Test the bilateral leg abductors by having the client hold position against medial pressure provided by you. These muscles should inhibit. If the test group remains concentrically contracted, chart the data.

A + A = Strong
B + B = Strong
A + B = Inhibit

K1

Control

Strong

K2

Strong

Control

K3

Inhibit

Control

K4

Control

Inhibit

K5

Intervention

Use massage methods to inhibit muscles that test as too strong by remaining in concentric contraction patterns when they should inhibit. Appropriate methods are slow compression, kneading, gliding, and shaking. Strengthen muscles that inhibit when they should hold strong. Appropriate methods are tapotement and rhythmic tensing of inhibited muscles. Then retest the pattern; it should be normal.

patterns. Whenever a pattern of overly short muscles exists, there is a pattern of inhibited and weak muscles. When the prime mover for a particular function does not respond appropriately, the synergist attempts to compensate, altering optimal movement. Synergistic dominance is a common form of neuromuscular dysfunction. These imbalances use energy and contribute to fatigue and pain in the client.

Muscle Group Interactions. Remember that most joints in the body have one-joint muscles (the muscle crosses a single joint) or two-joint muscles (the muscle crosses two joints). Muscles are tested in groups because isolating a single muscle is almost impossible; the brain does not process movement of individual muscles. It is more important to work with muscles in patterns of flexion and extension, adduction and abduction, or elevation and depression than to be concerned with the function of individual muscles. The movement pattern of each synovial joint is based on the flexion and extension principle. To move in gravity, each joint must be stabilized by some sort of diagonal pattern that functions as a counterbalance. Therefore the entire body is involved in all movement patterns.

Muscle Activation Sequences/Firing Patterns. Muscles also contract, or fire, in a neurologic sequence to produce coordinated movement. If the optimal muscle activation sequence is disrupted and muscles fire out of sequence or do not contract when they should, labored movement and postural strain result. Firing patterns can be assessed by initiating a particular sequence of joint movements and palpating for muscle activity to determine which muscle is responding first, second, or third to the movement.

The central nervous system recruits the appropriate muscles in specific activation sequences to generate the appropriate muscle function of acceleration, deceleration, or stability. If these firing patterns are abnormal and the synergist becomes dominant, efficient movement is compromised and the joint position is strained. The general firing pattern is prime movers, then stabilizers, then synergists. If the stabilizer must also move the area (acceleration) or control movement (deceleration), it typically becomes short. If the synergist fires before the prime mover, the movement is awkward and labored (Proficiency Exercise 10-6).

If one muscle is short and has increased motor tone, *reciprocal inhibition* typically occurs. Reciprocal inhibition exists

---

 PROFICIENCY EXERCISE 10-6

Common Muscle Activation Sequences/Muscle Firing Patterns

Trunk Flexion (Figures A1, A2)
Palpate either side of the rectus abdominis to assess contraction of the obliques and the transverse abdominis abdomen.
1. Normal firing pattern
   a. Transverse abdominis
   b. Abdominal obliques
   c. Rectus abdominis
2. Assessment
   a. Position the client supine with the knees and hips in approximately 90 degrees of flexion.
   b. Instruct the client to perform a normal curl up.
   c. Assess the abdominal muscles' ability to functionally stabilize the lumbar-pelvic-hip complex by having the

client draw the abdominal muscle in (as when bringing the umbilicus toward the back) and then do a curl just lifting the scapula off the table while keeping both feet flat. Inability to maintain the drawing-in position and/or to activate the rectus abdominis during the assessment demonstrates an altered firing pattern of the abdominal stabilization mechanism.
3. Altered firing pattern
   a. Weak agonist—abdominal complex
   b. Overactive antagonist—erector spinae
   c. Overactive synergist—psoas, rectus abdominis
4. Symptoms
   a. Low back pain
   b. Buttock pain
   c. Hamstring shortening

Hip Extension (Figures B1, B2)

1. Normal firing pattern
   a. Gluteus maximus
   b. Opposite erector spinae
   c. Same-side erector spinae and hamstring
   or
   a. Gluteus maximus
   b. Hamstring
   c. Opposite erector spinae
   d. Same-side erector spinae
2. Assessment
   a. Place the client in the prone position.
   b. Palpate the erector spinae with the fingers of one hand while palpating the muscle belly of the opposite gluteus maximus and hamstring with the little finger and thumb of the other hand.
   c. Instruct the client to raise the hip more than 15 degrees off the table.
3. Altered firing pattern
   a. Weak agonist—gluteus maximus
   b. Overactive antagonist—psoas
   c. Overactive stabilizer—erector spinae
   d. Overactive synergist—hamstring
4. Symptoms
   a. Low back pain
   b. Buttock pain
   c. Recurrent hamstring strains

B1

B2

Hip Abduction (Figures C1, C2)

1. Normal firing pattern
   a. Gluteus medius
   b. Tensor fasciae latae
   c. Quadratus lumborum
2. Assessment
   a. Place the client in the side-lying position.
   b. Stand next to the client and palpate the quadratus lumborum with one hand and the tensor fasciae latae and gluteus medius with the other hand.
   c. Instruct the client to abduct the leg from the table.
3. Altered firing pattern
   a. Weak agonist—gluteus medius
   b. Overactive antagonist—adductors
   c. Overactive synergist—tensor fasciae latae
   d. Overactive stabilizer—quadratus lumborum
4. Symptoms
   a. Low back pain
   b. Sacroiliac joint pain
   c. Buttock pain
   d. Lateral knee pain
   e. Anterior knee pain

C1

C2

Continued

Knee Flexion (Figures D1, D2)

1. Normal firing pattern
   a. Hamstrings
   b. Gastrocnemius
2. Assessment
   a. Place the client in the prone position.
   b. Place your fingers on the hamstring and the gastrocnemius.
   c. Instruct the client to flex the knee.

3. Altered firing pattern
   a. Weak agonist—hamstrings
   b. Overactive synergist—gastrocnemius
4. Symptoms
   a. Pain behind the knee
   b. Achilles tendinitis

Knee Extension (Figures E1, E2)

1. Normal firing pattern
   a. Vastus medialis
   b. Vastus intermedius and vastus lateralis
   c. Rectus femoris
2. Assessment
   a. Place the client in the supine position with the leg flat.
   b. Instruct the client to pull the patella cranially (toward the head).

   c. Place your fingers on the vastus medialis oblique portion, vastus lateralis, and rectus femoris.
3. Altered firing pattern
   a. Weak agonist—vastus medius, primarily oblique portion
   b. Overactive synergist—vastus lateralis
4. Symptoms
   a. Knee pain under the patella
   b. Patellar tendinitis

PROFICIENCY EXERCISE 10-6—cont'd

Shoulder Flexion (Figures F1, F2)

1. Normal firing pattern
   a. Supraspinatus
   b. Deltoid
   c. Infraspinatus
   d. Middle and lower trapezius
   e. Contralateral quadratus lumborum
2. Assessment
   a. Place the client in the seated position. Stand behind the client and put one hand on the client's shoulder and the other on the contralateral quadratus area.
   b. Instruct the client to abduct the shoulder to 90 degrees.

3. Altered firing pattern
   a. Weak agonist—levator scapulae
   b. Overactive agonist—upper trapezius
   c. Overactive stabilizer—ipsilateral quadratus lumborum
4. Symptoms
   a. Shoulder tension
   b. Headache at the base of the skull
   c. Upper chest breathing
   d. Low back pain

Intervention for Altered Firing Patterns

Use appropriate massage applications to inhibit the dominant muscle, then strengthen the weak muscles.

F1

F2

when a tight muscle decreases nervous stimulation to its a functional antagonist, causing it to reduce activity—i.e., inhibition. For example, a short psoas reduces the function of the gluteus maximus. The activation and force production of the prime mover (the gluteus maximus) are decreased, leading to compensation and substitution by the synergists (hamstrings) and stabilizers (erector spinae), creating an altered firing pattern.

The most common firing pattern dysfunction is *synergistic dominance,* in which a synergist compensates for a prime mover to produce the movement. For example, if a client has an inhibited gluteus medius, synergists (the tensor fasciae latae, adductor complex, and quadratus lumborum) become dominant to compensate for the weakness. This alters normal joint alignment, which further alters the normal length-tension relationships of the muscles around the joint. (See Proficiency Exercise 10-6 for the most commonly used assessment procedures and the intervention for altered firing patterns.)

Postural (Stabilizer) and Phasic (Mover) Muscles. The two basic types of muscle are those that support the body in gravity (**postural muscles**) and those that move it through gravity (**phasic muscles**) (Table 10-1).[7] Muscles can perform both functions.

TABLE 10-1

Major Postural and Phasic Muscles

Main Postural Muscles	Main Phasic Muscles
Gastrocnemius	Neck flexors
Soleus	Deltoid
Adductors	Biceps
Medial hamstrings	Triceps
Psoas	Brachioradialis
Abdominals	Quadriceps
Rectus femoris	Hamstrings
Tensor fascia lata	Gluteus maximus
Piriformis	Anterior tibialis
Quadratus lumborum	
Erector spinae group	
Pectorals	
Latissimus dorsi	
Neck extensors	
Trapezius	
Scalenes	
Sternocleidomastoid	
Levator scapulae	

These two types of muscle are made up of different kinds of muscle fibers. Postural muscles have a higher percentage of slow-twitch red fibers, which can hold a contraction for a long time before fatiguing. Phasic muscles have a higher percentage of fast-twitch white fibers, which contract quickly but tire easily. These two types of muscle are tested differently and develop different types of dysfunction.

Postural Muscles. Postural (stabilizer) muscles are relatively slow to respond compared with phasic (mover) muscles. They do not produce bursts of strength if asked to respond quickly, and they may cramp. They are the deliberate, slow, steady muscles that require time to respond. Using the analogy of the tortoise and the hare, these muscles are the tortoise. Inefficient neurologic patterns, muscle tension, reorganization of connective tissue with fibrotic changes, and trigger points are common in postural muscles.[7]

If posture is not balanced, postural muscles must function more like ligaments and bones to provide stability. When this happens, trigger points and additional connective tissue can develop in the muscle to provide the ability to stabilize the body in gravity. The problem is that the connective tissue freezes the body in the dysfunctional position, because unlike muscle, which can actively contract and lengthen, connective tissue is a more static tissue.

Postural muscles tend to shorten and have increased motor tone when under strain. This is an important consideration when massage practitioners attempt to assess which muscles are short, apt to develop trigger points and connective tissue changes, and require lengthening and stretching. (Chapter 11 discusses these issues in greater detail.) Connective tissue shortening is dealt with mechanically through forms of stretch. Trigger points usually respond to muscle energy methods and inhibitory pressure. Short concentric contraction muscles are dealt with through muscle energy methods and reflexive lengthening procedures (see Chapter 9).

Phasic Muscles. Phasic (mover) muscles jump into action quickly and tire quickly. Musculotendinous junction problems are more common in phasic muscles. The four most common problems are microtearing of the muscle fibers at the tendon, inflamed tendons (tendinitis), adherence of muscles and tendons to underlying tissue, and bursitis.

Phasic muscles usually are inhibited (weaker) in response to postural muscle shortening. Sometimes the inhibited muscles also shorten as a form of compensation, which allows the weak muscle the same contraction power on the joint. It is important not to confuse this condition with hypertense muscles. These muscles are inhibited and weak.

Phasic muscles occasionally become short. This almost always results from some sort of repetitive behavior and is a common problem in athletes. Phasic muscles also become short in response to a sudden posture change that causes the muscles to assist the postural muscles in maintaining balance. These common, inappropriate muscle patterns often result from an unexpected fall or near fall, an automobile accident, or some other trauma. Basic massage methods discussed in this text can be used to reset and retrain out-of-sync muscles (Proficiency Exercise 10-7).

PROFICIENCY EXERCISE 10-7

Have three other students do a muscle testing assessment on you. Include all the postural and phasic muscles listed for both strength and neuromuscular function. Compare the information they gather with what you gathered. As a group, compare the information gathered for similarities and differences. Take turns so that each student is assessed.

The Kinetic Chain

Neurologic Interaction Patterns and Mechanisms of Dysfunction. The muscular and skeletal systems coordinate function through the nervous system. Movement occurs through a series of patterns that are both inherent (e.g., reflexes) and learned (e.g., tying shoelaces). The patterns most relevant to the massage therapist are related to posture and gait. No set system exists for figuring out neuromuscular patterns. These patterns are activated in response to a disruption of balance in gravity, such as a fall or repetitive movement. Usually the body's response is to correct the disruption and then return to normal. Sometimes the body does not resume normal function, and dysfunction occurs. A general pattern of dysfunction can be detected during the assessment, and modification methods can be initiated during the massage intervention.

Gait patterns have a powerful influence. Additional powerful determinants of normal function are righting reflexes in the neck. These reflexes, when coordinated with the eyes, keep the body oriented perpendicular to a horizontal plane. Balance mechanisms of the inner ear also are a factor. Any inner ear difficulties or visual distortion affects neuromuscular interactions and postural balance patterns.

A common and often undiagnosed eye and ear problem is benign paroxysmal (or vestibular) positional vertigo, which occurs when otolith crystals in the inner ear become displaced and send erroneous positional information to the balance and muscle coordination centers in the lower brain. The eyes are linked through the righting reflex mechanism. Various muscle tension patterns can be linked to this and other similar conditions. Referral to the appropriate health care professional is important for proper diagnosis.

Postural Influence. The body is a circular form divided into four quadrants: a front, a back, a right side, and a left side. With divisions on the sagittal and frontal planes, the body must be balanced in three dimensions to withstand the forces of gravity and maintain normal function.

The body moves and is balanced in gravity in the following skeletal areas through the transverse plane: the atlas; the C6 and C7 vertebrae; the T12 and L1 vertebrae (the thoracolumbar junction); the L4, L5, and S1 vertebrae (the sacrolumbar junction); and at the hips, knees, and ankles, with stabilization at the shoulder (Figure 10-19). If a postural distortion exists in any of the four quadrants or within one of the jointed areas (i.e., the tissue between the atlas and the axis or the hip and the knee), the entire balance mechanism must be adjusted to maintain upright posture and keep the eyes horizontal. This

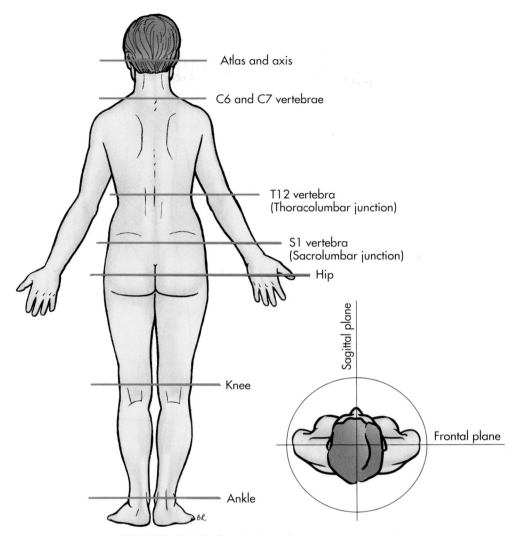

Atlas and axis

C6 and C7 vertebrae

T12 vertebra
(Thoracolumbar junction)

S1 vertebra
(Sacrolumbar junction)

Hip

Knee

Ankle

Sagittal plane

Frontal plane

FIGURE 10-19 Quadrants and movement segments.

occurs as a pinball-like effect that jumps front to back and side to side in the soft tissue between the movement lines at the joints (see Figure 10-18). Therefore, if one segment, such as the area between L1 and L4-5 and S1 (lumbar, low-back area) becomes altered (e.g., tipped or rotated), the segments above and below must tip or twist in the opposite direction to provide counterbalance and maintain the eye position and center of gravity. As expected, the next segments up and down also adjust, and the eventual result is distortion from head to toe.

The following demonstration can help you gain an understanding of postural balance.

First, get a pole of some type (a broom handle without the broom portion will work). Tie a string around the pole. Now, try to balance the pole on its end with the string. Note that in trying to counter the fall pattern of the pole, you work opposite that fall pattern. If the pole tends to fall forward and to the left, you apply a counterforce back and to the right.

This concept can be explained in another way. That is, the body is made up of many different poles stacked on top of one another. The poles stack at each of the jointed areas previously

mentioned. Muscles and other soft tissue between the joints form movement segments that must be three dimensionally balanced in all four quadrants to support the pole in that area. Each area needs to be balanced. If one pole area tips a bit to the right, the body compensates by tipping the adjacent pole areas (above and/or below) to the left. If a pole area is tipped forward, adjacent poles are tipped back. A chain reaction occurs, such that when compensating poles tip back, their adjacent areas must counterbalance the action by tipping forward. As explained previously, this is how the bodywide compensation pattern is set up.

Whether the pole areas sit nicely on top of each other with evenly distributed muscle and other soft tissue action or whether they are tipped in various positions and counterbalanced by compensatory muscle and fascial actions, the body remains balanced in gravity. However, the "tippy pole" pattern is much more inefficient than the balanced pole pattern (Figure 10-20). Tippy poles create caves (concave areas) and hills (convex areas); caves have short tissue, and hills have long tissue. Because massage affects short tissue most and supports elongation and relaxation, most massage intervention occurs

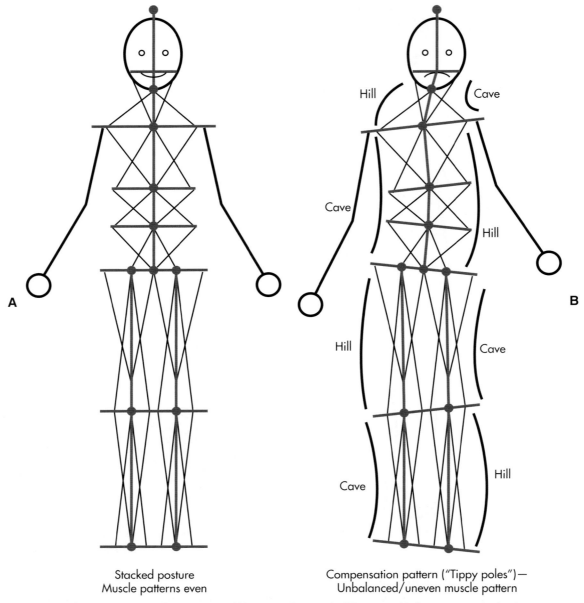

Stacked posture
Muscle patterns even

Compensation pattern ("Tippy poles")—
Unbalanced/uneven muscle pattern

FIGURE 10-20 Stacked pole **(A)** versus tippy pole **(B)** postural influences on the body.

in the concave areas, and tissues that are long (hills) need to be exercised.

Intervention plans attempt to normalize the balance process by relaxing short, tight areas and strengthening muscles in corresponding long, taut, but weak areas, allowing the poles to straighten out. If a pole is permanently tippy, such as with scoliosis or kyphosis, intervention plans attempt to support the appropriate compensation patterns and prevent them from increasing beyond what is necessary for postural balance.

Functional Biomechanical Assessment

Typical dysfunction includes local joint hypermobility or hypomobility, altered firing patterns (activation sequences), and postural imbalance (tippy pole), all of which lead to

changes in motor function and are accompanied by temporary or chronic joint, muscular, and nervous system disorders.

Functional assessment defines mobility through active and passive movements of the body, using palpation and observation to detect distortion in these movements. Muscle testing and identification of the functional relationships of muscles are also performed.

Distortion Categories

Distortions in functioning often are measured and categorized as follows:

■ *First-degree distortion:* Shortening or weakening of some muscles or the formation of local changes in muscle and motor tone. The person must use additional muscles from different parts of the body for usual and simple movements. As a result, movement becomes uneconomical and labored.

- *Second-degree distortion:* Moderately expressed shortening of postural muscles and inhibiting and weakening of antagonist muscles. Moderately peculiar postures and movements of some parts of the body are present. Postural and movement distortion, such as altered firing patterns, begin to occur.
- *Third-degree distortion:* Clearly expressed shortening of postural muscles and weakening of antagonist muscles occur, and specific, nonoptimal movement develops. Significantly expressed peculiarity in postures and movement occurs. Increased postural and movement distortions result in defined changes in muscle and motor tone.

It is very important to determine which muscles are shortened and which are inhibited in order to choose the appropriate therapeutic intervention.

Based on the three levels of distorted function, the development of postural and movement pathology is divided into three stages:

- *Stage 1—Functional tension:* In stage 1, the person tires more quickly than normal. This fatigue is accompanied by first- or second-degree limitation of mobility, painless local myodystonia (changes in the muscle tension/length relationship), postural imbalance in the first or second degree, and nonoptimal motor function of the first degree. An easy way to understand stage 1 is this: the person can do what he or she wants, but it takes more energy.
- *Stage 2—Functional stress:* Stage 2 is characterized by a feeling of fatigue from moderate activity, discomfort, slight pain, and the appearance of singular or multiple degrees of limited mobility that is painless or that results in first-degree pain. It may be accompanied by local hypermobility. Functional stress is also characterized by reflex vertebral-sensory dysfunction, fascial/connective tissue changes, and regional postural imbalance. It is also accompanied by distortion of motor function in the first or second degree and firing pattern alterations. An easy way to understand stage 2 is this: the person can still do most things but maybe not as easily. The individual eventually begins to avoid certain activities and uses more energy to achieve reduced function.
- *Stage 3—Connective tissue changes in the musculoskeletal system:* The reasons for connective tissue changes are overloading, disturbances of tissue nutrition, microtrauma, microhemorrhage, unresolved edema, and other *endogenous* (inside the body) and *exogenous* (outside the body) factors. Hereditary predisposition is also a consideration. In stage 3, changes in the spine and weight-bearing joints may appear, with areas of local hypermobility and instability of several vertebral motion segments, hypomobility, widespread painful muscle tension, fascial and connective tissue changes in the muscles, regional postural imbalance in the second or third degree in many joints, and temporary nonoptimal motor function with second- or third-degree distortion. Visceral disturbances may be present. Individuals in stage 3 have significantly reduced function. Stage 1 (functional tension) can often be managed effec-

tively by massage methods and by practitioners with training equivalent to 500 to 1,000 hours that includes an understanding of the information presented in this text. It is important that the client have all symptoms evaluated by the appropriate health care professional, because the early phases of many serious conditions present the same symptoms as those in stage 1 postural conditions. Working with stage 2 and stage 3 conditions (functional stress and connective tissue changes) usually requires more training and proper supervision within a multidisciplinary approach.

Resourceful Compensation. Assessment also identifies areas of resourceful and successful compensation. Resourceful compensation patterns develop when the body has been required to adapt to some sort of trauma or repetitive use pattern. Permanent adaptive changes, although not as efficient as optimal functioning, are the best pattern the body can develop in response to an irreversible change in the system. Resourceful compensation must be supported, not eliminated.

Performing a Functional Assessment

Remember that each individual joint movement pattern is part of an interconnected aspect of the neurologic coordination pattern of muscle movement, called the kinetic chain, and of the tensegrity of the body's design. Both posture and movement dysfunctions identified in an individual joint pattern must be assessed and treated in broader terms of kinetic chain interactions, muscle length relationships, and the effects of stress and strain on the entire system and the person's ability to adapt and respond to intervention.

When a movement pattern is evaluated, two types of information are obtained in one functional assessment.

First, when a jointed area moves into flexion and the joint angle is decreased, the prime mover and synergists concentrically contract, antagonists eccentrically function with controlled lengthening, and the fixators isometrically contract and stabilize. Bodywide stabilization patterns also come into play to assist in allowing the motion. During assessment, resistance, applied to load the prime mover groups and synergists, is used to assess for neurologic function of strength and, to a lesser degree, endurance as the contraction is held. At the same time, the antagonist pattern or the tissues that are lengthened when positioning for the functional assessment can be assessed for increased muscle or connective tissue shortening. Dysfunction shows itself in limited range of motion by restricting the movement pattern. Therefore, when placing a jointed area into flexion, the examiner assesses the extensors for increased motor tone and muscle tone, which can cause shortening that would limit movement. When the jointed area moves into extension, the opposite becomes the case. The same is true for adduction and abduction, internal and external rotation, plantar and dorsal flexion, and so on.

Each movement pattern (e.g., flexion and extension of the elbow and knee, circumduction and rotation of the shoulder and hip, movement of the trunk and neck) is assessed by sequence positioning in each area in all available movement patterns and by testing for strength, range, and ease of movement.

Resistance (pressure against) that is applied to the muscles is focused at the end of the lever system. For example, when the function of the shoulder is assessed, resistance is focused at the distal end of the humerus, not at the wrist. Elbow function is assessed with resistance at the wrist, not the hand. When extension of the hip is assessed, resistance is applied at the end of the femur. When flexion of the knee is assessed, resistance is applied at the distal end of the tibia. Resistance is applied slowly, smoothly, and firmly at an appropriate intensity, as determined by the size of the muscle mass.

Stabilization is essential for assessing movement patterns accurately. Only the area assessed is allowed to move. Movement in any other part of the body must be stabilized. The massage therapist usually applies a stabilizing force. As one hand applies resistance, the other provides the stabilization. Sometimes the client can provide the stabilization. Some methods use straps to provide stabilization. The easiest way to identify the area to be stabilized is to move the area to be assessed through the range of motion. At the end of the range, some other part of the body begins to move; this is the area where stabilization is applied. Return the body to a neutral position. Provide the appropriate stabilization to the area identified and begin the assessment procedure.

During assessments, muscles should be able to hold against appropriate resistance without strain or pain from the pressure and without recruiting or using other muscles. Appropriate resistance is applied slowly and steadily and with just enough force to induce the muscles to respond to the stimulus. Large muscle groups require more force than small ones. The position should be easy to assume and comfortable to maintain for 10 to 30 seconds. Contraindications to this type of assessment include joint and disk dysfunction, acute pain, recent trauma, and inflammation.

Assessment Results

The results of the assessment identify either appropriate function of each area or dysfunction, which is rated as first, second, or third degree. When all assessments have been completed, the overall result is described as normal or as stage 1, stage 2, or stage 3 dysfunction, as described previously. First-degree and stage 1 dysfunction usually can be managed by general massage application. (Remember to make sure the client has no underlying serious conditions.) Clients with stage 2 or stage 3 dysfunction should be referred to the appropriate health care professional, and cooperative multidisciplinary treatment plans should be developed (Figure 10-21).

INTERPRETATION AND ANALYSIS OF ASSESSMENT INFORMATION

SECTION OBJECTIVES

Using the information presented in this section, the student will be able to perform the following:

- Interpret assessment information to design a basic full-body massage session that focuses on the specific outcome desired by the client
- Refer clients for care when the assessment information indicates the need for specific diagnosis and treatment
- Use the clinical reasoning model to choose specific massage approaches to serve as intervention methods during the massage session

FIGURE 10-21 Postural and functional movement assessment. Example of dysfunction patterns.
Curved arrow→: Rotation
Curved line–: Short tissue
Straight line-: Long tissue
X: Reduced ROM

FIGURE 10-21, cont'd

Poor balance

Good balance

FIGURE 10-21, cont'd

After the assessment information has been gathered, it is time to connect all the pieces in an interpretation and analysis process to develop the best massage treatment plan for the individual client. This requires clinical reasoning and problem-solving skills.

Massage technicians typically do not develop a plan for the massage. They provide a massage based on a predetermined protocol, following the sequence without specific attention to the client's individual outcome. This type of massage often is based on a particular system, such as Swedish massage, a hot stone session, or a pre-event sports massage as a member of a sports massage team at an event. The application is geared more to the method than to the client outcome. There is nothing wrong with this approach, but it is very limited in terms of the client's unique circumstances.

A massage therapist performs outcome-based massage. After the assessment data have been collected in an organized manner and outcomes have been determined for the client, the massage application is adapted to meet the client's specific needs. The massage does not depend on a modality or protocol; rather, it is an individualized approach based on care/treatment plans.

The main purpose of intervention is to help the body regain homeostasis, symmetry, ease of movement, and optimal function. Therefore, when observing gait or posture, the practitioner notes areas that seem pulled, twisted, or dropped. The massage therapist's job is to use massage methods to lengthen shortened areas, untwist twisted areas, raise dropped areas, drop raised areas, soften hard areas, firm up soft areas, warm cold areas, and cool hot areas.

After rapport has been established, the client will be comfortable and will trust the massage therapist enough to let her guard down. She will communicate a variety of information during the discussion or the massage session. The practitioner should listen for repeated phrases, such as "It's a real pain in the neck" or "I can hardly stand up to it." The massage therapist should not counsel or explain the ramifications of the information, only notice the pattern and keep general clinical notes.

Careful attention should be paid to the order of priority in which the client relays the information. If the headache is mentioned first, the knee ache second, and the tight elbow last, the areas should be dealt with in that order, if possible, in the massage flow. A client typically says, "It's tight there" if a motor tone problem is the trouble. "Stiff" can apply either to a connective tissue problem or a fluid retention problem (muscle tone), and "stuck" often indicates a joint problem.

The importance of listening to understand is paramount. Many experienced professionals have learned that if we listen to our clients, they will tell us what is wrong and how to help them restore balance. Slow down, do not jump to conclusions, pay attention, and let the information unfold. Realize that each client is the expert about himself or herself. Clients are your teachers about themselves, and in teaching you they often begin to understand themselves better. In every session, approach each client with fascination about what you will learn from him. *No textbook, class, or instructor can equal the teaching provided by careful attention to the client.*

General Presence

In general, excessive sympathetic activation would be balanced by a relaxing, full-body rhythmic massage with a general nonspecific approach, and excessive parasympathetic activation would be balanced by a stimulating massage with a specific focus. However, it is not quite that easy. In the discussion of rapport, it was recommended that the practitioner work with a client by meeting the client's current state; this is also true in deciding whether the general massage approach will be stimulation or relaxation.

If the client is functioning from sympathetic nervous system dominance, and if relaxation methods such as rocking and slow gliding are used initially, the work often seems irritating to the client. If the session is begun with a more stimulating approach, using such strokes as rapid compression, muscle energy methods, lengthening, and percussion, the design of the massage fits the client's physiologic level. After some of the nervous energy has been discharged, the client is ready for more relaxing methods.

The same is true with parasympathetic dominance patterns. If the client is "down" that day, beginning with a stimulation approach may feel like an attack. The better course is to begin with the more subtle relaxation methods (e.g., oscillation, slow gliding and rocking, and shaking) and progress slowly into the stimulation approaches to encourage balance.

If the client seems "out of sorts," operating more as a collection of parts than the sum of the parts, entrainment processes may be off. The centered, coordinated presence of the professional providing a harmonized, rhythmic approach to the massage is beneficial.

Gesturing

The general guidelines for gestures that are listed in this section are not written in stone. Professional experience indicates that these guidelines are fairly dependable starting points until the student is more experienced with interpreting body language.

People tend to be consistent with their gestures and word phrases within their internal body language system. However, body language is as individual as the person. Particular gestures or styles of body language cannot be generalized to mean one specific thing. It is the professional's responsibility to understand what a gesture means for a particular individual.

Because of nervous system patterns and basic universal body language connected with survival emotions such as fear, anger, distress, and happiness, some body language is fairly consistent from person to person. However, the massage practitioner cannot assume that a certain gesture means the same thing with every person. It takes time and careful observation to decipher an individual's body language code. This is done by watching for repetitive body language and connecting the particular gesture or posture to the client's mood and state and the content of the conversation. Eventually the client repeats the body language patterns often enough that the individual pattern is evident.

Common gestures and indications include the following:

- If a finger is pointed to a specific area, this suggests hyperactivity of an acupressure or a motor point or possibly a joint problem. The meaning of the pointing depends on the area indicated.
- If a finger is pointed to a specific area but the hand then swipes in a certain direction, a trigger point problem may be the issue.
- If an area is grabbed, pulled, or held and moved as if being stretched, this often indicates muscle or fascial shortening.
- If movement is needed to show the area of tightness, the area may need muscle lengthening combined with muscle energy work to prepare for stretching and for resetting of neuromuscular patterns.
- If the client moves into a position and then acts as if stuck, the area may need connective tissue stretching.
- If the client draws lines on the body, this may indicate nerve entrapment in the fascial planes or grooves.

Posture Assessment

The focus of massage application is symmetry. When applying massage, the practitioner should honor what the body is doing. This can be done by creating a slight exaggeration of the asymmetric pattern found and then slowly encouraging the body to shift to a more symmetric pattern.

Misalignment of body areas can be caused by muscles that pull or that do not stabilize, by connective tissue shortening or laxity, or, more likely, by a combination of these. The best course is to follow the lead provided by the client's body. Determining whether one shoulder is too high or the other one is dropped may be difficult. Instead, the massage therapist should exaggerate the pattern and have the client push or pull out of the stabilizing pressure (the integrated muscle energy approach explained in Chapter 9 is effective in these situations). Attention should be paid to the pattern in which the client uses the most effort when pushing or pulling; this indicates where to look for further dysfunction.

For example, a client has a long left leg with an externally rotated foot. As part of the massage, a good approach is to pull (tension force) on the long leg to increase the pattern and externally rotate the foot even more. Then the corrective pattern can be encouraged by having the client pull and rotate the leg in the opposite direction against stabilizing pressure. As the client finishes this move, the lengthening and stretch should be continued in the same direction as the client's pulling force. All the shortened areas (caves) should then be massaged to support length, and the overstretched areas (i.e., long and taut [hills]) should be stimulated.

This method works well for neuromuscular problems. It is not as effective for altering connective tissue dysfunction, but it does prepare the body for connective tissue work. If the areas of contracted and shortened connective tissue are stretched without this preparation, the body may respond with protective spasms.

Working with connective tissue often requires slow, sustained stretching (15 to 30 seconds) that puts sufficient

mechanical force into the tissue, as well as specific application of friction (shear force) massage manipulations. Connective tissue approaches normalize the twists and pulls of shortened connective tissue.

Asymmetry usually results when short muscles (increased motor tone) or shortened connective tissue pulls the body out of alignment. Direct trauma pushes joints out of alignment. Weak stabilizing mechanisms, such as overstretched ligaments or inhibited antagonist muscles, contribute to the problem. In these situations a chiropractor, an osteopath, or another trained medical professional skilled in skeletal manipulation is needed. Often a multidisciplinary approach to client care is necessary (Figure 10-22).

Gait Assessment

When interpreting the information gathered from gait assessment, the massage practitioner should focus on areas that do not move easily when the client walks and areas that move too much. Areas that do not move are restricted; areas that move too much are compensating for inefficient function. By releasing the restrictions through massage and re-educating the reflexes through neuromuscular work, such as correcting gait reflex and exercise, the practitioner can help the client improve the gait pattern (see Proficiency Exercises 10-5 and 10-6).

The techniques followed are similar to those for postural corrections. The shortened and restricted areas are softened with massage, then the neuromuscular mechanism is reset with muscle energy techniques, muscle lengthening, and stretches.

The client should be taught slow lengthening and stretching procedures for the short areas (caves). After stimulating the muscles in weakened areas, the practitioner can teach the client strengthening exercises for the long areas (hills). The therapist must make sure to incorporate the adaptation methods into a complete, full-body massage rather than doing spot work on isolated parts of the body to support adaptation and integration. Suggestions could be made to the client to evaluate factors that may contribute to identified dysfunctions, such as posture, footwear, chairs, tables, beds, clothing, shoes, work stations, physical tasks (e.g., shoveling), and repetitive exercise patterns.

Proper functioning of the SI joint is an important factor in walking patterns. Because SI joint movement has no direct muscular component, it is difficult to use any kind of muscle energy lengthening when working with this joint. The joint is embedded deep in supporting ligaments. To keep the surrounding ligaments pliable, direct and specific connective tissue techniques are indicated unless the joint is hypermobile. If that is the case, external bracing combined with rehabilitative movement may be indicated. Sometimes the ligaments restabilize the area. Stabilization of the jointed area should be interspersed with massage and gentle stretching to ensure that the ligaments remain pliable and do not adhere to each other. This process takes time.

The diagnosis of specific joint problems and fitting for external bracing are outside the scope of practice for therapeu-

FIGURE 10-22 Learning posture assessment.

tic massage, and the client must be referred to the appropriate professional.

Range of Motion Assessment

Active and passive range of motion can identify limits of movement. If an empty capsular or hard end-feel is identified, the joint is damaged. Referral is needed for acute conditions. Range of motion limited by muscle contraction may indicate an underlying problem with joint laxity or injury, and caution is indicated before muscle guarding is reduced. Proceed slowly until a balance between increased range of motion and maintaining joint stability is achieved. If joint stability is reduced, the client usually experiences pain in the joint for a day or two after the massage; the person also may have increased stiffness in the area as stability is restored. Simple edema around a joint is managed with lymphatic drainage (see Chapter 11). If any unexplained edema develops, the client should be referred for diagnosis.

Range of motion should improve as the client's tissues normalize with general massage. Normalization in range of motion is an indication of improved function. Never force an increase in range of motion; instead, allow it to occur as a natural outcome of effective massage application to the soft tissues of the body.

Palpation Assessment

Palpation assessment becomes part of the massage. In any massage, about 90% of the touching is also assessment developed as part of gliding, kneading, or joint movement. Palpation assessment contacts the tissue but does not override it or encourage it to change. This type of work generally relaxes or stimulates the client, depending on the type of strokes used and the rhythm, duration, and speed of application.

Hot and Cold Areas

Hot areas may be caused by inflammation, muscle spasm, or increased surface circulation. When the focus of intervention is to cool the hot areas, a method such as application of ice can be used (see the section on hydrotherapy in Chapter 11). A hot area can also be cooled by reducing the muscle spasms and encouraging more efficient blood flow in the surrounding areas.

Cold areas often are areas of diminished blood flow, increased connective tissue formation, or muscle flaccidity. Heat can be applied to cold areas. Stimulation massage techniques increase muscle activity, heating up the area. Connective tissue approaches soften connective tissue, help restore space around the capillaries, and release histamine, a

FIGURE 10-23 Dehydration test. (From Seidel HM et al: *Mosby's guide to physical examination*, ed 5, St Louis, 2003, Mosby.)

vasodilator, to increase circulation. These approaches can warm a cold area.

Skin

Skin should be contained, hydrated, resilient, elastic, and even and have rich coloring. Skin that does not spring back into original position after a slight pinch may be a sign of dehydration (Figure 10-23). The skin should have no blue, yellow, or red tinges. Blue coloration suggests lack of oxygen; yellow indicates liver problems, such as jaundice; and redness suggests fever, alcohol intake, trauma, or inflammation. Color changes are most noticeable in the lips, around the eyes, and under the nails.

Bruises must be noted and avoided during massage except for simple lymphatic drainage, which is explained in Chapter 11. If a client's body shows any hot redness or red streaking, the person should be referred to a physician immediately. This is especially important with the lower leg because of the possibility of deep vein thrombosis (blood clot).

The skin should be watched carefully for changes in any moles or lumps. As massage professionals, we often spend more time touching and observing a person's skin than anyone else, including the person. If we keep a keen eye for changes and refer clients to physicians early, many skin problems can be treated before they become serious.

Depending on the area, the skin may be thick or thin. The skin of the face is thinner than the skin of the lower back. The skin in each particular area, however, should be similar. The skin loses its resilience and elasticity over areas of dysfunction. It is important to know the visceral referred pain areas on the skin. If changes occur in the skin in these areas, the client should be referred to a physician (see Chapter 5).

The superficial skin is a blood reservoir. At any particular time it can hold 10% of the available blood in the body. The connective tissue must be pliable to allow the capillary system to expand to hold the blood. Histamine, which is released from mast cells found in the connective tissue of the superficial fascial layer, dilates the blood vessels. Histamine is also

responsible for the client's reported sense of "warming and itching" in an area that has been massaged.

Damp areas on the skin are indications that the nervous system has been activated in that area. This small amount of perspiration is part of a sympathetic activation called a *facilitated segment*. Surface stroking with enough pressure to drag over the skin elicits a red response over the area of a hyperactive muscle. Deeper palpation of the area usually elicits a tender response. The small erector pili muscles attached to each hair also are under the control of the sympathetic autonomic nervous system. Light fingertip stroking produces goose bumps over areas of nerve hyperactivity. All of these responses can indicate potential activity, such as trigger points in the layers of muscle under the indicated area.

Hair and Nails

The hair and nails are part of the integumentary system and can reflect health conditions. The hair should be resilient and secure; hair loss should not be excessive when the scalp is massaged.

The nails should be smooth. Vertical ridges can indicate nutritional difficulties, and horizontal ridges can be signs of stress caused by changes in circulation that affect nail growth. Clubbed nails may also indicate circulation problems. The skin around the nails should be soft and free of hangnails.

During times of stress, the epithelial tissues are affected first. Hangnails; split skin around the lips and nails; mouth sores; hair loss; dry, scaly skin; and excessively oily skin are all signs of prolonged stress, medication side effects, or other pathologic conditions. Only a physician can diagnose the cause of the condition (refer to the contraindications in Appendix A for more information).

Superficial Connective Tissue

Methods of palpation that lift the skin, such as kneading and skin rolling, provide much information. Depending on the area of the body and the concentration of underlying connective tissue, the superficial fascia should lift and roll easily. Loosening and increasing the pliability of these areas are very beneficial, and the practitioner can achieve this by applying the assessment methods more slowly and deliberately, allowing for softening in the tissues.

Any areas that become redder than the surrounding tissue or that stay red longer than other areas are suspect for connective tissue changes. Usually, lifting and stretching (bend, shear, and torsion forces) of the reddened tissue or use of the myofascial approaches presented in Chapter 11 normalizes these areas.

Vessels, Pulses, and Lymph Nodes

Vessels should feel firm but pliable and supported. If any areas of bulging, mushiness, or constriction are noted, the practitioner should refer the client to a physician.

The practitioner should compare the pulses by feeling for a strong, even, full pumping action on both sides of the body. If differences are perceived, the client should be referred to a physician. Sometimes the differences in the pulses can be attributed to soft tissue restriction of the artery or a more serious condition that can be diagnosed by the physician. Refill of capillaries in the nail beds should take approximately 3 to 5 seconds and should be equal in all fingers.

Enlarged lymph nodes may indicate local or systemic infection or more serious conditions. The client should be referred to a physician immediately if these are noted. Tissue should not be boggy and taut from water retention. It is important to refer the client to a physician if the person has unexplained and persistent edema. General massage supports fluid movement. (Specific applications that affect blood and lymph circulation are presented in Chapter 11.)

Skeletal Muscle

Skeletal muscle is assessed for both texture and function. It should be firm and pliable. Soft, spongy muscle or hard, dense muscle indicates connective tissue and fluid dysfunction (muscle tone problems). Muscle atrophy results in a muscle that feels smaller than normal. Hypertrophy results in a muscle that feels larger than normal.

Muscles lie on top of each other in layers, typically known as the superficial, intermediate, and deep layers. Each layer must slide a bit over the one beneath it. If a muscle layer becomes adherent (stuck to) to the one beneath it, movement is limited to the available movement of the tissue it is attached to.

Application of the appropriate techniques can normalize the connective tissue component of the muscle, and circulation methods can address fluid movement. Excessively strong or weak muscles can result from problems with neuromuscular control or imbalanced work or exercise demand. Weak muscles can be a result of wasting (atrophy) of the muscle fibers or a result of neurologic inhibition (reciprocal inhibition). Tension can be felt in muscles that are either concentrically short or eccentrically long. Tension that manifests in short muscles that are concentrically contracted results in tissue that feels hard and bunched (caves). When muscles are tense from being pulled into an extension pattern, they feel like long, taut bundles with some contraction and shortened muscle fiber groups (hills). Usually, flexors, adductors, and internal rotators become short, whereas extensors, abductors, and external rotators palpate tense and taut but are long and have eccentric dysfunctional patterns.

Massage treatment addresses the short concentrically contracted muscles (caves) to lengthen them, rather than the long muscles (hills) because massage methods usually result in longer tissues. Remember, massage is effective at making tissues longer and more pliable; it is not very effective at making long tissues shorter. Therapeutic exercise is necessary to restore normal tone to the "long" muscles.

Important target areas are the musculotendinous junction and the muscle belly, where the nerve usually enters the muscle. Motor points cause a muscle contraction with a small stimulus, somewhat like a pilot light for a gas stove (motor tone). Disruption of sensory signals at the motor point causes many problems, including trigger points and referred pain (see Chapter 11), hypersensitive acupressure points (see Chapter 11), and restricted movement patterns caused by the increase in the physiologic barrier and the development of

pathologic barriers. Typically compression to create inhibitory pressure is used either at the muscle attachment or the muscle belly, or both, to reduce motor tone and restore normal resting length.

The skeletal muscle condition that develops depends on the person's heredity, activity level, and general health. It would be nice to give suggestions on how to proceed, but in this case, careful assessment of the entire pattern, use of clinical reasoning and problem-solving skills, and good general massage that addresses all tissue components are the best recommendations.

It is amazing what sorts itself out during a thorough generalized massage when the entire body is addressed. Do not discount the effectiveness of this type of massage when skeletal muscle imbalances are detected. Spot work on isolated areas is seldom effective. Neurologic muscle imbalances interfere with the kinetic chain (linked reflex patterns), most notably the gait reflexes and the interaction between postural and phasic muscles. A general full-body approach is the best intervention.

Tendons

Tendons should feel elastic and mobile. If a tendon has been torn (sprain), it may adhere to the underlying bone during the healing process. Some tendons, such as those of the fingers and toes, are enclosed in a sheath and must be able to glide within the sheath. If they cannot glide, inflammation builds, and the result is tendinitis. Overuse also can cause inflammation. Inflammation signals the formation of connective tissue, which can interfere with movement and cause the tendons to adhere to surrounding tissue. Frictioning techniques help these conditions. Usually, tight tendon structures normalize when the muscle's resting length is normalized.

Deep Fascia

Deep fascial sheaths should be pliable, but because they are stabilizers, they may be more dense than tendons in some areas. Problems arise if the tissues that are separated or stabilized by these sheaths become stuck to the sheath.

Myofascial approaches are best suited to dealing with the deep fascia. This type of bodywork is not usually included in basic massage training, but an introduction to the methods is provided in Chapter 11.

Mechanical work, such as slow, sustained stretching, and methods that pull and drag on the tissue are used to soften deep fascia. Because it often is uncomfortable, the work should not be done unless the client is committed to regular appointments until the area is normalized. This may take 6 months to 1 year.

Chronic health conditions almost always show dysfunction with the connective tissue. Any techniques discussed as connective tissue approaches are effective as long as the practitioner proceeds slowly and follows the tissue pattern. The massage therapist should not override the tissue or force the tissue into a corrective pattern. Instead, the tissue must be untangled or unwound gradually.

Fascial separations between muscles create pathways for the nerves and blood vessels. When palpated, these pathways feel like grooves running between muscles. If these areas become narrow or restricted, blood vessels may be constricted and nerves impinged. A slow, specific, stripping gliding along these pathways can be beneficial. The nerves run in these fascial pathways, and the nerve trunks correlate with the traditional meridian system. Therefore most meridian and acupressure work takes place along these fascial grooves. Muscle layers are also separated by deep fascia, and because muscles must be able to slide over each other, the practitioner must make sure there is no adherence between muscles. This situation often occurs in the legs. If assessment indicates that the muscles are stuck to each other, kneading and gliding can be used to slide one muscle layer over the other (Figure 10-24).

Water is an important element of connective tissue. To keep connective tissue pliable, the client must rehydrate the body by drinking a minimum of eight 8-ounce glasses of clean, pure water daily, as recommend by nutritionists and physicians.

Highly developed assessment and palpation skills are a must for working specifically with connective tissue dysfunction. General massage methods that are applied slowly and that generate a drag to introduce bend, shear, and torsion forces on tissues that are short and stuck should be used until more specific training is obtained.

When an emotional component is involved in the client's physical pattern, that component often surfaces while the practitioner is dealing specifically with the connective tissues. It seems that emotional chemicals and residue from trauma, addictions, and toxicity are stored in this tissue (see state-dependent memory and post-traumatic stress in Chapter 12). Because of this, the effects of connective tissue work can influence emotional states. Mental health support often is indicated, and these clients should be referred to a professional in that field.

Ligaments, Joints, and Bones

Movement of the joints through comfortable ranges of motion can be used as an evaluation method. Comparison of the symmetry of range of motion (e.g., comparing the circumduction pattern of one arm against that of the other) is effective for detecting limitations of a particular movement.

Muscle energy methods, as well as all massage manipulations, can be used to support symmetric range of motion functions.

Dealing specifically with ligaments, joints, and bone is out of the scope of practice of basic massage therapy as presented in this text. With additional education, a massage practitioner can learn applications that are beneficial for ligaments, joints, and bones.

All these tissues and structures are supported by general massage applications, which result in increased circulation, increased pliability of soft tissue, and normalized neuromuscular patterns.

Massage can positively affect the normal limits of the physiologic barrier. When joints are traumatized, the surrounding tissue becomes "scared," almost as if saying, "This joint will never get in that position again." When this happens, all the proprioceptive mechanisms reset to limit the range of motion, setting up a pathologic barrier. Massage and appropriate muscle lengthening and general stretching, combined with muscle energy techniques and self-help, can have a beneficial effect on ligaments, joint function, and bone health. Ligaments are relatively slow to regenerate, and it takes time to notice sustained improvement.

Application of various mechanical forces (e.g., kneading) to the soft tissue around joints can increase tissue pliability; however, the most common soft tissue dysfunction around joints is laxity, not shortening. Lax (loose) joint structures should not be massaged directly; instead, the muscles around the joint should be the main target.

Abdomen

Refer the client to a physician if any hard, rigid, stiff, or tense areas are noted in the abdomen. Close attention must be paid to the visceral referred pain areas (see Chapter 5). If tissue changes are noted, the practitioner must refer the client to a physician.

The skin often is tighter in areas of visceral referred pain. As a result of cutaneous and visceral reflexes, benefit may be obtained by stretching the skin in these areas. There is some indication that normalizing the skin over these areas has a positive effect on the functioning of the organ. If nothing else, circulation is increased and peristalsis (intestinal movement) may be stimulated.

In accordance with the recommendations for colon massage (see Chapter 9), repetitive stroking in the proper directions may stimulate smooth muscle contraction and can improve elimination problems and excessive intestinal gas. An understanding practitioner is prepared for the results and will point the way to the restroom.

Body Rhythms

The body rhythms are assessed before and after the massage. An improvement in rate and evenness should be noticed after the massage. Massage offered by a centered practitioner with

FIGURE 10-24 Sliding one layer of muscle over the layer beneath it.

a focused, rhythmic intent provides patterns for the client's body to use to entrain its own rhythms. The massage practitioner must remain focused on the natural rhythm of the client. Although the entrainment pattern of the practitioner and the massage provides a pattern for the client, it should not superimpose an unnatural rhythm on the client. Any foreign patterns ultimately will be rejected by the client's body. Instead, the practitioner should support the client in re-establishing her innate entrainment rhythm. Supported by rocking methods and a rhythmic approach to the massage and the appropriate use of music, the body can re-establish synchronized rhythmic function.

Breathing. Improved breathing function helps the entire body. The muscular mechanism for inhalation and exhalation is designed like a simple bellows system and depends on unrestricted movement of the musculoskeletal components of the thorax. The muscles of respiration include the scalenes, intercostals, anterior serratus, diaphragm, abdominals, and pelvic floor muscles. If a breathing pattern disorder (see Chapter 4) is a factor and the person is prone to anxiety, massage intervention can help normalize the upper body and support the breathing mechanism.

Because of the whole body interplay between muscle groups in all actions, tight lower leg and foot muscles often are found to interfere with breathing. By contracting the lower legs and feet and taking a deep breath, a person can discover for himself that breathing is a whole body function.

Disruption of function in any of these muscle groups inhibits full and easy breathing. (For additional information on breathing, see Chapter 13.)

General relaxation massage and stress reduction methods seem to help breathing the most. The client can be taught slow lengthening and stretching methods and the breathing retraining pattern found in Chapter 13. The client also can be advised to avoid wearing restrictive clothing.

Muscle and Joint Imbalance, Muscle Testing, Functional Assessment, and Range of Motion

Muscle dysfunction, discovered through muscle testing procedures, often indicates how the body is compensating for postural and movement imbalances. Muscle testing also can locate the main muscle problems. When the primary dysfunctional group of muscles is tested, the main compensatory patterns are activated, and the other body compensation patterns activate and exaggerate. The massage professional must become a detective, looking for clues to unwind the pattern. By concentrating on methods that restore symmetry of function, the practitioner helps the client's body work out the details.

A major muscle problem is short muscles with increased motor tone. If these muscles can be relaxed, lengthened and, if necessary, stretched to support connective tissue changes, the rest of the dysfunctional pattern often resolves.

If the extensors and abductors are stronger than the flexors and adductors, major postural imbalance and postural distortion result. Similarly, if the extensors and abductors are too

weak to balance the other movement patterns, the body curls into itself, and nothing works properly.

If gait and kinetic chain postural patterns are inefficient, more energy is required for movement, and fatigue and pain can result.

Shortened postural (stabilizer) muscles must be lengthened and then stretched. This takes time and uses all the massage practitioner's technical skills. Because of the fiber configuration of the muscle tissue (red or white twitch fibers), techniques must be sufficiently intense and must be applied long enough to allow the muscle to respond.

Shortened and weak phasic (mover) muscles must first be lengthened and stretched. Eventually, strengthening techniques and exercises are needed.

If the hypertense phasic muscle pattern is caused by repetitive use, the muscles can be normalized with muscle energy techniques and then lengthened. Overworked muscles often increase in size (hypertrophy). The client must reduce the activity of that muscle group until balance is restored, which usually takes about 4 weeks. Muscle tissue that has undergone hypertrophy begins to return to normal if it is not used for the excessive activity during that time. Athletes often display this pattern and very likely will resist complete inactivity. A reduced activity level and a more balanced exercise program, combined with flexibility training, can be beneficial for them. Refer these individuals to appropriate training and coaching professionals if indicated.

Inappropriate muscle activation sequences (firing patterns) can be addressed by inhibiting the muscles that are contracting out of sequence and stimulating the appropriate muscles to fire. Using compression at the attachment and in the muscle belly inhibits motor tone. Tapotement is a good technique to stimulate muscles. If the problem does not normalize easily, referral to an exercise professional may be indicated.

People usually complain of problems in the taut but long eccentrically functioning and inhibited muscle areas (hills). Massage in these areas makes the symptoms *worse*. Instead, identify the short tissues (caves) and apply massage to lengthen and stretch short areas. Assessment must identify the concentrically contracted shortened areas (caves) so that correction can be applied. Use surface massage to create counterirritation to reduce the pain sensation in the long areas.

Each jointed area has an ideal movement activation sequence (firing pattern). The movement is a product of the entire mechanism, including bones; joints; ligaments; capsular components and design; tendons; muscle shapes and fiber types; interlinked fascial networks; nerve distribution; myotatic units of prime movers, antagonists, synergists, and fixators; neurologic kinetic chain interactions; the bodywide influence of reflexes, including the positional and righting reflexes of vision and the inner ear; circulatory distribution; general systemic balance; and nutritional influences. Assessment of a movement pattern as normal indicates that all parts are functioning in a well-orchestrated manner. When a dysfunction is identified, the causal factors can arise from any one or a combination of these elements. Often a multidisciplinary diagnosis is necessary to identify clearly the interconnected nature of the pathologic condition (Box 10-4).

BOX 10-4

Muscle Tone/Motor Tone

The term *muscle tone* describes the density and length of a muscle structure with regard to connective tissues and the amount of fluid present (blood, interstitial fluid, lymph). The term *motor tone* describes how long or short a muscle is based on nervous system functions, such as agonist-antagonist interplay and other relationships.

Range of Motion

The range of motion of a joint is measured in degrees. A full circle is 360 degrees. A flat horizontal line is 180 degrees. Two perpendicular lines (as in the shape of a capital L) create a 90-degree angle. Various ranges of motion are possible. For example, when the range of motion of a joint allows 0 to 90 degrees of flexion, anything less is hypomobile and anything more is hypermobile. A great degree of variability exists among individuals as to the actual normal range of motion; the degrees provided are general guidelines. Range of motion is measured from the anatomic position. Whether the client is standing, supine, or side-lying, anatomic position is considered 0 degrees of motion.

Guidelines for analyzing problems found through the functional biomechanical assessment include the following:

- If an area is hypomobile, consider increased motor or muscle tone or shortening in the antagonist pattern as a possible cause.
- If an area is hypermobile, consider instability of the joint structure or muscle weakness in the fixation pattern or problems with antagonist/agonist co-contraction function as possible causes.
- If an area cannot hold against resistance, consider weakness from reciprocal inhibition of the muscles of the prime mover and synergist pattern and tension in the antagonist pattern as possible causes.
- If pain occurs on passive movement, consider joint capsule dysfunction and nerve entrapment syndromes as possible causes.
- If pain occurs on active movement, consider muscle firing patterns and fascial involvement as a possible cause.
- Always consider bodywide reflexive patterns, as discussed in the section on posture and gait and kinetic chain, as possible causes.

The following guidelines also are important:

- The ability to easily resist the applied force should be the same or very similar bilaterally.
- Opposite movement patterns should be easy to assume.
- Bilateral asymmetry, pain, weakness, inability to assume the isolation position or to move into the opposite position, fatigue, or a heavy sensation may indicate dysfunction.
- Intervention or referral depends on the severity of the condition (stage 1, 2, or 3) and whether the dysfunction is related to joint, neuromuscular, or myofascial problems.

Intervention plans need to work toward the client's goals. It is important to relate benefit derived from the methods to daily function. For example, a plan based on the client goal of more effective shoulder movement would read: "Improved shoulder movement would be encouraged with the use of weekly therapeutic massage and daily yoga practice. Client indicates that more effective shoulder movement could result in increased golf performance and the reduction of shoulder stiffness after the game."

A plan based on efficient biomechanical movement would focus on re-establishing or supporting effective movement patterns. Biomechanically efficient movement is smooth, bilaterally symmetric, and coordinated, with an easy, effortless use of the body. Functional assessment measures the efficiency of coordinated movement. During assessment, noticeable variations need to be considered.

Compensation Patterns

Compensation patterns are the result of a person adjusting to some sort of dysfunction. Years of clinical experience have taught many therapists that most symptoms are compensatory patterns. Some problems are recent, and some qualify for archeologic exploration, having developed in early life and been compounded through time. Compensatory patterns often are complex, but the client's body frequently can show us the way if we can listen to the story it tells.

The importance of compensation must be considered. Resourceful compensation, the adjustments the body makes to manage a permanent or chronic dysfunction, is common. Protective muscle spasm (guarding) around a compressed disk is an example. The splinting action of the spasms protects the nerves and provides additional stability in the area.

Decisions must be made regarding how and to what degree the compensatory pattern should be altered. It seems prudent to assume that the body knows what it is doing. The wise therapist spends time coming to understand the reasons for the compensatory patterns presented by the body. When resourceful compensation is present, therapeutic massage methods are used to support the altered pattern and prevent any more increase in postural distortion than is necessary to support the body change (compensation).

Some compensatory patterns are also set up for short-term situations that do not require permanent adaptation. Having a leg in a cast and walking on crutches for a time is a classic example. The body catching itself during an "almost" fall is another classic setup pattern. Unfortunately, the body often habituates these patterns and maintains them well beyond their usefulness. Over time the body begins to show symptoms of pain or inefficient function, or both.

Many compensatory patterns develop to maintain a balanced posture, and even though the posture becomes distorted during compensation (tippy poles), the overall result is a balanced body in a gravitational line. It also is important to consider the pattern of muscle interactions, such as the ones that occur when walking, and to recognize that gait has a certain pattern for the most efficient movement that the body can manage.

No set system exists for figuring out the compensatory patterns and deciding which ones to reverse and which to support. All these factors must be considered in devising a plan that best serves the client, assuming appropriate massage is performed. A simple (but not always accurate) measure of resourceful versus unresourceful compensation is as follows:

1. If immediately after the massage the client reports improvement and at least 50% of the improvement remains 24 to 48 hours later, the compensation pattern likely is reversible. Massage application is therapeutic change (see Chapter 5).

2. If immediately after massage the client reports improvement, but 24 to 48 hours later symptoms return at the same or increased intensity, the compensation pattern likely is resourceful and cannot be reversed at this time. Massage application becomes condition management.

3. If immediately after massage the client has no significant reduction in symptoms (adaptive capacity is exhausted), only palliative care is appropriate.

Dysfunction as a Solution

No education on assessment is complete without a discussion of whether the pattern discovered is a problem or a solution. The previous section defined resourceful compensation as the best that can be expected under the circumstances. The concept of dysfunction as a solution is similar to the patterns of resourceful compensation. If all the information gathered during assessment can be viewed as *an attempt at a solution*, a broader perspective in the decision making required for effective massage care plans is created. As discussed in Chapter 5, it is important to consider the client's whole situation in determining whether a condition is a dysfunction or a solution. For example:

- A workaholic client has continual tension headaches. When the client has a headache, she tends to slow her pace and work fewer hours. Is the headache a problem or a solution?
- A massage therapist who regularly provides massage sessions for 30 to 40 clients a week develops a low back condition that prevents her from working with more than 10 clients a week. Management of the low back condition requires the massage professional to receive regular massages, exercise regularly, and manage stress. She has to cut her workload, which opens time for teaching and community service. Is the low back dysfunction a problem or a solution?

Understanding the bigger picture when analyzing assessment information adds a very important dimension for the development of essential and appropriate massage care plans. If you can view each pattern as a solution and realize that problems are solutions that no longer provide benefit, a respect for the adaptable human being evolves. Solutions are to be supported. Problems must be understood and other possibilities offered for a solution. Massage effectively provides both for the body.

CLINICAL REASONING AND PROBLEM SOLVING TO CREATE MASSAGE CARE/TREATMENT PLANS

SECTION OBJECTIVE

Using the information presented in this section, the student will be able to perform the following:

- Use the clinical reasoning model as a decision-making tool in the development of massage care/treatment plans

Specific protocols (recipes) or modalities for therapeutic intervention seldom work without modification because each person is different. Protocols provide a model of how to begin a therapeutic process, but the massage professional must modify applications of methods based on the client's individual needs and circumstances. The ability to process information effectively in the development of a therapeutic plan is based on a clinical reasoning approach rather than protocols.

The ability to apply what is learned comes from a clinical reasoning/problem-solving process. Effective work with clients becomes a continual learning process of performing a premassage assessment, determining intervention procedures, analyzing their effectiveness through postmassage assessment, and recognizing progress made from session to session. Even in the most basic sessions with a client, when the goals are pleasure and relaxation, decisions must be made about the best way to encourage the body to respond to meet the particular client's goals.

After a history has been completed and an assessment performed, the information gathered is analyzed and interpreted. The next step is to make decisions about what to do and how to develop the process into a coordinated, effective plan for achieving the client's goals. This information was first presented in Chapter 3; now we put it all together.

Effective assessment, analysis, and decision making are essential to meeting the needs of the individual client. Routines, isolated modalities, or recipe-type applications of therapeutic massage methods often are limited and ineffective in attempts to individualize sessions for clients because each person has a different set of presenting circumstances and outcome goals. The mark of an experienced professional is the ability to use clinical reasoning effectively.

As noted in Chapter 3, sessions with massage professionals are goal oriented. Goals describe desired outcomes. A primary reason for developing care/treatment plans is to set achievable goals and outline a general plan for reaching them. It is important to develop measurable, activity-based (functional) goals that are meaningful to the client. Goals must be *quantifiable* and *qualifiable*.

The database developed in history taking and assessment procedures, combined with any health care treatment orders from other professionals, provides the foundation for clinical reasoning and decision making. Decisions are based on an analysis of the database information. The analysis process (which follows) has been presented in many ways throughout this text.

1. **Review the facts and information collected.**

   Questions that can help with this process include the following:
   - What are the facts?
   - What is considered normal or balanced function?
   - What has happened? *(Spell out events.)*
   - What caused the imbalance? *(Can it be identified?)*
   - What was done or is being done?
   - What has worked or not worked?

2. **Brainstorm the possibilities.**

   Questions that can help with this process include the following:
   - What are the possibilities? *(What could it all mean?)*
   - What is my intuition suggesting?
   - What are the possible patterns of dysfunction?
   - What are the possible contributing factors?
   - What are possible interventions?
   - What might work?
   - What are other ways to look at the situation?

3. **Consider the logical outcome of each possibility.**

   Questions that can help with this process include the following:
   - What is the logical progression of the symptom pattern, contributing factors, and current behaviors?
   - What is the logical cause and effect of each intervention identified during brainstorming?
   - What are the pros and cons of each intervention suggested? (Remember to look at both sides of the issue.)
   - What are the consequences of not acting?
   - What are the consequences of acting?

4. **Consider how the people involved would be affected by each possibility.**

   Questions that can help with this process include the following:
   - In terms of each intervention being considered, what is the impact on the people involved: client, practitioner, and other professionals working with the client?
   - How does each person involved feel about the possible interventions?
   - Is the practitioner within his or her scope of practice to work with such situations?
   - Does the practitioner feel qualified to work with such situations?
   - Is there a feeling of cooperation and agreement among all parties involved?

Based on your analysis, answer the following questions:

1. Does the client need referral? If so, to which professionals?
2. What are the measurable function goals for the care/treatment plan?
3. What interventions would you choose to achieve those goals?
4. How would you use them to address the various imbalances?
5. What results do you expect?
6. How long do you think it will take to achieve the goals?

Care or Treatment Plan

The development of a care or treatment plan is based on the four-part analysis of the information. After the analysis has been completed, the practitioner can make a decision about what will be involved in the care or treatment plan. Methods are chosen to achieve the agreed-on goals for the session. The plan is not an exact protocol set in stone, but rather a guideline. The care/treatment plan may evolve over the first three or four sessions and may be altered if a change occurs in the therapeutic goals or the client's status.

Decision making becomes a part of each session. As the care/treatment plan unfolds with each successive session, an update on effects, progress, and setbacks is discussed with the client before the massage begins. An updated targeted assessment based on goals is performed, and clinical reasoning and problem solving are used to choose the most effective methods for achieving the best results for the current session. As the plan is implemented, it is recorded sequentially, session by session, in some form of charting or documentation process (e.g., SOAP notes [see Chapter 3]).

An analysis of the effectiveness (or ineffectiveness) of intervention procedures is compared with previous sessions. Review of the charting notes from previous sessions becomes the foundation for this analysis. The plan is refined, reevaluated, and adjusted as necessary as the sessions progress (Proficiency Exercise 10-8). (See the Evolve Web site for a summary of the physiologic mechanisms of massage benefits.)

During the massage, assessment and intervention intermingle. It is difficult to differentiate the two except through careful observation. For the experienced massage therapist, assessment and intervention dance with each other in the context of the massage session. An area of imbalance is discovered through various methods of palpation and passive and active range of motion. Assessment leads into intervention, often simply by gently increasing the intensity or duration of the original evaluation method and repeating the methods three or four times.

Reassessment

After the massage is complete, a reassessment must be done to determine what changes the body has made. This can be done efficiently by targeting a few major areas that were the core focus of the massage. The reassessment process helps the client integrate the body changes. The before-and-after awareness also is a reinforcing factor for the client regarding the benefits of massage.

The entire process of massage is an assessment, an intervention for adaptation, and then a reassessment to see whether the approach was beneficial. This takes practice. During the learning process, assessment and reassessment can feel choppy. The skilled massage therapist learns through practice to flow between the three steps of assessment, intervention/adaptation, and reassessment during the massage, providing a sense of continuity and fluidity to the session (Proficiency Exercise 10-9).

PROFICIENCY EXERCISE 10-8

The following case studies can help students begin to make decisions about what the information gathered during assessment procedures might mean. They also can teach students how to make decisions on ways to achieve the client's goals. Remember, decision making is always a process. There are no right answers for this activity; effective applications are those that benefit the client.

This decision-making process should feel familiar by now. It was introduced in Chapter 2 to help you learn ethical decision making, and it is a thread that winds throughout the text. The same process is used to make decisions on interventions and ways to apply the best approach for a massage session. (For additional case studies, see Chapter 15.)

Case Study 1

A 54-year-old man seeks massage to deal with a nagging catch in his low back. No medical reason for the problem has been identified, and the physician states that age, an old injury, and flat feet are the probable culprits. The client was fitted with orthopedic shoes, and massage was suggested as an adjunct strategy.

The client's history revealed that the problem has been worsening over the past 2 years. The client played many high school and college sports, particularly football, and had many injuries that he did not allow to heal before playing again. He was an Air Force jet pilot for many years, which required long periods of sitting in confined areas and body positioning to accommodate for the gravitational forces of aerial combat maneuvers.

The client's current profession requires long hours of sitting and being attentive to people. Because of a change in physical activity, he gained 40 pounds over the past 4 years, and he had practically eliminated any physical exercise program. However, in the past 6 months he has lost the weight and begun exercising regularly.

The client had broken his foot 6 years ago, and 4 years ago it was rebroken and pinned to correct difficulties with the original healing process.

He has been under increased emotional stress for both professional and personal reasons. His sleep has been disrupted off and on for the past 2 years.

The client shows symptoms of adult attention deficit disorder but chooses not to use medication to treat it. He has no other health concerns. His last physical examination indicated normal functioning.

During the interview the client poked at his low back on the right, pulled at his neck, moved his left shoulder around, and pointed to the glenohumeral joint numerous times.

The physical assessment showed the following:
- The head is held in a forward position, with the chin elevated and the posterior neck area shortened.
- The shoulders are rolled forward, more so on the left.
- A slight lordosis is present.
- The most notable deviation is flat feet and a rolling to the outside of the heel of the foot, more so on the left.

Gait assessment indicated reduced arm and leg movement on the left side. The entire right side of the body seemed to lunge forward during walking. This assessment also revealed the following:
- The sacroiliac joint was more fixed on the right side.
- The weight is carried mostly on the heels and to the outside of the foot.
- The shoes show an uneven wear pattern.

Palpation indicated areas of cold on the back of the neck and a thickened skin texture, as well as the following:
- The right lumbar area was warmer than surrounding tissue, with a damp area and exaggerated reddening just below the last rib.
- The superficial connective tissue all seemed short and thick, and lifting the skin in any area was difficult.
- The muscle mass in the legs seemed overdeveloped in relation to the muscle mass of the upper body.
- The left shoulder had restricted range of motion and a hard end-feel in all directions.
- The left foot and ankle were restricted and had limited range of motion compared with the right foot and ankle.
- The breath was even but seemed out of sync with the rest of the rhythms.

Muscle testing indicated bodywide imbalance in adduction/abduction patterns, with the adductors short and the abductors weak, taut, and long. The quadratus lumborum fired first during abduction.

The client seemed edgy and spoke rapidly. He seemed impatient with the pain in his back. He kept saying that he was too busy to deal with this and that he wished he could ignore it.

Using the above information, complete the clinical reasoning process and develop a series of massage interventions and referrals to help this client. It can be helpful to puzzle through the information individually and then work together in groups to compare analysis processes and decisions.

1. **Review the facts and information collected.**

   Questions that can help with this process include the following:
   - What are the facts?

   - What is considered normal or balanced function?

Continued

PROFICIENCY EXERCISE 10-8—cont'd

■ What has happened? (Spell out events.)

■ What are the possible contributing factors?

■ What caused the imbalance? (Can it be identified?)

■ What are possible interventions?

■ What was done or is being done?

■ What might work?

■ What has worked or not worked?

■ What are other ways to look at the situation?

■ What do the data suggest?

2. **Brainstorm the possibilities.**
   Questions that can help with this process include the following:
   ■ What are the possibilities? (What could it all mean?)

3. **Consider the logical outcome of each possibility.**
   Questions that can help with this process include the following:
   ■ What is the logical progression of the symptom pattern, contributing factors, and current behaviors?

■ What is my intuition suggesting?

■ What are the possible patterns of dysfunction?

PROFICIENCY EXERCISE 10-8—cont'd

- What is the logical cause and effect of each intervention identified?

- What are the pros and cons of each intervention suggested? (Remember to look at both sides of the issue.)

- What are the consequences of not acting?

- What are the consequences of acting?

- Is the practitioner within his or her scope of practice to work with such situations?

- Is the practitioner qualified to work with such situations?

- Does the practitioner feel qualified to work with such situations?

- Is there a feeling of cooperation and agreement among all parties involved?

4. **Consider how the people involved would be affected by each possibility.**
   Questions that can help with this process include the following:
   - In terms of each intervention being considered, what is the impact on the people involved: client, practitioner, and other professionals working with the client?

   - How does each person involved feel about the possible interventions?

Based on your analysis, answer the following questions:
1. Does the client need referral? If so, to which professionals?

2. What are the measurable functional goals for the care/treatment plan?

3. What interventions would you choose to achieve those goals?

Continued

PROFICIENCY EXERCISE 10-8—cont'd

4. How would you use them to address the various imbalances?

5. What results do you expect?

6. How long do you think it will take to achieve the goals?

Case Study 2

The client, a 16-year-old female, displays atypical seizure patterns daily, but neurologic tests do not indicate an abnormality. The neurologist referred the patient to a mental health professional, suggesting stress as the causal factor. Physiologic evaluation indicates several emotional stressors, including the life-threatening illness of a family member, the recent relocation of a special friend, relationship problems, learning difficulties, and a tendency for obsessive-compulsive behavior. A breathing pattern disorder is evident. The client's self-esteem is low.

In the past 2 years the client has had two car accidents. She is taking several medications to try to control the seizure activity. Her diet is low in vitamins and minerals, and medications and counseling have had minimal benefit. A mental health professional referred the client for massage as part of a comprehensive treatment plan monitored by the neurologist.

The physical assessment indicated restricted breathing, with primarily an upper chest pattern, shortened muscles, and an elevated scapula on the left with trigger points that generate the suspected seizure activity when palpated. No other indications were evident on the physical and gait assessments.

During the assessment procedures the client seemed cooperative but distant and distracted. Her mother was supportive but overwhelmed. Both seemed somewhat desperate for an answer to what is happening.

Using the above information, complete the clinical reasoning process and develop a series of massage interventions and referrals to help this client. It can be helpful to puzzle through the information individually and then work together in groups to compare analysis processes and decisions.

1. Review the facts and information collected.
   Questions that can help with this process include the following:

▪ What are the facts?

▪ What is considered normal or balanced function?

▪ What has happened? (Spell out events.)

▪ What caused the imbalance? (Can it be identified?)

▪ What was done or is being done?

▪ What has worked or not worked?

2. Brainstorm the possibilities.
   Questions that can help with this process include the following:
   ▪ What are the possibilities? (What could it all mean?)

PROFICIENCY EXERCISE 10-8—cont'd

- What is my intuition suggesting?

- What are the possible patterns of dysfunction?

- What are the possible contributing factors?

- What are possible interventions?

- What might work?

- What are other ways to look at the situation?

- What do the data suggest?

3. **Consider the logical outcome of each possibility.**
   Questions that can help with this process include the following:
   - What is the logical progression of the symptom pattern, contributing factors, and current behaviors?

   - What is the logical cause and effect of each intervention identified?

   - What are the pros and cons of each intervention suggested? (Remember to look at both sides of the issue.)

   - What are the consequences of not acting?

   - What are the consequences of acting?

4. **Consider how the people involved would be affected by each possibility.**
   Questions that can help with this process include the following:
   - In terms of each intervention being considered, what is the impact on the people involved: client, practitioner, and other professionals working with the client?

Continued

PROFICIENCY EXERCISE 10-8—cont'd

- How does each person involved feel about the possible interventions?

- Is the practitioner within his or her scope of practice to work with such situations?

- Is the practitioner qualified to work with such situations?

- Does the practitioner feel qualified to work with such situations?

- Is there a feeling of cooperation and agreement among all parties involved?

Based on your analysis, answer the following questions:

1. Does the client need referral? If so, to which professionals?

2. What are the measurable functional goals for the care/treatment plan?

3. What interventions would you choose to achieve those goals?

4. How would you use them to address the various imbalances?

5. What results do you expect?

6. How long do you think it will take to achieve the goals?

Case Study 3

The client is a 40-year-old woman. Today is her birthday, and she received a gift certificate for a massage from her daughter. Her history does not indicate any contraindications. The client has no particular goals for the session and is not sure whether she will have any other massage sessions. The physical assessment does not reveal any major deviations of symmetry.

Using the above information, complete the clinical reasoning process and develop a series of massage interventions and referrals to help this client. It can be helpful to puzzle through the information individually and then work together in groups to compare analysis processes and decisions.

PROFICIENCY EXERCISE 10-8—cont'd

1. **Review the facts and information collected.**
   Questions that can help with this process include the following:
   - What are the facts?

   - What is considered normal or balanced function?

   - What has happened? (Spell out events.)

   - What caused the imbalance? (Can it be identified?)

   - What was done or is being done?

   - What has worked or not worked?

   - What is my intuition suggesting?

   - What are the possible patterns of dysfunction?

   - What are the possible contributing factors?

   - What are possible interventions?

   - What might work?

   - What are other ways to look at the situation?

   - What do the data suggest?

2. **Brainstorm the possibilities.**
   Questions that can help with this process include the following:
   - What are the possibilities? (What could it all mean?)

Continued

PROFICIENCY EXERCISE 10-8—cont'd

3. Consider the logical outcome of each possibility.

Questions that can help with this process include the following:

- What is the logical progression of the symptom pattern, contributing factors, and current behaviors?

- What is the logical cause and effect of each intervention identified?

- What are the pros and cons of each intervention suggested? (Remember to look at both sides of the issue.)

- What are the consequences of not acting?

- What are the consequences of acting?

4. Consider how the people involved would be affected by each possibility.

Questions that can help with this process include the following:

- In terms of each intervention being considered, what is the impact on the people involved: client, practitioner, and other professionals working with the client?

- How does each person involved feel about the possible interventions?

- Is the practitioner within his or her scope of practice to work with such situations?

- Is the practitioner qualified to work with such situations?

- Does the practitioner feel qualified to work with such situations?

- Is there a feeling of cooperation and agreement between all parties involved?

PROFICIENCY EXERCISE 10-8—cont'd

Based on your analysis, answer the following questions:

1. Does the client need referral? If so, to which professionals?

2. What are the measurable functional goals for the care/ treatment plan?

3. What interventions would you choose to achieve those goals?

4. How would you use them to address the various imbalances?

5. What results do you expect?

6. How long do you think it will take to achieve the goals?

PROFICIENCY EXERCISE 10-9

Design and conduct five massage sessions, following the assessment guidelines provided in this chapter.

evolve

10-1 Read an additional case study on posture assessment and answer a few questions.

10-2 Watch an additional video clip on gait assessment.

Don't forget to study for your certification and licensure exams! Review questions for this chapter are located on Evolve.

■■■ SUMMARY

Massage is a whole body discipline. Assessment skills are the basis for developing intuition; this is done by learning to pay closer attention and becoming more skilled in the interpretation of the assessment information. With practice and experience, these skills become almost second nature.

Trained massage professionals who consider themselves therapists modify methods to best address the client's needs. Massage therapists not only perform massage "routines," as does the massage technician, they also adjust and adapt massage applications in an outcome-based approach. Massage methods are simple; however, when they are applied with the right intensity and in the right location, the body recognizes the stimulation and can respond resourcefully. This is the approach used by a competent massage therapist. This learning is continuous; the client never stops teaching the therapist.

The more reliable the assessment information, the more likely it is to be accurately interpreted. The more accurate the interpretation, the more specific the application of massage methods. Massage and bodywork techniques are relatively basic. Soft tissue can be pushed, pulled, shaken, stretched, and pounded, regardless of the bodywork system. Forces applied to accentuate change are tension, bend, shear, compression, and torsion. The only variables are the location of the application; the intensity, including drag, depth of pressure, and rhythm; the direction; the frequency; and the duration. The detective work and skills required to assist the client in figuring out each individual pattern prevents the massage therapist from becoming bored, which can occur if the same protocol is administered over and over.

After completing 1,000 massage sessions, the massage professional begins to own the information learned in school. After 5,000 massage sessions, the massage professional has enough experience to begin to trust the process of massage. After 10,000 massages, the massage therapist allows the massage to happen. A master of massage has learned to respect the client and follow the client's lead. This takes years of practice.

The bottom line is, the client knows his or her body best. The practitioner's job is to understand what the client says verbally, visually, through body language, and in the tissues and movement patterns. Each person's body language is unique. It takes time to learn it. Only through listening, observing, touching, and then using effective clinical reasoning skills can the massage therapist begin to recognize the patterns, which ultimately allows solutions to be found for the individual.

The massage therapist should not hesitate to ask for help and should refer a client when the problem is beyond the professional skills determined by the scope of practice for massage therapy and the professional's individual training. By joining in the team approach with other health professionals, the massage practitioner can become an important part of the complex client treatment process.

Practice enables the massage professional's skills to grow. Students are surprised at how perceptive and sensitive the body actually is once we learn to pay attention.

Robert Fulghum tells a story about hiccups that epitomizes massage:

The reason most cures work, at some time on some people, is that hiccups usually last from between seven and 63 hicks before stopping of their own accord. Whatever you do to pass the time while the episode runs its course seems to qualify as a cure, so the more entertaining the cure is, the better. The hiccuper will be treated with great solicitation while in the throes of these miniconvulsions, and the shaman who has come up with the winning cure will be looked upon with respect.[8]

Applications of therapeutic massage certainly are "entertaining" for the body, and conditions often do improve with therapeutic massage. When a massage intervention allows more efficient functioning for a client, massage professionals must be mindful that they are not shamans; rather, they should focus on educating the client about the body's responses so that the client begins to experience personal empowerment and recognizes the body's own healing potential. We also must learn not to judge ourselves according to the "success" of the client's outcome. Continual analysis of our own professional growth provides more accurate information for self-assessment.

REFERENCES

1. Melzack R: The McGill Pain Questionnaire. In *Pain measurement and assessment*, New York, 1983, Raven Press.
2. Melzack R: The short-form McGill pain questionnaire, *Pain* 30:191-197, 1987.
3. Wolfe F et al: The American College of Rheumatology: 1990 criteria for classification of fibromyalgia, *Arthritis Rheum* 33:160, 1990.
4. Norkin CC, Levangie PK: *Joint structure and function: a comprehensive analysis,* ed 4, Philadelphia, 2005, FA Davis.
5. Smith LK, Weiss E, Lehmkuhl L: *Brunnstrom's clinical kinesiology,* ed 5, Philadelphia, 1996, FA Davis.
6. Greenman PE: *Principles of manual medicine,* ed 3, Baltimore, 2003, Williams & Wilkins.
7. Chaitow L: *Soft-tissue manipulation: a practitioner's guide to the diagnosis and treatment of soft-tissue dysfunction and reflex activity,* ed 4, Rochester, Vt, 1988, Healing Arts Press.
8. Fulghum R: *Uh-oh,* New York, 1991, Villard Books.

Workbook Section

Answers for the Workbook Section for Chapter 10 are provided on p. 769.

■ ■ ■ SHORT ANSWER

1. What is an assessment?

   _____

   _____

   _____

2. Why does the massage practitioner perform an assessment?

   _____

   _____

   _____

3. What or who is the most important source of information during the assessment process?

   _____

   _____

   _____

4. What is rapport?

   _____

   _____

   _____

5. What is considered when observing the general presence of the client?

   _____

   _____

   _____

6. What information can be gathered by watching a person's gestures?

   _____

   _____

   _____

7. What is the importance of open-ended questions?

   _____

   _____

   _____

8. Why is it important to repeat what the client has told you?

   _____

   _____

   _____

9. What interferes with the ability to listen?

   _____

   _____

   _____

10. What is the importance of measurement during assessment?

    _____

    _____

    _____

11. What are the three factors that influence posture, and which one is easiest to affect?

    _____

    _____

    _____

12. What is the essence of mechanical balance?

    _____

    _____

    _____

13. What is required to stand?

    _____

    _____

    _____

14. What is the "screw home" mechanism of the knee?

    _____

    _____

    _____

15. What is the position of the client during assessment of the standing position?

    _____

    _____

    _____

16. What is the importance of bony landmarks in the assessment process?

    _____

    _____

    _____

17. Why assess for efficient gait patterns?

    _____

    _____

    _____

18. What is the importance of the sacroiliac joint during walking?

    _____

    _____

    _____

Workbook Section—cont'd

19. What are the two main factors to look for during the assessment of gait?

_____

_____

_____

20. What are the most common reasons for dysfunctional walking patterns?

_____

_____

_____

21. Why is full-body massage beneficial for efficient gait patterns?

_____

_____

_____

22. What is palpation?

_____

_____

_____

23. Why is the hand such an effective assessment tool?

_____

_____

_____

24. Are palpation skills limited to the hand?

_____

_____

_____

25. Why is it important to trust first impressions during palpation?

_____

_____

_____

26. Why can we feel something that does not touch us?

_____

_____

_____

27. What is intuition?

_____

_____

_____

28. What type of information is gathered with near-touch, or palpation that does not actually touch the body?

_____

_____

_____

29. What types of things are noticed when one palpates the skin?

_____

_____

_____

30. What does the superficial connective tissue layer feel like?

_____

_____

31. Where are the superficial blood and lymph vessels located?

_____

_____

_____

32. Why refer clients with enlarged lymph nodes to a physician?

_____

_____

_____

33. How can you tell if you are feeling skeletal muscle?

_____

_____

_____

34. What is the importance of the musculotendinous junction?

_____

_____

_____

35. Do tendons attach only to bone? Why or why not?

_____

_____

_____

36. What is the function of deep fascia?

_____

_____

_____

37. Why is it important for the massage therapist to be able to palpate and recognize a ligament?

_____

_____

_____

38. What is joint end-feel?

_____

_____

_____

39. What should a normal joint feel like?

_____

_____

_____

40. What is the basic configuration of muscles around a joint?

_____

_____

_____

41. What would pull the alignment of a joint out of its anatomic position?

_____

_____

_____

42. Why is it important to differentiate between joint and soft tissue dysfunction?

_____

_____

_____

43. Explain why you palpate bone.

_____

_____

_____

44. What are the important things to look for when palpating the abdomen?

_____

_____

_____

45. What are body rhythms?

_____

_____

_____

46. What are the three basic types of muscle testing?

_____

_____

_____

47. What is the difference between strength testing and neurologic muscle testing?

_____

_____

_____

48. When muscles are evaluated both for strength and neurologic function, what is the importance of the firing pattern (muscle activation sequence)?

_____

_____

_____

49. What are the two basic types of muscles?

_____

_____

_____

50. Typically, how do muscle imbalances set up dysfunctional patterns?

_____

_____

_____

51. When is the information from the assessment interpreted?

_____

_____

_____

52. What are some key elements in developing a treatment plan?

_____

_____

_____

53. What is the purpose of the treatment plan?

_____

_____

_____

54. How does the massage therapist decide which method to use for intervention?

_____

_____

_____

55. What is the importance of reassessment?

_____

_____

_____

56. How does the quote from Robert Fulghum on p. 426 pertain to massage?

_____

_____

_____

Workbook Section—cont'd

ADDITIONAL ACTIVITY

DOING THE PAPERWORK

The following is an example massage session, from initial interview to completion of the massage. Read the example carefully. Then complete the

physical assessment form (Figure 10-25). It helps if you assume the different postures as indicated in the example and then assess yourself in a mirror. Next, complete the care/treatment plan form (Figure 10-26). Finally, complete the SOAP notes form (Figure 10-27) using only the information given in the example. Remember that much of this information is recorded

MASSAGE ASSESSMENT/PHYSICAL OBSERVATION/PALPATION AND GAIT

PRE

POST

Client Name: _____   Date: _____

OBSERVATION & PALPATION		
ALIGNMENT	**RIBS**	**SCAPULAE**
Chin in line with nose, sternal notch, navel	Even	Even
Other:	Springy	Move freely
HEAD	Other:	Other:
Tilted (L)	**ABDOMEN**	**CLAVICLES**
Tilted (R)	Firm and pliable	Level
Rotated (L)	Hard areas	Other:
Rotated (R)	Other:	**ARMS**
EYES	**WAIST**	Hang evenly (internal) (external)
Level	Level	(L) rotated ☐ medial ☐ lateral
Equally set in socket	Other:	(R) rotated ☐ medial ☐ lateral
Other:	**SPINE CURVES**	**ELBOWS**
EARS	Normal	Even ☐
Level	Other:	Other:
Other:	**GLUTEAL MUSCLE MASS**	**WRISTS**
SHOULDERS	Even	Even
Level	Other:	Other:
(R) high / (L) low	**ILIAC CREST**	**FINGERTIPS**
(L) high / (R) low	Level	Even
(L) rounded forward	Other:	Other:
(R) rounded forward	**KNEES**	**PATELLA**
Muscle development even	Even/symmetrical	(L) ☐ movable ☐ rigid
Other:	Other:	(R) ☐ movable ☐ rigid

FIGURE 10-25 Physical assessment form.

ANKLES		TRUNK		LEGS	
Even		Remains vertical		Swing freely at hip	
Other:		Other:		Other:	
FEET		**SHOULDERS**		**KNEES**	
Mobile		Remain level		Flex and extend freely through stance and swing phase	
Other:		Rotate during walking		Other:	
ARCHES		Other:		**FEET**	
Even		**ARMS**		Heel strikes first at start of stance	
Other:		Motion is opposite leg swing		Plantar flexed at push-off	
TOES		Motion is even (L) and (R)		Foot clears floor during swing phase	
Straight		Other:		Other:	
Other:		(L) swings freely		**STEP**	
SKIN		(R) swings freely		Length is even	
Moves freely and resilient		Other:		Timing is even	
Pulls/restricted		**HIPS**		Other:	
Puffy/baggy		Remain level		**OVERALL**	
Other:		Other:		Rhythmic	
HEAD		Rotate during walking		Other:	
Remains steady/eyes forward		Other:			
Other:					

FIGURE 10-25, cont'd

on the client history form. Record only the information relevant for SOAP notes.

Sue Williams, who is 37 and a new client, arrives for her first massage with you. She has received bodywork before while a member of a health spa. She says the massages were light and relaxing. At work she is a middle management supervisor for a local manufacturing company. Her job requires time on the phone and many hours of meetings. The company is in the process of downsizing. She has been experiencing tingling in her arms and also headaches (which she rates usually as 6 to 8 on a pain scale of 1 to 10), mainly at the back of her head. You notice that she squeezes the occipital area and pulls her hair in that location as she explains the headaches. She has had some shortness of breath and lately has not been sleeping well. She had a full physical checkup in which nothing untoward was found. Her physician told her that she was stressed and needed to find some ways to relax. Massage and exercise were suggested as options. She is in a long-term relationship and has two children, a 16-year-old and a 9-year-old. She was in a car accident 4 years ago and suffered minor head trauma and whiplash. She broke her left ankle while cheerleading in high school and tends to walk on the outside of that foot.

You notice that she also tends to roll her shoulders while breathing and that she sighs a lot. During the physical assessment, you find that she swings her left leg farther than the right leg when walking and that her right shoulder is high. She definitely is using shoulder muscles when she breathes. Her head is tilted toward her right shoulder. She has a very mild kyphosis and is pulled forward in the chest area, more so on the right, so that a rotation is present at the thoracolumbar junction. You note limited movement in her right scapula and the right side of her rib cage. Palpation and muscle testing reveal that the upper thorax is rigid. Her lower leg muscles are short, and her abdominals are weak.

You give Sue a general massage using muscle energy methods to lengthen the shoulders, lower legs, and upper posterior neck. You explain to her that she has some connective tissue shortening in the upper chest, low back, and posterior neck areas. You teach her lengthening exercises for the shoulders and lower leg. You also suggest weekly massage sessions for about 6 weeks and then a re-evaluation.

Sue agrees. She also says after the session that her headache is better (a 3 on a 1 to 10 scale) but not entirely gone and she thinks she can breathe better. Overall she feels more relaxed and wants to go home and take a nap.

After Sue leaves, you review her chart and wonder about the pattern between the broken ankle, the whiplash, and the short lower legs, shoulders, chest, and neck structures. You also wonder whether the fact that she wears high heels a lot, in addition to the considerable amount of sitting in meetings and talking on the phone that she does, may have something to do with the pattern.

Workbook Section—cont'd

TREATMENT PLAN

Client Name:_____ Date: 00/00/0000_____

Choose One: ✓Original plan   Reassessment date _____

Short-term client goals:
_____
_____

Long-term client goals:
_____
_____

Therapist objectives:
_____
_____

1) Frequency, 2) length, and 3) duration of visits:
1) _____   2) _____   3) _____

Progress "measurements" to be used: (Ex.—pain scale, range of motion, increased ability to perform function)
_____
_____

Dates of reassessment:
00/00/0000_____

Categories of massage methods to be used: (Ex.— relaxation, stress reduction, lymphatic, neuromuscular, connective tissue, neurochemical, etc.)
_____
_____

Additional notes:
_____
_____
_____

Client Signature:_____   Date: 00/00/0000_____

Therapist Signature:_____   Date: 00/00/0000_____

FIGURE 10-26 Care/treatment plan form.

SESSION NOTES
SOAP CHARTING FORM

Client Name: _____ Date: _00/00/0000_____

Subjective

CLIENT STATUS
- **Information from client, referral source or reference books:**
1) Current conditions/changes from last session: _____
_____
_____

2) Information from <u>assessment</u> (physical, gait, palpation, muscle testing): _____
_____
_____

Objective

CONTENT OF SESSION
- **Generate goal (possibilities) from analysis of information in <u>client status</u>.**
1) Goals worked on this session. (Base information on client status this session and goals previously established in Treatment Plan):
_____
_____

What was <u>done</u> this session:
_____
_____
_____

Analysis

RESULTS
- **Analyze results of session in relationship to what was done and how this relates to the session goals. (This is based on <u>cause</u> and <u>effect</u> of methods used and the effects on the persons involved).**
1) What worked/what didn't: (Based on measurable and objective post assessment)
_____
_____
_____

Plan

PLAN: Plans for next session, what client will work on, what next massage will reassess and continue to assess:
_____
_____
_____

CLIENT COMMENTS:
_____

Time In: _____ Time Out: _____

FIGURE 10-27 SOAP notes form.

Workbook Section—cont'd

■ ■ ■ PROBLEM-SOLVING EXERCISES

1. A client is obviously stressed and tense after a traffic tie-up on the freeway. She is pacing and talking loudly and fast. How would you begin the massage?

_____

_____

_____

2. A client complains of a leg problem and shows you a spot on his knee. He keeps pointing to a particular area and drilling into the spot. What kinds of problems could be present in that area?

_____

_____

_____

3. A client has a damp area by her scapula that gets goose bumps when it is lightly touched. It also gets very red when massaged. What could be happening to cause these signs?

_____

_____

_____

4. When comparing the pulses in a client's foot, you notice that the right side is not as strong as the left side. The client says his right leg has been tingling. What should you do?

_____

_____

_____

5. A factory worker has very short pectoralis muscles and taut trapezius muscles on the right side. His left hip recently has begun to ache and spasm. What might be going on?

_____

_____

_____

■ ■ ■ ASSESS YOUR COMPETENCIES

Now that you have studied this chapter, you should be able to:

1. Conduct an effective client interview.

2. Perform a basic physical assessment.

3. Interpret assessment information and develop a care/treatment plan.

On a separate sheet of paper, write a short summary of the content of this chapter based on the competencies listed above. When writing this paper, assume you are speaking to someone—a client, prospective employer, co-worker, or other interested person. Write the paper as if you were having a conversation and explaining the importance of the information and skills to professional massage development.

Next, in small student discussion groups, share the papers and compare and contrast how the information was presented. Discuss the content, looking for similarities, differences, potential misunderstanding of the information, and clear and concise methods of description.

■ ■ ■ PROFESSIONAL APPLICATION EXERCISES

You are being considered for a massage position with a chiropractor. The chiropractor wants to expand the wellness program currently provided by her office, and she believes that massage would be a wonderful health service to offer. A major concern of all the staff members is the ability of another person to work effectively as part of the team. How will assessment skills be an important influencing factor for this job?

Complementary Bodywork Systems

CHAPTER OBJECTIVES

After completing this chapter, the student will be able to perform the following:

- Understand the physiologic mechanisms of complementary bodywork systems
- Identify overlap in the technical skills used in the various systems and integrate concepts of these systems into therapeutic massage
- Consider a direction of interest for further study

CHAPTER OUTLINE

KEY TERMS

Acupressure
Ayurveda
Deep transverse frictioning
Hydrotherapy
Lymphatic drainage
Myofascial approaches
Polarity
PRICE first aid
Reflexology
Systemic massage
Trigger point

This chapter introduces systems of structured touch other than therapeutic massage. The many different systems of bodywork are far too extensive to be covered individually in this text. However, they cluster into six categories:

- Eastern and Asian methods involving vital energy, chakras, meridians, and points
- Reflex systems (e.g., hydrotherapy and reflexology)
- Energetic systems (e.g., polarity)

- Structural systems (e.g., Rolfing and myofascial release)
- Neuromuscular methods (e.g., trigger point therapy)
- Fluid movement systems (e.g., lymphatic drainage)

All these systems have in common with therapeutic massage the application of touch, in a structured way, to introduce various forms of sensory and mechanical information to the body so as to effect positive physiologic change. The language of each system is different, and the theory bases vary. The methods of assessment for each approach differentiate style variations more than any other part of the systems.

It is important to appreciate the similarities and differences of various bodywork approaches without becoming too concerned with or overwhelmed by the different terminologies, which tend nonetheless to describe the same elements of anatomy and physiology.

COMPLEMENTARY BODYWORK SYSTEMS

SECTION OBJECTIVE

Using the information presented in this section, the student will be able to perform the following:

- Identify similarities in bodywork methods

In their book, *Zen Shiatsu: How to Harmonize Yin and Yang for Better Health,* Shitzuto Masunaga and Wataru Ohashi describe the interface of various bodywork methods as follows:

> Some professional therapists insist that a great difference exists among the three (anma [Chinese], Western massage, shiatsu [Japanese]) forms of treatment. I believe that a great difference cannot exist within a general field, in this case, manually applied stimulation to the human body. Of course, there are a variety of methods and schools, but basically they are similar. It is important to note that effectiveness of any treatment depends on both the practitioner and the method working together. So the effectiveness of any treatment can vary greatly from one practitioner to another. All three methods of manipulation aim at stabilizing the functioning of the human body, the difference being whether they stimulate blood circulation and nerve interactions directly or indirectly. The effectiveness of manipulative therapy has been proven by modern scientific experiments involving cutaneous stimulation. From this point of view, no difference exists among the basic three techniques, though they were developed from different principles. The purpose of manipulative therapy is to work with a person's natural healing force to correct any internal malfunctioning particular to that person.[14]

Many massage professionals continue their learning through the comprehensive study of one other bodywork approach. Other practitioners study many different bodywork modalities, some in considerable depth and others more superficially. They then integrate the information into therapeutic massage, variations, concepts, and an expanded look at the body.

This text does not attempt to describe the varied systems in depth; rather, it is devoted to the professional practice of therapeutic massage. Providing only a brief description of these other systems would do an injustice to both the rich and complete massage system and the rich and complete complementary bodywork systems, each of which are textbooks and lifetime studies in their own right.

Expertise in any of the systems requires specific study. Massage students have enough to learn about therapeutic massage; they should not also be expected to develop expertise in the other various styles. Nor does it seem necessary to attempt to become proficient in multiple bodywork styles, because the ultimate result of the application for all of them is essentially the same. In simple terms, pick one (maybe two) and learn it (them) well.

It is important for massage practitioners to understand the basis of other methods because a client may respond better to a manual system other than therapeutic massage, and informed referral is important. Methodologies and technical skills overlap among the systems, and it is helpful to be able to identify and use these overlapping skills.

This chapter presents a brief overview of the basic bodywork systems, suggestions for implementing the basic concepts and techniques that overlap well with massage therapy, and guidance for the development of an integrated system.

The information in this chapter is not sufficient training to enable the practitioner to understand and use these methods purposefully and intelligently for anything other than general enhancement of the skills already developed. However, with a commitment to further education, these methods can add efficiency, effectiveness, and enthusiasm for the benefits that therapeutic massage has to offer with regard to wellness, prevention, rehabilitation, and client-directed healing. As you practice the various methods presented, pay attention to areas in which you display a particular interest and talent; this can help direct you to specific avenues for continuing education.

The Basis of Bodywork

You can apply pressure, lift and stretch tissue, rock the body, stroke the skin, entrain the rhythms, move the joints, generate tissue repair by creating therapeutic inflammation, stimulate reflex responses, soothe the energy field, and provide the client with interpersonal and professional support, compassion, and acceptance. Regardless of the theoretical, historical, and cultural base, all the bodywork systems, including therapeutic massage, are built on this foundation.

Expertise in any bodywork system consists of quality assessment for the purpose of making effective decisions about the application of treatment to provide a service that benefits the client. Benefits range from pleasure and comfort care to ongoing management of chronic conditions and stress, as well as a therapeutic change process. All these factors in some form are covered in this text.

Body, Mind, and Spirit

Bodywork—therapeutic massage as a complete system within the broader realm—serves the wholeness of the individual through a direct influence on the body and a respect for the mind and spirit. The concept of the body/mind/spirit connection found in many complementary systems of bodywork leads to the acceptance of the unity and integrity of the individual. Consideration must include different aspects of the person, although never separate from the whole. As discussed at the beginning of this textbook, the skin is not separate from the emotions, nor the emotions separate from the organs, nor the organs separate from the muscles. No part is separate from the spirit or the context of our influence on others, society, culture, and the larger expanse of the universe.

In bodywork traditions, this interconnectedness is also apparent. For example, the Ayurvedic medicine of India is similar to Asian medicine. These practices are similar to the tribal medicine of Native Americans and other indigenous peoples. In Thailand, Tibet, Russia, and other parts of the world, the ancient traditions of medicine and folk health wisdom share a common difference with Western scientific thought: these systems identify body/mind/spirit lifestyle imbalance, a concept referred to in this text as *dysfunction* or "almost sick and not quite well." They introduce interventions to reverse this process before it cycles into body/mind/spirit disease. Western health care is beginning to embrace this concept of wholeness through prevention, and whole personal care is now a consistent component of health care.

Wellness Massage Versus Medical Massage

Let's clear up one thing: there is no such thing as wellness massage, sports massage, medical massage, prenatal massage, geriatric massage, and so forth. There is only appropriate massage based on the unique circumstances of the client. (This concept is developed further in the next chapter.) The main purpose of this textbook is to train the massage professional to use massage methods intelligently to promote health and well-being. Massage is best used in the prevention of disease and the support of optimal health. Generally healthy people can benefit from the normalizing physiologic effects of hydrotherapy, connective tissue massage, lymphatic and blood circulation massage, trigger point work, acupressure, reflexology, and so forth. These methods, when integrated into the massage methods already used, can add another dimension to the effectiveness of the massage. The current trend in the expanding role of the massage profession is the spa industry. Typically, this setting reflects the integrated approach and offers clients many modalities in various combinations of service menus. For example, a hydrotherapy application, including the use of essential oils, mud and clay packs, and salt scrubs, may be combined with massage. (Specific information on spa applications is presented in Chapter 12.)

Sometimes the client may present the massage professional with minor problems that can be helped by the use of the techniques discussed in this chapter. These same methods can be used in various forms of health care and rehabilitative procedures or with athletes. To use the methods in a more specific way, massage professionals require additional training, especially in pathophysiology, pharmacology, and medical treatment protocols, so that they can understand the integra-

tion of massage therapy into these approaches. Even when the massage practitioner deals with medical conditions and works in the health care environment (see Chapter 12), the methods (i.e., massage manipulations and techniques as described in Chapter 9 or any of the methods described in this chapter) do not change. Some methods are more appropriate for certain conditions, and others are chosen for different outcomes. The difference is the condition of the person receiving the massage. Additional education does not focus on learning new methods, but rather on learning how to choose and apply methods with clients who have various complex circumstances.

Massage professionals who work with a client in the sports and fitness or health care setting need to increase their knowledge based on the function, dysfunction, or disease being addressed. For example:

- Serving the athlete requires an understanding of training protocols, common stress patterns, and injury rehabilitation of that particular sport.
- Working with stroke rehabilitation requires increased knowledge of stroke etiology, rehabilitation, and the use of massage as part of the overall rehabilitation and management process.
- Working with clients who suffer from depression is enhanced by an understanding of the manifestations of depression, mental health interventions, and psychotropic pharmacology.

The massage professional should confer with the medical team when dealing with clients who are undergoing medical intervention (e.g., medications, physical therapy, psychotherapy, chiropractic therapy). The massage should be integrated into the entire treatment protocol. Supervision by a licensed medical professional can help ensure that methods used for a client are monitored and evaluated for effectiveness and safety.

Whether the massage professional is working in the wellness setting, in the sports and fitness setting, or in the health care environment, the attractiveness of therapeutic massage and complementary bodywork systems lies in their totality and the simple disciplines inherent in them that support healthy lifestyles. Chapter 13 explores this concept in greater depth.

HYDROTHERAPY

SECTION OBJECTIVES

Using the information presented in this section, the student will be able to perform the following:

- Explain the general effects of hot and cold water applications
- Incorporate simple hydrotherapy methods into the massage setting
- Suggest easy self-help techniques for clients using basic hydrotherapy
- Identify the appropriate hydrotherapy application for the spa, sports and fitness, and health care settings

Hydrotherapy is a distinct form of treatment that combines well with massage. Water can be used in many different ways, depending on the health needs and condition of the client and the facilities available for therapy. Hydrotherapy is a component of the spa environment, sports treatment, and health care.

Water therapy is as old as the human race. One of the first recorded mentions of the use of water as medicine involves the temples of the Greek god of medicine, Aesculapius. At the temples, bathing and massage were part of the treatment of the sick. Hippocrates used water as a beverage for reducing fever and treating many diseases. He also stressed the value of using various types of baths, each with a different temperature, as a therapeutic tool to combat illness. Later, the ancient Roman physicians Galen and Celsus also recommended specific baths as an integral part of their remedies. Almost every warm-climate civilization has at some point in its history used baths for therapeutic purposes.[1]

Skillful use of hydrotherapy methods requires long-term study. The advanced level massage therapist should be well trained in hydrotherapy. These methods have very powerful physiologic effects and have been used for centuries as part of the healing process. Before the development of antidepressant and stimulant medications, hot, warm, and cold applications were used to stimulate or sedate the autonomic nervous system. Cold shock was used instead of electric shock to treat depression. Warm baths of long duration were used to calm anxious individuals. For centuries, herb and mineral additives were used to enhance the effects of water treatments.

Overview

Water is a near-perfect natural body balancer and is necessary for life. It accounts for the largest percentage of our body weight. A universal solvent, it is a perfect detoxifier for the body. It is available in many forms, all of which are therapeu-tically beneficial. Water can relax or stimulate, anesthetize, and reduce or increase circulation. It works naturally and is nonallergenic, tissue tolerant, inexpensive, and readily available.

Water's three forms (liquid, steam, and ice) allow it to be used at a variety of temperatures. As a liquid, water can be pressurized and used as a relaxing massage shower or in a whirlpool for muscle and joint therapy. As steam, it provides relaxation and cleansing in a steam bath, humidifies a winter home, and can serve as a breathing aid to a congested child or older person. It can be used as an antiseptic as steam or when boiling. When heated, water can increase body temperature and circulation; when cool, it can decrease these functions. As ice, it is an effective anesthetic and can minimize edema. In a flotation tank or soaking bath, water can reduce sensory stimulation and support relaxation.

Water can be used internally by drinking it or by forcing streams of water into orifices, as in an enema, bidet, or nose or ear bath. Water can be used externally in full or partial baths, showers, compresses, packs, hot water bottles, frozen ice bandages, and wrapped ice, and as steam it can be used in several different ways (Box 11-1).

Primary Effects of Hydrotherapy

The effects of water are primarily reflexive and focus on the autonomic nervous system. The addition of heat energy or the dissipation of heat energy from tissues can be classified as a mechanical effect. In general, cold stimulates sympathetic responses, and warmth activates parasympathetic responses. Short- and long-term applications of hot or cold differ in effect. For the most part, short cold applications stimulate and

BOX 11-1

Therapeutic Uses of Water

Analgesic (relieves pain)	Hot, warm, and cold applications
Anesthetic (reduces sensation)	Cold application
Antiedemic (reduces swelling)	Cold application
Antipyretic (reduces fever)	Cool to cold application
Antiseptic (kills pathogens)	Boiling water, high-pressure steam (not for use on the body)
Antispasmodic (reduces muscle spasms)	Hot, warm, and cold applications
Astringent (causes tissues to contract)	Cold application
Burn treatment (first-degree and mild second-degree burns only)	Cool application
Diaphoretic (produces sweating)	Hot application
Diuretic (increases urine formation)	Drinking water
Emetic (produces vomiting)	Drinking warm water
Expectorant (loosens mucus)	Hot and steam applications
Immunologic enhancement (increases white cell production)	Cold application
Laxative (promotes peristalsis of the bowel)	Drinking cold water or use of an enema
Purifier (eliminates toxins)	All forms of water
Sedative (reduces sympathetic arousal and encourages sleep)	Drinking warm water
Stimulant (increases sympathetic arousal)	Short hot and cold applications
Tonic (increases muscle tone)	Cold and alternating hot and cold applications

Modified with permission from Nikola RJ: *Creatures of water: hydrotherapy textbook*, Salt Lake City, 2005, EUROPA Utah PUBLISHING.

vasoconstrict, with a secondary effect of increased circulation as blood is channeled to the area to warm it. Long cold applications depress and reduce circulation. Short applications of heat vasodilate vessels and depress and deplete tone, whereas long heat applications result in a combined depressant and stimulant reaction.

Visceral Reflex

Cutaneous and Somatic Effects. Stimulation of certain nerve endings in organs results in both a muscle and skin response in a reflex loop. Usually the muscles spasm or increase in tension, and the skin becomes more taut. This reflex is responsible for visceral referred pain patterns (see Chapter 5). Theoretically the reflex is a loop, therefore stimulation of muscle and skin can reflexively affect the corresponding organ. In general, an organ is in a reflex pattern with the muscles and skin over it. Applications of hydrotherapy seem to have either sedative or stimulating effects on the specific organ.

Mechanical Effects. Different water pressures can exert a powerful mechanical effect on the nerve and blood supplies of the skin. Techniques that are used include a friction rub with a sponge or wet mitten and pressurized streams of hot and cold water directed at various parts of the body (Box 11-2).

Diffusion is a principle of hydrotherapy by which water moves across a permeable or semipermeable membrane from a mineral salt concentration that is low to a high concentration to equalize solution consistency. If the water used for hydrotherapy application is lower in salt content than body fluids, water moves from the outside of the body to the inside through the semipermeable superficial tissue of the skin and superficial fascia. If the salt content of the water external to the skin is higher, such as when mineral salt baths are used, water from the body moves into the external soak water. When this happens, surface edema is reduced.

Specifics of Hydrotherapy

Water is unique in that it is universally available, readily accessible, and applied with relatively simple and inexpensive equipment. The therapeutic properties of hydrotherapy are based on its mechanical and/or thermal effects and the body's reaction to hot and cold stimuli. Therapeutic effects also occur in response to the hydrostatic pressure exerted by the water when the body (or body part) is immersed in (surrounded by) water, as well as in response to the sensation of the water against the skin. The peripheral nerves are stimulated by the temperature or pressure of the water, and impulses from the sensation on the skin are carried deeper into the body, stimulating the central nervous system, the autonomic nervous system, and, indirectly, all the other systems in the body.

Generally, heat quiets and soothes the body, slowing the activity of internal organs. Cold, in contrast, stimulates and invigorates, increasing internal activity. When the body is submerged in water, such as a bath, a pool, or a whirlpool, the constant pull of gravity is reduced. Water also has a hydrostatic pressure effect; it has a massagelike effect, because water in motion stimulates touch receptors on the skin.

Water is effective as a therapeutic agent for several reasons:

- It has the ability to store and transmit heat.
- Is a good conductor of heat.
- It has solvent properties.
- It is nontoxic and therefore can be used both internally and externally.
- It can change states within a narrow, easily obtainable temperature range.
- In its solid form (ice), it is an effective cooling agent.
- It its liquid form (water), it may be applied using many pressures and temperatures, as well as methods ranging from total immersion to local compression.
- In its gaseous form (steam), it may be used in vapor or steam baths or for inhalation treatments.
- The density of water is near that of the human body, therefore it supports exercise for clients with joint disease, paralysis, or atrophy.
- The hydrostatic pressure exerted on the body surface during immersion increases urine output, as well as venous and lymphatic flow from the periphery.

Physiologic Effects

The physiologic effects of hydrotherapy can be thermal, mechanical, or chemical.

- Thermal effects are produced when the water temperature is higher or lower than the current body temperature. When the temperature difference is small, the effect is mild; when the temperature difference is large, the effect is strong.
- Mechanical effects occur from the pressure of the water on the body, such as occurs in showers or whirlpools, and hydrostatic pressure forces that occur in baths.
- Chemical effects occur by drinking water or irrigating a body cavity, such as the large colon.

In hydrotherapy, heating and cooling effects occur when heat from the water is transferred to the body or vice versa.

Importance of Drinking Water. Drinking pure, fresh water is essential to health and well-being. It is very important to drink sufficient water each day to make up for water that is lost throughout the day. Although the benefits of drinking water are widely recognized, many people still do not drink sufficient quantities of water for optimal health. It is important to remember that the need to drink cannot be determined by the sensation of thirst. People typically feel thirsty only when they are becoming dehydrated; therefore, water should be consumed before a person feels thirsty and regularly throughout the day. Water requirements increase as a person ages, because the mucous membranes become thinner and lose more water, and the kidneys function less efficiently.

Circulation Enhancement with Hydrotherapy. To promote healing, it is important to support circulation. Circulation can be enhanced very effectively with hydrotherapy. Massage is also very effective for moving blood in the body. The combined effects of massage and hydrotherapy can increase the rate of blood flow, decrease the rate of blood, increase blood flow to an ischemic area (an area with too little

BOX 11-2

Effects of Hydrotherapy Using Heat, Cold, and Ice Applications

Effects of Heat
- Increases circulation
- Increases metabolism
- Increases inflammation
- Increases respiration
- Increases perspiration
- Decreases pain
- Decreases muscle spasm
- Decreases tissue stiffness
- Decreases white blood cell production

Applications of Heat Hydrotherapy
- As a *sedative:* Water is a very efficient, nontoxic, calming substance. It soothes the body and promotes sleep.
  Techniques: Use hot and warm baths to quiet and relax the entire body. Salt baths, neutral showers, or damp sheet packs can be used to relax certain areas.
- For *elimination:* The skin is the largest organ of the body, and simple immersion in a long, hot bath or a session in a sauna or steam room can stimulate the excretion of toxins through the skin. Inducing perspiration is useful for treating acute diseases and many chronic health problems.
  Techniques: Use hot baths, Epsom salt or common salt baths, hot packs, dry blanket packs, and hot herbal drinks.
- As an *antispasmodic:* Water effectively reduces cramps and muscle spasm.
  Techniques: Use hot compresses (depending on the problem), herbal teas, and abdominal compresses.

Effects of Cold and Ice

Cold
- Increases stimulation
- Increases muscle tone
- Increases tissue stiffness
- Increases white blood cell production
- Increases red blood cell production
- Decreases circulation (primary effect); increases circulation (secondary effect)
- Decreases inflammation
- Decreases pain
- Decreases respiration
- Decreases digestive processes

Ice
- Increases tissue stiffness
- Decreases circulation
- Decreases metabolism
- Decreases inflammation
- Decreases pain
- Decreases muscle spasm

Types of Applications
- Ice packs
- Ice immersion (ice water)
- Ice massage

- Cold whirlpool
- Chemical cold packs
- Cold gel packs (use with caution)

Contraindications to Use of Ice
- Vasospastic disease (spasming of blood vessels)
- Cold hypersensitivity; signs include:
  - *Skin:* Itching, sweating
  - *Respiratory:* Hoarseness, sneezing, chest pain
  - *Gastrointestinal:* Abdominal pain, diarrhea, vomiting
  - *Eyes:* Puffy eyelids
  - *General:* Headache, discomfort, uneasiness
- Cardiac disorder
- Compromised local circulation

Precautions for Use of Ice
- Do not use frozen gel packs directly on the skin.
- Do not use ice applications (cryotherapy) for longer than 30 minutes continuously.
- Do not do exercises that cause pain after cold applications.
- Do not use cryotherapy on individuals with certain rheumatoid conditions or those who are paralyzed or have coronary artery disease.

Applications of Cold Hydrotherapy
Ice is a primary therapy for strains, sprains, contusions, hematomas, and fractures. It has a numbing, anesthetic effect and helps control internal hemorrhaging by reducing circulation to and metabolic processes within the area.
- For *restoring and increasing muscle strength and increasing the body's resistance to disease:* Cold water boosts vigor, adds energy and tone, and aids in digestion.
  Techniques: Use cold water treading (standing or walking in cold water), whirlpool baths, cold sprays, alternate hot and cold contrast baths, showers and compresses, salt rubs, apple cider vinegar baths, and partial packs.
- For *injuries:* The application of an ice pack controls the flow of blood and reduces tissue swelling.
  Technique: Use an ice bag in addition to compression and elevation.
- As an *anesthetic:* Water can dull the sense of pain or sensation.
  Technique: Use ice to chill the tissue.
- For *minor burns:* Water, particularly cold and ice water, has been rediscovered as a primary healing agent.
  Technique: Use ice water immersion or saline water immersion.
- To *reduce fever:* Water is nature's best cooling agent. Unlike medications, which usually only diminish internal heat, water both lowers temperature and removes heat by conduction.
  Technique: Use ice bags at the base of the neck and on the forehead and feet; cold water sponge baths; and drinking cold water.

BOX 11-3

Classifying Water Temperatures

Very cold	32° to 56° F	Painful
Cold	56° to 65° F	Uncomfortable
Cool	65° to 92° F	Goosebumps
Neutral	92° to 98° F	Normal skin temperature
Warm to hot	98° to 104° F	Comfortable
Very hot	104° to 110° F	Reddened skin

Temperatures higher than 110° F should not be used.

blood), and decrease blood flow in a congested area (an area with too much blood).

To accomplish these changes in blood flow, three physiologic effects are necessary:

- The revulsive effect
- The derivative effect
- The collateral circulation effect

Revulsive Effect. The revulsive effect occurs when there is an increase in blood flow through an area. The most effective means of accomplishing this is to use alternating hot and cold applications. The revulsive effect is dependent on repeated application. A series of three hot/cold applications is typical. The cold application should last for 20 to 30 seconds, which is long enough to produce vasoconstriction. The warm application is typically administered for twice as long as the cold application.

The revulsive effect is most beneficial for conditions involving tissue congestion. For example, if the massage client is experiencing sinus congestion, alternating hot and cold compresses over the face can reduce sinus pressure.

Derivative Effect. The derivative effect is the opposite of the revulsive effect. Instead of encouraging blood flow to an area or through an area, the goal is to shift blood flow away from an area, thereby creating blood volume changes from one area of the body to another. An example of the derivative effect is application of heat to the feet to reduce congestion in the head. Vascular headaches, in which too much blood in the vessels is causing pressure, may also respond to this type of intervention.

The applications of cold or heat can be applied for long time periods (up to 30 minutes) and at varying temperature extremes, depending on the size of the treated area and desired effect.

Collateral Circulation Effect. In the body, both superficial and deep tissues receive blood through the same arteries as they branch. These branches are called *collateral arteries.* The collateral circulation effect creates change in the deep, rather than superficial, collateral branches of the same artery. Application of heat to an area will cause surface vessels to dilate, increasing blood flow to the superficial tissues and at the same time reducing blood flow to the deep tissues. Application of cold will have the opposite effect. Local application of hydrotherapy techniques (generally by compress or pack) is used to produce collateral circulatory changes in a specific area of the body.

Indications and Contraindications for Hydrotherapy

Hydrotherapy techniques with heat and cold produce physiologic effects that help to improve circulation, stimulate the immune system, provide relief from pain, reduce stress, and tone the body. Water itself helps to restore and rejuvenate the body.

Effects of Cold Applications

In the skin, cold receptors are more numerous than heat receptors. The temperature-regulating mechanism in the hypothalamus responds to signals by attempting to prevent cooling or overheating. The primary or direct effect of cold applications is depressant. A decrease in function can occur locally if cold is applied to an area of the body or systemically if the entire body is exposed to cold. When the application of cold lasts a long time and the temperature is significantly colder than body temperature, the effects require a more adaptive response from the body. Caution is required for those who do not have sufficient adaptive capacity to respond to cold.

Cold applications consist of ice, cold water, cold air, or evaporation of water from the surface of the body. These forms can be applied singly or in combination with other forms. Regardless of the method used, the effects of cold application are similar. Cold applications typically cause shivering, goose bumps, increased pulse and respiration, dilation of blood vessels, and increased muscle tone. These effects are referred to as a *tonic,* a stimulating reaction to cold. As the body responds to the cold application, the return to normal function results in the secondary, or indirect, effect of cold, called the *reaction.* The secondary effect, or reaction, occurs only when the body has the adaptive capacity to respond to the cold by warming the area by increasing blood flow. In general, the colder the application is, the greater the reaction is. Many hydrotherapy techniques are directed at producing the reaction to the cold application.

Effects of Hot Applications

Hot applications stimulate the body to eliminate heat to prevent tissue damage. Heat applications will have different effects, depending on the temperature, length of application, and the method used. Water temperatures between 98° F and 104° F are generally considered "hot." Above 104° F is considered very hot. Hot air, such as in a sauna, may be tolerated by many individuals for fairly long periods. Temperatures in a sauna may reach as high as 200° F, which is well above an individual's tolerance for heat in water. Often, after exposure to heat, cold will be applied, such as a cold shower. Exposure to the high temperatures of hot tubs and saunas has become popular, but it can be dangerous. Prolonged use may weaken the individual or trigger dangerous changes in respiratory and cardiac function. In pregnant women, prolonged exposure to hot temperatures may harm the fetus.

Water may be applied to the human body in a variety of ways to achieve a therapeutic effect. To apply hydrotherapy successfully, the practitioner must be familiar enough with the procedure to use it efficiently and competently. For example, the equipment required for techniques must be sanitized and maintained properly. However, it is the comfort of the client that increases the effectiveness of the treatments.

Rest and relaxation are potential benefits of hydrotherapy; it is useful for some anxious clients because it promotes general relaxation of the nervous system. Hydrotherapy usually is one component of an overall health and wellness program. It also can offer specific relief to people with a number of conditions, such as:

- Arthritis problems
- Back and neck pain
- Sports injuries
- Work-related injuries
- Cerebral palsy
- Orthopedic injuries

Used correctly, hot and cold applications are probably the most powerful antiinflammatory treatments, and they have essentially no side effects.

Risks, Cautions, and Contraindications

- An impaired ability to sense temperature changes will put a person at risk for burns, scalding, or frostbite because they are unable to determine if tissue is being damaged.
- Clients with diabetes should avoid hot applications to the feet or legs and full body heating treatments such as hot baths and body wraps.
- Cold applications should not be used if the client has been diagnosed with Raynaud's disease.
- Elderly people and young children may not be able to adapt to long exposure to heat and should avoid long, full-body hot treatments such as whirlpools and saunas.
- Long-duration exposure to hot treatments such as immersion baths and hot saunas are not recommended for individuals with multiple sclerosis, women who are pregnant, anyone with high or low blood pressure, or individuals with any type of heart condition.
- Temperatures higher than 106°F should not be used on any person, because the body temperature increases very quickly and cannot adapt.

Specific indications and contraindications are discussed with each particular application.

Hydrotherapy Supplies, Treatments, and Common Techniques

Using hydrotherapy as an adjunct to massage is possible using a few basic supplies, including:

- Various sizes of tubs, bowls, and other containers to hold water
- Thermometer
- Large watering can
- Hot plate, large pot or crockpot, or electric roaster to heat water
- Small refrigerator to cool water and make ice
- Cotton sheets
- Wool or acrylic blankets
- Flannel material or towels and washcloths

- Some sort of waterproof sheeting (i.e., tarp, vinyl, or plastic tablecloth)
- Plastic sheeting
- Classic hot water bottle
- Elastic bandages used to wrap around an area to hold a compress or pack in place
- Rice-filled bags
- Microwave oven
- Access to a tub and shower if you want to use immersion methods

Many techniques can be used for hydrotherapy applications. These include baths, showers, douches, friction rubs, wraps, compresses, packs, and steam inhalation.

Baths, Showers, and Douches

Hydrotherapy Baths. A bath is a full or partial immersion of the body into water. Water temperature and the duration of the bath depend on the desired outcome. Substances can be added to the water to generate specific results. Additives most commonly used are salts, essential oils, milk, oatmeal, and seaweed preparations. The water may be moving, as in a whirlpool, or still.

Hot Full Immersion Bath. Water temperature range of 100°F to 106°F
Bath duration up to 20 minutes

Indications for a hot full immersion bath include:

- Muscular spasms
- Detoxification through sweating
- Relaxation and stress reduction

NOTE: Hot baths are typically followed by a brief, cool treatment such as a cool shower.

CAUTION: Prolonged hot immersion baths are contraindicated for the elderly, infants, young children, immunosuppressed individuals, pregnant women, and people with cardiac or kidney disease.

Neutral Full Immersion Bath. Average temperature of the skin, 92° to 95°F
Bath duration 15 minutes to 4 hours.

NOTE: If the bath lasts longer than 20 minutes, warm water must be added to maintain the temperature.

Indications for Neutral Full Immersion Bath

- Supporting parasympathetic dominance considered a sedative effect
- Creating increased urinary output (a result of the absorption of water into the body during prolonged immersion and hydrostatic pressure of the water against the body)
- Treating peripheral edema
- Decrease in the surface temperature of the body as a result of lack of the normal heat-producing stimulus of cool air on the skin
- Anxiety and Irritability
- Exhaustion from Insomnia
- Chronic pain

CAUTIONS
Clients commonly feel chilled after a neutral bath, and care must be taken to keep them warm.

Variations of Full Immersion Baths

- **Jacuzzi:** a tub with air jets to move the water to stimulate the tissues. Generally, the water temperature is hot. Jacuzzis open pores and promote sweating. It also promotes psychological and mechanical muscular relaxation
- **Mud bath:** a combination of volcanic ash or clay, peat moss, and natural spring water used to draw out the body's toxins and exfoliate and nourish the skin
- **Herbal bath:** herbs are added to the water and combine the therapeutic properties of the herbs with those of the water.

Preparation of the Herb Bath

Method 1. Place a cup of herbs in 2 quarts of water and simmer for 15 minutes to create an *infusion*. Strain the herbs from the water and then add the liquid to the bath water.

Method 2. Fill a thin cloth or mesh bag with about a cup of herbs and place it in the bath water or tie it to the spigot so that the hot water runs through it as the tub fills.

- Cold foot bath

The feet are placed in a tub filled calf deep with cold water. The client should stop soaking the feet when the water is no longer perceived as cold.

Indications for a cold foot bath:

- Varicose veins
- Edema
- Vascular headaches
- Low blood pressure
- Circulatory problems
- Ankle sprain, strain, or bruise
- Sweaty feet
- Aching feet

CAUTIONS

Cold foot baths are not used for clients who suffer from cold feet, very high blood pressure, diabetes, or peripheral vascular disease.

Rising temperature or warm foot bath

The feet are immersed in a foot bath filled with water at body temperature (Figure 11-1, *A*). Hot water is added gradually to produce a final temperature of 103° to 104° F.

For warm foot baths, the water is already at 100° to 104° F. The foot bath should last 10 to 15 minutes and can be done daily.

Indications for a rising temperature or warm foot bath:

- Cold feet
- Onset of a common cold
- Relaxation

CAUTIONS

Do not use when the client has varicose veins, lymphostasis, or edema.

Cold arm bath:

A tub filled with cold water until it reaches a depth several inches above the immersed elbow (Figure 11-1, *B*).

Indications for a cold arm bath:

- Headaches
- Shoulder, elbow, wrist, and hand pain

CAUTIONS

Do not use when client has heart or circulatory problems.

Rising temperature or warm arm bath

The arm is immersed in a tub filled with water at body temperature. Hot water is added gradually to produce a final temperature of 103° to 104° F.

For warm arm baths, the water is already at 100° to 104° F. The bath should last 10 to 15 minutes and can be done daily.

Indications for a rising temperature or warm arm bath:

- Bronchitis
- Asthma
- Respiratory infection
- Circulatory conditions

Sitz bath

An immersion bath of the pelvic region is typically performed using a specially constructed tub, but it may also be done in

FIGURE 11-1 A, Foot bath. **B,** Arm bath.

a regular bathtub. A sitz bath may be hot, neutral, cold, contrasting hot and cold, rising temperature, or warm. Before a sitz bath, the feet should be warmed with a warm foot bath

Variations of sitz baths

A hot sitz bath generally is given at a water temperature of 105° to 110°F and lasts 3 to 10 minutes. The primary effect is analgesic. Effects require a more adaptive response from the body. Caution is required for those who do not have sufficient adaptive capacity to respond to cold. Cold temperatures range from 55° to 65°. Anything colder, such as ice, is considered very cold. Anything warmer is considered cool.

- A neutral sitz bath is given at a water temperature of 92° to 95°F and lasts 15 minutes to 2 hours. To manage inflammation, the client needs to be kept warm during treatment.
- A cold sitz bath is given at a water temperature of 55° to 75°F and lasts 30 seconds to 5 minutes to increase the tone of the smooth muscles of the uterus, bladder, and colon.
- Contrast sitz baths usually are given in groups of three (i.e., three repetitions of hot to cold). Two separate tubs are necessary. For the hot bath, the water temperature is 105° to 115°F; for the cold bath, it is 55° to 85°F. The client is in the hot bath for about 3 minutes and then 30 seconds in the cold bath. The water level in the hot tub is slightly higher than the cold tub. The client must be kept warm. A contrast sitz bath increases pelvic circulation and the tone of the smooth muscles in the area.

Indications for a sitz bath:
- Cramps of the uterus
- Hemorrhoids or inflammation (cold sitz bath)
- Irritable bladder (warm or rising temperature sitz bath)

CAUTIONS

A warm or rising temperature sitz bath should not be used for hemorrhoids. Hot sitz baths are not indicated in cases of acute inflammation.

NOTE: All contrast hydrotherapy treatments finish with the cold application.

Saunas and Steam Baths

Saunas and steam baths have similar effects. A sauna is dry heat, and the heat acts more quickly to eliminate toxins through the skin as the body sweats. The moist air of a steam bath seems to have a greater effect on the respiratory system. The client should spend no more than 15 to 20 minutes at a time in a sauna and should wipe the face frequently with a cold cloth and drink cool water to prevent overheating.

Indications for saunas and steam baths:
- Increase blood flow
- Increase heart rate
- Support immune system
- Encourage secretions in the respiratory system and open the airways
- Support relaxation
- Reduce muscle aching from overexertion

CAUTIONS

Clients should not use a sauna, unless supervised by a physician, if they have any of the following conditions: rheu-matoid arthritis, acute infection, acute or chronic inflammation, vascular changes in the brain or heart, circulatory problems, or cancer.

Douches. Douches are a gentle flow of water over the area and can be applied with a watering can or hose. The water should not splash, but rather gently surround and flow over the area. The water stream is directed from distal to the proximal. Excess water is stroked off with the hands.

Douche Variations
- **Knee douche.** The water stream begins at the lateral side of the foot and moves along the outside of the lower leg to the back of the knee, then back along the inside and over the sole of the foot. The process is then repeated for the left leg (Figure 11-2, *A*).
  1. Indications for a knee douche:
     - Headaches and migraines
     - Low blood pressure
     - Insomnia
     - Contusions
     - Varicose veins
     - Knee pain
- **Thigh douche.** The procedure for a thigh douche is the same as a knee douche but includes the upper thigh.
- **Lower trunk douche.** The procedure is the same as for a thigh douche, but the lower abdomen and gluteal area is included.
  Indications for a thigh and lower trunk douche:
  - Poor circulation
  - Varicose veins
  - Muscle aches
- **Arm douche.** The water stream begins on the outside of the right hand to the shoulder, then back on the inside of the arm. The process then is repeated for the left arm (Figure 11-2, *B*).
  2. Indications for an arm douche:
     - Cold hands
     - Anxiety
     - Muscle ache of the arms
     - Headaches
  3. **Upper trunk, back, and neck douche.** This type of douche involves the upper torso and arms. It can be used to improve blood flow to the lungs, heart, and pleura.
  4. Indications for an upper trunk, back, and neck douche:
     - Bronchitis
     - Upper respiratory conditions
     - Headaches
     - Nervous excitability
     - Toning up
     - Weakened back muscles
     - Back pain
     - Shoulder and neck pain
  5. **Face douche.** The water stream begins at the right temple and moves downward to the chin, upward to the left temple, from right to left over the forehead, and repeatedly from the forehead to the chin, then in circles over the face. Make sure the client keeps the eyes closed
  6. Indications for a face douche:

FIGURE 11-2 Examples of douches. **A,** Knee douche. **B,** Arm douche.

- Headaches
- Tension and migraines
- Tired eyes

Compresses and Packs

The difference between a bath and a compress or a pack can be understood thus: with baths, the body is in the water; with a compress or pack (a material or bag that holds the water), it is layered on the body. The three basic types of compresses are hot, cold, and alternating hot and cold (Figure 11-3).

Compresses and packs are applied using cloth, or some other compress material, which is wrung out to the desired amount of moisture and then applied to any surface of the body. A single compress consists only of layers of the wet material. A double compress is a wet cloth is completely covered by dry material (usually wool), which prevents cooling by evaporation or heat loss. With a cold double compress, the body warms the area, producing a secondary reaction to the cold. A water bottle filled with hot or cold water or ice can also be used.

Compresses are named by the area of the body to which they are applied such as a head or knee compress.

Cold Compresses For a cold compress, a cloth is immersed in cold water (sometimes ice water), wrung out, and then placed on the body. Substances are often added to the water, such as baking soda, Epsom salts, boric acid, herbs, or cider vinegar. A cold compress can remain on the body 1 to 5 minutes before losing its temperature, at which time a new cloth should be applied, thereby maintaining the cold effect. The temperature of a cold compress depends on the issue, the desired outcome, and the client's adaptive capacity. In general, the colder the temperature, the less time is required. A cold double compress is achieved by covering a cold compress with several layers of dry material, such as flannel, wool, or other heavy fabrics. These layers of dry material trap heat and

prevent any heat loss by evaporation. The double compress remains on the area until it is warmed by the body.

The cold single compress has a primarily vasoconstrictive effect, both locally and distally. The primary effect of cold double compresses is to increase the local circulation and the elimination of metabolic waste from the area. The temperature of the initial application depends on the client's adaptive capacity and the reason for use. In general, the colder the application, the stronger the secondary reaction to the cold.

7. **Cold packs.** Crushed ice in a plastic bag is the most common cold pack. It can be left in place for up to 20 minutes and then removed, or it may be repeatedly applied for 1 minute and then removed for 5 minutes. Reusable cold packs that contain gel can be used. A bag of frozen peas or corn makes an effective cold pack

Indications for a cold compress or pack:

- Reduce edema after injury
- Inhibit inflammation
- Relieve pain caused by congestion
- Reduce body temperature such as fever, especially when applied over a large area
- Upper respiratory infections
- Sore throat
- Swollen lymph nodes

CAUTIONS

Do not use a cold compress for pleurisy, or acute asthma, because these conditions may be seriously aggravated. Cold compresses should not be used for very ill or weak individuals, because they are unable to generate a secondary response to cold and warm the area.

When using ice packs, place a thin cloth between the pack and the skin to prevent frostbite.

Hot Compresses A hot compress is a prolonged application of moist heat, generally to a local area of the body, which may

FIGURE 11-3 Examples of ways to apply a compress. **A,** Wet the compress with hot or cold water and wring it out. **B,** Apply it to the area. **C,** Cover the compress with a towel.

create an analgesic effect, especially for pain caused by muscle spasm and intestinal or uterine cramping. Fairly hot compresses may be applied directly to the skin surface, with care taken to avoid burning the client.

A *fomentation* is a special type of hot compress that provides prolonged exposure at a higher temperature. Fomenta-

tions must be applied over a bath towel placed on the affected area, because they are at temperatures that cannot be tolerated when applied directly to the skin.

8. **Warm packs.** A warm pack can be created by soaking wrapping cloth in a hot infusion or decoction of herbs, wringing it out, and then applying it to the client's body.

9. Alternatively, various sizes of bags can be filled with rice and then heated in a microwave oven. The typical heating time is 1 minute per pound, not to exceed 5 minutes. This type of pack stays warm longer than a water-based pack. Make sure the client is not burned.

Indications for hot compresses or packs
- Increasing blood flow to the periphery
- Reducing internal congestion
- Producing tissue warming and relaxation
- Insomnia
- Nervous tension
- Mild muscular spasms
- Arthrosis
- Sluggish blood flow
- Headaches (muscle tension type)

CAUTIONS

Hot applications are contraindicated on the extremities of diabetic individuals. Special precautions must also be observed when treating the elderly, infants, and individuals with impaired neurologic function, edema, or decreased circulation. It is important to make sure that the client is not burned.

NOTE: extreme caution is required when electric heating pads are used. Burns are common since the device does not cool down like a hot pack or hot water bottle.

10. **Wet sheet pack.** Treatment with a wet sheet pack is one of the most useful of all hydrotherapy procedures. It requires 1 to 3 hours, depending on the client's condition (Figure 11-4).

    1. Place two wool or acrylic blankets lengthwise on the table with a small pillow at the head and a small bolster under the knees for comfort. The blankets must be large enough to cover the person being treated

    2. Have the client take a warm shower or bath before applying the method. Soak a clean white cotton sheet in cold water and then wring it out as dry as possible. Open the sheet and place it lengthwise along the table with equal amounts draped over each side. The sheet should be slightly smaller than the blankets.

    3. Have the client remove his or her clothing (underwear can be left on) and lie down on the wet sheet. The shoulders should be 4 to 6 inches below the top of the sheet. Have the client raise both arms over the head. Wrap one side of the sheet around the client's body, tucking it in snugly on the opposite side. Below the hips, wrap the sheet around the leg on the same side.

    4. Have the client lower the arms. Then, bring the opposite side of the sheet over the body, covering both arms, and wrap the opposite leg.

    5. Smooth the wet sheet over the body to ensure complete contact and tuck it in around the feet.

6. Quickly pull the blankets on the table over the client's body and tuck them in firmly, making sure there are no drafts around the client's neck or feet.

7. Additional blankets may be placed over the client, and a stocking cap can be pulled over the head to increase the heating effect.

The client is closely supervised at all times. If the person feels claustrophobic or anxious, first remove the sheet from the feet. If this is unsuccessful, it may be necessary to stop the procedure. If the client complains of chilliness, add blankets, place a hot water bottle on the feet, or provide warm drinks. The wet sheet pack proceeds through four stages: tonic (cooling), neutral, heating, and eliminative. Depending on the desired effect, the therapist may wish to prolong any one specific stage.

■ *Tonic stage.* This stage lasts 2 to 15 minutes and is finished when the client no longer perceives the sheet as being cold. The tonic stage creates an intense thermic reaction. The length of this stage depends completely on the amount of water left in the sheet. For shorter duration, the sheet should be wrung out as completely as possible and used for those who are ill or fragile. More moisture can be left in the sheet to prolong this stage if the person is relatively healthy.

■ *Neutral stage.* The neutral stage begins when the client is no longer cold. This stage may last 15 minutes to 1 hour, depending on the client's adaptive capacity. During this phase the client experiences a sense of calm that is similar to that experienced during a neutral bath. Very often the client falls asleep during this phase.

■ *Heating stage.* Heat from the client accumulates beneath the blankets, and light perspiration eventually begins to appear on the forehead; the interval between the sense of feeling warm and the appearance of perspiration is the heating stage. This stage may last 15 minutes to 1 hour.

11. *Elimination stage.* In the elimination stage, the client begins to perspire. This stage is especially beneficial for clients who need detoxification.

The entire procedure can take up to 3 hours. If an individual cannot remain confined (e.g., needs to use the restroom frequently), *do not* use this technique.[5]

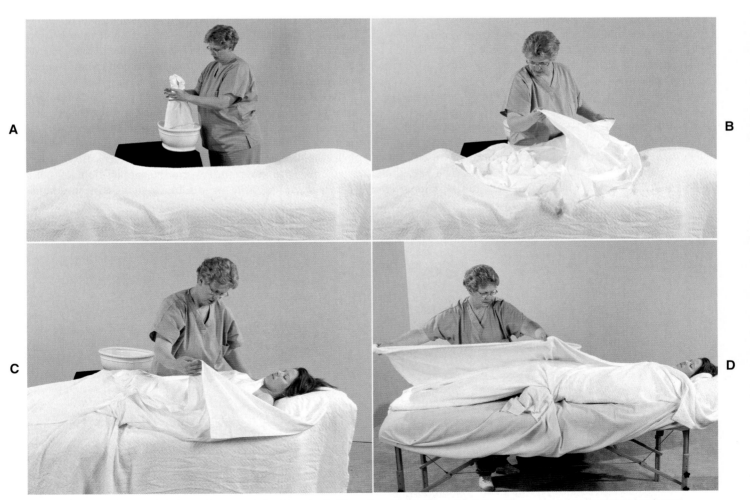

FIGURE 11-4 Procedure for using a wet sheet pack. **A,** Place two blankets on the table. Then wet a sheet and wring it out. **B,** Place the wet sheet over the blanket. **C,** Have the client lie down on the wet sheet. Then wrap the sheet around the person. **D,** Wrap the blanket around the client.

Integrating Hydrotherapy into Therapeutic Massage

The basic techniques of hydrotherapy can be taught to clients as self-help measures. Although many massage therapy facilities do not have access to hydrotherapy equipment, simple hot and cold compresses or packs can be used. A warm foot bath is easy to incorporate into a massage and serves the dual purpose of relaxing the client and freshening "stale" feet before the massage. A bag of frozen peas makes a great cold pack because it can mold to almost any area. Hot water bottles or seed bags warmed in a microwave oven are safer to use than electric heating pads, because they naturally cool down before they can cause a burn. Water frozen in a paper cup with a stick stuck in it (Figure 11-5) makes an effective massage tool, especially when the practitioner uses ice as a counterstimulant to assist in lengthening and stretching procedures. Clean, pure drinking water should be available for both the client and the therapist. Meticulous attention to sanitation is necessary when water applications are used (Box 11-4).

PRICE First Aid

Everyone should understand basic first aid. The PRICE first aid application includes hydrotherapy and is appropriate for most soft tissue injuries, especially sprains and strains. Always refer serious injuries to a medical doctor.

The acronym PRICE stands for the following:

P—Protection
R—Rest
I—Ice
C—Compression
E—Elevation

Protection reduces the risk of further injury. Muscles surrounding the injured area tend to contract in a splinting action called *guarding*. The injured area can be supported through short-term use of protective wraps.

Rest allows the injured area or areas or the entire body to best use regenerative energy to heal. Ice slows the metabolism, resulting in less secondary injury caused by swelling from the primary injury. Ice does not affect the original injury but keeps body processes from making the injury worse.

Compression increases pressure outside the vasculature. This helps control edema by promoting the resorption of fluids.

Elevation reduces blood and fluid flow to injured areas.

PRICE shortens recovery time by reducing the secondary injury to tissue caused by the inflammatory response. Less total damage results, reducing the need for repair. A decrease in pain and muscle spasms results in a more normal range of motion and muscular strength. The client therefore can return to activity much more quickly, reducing other complications set up by the injury.

A wrapped ice bag is the most effective initial therapy for many injuries, especially sports injuries. An ice bag held close to the injury site with an elastic bandage is ideal because the resulting compression reinforces the physiologic action of the application. An ice bath or ice massage is also effective.

To prevent frostbite, place a layer of fabric between the ice and the skin. Ice therapy varies with the injury and its severity. Most injuries respond within 24 to 48 hours. Ice bag compression should be used for 20 minutes twice a day or for shorter applications four times a day. Apply ice periodically, not continuously. Between ice applications, rub the body part briskly with the hand. When heat is ineffective for muscle spasms, use ice. Often a sciatica attack that does not respond to moist heat will respond to one or two frozen bandages.

Be sure the injury has been evaluated by a physician. Apply ice to the injured area by immersion in ice water (ice bath) and massage with ice cubes or pops, an ice bag, or ice packs.

Ice application continues through four sensations (over a 10- to 15-minute time period): appreciation of cold (pain), warming, ache or throbbing, and skin anesthesia (numbness).

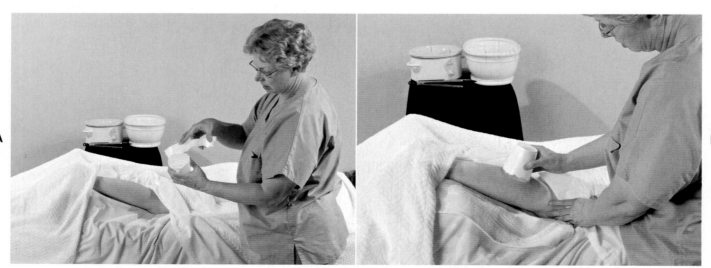

A   **B**

FIGURE 11-5 Ice massage. **A,** Ice in a cup. Peel away the edge of the cup, or freeze the ice with a stick inserted. **B,** Use ice to massage local area. Catch dripping water with a towel.

BOX 11-4

Rules of Hydrotherapy

Hydrotherapy has a powerful effect on the body. The following rules, taken from the Ontario, Canada, curriculum guidelines for massage therapy, should be followed when hydrotherapy is used in the massage setting.

1. Always take a thorough case history to check for possible contraindications. Contraindications include various circulatory and kidney problems, as well as skin conditions.
2. Always adapt the method to the individual, not vice versa. The time, temperatures, and other variables used in procedures should be considered guidelines, not absolutes.
3. Have the client go to the bathroom before treatment begins.
4. Stay with the client during treatment or have some way for the client to contact you, such as by using a bell.
5. Explain the complete treatment to the client beforehand so that he or she knows what to expect and what is expected.
6. Make sure the room is draft free, clean, and quiet. All equipment should be sanitary and in good working condition. Each client should have clean towels and sheets.
7. Keep the client from becoming chilled during or after the treatment.
8. For cold water treatments, the water should be as cold as possible, within the client's tolerance. A 10° difference is the minimum needed to produce stimulation and change in the circulation.
9. For warm water treatments, the water should be as warm as necessary, within the client's tolerance. A temperature that is too hot can be debilitating.
10. More is not better. It is not always more effective to use greater extremes in temperature or greater lengths of time. The aim is to achieve a positive change, and too much can overtax, damage, or set back the condition.
11. Ask pertinent questions during the treatment, including questions about comfort level and thirst, but keep talking to a minimum to allow the client to relax.
12. Check the client's respiratory rate and pulse before, during, and after treatments as required, especially with prolonged hot treatments. The pulse should stay fairly even.
13. Watch for discomfort and/or negative reactions to the treatment.
14. Stop the treatment if a negative reaction occurs.
15. Generally, short cold treatments are followed by active exercise. Prolonged cold and hot treatments are followed by bed rest and then exercise.
16. Apply cold compresses to the head with hot treatments and prolonged cold treatments.
17. Never give a cold treatment to a cold body. Always warm the body first. The easiest method for this is a warm foot bath.

(See Box 11-4 for classification of water temperatures for treatments.)

Water Applications for Health Purposes

1. Local heat: Apply heat to a specific area of the body, such as a joint, the chest, throat, shoulders, or spine. Use a hot, moist compress or a hot water bottle.
2. Local cold: Apply cold to a specific area of the body. Use a cold compress, ice bag, ice pack, ice hat, or frozen bandage.
3. Sponging: Use alcohol, water, or witch hazel applied with a sponge to wash the body.
4. Tonic friction: Combining water sponging and washing with some form of friction, either from the hand or a rough wash cloth, produces a tonic effect in the body. Use cold friction massage or a cold sponge rub.
5. Baths: Baths involve immersion of the body in cold, hot, or tepid water. Use foot, sitz, full, mineral, or herb baths. Any part of the body may be partly bathed, as in an arm, eye, or finger bath. A whirlpool is a bath in which the water is moving under pressure.
6. Compresses and packs: Compresses and packs are folded cotton, flannel, or gauze soaked in water or liquid medications or herbs. A pack covers a larger area than a compress.
7. Showers: Several kinds of water streams can be directed against the body. Alternate streams can also be directed against the body, or large amounts of water can be poured from a height.
8. Shampoo: Using soap and water together on one or all parts of the body creates a shampoo. Use shampoos to cleanse the hair or after a sauna or steam room session.
9. Steam: A vaporizer can cleanse the upper respiratory system, and a steam room or sauna increases body perspiration and releases many stored toxins. Cold steam, as from a humidifier, moistens dry rooms in winter and is important in preventing colds and sinus headaches.
10. Sauna (dry heat): A sauna is an intense but tolerably heated room. A tepid or cold shower should be taken after a sauna treatment.

The effects of alternating hot and cold include constriction and dilation of vessels and decreased congestion. Techniques include hot and cold compresses, ice bags, warm or hot baths, hot packs, whirlpool baths, and alternating hot and warm or hot and cold showers. Do not use heat on a fresh injury; it increases the blood flow and inflammation and therefore produces tissue swelling (Proficiency Exercise 11-1).

Hot and Cold Stones and Other Thermal Applications

The use of stones is an ancient healing art that has been rediscovered, particularly in the spa setting. Its modern form came in the early 1990s, when massage therapist Mary Hannigan of Tucson trademarked her particular style and called it LaStone

PROFICIENCY EXERCISE 11-1

Visit a whirlpool, a sauna, and a steam room (hotels may have this equipment available). Use the equipment and pay attention to how your body feels.

Therapy. Since then, it very quickly became a popular treatment in the spa industry in North America, and it has taken many forms. Most spas offer their own versions.

Stone therapy is a type of thermotherapy. It uses deep penetrating heat from smooth, heated stones and alternating cold from chilled stones. As shown in the hydrotherapy section, the physiologic benefits of applying alternating temperatures to the body have long been scientifically investigated and validated. The weight of the stones also has value for providing a sustained compressive force against the tissue while the stone is in place.

There is nothing magical about stones. The simple fact is that stones have an innate ability to hold heat well. Basalt stones are commonly used. Basalt is an igneous rock (this is explained later in the chapter) and holds heat well, but many other types of stone work just fine. The size, weight, and shape of the stone are more important than the type of stone. When the stones are wet or oiled, they change color, becoming darker and acquiring a satinlike appearance.

Types of Stones Commonly Used for Massage

River rock is commonly used for stone thermal applications in massage. River rocks have smooth rounded edges from movement in river and stream beds. It is also important that the river rock used have some flat surfaces. Quality is determined by the type of parent rock (e.g., sandstone, granite, basalt) and the distance the rock has traveled in the river. Some stones will be smoother than others and color will vary—not all river rock is smooth and black. The ability for a stone to hold heat depends on the amount of ore in the stone. Ore can appear in the rock as tints of green, grey, rust, blue, and other colors. Black stones will not necessarily hold heat better than lighter colored ones. Another rock commonly used for stone massage is jade. Jade is a nephrite stone and is composed of calcium, magnesium, and iron silicate. Nephrite is unique and versatile as it can hold heat just as well as it can hold cold.

Use of Stones During Massage

Gliding Tool. The smoothness and shape of stones allow some to be used for gliding techniques. A little oil applied to the stone allows a smooth gliding movement as the muscle is warmed; this is similar to "ironing" a muscle. However, some body mechanics concerns arise with regard to gripping the stone. When the massage therapist holds the stone, the muscles in the forearm are activated, which has the potential to cause damage. The use of stones for actual massage should be limited or avoided entirely.

Pressure Point Tool. Stones of a certain shape can be used for compression. For example, reflexology trigger point treatments can be provided with stones. Client safety is always a concern when using implements, and caution is necessary.

Compression Tool. The weight of the stones provides physical and mental comfort and enhances compression applications. As the stones cool, they can remain on the body while massage is applied to other parts of the body; this is the preferred application and has the primary therapeutic benefit.

Thermotherapy Tool. Because of their ability to hold heat and cold, stones make excellent thermotherapy tools. Warm stones transfer heat to the client's muscles and cause relaxation. When frozen or chilled, the stone can be used in all cases in which ice would be appropriate. Alternating applications of heat and ice is a well-practiced method of increasing circulation. Stones provide a uniform element to apply the heat and cold while preventing cold drips from the ice bag.

Justifying the Use of Stones with Massage

It is important for massage therapists to avoid using gimmicks, fads, and buzz words, because these compromise the practitioner's professionalism and the validity of the treatment. Some may question whether the use of stones can be justified in the massage setting. A case can be made for using stones as an adjunct therapy, but this reasoning is based on the properties of the stones.

If you are going to use stones during massage, you should do some research about stones. *Petrology* is the study of the classification and mineralogic and chemical composition of rocks (the term *petrology* is derived from the word *petroleum*). The terms *stones* and *rocks* can be used interchangeably.

Rocks generally are classified into three main groups:
- Sedimentary rock
- Metamorphic rock
- Igneous rock

Sedimentary rock is formed from sediments, such as gravel, sand, clay, or organic material, that have become cemented together naturally. *Metamorphic rock* is formed when heat, pressure, or both change or rearrange the composition of sedimentary, igneous, or other metamorphic rocks. *Igneous rock* is formed from magma, or molten rock, as it cools and solidifies, either deep inside the earth or on the surface when it is extruded as lava from volcanoes.

A rock is an aggregate of one or more minerals (rocks may also include organic remains). The specific mineralogic makeup of rocks can vary considerably. Some minerals are common (e.g., quartz, mica, and feldspar), whereas others are found in only one or two locations in the world.

Rocks and Minerals: Classification of Rocks

Minerals. Minerals are natural compounds formed through geologic processes. They range in composition from pure elements and simple salts to very complex silicates with thousands of known forms (organic compounds are usually excluded). The study of minerals is called *mineralogy*.

To be classified as a true mineral, a substance must be a solid and must have a crystal structure. It must also be an inorganic, naturally occurring, homogenous substance with a defined chemical composition. The chemical composition and crystal structure together define a mineral. In fact, two or more minerals may have the same chemical composition but different crystalline structures (these are known as *polymorphs*). Similarly, some minerals have different chemical compositions but the same crystalline structure.

The crystalline structure greatly influences a mineral's physical properties. For example, although diamond and graphite have the same composition (both are pure carbon), graphite is very soft, whereas diamond is the hardest of all known minerals.

Currently there are just over 4,000 known minerals, according to the International Mineralogical Association, which is responsible for approving and naming new mineral species found in nature.

Physical Properties of Minerals
- Crystal structure and habit: A mineral may show good crystal habit, or form, or it may be massive, granular, or compact with only microscopically visible crystals.
- Hardness: The physical hardness of a mineral usually is measured according to the Mohs scale of mineral hardness.
- Luster: Luster is the way a mineral's surface interacts with light; this can range from dull to glassy (vitreous).
- Color: Color is the appearance of the mineral in reflected light or, for translucent minerals, transmitted light (i.e., what it looks like to the naked eye).
- Streak: Streak is the color of the powder a mineral leaves when it is rubbed on an unglazed porcelain streak plate.
- Cleavage: Cleavage is the way a mineral may come apart, or cleave. In thin section, cleavage is visible as thin parallel lines across a mineral.
- Fracture: Fracture is how a mineral breaks when it is broken contrary to its natural cleavage planes.
- Specific gravity: The specific gravity relates the mineral mass to the mass of an equal volume of water; it is, therefore, the density of the material.
- Other properties: Fluorescence (response to ultraviolet light), magnetism, radioactivity, tenacity (response to mechanically induced changes in shape or form), and reactivity to dilute acids are other properties used to classify minerals.[26]

Healing Properties of Minerals.
The properties of the crystalline structures of minerals have led to a belief in the healing qualities of various stones. The rarer the stone, the greater its value, and therefore the more healing properties or mystical qualities that are attributed to the mineral.

Gemstones and crystals exhibit rather unusual electrical properties. Four types of electrical gemstone phenomena have been described.

- Frictional electrical charges. Certain gemstones develop an electrical charge when rubbed by a particular material. Thales recognized this quality in amber around 600 BC; in fact, the Greek word for amber is *electron*. In essence, the outer layers of electrons are exchanged between the two materials, and the charge generated depends on the materials. For instance, glass develops a positive charge when rubbed with silk and a negative charge when rubbed with flannel. Diamond, tourmaline, and topaz can be electrically charged by friction.
- Pyroelectricity. Pyroelectricity is electrical forces induced by heat. Tourmaline and quartz exhibit this effect, which is the reason they attract dust in a display case if they are located near a heat source, such as a light bulb. This effect was first recognized in tourmaline by Theophrastus in 315 BC and was fully researched during the eighteenth century. The German name for tourmaline originally was *aschentrekker*, which means "ash drawer," a reference to the gem's tendency to attract dust when charged. The color of the tourmaline seems to make a difference; black is the least chargeable, and red is the most chargeable.
- Piezoelectrical charges. Piezoelectrical charges are created by mechanical compression of a material; that is, the electrical charge is generated by squeezing, pulling, or compressing the material. Quartz and tourmaline show this property. Even more important is the reverse effect; that is, when an electrical current is passed through the material, it thickens or lengthens. This is the process by which quartz is used to regulate a clock. An electric current causes the quartz to oscillate (vibrate) at a very consistent rate. The same principle was used in submarine detection as early as 1918 and in radio broadcasting frequency control in 1922. An intriguing and still unanswered question is whether piezoelectric forces in certain of the earth's minerals may be what animals sense, either in their systems or on the ground, when they "predict" earthquakes by exhibiting strange behavior. Strong changes in atmospheric pressure may cause this effect. Piezoelectrical forces are known to exist in the bones, cartilage, and tendons of vertebrates.
- Some gemstones also conduct electricity.

Stones used therapeutically have to have a weight and shape that are conducive to body placement. Typically, a flat, oval shape lies on the body without rolling off. River rock often has shapes that fit these criteria. Different sizes of stones can be used on different areas. For example, a stone for the forehead would be flat, rectangular, approximately 3 inches by 5 inches, and $1/2$ inch thick. A stone used for placement on the sacrum could be flat, triangular, and about the size of your hand.

Body parts that can be treated with stones include the following:
- Forehead
- Area between the toes
- Thigh and back of calf
- Arm (elbow joint, forearm)
- Sternum, stomach
- Back
- Shoulder
- Neck

- Lumbar area
- Gluteals
- Scapula

Stones typically are placed on areas of the body with concentrated neurovascular activity; joints, nerve plexuses, acupuncture points, and meridians, as well as chakras, respond to the compressive thermal influence.

Make the stone selection process unique by searching for your own or, for convenience, purchase a set from a distributor. To select stones, you can go to a quarry, the beach, a landscaper, or your garden. Many distributors sell crystals. You can find smooth or tumbled stones in many places. Make it a fun practice to search for stones that intrigue you and begin your collection.

Keep in mind that stones used during massage must be able to withstand constant immersion in hot or cold water and must be sanitized by boiling them in a sanitizing agent (e.g., 10% bleach solution) after each use. The stones must be fairly flat so that they do not roll around on the body, and they should be fairly smooth so that they do not cause injury. Stones can be warmed in a slow cooker. A cooking thermometer is necessary to achieve a beneficial and safe temperature.

Some applications of stone massage include holding the stone in the hand and using it to apply the method of gliding or compression pressure on a trigger point or acupuncture point. As previously explained, body mechanics concerns arise with this process. The need to grip the stone while using it to apply pressure strains the practitioner's forearm muscles. The hand must remain relaxed during the massage application, or the muscles in the forearms will be strained. Even if the stone is not gripped but rather slid around the body, just using the palm of the hand tends to activate the forearm muscles. Another safety concern when using stones, or any object, to apply compression is that the massage practitioner's hand is not in direct contact with the client's body, monitoring feedback and pressure depth, therefore injury might occur.

Simply allowing the stones to rest on the body is beneficial. The therapeutic quality of the stone, coupled with the sustained compressive force from the weight of the stone and possibly the energy influence from the crystal structure and color, is sufficient to achieve a therapeutic effect, and the practitioner avoids the potential for repetitive strain injuries caused by using the stones to apply the massage (see Figure 12-1 on p. 522).

Procedures for Using Stones During Massage

- Before the client arrives, sanitize the stones and heat them in water at a temperature of 120° to 150° F.
- Use gliding strokes with the heated stone. When the stone loses heat, replace it with another. Observe precautions for body mechanics.
- Preferably, use the warm stone to heat your hands. Use your hands for massage and place the stone as described in the next step.
- Place heated stones at specific points along the body meridians, the spine, in the palms of the hand, or between the toes (anywhere they will stay) to improve the flow of energy in the body.
- When there is inflammation or muscle injury, use cold stones.
- Instruct the client to speak up if the stones are too warm or the pressure is too intense.
- Cover the area with a sheet and then place the stones on the sheet rather than directly on the skin; this is the safest and most sanitary method. With direct application to the skin, the most serious concern is burning the client if the stone is too hot for the individual's skin and/or if it is left on too long. *Always use warm, not hot, stones.*
- Apply the stones with an intentional, centered approach.
- Placement of stones can be combined with general massage. If the therapeutic benefit of stone application depends on temperature and weight, cloth bags filled with rice or other grains can be used. A pair of socks makes a great bag for this purpose. Fill one sock with the grain (the most inexpensive rice you can buy works fine) and tie the end tightly with string. Then slip the other sock over the filled one and tie it off with a string in a bow that can be tied and untied. The top sock can easily be removed and laundered. Various sizes and shapes of bags can be made using different sizes of socks.

Different colors of socks can be used to add a color element to the process. If appropriate, an essential oil can be placed on the surface sock. These bags—rice, socks, and string—cost less than $5 to make. Sock bags can be heated in the microwave or cooled in the freezer. They also can be molded to the area where they are placed, and they tend to stay put. These grain bags provide all the same therapeutic elements as stones except piezoelectric qualities. It might be fun to have a selection of stones to give clients for self-help methods. However, make sure the client understands the importance of safe temperature.

LYMPH, BLOOD, AND CIRCULATION ENHANCEMENT

SECTION OBJECTIVES

Using the information presented in this section, the student will be able to perform the following:

- Explain the general effects of lymphatic and circulation enhancement massage
- Incorporate the principles of lymphatic and circulation massage into the general massage session

One of the well-documented benefits of massage is stimulation of the lymphatic and circulatory systems. Many variations and styles of massage are used to stimulate lymph and blood circulation. When the massage is focused to stimulate the lymphatic or circulatory system specifically, a special type of massage is necessary. Because an entire body system is being stimulated, the approach is called systemic massage. In this section we discuss the important physiology and methods of focusing the massage to enhance lymph and blood circulation.

Lymphatic Drainage

Various styles of bodywork are used for lymphatic drainage. One style is manual lymph drainage, which was developed by Emil Vodder. Another style, described by Eyal Lederman, an osteopathic physician, takes a somewhat different approach. Recently, a third approach was added, taught by Bruno Chickly through the Upledger Institute. These three methods provide the foundation for this section. Lymphatic drainage is a specific therapeutic method. As with all the methods presented in this chapter, specialized training is required to use it successfully.

All massage stimulates the circulation and lymph movement, but structuring a massage to focus on this system is a specific therapeutic intervention. When the massage treatment focuses on an individual body system and the effects of the massage are concentrated on a certain response, the client often feels the effects of the methods more than with a general or local massage.

After undergoing massage involving the precise movement of lymph, the client may feel listless, fatigued, or achy for 48 hours. Some have described this feeling as a massage "hangover." The physiologic effects of toxin overload are similar to those of an alcohol hangover. To counter this effect and to support detoxification, the client should increase his or her water intake for 24 hours after the massage.

The Lymph System

The lymph system is a specialized component of the circulatory system that is responsible for waste disposal and immune response. The lymphatic system transports fluid from around the cells through a system of filters. Lymph and blood are very similar, except that lymph does not have red blood cells or platelets, it has a slightly higher protein content, and it carries large molecules, such as proteins, lipids, and bacteria, and other debris. Lymph is the interstitial fluid (i.e., the fluid that surrounds the cell). It is generated when plasma is forced out of the blood capillaries into cellular spaces to bathe and nourish the cells (Figures 11-6 and 11-7).

The lymphatic system permeates the entire tissue structure of the body in a one-way drainage network of vessels, ducts, nodes, lacteals, and lymphoid organs such as the spleen, tonsils, and thymus. Lymph tissue is a specialized type of fibrous connective tissue that contains lymphocytes.

The spleen, the largest organ of the lymphatic system, filters the blood. It manufactures lymphocytes, stores red blood cells, releases blood to the body in cases of extreme blood loss, and removes foreign substances and dead red blood cells. The spleen contains red and white pulp. The white pulp contains white blood cells and surrounds arteries that enter the spleen, and the red pulp surrounds veins that leave the spleen. Macrophages in the red pulp remove foreign substances and worn out or dead red blood cells.

The tonsils form a ring of lymphatic tissue that surrounds the opening to the digestive and respiratory tracts, an area where harmful substances can easily enter the body. The three pairs of tonsils are the pharyngeal, palatine, and lingual tonsils.

The thymus forms antibodies in newborns and is involved in the initial development of the immune system. Lymphocytes that are produced in the red bone marrow migrate to the thymus, where they develop into T cells. The thymus also produces the hormone thymosin. The activity of the thymus gland declines with age.

Aggregated lymph nodules are collections of lymphatic tissue in mucous membranes that are continuous with the skin; some examples of these nodules are the tonsils, the bronchi of the respiratory tract, the small intestine, and the appendix. Aggregated lymph nodules respond to antigens in those areas and create antibodies.

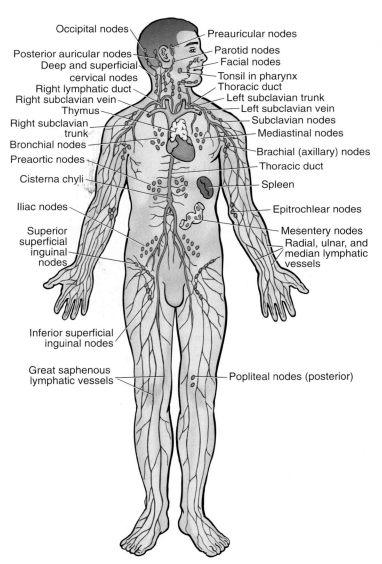

FIGURE 11-6 The lymphatic system and lymphatic drainage pathways throughout the body.

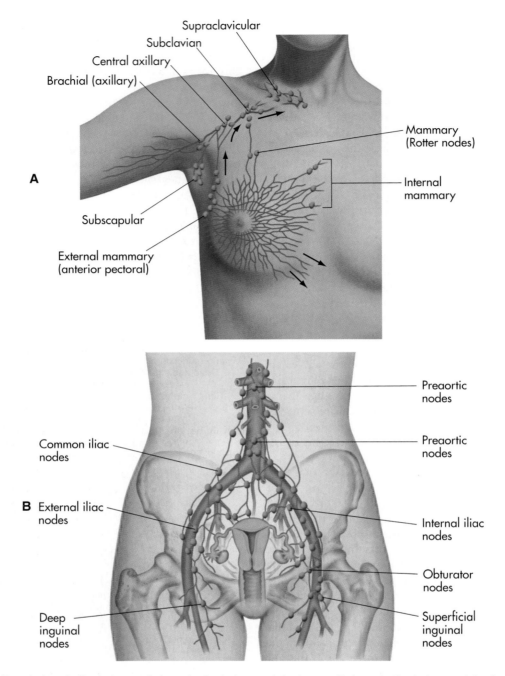

FIGURE 11-7 Female lymphatic drainage. **A,** Lymphatic drainage of the breast. **B,** Lymphatic drainage of the female genital tract. (From Seidel HM et al: *Mosby's guide to physical examination,* ed 6, St Louis, 2006, Mosby.)

To get an idea of the extensive lymph network, visualize the roots on a plant. Tiny lymph vessels, known as *lymph capillaries,* are distributed throughout the body, except in the eyes, brain, and spinal cord. Fluid collects in the lymph capillaries in a manner somewhat similar to the way water is drawn up into a plant's roots. Segments of lymph capillaries are divided by one-way valves and a spiral set of smooth muscles called *lymphangions.* This system moves fluid against gravity in a peristalsis-type undulation.

The lymphatic tubes merge into one another until major channels and vessels are formed. These vessels run from the distal parts of the body toward the neck, usually alongside veins and arteries. Valves in the vessels prevent the back flow of lymph.

Lymph nodes are enlarged portions of the lymph vessels that generally cluster at the joints. This arrangement assists movement of the lymph through the nodes by means of the pumping action from joint movement. These nodes filter the fluid and produce lymphocytes.

All the body's lymph vessels converge into two main channels, the thoracic duct and the right lymphatic duct. Vessels from the entire left side of the body and from the right side

FIGURE 11-8 Assessment for edema.

of the body below the chest converge into the thoracic duct, which in turn empties into the left subclavian vein, situated beneath the left clavicle. The right lymphatic duct collects lymph from the vessels on the right side of the head, neck, upper chest, and right arm. It empties into the right subclavian vein beneath the right clavicle. Waste products are then carried by the bloodstream to the spleen, intestines, and kidneys for detoxification.

The movement of lymph occurs along a pressure gradient from areas of high pressure to areas of low pressure. Lymph moves from the interstitial space (high pressure) into the lymph capillaries (low pressure) through a pressure mechanism exerted by respiration, peristalsis of the large intestine, the compression of muscles, and the pull of the skin and fascia during movement. This action is especially prominent at the plexuses in the hands and feet. Major lymph plexuses are found on the soles of the feet and the palms of the hands. The rhythmic pumping of walking and grasping probably facilitates lymphatic flow. As mentioned in Chapter 4, recent research indicates the existence of a primary intrinsic pumping mechanism in the lymphatic system.

Lymph circulation involves two steps:
- First, the lymph is absorbed into the lymphatic capillaries. Plasma is forced out of blood capillaries and around the cell walls. As fluid pressure increases between the cells, the cells move apart, pulling on the microfilaments that connect the endothelial cells of the lymph capillaries to tissue cells. The pull on the microfilaments causes the lymph capillaries to open like flaps, allowing tissue fluid to enter the lymph capillaries.
- Next, the lymph moves through the network of contractile lymphatic vessels. The lymphatic system does not have a central pump like the heart. Various factors assist the transport of lymph through the lymphatic vessels.

The "lymphatic pump" is the spontaneous contraction of lymphatic vessels as a result of the increase in pressure of lymphatic fluid. These contractions usually start in the lymphangions adjacent to the terminal end of the lymph capillaries and spread progressively from one lymphangion to the next, toward the thoracic duct or the right lymphatic duct. The contractions are similar to abdominal peristalsis and are stimulated by increases in pressure inside lymphatic vessels. Contractions of the lymphatic vessels are not coordinated with the heart or breath rate. If the pressure inside the lymphatic vessels exceeds or falls below certain levels, lymphatic contractions stop.

During inhalation, the thoracic duct is squeezed, which pushes fluid forward and creates a vacuum in the duct. During exhalation, fluid is pulled from the lymphatics into the thoracic duct to fill the partial vacuum.

Edema

Edema, which is an increase in interstitial fluid, can be caused by a variety of factors (Figure 11-8 and Box 11-5).
- *Lack of exercise.* Exercise, in which muscles alternately contract and relax, stimulates lymph circulation and cleans muscle tissue. If the muscles stay contracted or flaccid, lymph circulation declines drastically inside the muscles, and edema can result.
- *Increase in exercise.* An increase in exercise can strain the lymph system by causing blood capillary permeability, resulting in an increase in fluid movement to the interstitial spaces. This is one cause of the delayed onset of muscle soreness.
- *Salt consumption.* The body retains a specific ratio of salt to fluids. The more salt a person consumes, the more water is retained to balance it, resulting in edema.
- *Heart or kidney disease.* These diseases affect blood and lymph circulation. Lymphatic massage stimulates the circulation of lymph. However, caution is indicated because the increase in fluid volume could overload an already weakened heart. Blood volume is regulated by the kidneys,

BOX 11-5

Assessment for Fluid Imbalance and Treatment

1. Ask the client if tissue feels taut, distended, fat, or stiff. If the answer is no, palpate to confirm that edema is not present and then proceed with the general massage. If the answer is yes, ask for the *history*.
2. The history would include any injury, swelling, bruising, static position, and unusual increase in physical activity followed by extended inactivity. If the client answers yes to any of these, then *observe*.
3. Observe for a decrease in muscle definition, bruising, tissue distention, and changes in color. If any of these are found, *palpate*.
4. Palpate for increased muscle tone, specifically tissue tautness and an increase in fluid (pitting edema) or venous congestion. If these are noted, *observe* and *palpate* for signs of inflammation.
5. Palpate for heat and observe for redness. Ask about *pain*.
6. If the area is swollen, hot, red, and painful, refer the client to a medical professional. If inflammation is present, massage the area only after the reason for the condition has been determined.
7. If the area is not hot or red, determine if the tissue is *congested* or *swollen*.
8. Congested tissue has increased blood in the veins and capillaries; the tissue feels dense and stiff but does not show pitting edema. Swollen tissue has increased interstitial fluid; this tissue pits when pressure is applied.
9. If the tissue is congested, massage methods that enhance venous return are indicated. Observe cautions for thrombosis, kidney disease, and heart disease.
10. If the tissue is swollen, lymphatic drainage is indicated. Observe cautions for infection, kidney disease, and heart disease.

therefore an increase in blood volume could overload already weakened kidneys as well.

- *Menstrual cycle.* Water retention and/or a swollen abdomen are common before or during the menstrual cycle.
- *Lymphedema.* Limbs affected with this condition become very swollen and painful, resulting in difficulty moving the affected limb and disfigurement. Lymphedema can be life threatening, because the interstitial fluid is contaminated, injuries to the skin do not heal, and even small abrasions and sores can become infected.
- *Inflammation.* Increased blood flow to an injured area and the release of vasodilators, which are part of the inflammatory response, can cause edema in the localized area.
- *Other causes.* Medications, including steroids, hormones, and chemotherapy for cancer, may cause edema as a side effect. Scar tissue and muscle tension can cause obstructive edema by restricting lymph vessels.

Contraindications and Cautions for Lymphatic Drainage Massage

Edematous tissues have poor oxygenation and reduced function, and they heal slowly after injury. Chronic edema results in chronic inflammation and fibrosis, which makes the edematous tissue coarse, thicker, and less flexible.

Lymphatic drainage massage can lower blood pressure. If the client has low blood pressure, the danger exists that it will fall further, and the client may be dizzy upon standing.

When a person is ill with a viral or bacterial infection and fever, circulation of lymph through the nodes slows, giving the lymphocytes more time to destroy the bacteria or virus. Because massage moves fluid through the lymphatic system more quickly, it can interfere with the body's efforts to defeat the attacking cells and can prolong the illness. During fever, white blood cells multiply more rapidly and bacteria and viruses multiply more slowly; fever therefore is part of the body's healing process. Because lymphatic drainage massage lowers the body temperature, it should not be given to a client with a fever.

Lymphatic drainage massage affects the circulation of fluid in the body and can overwhelm an already weak heart or kidneys. Do not give lymphatic drainage massage to anyone with congestive heart failure or kidney failure or anyone undergoing kidney dialysis unless it is specifically ordered by the physician.

Indications for Lymphatic Drainage Massage

Simple edema, with screening for contraindications, responds well to massage focused on the lymphatic system. This approach is helpful for soft tissue injury, which includes surgery (with supervision), because it speeds healing and reduces swelling.

Traveler's edema is the result of enforced inactivity, such as sitting in an airplane or a car for several hours. The same is true for anyone who sits for extended periods. Interstitial fluid (tissue fluid) responds to gravity, causing swelling in the feet, hands, and buttocks of a person who has to sit without moving very much for a few hours. Lymphatic drainage massage can move the fluid and reduce the pain and stiffness caused by the edema. Caution is indicated because of the possibility of the formation of blood clots with prolonged activity.

Exercise-induced, delayed-onset muscle soreness is partly caused by increased fluid pressure in the soft tissues. Lymphatic drainage massage is effective for reducing the pain and stiffness of this condition.

Principles of Lymphatic Drainage Massage

The pressure provided by massage mimics the drag and compressive forces of movement and respiration and can move the skin to open the lymph capillaries. The pressure gradient from high pressure to low pressure is supported by creating low-pressure areas in the vessels proximal to the area to be drained. The depth of pressure, speed and frequency, direction, rhythm, duration, and drag are adjusted to support the lymphatic system.

- **Depth of pressure.** According to Vodder, the softer the tissue or the greater the edema, the lighter the pressure that should be used. Vodder estimated the proper pressure for lymphatic drainage to be 8 to 12 ounces per square inch, with the pressure in the peripheral lymphatics even lighter (less than 1 to 8 ounces per square inch). You can develop a sense of these levels of pressure by stroking the surface of a postage scale until you can easily keep the pressure within the recommended range. This pressure is just enough to move the skin. The lymphatics are located mostly in superficial tissues, in the outer 0.3 mm of the skin, and surface edema occurs in those superficial tissues, not in the deep tissue.

  Simple muscle tension puts pressure on the lymph vessels and may block them, interfering with efficient drainage. Massage can normalize this muscle tension. As the muscles relax, the lymph vessels open, and drainage becomes more efficient. Work on the areas of muscle tension first, using appropriate massage methods and pressure, and then finish the area with lymphatic drainage.

  Disagreement exists about the intensity of the pressure used. Some schools of thought recommend very light pressure, such as that described by Vodder. Other methods, such as the technique described by Lederman, use a deeper pressure. Lederman holds that the stronger the compression used, the greater the increase in the flow rate of lymph. Light pressure is used initially, and the pressure is methodically increased as the area is drained.[13] Moving the skin moves the lymphatics. Stretching the lymphatics longitudinally, horizontally, and diagonally stimulates them to contract.

- **Speed and frequency.** The greater the amount of fluid in the tissue, the slower the massage movements. Massage strokes are repeated at a rate of approximately 10 per minute in an area, the approximate rate at which the peripheral lymphatics contract.

- **Direction.** The lymph is moved toward the closest cluster of lymph nodes, which are located in the neck, axilla, and groin for the most part. Massage near nodes first, then move fluid toward them, working proximally from the swollen area toward the nodes. Massage the unaffected side first, then the obstructed side. For instance, if the right arm is swollen because of scar tissue from a muscle tear, massage the left arm first.

- **Rhythm.** Slow, rhythmic repetition of the massage movements stimulates a wave in the lymph fluid similar to intestinal peristalsis (a pump would be an example).

- **Duration.** Full-body lymphatic drainage massage lasts about 45 minutes. Focus on local areas for about 5 to 15 minutes.

- **Drag.** Drag on the tissue pulls open the terminal ends of the lymphatic capillaries (flap), allowing interstitial fluid to enter. Drag moves the superficial tissues (skin and superficial fascia) into and out of bind.

Application of Lymphatic Drainage Massage

The massage approach described next specifically targets the lymphatic system and is appropriate for clients who are generally healthy. People commonly develop a somewhat sluggish lymphatic flow. The usual culprits are inactivity, consumption of junk food and beverages, and reduced water intake. All these factors stress the lymphatic system. General massage with a focus as presented in this section, coupled with corrective action by the client (i.e., increased water intake, increased activity, and reduced junk food intake) can reverse the problem.

Additional training and medical supervision are required for professionals who intend to work with clients with lymphatic conditions (Proficiency Exercise 11-2).

Although disagreement exists about methodology, all approaches have some validity. Therefore the method described in this text combines the various methods to support lymphatic movement in the body.

The massage session begins with a pumping action on the thorax. Place both hands on the anterior surface of the thoracic cage. As the client exhales completely, allow your hands to passively follow the movements of the thorax. When the client starts to inhale, resist the movement of the thorax with counterpressure for 5 to 7 seconds. Repeat this procedure four or five times. Pumping action on the thorax increases lymphatic drainage through the lymph ducts by additionally lowering intrapleural pressure and exaggerating the action of inhalation and exhalation.

The massage application consists of a combination of short, light, pumping, gliding strokes beginning close to the torso at the node cluster and directed toward the torso; the strokes methodically move distally. The stroke does not slip, but rather drags the tissue to bind. The phase of applying pressure and drag must be longer than the phase of pressure and drag release. The releasing phase cannot be too short, because the lymph needs time to drain from the distal segment. Therefore the optimal duration of the pressure and drag phase is 6 to 7 seconds; for the release phase, it is about 5 seconds. Traditionally, this application was described as stationary circles, which essentially produces a bind/release movement. This pattern is followed by long surface gliding strokes with a bit more pressure to influence deeper lymph vessels. The

PROFICIENCY EXERCISE 11-2

1. *Fill a long balloon with water. Leave an air bubble in it. Use short gliding strokes with a drag component to move the bubble. Notice the level of pressure that moves the bubble most effectively.*

2. *Design a lymphatic self-massage. Incorporate deep breathing movement and compression action at the joints, palms, and soles of the feet.*

FIGURE 11-9 Direction of strokes for facilitating lymphatic flow.

direction is toward the drainage points (following the arrows in Figure 11-9; also see Figure 11-10).

The focus of the initial pressure and finishing strokes is the dermis, just below the surface layer of skin, and the layer of tissue just beneath the skin and above the muscles. This is the superficial fascial layer, which contains 60% to 70% of the lymphatic circulation in the extremities. Not much pressure is required to contact the area. If too much pressure is applied, the capillaries are pressed closed; this nullifies any effect on the more superficial vessels. With lymphatic massage, generally light pressure is indicated initially, which increases to a moderate level (including kneading and compression as well as gliding) during repeated application to the area to reach the deep lymphatic vessels; the technique then returns to lighter pressure over the area.

Drag is necessary to affect the microfilaments and to open the flaps at the ends of the capillary vessels. A pumping, rhythmic compression on the soles and palms supports lymph movement.

Rhythmic, gentle, passive and active joint movement reproduces the body's normal means of pumping lymph. The client helps the process by deep, slow breathing, which stimulates lymph flow in the deeper vessels. When possible, position the area being massaged above the heart so that gravity can assist lymph flow. This approach is very methodical and repetitious. Drinking clean water supports the system.

Circulatory Massage

The purpose of circulatory massage is to stimulate the efficient flow of blood through the body. As with lymphatic massage, specific application for circulatory impairment disease is out of the scope of practice for the massage professional unless the massage is performed under appropriate supervision. In this situation, massage can be beneficial as part of the overall treatment plan.

Clients who are not sick can benefit greatly from increased efficiency in the circulatory system. This type of massage tends to normalize blood pressure, tone the cardiovascular system, and undo the negative effects of occasional stress. It is an excellent massage approach to use with athletes and anyone else after exercise. Circulatory massage also supports the inactive client by increasing blood movement mechanically; however, it in no way replaces exercise. Both the circulatory and lymphatic types of massage are very beneficial for a client who is unable to walk or exercise aerobically.

The Circulatory System

The circulatory system is a closed system composed of a series of connected tubes and a pump. The heart pump provides pressure for the blood to move through the body via the arteries and eventually into the small capillaries, where the actual blood gas and nutrient exchange happens. The blood returns to the heart by way of the veins. Venous blood flow is not under pressure from the heart. Rather, it relies on muscle compression against the veins to change the interior venous pressure. As in the lymphatic system, back flow of blood is prevented by a valve system.

Massage Methods for the Circulatory System

Massage to encourage blood flow to the tissues (arterial circulation) is different from massage to encourage blood flow from the tissues back to the heart (venous circulation). Because the veins and lymph vessels have a valve system, deep, narrow-based stroking over these vessels from proximal to distal (from the heart outward) is contraindicated. A small chance exists of breaking down the valves if this is done. Compression, which does not slide, as does gliding or stripping, is appropriate for stimulating arterial circulation.

Compression is applied over the main arteries, beginning close to the heart (proximal) and moving systematically toward the tips of the fingers or toes (distal). The manipulations are applied with a pumping action at a rhythm of approximately 60 beats per minute, or at a rhythm that matches the client's resting heart rate. Compressive force changes the internal pressure in the arteries, stimulates the

FIGURE 11-10 Examples of lymphatic drainage methods. **A,** Skin drag method, back (stationary circles). **B,** Skin drag method, back. **C,** Rhythmic pumping, upper thorax. **D,** Rhythmic pumping, ribs. **E, F,** Skin drag method, arm (draining process).

Continued

FIGURE 11-10, cont'd G, Rhythmic joint movement. **H,** Stationary circles, calf. **I, J,** Skin drag method, thigh. **K,** Kneading. **L,** Continue with skin drag.

FIGURE 11-10, cont'd **M,** Rhythmic pumping at hip. **N,** Rhythmic compression on plexus, sole of foot.

intrinsic contraction of arteries, and encourages the movement of blood out to the distal areas of the body. Compression also begins to empty venous vessels and forms an arteriovenous pressure gradient, encouraging arterial blood flow (Figures 11-11 and 11-12).

Rhythmic, gentle contraction and relaxation of the muscles powerfully encourage arterial blood flow. Both active and passive joint movements support the transport of arterial blood.

The next step is to assist venous return flow. This process is similar to lymphatic massage in that a combination of short and long gliding strokes is used in conjunction with movement. The difference is that lymphatic massage is done over the entire body and the movements usually are passive. With venous return flow massage, the gliding strokes move distal to proximal (from the fingers and toes to the heart) over the major veins, and the strokes actually slide somewhat like a squeegee washing a window. Also, the gliding stroke is short, only about 3 inches long; this enables the blood to move from valve to valve. Long gliding strokes carry the blood through the entire vein. Both passive and active joint movements encourage venous circulation. Placing the limb or other area above the heart brings gravity into assistance (Figures 11-13 and 11-14) (Proficiency Exercise 11-3).

REFLEXOLOGY   11-3

SECTION OBJECTIVES

Using the information presented in this section, the student will be able to perform the following:

* Explain the physiologic benefits of foot and hand massage
* Incorporate the principles of reflexology into the general massage session

Reflexology is the stimulation of areas beneath the skin to improve the function of the whole body or of specific body areas away from the site of the stimulation. Eunice Ingham

FIGURE 11-11 Direction of compression over arteries to increase arterial flow.

FIGURE 11-12 Examples of arterial support.

FIGURE 11-13 Direction of short gliding strokes to facilitate venous flow.

PROFICIENCY EXERCISE 11-3

1. *Hook up a hose to a faucet and barely turn on the water; this simulates the heart pump. Use compression to facilitate the movement, or "circulation," of the water in the hose.*
2. *Obtain a 3-foot piece of clear, soft plastic tubing. As if sucking on a straw, draw up a small amount of water into the tubing. Massage the water to the other end of the tube; this is similar to venous return massage.*

ducted through neural pathways in the body that initiate the body's electrical and biochemical activities.

The medical definition of *reflexology* is "the study of reflexes." *Reflexotherapy* is treatment by manipulation applied to an area away from the disorder. In physiologic terms, a *reflex* is an involuntary response to a stimulus.

This discussion of reflexology attempts to explain why foot and hand massage is beneficial in terms of standard physiology; it avoids the issue of whether actual corresponding points exist on the foot or hand that relate directly to other body areas. An explanation based on standard anatomy and physiology is better suited to the format of this textbook and may be better accepted by the public.

Physiologic Reflexes of the Foot

The foot is a very complex structure. The ankle and foot consist of 34 joints, with many joint and reflex patterns (Box 11-6). The nerve distribution to the feet and hands is extensive. The position of the foot sends considerable postural information from the joint mechanoreceptors through the central nervous system. The sensory and motor centers of the brain devote a large area to the foot and hand.

It seems logical to assume that stimulation of the feet activates the responses of the gate control mechanism and hyperstimulation analgesia, with activation of the parasympathetic autonomic nervous system. Bodywide effects are the result. This fact alone is helpful in explaining the benefits of foot and hand massage. In addition, many nerve endings on the feet and hands correlate with acupressure points, which trigger the release of endorphins and other endogenous chemicals when stimulated. In addition, major plexuses for the lymph system are located in the hands and feet. Rhythmic compressive forces in these areas stimulate lymphatic movement.

Reflex Phenomena

Reflex phenomena must be put into perspective. Reflex points are located throughout the whole body, including the hands, head, ears, and torso. If you consider all the reflexology points, acupuncture points, neurolymphatic points, motor points, and other reflex points, the body itself can be seen as a point.

has been credited with formalizing the system, which is based on the theory that certain points in the foot and hand affect other body organs and areas. Historically, the approach seems to have originated in China. Foot reflexology is the most popular type of reflexology.

Another approach to reflexology is referred to as *zone therapy*. This method is based on the theory that 10 zones run through the body, and reflex points for stimulation are located within these zones.

Reflexology applies the stimulus/reflex principle to healing the body. The foot has been mapped to show the areas to contact to affect different parts of the body. Charts mapping these areas vary somewhat (Figure 11-15). Typically, the large toe represents the head, and the junction of the large toe and the foot represents the neck. The next toes represent the eyes, ears, and sinuses. The waist is about midway on the arch of the foot, with various organs above and below the line. The reflex points for the spine are along the medial longitudinal arch. It is thought that this stimulus/response reflex is con-

FIGURE 11-14 Examples of venous return.

Because of the reflex nature of the body and its inherent ability to self-regulate in response to stimulation, it usually is not necessary to overly focus on a particular system's name and use for a point.

More important is the ability to identify these various points during assessment procedures, to analyze the body context of the point, and to choose effective treatment for it. Assessment usually indicates an area tender to palpation if the point is hypersensitive or if the reflex structure associated with the particular point is hyperreactive. The opposite is true if the point area feels empty, numb, or disconnected from the surrounding tissue.

There are two basic treatment processes: if a reflexive point is tender and therefore likely to be overactive, relaxation and sedating methods are used; if the point is underactive, stimulation methods are applied. If you are not sure which application is appropriate, trust the innate balancing ability of the body. Alternately use both approaches, allowing the body to choose.

The professional can truly become overwhelmed with so many different names for the same phenomenon. The simplicity of the body response patterns is uniquely profound. Complicated methodology need not confuse the issue of generation of healing energy.

FIGURE 11-15 Generalized reflexology chart.

Methods of Massage for the Foot

An excellent way to massage the foot is to apply pressure and movement systematically to the entire foot and ankle complex. The pressure stimulates the circulation, nerves, and reflexes. Moving all the joints stimulates large-diameter nerve fibers and joint mechanoreceptors, initiating hyperstimulation analgesia. The result is a shift in proprioceptive and postural reflexes. The sheer volume of sensory information flooding the central nervous system has significant effects in the body that support parasympathetic dominance.

Foot massage usually is boundary safe; that is, most people accept foot or hand massage when the idea of removing the clothing is objectionable. Hand and foot massage is likely to be the most effective form of self-massage. The hand and foot have similar motor cortex distribution patterns. Stimulation of the hands during the massage does not override the sensations to the feet being massaged. The hands are massaged while they massage the feet (Figures 11-16 and 11-17) (Proficiency Exercise 11-4).

CONNECTIVE TISSUE APPROACHES

 11-4

SECTION OBJECTIVES

Using the information presented in this section, the student will be able to perform the following:

- Modify massage methods to address the connective tissue specifically
- Explain the principles of deep transverse friction massage

Methods that affect the connective tissue of the body have been discussed throughout the text. Connective tissue systems range from the very subtle, light work of craniosacral and fascial release concepts to the very mechanical deep transverse frictioning of Cyriax. This section provides specific introductory information about deep transverse friction and myofascial approaches. Refer to Chapters 4, 5, and 9 to review the information presented on connective tissue treatment, anatomy, physiology, and methodology.

The basic connective tissue approach consists of mechanically softening the tissue by introducing various mechanical forces that result in pressure, pulling, movement, and stretch on the tissues; this allows the tissue to rehydrate and become more pliable. The process is similar to softening gelatin by warming it. For connective tissue to stay soft, water must be added. This is one reason it is important that the client drink water before and after the massage.

PROFICIENCY EXERCISE 11-4

1. *Exchange foot massages with another student or visit a professional reflexologist for a foot massage. Compare the effects with those of a full-body massage.*
2. *Using a skeletal model, move each of the joints of the foot. Then move each of the joints of your foot.*
3. *Massage your feet daily for 15 minutes for a period of 2 weeks and take note of the effects.*

BOX 11-6

Reflexes Associated with the Foot

Achilles tendon reflex: Plantar flexion/extension of the foot resulting from the contraction of calf muscles after a sharp blow to the Achilles tendon; similar to the knee jerk reflex

Extensor thrust: A quick, brief extension of a limb after application of pressure to the plantar surface

Flexor withdrawal: Flexion of the lower extremity when the foot receives a painful stimulus

Mendel-Bekhterev reflex: Plantar flexion of the toes in response to percussion of the dorsum of the foot

Postural reflex: Any reflex concerned with maintenance of posture

Proprioceptive reflex: Reflex initiated by movement of the body to maintain the position of the moved part; any reflex initiated by stimulation of a proprioceptor

Rossolimo's reflex: Plantar flexion of the second to fifth toes in response to percussion of the plantar surface of the toes

Connective Tissue Dysfunctions

People can develop several basic connective tissue dysfunctions. Connective tissue may shorten, lose fluidity, and adhere, causing binding, pulling, and restricted movement. Another common problem is overstretched connective tissue at the joint, resulting in laxity and destabilization of the joint. This sets the stage for protective muscle spasms, which reduce joint space.

Normalization of connective tissue may allow the joint to function properly; however, this process may become problematic. The purpose of the connective tissue is to stabilize; stabilization may require that the joint remain out of optimal alignment. As explained by Dr. David Gurevich, a Russian physician, the pattern of degeneration usually begins with *dystonia,* or disruption of motor tone. (Sometimes direct trauma to a joint may cause misalignment, rather than increased or decreased muscle tension pulling joints out of alignment.) Bones are designed to fit at the joint in a specific way. When this fit is disrupted, the next step is a protective muscle spasm, followed by connective tissue reorganization to stabilize the area. Areas of disruption in joint play or joint alignment eventually include a connective tissue component in the dysfunction.[12]

Gurevich taught that the treatment sequence is first massage, including connective tissue approaches; then mobilization (movement of jointed areas within a comfortable range of motion); and finally joint manipulation. Massage and mobilization are within the scope of bodywork practice, whereas joint manipulation is not. The services of a chiropractor, osteopath, or other professional trained in joint manipulation are needed for problems that require direct manipulation of the joint.

Professional experience suggests that the longer the problem has existed, the more mechanical the techniques

FIGURE 11-16 Examples of foot massage.

required initially. Mechanical techniques include all gliding, kneading, skin rolling, and compression styles of bodywork, as long as the contact slowly elongates and drags or pulls on the tissue for sustained periods. The connective tissue responds relatively slowly, sometimes taking 30 seconds. Conversely, neuromuscular techniques usually elicit a response in 15 seconds.

The stretching, pulling, or pressure on the connective tissue is a little different from that of neuromuscular methods. Neuromuscular techniques usually flow in the direction of the fibers to affect the proprioceptive mechanism and create a quick response. Connective tissue approaches are slow and involve deliberate drag, usually against or across the fibers. Connective tissue stretching is elongated or telescoped at the

FIGURE 11-17 Methods of compression for reflexology. **A,** Braced fingers. **B,** Knuckle. **C,** Thumb.

point of the bind.[3,4] In chronic conditions, it is important to induce a small inflammatory response in the dysfunctional area. This process initiates the reorganization of tissue by stimulating tissue repair mechanisms.[5,13]

Another of the body's responses to inflammation is the generation of healing potentials through controlled injury. Injured tissue also yields a current known as the *current of*

injury. First detected by Galvani in 1797, this current can encourage healing processes for days until the miniature wound heals.[9] In acupuncture the insertion of a needle into a muscle generates a burst of electrical discharges, which can cause a shortened or hypertonic muscle to relax instantly or within minutes.

Deep Transverse Frictioning

The most specific localized example of connective tissue work is Dr. James Cyriax's cross-fiber frictioning method. This method is especially effective around joints, where the tendons and ligaments become bound. Deep transverse frictioning is always a specific rehabilitation intervention; it introduces therapeutic inflammation through the creation of a specific and controlled reinjury of the tissues. Cyriax asserts that the essential component of a transverse friction massage is the application of concentrated therapeutic movement over a very small area. The key element is the use of friction to move the tissue against its grain. In Cyriax's words:

> During treatment by deep friction, great precision in seating (positioning) of the patient and of the physiotherapist's hand is essential; throughout the session the physiotherapist keeps her mind on her fingertip. This type of work involves much more concentration and care than most of the physiotherapist's other work. Nothing about it is routine; each patient and each lesion must be assessed and given expert and individual attention.[8]

Although mastery of this type of deep transverse friction is beyond the scope of the technical development of this textbook, it is a valuable form of rehabilitative massage. Any massage practitioner working in a medical or sports setting should be trained in the techniques. The additional skills required are not so much in the delivery of the methods, which are fairly straightforward, but in the assessment of where to friction and how to incorporate it into a comprehensive rehabilitation plan. Specific anatomic knowledge is required for the precision of which Cyriax speaks.

The frictioning can last as long as 15 minutes to create the controlled reinjury of the tissue, which introduces a small amount of inflammation and traumatic hyperemia to the area. The result is the restructuring of the connective tissue, increased circulation to the area, and temporary analgesia.[8]

Proper rehabilitation after the massage is essential for the friction technique to be effective and to produce a mobile scar on rehealing of the tissue. The frictioned area must be contracted painlessly, without any strain put on the frictioned tissue. This is done by fixing the joint in a position in which the muscle is relaxed and then having the client contract the muscle as far as it will go. This is sometimes called a *broadening contraction* (Figure 11-18).

As Cyriax has said:

> Deep transverse friction restores mobility to muscle in the same way as manipulation frees a joint. Indeed, the action of deep transverse friction may be summed up as affording a mobilization that passive stretching or active exercises cannot achieve. After the friction has restored a full range of painless broadening to the muscle belly, this added mobility must be maintained. To this

end, the patient should perform a series of active contractions with the joint placed in a position that fully relaxes the affected muscle, that is, the position that allows the greatest broadening. Strong resisted movement should be avoided until the scar has consolidated itself; otherwise, started too soon, [such movements] tend to strain the healing breach again.[8]

Methods of Deep Transverse Frictioning

Cyriax teaches that when massage is given to a muscle, tendon, ligament, or joint capsule, the following principles must be observed (Figure 11-19):

1. The right spot must be found.
2. The therapist's fingers and the client's skin must move as one. Care must be taken not to cause a blister. The client must understand that deep friction massage to a tender point can be painful.
3. The friction must be given across the fibers composing the affected structure.
4. The friction must be given with sufficient sweep. Pressure only accesses the tender area; it does not replace the friction. Circular friction is not recommended. Only a back-and-forth friction is effective.
5. The friction must reach deep enough. If it does not reach the lesion, it is of no value.

6. The client must be placed in a suitable position that ensures the appropriate degree of tension or relaxation of the tissues to be frictioned.
7. Muscles must be kept relaxed while being frictioned. Because the connective tissue of the muscle is affected, the massage must penetrate into the muscle and not stay on the surface.
8. Tendons with a sheath must be kept taut during friction massage.
9. Broadening contractions are used between sessions to promote circulation and mobile scar development during the healing process.

Using Cyriax's principles, this textbook introduces a modified version of these methods that can be incorporated into a general massage session for small areas of adhered tissue. The modified version of deep transverse friction does not have the same effects on an area of adhesion, but the ability to move the tissue in a transverse way may keep the development of adhesions in check when a person develops minor soft tissue tears from overstretching or minor muscle pulls.

To accommodate the lack of precise location of the anatomic structures, the friction suggested is done over a broader area for a shorter time, using the following procedure:

1. Locate the area to be frictioned.

FIGURE 11-18 Broadening contraction. **A,** Beginning point. **B,** Contract the muscle by flexing the joint.

FIGURE 11-19 **A,** Deep transverse friction. **B,** Deep transverse friction = compression + movement.

2. Place the muscle in a relaxed position.
3. Provide friction as described in Chapter 9.

Myofascial Approaches

Other forms of connective tissue massage also can be used. Bindegewebmassage, developed by Elizabeth Dickie, consists of light strokes without oil with a focus on the superficial fascial layer (between the skin and muscles). The method involves movement of the superficial fascial layer in a specific pattern. The results are both reflexive and mechanical. The depth of pressure is sufficient to move the superficial fascia on top of the muscle layer in the direction of the arrows shown in Figure 11-20.

Rolfing, developed by Ida Rolf, and its various offshoots, such as Hellerwork, are methods of structural integration focused to bring the physical structure of the body into an efficient relationship with the perpendicular alignment of the body in gravity. The focus is normalization and redirection of the deeper fascial components of muscles and fascial sheaths. Osteopathy and physical therapy theory and practice contribute to the body of knowledge for **myofascial approaches**.

These styles of bodywork are often called *soft tissue manipulation* or *myofascial release*. The procedures described in this textbook are only a portion of these systems, and additional training is required to learn these valuable methods in more detail. Craniosacral therapy, which is a subtle connective tissue approach that reaches many structures deep within the body, is a valuable technique to perfect. John Barnes' Myofascial Release Seminars and the Upledger Institute's CranioSacral Therapy Seminars are reliable sources of additional training. In October 2007, the First International Fascia Research Congress was held at Harvard Medical School in Boston (www.fascia2007.com). The information shared and the global and interdisciplinary interaction was groundbreaking. The information presented in this textbook was confirmed, and even more exciting is the bright outlook for more conferences and ongoing research in the extremely important area for those professionals who work with soft tissue.

Nature of the Fascia

The nature of connective tissue has been addressed in Chapters 4, 5, 9, and 10. Fascia, which is a form of connective tissue, is the specific focus of myofascial approaches.

Fascia is loose, irregular connective tissue with a loose, multidirectional network of collagen and elastin fibers. It has a large percentage of ground substance. The fascia is embedded with bundles of smooth muscle that add to the supportive nature of fascia and can respond to neurologic signals, making the fascial tissue respond to sensory input. As was explained in Chapter 4, ground substance is thixotropic (i.e., it becomes pliable when manipulated) and a colloid substance, therefore fascia has many thixotropic and colloid qualities.

FIGURE 11-20 Application of connective tissue massage, modified from Bindegewebmassage. This system primarily introduced the mechanical forces of tension, bend, shear, and torsion.

Fascia in some form surrounds and separates almost every structure and cell in the body. It forms the interstitial spaces (space between individual cells). Fascia is involved in structural and visceral support, as well as separation and protection, and therefore influences respiration, elimination, metabolism, fluid flow, and the immune systems. Fascia is stress responsive, becoming thicker in response to real or perceived threats, as well as any other activation of the sympathetic autonomic nervous system. This emotional response of the fascial guarding system is sometimes called *body armoring*. It is an important factor in the relationship between body and emotional expression. This factor is often a component of body/mind approaches.

According to Tom Myers, the term *tensegrity* was coined from the phrase "tension integrity" by the architect R. Buckminster Fuller. Tensegrity refers to structures that maintain their integrity primarily because of a balance of continuous tensile forces through the structure, as opposed to leaning on continuous compressive forces. Although every structure is ultimately held together by a balance between tension and compression, tensegrity structures, according to Fuller, are characterized by continuous tension and local compression.[15]

The geometry of tensegrity is not confined to the body, by any means. An astonishingly wide variety of natural systems, including carbon atoms, water molecules, proteins, viruses, cells, tissues, and other living creatures, are constructed on the principles of tensegrity. Tensegrity structures are efficient. Tension forces naturally transmit over the shortest distance between two points, therefore these structures offer a maximum amount of strength for a given amount of material.

A tensegrity model of the body combines the tension (muscle or fascia) and compression (bones) factors of a mechanical model of the musculoskeletal display, but the compression members are islands, floating in a sea of continuous tension. The compression members push outward against the tension members, which pull inward. As long as the two sets of forces are balanced, the structure is stable. A tent constructed of canvas, poles, and tension supplied by ropes is a good example.

A tensegrity structure generally is less stiff and more resilient than a continuous compression structure. Load one "corner" of a tensegrity structure, and the whole structure gives a little to accommodate. Load it too much, and the structure ultimately breaks, but not necessarily anywhere near where the load was placed. Because strain is distributed throughout the structure along the lines of tension, the tensegrity structure may "give" at a weak point remote from the area of applied strain. All the interconnected structural elements of a tensegrity model rearrange themselves in response to a local stress. As the applied stress (load) increases, more of the structures come to lie in the direction of the applied stress, resulting in a linear stiffening of the material. Tensegrity structures, therefore, are resilient, becoming more stable the more they are loaded. These concepts are used to design buildings that can withstand earthquakes.

Because the body is a tensegrity structure, an injury at any given site often begins as long-term strain in other parts of the body. The injury manifests where it does because of inherent weakness or previous injury, not purely and always because of local strain or a direct impact. Discovering these points of tension and easing chronic strain in the body become a natural part of restoring balance in the structure and tend to prevent future injuries.

As mentioned previously, in the body the bones are compressing structures and the myofascial tissues are surrounding tension structures. In this model the bones are seen as "spacers" that push out into the soft tissue, and the tone of the tensile myofascia becomes the determinant of balanced structure. To change the relationships among the bones, the tensional balance through the soft tissue must be changed, and the bones will rearrange themselves.

The ground substance and adhesive matrix proteins are linked into the system of the intracellular cytoskeleton in a tensegric form to hold the body together. Individual body cells are connected and responsive to an actively changing connective tissue matrix. This matrix communicates with the individual cells, creating a mechanical communication link throughout the body by means of vibration along the fiber matrix of the connective tissues.

Whenever movement occurs in the body, the extracellular matrix extends, cells distort, and the interconnected molecules that constitute the internal framework of the cell feel the pull. The mechanical restructuring of the cell and cytoskeleton apparently tells the cell what to do. Very flat cells, with their cytoskeletons stretched, sense that more cells are needed to cover the surrounding area, as in wound repair, and that cell division is needed. Rounding indicates that too many cells are competing for space on the matrix and that cells are proliferating too rapidly; some must die to prevent tumor formation. In between those two extremes, normal tissue function is established and maintained.

This research points the way toward a holistic role for the mechanical distribution of strain in the body that goes far beyond merely dealing with localized tissue pain. Creating a balance across the bones, myofascial component and, further, across the entire fascial net, could have profound implications for health, both cellular and general. The goal for massage is to support balance in the myofascial systems.[15]

Location of the Fascia

Anatomically, fascia can be classified as superficial (subcutaneous) fascia or deep fascia. Superficial fascia lies between the skin and the muscles. Deep fascia surrounding the muscles weaves diagonally through the body, creating fascial sheaths (see Chapter 10). Subserous fascia lies between the deep fascia and the membranes lining the body cavities. A deep level of fascia interconnects the cranium, spine, and sacrum, joining the connective tissue coverings of the central nervous system with the unity of the body. The body also has three or four transverse fascial planes. These are located in the cranial base, cervical thoracic area, diaphragm, and lumbar and pelvic floor areas. Transverse planes exist for joints as well. These classifications of fascial layering are artificial, because as previously described, the tensegric nature of fascia is one large, interconnected, three-dimensional microscopic dynamic grid structure that connects everything with everything. Through the fascial system, if you pull on the little toe, you affect the nose, and if the structure of the nose is dysfunctional, it can pull anywhere in the body, including the little toe.

Although fascia generally orients itself vertically in the body, it will orient in any directional stress pattern. For example, scar tissue may redirect fascial structures, as can trauma, repetitive strain patterns, and immobility. This redirection of structural forces occurs as a result of compensation patterns (see Figure 10-20, the tippy pole pattern). During physical assessment the body appears "pulled" out of symmetry or stuck.

Myofascial Dysfunction

Dysfunction in the fascial network compromises the efficiency of the body, requiring an increase in energy expenditure to achieve functioning ability. Fatigue and pain often result. Fascial shortening and thickening restrict movement, and the easy undulation of the expression of body rhythms and entrainment mechanisms is disturbed. Twists and torsions of the fascia bind and restrict movement from the cellular level outward to joint mobility. This bind can be likened to ill-fitting clothing or, more graphically, "fascial wedgies." The dysfunctions are difficult to diagnose medically, are not apparent with standard medical testing, and are a factor in many elusive chronic pain and fatigue patterns. Adhesions result when fascia attempts to stabilize itself by attaching to surrounding tissue. Stabilizing formations can orient in any direction. Breakdown of the fascial system is a primary factor in the aging process.

Fascial dysfunction is seldom simple and almost always multidimensional, often encompassing body and emotional phenomena because body armoring is an effective coping strategy. As was explained in Chapter 5, introducing corrective intervention is a therapeutic change process akin to remodeling a house. If the person is unable to respond effectively to a change process, management approaches can be offered, but the result is more symptom management than structural change.

The methods themselves are deceptively simple in relation to the degree of change that can be experienced. Therefore a solid respect for myofascial approaches is in order. Use them wisely after considering the broader picture of the client's state of being and ability to cope with active change.

Myofascial Massage Methods

In most cases a lubricant is not used with myofascial approaches because the drag quality on the tissue is necessary to produce results, and lubricant reduces drag.

Methods that affect primarily the ground substance require a quality of slow, sustained pressure and agitation. Most massage methods can soften the ground substance as long as the application is not abrupt. Tapotement and abrupt compression are less effective than slow gliding methods that have a drag quality. Kneading and skin rolling that incorporate a slow pulling action are effective as well. The appropriate application introduces one or a combination of the mechanical forces of tension, compression, bind, shear, and torsion to achieve results.

The fiber component is affected by stretching methods that elongate the fibers past the normal give of the fiber and enter the plastic range past the bind (see Chapter 9). This creates either a freeing and unraveling of fibers or a small therapeutic (beneficial and controlled) inflammatory response that signals for change in the fibers.

Tissue Movement Methods Specific for the Superficial Fascia. To apply the more subtle connective tissue approaches, the practitioner must develop the skill to follow tissue movement under the skin.

1. Make firm but gentle contact with the skin.
2. Increase the downward (vertical) pressure slowly until resistance is felt; this barrier is soft and subtle.
3. Maintain the downward pressure at this point; now, add horizontal pressure until the resistance barrier (bind) is felt again.
4. Sustain the horizontal pressure and wait.
5. The tissue will seem to creep, unravel, melt, slide, quiver, twist, or dip, or some other movement sensation will be apparent.
6. Follow the movement; stay at bind.
7. Close your eyes; do not interpret the process. Become fascinated with the journey. Eventually the tissue will become still.
8. Wait and sustain the stillness.
9. Slowly and gently release first the horizontal force and then the vertical force.

Following tissue movement becomes simple once the practitioner stops thinking about the process and begins to experience it. A curious result of this type of work is the development of vasomotor responses on parts of the skin not directly addressed during the fascial tissue movement method. One theory suggests that these are areas with internal fascial connections that were pulled during the method. To continue the process, introduce vertical pressure over the vasomotor reddening and begin again.

Fascial Restriction Method. Fascial restriction involves an area larger than a small, localized spot. A restricted area is palpated as a barrier or an area of immobility within the tissue. The area is worked initially using routine massage techniques; if it does not soften, the pressure must be more specific.

1. Stabilize the tissue with one hand.
2. With the fingers of the other hand, pull the tissue in the direction of the restriction.
3. Use the heel of the hand or the arm to separate the tissue.
4. Maintain the pressure until a softening occurs.

Twist-and-release kneading and compression applied in the direction of the restriction can also release these fascial barriers (Figures 11-21 and 11-22).

The important consideration for all connective tissue massage methods is that the pressure exerted vertically and horizontally must actually move the tissue to create tension, torsion, shear, or bend; in addition, these forces must alter the ground substance long enough for energy to build up, soften the ground substance, and influence the smooth muscle

FIGURE 11-21 Light compressive force is applied, molding the hand to the skin. The hands then are separated without additional compressive force, providing for a fascial stretch.

bundles. The development of connective tissue patterns is highly individualized, therefore systems that follow a precise protocol and sequence often are less effective for dealing with these complex patterns (Figure 11-23) (Proficiency Exercise 11-5).

TRIGGER POINT THERAPY

SECTION OBJECTIVES

Using the information presented in this section, the student will be able to perform the following:

- Describe a trigger point
- Locate a trigger point
- Use two methods to massage a trigger point

Dr. Janet Travell did extensive research on myofascial pain involving trigger points and was considered the foremost authority in this area.[21] The research of Dr. Leon Chaitow has

FIGURE 11-22 Myofascial application. **A,** Begin with ease. **B,** End with bind. **C,** Bind. **D,** Lift to bind.

FIGURE 11-23 Using connective tissue methods to increase the pliability of scar tissue. **A,** Old scar on abdomen. **B,** Tension force. **C,** Bend and shear.

provided additional information about trigger point therapy.[3-5] These two experts are the resources for the information in this section about trigger point therapy.

Some confusion exists about the synonymous use of the terms *neuromuscular therapy* and *trigger point therapy*. *Neuromuscular therapy* is an umbrella term that encompasses a variety of treatment approaches, one of which is trigger point therapy. *Trigger point therapy* is one of many techniques useful in the treatment of myofascial problems. As with most of the methods discussed in this chapter, massage therapists require additional training to use trigger point methods specifically and efficiently. However, in general massage applications, the practitioner can deal with mild trigger point activity effectively by using the methods discussed in this section.

Definition of a Trigger Point

A trigger point is an area of local nerve facilitation of a muscle that is aggravated by stress of any sort that affects the body or mind. Trigger points are small areas of hyperirritability within muscles (Box 11-7). If these areas are located near motor nerve points, the person may experience referred pain caused by nerve stimulation. The area of the trigger point often is the motor point where nerve stimulation initiates a contraction in a small, sensitive bundle of muscle fibers that in turn activates the entire muscle.[5,21]

A trigger point area often is located in a tight band of muscle fibers. Palpation across the band may elicit a twitch response, which is a slight jump in the muscle fibers. This is difficult to detect when the trigger point is in the deeper muscle layers.

Any of the more than 400 muscles in the body can develop trigger points. The development of trigger points is accompanied by the characteristic referred pain pattern and the restriction of motion associated with myofascial pain. With classic trigger points the referred pain pattern can be traced to its site of origin. The distribution of the referred trigger point pain does not usually follow an entire distribution of a peripheral nerve or dermatomal segment (Figure 11-24).[21]

Perpetuating Factors

The development of trigger points can be perpetuated by reflexive, mechanical, and systemic factors. Reflexive perpetuating factors include the following:
- Skin sensitivity in the area of the trigger point
- Joint dysfunction
- Visceral dysfunction in the viscerally referred pain pattern
- Vasoconstriction
- A facilitated nerve segment

Mechanical perpetuating factors include the following:
- Standing postural distortion
- Seated postural distortion
- Gait distortion
- Immobilization
- Vocational stress
- Restrictive or ill-fitting clothing and shoes
- Furniture

PROFICIENCY EXERCISE 11-5

1. *Make some gelatin using only half the required water. Let it set. Massage it into liquid form. Pay attention to the type of massage you use.*
2. *Get some plastic wrap and twist and wad it into a ball. Smooth it out. What methods did you need to use?*
3. *Take the same plastic wrap and pull it. Take out all the slack, and telescope and elongate the tissue. What did you have to do to accomplish the stretch?*

BOX 11-7

Theory of Trigger Point Formation

The following progression has been proposed to explain the formation of trigger points.

1. Dysfunctional endplate activity occurs, commonly associated with a strain, overuse, or direct trauma.
2. Stored calcium is released at the site as a result of overuse or of tearing of the sarcoplasmic reticulum.
3. Acetylcholine (Ach) is released excessively at the synapse because of calcium-charged gates.
4. High calcium levels present at the site keep the calcium-charged gates open, and the release of Ach continues.
5. Ischemia develops in the area, resulting in an oxygen and nutrient deficit.
6. A local energy crisis develops.
7. Because adenosine triphosphate (ATP) is no longer available, the tissue is unable to remove the calcium ions, and Ach continues flowing.
8. Removal of the superfluous calcium requires more energy than sustaining a contracture, therefore the contracture remains.
9. The contracture is sustained not by action potentials from the spinal cord but by the chemistry at the innervation site.
10. The actin/myosin filaments slide to a fully shortened position (a weakened state) in the immediate area around the motor endplate (at the center of the fiber).
11. As the sarcomeres shorten, a contracture knot forms.
12. The contracture knot is the "nodule," a palpable characteristic of a trigger point.
13. The remainder of the sarcomeres of that fiber are stretched, creating the usually palpable taut band that also is a common trigger point characteristic.
14. Attachment trigger points may develop at the attachment sites of these shortened tissues (periosteal, myotendinous) where muscular tension provokes inflammation.

Modified from Chaitow L, Delany J: *Clinical application of neuromuscular techniques,* vol 1, *The upper body,* London, 2001, Churchill Livingstone.

Systemic perpetuating factors include the following:

- Enzyme dysfunction
- Metabolic and endocrine dysfunction
- Chronic infection
- Dietary insufficiencies
- Psychological stress

Assessment for Trigger Points

Determining whether a tender spot is really a trigger point, a point of fascial adhesion requiring friction, a motor point, or some other irritable reflex point, including any active acupuncture points, can be difficult. However, stretching of trigger point areas is essential to effective treatment, therefore if doubt exists about the nature of the point, it should be treated as a trigger point.

The massage therapist usually finds trigger points during palpation or general massage using both light and deep palpation consisting of gliding strokes (Box 11-8). Chaitow recommends that gliding strokes cover a region of 2 to 3 inches at a time.

Travell and Chaitow agree that some pain is elicited during assessment and treatment; however, *the pain elicited during treatment should be well within the client's comfort zone,* so that the client is aware of the trigger point but does not initiate protective mechanisms such as guarding (tightening up), breath holding, or flinching. The muscle must be relaxed to be examined effectively. If the pressure is too great, severe local pain may overwhelm the referred pain sensation, making accurate evaluation impossible. Trigger points that are so active that referred pain is already produced have no need of exaggerated pressure.

Only muscles that can actually be treated at the same visit should be examined. Palpation for trigger points can aggravate their referred pain activity, therefore only areas intended for treatment should be palpated.

Methods of Treating Trigger Points

Trigger point therapy must not be done for extended periods. Because of the nature of the syndrome and the irritation involved, 15 minutes is a sufficient amount of time to spend on trigger points. On some occasions 30 minutes of therapy can be tolerated, but this should not become a standard practice, and it should be incorporated into a more general approach, such as full-body massage.

All the basic neuromuscular techniques, including the muscle energy techniques (see Chapter 9), deal effectively with trigger points *if* the hyperirritable area within a muscle is hyperstimulated and then lengthened, and the connective tissue in the area is softened and stretched. Travell and other professionals in the field suggest direct pressure, dry needling (acupuncture), and ice massage for trigger point areas. Direct manipulation of proprioceptors by pushing or pulling on a muscle belly or its attachments is also very effective. Positional release with the appropriate stretching is one of the most effective ways to treat trigger points.

After a trigger point has been identified, the massage therapist uses a pressure technique, muscle energy, or a direct manipulation and stretch method to eliminate the point. Positional release and lengthening and direct manipulation are the least invasive and gentlest methods. The integrated muscle energy method is more aggressive than positional release or direct manipulation but less aggressive than pressure or pinch-

Sternomastoid   Splenius capitis   Temporalis   Masseter   Lower trapezius

Upper trapezius   Levator scapulae   Posterior cervical   Adductor pollicis   First interosseus

Infraspinatus   Supraspinatus   Scaleni

Iliocostalis   Multifidus   Gluteus medius

FIGURE 11-24 Common trigger points. (From Chaitow L: *Modern neuromuscular techniques,* ed 2, Edinburgh, 2003, Churchill Livingstone.)

Continued

Tibialis anticus

Long extensors

Gastro-cnemius

Soleus

Peroneus longus

Abductor hallucis

Short extensors

Subscapularis

Deltoid

Middle finger extensor

Extensor carpi radialis

Supinators

Pectorals

Pectoralis major

Sternalis

Serratus anterior

Longissimus

Vastus medialis

Biceps femoris

Gluteus minimus

Vastus medialis

FIGURE 11-24, cont'd

ing methods. These methods often are effective and are worth trying before the more intense pressure or pinching techniques.

As a reminder, positional release consists of identifying the painful point and positioning the body in the easiest position that reduces the pain at the point. Positional release is the first step in the integrated muscle energy method, which then introduces muscle contraction before lengthening (see Chapter 9).

Direct manipulation methods consist of pushing together at the belly of a muscle to affect spindle cells and pushing apart on tendons to affect tendon receptors. If the belly of the muscle is pressed together and the desired effect is not experienced, the next step should be to separate the tissue from the middle of the muscle belly toward the tendons. The local area must be lengthened. This lengthening is performed either directly on the tissues or through movement of a joint (Figure 11-25).

BOX 11-8

Palpation for Trigger Points

In performing light palpation, the therapist may notice trigger points from the following responses.

Skin changes: The skin may feel tense and show resistance to gliding strokes. It may be slightly damp as a result of perspiration from sympathetic facilitation, causing the therapist's hand to stick or drag.

Temperature changes: The temperature in a local area increases with acute dysfunction but decreases with ischemia, which indicates fibrotic changes within the tissues.

Edema: Edema is an impression of fullness and congestion within the tissues. With chronic dysfunction, edema is gradually replaced by fibrotic (connective tissue) changes.

Deep palpation: During deep palpation, the therapist establishes contact with the deeper fibers of the soft tissues and explores them for any of the following:

- Immobility
- Tenderness
- Edema
- Deep muscle tension
- Fibrotic changes
- Interosseous changes

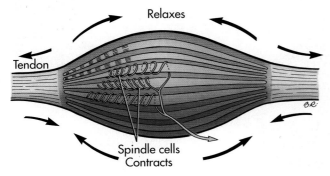

FIGURE 11-25 Direct manipulation of proprioceptors.

If the trigger point remains after the less invasive methods have been attempted, pressure techniques (i.e., inhibitory pressure) should be tried. The pressure may take the form of direct pressure, in which the trigger point is pressed by the therapist against an underlying hard structure (bone), or pinching pressure, when no bony tissue lies underneath, as in the "squeezing" of the sternocleidomastoid muscle.

Pressure techniques can end the hyperirritability by mechanical disruption of the sensory nerve endings mediating the trigger point activity. When using the direct pressure technique, the therapist must hold the compression long enough to stimulate the spindle cells.

The pressure technique must be done properly. Travell has pointed out that referred pain usually is sensed by the client within 10 seconds of pressure being applied. Therefore the practitioner need not maintain pressure longer than 10 seconds when trying to locate the trigger.

After the trigger has been located, the *time of applied pressure* is different from the time used to locate the trigger. Chaitow recommends a procedure of gradually intensifying pressure, building up to 8 seconds, then repeating the process for up to 30 seconds or as long as 2 minutes. The procedure should end when the client reports that the referred pain has stopped or when the therapist feels a "release" in the trigger point tissue.

Sufficient duration is determined by the fiber construction of the muscle. Muscles are made up of red or white fibers, which can be slow twitch or fast twitch. The type of fiber that makes up a muscle is determined by whether the muscle functions as a postural (stabilizer) muscle or a phasic (mover) muscle and the demands of the client's lifestyle. Phasic muscle fibers are easier to fatigue than postural muscle fibers. After the muscle is fatigued, a period of recovery ensues in which the fibers will not contract, and the muscle can be lengthened effectively and stretched if necessary.

Chaitow also recommends variable pressure, rather than constantly held pressure from beginning to end, to avoid further irritation of the trigger area. Students should not misinterpret this idea of variable pressure; it is not a "bouncing" in and out of the tissue, but rather a carefully changing pressure for a specific purpose. The pressure used reflects the therapist's sensitivity to what is happening as the tissue responds; the therapist applies more pressure as the tissue shows that it is relaxing and accepting more pressure. When the massage therapist senses that the tissues are becoming tense, pressure is reduced.

As an alternative, deep cross-fiber frictioning over the trigger point can be effective, followed by lengthening and stretching. This method is beneficial if the massage therapist suspects that the connective tissue around the trigger point has become immobile.

Travell recommends that after treating the trigger point with pressure methods, the practitioner again stimulate circulation to the local area with circular friction, kneading, and/or vibratory massage techniques. Localized treatment of the muscle should always end with lengthening and stretching, whether passive or active, of the affected muscle.

Travell and Chaitow agree that gradual, gentle lengthening to reset the normal resting length of the neuromuscular mechanism of a muscle and stretching to elongate shortened connective tissue of the treated (involved) muscle must follow any other interventions. Incomplete restoration of the full length of the muscle means incomplete relief of pain. Failure to lengthen and stretch the area results in the eventual return of the original symptoms. Muscle energy approaches are more effective than passive stretching in achieving the proper response. They enable the muscle to "learn" that it can now return to a fuller resting length and more complete range of motion. Trigger points in deep layers of muscle or in a muscle that is difficult to lengthen by moving the body are addressed with local bend, shear, and torsion techniques.

After treating a trigger point, the practitioner should search the target (referred) area to uncover and deal with satellite or embryonic triggers. Immediately after treatment, moist heat (a hot towel) over the region is soothing and useful. The area requires rest for a few days and avoidance of all stressful activity.

Trigger points in the muscle belly usually are found in short, concentrically contracted muscles. Trigger points located near the attachments usually are found in eccentric patterns and in long, inhibited muscles acting as antagonists to concentrically contracted muscles. Muscle contractions may serve as a response for compensation purposes. The best course is to address the trigger point activity in the short tissues first and wait to see whether the trigger points in the long muscles and at the attachments resolve as the posture of muscle interaction normalizes. The sequence for addressing trigger points is as follows:

1. Those that are most painful and that reproduce familiar symptoms
2. Those most medial
3. Those in the short tissue
4. Those in the muscle belly

As seen with the previous skills, the actual application of trigger point methods is fairly basic. The trained professional's skill is required more in the assessment, in decision making about the appropriateness and intensity of treatment, and in the choice of methods. As with myofascial methods, the appli-

cation of treatment protocols is deceptively simple, especially when the client's condition is multifaceted and complex. Often more than one method is required in these cases. Trigger point release is a good example of the integration of multiple methods, because effective intervention involves the use of several treatment protocols, massage manipulations, muscle energy methods, stretching methods, and hydrotherapy methods (Figure 11-26) (Proficiency Exercise 11-6).

ASIAN BODYWORK METHODS

SECTION OBJECTIVES

Using the information presented in this section, the student will be able to perform the following:

- Explain the basic physiology of acupuncture points and the effects of acupuncture
- Locate an acupuncture point
- Use simple methods to normalize acupuncture points

The richness of Asian health theory and the unity of its body/mind/spirit connection are based on the energy of life. Life force, called *Chi* (or *Qi/Ri*) *energy,* flows through the body through interconnected pathways as water flows through the streams, rivers, lakes, and oceans of the earth. When Chi energy flows through the body like pure water, all of life's processes are balanced. However, if obstruction or stagnation in the life force develops, it becomes the basis for disease.

The Tao, or "Way," supports the balanced functioning of all the senses and teaches a lifestyle of moderation that avoids both deprivation and excess. Chi energy is the vital force of life, and Tao is the path or way to sustain the Chi energy.

Some are concerned about taking pieces from the totality of being expressed in the Tao. Western science has lifted techniques from this simultaneously simple and complex, all-encompassing system. Very often, a technique separated from its theoretical basis is less effective. Although techniques can stimulate physiologic functions, they cannot support the human experience. The small section presented in this textbook is based on a very limited part of the total Asian medi-

FIGURE 11-26 Methods of addressing trigger points. **A,** Direct manipulation. **B,** Pinching compression of the trigger point.

FIGURE 11-26, cont'd C, Move and hold area at ease. **D,** Positional release. **E,** Direct tissue stretching.

 PROFICIENCY EXERCISE 11-6

1. *Place a dried pea under a ¹/₂-inch piece of foam. Locate the pea with light and deep palpation.*
2. *Working with a partner, use light palpation to locate an area of suspected trigger point activity. After an area has been found, use deep palpation to find the exact area of the trigger point. Then use the methods described in this section to normalize the area.*

cine system. As you begin to develop an understanding of these methods, be mindful and respectful of the larger body of knowledge from which they have been taken. [9,10,14,16,19,22,23,25]

Shiatsu

Shiatsu (finger pressure), which was developed in Japan, is one of the more familiar Asian bodywork systems. Shiatsu and acupressure sometimes are considered the same method. However, shiatsu is much broader in its application of methods and diagnosis. Shiatsu was recognized in Japan as a manipulative therapy about 70 years ago. Basically, it is a form of massage in which the fingers are pressed onto particular points of the body to ease aches, pain, tension, fatigue, and symptoms of disease. These points, called *tsubo,* or *acupuncture points,* are located along the meridians described later in this section. One distinguishing method of shiatsu diagnosis is done through areas on the *Hara* (abdomen or center) and the back. Pressure in these areas or along the meridians identifies energy flow (in Japanese, *Ki*) as either *kyo* (under energy) or *jitsu* (over energy). Shiatsu restores balance by strengthening or stimulating (toning) the kyo and sedating the jitsu.

The traditional meridian system is the foundation of the shiatsu system (Figure 11-27). The following list describes each meridian function, as well as imbalances that manifest as kyo and jitsu symptoms.[14] It is interesting to compare these meridian descriptions to those most closely identified with Chinese theory (see p. 485).

- **Lung meridian:** Functions with the intake of Ki energy from the air to build up strength and to eliminate unneeded gases through exhalation.
  Kyo imbalances: Hypersensitivity, anxiety, breathing difficulties, antisocial demeanor, shortness of breath, coughing;

FIGURE 11-27 The main meridians pathways of shiatsu. (From Anderson SK: *The practice of shiatsu,* St Louis, 2008, Mosby.)

also excess body weight, elimination difficulties, upper body fatigue, susceptibility to respiratory infection, shoulder pain.

Jitsu imbalance: Anxiety over small details; tendency to sigh and choke while breathing; susceptibility to nasal congestion, colds, constipation, shoulder pain, bronchitis, asthma, excess production of mucus, thumb pain, and tightness in the chest muscles.

- **Large intestine meridian:** Assists functioning of the lung; secretes and excretes from inside and outside the body; eliminates the stagnation of Ki energy.

Kyo imbalances: Lack of determination, disappointment, overdependency, negative thinking; dry or congested nasal passage; weak bronchial tubes, constipation; prone to diarrhea when digesting coarse foods; poor circulation in the lower abdomen; tendency to shiver; malfunctioning of the large intestine; fatigue in the lower body below the hips; lack of vitality, susceptibility to inflammation.

Jitsu imbalances: Perpetual dissatisfaction; headaches, flushed complexion; runny nose, nasal congestion, nose bleed, prone to respiratory infection; painful sensation in the lower teeth; shoulder pain; tension in the chest and arm

muscles; constipation but occasional diarrhea; tendency to overeat; itchy skin, puffiness in lower abdomen and hemorrhoids; epilepsy.

- **Spleen meridian:** In modern terms the spleen is considered to be the pancreas. It supports digestion, including the secretion of saliva and gastric bile, secretions from the small intestine, and secretion of reproductive hormones related to the breasts and ovaries. Mental fatigue adversely affects the spleen meridian, and lack of exercise causes malfunctioning digestion and hormone secretion.

Kyo imbalances: Obsession with details; restless, anxious, and dissatisfied; tendency to overeat and eat quickly; busy brain, memory loss; sleepiness; diminished gastric acid and saliva; sticky, dry taste in the mouth, thirst; inability to consume food without liquid; diminished taste sensations, poor digestion, inability to taste food; brownish cast of the face, lack of energy for exercise, poor circulation in the legs and feet.

Jitsu imbalances: Tendency to be isolated; hesitant, timid, and thinks too much; cautious and anxious; eats quickly with craving for sweets; thirsty, sticky feeling in the mouth; no appetite, no appreciation for tasting foods; gastric hyperacidity, overeating, obesity; heaviness in the legs, no strength, and stiffness in the shoulders and arms.

- **Stomach meridian:** Related to functioning of the stomach, esophagus, and duodenum, as well as functioning of the reproductive and menstrual cycles, lactation, ovaries, and appetite mechanism.

Kyo imbalances: Busy brain with tendency to want to lie down; craves cold and soft food; emotional eating, lack of chewing with tendency to eat while doing something, and irregular meal intake; chronic gastric problems, eats with no appetite; shoulder pain caused by problems with ovaries; yawning; fat legs; fatigue, coldness felt in the front part of the body; lack of flexibility in the muscles.

Jitsu imbalances: Nervous about details; frustrated, lacking in affection; overeats; time urgency, neurotic; gastric hyperacidity; cold sores; thirst; stiffness in the shoulder, pain and stiffness in the solar plexus and the heart; prone to upper respiratory infections; poor circulation in the legs; rough, dry complexion; intestinal gas; yawning; redness on top of the nose; tendency to be anemic; female reproductive system problems.

- **Heart meridian:** Related to functions of compassion and emotions, as well as blood circulation. Also the mechanism that adapts external stimuli to the body's internal environment.

Kyo imbalances: Mental fatigue, shock, nervous tension, stress, neurosis, poor appetite, restlessness, memory loss; timidity, tendency to be disappointed, no will power; upper abdomen weakness, tightness in the solar plexus area; strong palpitations, heart organ problems; abdominal tension; sweaty palms; fatigue, angina, coated tongue, myocardial infarction.

Jitsu imbalances: Chronic tension and stiffness in the chest; tries to contain anxiety and restlessness; perpetual fatigue; tendency to stammer; stiffness in the solar plexus area; thirst; laughing; always clearing the throat; tightness in the heart area; stiff body; hysteria; sweaty palms, perspires easily, sensitive skin; shoulder pain; desire for cold drinks; nervous stomach; palpitations.

- **Small intestine meridian:** Exerts a total body influence through digestion of food.

Kyo imbalances: Narrow focus, oversensitivity to small details, anxiety; strong determination, decreased ability to control deep emotional sadness, emotional shock; anemia caused by poor nutrition and digestion; blood stagnation and poor circulation and heaviness in the hips and legs; fainting; dysfunction of the intestinal organs; easily fatigued in the hip area, low back problems, weak abdominal muscles; hearing difficulty; eye fatigue; abnormal menstrual cycle; pain in the ovaries; shoulder pain; migraine headaches.

Jitsu imbalances: Patient, determined, overworked; restless rapid eye movements, headaches; stiffness of the cervical vertebrae; puffiness of the eyes and ears; feeling of having a chilled body and heat in the head; redness in the cheeks; bladder and bowel urgency; poor circulation in the extremities; poor digestion, constipation; ovary malfunctioning; lower back ache; shoulder pain; pain in the upper part of the teeth; dry mouth, lack of saliva.

- **Kidney meridian:** Functions to control the spirit and energy to the body and to promote resistance against mental stress through control of hormone secretions, including cortisol; detoxifies and purifies the blood, preventing acidosis.

Kyo imbalances: Anxiety, fear, restlessness, nervousness, pessimism; family stress, lack of patience and determination, mental fatigue; dry, puffy, inelastic skin; poor circulation in the hips and abdomen; bladder frequency; low back ache; malfunctioning of hormone secretions; insomnia; sexual dysfunction, reproductive organ problems; cracks in the nails; prone to bone fractures; tendency to stumble; stiffness in the abdominal and torso muscles.

Jitsu imbalances: Impatient, "workaholic," nervousness, restlessness, constant complaining, overfocuses on details, lack of determination; blackish cast to face; vomiting, blood in the saliva; prone to nose bleeds and fainting; thirst; ringing in the ears; back stiffness; tension in the torso muscles; abnormal hormone secretion; dark urine; bad breath and bitter taste in the mouth; prone to inflammation; work-related burnout.

- **Bladder meridian:** Connected to midbrain; function is to support kidney hormone system and pituitary gland; also connected to the autonomic nervous system, especially reproductive and urinary organs; eliminates urine.

Kyo imbalances: Strained nerves, stiff body; complains and is easily frightened, night sweats, anxiety; nasal congestion; heaviness and pain in the eyes; migraine headache; malfunctioning of the autonomic nervous system, poor circulation, especially in the lower back; frequent urination, bladder inflammation and pain.

Jitsu imbalances: Worry and oversensitivity; stiff neck pain, head and eye heaviness, shoulder muscle tension; tightness in the backs of the legs; nasal congestion; frequent urination; inflammation or pain in the bladder or prostate area; autonomic nervous system strain.

- **Heart constrictor meridian:** Supports and assists functioning of the heart related to the circulatory system; also controls total nutrition.

Kyo imbalances: Absent-mindedness; insomnia and vivid dreams, heart palpitations and shortness of breath, squeezing sensation around the chest; swallowing problems; heart dysfunctions, easily fatigued; low blood pressure; dropsy, poor circulation; pain in the stomach and duodenum; abnormal blood pressure; pain in the chest and rib cage.

Jitsu imbalances: Restless when asleep or awake; social anxiety; difficulty focusing on tasks; inappropriate emotions and hypersensitivity; strong heart palpitations; high blood pressure; dizziness, easily fatigued; poor circulation; headache; tightness in the abdomen, stomach pain; tingling in the fingers; hot palms; colitis; coated tongue.

- **Triple heater meridian:** Supports functioning of the small intestine; controls visceral organs circulating energy to the entire body; supports functions of the lymphatic system.

Kyo imbalances: Mental obsessions; headaches, ringing in the ears, heaviness and dizziness in the head; sensitivity to heat, cold, and dampness; weak and strained lymphatic system; nasal problems; sensitivity to humidity and temperature change, easily catches cold; tired eyes; sensitive skin, allergy; tightness in the chest and abdomen; abnormal blood pressure, pain in the back of the head and in the temples.

Jitsu imbalances: Extremely cautious with tendency to be hypervigilant; nervous reaction to external changes in heat, cold, and humidity; heaviness in chest (upper heater), stomach (middle heater), and lower abdomen; sensitivity; foggy brain; eye pressure; neck, shoulder, and arm pain; lymphatic inflammation; itchy skin; poor circulation in the legs; susceptible to humidity; ticklish.

- **Liver meridian:** Stores nutrients and energy for physical activity; supports resistance against disease and maintains blood for physical energy.

  Kyo imbalances: Lack of determination; easily upset, inconsistent; inability to gain weight; weak joints, easily fatigued; dizziness, tendency to stumble, tired eyes; body system easily poisoned because of poor detoxification; fever; lack of appetite; stiff muscles; sexual dysfunction.

  Jitsu imbalances: Stubbornness, works impatiently and impulsively until exhausted; easily affected emotionally, displays emotion and then controls it; burnout; overeating (especially sweets), excessive drinking; swollen chest and stomach; headaches; poor digestion; lack of exercise; dizziness; high fever without cause; liver organ malfunction; hemorrhoids; prostate problems; pain in the sacrum and coccyx; general bending stiffness; flatulence; prone to inflammations.

- **Gallbladder meridian:** Distributes nutrients and balances energy, supporting internal hormones and secretions such as bile, saliva, gastric acid, insulin, and intestinal hormones.

  Kyo imbalances: Susceptible to emotional excitement; sudden fatigue after stress; timid, lack of determination, strained nerves, light sleeper, lack of energy; tired, weak eyes, lack of energy caused by deficiency of nutrients, tired legs; poor digestion of fats, prone to diarrhea and constipation; neuralgia; dizziness; pale complexion; obesity despite poor appetite, accumulation of fatty tissues without consumption of greasy foods, gastric hyperacidity; improper nutritional distribution.

  Jitsu imbalances: Takes on too much responsibility; fatigued, impatient, time urgency; lack of sleep, causing tired eyes; bloated stomach, loss of appetite; yellowish tinge in white part of eye and skin; tendency to blink frequently; stiffness in the extremities; bitter taste in the mouth; gallstones and spasms in the gallbladder; shoulder pain; heaviness in the head; migraine headache; mucosal stagnation; coughing; excessive intake of sweets; lack of sour food consumption.

Acupuncture

Acupuncture increasingly is gaining acceptance by Western science. It is a branch of Chinese medicine that has been proven effective in the treatment of many diseases and dysfunctions. The exact origin of acupuncture is unknown. Although the process remains a mystery in some respects, Western science is close to validating its phenomena. Whatever physiologic factors underlie acupuncture, the beneficial

changes that occur clearly provide a sound basis for acupuncture treatment.

Acupuncture can be defined as the stimulation of certain points with needles inserted along the meridians (channels) and *AhShi* (meaning "ouch") points outside the meridians. Interestingly, AhShi and traditional acupuncture points have a high degree of correlation with trigger points. The purpose of acupuncture is to prevent and modify the perception of pain (analgesia) or to normalize physiologic functions.

Acupressure is a modified version of acupuncture that substitutes pressure for needle insertion (Figure 11-28). The results of acupressure are not as dramatic as those of acupuncture, but the technique is still effective, especially if it is repeated often with the pressure held long enough. The human body has hundreds of acupuncture points. Approximately 360 of the most used points are located on 12 paired and two unpaired centrally located meridians. These meridian patterns are very similar to the meridians used in shiatsu.

Meridians in Chinese Bodywork Systems

According to Chinese theory, the meridians are internally associated with organs and externally associated with the surface of the head, trunk, and extremities. Meridians seem to be energy flows from nerve tracts in the tissue and are located in the fascial grooves.[7]

Yin and Yang. The Chinese perspective considers body functions in terms of balance between complementary forces. These complements, which are often thought of as opposites, are actually parts of a continuum. A circle is a good example; no matter where you stand on a circle, you can look across and see the other side. In this idea of duality, we often forget that a circle is one concept; it is broken into sections only through the limitation of our perceptions. *Yin* and *yang* are representations of this concept. Yin and yang functions are complementary pieces of the whole (Figure 11-29). When all parts of the continuum function equally and in harmony, the natural balance of health exists in all areas of the body, mind, and spirit. Conversely, if part of the continuum becomes out of sync with the rest, stress is put on the entire circle. Thus imbalances and symptoms might occur in many areas.

Physiologically, the body is a closed system. There cannot be areas of "too much" energy in the body without reciprocal areas of "not enough" energy. Just as muscles work in pairs and facilitate and inhibit each other, so do meridians. The body has yin meridians, or channels, and yang meridians, or channels.

Yin meridians are associated with parasympathetic autonomic nervous system responses and functions of the solid organs essential to life (e.g., the heart). The energy is considered "female" and a "negative" charge. (Terminology and metaphor tend to become confused with the terms *female* and *negative*. In this context the terms mean that the functions draw energy of sustenance and nurturing in and restore or reproduce.) Yin meridians are located on the inside soft areas of the body and flow from the feet up (Chinese anatomic position with the arms lifted into the air).

Yang meridians are associated with sympathetic autonomic nervous system responses and with hollow organs that support

FIGURE 11-28 Acupressure is based on the aspect of Chinese medicine that concerns stimulation of various points on the body that are organized into patterns called *meridians.* Chinese medicine is a very complex system that requires long-term study and practice. Simple application of acupressure can be integrated into massage. **A,** Measure to find the correct point. **B,** Apply compression. **C,** Inside wrist. **D,** Hand. **E,** Between the lip and the nose. **F,** At the temples.

Yang (Sympathetic— using intermittent function, protective and supportive function)

Yin (Parasympathetic— restoring constant function, vital function)

FIGURE 11-29 Yin and yang.

life but are not essential (e.g., the stomach). The energy is considered "male" and a "positive" charge. (Again, in metaphor these terms mean that the energy of transformation and transportation is expended in short bursts as necessary and moves out from the body). Chinese philosophy teaches that a balance must exist between the forces of yin and yang for health to exist. This balance changes according to the weather, seasons, and other rhythms of nature (Box 11-9).

The patterns that acupuncture points make on the body's surface have been charted by practitioners of acupuncture for centuries. They have been grouped together in lines (called *channels,* or *meridians*) and have been allocated to the organs or functions upon which they appear to act. In addition to the 12 pairs of bilateral meridians, two meridians lie on the anterior and posterior midline of the trunk and head. Various extra meridians appear to relate to the body's organs and functions. Other points in the ear surfaces, the hands, and the face have specific reflex effects (Figure 11-30).

The 12 Main Meridians. The 12 main meridians are bilateral, symmetrically distributed lines of acupuncture points with affinity for or effects upon the functions or organs for which they are named (Box 11-10).

BOX 11-9

Meridians

Yin Meridian	Yang Meridian
Pericardium	Triple heater
Liver	Gallbladder
Kidney	Bladder
Heart	Small intestine
Spleen	Stomach
Lung	Large intestine

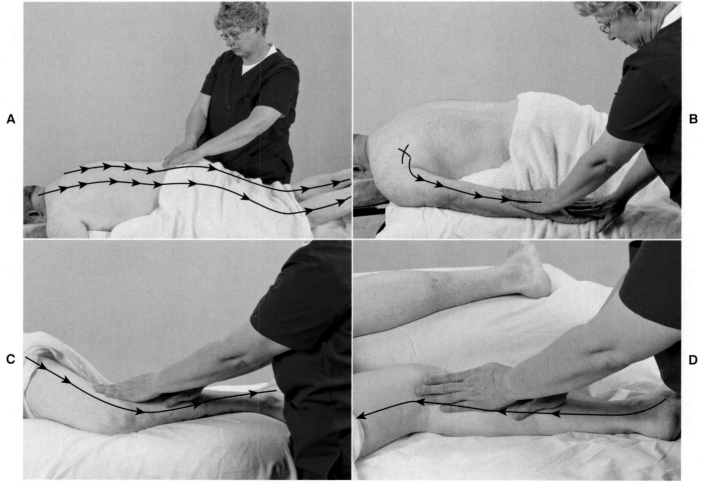

FIGURE 11-30 Examples of meridian therapy. **A,** Bladder meridian (yang). **B,** Arm yin meridian. **C,** Gallbladder meridian (yang). **D,** Yin meridians of the leg.

BOX 11-10

The 12 Main Meridians and Associated Acupuncture Points

1. **Lung (L) meridian** (yin) begins on the lateral aspect of the chest, in the first intercostal space. It then passes up the anterolateral aspect of the arm to the root of the thumbnail. (11 acupuncture points.)
   Pathologic symptoms: Fullness in the chest, cough, asthma, sore throat, colds, chills, and aching in the shoulders and back.

2. **Large intestine (LI) meridian** (yang) starts at the root of the fingernail of the first finger. It passes down the posterolateral aspect of the arm over the shoulder to the face. It ends at the side of the nostril. (20 acupuncture points.)
   Pathologic symptoms: Abdominal pain, diarrhea, constipation, nasal discharge, pain along the course of the meridian.

3. **Stomach (ST) meridian** (yang) starts below the orbital cavity and runs over the face and up to the forehead, then passes down the throat, the thorax, and the abdomen and continues down the anterior thigh and leg to end at the root of the second toenail (lateral side). (45 acupuncture points.)
   Pathologic symptoms: Bloating, edema, vomiting, sore throat, pain along the course of the meridian.

4. **Spleen (SP) meridian** (yin) originates at the medial aspect of the great toe. It travels up the internal aspect of the leg and thigh to the abdomen and thorax, where it finishes on the axillary line in the sixth intercostal space. (21 acupuncture points.)
   Pathologic symptoms: Gastric discomfort, bloating, vomiting, weakness, heaviness of the body, pain along the course of the meridian.

5. **Heart (H) meridian** (yin) begins in the axilla and runs up the anteromedial aspect of the arm to end at the root of the little fingernail (medial aspect). (9 acupuncture points.)
   Pathologic symptoms: Dry throat, thirst, cardiac area pain, pain along the course of the meridian.

6. **Small intestine (SI) meridian** (yang) starts at the root of the small fingernail (lateral aspect) and travels down the posteromedial aspect of the arm and over the shoulder to the face, where it terminates in front of the ear. (19 acupuncture points.)
   Pathologic symptoms: Pain in the lower abdomen, deafness, swelling in the face, sore throat, pain along the course of the meridian.

7. **Bladder (B) meridian** (yang) starts at the inner canthus, then ascends and passes over the head and down the back and the leg to terminate at the root of the nail of the little toe (lateral aspect). (67 acupuncture points.)
   Pathologic symptoms: Urinary problems, mania, headaches, eye problems, pain along the course of the meridian.

8. **Kidney (K) meridian** (yin) starts on the sole of the foot. It ascends the medial aspect of the leg and runs up the front of the abdomen to finish on the thorax just below the clavicle. (27 acupuncture points.)
   Pathologic symptoms: Dyspnea, dry tongue, sore throat, edema, constipation, diarrhea, motor impairment and atrophy of the lower extremities, pain along the course of the meridian.

9. **Circulation (C) meridian** (yin) (also known as heart constrictor or the pericardium) begins on the thorax lateral to the nipple. It runs up the anterior surface of the arm and terminates at the root of the nail of the middle finger. (9 acupuncture points.)
   Pathologic symptoms: Angina, chest pressure, heart palpitations, irritability, restlessness, pain along the course of the meridian.

10. **Triple heater (TH) meridian** (yang) begins at the nail root of the ring finger (ulnar side) and runs down the posterior aspect of the arm, over the back of the shoulder, and around the ear to finish at the outer aspect of the eyebrow. (23 acupuncture points.)
    Pathologic symptoms: Abdominal distortion, edema, deafness, tinnitus, sweating, sore throat, pain along the course of the meridian.

11. **Gallbladder (GB) meridian** (yang) starts at the outer canthus and runs backward and forward over the head, passing over the back of the shoulder, and down the lateral aspect of the thorax and abdomen. It passes to the hip area and then down the lateral aspect of the leg to terminate on the fourth toe. (44 acupuncture points.)
    Pathologic symptoms: Bitter taste in the mouth, dizziness, headache, ear problems, pain along the course of the meridian.

12. **Liver (LIV) meridian** (yin) begins on the great toe, runs up the medial aspect of the leg, up the abdomen, and terminates on the costal margin (vertically below the nipple). (14 acupuncture points.)
    Pathologic symptoms: Lumbago, digestive problems, retention of urine, pain in the lower abdomen, pain along the course of the meridian.

The Midline Meridians

There are two midline meridians.

- The **conception** (or **central**) **vessel (CV) meridian** (yin) starts in the center of the perineum and runs up the midline of the anterior aspect of the body to terminate just below the lower lip (24 acupuncture points); it is responsible for all yin meridians.

- The **governor vessel (GV) meridian** (yang) starts at the coccyx and runs up the center of the spine and over the midline of the head, terminating on the front of the upper gum (28 acupuncture points); it is responsible for all yang meridians.

Clinically, abundant evidence indicates the existence of reflex links between acupuncture points and specific organs and functions. In fact, no one really knows what an acupuncture point is. A body of information about acupuncture points, their nature, structure, function, interrelationships, and interactions also exists, and we have the experience derived from thousands of years of using acupuncture points to treat illness. Nevertheless, the most reliable authorities in Chinese medicine seem to agree that there is something mysterious about acupuncture points. An acupuncture point is a component of a system. Acupuncture points possess a reflexive characteristic in relation to this system. They reflect information, energy, states of being, conditions of existence of the body and the mind, of the being as a whole and its component parts. The system that comprises the acupuncture points is likewise a reflexive system of information generation and conveyance. In traditional Chinese medicine this system is known as *jing luo*, usually translated into English as either "meridians" or "channels and network vessels."

Thus the system of acupuncture points can be visualized as a matrix that passes through the body, connecting all its parts and serving as an energy and communications grid that generates, propagates, stores, and releases information and force related to the body and its various components. Every place in the body is permeated by and connected with every other place in the body by means of the jing luo system, which is, in short, the fundamental infrastructure of Chinese anatomy and physiology. The similarity between this description and current research on the fascial network is exciting.

The Chinese word-concept that we translate into English as "acupuncture point" is composed of elements conveying the sense of "body transport (of communications) hole." It is written *shu xue*. Functionally, acupuncture points seem to have two most basic actions: they open, and they close. The names of the many points include words that mean *gate, pass,* or *door*. In opening, they release information and energy. In closing, they store it.

The channels contain and convey Qi and *xue* (blood). The basic nature of Qi is the manifestation of transformation. From the Chinese viewpoint, everything that is sensed or experienced is a form of Qi.

Yin-yang theory is one of the oldest doctrines in Chinese culture. The words *yin* and *yang* originally were pictographic representations of the shady and sunny sides, respectively, of a mountain or a hill. They came to represent two primordial forces that were the fundamental constituents of the universe and everything in it.

Qi is the result of the interplay between yin and yang. Yin and yang mix together, and Qi issues forth; when yin and yang were separated from the singularity at the beginning of existence, the resulting potential gave rise to Qi.

The Five Elements

Chinese medical thinking is based on the relationship of the human being with nature. The five elements of nature become a basis for examination, diagnosis, and treatment to support health and relieve disease. The concepts of health parallel natural occurrences of life force energy as represented in the

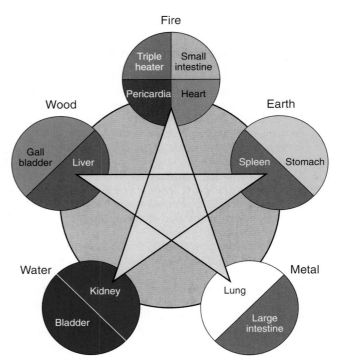

FIGURE 11-31 Wheel showing the relationship between the five elements and organs of the body. The center depicts the *ko,* or control cycle. Wood controls earth by covering it or holding it in place with roots. Earth controls water by damming it or containing it. Water controls fire by dousing or extinguishing it. Fire controls metal by melting it. Metal controls wood by cutting it. The next set of lines that form a circle depict the *sheng,* or creative cycle. Water engenders wood. Wood fuels fire. Fire creates earth (ashes). Earth engenders metal. Metal engenders water. The two rings indicate the solid *(yin)* and hollow *(yang)* organs that are associated with the elements.

five elements. The five elements are wood, fire, earth, metal, and water. Each organ is represented by an element, and each element has qualities of colors, sounds, smells, fluid secretion, anatomy, emotions, time, seasons, numbers, flavor, foods, planets, moon phases, dreams, and more (Figure 11-31 and Table 11-1).

The human being is a reflection of the universe, and the five elements become a metaphor for the life processes of people. The qualities of the five elements become the basis for life. As mentioned previously, in Chinese medicine the five elements are the basis for examination, diagnosis, and treatment. Each element is a yin-yang relationship of two meridians.

Earth—Spleen/stomach
Metal—Lung/large intestine
Water—Kidney/bladder
Wood—Liver/gallbladder
Fire—Heart/small intestine, pericardium/triple heater

The outside circle of the five-element figure (see Figure 11-31) represents the *sheng,* or creative cycle. The metaphor is as follows: during the birth phase of the universe, wood came to represent all that grows. As wood grows, it surges out to fire and matures as earth. As continued breakdown occurs, the metal, or inorganic, separates from the organic, with water representing death and rebirth of wood, and so the cycle continues. On the inside, a five-pointed star represents the *ko,* or

TABLE 11-1

Qualities of the Five Elements

Phase	Element				
	Metal	**Earth**	**Fire**	**Water**	**Wood**
Yin	Lung	Spleen	Heart	Kidney	Liver
Yang	Large intestine	Stomach	Triple-heater	Bladder Small intestine	Gallbladder
Sense	Smell	Taste	Speech	Hearing	Sight
Organ	Nose	Mouth, lips	Tongue	Ears	Eyes
Liquid	Mucus	Saliva	Sweat	Urine	Tears
Color	White	Yellow	Red	Blue/black	Green
Expression	Weeping	Singing	Laughing	Groaning	Shouting
Extreme emotion	Grief, anxiety	Worry, reminiscence	Shock, overjoy	Fear	Anger
Balanced emotion	Openness, receptivity	Sympathy, empathy	Joy, compassion	Resolution, trust	Assertion, motivation
Taste	Pungent, spicy	Sweet	Bitter, burned	Salty	Sour
Season	Fall	Indian summer	Summer	Winter	Spring
Related activity	Releasing	Thinking	Inspiration	Willpower and intimacy	Planning and decision making
Times	Lung, 3-5 am	Stomach, 7-9 am	Heart, 11 am-1 pm	Bladder, 3-5 pm	Gallbladder, 11 pm-1 am
	Large intestine, 5-7 am	Spleen, 9-11 am	Small intestine, 1-3 pm	Kidney, 5-7 pm	
				Triple-heater, 9-11 pm	Pericardium, 7-9 pm Liver, 1-3 am

control cycles. The dynamic balance between creation and control is representative of homeostatic mechanisms in Western science and is explained in the metaphor as follows:

Wood controls earth by penetrating it with roots.

Earth controls water by containing it (a pond or lake).

Water controls fire by extinguishing it.

Fire controls metal by melting it.

Metal controls wood by chopping it.

These elegant metaphors in relation to the natural world are easy to understand and become the basis for understanding health and well-being, as well as methods for assessment and treatment. If processes become disturbed in either the creative or the control cycle, homeostasis is disrupted.

Like yin and yang, the five elements are categories of quality and relationship. The ancient Chinese saw phenomena in the universe as the products of the movement and mutation of the five entities. These elements represent qualities that relate to each other in specific ways. They function metaphorically, providing images that ancient theorists used to organize their thinking about the physical world.[23]

Si shi is the term for the four seasons—spring, summer, autumn, and winter—in which the third month of summer (the sixth month of the Chinese lunar year) is called *long summer*. The four seasons correlate with the five elements: spring/wood; summer/fire; long summer/earth; autumn/metal; winter/water.

Shen is the spirit, seen as a general term for vital activities, especially as reflected in the external appearance of the internal (physiologic and/or psychological) condition of the body. As such, it is the primary criterion for diagnosis and progno-

sis. The word *shen* refers to the eternal dimension of life, to the magical or heavenly aspects of being alive. It means, "god, deity, divinity or divine nature; supernatural; magical expression, look, appearance; smart, clever."

Xue is the blood, described as an essential component of the body derived from the refined foodstuff that is consumed and made capable of being assimilated through the processes of digestion and metabolism. It is the liquid substance that circulates in the blood vessels to deliver nourishment to all parts of the body. The word *xue* is used to mean the blood itself in the same sense as it is understood in modern physiology. It is also used to mean something specific to Chinese medicine: the substantial fraction of the circulatory system in a unique relationship with the circulation of Qi.

Ying is an essential ingredient of the blood and is responsible for the production of blood and the nourishment of body tissues. The blood and the *ying* are inseparable, thus they often are referred to as *ying xue*.

Jin ye is a general term for all fluids of the body other than the blood. It is one of the basic substances that transforms into blood. It exists extensively within the human body, between organs and tissues, and serves a nutritive function. It is composed of two categorically different substances that form a single entity and that can transform one into the other.

Wu zang describes the five viscera, the so-called solid organs. This is a name given collectively to the heart, liver, spleen, lungs, and kidneys. These organs constitute one category that is distinguished from the six *fu* organs in both structure and function. The *zang* organs are thought of as solid, essence-containing organs. *Liu fu* is the word for the six bowels, the six hollow organs; it is a term given collectively to the gallbladder, stomach, large intestine, small intestine, urinary bladder, and the difficult to define "triple burner" *(san jiao)*. In contrast to the five *zang* organs, the six *fu* organs are considered to be involved in the transportation of substances rather than the storing of essential substances. The word *liu* means "six." The word *fu* means "bowel." Like *zang,* it is a special term of Chinese medicine.

Qi heng zhi fu literally means "extraordinary organs." This designation is given to a group of organs that resemble the *fu* organs in structure and the *zang* organs in function; they include the bones, blood vessels, gallbladder, and uterus. The brain and bone marrow are also in this category. These extraordinary organs are distinguished from the bowels on the grounds that they do not decompose food or convey waste and from the viscera on the grounds that they do not produce or store excess. The gallbladder is an exception, because it is classified both as a bowel and as an extraordinary organ. It is considered a bowel because it plays a role in the processing and conveyance of food and stands in interior-exterior relationship with its paired organ, the liver. However, the bile that it produces is regarded as a "clear fluid" rather than waste; hence it is also classified among the extraordinary organs.

Liu qi comprises the six excesses, referring to wind, cold, summer heat, dampness, dryness, and fire. This term is used to describe the environmental conditions that ancient theorists identified as pathogenic factors. When changes in weather exceed an individual's tolerance, disease results. Identifying which of the six *qi* are involved in the pathogenesis of a disease is an important step in diagnosis. Wind diseases are most common in spring, summer heat diseases in summer, damp diseases in long summer, dryness diseases in autumn, and cold diseases in winter.

Qi qing, or the seven affects, refers to emotional as well as mental activities in general and their potential as pathogenic factors in the onset and progress of disease. Ancient theorists recognized that intense or prolonged emotional disturbance can act as a pathogenic factor, and they identified seven such states: anger, melancholy, anxiety, sorrow, terror, fright, and excessive joy. Each of these can act to disturb the normal function of the *qi,* blood, and viscera, resulting in disease. This notion embraced thinking itself, which is understood as having the potential to exhaust the *qi* of the spleen if one thinks (or worries) excessively. The word *qi* means "seven." The word *qing* means "feeling, affection, sentiment, emotional."

Xu shi means vacuity and repletion or deficiency and excess, insubstantial and substantial (particularly in the martial arts), replete and deplete, full and empty. *Xu shi* refers to two principles for estimating the condition of both the person's resistance and the pathogenic factors present. *Vacuity* generally refers to a general insufficiency of vitality, energy, and functioning of the body and is usually expressed in terms of yin, yang, Qi, and blood. *Repletion* typically is used to refer to the hyperactivity of pathogenic factors and the resulting symptoms of conflict between the body's healthy resistance and these pathogenic factors.

Han re describes cold and heat and is considered the primary manifestation of yin and yang (i.e., symptoms that evidence predominance of cold or heat). These two signs of disease are considered of primary importance in the selection of herbal ingredients for prescriptions to treat illness. The word *han* means "cold." The word *re* means "heat."[2,3,9] *Zhen* is the term for the four examinations, which are the four traditional methods of physical examination:

Wang zhen—Visual inspection (looking at the patient)

Wen zhen—Listening and smelling (not only to what the patient says but to other sounds present in the patient's body)

Wen zhen—Inquiry

Qie zhen—Palpation

The four examinations (inspection, listening and smelling, inquiry, and palpation) provide the raw data for diagnosis. It is essential that the data from all four examinations be correlated to arrive at a complete diagnosis. The four examinations are followed by pattern identification.

The first and most fundamental method of gathering diagnostic information consists of looking at the patient's physical appearance, posture, mental and emotional status (as reflected in outward signs), color, and so forth. This includes inspection of urine, stool, and other secretions and excretions. For the well-trained Chinese doctor, it includes a comprehensive inventory of all relevant data that can be gathered through observation. The word *wang* means "inspection; looking with the eyes." Special attention focuses on the complexion and tongue, which are important indicators of the bowels and viscera. Listening and smelling consists of gathering data by means of the olfactory and auditory organs. The doctor of Chinese medicine listens to the various sounds the person makes, such as voice, breathing, coughing, moaning, and notes any particular odors.

Shi wen, the 10 questions, refers to the 10 basic aspects of a patient that a doctor inquires about in gathering diagnostic information. These include feelings of heat or coldness; perspiration; the condition of the head, trunk, and limbs; urination and defecation; appetite; the condition of the chest and abdomen; hearing and sleeping; thirst; menstruation, leukorrhea, and so forth, including the growth and nourishment of children; the past history; and the cause of disease.

Wu se, or the five colors, refers to the colors associated with the five elements and the five *zang* organs. These are green (a greenish-blue associated with wood, liver); red (fire, heart); yellow (earth, spleen); white (metal, lungs); and black (water, kidneys). Observation of these colors as they appear in the body is taken together with other clinical data and forms an important aspect of diagnosis.

San yin describes a method of classifying pathogenic factors, in terms of their point of origin, as endogenous, exogenous, or neutral (literally non-external-internal). These three categories are *nei yin,* endogenous pathogenic factors, which include abnormal emotional activities; *wai yin,* exogenous pathogenic factors, including wind, cold, summer heat, damp, dry, and fire; and *bu nei wai yin,* improper diet, trauma, animal bites, insect stings, and fatigue. The word *yin* means "cause, because of, as a result of." The word *nei* means "inner, within, inside." The word *wai* means "outer, outward, outside, external."

External factors are the six excesses. Internal causes are the *seven effects.* Neutral causes ("non-external-internal") include eating too much or too little, falls, crushing, drowning, and animal injuries.

A *thousand sufferings* fall into just three categories. First, the evil invades the *jing luo* and enters the *zang fu;* this is known as external causes. Second, blood and vessels connect the four limbs and nine orifices. When these become congested, illness follows; these are called *internal causes.* The third category contains such aspects as sexual life, wounds from knives, bites from insects, and beasts; these are "neither internal nor external."

Si qi si xing refers to the essential synergistic characteristics of medicine or treatment. The four natures are cold, hot, cool, and warm. They are categorized according to yin and yang. Hot and warm are in the yang category; cold and cool are in the yin category. The purpose of categorizing medicinal substances in this fashion is to permit herbal practitioners to follow a basic precept of Chinese herbal medicine: "Use heat to overcome cold pathogenic factors; use cold to overcome hot pathogenic factors." Herbs with a cold nature are typically used to clear hot or warm pathogenic factors, as well as internally generated heat. They are used to treat heat patterns and yang patterns. Herbs with a hot nature are used to dispel cold pathogenic factors by warming the interior, invigorating yang, and nourishing qi. They are used in the treatment of cold patterns and yin patterns.

Wu wei, the five flavors, refers to the tastes of herbs: acrid, sweet, sour, bitter, and salty. These flavors are understood to correspond with the five *zang* organs according to the following arrangement:

Heart—Bitter
Liver—Sour
Spleen—Sweet
Lungs—Acrid
Kidney—Salty

The flavors can be classified as yin and yang. Acrid and sweet effusing (i.e., diaphoretic) and dissipating medicinals are yang; sour and bitter upwelling (i.e., emetic) and discharging (i.e., draining) medicinals are yin; salty upwelling and discharging medicinals are yin; bland percolating and discharging medicinals are yang.

Zhen jiu translates as "needle" and "long-lasting fire." Together, these two words form the term that is typically translated in English as "acupuncture and moxibustion" or "acumoxa therapy," commonly referred to simply as *acupuncture.* The term refers to two allied forms of therapy, *zhen fa* and *jiu fa. Zhen fa* refers to the therapeutic method of applying any of a variety of types of needles, including filiform needles, three-edged needles, plum-blossom needles, and intradermal needles, among others. The needles are applied to stimulate certain points that lie among channels for the treatment of disease. *Jiu fa* consists of the application of an herb, artemisia, which is prepared in various ways and then burned either near or on certain points to warm and thereby stimulate the movement of Qi.

Shu xue, or *in bach shu,* means transport point and is a term for a category of acupoints found on the back in two lines, one approximately 11 inches lateral to the spine and the other at about 3 inches lateral to the spine. These points are related to the functioning of the internal organs and various other aspects of physiology.

Mu xue means an alarm point and refers to a group of points on the anterior surface of the body that have both diagnostic and therapeutic interrelationships. Because changes in the Qi frequently precede any other clinical symptoms or signs, *mu xue* points can "sound an alarm" prior to the onset of disease. The word *mu* means to "collect, gather, or muster together."

Wu shu xue is the Chinese term for the five transport points, referring to a group of points on each of the 12 primary channels. These points include well points, spring points, stream points, river points, and uniting (sea) points. Here the word *shu* means "transportation or communication."

Tui na is a general name for massage. The word *tui* means "push, push forward, promote." The word *na* means to "hold, to grasp." *Tui na* thus means pushing and holding (i.e., massage).

An mo is another general term for massage. The word *an* means "press, push down, keep one's hand on (something)." The word *mo* means "to rub, scrape, touch." *An mo* is a method of preventing and treating diseases using various massage techniques and methods, as well as undertaking manipulation and adjustment of the joints and of the extremities. More specifically, *an mo* is one of the eight manipulations used in bone setting in order to relax muscle tissue, dissipate blood stasis, and reduce swelling.

Health Preservation and Exercise

An important part of Chinese medicine is the discipline of preserving health and extending life. Foremost among the various methods that fall in this category are exercise and disciplines aimed at cultivating the inborn treasures of the body, mind, and spirit.

- **Qi gong.** Qi gong, or breathing exercise, refers to a variety of traditional practices consisting of physical, mental, and spiritual exercises. The regulation of the breath *(qi)* is a common feature of such exercise methods. The word *gong* means "achievement, result; skill; work; exercise." It is composed of two radicals. The radical on the left is also pronounced *gong* and means "work." The radical on the right is the word *li* and means "strength or force." Qi gong can be understood as exercise designed to strengthen and harmonize the Qi, regulate the body and mind, and calm the spirit.

- **Tai ji quan.** Tai ji quan (tai chi) is a martial as well as a meditative art. Thus it has complementary aspects that combine in a comprehensive discipline of physical culture and mental and spiritual discipline. The word *quan* means "fist; boxing; punch."

- **Dao yin.** This discipline involves meditation and breathing exercises that seek to develop the ability to lead and guide the Qi throughout the body for the benefit of the spirit, mind, and body. Dao yin exercises have a long history in China. They consist of bending, stretching, and otherwise mobilizing the extremities and the joints to free the flow of

Qi throughout the whole body. Like Qi gong, dao yin emphasizes control of the breath (Qi). Dao yin also includes self-massage techniques that relieve fatigue and prolong life by activating and harmonizing the circulation of blood and Qi. These techniques also stress the development of strength in the muscles and bones.

The vastness of the Asian medicine model and its elegance are far beyond the scope of this textbook, therefore no attempt is made to present scaled-down versions of these systems. The student is directed to the reference list for sources of further study. Students who are drawn to these concepts are encouraged to explore them in depth as they continue on their path of knowledge.

During the natural course of therapeutic massage, the physical aspects of meridians and points are addressed. The following section briefly investigates methods of incorporating this approach into therapeutic massage.

Methods of Treating Acupuncture Points

Acupuncture points usually lie in a fascial division between muscles and near origins and insertions. A point feels like a small hole, and pressure elicits a "nervy" feeling. Unlike a trigger point, which may be found only on one side of the body, acupuncture points are bilateral (i.e., found on both sides of the body) and are located on the central, or governing, meridian. To confirm the location of an acupuncture point, locate the point in the same place on the other side of the body (Figure 11-32).

To stimulate a hypoactive acupuncture point (one with insufficient energy), use a short vibrating or tapping action. This method is effective if the area is sluggish or if a specific body function needs to be stimulated.

To sedate a hyperactive acupuncture point (one with too much energy) to reduce pain, elicit the pain response within the point itself. Use a sustained holding pressure until the painful overenergy dissipates and the body's own natural painkillers are released into the bloodstream.[19] The pressure techniques are similar to those used for trigger points; however, an acupuncture point does not need to be lengthened and stretched after treatment.

As with other reflex points, if you are unsure whether the acupuncture point is hypoactive or hyperactive, alternately apply both techniques and allow the body to adjust to the intervention.

Determining whether you are dealing with a trigger point or an acupressure point often is difficult, because the two often overlap. It may be wise to lengthen and stretch the area gently after using direct pressure methods; this does not interfere with the effect on an acupressure point, but without it a trigger point cannot be treated effectively (Proficiency Exercise 11-7).[2]

Asian methods work for sound physiologic reasons through the neuroendocrine system. Particular effects can be demonstrated after acupuncture treatment. Some of these effects involve alteration of the function of organs or systems. An analgesic effect and an anesthetic effect also are seen. It is not necessary to hold that imbalance between yin and yang (the two equal and opposite forces of the universe, which act through Qi) causes disease. Instead, the acupuncture benefit can be framed in terms of the body's homeostatic tendency, whereby a stable internal environment is maintained through the interaction of the various body processes and systems. For many years osteopaths and chiropractors have used reflex pressure techniques to assist the body in its efforts toward health. Many of the points used correspond with acupuncture points.

If one accepts that the body constantly strives for health, then one must agree that the body will use all helpful stimuli to that end. If this function can be assisted through acupuncture or manual pressure, the homeostatic interplay of organ systems will carry on the work to the extent possible at that time (Figure 11-33).

Acupuncture successfully induces the desired feeling of soreness and fullness that is a forerunner of the anesthetic effect (pain modulator). Electrophysiologic studies have shown that deep pressure applied to muscles and tendons has a definite inhibitory effect on the unit discharge of neurons in the nonspecific nucleus of the thalamus, which would support the claimed benefit of acupressure.

Pain relief might well be the result of neurally mediated changes in the brain's receptivity to pain impulses, as well as an effect of biochemical changes caused by the release of hormonelike substances both locally and generally.

Western research so far has produced no great breakthrough in our understanding of acupuncture, although Melzack and Wall have proposed the gate control theory, and endogenous polypeptides that link to opiate receptors in the brain and central nervous system offer an explanation of the acupuncture phenomenon. Regardless, skillful application of

FIGURE 11-32 Chinese methods of exercise.

PROFICIENCY EXERCISE 11-7

1. *Working with a partner, perform a massage that incorporates running the hand down each of the meridian grooves in the body. Stop at each hole or point you feel.*
2. *When you locate a point while performing this massage, decide whether the point needs to be stimulated with vibration or tapping, or sedated with sustained direct pressure. How did you decide?*

FIGURE 11-33 Treatment of acupuncture points. **A,** Press, sedate. **B,** Tap, stimulate.

the method provides benefits and can easily be integrated into therapeutic massage.

AYURVEDA

SECTION OBJECTIVE

Using the information presented in this section, the student will be able to perform the following:

* Identify and understand introductory Ayurvedic terminology

Ayurveda is a system of health and medicine developed in India. The foundation of its theory base is similar to that of Asian systems. As with all the complementary systems presented in this chapter, Ayurveda is a distinct and rich body of knowledge. The language of Ayurveda is being used more often in Western society, and massage professionals should be familiar with some of the terms that describe Ayurvedic principles of thought.[11]

The word *Ayurveda* means life knowledge or right living. Ayurveda is grounded as a body/mind/spirit system in the Vedic scriptures. The *tridosha* theory is unique to this system. A *dosha* is a body chemical pattern. When the doshas combine, they constitute the nature of every living organism. The three doshas are *Vata* (wind), *Pitta* (bile), and *Kapha* (mucus). These three combine to form the five elements (similar to Asian theory) of ether, air, fire, water, and earth.

Bones, flesh, skin, and nerves belong to the *earth element*. Semen, blood, fat, urine, mucus, saliva, and lymph belong to the *water element*. Hunger, thirst, temperature, sleep, intelligence, anger, hate, jealousy, and radiance belong to the *fire element*. All movement, breathing, natural urges, sensory and motor functions, secretions, excretions, and transformation of tissues belong to the *air element*. Love, shyness, fear, and attachment belong to the *ether element*.

People display temperament based on the degree of influence or dominance of a particular dosha; this is considered an inherited genetic quality that influences a person through his or her entire life. The balance of function within the dosha system equates with health.

The points connected with this system are called *marmas.* There are about 100 marmas, which are concentrated at the junctions of muscles, vessels, ligaments, bones, and joints. These junctions form the seat of vital life force (in Hindi, *Prana*). Marmas have a strong correlation with common trigger points and the location of the traditional meridians (Figure 11-34).

In Ayurveda, chakras (Figure 11-35) are considered the seven centers of the Prana. They are located along the spinal column, interrelated with the nervous system and endocrine glands. These are subtle centers of consciousness that are the link between the universal source of intelligence and the human body. Chakras are wheels of energy, and they govern the various physical organs, as well as etheric bodies, such as the emotional body (the feelings). Within every living body, although on the subtle rather than the gross or the physical level, there is said to be a series of energy fields or centers of consciousness, which in traditional Tantric teachings are called *chakras* (wheels) or *padmas* (lotuses). They are said to be located either along or just in front of, the backbone, even though they might express themselves externally at points along the front of the body (e.g., navel, heart, throat). Associated with the chakras is a latent subtle energy, called *kundalini* in Shaktism and *tumo* in Tibetan Buddhist Tantra.

The massage methods of Ayurveda are tapping, kneading, rubbing, and squeezing. The use of specialized oil preparations is integral to the systems.[11]

POLARITY THERAPY

SECTION OBJECTIVES

Using the information presented in this section, the student will be able to perform the following:

* Explain the basic theory of polarity therapy
* Incorporate the principles of polarity therapy into the massage session

A

B

- ● Ayurvedic marmas
- ○ Common trigger points
- ◎ Overlap of ayurvedic marmas and common trigger points
- ⬭ Meridians where acupuncture points are located

FIGURE 11-34 Comparison of Ayurvedic marmas, common trigger points, and traditional meridians where acupuncture points are located. Anterior **(A)** and posterior **(B)** views of overlapping locations of various points suggest that the points have a common anatomy and physiology.

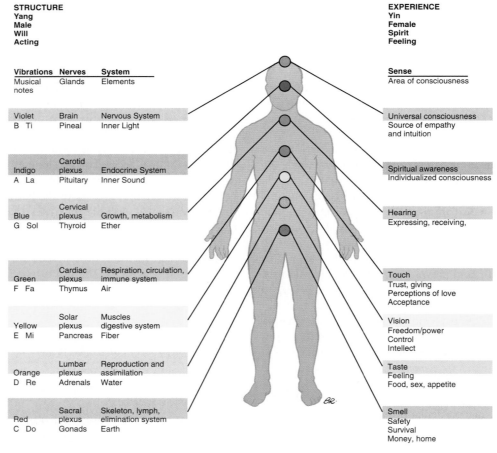

STRUCTURE
Yang
Male
Will
Acting

Vibrations	Nerves	System
Musical notes	Glands	Elements
Violet B Ti	Brain Pineal	Nervous System Inner Light
Indigo A La	Carotid plexus Pituitary	Endocrine System Inner Sound
Blue G Sol	Cervical plexus Thyroid	Growth, metabolism Ether
Green F Fa	Cardiac plexus Thymus	Respiration, circulation, immune system Air
Yellow E Mi	Solar plexus Pancreas	Muscles digestive system Fiber
Orange D Re	Lumbar plexus Adrenals	Reproduction and assimilation Water
Red C Do	Sacral plexus Gonads	Skeleton, lymph, elimination system Earth

EXPERIENCE
Yin
Female
Spirit
Feeling

Sense
Area of consciousness

Universal consciousness
Source of empathy
and intuition

Spiritual awareness
Individualized consciousness

Hearing
Expressing, receiving,

Touch
Trust, giving
Perceptions of love
Acceptance

Vision
Freedom/power
Control
Intellect

Taste
Feeling
Food, sex, appetite

Smell
Safety
Survival
Money, home

FIGURE 11-35 The major chakras.

Polarity is a holistic health practice that encompasses some of the theory bases of Asian medicine and Ayurveda. Polarity therapy was developed by Dr. Randolph Stone in the middle 1900s. It is an eclectic, multifaceted system.

Life force energy (e.g., Chi, Qi, and Prana) has not been a popular subject of Western scientific research. The abstract quality and esoteric nature of the concept are still primarily held in the knowledge base of "spiritual truth." Many spiritual disciplines practice the "laying on of hands." Polarity therapy is also a respectful, compassionate, and intentional laying of the hands on the body.

A physiologic explanation can be postulated as to the result of this therapeutic "laying on of hands" process. Entrainment is one of the most plausible of the physiologic responses. Because some polarity techniques involve rocking motions, all physiologic benefits of rocking (as discussed in Chapter 9) apply. Gentle stimulation through application of polarity methods to joint receptors generates reflex responses to the associated muscles.

As with all methods of healing touch, something exists beyond the physiologic explanation for the benefit. This "something" is intangible but very real in the experience of it. Therein remains the mystery.

The bodywork principles of polarity blend easily with massage. The intention of the touch is the same as that of therapeutic massage, explained in Chapters 1 and 2 and as a theme throughout this text. Nothing is ever forced. The experience belongs to the client. The practitioner offers the methods not by protocol but through a practiced development of decision making guided by intuition. When the professional feels no attachment to the outcome for his or her own sense of achievement, the methods become "free" to influence the experience of the client (Figure 11-36).

As with the other methods discussed in previous sections of this chapter, the application of polarity methods is simple. However, for those interested in pursing advanced learning, the goal is to develop the ability to deliver the methods in a purposeful and individualized way, detached from expecta-

tion but fascinated with the outcome. Eventually the practitioner learns that the more complex the client situation, the simpler the methods used. The simplicity of polarity make it one of the gifts to bodywork.

Principles and Applications of Polarity Therapy

The purpose of polarity therapy is to locate blocked energy and release it, using the principles outlined here. When blocked energy is released, body systems and organs can function normally, and healing can take place naturally.

Polarity therapy does not treat illness or disease; it affects the body (life) energy, which flows in invisible electromagnetic currents through the body's organs and tissues. It stimulates the energy that is inactive in a diseased body part. The following principles apply:

1. The head and spinal column form the central neutral (0) energy axis of the body.
2. Long vertical currents of energy travel from head to foot on the right side of the body, flowing down the front and up the back. Positive (1) outward energy is expressed through the right side. The right side represents the following:
Warmth
Heat
Sun
Yang
Positive, expanding energy
3. On the left side of the body, the vertical currents flow up the front and down the back. Negative (2) inward energy is expressed through the left side. The left side represents the following:
Cooling
Contracting
Moon
Yin
Negative, receptive energy
4. Five electromagnetic currents are present on each side of the body. Each current is related to an element. The elements are ether, air, fire, water, and earth. Each current relates to the organs and functions of its area (Figure 11-37).

The Five Major Body Currents

The five major body currents are ether, air, fire, water, and earth.

- *Ether* is associated with hearing, the voice, the throat, and the quality of nothingness. The core current of the torso flows from north to south (head to pelvis to back). The ether element represents pure vibration and responds to gentleness and love.
Color: Sky blue
Sense: Hearing
Food: Pure air
- *Air* is associated with respiration, circulation, the heart, the lungs, and speed. It flows from east to west (from front to back in a circular pattern).With a balanced air element, we are calm and relaxed.

FIGURE 11-36 Energy modality.

FIGURE 11-37 Electromagnetic currents traveling vertically on the body.

Color: Emerald green
Sense: Touch
Food: Fruits and nuts

■ *Fire* is associated with digestion, the stomach, the bowels, warmth, and the heat of the body. A diagonal current found on both sides of the body, it starts at the shoulders and goes to the opposite hip. It is part of the figure-eight energy and is activated by touch, food, and exercise.
Color: Yellow
Sense: Sight
Food: Grains

■ *Water* is associated with generative power, creativity, the pelvic organs, sexuality, glandular secretions, emotional drive, equilibrium, and balance. A long current that splits the body in half, it extends from the head to the foot, including the arms and legs. The right side moves clockwise, the left side counterclockwise.
Color: Orange
Sense: Taste
Food: Leafy green vegetables, seaweed, watery foods

■ *Earth* is associated with the elimination of solids and liquids, the bladder, the rectum, the formation of bone,

structure, and support. A zigzag current is formed by solid straight lines from one side to the other.
Color: Red
Sense: Smell
Food: Tubers, meat, dairy

Each of the five electromagnetic currents passes through a corresponding finger and toe, giving its name to the finger and toe (e.g., the middle, or fire, finger) (Figure 11-38).

The polarity (positive [+] or negative [−]) of these electromagnetic currents is shown in Figure 11-38. Positive and negative are opposites. However, the use of positive and negative labels is only relative; it is a way of showing relationships.

The right side of the body is positive (+), whereas the left side of the body is negative (−). The head is positive, whereas the feet are negative. The front of the body is positive, whereas the back is negative. The top is positive, whereas the bottom is negative. Each joint is neutral and is a crossover for energy currents, which change polarity at the crossover. The neutrality of the joints allows them to be flexible. Each finger and toe has an individual polarity (see Figure 11-38).

Blocked energy usually registers as soreness, tenderness, or pain. A simple way to bring energy to an area where it is blocked is to place your left hand on the pain and your right hand opposite that area—on the back, front, or side of the body.

Reflexes

Reflexes are points along an energy current that connect with other points along that current. When stimulated, a reflex point can affect the other reflexes on the same energy path. Manipulations that stimulate the foot and hand poles use the reflex principles located there (Figure 11-39).

Positive and Negative Contacts

Because all polarity contacts are bipolar, both hands must be in contact with the body so that energy can move from one hand to the other through the blockage. If the energy blockage is on the front of the body, place the left hand over the painful, blocked area and the right hand on the back of the body directly opposite the left hand. This double contact draws energy through the body from front to back, side to side, and top to bottom contacts.

In practice, a positive contact (e.g., the right hand or fire finger) activates and gives energy. The opposite is also true; a negative contact (e.g., the left hand or air finger) is relaxing and receives energy.

Figure 11-39 shows the foot reflexes as they relate to the rest of the body. In addition to those in the feet, reflexes are present in the hands, arms, legs, and head. Alternately stimulating a reflex and then its corresponding body part can free blocked energy and allow normal functioning. The negative poles of the body are most frequently obstructed. The negative pole is stimulated first, then the positive pole, to send currents over the entire body.

The use of diagonal contacts on the body activates the serpentine brain wave currents shown in Figure 11-40.

Applying a Polarity Method

- With most procedures, stimulate the area (rub briskly) for a few minutes, then hold and feel the energy. Hold for 30

FIGURE 11-38 The finger and toe chart.

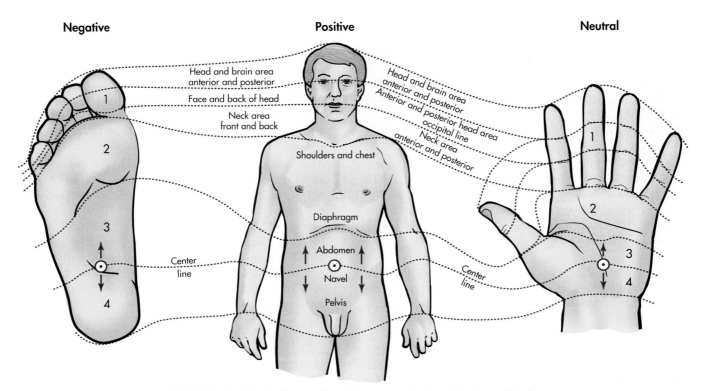

FIGURE 11-39 Reflex relationships among the hand, foot, and body.

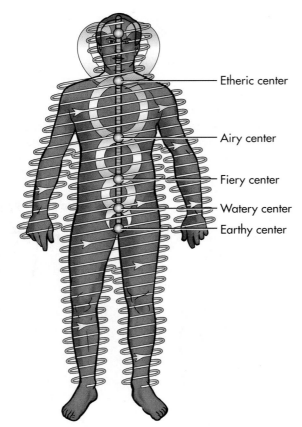

Etheric center

Airy center

Fiery center

Watery center

Earthy center

FIGURE 11-40 Brain wave currents crisscrossing the spine from the brain to the coccyx. These currents resemble the caduceus, the ancient Greek symbol for medicine. Each crossover point is known as a *chakra,* or energy center.

to 60 seconds. If you feel no energy after stimulating for 2 minutes, hold for 1 minute longer and then move on.

- When possible, keep the client's body centered between your hands.
- Be careful not to cross your hands on your client's body.
- When stimulating points, use the fleshy pads of your fingers.
- Be gentle; never force. Forcing creates tension, which blocks energy. A light, gentle touch moves energy.
- When you feel the energy, the blocked energy is released. Life energy has intelligence. After it is moving, it knows what to do and where to go.
- People heal at different rates; do not expect a physical result after completion of a procedure. Be neutral when working with a client. Don't let your expectations be a part of the energy.
- If the manipulations are ineffective, place your hand on your client's body and send love. Visualize energy flowing through your hands to your client (Proficiency Exercise 11-8).

COLOR THERAPY

Light can be used therapeutically. When the light spectrum is spread, a rainbow appears. Each color has a specific frequency

 PROFICIENCY EXERCISE 11-8

1. *Design three original massage sessions that incorporate a principle from each topic covered in this chapter.*
2. *Exchange massage with three students using one of the massage sessions developed in this chapter.*
3. *While giving 10 general massages to "practice" clients, mentally note each time you use one of the methods in this chapter.*
4. *Using professional journals and massage school catalogs, find a continuing education opportunity for each method discussed in this chapter.*

that is thought to influence the body. Color can be incorporated into massage in the color of uniforms, linens, or tinted lighting. The traditional Chinese medicine system also relies on color. Chakra therapy often is related to color. The following is a brief, basic discussion of the individual chakras and the color relationship (Box 11-11; see also Figure 11-35).

- The chakras are numbered, beginning with the lowest vibration as the first chakra, or **root** chakra. Located at the base of the spine, the first chakra is associated with the color **red.** Energy is tied to the element of earth, grounding us and connecting us to the physical plane. Glandular system: gonads.
- The second chakra, or **sacral** chakra, sits in the area of the reproductive organs and vibrates to the color **orange.** The sacral chakra controls emotions and sexuality. Glandular system: adrenal.
- The third chakra, or **solar plexus** chakra, is tied to the color yellow and is located just below the diaphragm. This chakra deals with intellect and ego. Glandular system: pancreas.
- The fourth chakra, or **heart** chakra, is located in the chest and is linked to the color **green.** It controls love and relationships, especially *agape,* or divine love. Glandular system: lymphatic.
- The fifth chakra, or **throat** chakra, radiates **blue** and holds sway over expression, helping to transmit the voice of the creative soul to the physical world. Glandular system: thyroid.
- The sixth chakra, or **brow** chakra, sits between and slightly above the eyes. Radiating **indigo,** it controls internal vision, intuition, and self-realization. Glandular system: pituitary.
- The seventh chakra, or **crown** chakra, lies directly atop the head and corresponds to the highest vibrations. It vibrates to the color **purple** and controls integration of the conscious and subconscious minds. Glandular system: pineal. It is interesting to rote that the color spectrum found in rainbows is the same as that found in the chakra system.

AROMATHERAPY

Aromatherapy involves the use of essential oils, which are distilled extracts from aromatic plants. Aromatic plants and infusions prepared from them have been employed in medi-

BOX 11-11

Color Therapy and Recognized Associations

Red
Enthusiasm,
passion, and vitality

Orange
Joyfulness, warmth, and
happiness

Yellow
Mental energy, creativity,
focus, and concentration

Green
Feelings, healing, and love

Blue
Expression, relaxing,
and serenity

Indigo
Intuition, meditation, and
spiritual awareness

Violet
Compassion, awareness of
spiritual self, letting go

---

cines and cosmetics for thousands of years, but the use of distilled oils dates back only 1000 years. Ancient civilizations used these oils to protect against disease, ward off evil, and aid in spiritual healing. As various societies came into contact with each other and shared these oils, knowledge spread. The term *aromatherapy* was coined in the early twentieth century and was recognized as a healing discipline.[17,18,20]

Modern aromatherapy is used in healing mind, body, and spirit and uses range from spiritual to relaxation to therapeutic. Essential oils can be directly inhaled or absorbed through the skin to achieve therapeutic effect. Massage can be combined with aromatherapy. This combination stems from the fact that essential oils, being lipids, are easily absorbed through the skin. Topical application also allows the client to benefit through inhalation for absorption through mucous membranes.

Medical aromatherapy is common in Europe, with physicians prescribing essential oils for the treatment of diseases and conditions. In the United States, nurses and other healthcare providers are often trained in aromatherapy. Because essential oils have antiseptic, antibacterial, and antibiotic properties, they complement most forms of healthcare.

Aromatherapy training ensures practitioners are prepared to take a client history, assess and be aware of contraindications, and create and treat the client with essential oil blends to address the client's concerns. This approach would be considered a medical treatment. Essential oils can also be used for many spa applications (particularly in relation to skin care) such as cleansing and reduction of pores, soothing burns, treating sensitive or cracked skin, detoxification, oil gland regulation, hair growth, and skin nourishment. These are common focuses in the spa setting.

How Essential Oils Work

Essential oils are beneficial both through inhalation of the scent, which affects the limbic system, and through lipid absorption of the oil through the skin. Aromatherapy is an extensive study, and care and caution are advised in the use

of essential oils. Only therapeutic grade (100%) essential oils should be used, and they should be diluted in a carrier oil (e.g., olive, jojoba, grapeseed, or almond oil) before being applied to the skin. Only three or four drops of essential oil are needed in 2 ounces of carrier oil. When a drop of oil is mixed with a small amount of salt ($1/4$ cup), it can be dissolved in a warm water immersion, such as a bath. Essential oils in the pure state should *never* be applied directly to the skin.

Only oils that are generally considered safe, such as the ones listed in this text, should be used. The following are some of the effects of essential oils:

- *Skin:* They can dissolve dead surface cells, increase cell turnover, stimulate metabolism, improve texture, add softness, give radiance, stimulate, and tone.
- *Nervous system:* They can calm, soothe nerve endings, cause a sense of euphoria, and promote relaxation.
- *Glands:* They can have a soothing and sedating effect, or a toning and stimulating effect.
- *Muscles:* They can relieve fatigue, reduce soreness and stiffness, and improve the resilience and elasticity of muscle.

Additives for an aromatherapy bath or massage oil might include the following:

- Relaxing: Lavender, clary sage, melissa, ylang ylang, bergamot, chamomile
- Stimulating: Rosemary, thyme, lavender (good for toning), pine, cypress
- Soothing: Chamomile, jasmine, geranium, rose
- Moisturizing: Orange blossom, neroli, patchouli, lavender

Essential Oils

Essential oils are subtle, volatile chemicals distilled from plants, shrubs, flowers, trees, roots, bushes, and seeds. They have hormonelike properties and are natural antiseptics. Each oil is thought to have a unique power on the body and mind, but the oil also can be easily classified as antiseptic, analgesic, antiinflammatory, detoxifying, regenerating, stimulating, and sedating. Essential oils are not oily; rather, they are more like water. They generally are transparent and can be various colors. Because essential oils are lipid (fat) based, they are soluble in alcohol, oils, and fats, but not water.

Degradation can be an issue with essential oils. It is best to store them in dark glass bottles, away from heat and sunlight. Storage in a cool dark place, such as a refrigerator, is recommended. Also, use of stoppered caps will help prevent oxidation, which can reduce efficacy or result in chemical changes of essential oils. Never store essential oils in plastic and make sure they are not within reach of children. It is recommended that most essential oils be used within 1 year of purchase, although refrigeration can at least double this lifespan. Some oils, such as orange, lemon, and lime degrade more readily and may only last 6 months without refrigeration.

Fragrance Oils. Essential oils are the organic constituents of fragrant plant matter and are extracted by distillation or cold pressing. They contain the true essence of the plant. Fragrance or perfume oils are blended synthetic aroma compounds diluted with carrier oils. These artificial oils are used most often in perfumes, cosmetics, and flavoring and are not as therapeutically effective as pure essential oils.

Because use of the term *aromatherapy* is not regulated by the U.S. government, caution is required when using products. Many beauty and skin care preparations, candles, and other products are improperly labeled with the term *aromatherapy*, although the scent actually is artificial, using fragrance oils. As mentioned, fragrance oils do not offer the therapeutic value of pure high-grade essential oils.

Distillation is a primary determinant of therapeutic grade status. The higher the pressure used in distillation, the higher the yield of oil; however, this also causes unnecessary fractionation of the oil molecules as a result of the higher temperatures created by increasing the pressure. Flavor and fragrance companies produce their oils this way because they are interested in the scent or flavor applications for food, soft drinks, and other beverages. Oils produced by high-pressure distillation work fine for flavor and fragrance; they just are not therapeutic grade. Therapeutic-grade oils are produced under lower pressure to preserve their molecular structures with the highest integrity. Lower pressure yields less essential oil, which is one reason therapeutic oils generally are more expensive than commercial-grade oils.[24]

Benefits of Aromatherapy

The physiologic effect of essential oils is primarily chemical. The chemistry of essential oils is very complex. Hundreds of components, such as terpenes, aldehydes, and esters, make up the oils. Lavender, for example, has antiseptic, antibacterial, antibiotic, antidepressant, analgesic, decongestant, and sedative properties. Essential oils also reach the bloodstream through inhalation. When inhaled, they pass through the tiny air sacs to the surrounding blood capillaries by the process of diffusion. Once in the bloodstream, the aromatic molecules interact with the body's chemistry.

In addition to essential oils' medicinal properties, smelling them can uplift the spirits, making clients feel better. The sense of smell is interrelated with the limbic system, an area of the brain primarily concerned with emotion and memory. This influence of aromas on the psyche has led many aromatherapists to practice a form of aromatherapy called *psychoaromatherapy,* in which essential oils are used to enhance the client's mood and emotions. The massage therapist needs to be cautious of the scope of practice and ethical boundaries when oils are used for specific treatment of physical or mental disorders.

When an essential oil is inhaled, the chemicals in it stimulate the olfactory center, which receives the odor and carries it to the limbic system. The signal passes between the pituitary and pineal glands, targeting the amygdala (memory center for fear and trauma). The olfactory system is used to bypass the blood-brain barrier. These areas of the brain influence mood, and the hippocampus and amygdala are specifically related to emotion and memory. Scent memory is longer than visual memory. The experience is one of déjà vu; that is, feeling as if the current experience is familiar and seems to be triggered by memory.

An aromatherapy massage can help a person deeply relax and let go of worries, even if only for a short time. Relaxation is powerful enough to activate the body's self-healing ability. Combining the physical and emotional effects of massage with the medicinal and therapeutic properties of essential oils can alleviate stress and improves a person's mood.

Essential oils can help with moderate anxiety and depression, insomnia, digestive disorders, headaches, and muscle aches and pains. Many essential oils are wonderful for skin care. They balance sebum (the skin's natural oil secretion) and can help tone the complexion in supporting capillary function. Essential oils can be used in hair and scalp products to improve circulation to the scalp, to prevent dandruff and promote healthy new hair growth. Essential oils can help heal many minor skin problems, such as athlete's foot, cold sores, ringworm, scabies, psoriasis, dry skin, and oily skin, when used with appropriate health care supervision. Steam or direct inhalation of essential oils can help reduce cold and flu symptoms such as coughs, tonsillitis, sore throats, sinusitis, and bronchitis.

Essential oils are highly concentrated and should be used topically only with extreme care and at the proper dilution in a carrier oil. Less is very effective, as opposed to more, which can be toxic or can cause skin irritation. Inhalation of essential oils should be used for the purposes suggested and also should be done with care and caution. To achieve the best aromatherapy benefits, the highest quality organic, therapeutic-grade essential oils should be used.

Safety Guidelines for the Use of Essential Oils

As mentioned, essential oils are highly concentrated, volatile substances and if used correctly, can have therapeutic benefit. While many oils are useful, some are not safe to use at all and proper safety guidelines must always be adhered to when using essential oils.

NOTE: The following cautions and information do not in any way replace medical and professional advice and may not include all cautionary information available.

- Always dilute essential oils in a carrier oil to prevent skin irritation and burning. Never use undiluted essential oils directly on the skin. Experienced aromatherapists may break with this rule but without extensive training, it is important to work with these substances with caution. Some clients can tolerate some oils, such as tea tree and lavender, in an undiluted form, but again, caution is advised as severe reactions and sensitivity are possible.

- When using a new oil on your client, it is important to patch test for sensitization and irritation. To patch test, apply a small amount of the diluted oil to the client's skin and leave for 24 to 48 hours to determine where there is a reaction. Even if working with an oil that does not commonly cause irritation, the patch test is important as a measure of safety.

- Be familiar with essential oils that are contraindicated during pregnancy or for those with diseases and illnesses such as asthma and epilepsy.

- Only small quantities of essential oils are needed, and you should use the smallest amount possible for effective treatment. If an additional drop is not necessary, do not use it.

- Many essential oils are not appropriate for use in aromatherapy. Do not assume that every essential oil can be used safely. Some oils, such as wormwood, onion, bitter almond, pennyroyal, camphor, horseradish, wintergreen, rue, and sassafras should only be used by a qualified aromatherapist. Some oils should not be used at all.

- Keep essential oils out of children's reach. These oils can be tempting, because the scents are appealing, and children may think they are lotions or even candy or sweet drinks (e.g., citrus oil). Treat these oils as medicines or poisons when considering storage.

- Keep essential oils away from animals.

- Do not eat, drink, or otherwise ingest essential oils. With extreme caution, a qualified aromatherapy practitioner may prescribe internal use of an essential oil, but only after detailed consultation with the client.

- Essential oils are flammable. Store properly and keep away from fire hazards.

- Keep oils away from the eyes. If a drop or so of oil accidentally gets in the eye, put some vegetable oil (e.g., almond oil) into the eye, which will absorb the essential oil, and then use a tissue to remove the oil. Do not use water, which will spread the oil. If burning or itching occurs, seek medical treatment.

- Do not use the same oils for a prolonged period.

- Use photosensitizing oils cautiously (i.e., bergamot, verbena, lime, angelica root, bitter orange, lemon, and grapefruit). Avoid sun exposure and the use of tanning beds for 12 hours after application of these oils. Photosensitization occurs when oils containing furanocoumarin compounds are applied to the skin and the skin is immediately exposed to sunlight or ultraviolet light. Furanocoumarin compounds allow the UV rays to penetrate the skin more readily, resulting in abnormal skin pigmentation or mild to severe burns. Remember, UV rays are present even on cloudy days.

- Store essential oils away from light and heat and keep the cap tightly closed. Essential oils are volatile and evaporate readily.

Potentially Hazardous Essential Oils

Some aromatherapy experts believe that certain essential oils should not be used unless administered by qualified aromatherapists, and some oils should not be used even by qualified practitioners. Do not assume that an oil is safe to use if it is not included in the following lists. This information is for general educational purposes only and is not considered complete nor is it guaranteed to be accurate.

Oils that should not be used include the following:

Bitter almond	Sassafras
Boldo leaf	Savin *(Juniperus sabina)*
Calamus	Southernwood
Camphor (yellow)	Tansy
Horseradish	Thuja
Jaborandi leaf	Western red cedar *(Thuja plicata)*
Mugwort	Wintergreen
Mustard	Wormseed
Pennyroyal	Wormwood
Rue	

The following oils should not be used on pregnant women:

Aniseed	Marjoram
Basil	Myrrh
Cinnamon	Rose
Clary sage	Origanum
Cypress	Peppermint
Fennel	Rosemary
Hyssop	Sage
Jasmine	Thyme
Juniper	

Individuals with epilepsy should not use the following oils:

Camphor
Fennel
Hyssop
Sage
Rosemary

Carrier Oils

As mentioned, essential oils are mixed with a carrier oil. Carrier oils are high-quality, fresh vegetable oils that are used to dilute essential oils. Carrier oils also have their own therapeutic properties. The most popular carrier oils are listed in Box 11-12. Make sure all carrier oils are fresh and not rancid.

Aromatherapy Applications

Essential oils can be used in various ways in combination with hydrotherapy and massage.

- *Aromatic bath, hot tub or sauna:* Put 4 to 10 drops of essential oil in the water just before the person gets into it. Gently stir the water to disperse the oil. For a sauna, dilute the oil with 70% to 90% water and spray it on the rocks and into the air. The bottle must be shaken continually to keep the oil in suspension in the water.

BOX 11-12

Common Carrier Oils

Apricot kernel oil (*Prunus armeniaca*)	Extremely moisturizing; use to help revitalize dry skin, delicate skin, mature skin, and sensitive skin and to help soothe minor skin inflammations.
Avocado oil (*Persea americana*)	Rich in vitamins A, B₁, and B₂; excellent for cases of extremely dry skin (e.g., calluses on the feet). Use on dry, cracked, chapped, and irritated skin and for eczema and psoriasis.
Corn oil	Soothing for all skin types.
Evening primrose oil (*Oenothera biennis*)	Reduces the appearance of wrinkles; also beneficial for sluggish skin, scarring, inflammation, eczema, acne, and minor skin irritations.
Grapeseed oil (*Vitis vinifera*)	Used in most cosmetics as a base oil; use for thin skin around the eyes and for normal to combination skin as a light moisturizer.
Hazelnut oil (*Corylus avellana*)	Helps to tone and tighten skin and to restore elastin to the skin; use to help promote cell regeneration; apply on oily and combination skin.
Hemp seed oil (*Cannabis sativa*)	Penetrates the skin to moisturize, stimulate, and repair cells damaged by the elements, sun, wind, and ultraviolet light; useful for any skin type.
Jojoba golden (*Simmondsia chinensis*)	Similar to sebum (the oil human skin produces). Skin absorbs it very quickly, and no oily residue is left on the surface; good for dry, chapped, and cracked skin.
Olive oil	A heavy oil used in cosmetics and soaps; for massage, it is best blended with a lighter vegetable oil
Rose hip seed (*Rosa mosqueta*)	Has the highest natural vitamin C content of all the carrier oils and is a renowned cell-renewal agent. Use rose hip seed oil for scars, stretch marks, wrinkles, cracked skin, dry skin, and sunburn and to support collagen in the skin.
Sesame oil (*Sesamum indicum*)	Nourishes damaged skin. Use it on dry, chapped, discolored, flaky, sun-damaged and burned skin
Soybean oil	Used for mature skin
Sunflower oil (*Helianthus annuus*)	Has excellent healing properties. Use as a treatment for acne on the body and for accelerating the process of healing wounds and insect bites
Sweet almond oil (*Prunus dulcis*)	A favorite of massage therapists due to its nutritive and moisturizing qualities. Great for sensitive skin, sweet almond oil is high in vitamins A, B₁, B₆ and E. Use for dry skin, itchiness, and irritated and inflamed skin
Wheat germ oil (*Triticum vulgare*)	Known for its high content of vitamins E and C. Use this product on mature skin, wrinkles, sun damage, dark spots, eczema, psoriasis, premature aging, and stretch marks

- *Aromatic compress:* Put 3 to 5 drops of oil into 1 to 2 cups of hot or cold water, depending on the need for a compress. Fold a clean cloth and submerge it in the water, then squeeze the excess water from the compress into the basin. Apply immediately to the treatment area.
- *Aromatic facial steam:* Use 1 to 2 drops of oil per 1 cup of boiling water. Place the oil in the bowl or basin after the water has boiled. Stir the water to disperse the oil. Immediately place a towel over the head and place the face as close as possible to the aromatic steam without causing any discomfort. The usual method is to add 5 to 7 drops of oil or an oil blend to about 2 cups of hot water. First, bring the water to a boil and then let it cool for about 5 minutes. Add the oil or oil blend and inhale the vapors for about 5 to 10 minutes.
- *Environmental and room fragrance:* Electronic diffusers are an easy, effective way to fragrance a room for esthetic and therapeutic purposes. Use only pure essential oils or synergies of pure essential oils. Never use essential oils cut with carrier oils in diffusers, because this will clog the diffuser.
- *Aroma lamps:* Aroma lamps are great for adding environmental fragrance. Add 10 drops of essential oils to 1 tea-spoon of water and place in the designated receptacle on the lamp. The heat of the light will disperse the fragrance.
- *Inhalation.* Another effective and simple way to inhale essential oils is to place a couple drops of an oil or blend on a handkerchief or cotton cloth and inhale throughout the day. This is a nice gift for the person who just received the massage.
- *Aromatic spray:* Mix about 100 drops of essential oil (a single oil or a blend of oils) with 4 ounces of vodka. This creates a concentrate that can be added to water to create the aromatic spray. Add about 100 drops of the concentrate to 2 ounces of distilled water and shake well. To create a spritzer for the face or body, use only water and essential oils. For the body, add about 40 to 50 drops of essential oil or a blend to 4 ounces of distilled water. For the face, add 8 to 10 drops to 4 ounces of water.
- Massage: Use a dilution of about 1% to 2.5% of essential oil to carrier oil when preparing the massage oil. This means approximately 5 to 15 drops of essential oil per 1 ounce of carrier oil. If you are using more than one essential oil, blend them together first and then add no more than 15 drops of the blend to the carrier oil. Remem-

BOX 11-13

Therapeutic Qualities of Individual Essential Oils

Bergamot	Conditions skin, soothes, antiseptic, phototoxic
Cajeput	Stimulates, mood enhancer, antiseptic
Cardamom	Muscle relaxant, skin conditioner, soothing agent
Carrot seed	Muscle relaxant, soothing agent, skin conditioner
Cedarwood	Antiseptic, skin conditioner, deodorant, soothing agent
Clary sage	Skin conditioner, astringent, soothing agent, muscle relaxant. Do not use if pregnant or if drinking alcohol
Eucalyptus	Antiseptic, soothing agent, skin conditioner, sinus clearing
Frankincense	Skin conditioner, soothing agent
Geranium	Skin refresher, muscle relaxant
Ginger	Astringent
Grapefruit	Soothing agent, astringent, skin conditioner
Jasmine absolute	Emollient, soothing agent, antiseptic
Juniper	Skin detoxifier, astringent, soothing agent. Flammable
Lavender	Muscle relaxant, skin conditioner, soothing agent, astringent
Lemon	Soothing agent, antiseptic
Lemongrass	Skin conditioner, soothing agent, muscle relaxant, antiseptic
Lime	Soothing agent, skin conditioner, astringent
Mandarin	Soothing agent, skin conditioner, astringent
Myrrh	Antiinflammatory, emollient, antiseptic. Use in moderation if pregnant
Neroli	Antiseptic, emollient
Nutmeg	Antiseptic, soothes irritated skin, muscle relaxant
Orange	Astringent, soothing agent, skin conditioner
Peppermint	Emollient, antiseptic, muscle relaxant
Pine	Antiseptic
Roman chamomile	Muscle relaxant, skin conditioner
Rose absolute	Skin conditioner
Rose otto	Astringent
Rosemary	Antiseptic, muscle relaxant, soothing agent, skin conditioner. Do not use if pregnant or have high blood pressure
Rosewood	Muscle relaxant
Sandalwood	Antiseptic, emollient, soothing agent, skin conditioner
Spearmint	Emollient, astringent, soothing agent. Use sparingly
Tea tree	Antiseptic, acne fighter, dandruff fighter
Ylang-ylang	Reduces stress and tension

BOX 11-14

Oils for Emotional Well-Being

Anger	Bergamot, jasmine, orange, patchouli, rose, ylang-ylang
Anxiety	Clary sage, frankincense, geranium, lavender, mandarin, rose, sandalwood
Confidence	Bergamot, grapefruit, jasmine, orange, rosemary
Depression	Bergamot, clary sage, frankincense, geranium, grapefruit, jasmine, lavender, lemon, mandarin, neroli, orange, rose
Fatigue, exhaustion, and burnout	Bergamot, clary sage, frankincense, grapefruit, jasmine, lemon, peppermint, rosemary, sandalwood
Fear	Clary sage, frankincense, grapefruit, jasmine, lemon, neroli, orange
Grief	Frankincense, neroli, rose
Happiness, peace	Frankincense, geranium, grapefruit, lemon, neroli, orange, rose sandalwood, ylang-ylang
Insecurity	Frankincense, jasmine, sandalwood
Irritability	Lavender, mandarin, neroli, Roman chamomile, sandalwood
Loneliness	Bergamot, clary sage, frankincense, rose
Memory, concentration	Lemon, peppermint, rosemary
Stress	Bergamot, clary sage, frankincense, geranium, grapefruit, jasmine, lavender, mandarin, neroli, Roman chamomile, rose sandalwood, ylang-ylang

From "Aromatherapy for Emotional Well-Being," copyright Aroma Web, LLC at http://www.aroma.com/articles/emotional/wellbeing.asp

ber, when creating a massage blend, less is more, and in fact the desired result can be achieved with very low dilutions.

Choosing Essential Oils to Complement Massage

A number of factors can affect the selection of essential oils to be used for massage. The choice can be based on the therapeutic quality of the oil or oils (Box 11-13), the client's emotional well-being (Box 11-14), or the presence of a specific condition (Box 11-15).

As a general rule:

- Blend no more than three oils together.
- Offer a selection of oils you can tolerate (no more than 10).

- Let the client choose the oil.

Let the client sniff each oil; have the person choose one or two he or she really likes and then the one the individual least likes. Create a unique blend for the client with 2 drops of each of the preferred oils (four drops total) and 1 drop of the least favorite oil. Then:

- Blend the mixture into a carrier oil that is chosen on the basis of the client's skin type and the qualities of the carrier oil.
- Look up the characteristics of the oils with the client (see Box 11-13) and see how they relate to the client's current condition.

BOX 11-15

Essential Oils for Common Physical Conditions

Abdominal cramps	Lavender, clary sage
Acne	Bergamot, chamomile, geranium, lavender, patchouli, sandalwood, tea tree
Aging skin	Carrot seed, frankincense
Arthritis	Chamomile, eucalyptus, ginger
Athlete's foot	Tea tree
Brain fog	Grapefruit, lemongrass, lime, orange
Colds, flu, bronchitis	Cajeput, eucalyptus, frankincense, ginger, lavender, peppermint, tea tree
Corns, warts	Lemon, tea tree
Bruises	Chamomile, lavender
Burns	Lavender
Children's tummy upsets	Mandarin, tangerine
Cold sores	Eucalyptus, tea tree
Coughs	Eucalyptus, ginger, tea tree
Dandruff	Lavender
Dermatitis	Chamomile, lavender
Dry skin	Geranium (especially skin with oily patches), sandalwood
Dysmenorrhea (painful periods/menstrual cramps)	Chamomile, clary sage, cypress, lavender
Edema	Carrot seed, grapefruit
Fevers	Eucalyptus, lemongrass
Flatulence	Lime
Headache	Chamomile, lavender, peppermint
Herpes	Tea tree
High blood pressure (hypertension)	Lavender, ylang-ylang
Indigestion	Chamomile, orange
Inflammation	Chamomile, lavender
Insect bites and stings	Chamomile, lavender, tea tree
Insect repellent	Lemongrass, lavender
Insomnia	Chamomile, lavender
Laryngitis, sore throat	Ginger, lavender, thyme
Muscle aches and pains	Chamomile, eucalyptus, ginger, grapefruit, lavender, rosemary
Nausea	Chamomile, lavender
Nervous exhaustion, fatigue	Peppermint, rosemary
Nervous tension, stress	Chamomile, clary sage, frankincense, lavender, sandalwood
Neuralgia	Chamomile
Premenstrual syndrome (PMS)	Geranium, lavender
Poor circulation	Ginger, rosemary
Scars	Frankincense, lavender
Sinusitis	Eucalyptus, pine
Sprains, strains	Chamomile, eucalyptus, lavender
Stretch marks	Mandarin, lavender
Vertigo	Lavender, peppermint

■■■ SUMMARY

Each bodywork system is complete within itself; however, extensive overlap exists in both the application of techniques and physiologic effects. Although further study of the methods presented will benefit the massage professional, the ability to become proficient in the application of any of the systems, including therapeutic massage, is a lifelong study. Just as studying a foreign language tends to improve proficiency in a person's primary language, the study of bodywork systems complementary to therapeutic massage improves the understanding and technical application of massage methods. All bodywork systems are forms of structured professional touch that complement, not replace, each other. As massage and various bodywork methods become increasingly popular, the establishment that is responding most quickly is the health spa, which is described in Chapter 12.

The addition of these methods to the massage professional's skills can provide a more specific focus during the massage. For example, a client could enjoy a relaxing foot bath and sip a cup of hot tea while waiting for the appointment. The client and the massage therapist may drink a glass of pure water together. A cold compress could be placed on the back of the neck, the forehead, or other area of the body during the massage. Essential oils can be used as a room fragrance or added to the massage lubricant.

Use of gliding could be focused to move lymph and blood in the veins, whereas compression could move down the arteries to stimulate arterial blood flow.

Gliding, specifically applied into the grooves of the body, may stimulate the meridians. Compression, vibration, and tapping of the acupuncture points may normalize body function.

Kneading, stretching, and friction methods applied slowly and deliberately to drag, pull, and elongate might soften and normalize the connective tissue.

The occasional trigger point might be treated with direct pressure or frictioning, with a hot compress or stone applied afterward. An ice pack may sometimes be a better choice after frictioning to control the amount of inflammation.

Every joint in the hands and feet may be moved and attention given to compression on the bottoms of the hands and feet to stimulate the flow of lymph. The client can be instructed in deep breathing to further encourage lymph movement.

Various colors of sheets or soft lighting can be offered.

Awareness of the energy patterns of the body and the compassionate "laying on of hands" becomes part of every technique. Warm stones or seed bags can be placed on the traditional energy centers.

As a result of the massage interaction, the client should experience a pleasant, relaxed, and alert state in response to the physiologic shifts in the body.

REFERENCES

1. Buchman DD: *The complete book of water therapy: 500 ways to use our oldest natural medicine,* New York, 1979, EP Dutton.
2. Chaitow L: *The acupuncture treatment of pain,* Rochester, Vt, 1990, Healing Arts Press.
3. Chaitow L: *Soft-tissue manipulation,* Rochester, Vt, 1988, Healing Arts Press.
4. Chaitow L: *Workshop notes,* trigger point assessment and treatment Lapeer, Mich, 1988, 1991, 1992, 1993.
5. Chaitow L, Delany J: *Clinical application of neuromuscular techniques,* vol 1, The upper body, London, 2000, Churchill Livingstone.
6. The *Audubon Society field guide to North American rocks and minerals,* New York, 1979, Knopf.
7. Cunningham S: *Cunningham's encyclopedia of crystal, gem and metal magic,* Woodbury, Minnesota, 2002, Llewellyn Publications
8. Cyriax J, Coldham M: *The textbook of orthopaedic medicine treatment by manipulation massage and injection,* ed 11, vol 2, East Sussex, England, 1984, Bailliere Tindall.
9. Gunn C: *Reprints on pain, acupuncture and related subjects,* Seattle, 1992, University of Washington.
10. Yu HZ, Rose K: *Who can ride the dragon?* Brookline, Mass, 1999, Harcourt.
11. Johari H: *Ayurvedic massage: traditional Indian techniques for balancing body and mind,* Rochester, Vt, 1996, Healing Arts Press.
12. Kreighbaum E, Barthels KM: *Biomechanics: a qualitative approach for studying human movement,* ed 4, New York, 1995, Benjamin Cummings.
13. Lederman E: *Fundamentals of manual therapy: physiology, neurology, and psychology,* ed 2, New York, 2005, Churchill Livingstone.
14. Masunaga S, Ohashi W: *Zen shiatsu: how to harmonize yin and yang for better health,* New York, 1977, Japan Publications.
15. Myers T: *Anatomy trains: myofascial meridians for manual and movement therapists,* New York, 2001, Churchill Livingstone.
16. Ohashi W: *Do-it-yourself shiatsu: how to perform the ancient Japanese art of acupuncture without needles,* New York, 1993, Penguin Books.
17. Price S, Price L: *Aromatherapy for health professionals,* London, 1999, Churchill Livingstone.
18. Schnaubelt K: *Advanced aromatherapy: the science of essential oil therapy,* Rochester Vt, 1998, Healing Arts Press.
19. Tappan F, Benjamin P: *Tappan's handbook of healing massage techniques: classic, holistic, and emerging methods,* ed 4, New York, 2004, Appleton & Lange.
20. Tissarand R, Balacs T: *Essential oil safety,* New York, 1995, Churchill Livingstone.
21. Travell JG, Simons DG: *Myofascial pain and dysfunction: the trigger point manual,* vol 2, Baltimore, 1999, Williams & Wilkins.
22. Yao JH: Acutherapy, 1984, Acutherapy Postgraduate Seminars, 808 Paddock Lane, Libertyville, Ill 60048.
23. Veith I, Rose K: *The yellow emperor's classic of internal medicine,* Berkeley, Calif., 2002, University of California Press.
24. Watt M: Plant aromatics: a data and reference manual on essential oils and aromatic plant extracts http://atlanticinstitute.com/safety.html retrieved 10/2/07
25. Wiseman N, Feng Y: *A practical dictionary of Chinese medicine,* Brookline, Mass, 1997, Harcourt.
26. http://en.wikipedia.org/wiki/Minerals

evolve

11-1: The Evolve Web site presents a 2-minute video of the Thia massage and a section on the history of Thia technique.

11-2: The Evolve Web site presents a 2-minute video of the shiatsu technique.

11-3: Categorize the effects of hydrotherapy.

11-4: Study the therapeutic uses of water with electronic flashcards.

Don't forget to study for your certification and llcensure exams! Review questions for this chapter are located on Evolve.

BIBLIOGRAPHY

Anderson SK: *The practice of shiatsu,* St. Louis, 2008, Mosby.
Gold R: *Thai massage: a traditional medical technique,* ed. 2, St. Louis, 2007, Mosby.

ADDITIONAL RESOURCE

The International Medical Spa Association 310 17th Street, Union City, New Jersey 07087

Workbook Section

Answers for the Workbook Section for Chapter 11 are provided on p. 772.

■ ■ ■ SHORT ANSWER

1. Why is continuing education required to use the methods presented in this chapter effectively?

   _____

   _____

   _____

2. What are the primary effects of hydrotherapy?

   _____

   _____

   _____

3. What are some simple hydrotherapy methods the massage practitioner can use that do not require special hydrotherapy equipment?

   _____

   _____

   _____

4. What are some important contraindications to and precautions for the use of ice?

   _____

   _____

   _____

5. What are safety precautions for incorporating stones into a massage?

   _____

   _____

   _____

6. What is systemic massage, and what results can be expected from this type of massage?

   _____

   _____

   _____

7. What are the basic procedures for lymphatic massage?

   _____

   _____

   _____

8. What are the basic procedures for circulatory massage?

   _____

   _____

   _____

9. What are the physiologic mechanisms that make reflexology a valuable massage approach?

   _____

   _____

   _____

10. What are the recommended methods for foot massage?

    _____

    _____

    _____

11. Why is hand and foot self-massage beneficial?

    _____

    _____

    _____

12. What are connective tissue approaches?

    _____

    _____

    _____

13. What is the intent of connective tissue massage?

    _____

    _____

    _____

14. Why is additional education so important before using connective tissue approaches?

    _____

    _____

    _____

15. What is a trigger point?

    _____

    _____

    _____

16. How are trigger points located?

    _____

    _____

    _____

17. What methods are used to normalize trigger points?

    _____

    _____

    _____

Workbook Section—cont'd

18. What types of therapy follow treatment of a trigger point?

_____

_____

_____

19. What is the Western terminology for acupuncture points, meridians, and yin and yang?

_____

_____

_____

20. What wisdom is offered by the Eastern and Asian approaches for the massage practitioner?

_____

_____

_____

21. Where are acupuncture points located?

_____

_____

_____

22. How are acupuncture points treated?

_____

_____

_____

23. How does polarity therapy combine the knowledge base of both Asian and Ayurvedic systems?

_____

_____

_____

24. How is color an aspect of healing systems?

_____

_____

_____

25. What are the safety precautions for including essential oils in a massage?

_____

_____

_____

■■■ MATCHING I

Match the term to the best definition.

1. Acupressure
2. Ayurveda
3. Cryotherapy
4. Hydrotherapy
5. Myofascial release
6. Polarity therapy
7. Reflexology
8. Shiatsu
9. Systemic massage
10. Trigger point
11. Yang
12. Yin

a. In Eastern thought, the part of the whole realm of function of the body, mind, and spirit that corresponds to the parasympathetic autonomic nervous system functions
b. In Eastern thought, the part of the whole realm of function of the body, mind, and spirit that corresponds to the sympathetic autonomic nervous system functions
c. an area of local nerve facilitation that results in hypertonicity of a muscle bundle and referred pain patterns
d. therapeutic use of various types and temperatures of water applications
e. methods of toning or sedating acupuncture points that do not involve the use of needles
f. a system of health care that uniquely developed the tridosha system
g. the therapeutic use of ice
h. massage primarily structured to affect one body system; an approach usually used for lymphatic and circulation enhancement massage
i. a system of bodywork that affects the connective tissue through various methods that elongate and alter the plastic component and ground substance of the connective tissue
j. an eclectic system that combines principles of Asian theory and Ayurveda
k. a massage system directed primarily at the feet and hands
l. an acupressure- and meridian-focused bodywork system

■■■ MATCHING II

Various reflexes are associated with the feet. Match the reflex with its description.

1. Achilles tendon reflex
2. Extensor thrust reflex
3. Flexor withdrawal reflex
4. Mendel-Bekhterev reflex
5. Postural reflex
6. Proprioceptive reflex
7. Rossolimo's reflex

a. plantar flexion/extension of the foot resulting from contraction of calf muscles after a sharp blow to the Achilles tendon; similar to the knee-jerk reflex

b. flexion of the lower extremity when the foot receives a painful stimulus
c. plantar flexion of the toes in response to percussion of the dorsum of the foot
d. a quick, brief extension of a limb on application of pressure to the plantar surface
e. a reflex initiated by movement of the body to maintain the position of the moved part; any reflex initiated by stimulation of a proprioceptor
f. any reflex concerned with maintenance of posture
g. plantar flexion of the second to fifth toes in response to percussion of the plantar surface of the toes

■■■ LABELING

Label the muscles in Figure 11-41 to show the locations of common trigger points.

A. Abductor hallucis
B. Adductor longus
C. Anterior serratus
D. Biceps femoris
E. Deltoid
F. Gastrocnemius
G. Gluteus medius
H. Gluteus minimus
I. Iliocostalis
J. Infraspinatus
K. Levator
L. Long extensors
M. Longissimus
N. Masseter
O. Multifidus
P. Pectoralis
Q. Peroneus longus
R. Soleus
S. Splenius capitis
T. Sternocleidomastoid
U. Subscapularis
V. Supinators
W. Supraspinatus
X. Temporalis
Y. Tibialis anterior
Z. Trapezius
AA. Upper trapezius
BB. Vastus medialis

Workbook Section—cont'd

FIGURE 11-41

ADDITIONAL EXERCISE

The massage therapist must know the effects of the various forms and temperatures of hydrotherapy to achieve the desired results. For each desired result listed, put an X in the column or columns of the effects that would produce that result.

Desired Result	Effect of Heat	Effect of Cold	Effect of Ice
1. Increased circulation			
2. Decreased circulation			
3. Increased metabolism			
4. Decreased metabolism			
5. Increased stimulation			
6. Increased inflammation			
7. Decreased inflammation			
8. Decreased pain			
9. Decreased muscle spasm			
10. Decreased tissue stiffness			
11. Increased tissue stiffness			
12. Increased muscle tone			

■ ■ ■ PROBLEM-SOLVING EXERCISES

1. How can you tell the difference between a trigger point and an acupuncture point?

2. A client wants a general relaxation massage but has some mild circulatory sluggishness. What style of massage would you use to best serve the client?

■ ■ ■ ASSESS YOUR COMPETENCIES

Now that you have studied this chapter, you should be able to:

1. Understand the physiologic mechanisms of complementary bodywork systems.

2. Identify overlap in the technical skills among the various systems and integrate concepts of the styles into the therapeutic massage system.

3. Consider a direction of interest for further study.

On a separate sheet of paper, write a short summary of the content of this chapter based on the competencies listed above. When writing this paper, assume you are speaking to someone—a client, prospective employer, co-worker, or other interested person. Write the paper as if you were having a conversation and explaining the importance of the information and skills to professional massage development.

Next, in small student discussion groups, share the papers and compare and contrast how the information was presented.

Discuss the content, looking for similarities, differences, potential misunderstanding of the information, and clear and concise methods of description.

■ ■ ■ PROFESSIONAL APPLICATION EXERCISES

1. You are a massage therapist who has been in practice for about 3 years. An increasing number of your clients seem to have connective tissue problems. What types of continuing education would help you to work most effectively with these clients?

2. You have the opportunity to work in a pain management clinic with a team of health care professionals that consists of an osteopathic physician, a nurse practitioner, a psychologist, a physical therapist, an acupuncturist, and a nutritionist. Based on the information in this chapter, develop a presentation explaining the integration of complementary bodywork methods into massage therapy. (Use a separate piece of paper.) Include recommendations for additional education for yourself. Justify or explain the benefit of continuing education in one of the modalities discussed in this chapter. Explain why you think this method would offer the most benefit combined with therapeutic massage. Also, consider what other modalities the other bodywork professionals may be using in the clinic. Use the clinical reasoning model as you prepare your presentation.

CHAPTER 12

Massage Career Tracks and Massage for Special Populations

CHAPTER OBJECTIVES

After completing this chapter, the student will be able to perform the following:

- Identify the three main career tracks for massage: spas, sports and fitness, and health care
- Develop a massage environment that will best serve individuals with special needs
- Demonstrate the communication skills that are important for working with a client with special needs
- Gather information on additional training that can help the practitioner better serve clients with special needs

CHAPTER OUTLINE

THERAPEUTIC MASSAGE IN THE SPA ENVIRONMENT
    History of the Spa
    The Spa Industry
    Massage Therapy in the Spa
    The Spa Language
    Hydrotherapy
    Aromatherapy
    Products

THERAPEUTIC MASSAGE IN THE HEALTHCARE
    ENVIRONMENT
    Clinical/Medical Massage
    Integrating Massage into the Healthcare Setting
    Best Practice
    Health Insurance
    Record Keeping (Documentation)
    Massage Career in Health Care
    Compatibility of Massage and Health Care

THERAPEUTIC MASSAGE IN THE SPORTS AND FITNESS
    ENVIRONMENT
    Common Goals and Outcomes for Massage in Sports
      and Fitness
    Types of Sports Massage
    The Sports Massage Team

SPECIAL POPULATIONS
ANIMAL MASSAGE
    Communication
    Massage Benefits for Animals
    Animals That Benefit from Massage
    Pain Management
    Rehabilitative Massage
    Providing Massage for Animals
    Body of Knowledge for Animal Massage

ATHLETES
    Common Sports Injuries
    Ongoing Care of the Athlete

BREAST MASSAGE
    Ethical Considerations in Breast Massage

CHILDREN

CHRONIC ILLNESS

THE ELDERLY

INFANTS

ON SITE MASSAGE

PHYSICALLY CHALLENGED INDIVIDUALS
    Personal Awareness
    Supporting Clients with a Visual Impairment
    Supporting Clients with a Speech Impairment
    Supporting Clients with a Hearing Impairment
    Supporting Clients with a Mobility Impairment
    Supporting Clients with a Size Impairment
    Supporting Clients with Burns and Disfigurements
    Barrier-Free Access

PSYCHOLOGICALLY CHALLENGED INDIVIDUALS
    The Importance of Informed Consent
    Addictions
    Chemical Imbalances in the Brain
    Developmental Disabilities
    Learning Disorders
    Psychiatric Disorders
    Post-traumatic Stress Disorder

KEY TERMS

Abuse
Acute illness
Alternative
Anxiety
Athlete

Chronic illness
Complementary
Complementary and alternative medicine (CAM)
Depression
Dissociation
Mental impairment
Pain and fatigue syndromes
Panic
Physical disability
Post-traumatic stress disorder (PTSD)
Recovery massage
Re-enactment
Remedial massage
Spa
State-dependent memory
Trauma

12-1

The three main career tracks for massage can be categorized as follows:

- Wellness/spa massage
- Health care (clinical/medical) massage
- Sports performance and fitness massage

These career tracks typically are defined more by the location where the massage is provided, common outcomes requested for the massage, and parameters that define a specific population. However, the massage application does not vary extensively; gliding remains gliding, joint movement is still joint movement, and ethics, professionalism, and concern and compassion for the client do not change.

The current kaleidoscope of massage practice can create much confusion for the massage student, the massage practitioner, potential employers, and the consumer. The trend is for all the outcomes, environments, and populations to overlap. For example:

- Scar tissue management for cosmetic surgery may be combined with general full-body massage in a medical spa; this appears to be a case of clinical/medical massage, but it takes place in the spa setting.
- Restorative massage with essential oils and soft music and lighting may be provided to support relaxation and sleep for an athlete after a competition; this appears to be spa focused, but the population is sports and fitness.
- Massage to increase flexibility, improve posture and gait, and provide lymphatic drainage may be done to address soreness after exercise for participants in a cardiac rehabilitation program; this appears to be sports and fitness targeted, but the massage is provided in the clinical/medical setting.

What determines the focus of the massage? The most obvious response is the domain. The health care/medical environment consists of health care professionals who work in various settings, such as hospitals, physical therapy clinics, and specialty centers (e.g., cancer treatment or dialysis); as private practice physicians; and in hospice and long-term care.

The sports and fitness environment consists of fitness centers, academic sports facilities (e.g., for high school track or collegiate gymnastics), and centers for professional or semiprofessional athletes (e.g., golfers, football players, soccer players, baseball players, and so on). These facilities are staffed by professionals, such as exercise specialists, athletic trainers, and coaches. In addition, the needs of individuals who exercise for fitness and those of recreational and mature athletes must be addressed.

The spa environment is extremely varied. It includes local day spas and chain spas in various resorts, hotel chains, and cruise ships. The focus of a massage in the spa setting can be:

- To serve as an adjunct to cosmetic procedures performed by professionals such as cosmetologists, estheticians, and nail technicians
- To serve as an adjunct to hydrotherapy treatments for the purposes of relaxation and detoxification
- To support antiaging programs
- To serve as part of the program at a retreat center
- To support a weight management program

Regardless of the setting, the spa environment has several consistent characteristics: ambience; a peaceful, pleasant location; pampering; and multiple services that can be selected from a spa menu. The spa environment is more commercial and entrepreneurial than the sports and fitness and health care environments. The spa environment deals with strategic marketing. The spa industry is extremely innovative in creating branded (also called *signature*) products and services that identify the uniqueness of the particular spa.

For each of these three main environments, the massage student must learn the particular focus, the roles of the various professionals, and how massage fits into and supports multidisciplinary care. Regardless of the environment, each client must be addressed according to his or her unique situation. For each of the populations discussed, the chapter describes the adaptations and accommodations that may be necessary for the individual client, regardless of the environment in which the massage is provided. The chapter first discusses the three basic environments of massage practice and then addresses the unique needs of special populations.

THERAPEUTIC MASSAGE IN THE SPA ENVIRONMENT

SECTION OBJECTIVES

Using the information presented in this section, the student will be able to perform the following:

- Describe various spa settings
- Describe the unique aspects of massage in the spa environment
- Use various massage and bodywork methods in the spa environment
- Alter fundamental massage training to the specific requirements of an individual spa

As mentioned, the spa industry is extremely innovative at creating signature products and services that become unique signifiers of the particular spa. Because the pressures of modern lifestyles and daily activities are becoming ever more stressful, the spa concept of a health retreat has mushroomed in popularity. Historically, American spas have not been as "cure" oriented as European spas; rather, they are more fitness and beauty oriented. However, American spas are converting quickly to an integrated system.

Of the three main career tracks, the spa track is the most difficult for therapeutic massage education and training. Although the basic massage procedures in this textbook form the foundation of the various styles of massage offered in the spa environment, each spa creates its own presentation by offering various combinations of services (see Chapter 11). For example:

- Aromatherapy massage may be provided with a signature blend of essential oils developed by the spa.
- The spa may provide a signature massage style that uses aspects of Eastern and Western methods and combine it with color therapy to promote deep relaxation and support rejuvenation of the body.
- Massage with hot stones may be combined with cold hydrotherapy and meditative music created specifically for the spa to provide relaxation and introspection for self-enlightenment.
- The spa may provide historical or culturally based massage (e.g., Amma, Lomi Lomi, Thai massage, shiatsu, or Swedish massage).

Massage students interested in the complex, ever-changing spa environment must understand the following:

- The underlying general themes of the spa industry
- How uniqueness in environment and services is developed and implemented
- The foundation of the general categories of massage application in the spa industry
- The application and benefits of spa services other than massage

With this knowledge and the appropriate skills, the massage graduate should be able to easily adapt to a specific spa and the in-house training it provides. The massage professional should be able to perform to the expectations of the spa.

Therapeutic massage as presented in this text is the foundation of spa-based massage. Practitioners also must understand the physical effects of hydrotherapy, the various common and safe essential oils, and the use of adjunct implements, products, and methods (e.g., stones, scrubs, muds and clays, magnets, vibration methods, color, and sound). They also must understand how these methods are combined to create the signature massage style offered by the spa. Much of this information was presented in Chapter 11.

It is important that the student understand the history of spas, the general types of spas, and the common populations drawn to various spa environments. The student also must learn about the professional behavior, ethics, and business strategies characteristic of the spa environment.

History of the Spa

Although the popularity of spas seems to have sprung up overnight, people have been visiting some form of spa for thousands of years. The word spa is rooted in the Latin language and means *salus per aquam*, or health from water. The use of water as therapy can be traced back to early civilizations (see Chapter 11). Throughout history, the different time periods brought different meanings and purposes for a bath or spa. Social bathing was an important cultural process practiced by the Mesopotamians, Egyptians, Minoans, Greeks, and Romans whenever they sought health and relief from pain and disease.[1] The natural hot springs in Bath, England, were used by the Romans and are recognized for their therapeutic properties. At Bath, the springs generate more than 1 million gallons of mineral water at a temperature of 120° F each day. This mineral water contains numerous elements, such as magnesium, potassium, sulfur, and calcium.

Native Americans also found medicinal waters and used them for regeneration and physical and spiritual health. Colonists often would build log cabins and wooden tubs for bathing near these sites. Eventually, baths and spas became more than just places near hot springs; they evolved into resorts.

Current trends in the spa environment indicate an interesting combination of ancient traditions from many cultures and modern scientific research. Recently many additions have been made to spa water therapies; these have come as a result of advances in technology that allow the therapeutic use of water in every spa willing to invest in the cost and maintenance of the various types of equipment available. For example, a hot tub can replace the hot spring. Nowadays hot water is common; in previous centuries, hot water in nature was rare, and the process of heating water was time-consuming and labor intensive.

During the eighteenth and nineteenth centuries, spas began to be staffed by medical professionals who prescribed and carefully monitored the treatments given to each visitor. The treatments primarily consisted of either soaking in the water or drinking it.

With the medical discoveries of the early twentieth century, hospitals replaced the spas. Existing spas changed focus and began offering luxury accommodations, and many eventually turned into vacation locations or clinics that concentrated on weight loss or catering to the wealthy. In recent years, the value of prevention, healthy lifestyles, and relaxation has been rediscovered, and the spa is again finding its place as a location uniquely qualified to address these needs. The spa industry is embracing holistic health care and wellness. Today the spa is returning to its roots; the medical spa is a growing industry.

The Medical Spa

A medical spa is a facility that operates under the full-time, on site supervision of a licensed health care professional. The facility operates within the scope of practice of its staff (e.g., dermatology, cosmetic surgery, weight loss) and offers traditional, complementary, and alternative health practices and treatments in a spalike setting.[2] Medical spas can be classified as integrative health and wellness spas or cosmetic medical spas. The cosmetic spa provides services related to beauty and appearance, whereas the wellness spa provides services related to education and guidance on choices affecting healthy living and longevity.

Medical spas and the use of alternative medical therapies have been increasing in popularity. Treatments at medical spas include herbal therapies, chiropractic treatments, self-help imagery, hypnosis, homeopathy, biofeedback, acupuncture, massage, and energy healing. Medical spas are also becoming very popular as adjuncts to plastic surgery, dentistry, chiropractic, dermatology, and antiaging medical practices.

Antiaging medicine is a major focus of the medical spa. It encompasses lifestyle change through education and counseling, hormone replacement therapies (as determined by a physician through laboratory testing), nutrition, antioxidants and vitamin supplements to reduce free radical damage, and clinical tests related to antiaging.

Medical cosmetic procedures include cellulite treatments; Botox injection; laser hair removal; microdermabrasion; waxing and sugaring; permanent makeup application; electrolysis; hydrotherapy; sclerotherapy/vein therapy; collagen injections and fillers; chemical peels; and photorejuvenation, such as ClearLight (a machine that uses different types of low-level lasers to treat acne) and Relume (a machine that uses different types of low-level lasers to treat stretch marks and remove scars).

Cosmetic surgical procedures offered at some medical spas include liposuction, liposculpture, lipoplasty, breast augmentation (breast implants), breast reduction, gynecomastia (reduction of enlarged, femalelike breasts in men), facelift, rhinoplasty (nose job), mastopexy (breast lift), lip augmentation, abdominoplasty (tummy tuck), blepharoplasty (eyelid surgery), brow lifts, forehead lifts, facial contouring, facial implants, scar revision, hair restoration, and thermage. Cosmetic dentistry is also popular.

Spa services at a medical spa include facials, massage, manicures and pedicures, waxing, body scrubs, body masks, wraps, muds, self-tanning, aromatherapy, reflexology, and Vichy showers and other hydrotherapy treatments.

Another component of the medical spa environment is the integrative health and wellness center. Integrative health centers incorporate all aspects of wellness, including body therapies, fitness, yoga and meditation, nutrition, and spirituality. A guest-centered approach, rooted in education, proactive wellness, and preventive wellness, is the cornerstone of programs that address the whole person. A comprehensive program that includes both Eastern traditions and Western scientific advances provides guests with a guided approach to personal well-being. A highly trained staff, under the guidance of a physician, creates customized programs based on the needs of the individual for optimum health and wellness. These centers use a multidisciplinary approach consisting of a medical team trained in complementary and alternative medicine and specialized service providers in preventive medicine, fitness, and spa services.

Massage is a very important aspect of the medical spa. It supports general healing responses and aids in the management of postprocedural pain. It also can manage postprocedural edema and support the development of supple scar tissue.

Concern recently has developed about appropriate practice in the medical spa. No statistics are available on exactly how many medical spas there are, because no official definition of a medical spa exists, and no single licensing body regulates them. Some are concerned that unlicensed professionals are performing medical procedures and that the environment may not be maintained in a medically appropriate, safe, and sanitary manner (Box 12-1).

Health Regulations and the Spa. In April, 2003, new regulations were issued under the Health Insurance Portability and Accountability Act (HIPAA) that may affect spa practice in some cases.

Essentially, HIPAA's health information privacy rules are designed to ensure the protection and security of medical records and other personal health information and to protect an individual's right to privacy in matters involving health care. The HIPAA rules apply to all "covered entities," defined as health plans, health care clearinghouses, and health care providers that transmit any health information in electronic form in connection with a list of specified transactions. In general, if the spa company does not bill or receive payment for health care in the normal course of business, the HIPAA requirement may not apply. Regardless, privacy and client confidentiality are essential aspects of ethical professional practice.

The Spa Industry

The spa industry is one of the fastest growing career options for massage therapists. Because of the increased pace and multiple stresses of modern life, people have both a need and a desire for effective relaxation to counteract or reverse life pres-

Courtesy of the International Medical Spa Association

BOX 12-1

Focus and Code of Ethics of the International Medical Spa Association

Recognizing the importance of bringing together the health care and spa industries in a way that will ensure the quality of care available to consumers, medical spa industry leaders, including licensed health care professionals, spa owners, spa consultants, medical spa facility designers, and product manufacturers, have come together to form the Medical Spa Association.

Our members, professionals with health care or spa experience, are working together to develop and implement programs that will help shape the future of the medical spa industry. They have decided to pool their expertise and resources to form an active, well-informed association that will assist its members in integrating the worlds of medicine and the spa.

The Medical Spa Association is dedicated to the creation of a positive industry image and the enhancement of those who serve it through the development, implementation, and continuous evaluation of a practical but strict code of ethics based on the highest standards of care and regulated peer review.

Code of Ethics

- A member of the Medical Spa Association and staff will provide competent care, delivered with respect for clients' dignity and rights.
- A member of the Medical Spa Association and staff will provide only those treatments, products, and services that are safe, effective, and of the highest quality.
- A member of the Medical Spa Association and staff will uphold the highest standards of professionalism, be

honest in all professional interactions, and shall not engage in fraudulent, deceptive, or unethical practices.

- A member of the Medical Spa Association and staff will make a commitment to ongoing education, to the application of that knowledge toward improving services and treatments, and to making the most accurate information available to its clients and the public as a whole.
- A member of the Medical Spa Association and staff will respect the rights of clients and staff to confidentiality and privacy.
- A member of the Medical Spa Association and staff will adhere to the laws, rules, and regulations governing the provision of treatments and services as required by the state in which the facility operates.
- A member of the Medical Spa Association and staff will respect and value the community in which the facility operates and look for opportunities to actively support and improve the health and well-being of that community.

The Medical Spa Association defines a medical spa as one that is operated by a licensed health care professional, a broad definition that can include physicians, registered nurses, physical therapists, nutritionists, and others. Most spas are licensed and regularly inspected by the state cosmetology board, the same agency that oversees hair and nail salons. However, even those in the spa industry acknowledge that cosmetology does not encompass all the high-tech treatments that spas often deliver.

---

sures. People go to spas for fitness, stress management, peace of mind, pampering and pleasure, and health and wellness (Box 12-2).

The wide range of treatments offered in spas includes wet treatments (e.g., wet table with Vichy shower and/or hydrotherapy), dry treatments (e.g., massage and body wraps), wellness therapies (e.g., oxygen inhalation), and health assessments, in addition to beauty treatments. Typically, a sauna, steam room, and spa pool are found at a spa. Although hydrotherapy is still regarded as an important treatment, spas no longer need to use or be near mineral water. Also, not all spas focus on hydrotherapy as a main component of treatment.

Spa Treatments

Spa treatments are basically the services that a spa provides. The most popular service in the spa is therapeutic massage. The second most popular service is the facial, which involves skin analysis, deep cleansing, massage, extractions (removal of blackheads and other impurities), toning, and moisturizing.

Body treatments basically are facials for the whole body. The most popular body treatment is a body scrub, an exfoliating treatment in which the technician rubs off the outermost

layer of dead skin cells, leaving the skin feeling soft and renewed. Medicinal salts typically are used as an abrasive to scrub the body.

A body wrap is a treatment in which products such as mud, algae, or seaweed are applied to the body, which is then wrapped in sheets, plastic, or some other covering. Wraps are thought to detoxify the body because they stimulate blood circulation and the lymphatic system. A rich cream or oil is used to soften and condition the skin and acts as a hydrating treatment.

Most but not all spas offer spa manicures and spa pedicures. Day spas with salons offer hair styling services.

You can do an Internet search to learn more about the spa industry. You will be surprised at the many different applications of the same procedures. Start by visiting the Web site www.spaassociation.com.

The Spa Signature

Spas offer a variety of treatments along with products to meet their clients' needs and expectations. Each spa approach tends to be unique to the spa (i.e., signature treatments, or branding). Services attempt to balance scientific advances and clinical treatments with ancient wisdom and alternative approaches

BOX 12-2

Spa Specifics

Spa environments address the senses of sight, smell, hearing, taste, and touch. Examples include:

Sight: Use of color and light
Smell: Essential oils and flowers
Hearing: Music and wind chimes
Taste: Herbal teas and juice drinks
Touch: Massage and fascial

Signature spa services feature unique combinations to target the five senses:

Product-related
Smell: product fragrance
Touch: texture and application of product

Hydrotherapy-related
Sight: scenery (i.e., mountain view)
Smell: smell of natural sulphur springs
Hearing: waterfall, fountain

Taste: mineral waters, flavored waters
Touch: whirlpool, showers

Culture-related
Sight: plants, ethnic dress
Smell: local flowers, incense
Hearing: ethnic music
Taste: ethnic food and drinks
Touch: cultural-based bodywork (i.e., shiatsu, lomi lomi)

Spa services and environments should be targeted to populations based on:
Geography (i.e., rural, agricultural, urban, resort)
Outcomes desired: pampering, fitness, skin care, detoxification, longevity, vacation
Age: adolescent, middle-aged, elderly
Gender-specific needs: athletes, pregnancy, cosmetic surgery

to total skin and body care. A spa should be staffed with people who are educated, licensed, or certified as necessary. As mentioned previously, this is the reason it is almost impossible for a therapeutic massage education program to train the graduate specifically for a career in the spa industry. Massage professionals who are successful in the spa environment have a solid foundation both in the fundamentals of massage application and in adjunct methods such as hydrotherapy and aromatherapy.

Trends. The spa industry currently is very fragmented, but it is beginning to show signs of stabilization (Box 12-3). An increasingly sophisticated consumer is requiring a more sophisticated spa experience. The industry is responding through a market-specific focus by creating spas with specialized services such as teen spas, men-only spas, spas for expectant mothers, and even spas that provide services for pets. A broader population is being introduced to spa services, primarily through the resort and day spa industry.

As mentioned, a *brand* is a collection of products created and marketed for a specific spa business. Building a brand becomes increasingly important both for independent spa businesses and for large chains, such as branded hotel companies. The users of both day spas and resort spas rely on the strength and reputation of the brand. The challenge for spa management is to maintain brand standards internationally in the new global economy. Standardization in service delivery is essential.

The development of clearly identifiable, branded spas will lead the way for consolidation in the spa industry. Chain spas

are becoming popular, therefore it is critical that throughout the process of brand development, companies consider targeting specific markets or appealing to a mass market. This trend is apparent with companies such as Stiener, Bliss, Starwood and Willow Stream, and Fairmont. The luxury-segment market leaders, such as Mandarin Oriental, Four Seasons, and Ritz-Carlton, can expand their spas internationally by creating an additional brand to support the spa operations. As consumers develop loyalty to specific spa brands, it will become increasingly crucial for each spa to develop its signature, consistently delivered regardless of location.

This need for consistency will influence many aspects of massage. With regard to massage education, the stated focus of this text is that massage application needs to be based on client goals and individualized for each client. In the spa environment, the massage therapist may be expected to perform standardized protocols that are based on the spa's signature approach rather than client goals. The massage therapist must learn these protocols and structure the massage application according to the spa's direction. At times this may be frustrating, such as when a client has chosen a specific type of massage and the massage therapist does not believe that the protocol best fits the client. The therapist may be tempted to change the protocol to meet the client's needs, only to discover that spa management expects consistency in the application of protocols.

Usually a middle ground can be found between massage-specific protocols and massage based on client outcomes. Massage therapists must be willing to modify their specific style of massage in order to replicate the spa-designed protocols; they must maintain a unique application for each client

BOX 12-3

International Spa Association 2004 Consumer Trends Report

Executive Summary
During the months of April through July, 2004, the Hartman Group conducted ethnographic and qualitative research among spa-going consumers in Los Angeles, Houston, Atlanta, Chicago, Minneapolis, Boston, and Seattle.

There emerged a segment of "core" spa goers who typically believe that spas are an integral part of health and wellness (physical, mental, emotional, and spiritual). They have become fluent in the ritual, language, and behaviors of the spa and have incorporated these philosophies into a way of living. However, these consumers represent a very small percentage of the total population. Instead, most spa goers are still infrequent day spa users interested in indulgence, an escape, and perhaps specific benefits associated with work such as relief of headaches, softening of tight shoulders, or stress reduction. They are thinking about the near-term benefits of spa services. These benefits usually are defined on their terms, which mean that they are most likely to approach spas with a "get in, get my pampering, get out" perspective as opposed to a long-term, holistic approach to overall health and well-being.

The following key findings, taken from the body of the report, affect massage therapy.

1. Consumers generally want "bread and butter" services (e.g., facials, pedicures and manicures, and basic massage) at day spas.
2. Consumers experiment more when at spas on vacation and expect a broader array of authentic, indigenous bodywork, as well as health- and wellness-oriented services.
3. Most spa consumers appreciate highly refined entrance and transition experiences in spas, regardless of their level of experience. Interior design and ritual are the keys to loyalty among all spa goers.
4. Spa goers are generally price sensitive when they consider services beyond the basics. Price is also a barrier when they receive services more than once a month.

Consumers motivated to visit spas incorporate one or more of the following into their spa experience:
- Indulgence (i.e., activities that are pleasurable, fun, and appealing to the senses)
- Escape (i.e., activities that relieve the pressures of everyday life)
- Self-improvement (e.g., individual work related to improvement of some aspect of the person's body, emotional state, or long-term spiritual and personal dispositions)

As the spa industry continues to grow and expand to include mainstream consumers and their health and wellness regimens, therapists' credentials, as well as the overall effectiveness of the spa experience (e.g., menus, pricing, environment, "extras") will come under greater scrutiny by all consumers. The desire for human interaction, personalization, and customization will become important factors in consumers' decision making. These factors often run counter to rapid industry growth.

Broader Cultural Trends in Spa Going
The following broad cultural trends intersect with the spa environment, and spas need to pay attention to them as they evolve and market themselves to the wider public.
- The reawakening of male grooming
- Mother-daughter bonding
- Gender-neutral interior design
- An interest in the local and the indigenous in food, furniture, design, and services
- Minimizing retail product choice and maximizing the purchase of signature products
- Customization

North American Spa Industry: Fast Facts

Spa Locations
An estimated 14,600 spas operate throughout the United States, and 2800 operate in Canada, and the numbers are growing. In the United States the largest spa category is the day spa. Geographically, the distribution of spas in the United States generally reflects the distribution of the population, with the Southwest being the largest region. In Canada, spas are concentrated in Ontario, British Columbia, and Quebec.

Spa Visits
Consumers made approximately 111 million spa visits in the United States in 2006; 60% of these were to day spas, and 27% were to resort or hotel spas.

Revenue
The U.S. spa industry generated an estimated $9.4 billion in revenue in 2003. On average, about half of a spa's revenue (52%) derives from massage treatments. Day spas account for more than half (56%) of the industry's revenues.

Square Footage
The U.S. spa industry occupies an estimated 56 million square feet of indoor space. Day spas account for 62% of industry space. On average, 48% of the space in U.S. and Canadian spas is occupied by treatment rooms.

Employment
An estimated 232,700 people are employed by the U.S. spa industry. Fifty percent of these are full-time employees, 31% are part-time employees, and 18% are on contract. Employee wages and salaries totaled approximately $4.9 billion in 2003.

Courtesy of the International Spa Association, Lexington, Kentucky, 2006.

based on focused intent and subtle shits in pressure, rhythm, and so on while maintaining the integrity of the spa protocol. Signature spas must be able to assure clients that regardless of who the massage therapist is, the product of massage will remain consistent. Recruitment, specific on site training for signature methods and products, and retention of massage therapists who find satisfaction in this career environment will become the ultimate challenges of the spa business.

Credentialing in the Spa Industry

Spa training and certification are in the very beginning stages. Spa Secure, introduced in July, 2004, is an international credentialing system. Spa Secure is a self-regulating organization that works in cooperation with state and federal agencies such as the Public Health Department and the Board of Barbers and Cosmetologists.

Spa Secure performs on site inspections of spas to check for unsafe practices and to evaluate sanitation procedures, health and safety measures, and scope of practice issues. A test is administered to the management and technical staff of the spa. Ongoing quality is monitored through unannounced mystery shopping of the facility to check for consistency in safety and the quality of operations (Box 12-3).

Massage Therapy in the Spa

Students who are competent in the application of the lessons in this text, as well as in anatomy and physiology, are prepared to enter spa employment upon graduation from a 500- to 1,000-hour therapeutic massage program. This text does not attempt to present specific spa procedures; however, the information prepares you to be easily and effectively trained in the signature treatments provided at individual spas. Little would be gained by trying to present specific spa massage applications in this textbook, because the spa industry is very competitive, and each spa is always trying to outdo the competition. This means that each spa makes up its own procedures, menus, and product use. To work in a spa, the massage practitioner must be able to figure out the underlying premise of the signature treatment. For massage practitioners, the foundation is solid application of full-body massage, as presented in this text. Many spa treatments that are not related to massage are based on hydrotherapy, therefore spending extra time studying this information (see Chapter 11) is a prudent course of action. In addition, many spa treatments target the skin, therefore the wise student will spend extra time studying the integumentary system and the lymph and blood circulations, as presented both in this text and in *Mosby's Essential Sciences for Therapeutic Massage* (or a similar science text).

Think of the career situation in massage as something like a sandwich. The "filling" is always the same (i.e., the information presented in this text and in *Mosby's Essential Sciences for Therapeutic Massage*); however, each practitioner may choose a different "bread" (i.e., clinical/medical massage, sports massage, or spa massage). When you graduate from a well-designed and well-implemented massage curriculum, you should have the "filling" in this professional sandwich; this chapter provides an overview of the "bread."

Massage Education Level

Massage therapists employed by the spa industry should be licensed by the appropriate government agency and/or should have national certification from the appropriate certifying agency. Sophisticated spas expect the massage therapists they employ to have educational credentials and practical experience, and they also expect their employees to pass standardized testing. A therapist's expertise typically is determined by the number of hours the technician attended school to obtain a license, the number of total years in practice, and the types and extent of continuing education obtained after graduation.

Types of Spas

There are many variations on the spa theme. Therapeutic massage is one of the unifying services found in almost all spa environments. The basic spa classifications are as follows:

- *Resort spas* are located on the property of a hotel, normally in a resort where other sports and activities are offered in addition to the spa program. Spa guests and hotel guests intermingle.
- *Amenity spas* are similar to resort spas in that the actual goal of management is to add the spa as an amenity to the hotel. Thus the spa is not necessarily viewed as a profit center as seriously as are some resort spas.
- *Destination spas* are a hotel property geared specifically to the spa guest and spa program. Outside guests are not normally part of the program. Everything is geared toward the spa and its program.
- *Fitness and beauty spas* are low- to high-priced spas that emphasize physical fitness, nutrition, beauty, and relaxation.
- *Luxury spas* are high-priced spas with posh surroundings that offer an array of state-of-the-art facilities and services.
- *Weight loss spas* cater specifically to those interested in losing weight, using a variety of methods, such as medically supervised dieting, behavioral modification, exercise, detoxification, fasting, and so on.
- *Medical wellness spas* enlist the services of physicians to assist guests in achieving optimal health and well-being. The emphasis in these spas is on prevention and lifestyle changes rather than on treatment of acute illness. Programs include back care, sports medicine, physical therapy, lifestyle education, stress management and risk reduction, smoking cessation, heart-healthy regimens, and so on.
- *New age spas* provide a wide range of alternatives to more traditional spas and focus on such elements as spiritual awareness, the body/mind connection, holistic health, yoga, vegetarianism, acupuncture, aromatherapy, reflexology, tai chi, transcendental meditation, and so on.
- *Adventure spas* focus on customers interested in various outdoor activities such as hiking, rafting, mountain biking, skiing, mountain climbing, and fishing.
- *Mineral spring spas* are built around naturally occurring hot or cold water springs rich in minerals. In addition

to mineral springs, some of these spas offer mud and thalassotherapy (sea water treatments), herbal wraps, saunas, and a host of other services typically found in spas.

- *Spas at sea* or *spa cruises* are a new category that recently has been added because of the increasing popularity of cruise vacations. Some large cruise ships offer spa services and packages as part of their regular voyages.
- *Day* (or *urban*) *spas* offer one-day service. The client spends the day receiving various spa treatments, breakfast and lunch are provided, and activities such as aerobics and yoga are included. These are local, "in and out" spas.

Spa Safety

Regardless of the focus of the spa, some aspects of the spa experience should be consistent to ensure the safety and comfort of the spa client. For example, spa sanitation considerations include the following:

- Clean, unused linens and spa wear
- Sanitized, clean, uncluttered work surfaces
- Sealed containers for implements such as cotton balls and facial pads
- Professional products that are single use or that have been taken from a larger container without coming in contact with an unsanitary or nonsterile surface
- Disposable tools and implements for any procedure that requires breaking the surface of the skin
- Cleaning of implements with a hospital-grade disinfectant, sanitization by ultraviolet (UV) light or a similar piece of equipment, or sterilization in an autoclave
- Requirement that technicians provide spa treatments with freshly washed and dried hands or while wearing surgical gloves
- Sealed and covered waste receptacles and laundry bins
- Tools and products that are clearly labeled and safely stored

All of the safety and sanitation requirements for massage therapists described in this text are applicable.

Spa Etiquette

Spa services should be provided as they are described in any promotional or informational materials and in a timely fashion. Furthermore, services should be provided in a safe, clean environment that respects privacy. Professional standards of behavior should be maintained at all times by the attending technicians, therapists, and staff. The staff must be sufficiently educated and experienced so that they can answer personal care and medical-related questions, provide guidance on appropriate treatments for specific needs, and make home care recommendations.

Spa service professionals, including massage therapists, usually are expected to wear a uniform specific to the organization. Massage therapists should always behave in an ethical and professional manner; they should be impeccably groomed, friendly, pleasant, and timely (i.e., maintain appropriate time management for sessions).

Other considerations are also important:

- A guest/client is expected to give at least 24 hours' notice of a cancellation and should arrive 5 to 10 minutes before the appointment time.
- Most spas require the client to fill out a medical evaluation form designed to reveal any concerns that might be contraindications to treatments. It is the client's responsibility (and it is in the person's best interest) to fill out this form as accurately as possible.
- Dress and conduct specifications should be indicated on informational materials. In most spas, spa wear (e.g., robe, slippers) and the necessary items for enjoying the visit are all provided by the spa. If the client is particularly modest and would like to remain clothed at all times, she may want to bring a swimsuit. Jewelry and valuables should always be left at home.

The spa setting is based on client service and satisfaction. The concept of pampering is an important aspect of spa services. Some aspects of service and pampering include the following:

- Greet the client with a warm handshake and a smile. If time allows, ask if the client would like to sit in the steam room, dry sauna, or even the hot tub before the treatment. Offer the client ice water while he or she is relaxing before the treatment.
- Make sure the client is completely comfortable and at ease. The atmosphere should be warm, quiet, and comfortable, with soft music and lighting.
- Use warm towels and warm or cold eye packs during treatments.
- When the treatment is finished, meet the client outside after he or she has put on a robe. Offer tea, cookies, fresh fruit, or water. If the client accepts, the spa staff should "serve" the client the refreshment. In this way, the client feels very special. If the client declines any refreshment, walk the person to the sauna area or locker room and bid him or her a fond farewell.

The Massage Practitioner's Responsibilities in the Spa Environment

Each spa has its own system and products for the various spa services. Any massage professional proficient in the content of this textbook, coupled with a strong background in science, can easily be trained in spa services. As with all the career tracks described in this chapter, additional training is necessary. For spa work, this training usually is provided by the spa, but various courses are available through continuing education.

The massage practitioner is one of many professionals and technicians who provide spa services. The responsibilities of the massage professional are to provide various types of massage, support other spa procedures, and provide education about spa services to clients. The following guidelines are important in the spa environment:

- Be punctual for appointments.
- Perform therapies and treatments in a courteous manner so that the client feels pampered and relaxed.
- Continually update your skills and education.

- Assist in educating and informing clients about spa products and services when the opportunity arises.
- Maintain a positive attitude and a professional, personal image.
- Maintain the physical environment of the spa to perfection.

The spa environment is a wonderful place to serve clients seeking massage. The spa industry has created one of the largest employment opportunities for massage practitioners. The spa concept is unique and requires the same professional commitment to learning as do all the career paths discussed in this chapter.

Pay Scales for Massage Therapists in the Spa Environment

Most spas hire all personnel as employees, typically on a wage plus commission basis. Spas are not known for paying high wages, but they typically pay fair wages. The average is $10 to $12 an hour plus commission and gratuities. Independent contractors usually get about 50% of the charge, but they have to supply most amenities and pay taxes.

A number of other expenses also must be factored in. For example, the environment of the spa is extremely important. Facility management is expensive. Marketing and advertising are essential aspects of the spa business plan. As a result, the overhead costs for a spa are high, typically at least 50% of gross income.

Employer or subcontractor wages therefore must be figured on the remaining 50% of gross receipts. In addition to the professional staff, spas require a sizable support staff, including maintenance workers, receptionists, managers, food service workers, and so on. These wages can easily account for 25% of the gross receipts left after overhead costs. Consequently,

technician and therapist wages must be provided from the remaining 25%. Also, the owner needs to make a profit.

Consider the following example:

Fee for massage with hot stones and aromatherapy:	$100 (i.e., gross receipts)

The expenses that must be deducted from this $100 are as follows:

Facility, supplies, and advertising and marketing overhead:	$50
Wages for support staff (typically $10 an hour):	$25
Amount left for technician and therapist wages and profit margin:	$25

The minimum profit should be 50% of the $25, or $12.50 per treatment.

Amount left for technician and therapist wages:	$12.50 per hour

This example should help you develop realistic expectations about guidelines and wages in the spa industry (Boxes 12-4 and 12-5).

The Spa Language

The spa environment has a language that employees must understand. These terms usually describe various services, which are listed on a spa menu from which the client chooses. Some of these methods may be performed by the massage practitioner, others may fall under the scope of practice of a cosmetologist or esthetician. Clients will ask questions about various services and treatments. You must understand the services, whether you perform them or not, so that you can educate the client and support the spa's business sales (Box 12-6).

BOX 12-4

Guidelines of the Day Spa Association

The Day Spa Association has set guidelines to help distinguish between a facility that offers spa services and a true day spa.

A true day spa has:

- A clean, safe, calming, and nurturing environment
- Private treatment rooms for each client receiving a personal service
- Separate showering and changing facilities for women and men
- Spa robes and shoes for all sizes
- Business licenses; professional, licensed estheticians and therapists on staff
- Professional spa products for which estheticians and therapists have received training in their use
- Massages: Swedish, lymphatic drainage, and reflexology (optional: shiatsu; polarity treatments; and sports, deep tissue, and deep muscle massages)
- Body treatments (one or more on the menu): body packs and wraps, exfoliation, cellulite treatments, body

toning/contouring, waxing, home care program (optional: electrical impulse body toning, heat treatments, Ayurveda treatments, laser hair removal, electrolysis, hand and foot care)
- Face: Cleansing facial, home care program (optional: medical facial, electrical toning, laser hair removal, electrolysis, cosmetics, makeup consultation)
- Aromatherapy: Personalized for body and/or face

One of the following:
- Hydrotherapy
- Steam bath and sauna

One of the following:
- Nutritional counseling/weight management
- Private trainer/yoga/meditation
- Spa cuisine

Optional:
- Hair: Full-service salon, scalp treatments, and hair packs
- Spa manicure and pedicure

Courtesy of the Day Spa Association

BOX 12-5

Sample Spa Menu

Eastern Practices

Ayurveda: "The science of life"
Ayurveda is an ancient Indian healing system and cleansing process that seeks to maintain the balance of the three doshas, each of which represent certain emotional and physical characteristics.

Shiatsu
Shiatsu is a style of Japanese acupressure massage in which the therapist's fingers, palms, and thumbs are applied to specific points on the body to stimulate inner healing.
30 minutes—$60
60 minutes—$100
90 minutes—$125

Reiki
An ancient method of healing that uses energy drawn from a higher source. Reiki is a very gentle yet powerful method of encouraging physical, emotional, and spiritual well-being.
60 minutes—$100
90 minutes—$125

Reflexology
This ancient Asian method of massage is applied to pressure points on the soles of the feet that correspond to internal organs of the body. Through stimulation, energy lines in the body are cleared.
30 minutes—$55
60 minutes—$90

Thai Massage
Using the hands, feet, knees, and elbows, the massage therapist applies pressure to important points along the energy lines in combination with assisted yoga stretches. An invigorating treatment that restores balance and energizes the body.
30 minutes—$60
60 minutes—$100
90 minutes—$125

Integrated Signature Massage
Experience the blending of Ayurvedic, Swedish, deep tissue, and Thai massage, combined for their unique actions and complementary benefits.
30 minutes—$55
60 minutes—$90
90 minutes—$120

Hot Stone Chakra Balancing
Hot stones are placed on the different chakra points to clear energy blockages and balance the body.
45 minutes—$85

Swedish Massage
Relieve built-up tension and alleviate stress with this classic and timeless favorite.
30 minutes—$55
60 minutes—$90
90 minutes—$120

Deep Tissue Massage
Especially beneficial for the physically active individual, this treatment provides a deep, strong massage to relieve tightness and strain.
30 minutes—$65
60 minutes—$100
90 minutes—$125

Myofascial Release
A therapeutic treatment using a gentle form of stretching that produces a profound healing effect on the body's tissues, helping to eliminate pain and restore motion.
30 minutes—$65
60 minutes—$100
90 minutes—$125

Craniosacral Treatment
With gentle support to the cranium and spine, this treatment encourages the release of adhesions and restrictions, promoting deep relaxation. It is especially beneficial for those with migraines, temporomandibular joint (TMJ) problems, and common joint dysfunction.
30 minutes—$60
60 minutes—$100

Prenatal Massage
Designed for the expectant mother, this massage uses specially designed body cushions to provide relief from swelling and cramping. Massage is provided after the first trimester.
30 minutes—$55
60 minutes—$90
90 minutes—$120

Hot Stone Therapy
Basalt lava stones are used to enhance a nurturing, head-to-toe massage. Heated stones glide over muscles, providing deeper penetration and allowing stress and tension to melt away.
60 minutes—$100
90 minutes—$125

Lomi Lomi
Considered the "dance of massage," this Hawaiian-inspired massage combines the use of breath energy and rhythmic movements for complete harmony.
30 minutes—$55
60 minutes—$90
90 minutes—$120

Aromatherapy Massage
A nurturing massage using therapeutic-grade essential oils from herbs, botanicals, and plant extracts blended for your individual needs.
30 minutes—$55
60 minutes—$90
90 minutes—$120

BOX 12-6

Bodywork Terms and Treatments Commonly Used in the Spa Setting

- *Bodywork exfoliation:* Exfoliation is the process by which the skin is rubbed, polished, or scrubbed or enzymes are used on it to remove dead skin cells, rancid oils, dirt, and debris.
- *Detoxification:* When the circulation and metabolism are stimulated, the body's own processing improves. This in turn improves the elimination process, helping the body to rid itself of wastes and toxins. In other words, this helps the body to detoxify itself. The end result is normally a more energetic, active individual who feels better.
- *Dry brush:* Dry brush involves the use of a luffa, brush, washcloth, or sponge to exfoliate dead surface skin. After this process, lotion is applied. The main purpose is to stimulate circulation.
- *Salt glow:* Special salt is mixed with oil or liquid soap to exfoliate the entire body or just an area for a spot treatment. Afterward, lotion is used on the client. A dry brush tool, such as a luffa, may be used with the salt mixture for added exfoliation. If salt is used, the client should not shave for 1 to 2 days before the treatment.
- *Body polish:* Salt or any abrasive substance or granular scrub can be used as a body polish. The product used is a cream base with granules of the abrasive substance added to exfoliate and condition or soften the skin at the same time.
- *Full-body seaweed mask:* Seaweed powders are normally mixed with water to a consistency resembling pancake batter. The mixture is applied over a conditioning lotion. The entire body may be covered, or the stomach, breasts, and buttocks may be left out, depending on the client's wishes. Essential oils are often added to full-body seaweed masks to achieve different effects on the body. The full-body seaweed mask treatment normally takes about 60 minutes.

- *Full-body mud mask:* Sea-based muds and clay muds, depending on the particular type, are said to cleanse and draw out impurities, to condition and mineralize the body, or just to soften and hydrate the skin. The mud is applied thickly to the body, which is then wrapped in plastic or foil. The client rests for 20 to 30 minutes. A full mud treatment normally takes about 60 minutes.
- *Herbal body wrap:* Linen or muslin sheets are heated and soaked in a machine called a *hydrocollator,* in which the temperature is 150° to 175° F. Herbal pouches or bags of herbs and essential oil essences are placed in the hydrocollator to achieve the desired effects. The body is first covered with towels or rubber sheets, and the linen or muslin sheets are laid over this. The body then is wrapped in sheets and blankets, and the client is allowed to rest for 20 minutes. A cool, wet cloth is applied to the client's forehead during the treatment and changed often. This treatment can be done in 30 minutes. The sheets are very hot. Thick, long rubber gloves must be worn by the technician when handling hot sheets.
- *Paraffin body wrap:* When applied to the body, paraffin forms a mask with heat. This helps the body perspire, and the trapped moisture is absorbed into the skin, along with nutrients that either have been put on the skin first or that are in the oils in the paraffin. The paraffin may be used alone, or it may be mixed with mud or seaweed. Paraffin can be painted on the body with a paint brush. Also, large gauze strips can be dipped in the paraffin and molded to different parts of the body. Several layers are applied, because the more layers (i.e., three to five), the greater the heat and the longer it will last. The body then is wrapped with foil or plastic, and the client is allowed to rest for 15 to 20 minutes. Paraffin is commonly used for the hands, feet, and face.

Massage Terms and Treatments Typically Found on Spa Menus

It is important that the massage therapist understand basic concepts related to signature services provided by spas. This section describes generic procedures to better help the student understand the services that other professionals are providing in the spa environment.

Swedish massage is general systematic massage of the soft tissues of the body to induce a state of deep relaxation. It works mainly on the muscles, ligaments, and tendons, and it increases the body's blood and lymphatic circulation. Swedish massage incorporates five main manipulations: effleurage (long gliding strokes), pétrissage (kneading), compression, vibration, and tapotement (see Chapter 9).

Stone therapy massage is a combination process that uses various types and sizes of stones, which are either heated or cooled. They then are placed on the body at strategic points or are coated with oils or lotions and rubbed on the body. The

hot and cold applications are a type of hydrotherapy method. The stones usually are placed over chakras, meridians, acupuncture points, and so on. The weight of the stone applies a compressive force on the point, and the stones either hold heat and slowly release it on the body or act like ice and absorb heat and cool the body. The various types of stones used are said to have healing properties that could be attributed to piezoelectric properties of the crystalline structure of the stones. The warmth and weight provided by warm stones can also be provided by rice bags (Figure 12-1).

Shiatsu (acupressure) is an Asian-based system of finger pressure massage that treats special points along acupuncture meridians. These meridians are invisible channels through which energy flows in the body. Physical discomforts are thought to be caused by blocks in the meridians; shiatsu releases those blocks and rebalances the energy flow (see Chapter 11).

Reflexology (zone therapy) is organized around a system of points on the hands and feet that are thought to correspond to the major joints and organs of the body (see Chapter 11).

FIGURE 12-1 Stone massage and use of rice bags. **A,** Stones and rice bags, which can be used for hot and cold applications. **B** to **I,** Applications of stone massage.

FIGURE 12-1, cont'd

Trigger point therapy (myotherapy or neuromuscular therapy) applies concentrated finger pressure to trigger points, which are painful, irritated areas in muscles, to break the cycle of spasm and pain. By working on key trigger points, the massage therapist often is able to relax an entire area (see Chapter 11).

Deep muscle/connective tissue massage releases the chronic patterns of tension in the body through slow strokes and deep pressure on contracted areas, by both following and moving across the grain of the muscles, tendons, and fascia (see Chapter 9).

Sports massage is designed specifically for athletes or people who engage in a sports, exercise, or fitness program. It usually is deeper and more vigorous than an average massage. Sports massage can be used to ready the muscles for strenuous activity or to help the body recover from the aftereffects of such an activity (see Chapter 9).

Cosmetic Treatments

The massage therapist typically does not perform cosmetic treatment. These procedures target the integumentary system (i.e., the skin), and cosmetologists, estheticians, and dermatologists are the experts in this area.

The Facial. A facial is given by a licensed esthetician or cosmetologist with special training in skin care. An esthetician is a skin care specialist who has undergone a professional train-ing program similar to cosmetology. A facial, which usually lasts 50 minutes, cleanses, tones, and hydrates the skin.

A facial involves some basic steps: cleansing, skin analysis, exfoliation, massage, extraction of blackheads and other impurities, and application of products targeted to the client's skin type (e.g., dry, oily, mixed, sensitive, or mature.) Variations on the classic European facial include the minifacial (cleansing without extractions) and specialty facials.

It is recommended that spa clients receive a facial once a month or every 6 weeks, because that is how long it takes the skin to regenerate (Box 12-7).

Peels. A peel involves the use of products to remove the surface layer of skin (dead skin) and expose the fresher tissue beneath.

An *enzyme peel* is a special enzyme-based exfoliating treatment that breaks down and removes the dead skin layer or layers from the face. Undergoing an enzyme peel from time to time forces the body to regenerate new skin, and this process makes the skin appear stronger and healthier.

Vitamin peels (i.e., vitamins A and C) are used to repair sun damage, lighten dark spots, rehydrate the skin, and encourage elasticity.[3]

Pedicures and Manicures. Spa pedicures and manicures moisturize the skin. The nails are trimmed, shaped, and painted.[3]

BOX 12-7

Types of Spa Facial Treatments

- **Microdermabrasion:** Microdermabrasion is a nonchemical, noninvasive procedure that removes the outermost layer of dry, dead skin cells to reveal younger, healthier-looking skin. Additional treatments encourage the production of a new layer of skin cells containing higher levels of collagen and elastin, both of which further improve the skin's appearance.
- **Facial contouring:** In facial contouring, a combination of therapies, including deep muscle massage and acupressure, is used to tone and tighten areas of the face and neck.
- **Facial oxygen therapy:** Facial oxygen therapy combines many different vitamins, minerals, amino acids, and enzymes, as well as pure oxygen, to cleanse, hydrate, and rejuvenate skin.
- **European deep suction cleansing:** European deep suction cleansing is a very deep cleansing procedure that uses enzymes and deep suction to remove impurities from the facial pores.
- **Photofacial:** This type of facial is performed only by trained medical professionals. Photofacial is a 30-minute procedure that uses a machine that releases intense pulses of light to penetrate all layers of the skin. This causes collagen and blood vessels under the top layer to constrict. For a complete treatment, five full-face light treatments must be done, spaced at three-week intervals. Clients report minimal discomfort, and the redness and facial swelling present after treatment are short-lived. The effects are gradual and are noticed over the few weeks following the treatment.

Courtesy Day Spa FYI at http://www.dayspafyi.com/day_spa_treatments.html

Waxing and Hair Removal Services. Most day spas offer a variety of waxing services to remove unwanted hair, such as:

- Leg waxing
- Arm waxing
- Eyebrow waxing
- Face and lip waxing
- Bikini waxes
- Brazilian waxes
- Laser hair removal[3]

Application of Permanent Makeup. Some day spas offer permanent makeup, a form of cosmetic tattooing.[3]

Tanning Services. Self-tanning services are offered by many day spas. With spray-on tanning, guests can achieve a summer tan without exposing the skin to damaging UV rays. Tanning booths are also available.[3]

Hydrotherapy

Hydrotherapy and hydrothermal therapy are traditional methods of treating disease and injury that have been used by many cultures, including ancient Rome, China, and Japan. Hydrotherapy is the external application of water for therapeutic purposes. The body or any of its parts may be immersed in water, or water may be applied to the surface, with or without the intermediary of absorbent materials. Hydrotherapy should be specified by type, temperature, duration, and frequency.

Water therapy has been used for centuries. The ancient Greeks took therapeutic baths. Water also is an important ingredient in the traditional Chinese and Native American healing systems. A Bavarian monk, Father Sebastian Kneipp, helped repopularize the therapeutic use of water in the nineteenth century. Nowadays, dozens of methods of applying hydrotherapy are available, including baths, saunas, douches, wraps, and packs (see Chapter 11 for specific information).

Specific Hydrotherapy Treatments in the Spa

A hydrotherapy tub treatment has many benefits. Hydrotherapy can:

- Relax the body
- Invigorate the body
- Equalize circulation and increase metabolism
- Enhance the penetration of other nutritional substances (additives in the water)
- Relieve stiffness, soreness, and pain
- Enhance the body's own detoxification process by improving circulation and elimination

Medical Concerns. Immersion in hot water is contraindicated for pregnant women, especially in the first trimester of pregnancy. Also, warm to hot water lowers the blood pressure and pulls blood into the extremities, slowing blood as it is redistributed back to the heart, lungs, and central circulatory system. This is great for relaxation but may cause lightheadedness, which can be dangerous for a client with a heart condition.

Types of Tub Treatments. The two primary types of bath treatments that may be given at a spa are:

- Plain water baths with no additives, with or without underwater massage
- Thalassotherapy baths, with additives of seaweed, seawater, sea salts, and sometimes sea mud

Additives for a relaxing bath might include the following:
Blue-green: Spirulina
Brown: Fucus, *Ascophyllum nodosum* (a type of seaweed)
Red: Chondrus, corallina

Spirulina is rich in vitamins and beta carotene and is effective for reducing fatigue and stimulating the metabolism. Fucus and *Ascophyllum nodosum*, which are rich in vitamins and amino acids, help relax the body and neutralize free radicals. Chondrus and corallina are both remineralizers and revitalizers.

Additives for an invigorating bath might include the following:
Blue: Spirulina
Brown: Laminaria, Fucus, Macrocystis
Green: Chlorella

Cleaning the Tub and Room. The tub must be cleaned and disinfected after each client (remember, the jets in the tub must also be cleaned out). The whole tub then is rinsed and dried. The room should be sanitized and wiped down with a towel. The floors should be sanitized and dried.

Other Hydrotherapy Treatments.

Vichy Shower. Originating in France, the Vichy shower consists of a row of shower heads suspended over a massage table. The client lies on the table, and the entire body is sprayed down from stem to stern on both sides. This usually is done as part of a body mud treatment, although it is both relaxing and stimulating on its own.[3]

Scrubs, Friction Rubs, and Ablutions. Scrubs and friction rubs help exfoliate and hydrate the skin. Scrubs usually use sugars, salts, and other natural ingredients and are applied by hand or with a special coarse mitten that helps remove dead, dull skin. Spas usually offer several different types of scrubs, such as the following[3]:

- *Salt glow:* Mineral-rich sea salts are used to exfoliate dry skin, revealing the healthier, younger skin beneath.
- *Aromatherapy scrubs:* These scrubs exfoliate the body and soothe the senses with therapeutic aromas.
- *Oatmeal scrubs:* Oatmeal scrubs exfoliate the body and help draw out impurities at the same time.
- *Cold rubbing (ablution):* To perform a cold ablution, soak a linen cloth in cold water, wring it out, and briskly rub the upper and lower trunk or the entire body. Relax until warm and dry. Cold ablutions are used to invigorate, to tone up the body, to promote blood flow, to address problems of circulation, or for infections of the respiratory system. The primary effect of a cold ablution is tonic, therefore it may be used for any condition in which a tonifying treatment is desired, such as fatigue after an illness or surgery, or after hot applications such as saunas, whirlpools, or hot baths. Cold ablution is an excellent hydrotherapy technique when used regularly along with saunas, hot tubs, and massage.
- *Whole body ablution:* A whole body ablution is performed with the client lying alternately supine and prone and covered completely; care must be taken to ensure that the person does not become chilled. Using cool to cold water, dip the mitt into the water and vigorously friction a portion of the body. Depending on the cooling effect desired, the mitt may either be saturated or wrung dry before the frictioning. The body part is frictioned until it reddens. If the client is weak, dry the area using a coarse, dry towel. If the client is strong and vigorous, wait to dry the person at the end of the treatment.

The sequence for an ablution treatment is as follows (only the part being frictioned is exposed at any time):

1. Position the client supine.
2. Perform the ablution on the chest.
3. Proceed from the chest to the arms.
4. Perform the ablution on the legs.
5. Turn the client over.
6. Perform the ablution on the legs and feet.
7. Perform the ablution on the buttocks.
8. Perform the ablution on the back.

Wraps. Body wraps help exfoliate, hydrate, and tone the skin. They are also used to detoxify the body and improve circulation. The basic body wrap is fairly simple; the body is covered with sea clay or a mineral or herbal solution and then wrapped with light sheets.

The effects of body wraps are based on two principles, absorption and compaction. Over time the body collects toxins from foods, water, and air. Body wraps are believed to work first by absorbing toxins (i.e., the solution rubbed into the skin opens the pores and collects impurities) and then by compressing, or tightening, the skin to achieve a more toned look.

Different body wraps provide different results. The most common types of wraps use sea clay, seaweed, herbs, minerals, and aloe vera. Overall, sea clay is said to be the most absorbent material.

- Enzymatic body wrap: This wrap combines fruit acids and an invigorating scrub to exfoliate and smooth the skin and cleanse the blemish-prone skin on the back.
- Herbal body wrap: Special herbs are used to soothe the body and muscles as impurities are drawn away.
- Aromatherapy wrap: This treatment involves the use of herbs and oils.
- Seaweed wrap: Seaweed has healing properties that can detoxify and energize the body.

The sequence for a body wrap is as follows:

1. Place the client in a relaxed position.
2. Moisten a linen cloth of the appropriate size with cold water (warm water for respiratory diseases), wring it out well, and wrap it tightly (but not tightly enough to cause constriction) around the appropriate part of the body.
3. Wrap a dry cotton or linen cloth around the moist cloth.
4. Wrap the client in a blanket or another cloth. The client should rest for 45 to 60 minutes or, if the intention is to induce sweating, for up to 3 hours.
5. If the wrap does not feel warm after 15 minutes, apply heat in the form of a hot water bottle or by giving the client warm tea. Remove the wrap immediately if the client complains of feeling unwell.

Steam Inhalation. Some spas use steam inhalation to help break up blockages in the chest after a cold or simply to open up the air passages. Specialized inhalation equipment can be used when using a small tub with hot water and a towel draped over the head.[3]

Aromatherapy

Spa regimens often make use of essential oils, commonly with various hydrotherapy and massage treatments. These oils also can be diffused into the air and inhaled (see Chapter 11 for a more detailed discussion). Each spa typically has its own signature essential oil blends, which are synergistic combinations of essential oils. Often these blends are premixed in a selected carrier oil, and this, too, may be a signature blend of the spa.

Keep in mind that a single oil or blend of oils should not be used consistently every day. Examples of blends (and individual oils) that are appropriate for massage include the following:

Sensual: Ylang-ylang, sandalwood and jasmine
Stimulating: Peppermint and rosemary
Mood lifter: Sweet orange, rose and geranium
Relaxing: Lavender, rose
Soothing (for muscle aches): Grapefruit and lemongrass

Products

Spas use many products to provide benefits, especially to treat the skin and detoxify the body (Box 12-8). *Cosmetologists* are professionals trained in cosmetic and wellness skin care; *dermatologists* are medical doctors who specialize in treating skin disease. The massage therapist needs to understand the reason a product is used and how various ingredients in the product work. Skin care products basically include cleansers, exfoliants, and moisturizers. The Evolve Web site provides a comprehensive list of product ingredients and their purposes.

Massage therapists who work in spas need to understand the specific products used in their spa. This information should be provided through in-house training after the massage practitioner is hired. Massage therapists may be required to use a certain product as a lubricant based on the spa's signature line, and they may be required to participate in the sales of products specific to the spa.

Students who commit to becoming competent in the lessons provided by this text, and who also are willing learners, will be well equipped to pursue successful careers in the spa environment.

A Day at the Spa

Now that you are familiar with spa-related therapeutic massage, study the photographs in Figure 12-2, which take you through an enjoyable, safe, and sanitary day at the spa.

THERAPEUTIC MASSAGE IN THE HEALTHCARE ENVIRONMENT

SECTION OBJECTIVES

Using the information presented in this section, the student will be able to perform the following:

- Explain the importance for massage practitioners of working under supervision in the health care setting
- Describe the written and verbal communication necessary for working in the health care environment
- List special considerations for working with clients undergoing medical treatment either in the health care environment or in the home health care setting

The term *medical massage* has been a source of confusion. Is medical massage a specific type of application, or is it the particular ability to work with people receiving medical care? Is medical massage a health care method used by more highly trained medical professionals and a massage specialty requiring additional training? Is medical massage a prescription or treatment for specific conditions? Is it massage applications that are eligible for third-party insurance reimbursement?

These questions have yet to be answered by the massage community.

Special considerations arise for massage therapists who work with clients in a health care environment (e.g., hospital, rehabilitation center, extended care facility, or mental health facility). Also, because people increasingly are being cared for in their homes by visiting nurses and home health workers, the massage professional in these situations functions as part of a health care team and works to meet the objectives of a comprehensively designed treatment plan. The overall treatment plan is supervised by a medical professional, usually a physician. The massage therapist often is supervised directly by a physician's assistant, nurse, physical therapist, occupational therapist, or some other qualified health care professional.

When working with a client undergoing medical intervention outside the organized health care environment, the massage therapist must pay attention to the total health care program, and effective interaction must be maintained between the supervising personnel and the massage professional. In these situations the client often is the main interface, but the massage practitioner occasionally may need to speak directly with the physician or psychologist.

The interaction with other health care professionals is very important. A balance must exist between professional exchange of information, with each member of the team carrying out his or her part of the treatment plan, and the expectation of extensive face-to-face communication. These professionals are very busy, and they are unlikely to be able to speak at length with the massage professional about a particular client. Although this may be unfortunate, it is the reality, and brevity, along with precise and concise information, becomes important. Most communication is done in written form through treatment orders and charting. The massage professional's documentation skills must be very effective to work in the health care environment.

Cooperative interaction is necessary to coordinate various home care situations. Independent action must be tempered by awareness of the client's total health care picture and by respect for the other health care professionals involved.

Other considerations arise as well. Universal precautions and other sanitation procedures must be followed precisely. The massage therapist often must work around various types of equipment and devices, such as intravenous lines. The massage often must be modified because the client is unable to assume the classic position of lying on a massage table. Many such clients are confined to a bed or wheelchair. Privacy often is compromised, and interruptions are common. The environment may be noisy and busy with other activity.

Various medications and their interaction with the effects of the massage must be considered. The effects of medical tests or preparation for tests can affect massage intervention. For example, many testing procedures require fasting before the test. This stresses the body, and in such cases the intensity of massage needs to be modified.

Therapeutic massage has much to offer in the health care environment. Clients are stressed, and the relaxation approaches of massage support the other medical interventions

BOX 12-8

Common Terminology for Spa Products

Allantoin: A substance derived from comfrey root that is believed to aid the healing of damaged skin by stimulating new tissue growth.

Aloe vera: A regenerating, soothing, softening, and reparative substance with antimicrobial and antiinflammatory properties. It is rich in more than 200 nutrients and is very healing and moisturizing.

Alpha-hydroxy acids: These acids, which include lactic acid and glycolic acid, are often used as peeling agents. At higher concentrations they also have a descaling or keratolytic action, thinning the stratum corneum.

Alpha-lipoic acid: A powerful water- and oil-soluble antioxidant, alpha-lipoic acid is 400 times more potent than vitamin C as an antioxidant. It also increases the level of glutathione, the body's most important antioxidant, and is a powerful antiinflammatory.

Bentonite: A substance that brightens dull, lifeless skin and leaves it with a fresh, renewed texture.

Borax: A cleansing agent that helps blend water and oil. A mild alkali, it cleanses without drying the skin.

Clay, kaolin: This substance draws out impurities and is used as a deep pore cleanser. It removes excess oil, dirt, and grime.

Cleanse: To clean and remove impurities from the skin's surface.

Cleansers and exfoliants: Products used to remove makeup and impurities on the skin's surface. They also remove sebum (oily secretions produced by the sebaceous gland) and dead skin cells.

Cream: A cream is a more occlusive, thicker barrier on the skin. Those that contain dimethicone are particularly useful for hand dermatitis.

Emollient: An ingredient that softens and soothes the skin. Emollients are used in moisturizers to correct dryness and scaling of the skin.

Glycerin: A humectant and emollient from plants. It absorbs moisture from the air and helps keep moisture in creams and other products.

Glyceryl stearate: A substance that helps produce a neutral, stable emulsion. It is also a solvent, humectant, and consistency regulator in water-in-oil and oil-in-water formulations. It is derived from palm kernel or soy oil for cosmetic use. It also is found naturally in the body.

Humectant: A substance that increases the water-holding capacity of the stratum corneum. It is particularly important in the management of ichthyoses (inherited or acquired scaly disorders of the skin).

Lanolin: A sebumlike product obtained from washing sheep's wool. It acts as an emollient and a humectant for the skin.

Lotion: A substance that is more occlusive than an oil. Lotions are best applied immediately after bathing to

retain the water in the skin and should be used at other times as necessary.

Mask: A mask draws impurities to the skin's surface. Masks also slough off dead skin cells and stimulate blood circulation, leaving the skin feeling smoother and softer. Masks are applied after cleansing but before toning and can be used once or twice a week.

Moisturizers and serums: Products that use advanced humectants to help the skin retain water; they also provide a protective barrier to prevent the evaporation of the skin's natural moisture.

Night creams: Creams that contain a higher concentration of nutrients that assist in the rebuilding of the molecular structure of the skin's underlying tissues. They also improve the skin's ability to retain moisture.

Ointments: Pure oil preparations (e.g., equal parts white soft and liquid paraffin or petroleum jelly), which are prescribed for drier, thicker, more scaly areas. Many clients find them too greasy.

Phospholipid: A substance derived from plants that reduces moisture loss from the skin and acts as a carrier for deep penetration.

Retinol: A vitamin A carotenoid with antioxidant and skin-renewing properties.

Rubefacient: A local irritant that reddens the skin.

Salicylic acid: A substance that softens the keratinized barrier cells, has antibacterial properties, and helps eliminate clogged pores

Salt: A substance that is good for drying, cleansing, drawing, and soothing. It also can be used as an exfoliant. It dilates pores, allowing the skin to absorb trace minerals, and it encourages the skin to secrete its natural oil. It soothes irritated skin and aching muscles.

Serum: An intense concentration for exceptional revitalization of aging skin.

Shea butter: A moisturizing, soothing emollient fat that has cellular renewal properties.

Silicone: A substance derived from silica, a naturally occurring mineral, that has a softening effect on the skin.

Skin lighteners: Products that help reduce the production of melanin, which causes coloration of the skin. These products are used to lighten the complexion. Skin lightening regimens include their own cleansers, masks, toners, moisturizers, and serums.

Sodium bicarbonate: A highly alkaline, gentle substance that cleans, soothes, and softens the skin. It also is deodorizing, and it draws out oil and impurities.

Toner: A toner removes any residue left by cleansers and returns the skin to its proper pH by maintaining the skin's natural acidic balance. Toners and lotions prepare the skin for the application of a moisturizer.

FIGURE 12-2 A day at the spa. **A,** The client is greeted warmly. The intake interview is conducted, and the client is presented with a spa menu. **B,** The client changes into spa wear and then is offered a cup of tea. **C,** The client's hair is protected with a cap. **D,** Signature aromatherapy oils and bath salts are used for the treatments. **E,** The client is encouraged to enjoy the hydrotherapy treatment. **F,** The client's feet are gently dried and then given a reflexology treatment. **G,** The client then is given a relaxation-based, full-body signature massage. **H,** A compress can be placed over the client's eyes.

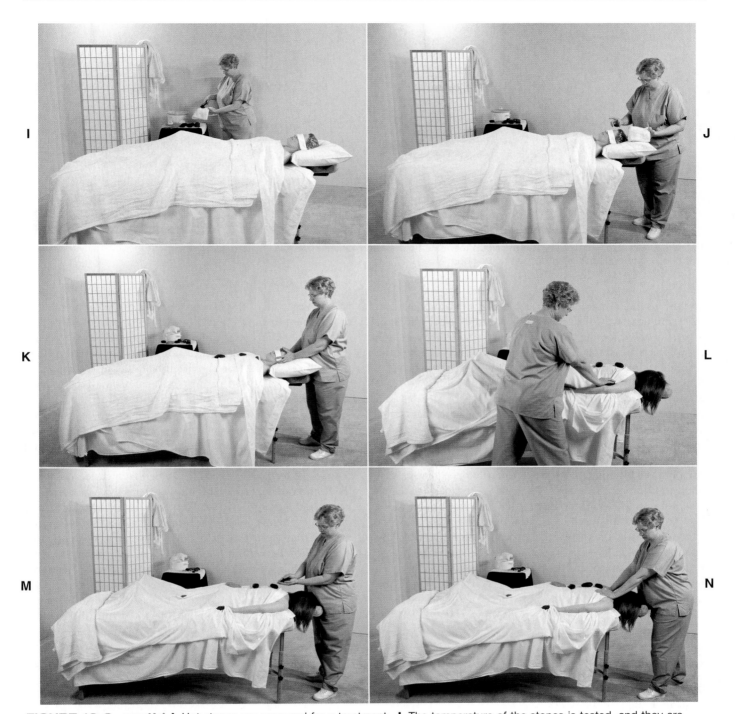

FIGURE 12-2, cont'd **I,** Hot stones are prepared for a treatment. **J,** The temperature of the stones is tested, and they are then gently placed at nodal points. **K,** A few stones can be placed on the chakras with focused energy intention. **L,** Massage can be performed with a hot stone. **M,** The massage therapist can warm the hands with the stone. **N,** The massage then is given with warm hands. *Continued*

FIGURE 12-2, cont'd **O,** The massage therapist finishes and focuses (compassionate energy). **P,** The therapist says good-bye and encourages the client to visit again soon.

and the healing process in general. Massage before surgery can help with anxiety. Comfort or palliative care before and after a person undergoes an invasive medical procedure can ease the discomfort somewhat. Massage provided during drug rehabilitation programs supports the recovery process. Massage for the medical staff promotes their ability to serve effectively, because the health care staff often is stressed and overworked. The possibilities for massage in the health care environment are numerous. Massage to manage chronic illness and pain are good examples.

The massage provided in the situations just described usually is very basic and focuses primarily on palliative care and condition management. The challenge for massage therapists who want to work in the health care environment is not how to work with specific diseases, but rather how to work effectively with the health care professionals serving the patient. The skill levels presented in this text are sufficient for this type of care, provided the professional is qualified to work in the complex health care environment. To function in the health care environment, the massage professional must be skilled and knowledgeable in the following areas:

- Clinical reasoning
- Problem solving
- Preparation of justifications for treatment
- Setting qualifiable and quantifiable goals
- Medical terminology
- Pathology
- Medical tests and procedures
- Medications
- Assessment
- Development of treatment plans
- Analysis of the effectiveness of methods used
- Charting
- Effective communication of information

These skills can be developed through continuing education for massage professionals or through comprehensive massage training for individuals who already have health care training (e.g., nurses and physical therapy assistants). For professionals who already have health care training, it is unreal-

istic to expect that simple exposure to massage is sufficient to enable them to work effectively with the vast knowledge base of massage. It is just as unrealistic to believe that a massage professional with an entry level education can function effectively in the health care environment. Because therapeutic massage falls within the paraprofessional realm, it seems most logical to extend the education of massage professionals who want to work in a health care setting and provide supervision of the massage professional by qualified health care personnel. Many of the case studies in Chapter 15 are examples of medical massage.

Various terms are used to describe therapeutic massage in the health care environment, most commonly *clinical massage* or *medical massage*. This text is based on the premise that all massage is therapeutic and that the terms *clinical massage* and *medical massage* can be used interchangeably. Both describe massage offered within the health care environment to serve people seeking preventive care and those who have diagnosed medical conditions and are being treated at some level by a medical professional. Increasingly, massage and other complementary therapies are being integrated into the medical environment.*

Methods and knowledge overlap significantly in the health care, sports and exercise, and spa career tracks, and all these methods are solidly grounded in the theory and practice of therapeutic massage.

In the health care setting, massage typically focuses on systemic illnesses (e.g., cancer, multiple sclerosis, diabetes) and on soft tissue dysfunctions that affect the general population. Most massage applications in the health care setting are general in nature, targeting restorative mechanisms, maintenance of homeostasis, and palliative care. Massage related to soft tissue dysfunction targets common conditions such as

---

*For specific information on how this is being accomplished, see *Integrating Complementary Therapies in Primary Care: a Practical Guide for Health Professionals,* by David Peters, Leon Chaitow, Gerry Harris, and Sue Morrison (Churchill Livingstone, 2002) and *Clinical Massage in the Health Care Environment,* by Sandy Fritz (Elsevier, 2007).

headaches, neck and shoulder pain, low back pain, tendinitis, bursitis, and arthritis. Pain and pain management are also important consideration. In addition, the massage therapist must understand how the inflammatory response is connected to seemingly unrelated diseases.

Massage therapists who want to work in the health care setting must have a basic understanding of the various medical tests and treatments so that they can make safe, beneficial decisions on ways to use massage to complement the medical treatments the patient is receiving.

As mentioned, massage now is offered in a variety of medical environments and with various health care professions (e.g., hospitals, physical therapy, private practice physicians, mental health, chiropractic, long-term care, and hospice care). Massage professionals who want to work in health care must be skilled in and knowledgeable about infection control, sanitation measures, HIPAA requirements, record keeping, and third-party insurance reimbursement requirements. They also must be willing to accept supervision and to function as a member of the health care team.

More and more, research is validating the effects of massage, making its inclusion in health care possible. (See the Evolve Web site for a link to massage-related research.) For massage practitioners, the health care environment is a unique place that requires a specific skill set and a professional set of behaviors. Recent developments in mental health and in general wellness and preventive care support the current trend toward a more holistic approach to health care.

The massage therapist who pursues a career in health care must understand all the aspects of clinical massage provided as part of an integrated medical practice.

Clinical/Medical Massage

Definitions are difficult. As was mentioned earlier, the massage community has not reached agreement on the knowledge base and scope of practice that define a career path in clinical/medical massage. However, for this chapter to make sense, a definition is necessary.

For the purposes of this textbook, *clinical/medical massage* (or simply *massage* in the remainder of the text) is an outcome-based treatment specifically targeted to address conditions that have been diagnosed by an appropriate health care professional. Massage is included as an aspect of a total treatment program. In clinical/medical massage, the focus is not on what kind of massage methods to use, but on massage application that supports the diagnosis, the prescribed treatment, and the determined outcomes for the patient.

Massage professionals typically call the people they work with *clients;* however, in the health care setting, the massage therapist works with the *patients* of the supervising health care providers (although this terminology may be changing). Massage therapists do not diagnose; rather, they typically work from a prescribed treatment plan, following the health professional's treatment orders. This is the nature of the health care environment. Health care settings are not the arena for independent practice by the massage professional or for

unproductive conflicts among members of a multidisciplinary team. This is an environment that requires a team spirit, as well as the ability to follow orders and relay information accurately (both written and verbal) and to contribute intelligently to the care of the patient.

The massage practitioner who chooses to pursue a career in the health care setting must develop a team player attitude and a willingness to accept supervision and instruction from medical professionals. Agreeing to work in this area means agreeing to defer to the supervising physician, nurse, or other health professional. Face it—they have a more comprehensive education than the typical massage therapist. They also shoulder the responsibility for the often serious and even life and death decisions that must be made in the course of health care. These professionals may not know as much about massage as you do, but in general, they know more about health care.

In choosing a career in the health care environment, the massage professional needs to understand the responsibility of providing service to those who face health challenges. This is not a decision that should be made lightly. In some situations, a massage therapist may receive health insurance reimbursement outside the traditional health care setting, in the context of private practice. In some cases a physician's referral and preauthorization may be required. Reimbursement through health insurance may be available if the patient has this coverage as part of his or her health care coverage. Even in private massage therapy practice, the components of team care, effective communication, and respect are essential.

Highly trained massage therapists are able to discuss the treatment plan intelligently with various medical professionals, to provide valid input, and, if disagreement arises, to state their position accurately and professionally and justify their recommendations to the supervising personnel. This is a world of ethical behavior and ethical decision making (see Chapter 2). Maintaining appropriate professional boundaries is important. The more complex a patient's condition and life circumstances are, the more balance the massage therapist must exercise between dedication to service and remaining somewhat neutral and objective in professional practice.

The term *medically fragile* sometimes is used to describe patients with serious and complicated medical conditions. *Fragile* is a good word; practitioners who choose to serve the ill or injured need to handle these people as if they were delicate glass globes. One of the biggest mistakes massage therapists make is to do too much too soon; this simply exacerbates the strain on the patient's adaptive mechanisms. Because of the patient's fragile condition, continual decisions must be made on whether the person will benefit from massage treatment or be excessively stressed by it. Supervision and sharing the responsibility of patient care help maintain this delicate balance.

Fortunately, massage application in this text is presented as an outcome-based process, which is necessary to develop and follow treatment plans and work effectively in the health care setting. Points to consider when offering massage in the health care environment include the following:

- Typically the target population is ill or injured; however, preventive care is increasing, as reflected in wellness programs and medical spas.
- The more injured or ill the patient, the more basic the massage application.
- Massage should support, not interfere with, medical treatment.
- Healing is a body, mind, and spirit process that requires a multidisciplinary approach; this honors the roles of various professionals and respects scope of practice.
- Healing does not necessarily mean cure. Successful coping is a healing process.
- Living well with hope and compassion, regardless of circumstances, is an important goal of healing.
- Massage is targeted to the body, and the appropriate scope of practice must be maintained; therefore the massage therapist respects and honors but does not cross over into the mind and spirit aspects of treatment.
- Respect for the patient and the health care team is paramount.
- Dying is an important part of living and should be treated with compassion and dignity.

Integrating Massage into the Healthcare Setting

The emerging trend in health care generally can be described as the *biopsychosocial model* of medicine. The concept of health has become a metaphor for wholeness.

By definition, the term **complementary** refers to approaches or therapies that are used in addition to conventional medical treatments; for example, the use of acupuncture or massage with physical therapy and medications in patients who have chronic pain syndromes. The term **alternative** refers to approaches or therapies that are used instead of or in place of conventional medicine; for example, the use of homeopathy and homeopathic remedies instead of pharmaceutical drugs. In everyday use, this clear distinction is lost. This text is based on the concept of massage as a complementary method, not an alternative approach to care.

The term **complementary and alternative medicine (CAM)** refers to the use of approaches, therapies, and treatments that are not considered part of the current biomedical model of medicine. The biomedical model is based on clearly defined philosophies and approaches to health and illness or injury that are based on the beliefs and values of Western scientific culture. CAM encompasses a broad range of philosophies and beliefs about the nature of health, healing, illness, and disease that are different from those on which the Western health care system is based. Many complementary and alternative approaches are derived from health care systems from other cultures and other countries, such as the use of the meridian system and the concept of Qi in the diagnosis and treatment of illness in traditional Chinese medicine. Others emerge from visionary ideas by individuals such as Milton Trager or Ida Rolf.

Complementary therapies or medicine are considered whole medical systems (e.g., Chinese medicine, Ayurvedic, therapeutic massage). The various systems differ somewhat in their philosophical approaches to the prevention and treatment of disease, but they have a number of common elements, such as:

- The body has the power to heal itself.
- Most health problems derive from a failure of the tissues, or the individual, to adapt to the biochemical, biomechanical, and/or psychosocial stressors of life.
- Healing often requires the use of multiple techniques that involve the mind, body, and spirit in order to enhance the individual's adaptive capacity (self-healing) or to reduce the adaptive load, or to minimize excessive symptomatic responses.
- Treatment often is individualized and depends on the patient's presenting symptoms, as well as the context from which they emerged and the processes involved.

Unfortunately, at this point the research efforts of the National Center for Complementary and Alternative Medicine have focused on individual therapies with an adequate experimental rationale, not on evaluating whole systems of medicine as they are commonly practiced. However, the whole-system approach to health care likely is more effective because the pieces of the system have synergistic influences. Even with this research limitation, complementary modalities have been shown to be beneficial in some instances.

For the sake of clarity, medical practices currently derived from a biomedical Western scientific model are referred to as *conventional health care.** Many conventional health care professionals are frustrated and concerned about the inability to treat lifestyle-related illnesses effectively, particularly those that are chronic, with standard approaches using medication, surgery, and other such methods. Unconventional approaches to treatment of these conditions (e.g., massage) have become more accepted because the intent is to emphasize care in a wider context of body/mind/spirit interconnectedness and the importance of supporting wellness as well as treating pathology. This is called *integrative medicine*. The health care community would be thankful if complementary methods could provide effective (and less potentially harmful) treatments for difficult conditions by stimulating and supporting the body's self-regulatory processes.

Because of our vast and growing ethnic diversity, it is important to be sensitive and respectful of cultural influences on peoples' behavior and beliefs. This respect extends to the historical and cultural bases of many complementary or alternative therapies. In previous years many of these intricate systems have been exploited and misused by people with insufficient training and appreciation of the depth and complexity of the system. Weekend classes in all sorts of methods have become available, leading practitioners to feel as if they could competently practice the system. This insults the extensive training and discipline of those who have dedicated themselves to years of education and experience to become proficient in a specific health practice. The most common example of this is separating acupuncture from the vastness of the entire Chinese medical system.

The existence, use, and popularity of complementary and alternative medicine are not new phenomena. In the past, because of the harsh approaches and unsuccessful outcomes offered by Western-educated physicians, more and more people chose "alternative" healers because the treatments were gentler and more natural, using herbs, lifestyle changes, nutrition, and an approach that incorporated the whole person. With the increasing popularity of alternative practices, and as Western-educated physicians began to use some of those practices themselves, conventional medical practice became more interested in alternative modalities.

In 1900, 20% of all practitioners of medicine were "alternative" physicians. The American Medical Association (AMA) was formed in 1848. In the early 1900s, the AMA issued a statement to its members saying that it was unethical for physicians and members of the AMA to consult, confer, or interact with "alternative" practitioners. This began the exclusion of any medical approaches or treatments that were not considered within the mainstream of medicine. Other factors also contributed to the near disappearance of alternative health approaches, including Rudolf Virchow's cell theory and Louis Pasteur's germ theory in the late 1800s, followed by the discovery of x-rays in the early 1900s and of penicillin in the late 1920s.

The discovery of antibiotics was a pivotal point for the emergence of conventional medicine, and the use of alternative medicine almost completely disappeared in the United States from 1920 to 1960. However, it continued as an important aspect of health care in other parts of the world, where chiropractors, naturopaths, and osteopaths remained active. For example, Dr. Leon Chaitow, who wrote the foreword to this text, qualified as a doctor of naturopathy (naturopath, or ND) and a doctor of osteopathy (osteopath, or DO) in 1960 and joined a thriving profession.

Beginning around 1970, alternative approaches to health and healing began to resurface in the United States. The health care culture was truly changed by the social upheaval of the 1960s. The cost of health care was becoming prohibitive. The new prominence of the field of psychology and the role of the mind in illness and disease were major influences, as was recognition of the debilitating and sometimes fatal adverse side effects of medications previously thought safe. Cardinal factors in the change were the emergence of resistant strains of bacteria, the human immunodeficiency virus (HIV) and acquired immunodeficiency syndrome (AIDS) epidemics, and the increasing inability to treat lifestyle diseases successfully with conventional medical approaches. Currently we are beginning to embrace and refine the concepts of multidisciplinary and interdisciplinary health care.

In 1991 Congress established the Office of Alternative Medicine (OAM) within the National Institutes of Health (NIH). (The OAM now is known as the National Center for Complementary and Alternative Medicine [NCCAM].) The purpose of the OAM was to facilitate the evaluation of alternative medical treatments and their effectiveness through research and other initiatives. The initial budget for this undertaking was $2 million.

Before it could begin the process of evaluation, the OAM needed a classification system that would allow better identification of the alternative treatments. Seven groups were established initially, but the system has since been revised to five major domains:

- *Alternative health systems:* Traditional Asian medicine, Ayurvedic (Indian) medicine, Tibetan medicine, Native American medicine, homeopathy, and naturopathy.
- *Mind/body interventions:* Meditation imagery, hypnosis, biofeedback, yoga, tai chi, Qigong, prayer, spiritual healing, soul retrieval, and intuitive diagnosis.
- *Biologically based therapies:* Herbal medicine, special diets (Ornish, Pritikin, Weil, Atkins, macrobiotic), orthomolecular medicine, and iridology.
- *Manipulative and body-based methods:* Chiropractic, osteopathy, craniosacral therapy, massage, reflexology, Pilates, Rolfing, structural integration, Trager body work, and Alexander technique.
- *Energy therapies:* Qigong, Reiki, polarity therapy, therapeutic touch, and electromagnetic therapies.

The focus of NCCAM is to make complementary alternative modalities safe and accessible to the American population. The agency recommended that the education of those studying conventional medicine include CAM instruction, and the education of CAM practitioners include studies in conventional medicine. The intended result is to train conventional providers who can discuss CAM with their patients, provide guidance on the use of CAM treatments, and collaborate with CAM practitioners, as well as CAM practitioners who can communicate and collaborate with conventional providers.

Some common complementary modalities that have moved into mainstream biomedical practice are massage, acupuncture, relaxation/stress management, and herbal treatments (Box 12-9). Massage is being incorporated into the conventional health care setting for three main reasons: low risk, low cost, and high patient satisfaction. Research into the physiologic mechanisms of massage benefits has demonstrated the *efficacy* (i.e., the ability to produce a desired effect) of massage.

Integrated Medicine

Integrated medicine incorporates complementary therapies into the structure of conventional medical care. The term is used to describe a system in which mainstream medical care and complementary therapies are integrated within a practice or an institution, enhancing each other. Lifestyle illnesses are increasing as a result of stress, fatigue, poor nutritional choices, obesity, and similar factors. Many people will come to recognize the overwhelming need to change their lifestyle, and these people will turn to integrated medicine as a means of change. The medical spa is a model of an integrated approach. The medical spa concept is one of relaxation, pleasure, and pampering combined with the treatment of medical conditions. The medical spa is an ideal environment for addressing health care conditions that require major lifestyle changes, such as weight management, chronic fatigue, some types of physical rehabilitation, and physical conditioning. Some medical spas also offer nutritional help to assist in a dietary lifestyle change, which in turn assists with disease, weight management, and some illnesses. A growing aspect of integrated health care can

BOX 12-9

Complementary Medicine Approaches

Treatment approaches that commonly are considered complementary medicine include the following health care practices.

Acupressure
Acupuncture
Alexander technique
Applied kinesiology
Aromatherapy
Autogenic training
Ayurveda
Chiropractic
Cranial osteopathy
Environmental medicine
Homeopathy
Hypnosis

Massage
Meditation
Naturopathy
Nutritional therapy
Osteopathy
Qi gong
Reflexology
Relaxation and visualization techniques
Shiatsu
Tai chi
Therapeutic touch
Yoga

From Paters D, Chaitow L, Harris G, Morrison S: *Integrating complementary therapies in primary care,* Edinburgh, 2002, Churchill Livingstone.

be seen in the increase in cosmetic surgery coupled with anti-aging modalities that primarily target control of inappropriate inflammation, supporting both physical fitness and mental health.

Beneficial and Safe Complementary Practice

People usually consult complementary practitioners with mild to moderate, long-term, painful, functional, and stress-related conditions and disorders, all of which occupy a great deal of the general medical practitioner's time. Conditions that often can be managed successfully with complementary therapies include undifferentiated illnesses and chronic structural and relapsing functional disorders. Good clinical trials suggest that for certain conditions, complementary therapies are the treatment of choice. Well-designed studies have been done on the effectiveness of complementary methods for a range of common problems, including anxiety, fibromyalgia syndrome, asthma, irritable bowel syndrome (IBS), eczema, and migraine. Microbiologists are studying the effects of nutrition and stress on the human body, and the results of these studies likely will provide a whole new realm of treatment knowledge.

The growing acceptance of complementary therapies coincides with an increased interest in lifestyle change, health promotion, and low-technology treatments. These approaches, integrated into conventional medical care, might provide inexpensive, safe ways to address conditions that currently do not respond well to conventional care.

Conventional medicine can be the best treatment for trauma and acute care. Conventional medicine can provide effective treatment for many common conditions, such as acute bacterial infection, congestive heart failure, and glaucoma. Alternative or adjunctive treatments support this care. Accepted modalities currently available in health care (e.g.,

nursing, physiotherapy, specialist referral, counseling, and medications) do not necessarily meet the needs of patients whose problems are not "fixable." Other people have long-term relapsing structural or functional disorders, for which medical treatment often is less than satisfactory. People with conditions that do not respond to conventional medical care alone might have better outcomes with the combined approach used in multiprofessional/multidisciplinary integrated health care. If this new type of health care approach is to succeed, those who practice complementary therapies must comply with various requirements to achieve integration into the current health care system.

The conventional health care community has concerns about the new approach, most of which are valid. If people are seen by unqualified practitioners, the risk of a missed or delayed diagnosis arises, possibly with tragic results. People may waste money on ineffective treatments and discontinue or not use effective conventional treatment. The mechanisms of benefit claimed for some complementary treatments are implausible, and many complementary therapies are scientifically unproven. Health care insurers must establish whether and how complementary therapies support health care before routine insurance coverage is authorized. Public expectation is growing that complementary therapies should be made available. Therefore it must be demonstrated that patients are being treated with a safe, effective therapy, by a qualified practitioner (Box 12-10), and that this approach is more acceptable and more cost effective than the conventional medical alternatives.

Practitioners of complementary therapies, including massage, must comply with the logical and attainable recommendations of conventional medicine before a unified move can be made toward integrated medicine. The main focus of this text is therapeutic massage, which is being integrated into health care, and the massage community is working to meet

BOX 12-10

Key Constituents for a Professional Practice Model for Complementary Medicine Practitioners

- **Qualifications:** Practitioners should have a recognized qualification from a training establishment that is accredited by a suitable regulatory body.
- **Registration license:** Practitioners must be registered with a recognized professional body that requires its members to abide by codes of conduct, ethics, and discipline.
- **Insurance:** Practitioners must have adequate professional liability insurance coverage that applies to the period of their employment.
- **Consent to treatment:** Patients must be fully informed about the nature of the therapy and its effects, including any side effects, and must have realistic expectations of its benefits. The informed consent of the patient or, in the case of young children, of the parent or guardian, must be gained and documented.
- **Medical responsibility:** Practitioners should be aware that patients referred to them for treatment remain the overall responsibility of the referring clinician. Complementary and alternative medicine (CAM) practitioners should not advise the client to discontinue existing treatments without the agreement of the referring clinician.
- **Documentation:** A written record should be kept by practitioners of the consultation and each episode of treatment. All written (and oral) information should be treated as confidential and should take into account the

requirements of the Health Insurance Portability and Accountability Act (HIPAA).
- **Refusal to treat:** Practitioners have a duty not to treat a patient if they consider the treatment unsafe or unsuitable.
- **Education and training:** Practitioners should take responsibility for keeping abreast of developments in the practice of their therapy.
- **Quality standards:** Practitioners, in conjunction with other health care professionals, should assist with the development of local standards and guidelines for practice.
- **Audits:** Practitioners should undertake a clinical audit and report the results to the employing or commissioning practice/PCG. They should be responsible for monitoring the outcome of therapy; clients' opinions should be actively sought and included in any evaluation.
- **Research:** Practitioners should be expected to agree to take part in research trials to support the evaluation and development of treatment programs.
- **Health and safety:** Practitioners should comply with the requirements of health and safety legislation and should adhere to good practice in the protection of staff, patients, and the public.
- **Control of infection:** Practitioners should adhere to regulations governing infection control and follow the procedure for reporting outbreaks of infection.

Adapted from the Scottish Department of Health 1996 Complementary Medicine and the National Health Service: Complementary medicine information pack for primary care groups, June, 2000.

these recommendations. Massage has come a long way, especially in the past 5 years. Evidence-based research supports the efficacy of massage, and avenues are available for appropriate education, licensure or certification, insurance coverage, and so forth.

The biggest hurdles to integrating massage into conventional heath care are (1) finding appropriately trained massage therapists (see *Clinical Massage in the Healthcare Setting,* by Sandy Fritz, Leon Chaitow, and Glenn Hymel) and (2) identifying the source of funds to pay for massage. Currently health insurance does not routinely cover therapeutic massage. Further research must be done to show that massage treatment is more cost-effective than conventional medical treatment for various conditions and that it has the same or better benefits without an increase in risk to the patient. Research can also document whether conventional medical treatment achieves better outcomes when combined with complementary methods. When this has been shown (and the massage community is confident that it will be), the final hurdle to full integration of massage into the health care community will be overcome. Massage therapists are unlikely to work and bill health insurance companies independently. More likely, qual-

ified massage therapists will be directly supervised by health care providers who can bill for the massage session.

The Role of Massage in Health Care

As integration progresses, massage therapists probably will fall into the category of technical specialist/paraprofessional. The education will be equivalent to at least 1 year of college but will be obtainable through vocational training schools. The model for this can be seen in programs for medical assistants, respiratory therapy assistants, and physical therapy aides. Education for massage therapists in health care would include about 36 credits (1,200 contact hours), which fits the current educational trend in massage. Currently, entry level education is 500 to 750 contact hours (approximately 20 credits). This level of education prepares the massage graduate for the wellness massage career path. The knowledge needed to work in a medical setting, a specialty, would require an additional 15 to 16 credits (300 to 500 contact hours). The educational requirements may rise as high as an associate's degree (64 credits). If this becomes the situation, massage would be ranked with other health care technical specialists, such as physical therapy assistants.

What Massage Realistically Can Do. Massage care is supportive, not curative, for those who are ill or injured. Massage effectively supports various forms of medical intervention (including mental health) as well as the body's innate ability to heal.

Some diseases and injures are cured with medical intervention. This is especially true of acute care situations, the area in which the science and practice of medicine shine. However, most people are not cured with health care interventions (e.g., medication, surgery); instead, their condition is managed, a situation that puts a major strain on the health care delivery system. Because most health conditions are managed, and therefore require long-term care, treatment is expensive. Massage offers benefits for the management of many chronic health conditions in a potentially cost-effective manner.

The doctor and highly trained support staff are best suited to handle acute situations. This is an important distinction in the health care environment. Massage therapists work most effectively with patients who have chronic conditions and those facing death, because there is no cure in these cases. We must also remember the contraindications to medical treatment for conditions that cannot be cured. Patients must look at the possible side effects of medications to make sure the drug's purpose outweighs any possible side effects. Sometimes the treatment is worse than the disease. The difficult health problems are the ones that medical science does not know how to fix, as well as those that occur because of certain lifestyle choices, which require the person to change behaviors (e.g., nutrition, exercise, diet modification).

Some health benefits of massage have been validated by research (see Chapter 4); others are based on clinical experience and/or are historically supported by the experience of many cultures over centuries of practice. The main focuses of massage in the health care environment are as follows:

- Breathing effectiveness
- Circulation support (blood and lymph)
- Comfort and pleasure
- Edema and fluid imbalance management
- Enhanced parasympathetic dominance
- Pain management
- Reduced sympathetic dominance
- Support for sleep and reduction of fatigue
- Soft tissue normalization (neuromuscular and myofascial)

These outcomes can overlap. For example, reducing sympathetic dominance should improve breathing, support sleep, and increase pain tolerance. Reducing edema could ease pain and increase circulation to an area. Neuromuscular balance allows for effective movement, and myofascial balance supports mobility and stability; together they support effective, efficient movement that encourages circulation, increases comfort, and supports productivity.

The Health Care Environment

Massage students must understand that they must acquire a comprehensive knowledge base and develop effective use of clinical reasoning to pursue a career in clinical/medical massage. Additional study in areas other than massage is a necessity.

The health care world is as dynamic as the human body. Demands on the system eventually change the structure. This is one reason for the greater role massage is playing as part of the health care delivery system. Demands from the public have begun the process of changing the form of health care. These changes do not happen quickly, and transitional times can be difficult, because the pre-existing structure is no longer as effective but the new form is not ready to assume function completely. This is the state of health care today. What seems like a mess is actually the dynamics of change based on demand. Massage therapists in this environment must understand what the pre-existing form was, what demands are causing the change, and what is needed from them to ease the transition. They must be patient as well as persistent in career development during these active transitional periods. It also is necessary to be progressive and to anticipate what skills and qualities will be required in the future and to train for them *now,* so that they are ready to respond when opportunities become available.

Currently healthcare is organized in what is called a *hierarchy,* which is a top-down system. At the top of the organization is the doctor; other levels of support professionals descend from this, typically based on training, with the least-trained at the bottom of the organization. As a result of changes in insurance coverage for health care and managed health care systems, the top role of the hierarchy is in question. When this type of power shift occurs, conflict is common until some sort of resolution is achieved. Health care administration (the management and business) is in a struggle with the doctor for the top position in the hierarchy. This is not a bad thing, but a different way of operating. The health care delivery system in the United States is trying to figure out how to do this, whereas other countries, such as Canada and the United Kingdom, are involved in their own struggles to be effective with government-administered health care delivery. It is not the goal of this text to solve this problem.

Various forms of complementary health methods are becoming part of the health care system, and the transition is clumsy. The biggest hurdle truly seems to be economic. As mentioned, health care insurance is still seeking ways to include methods such as therapeutic massage in its reimbursement policies. Because few studies have confirmed the cost-saving benefits of massage, the justification for payment is elusive. Again, this text is not going to resolve this issue; in time, the problem will resolve itself. The massage professional needs to prepare now to be ready as the transition occurs.

Massage is part of the distant past, the current transition, and the future of health care. If you are going to be part of this environment, you must understand not only those with and for whom you work, but also your place in the system.

Therapeutic massage can be provided at various locations, from hospitals to nursing homes, sporting institutions to spas. The rules and preferences of all organizations are not the same. Similarities will exist, but as a massage therapist, you must comply with the policies of the organization for which you work. Its policies are intended to protect the patient, the organization, and you. Also, they may arise from health insurance or occupational safety regulations. If you have questions, ask.

In addition, massage therapists must remain current, continually enhance their training, and be ready to assume more of a team and peer role as the inevitable evolution takes place.

Massage is historically rooted in health care; this is not a new world for massage. Massage returning to its roots seems novel for this era. The following discussion will help you understand the organization of the health care environment as it currently operates; it also will help prepare you to become a contributing and productive member of the evolutionary process (Box 12-11).

Becoming Part of the Health Care Team. How will you work and behave with other health care professionals? In 1994, the Bureau of Health Professions released the findings of a task

---

BOX 12-11

The Patient Care Partnership: Understanding Expectations, Rights and Responsibilities

When you need hospital care, your doctor and the nurses and other professionals at our hospital are committed to working with you and your family to meet your health care needs. Our dedicated doctors and staff serve the community in all its ethnic, religious and economic diversity. Our goal is for you and your family to have the same care and attention we would want for our families and ourselves.

The sections explain some of the basics about how you can expect to be treated during your hospital stay. They also cover what we will need from you to care for you better. If you have questions at any time, please ask them. Unasked or unanswered questions can add to the stress of being in the hospital. Your comfort and confidence in your care are very important to us.

What to Expect During Your Hospital Stay

- **High quality hospital care.** Our first priority is to provide you the care you need, when you need it, with skill, compassion, and respect. Tell your caregivers if you have concerns about your care or if you have pain. You have the right to know the identity of doctors, nurses and others involved in your care, and you have the right to know when they are students, residents or other trainees.
- **A clean and safe environment.** Our hospital works hard to keep you safe. We use special policies and procedures to avoid mistakes in your care and keep you free from abuse or neglect. If anything unexpected and significant happens during your hospital stay, you will be told what happened, and any resulting changes in your care will be discussed with you.
- **Involvement in your care.** You and your doctor often make decisions about your care before you go to the hospital. Other times, especially in emergencies, those decisions are made during your hospital stay. When decision-making takes place, it should include:
- *Discussing your medical condition and information about medically appropriate treatment choices.* To make informed decisions with your doctor, you need to understand:
- The benefits and risks of each treatment.
- Whether your treatment is experimental or part of a research study.

- What you can reasonably expect from your treatment and any long-term effects it might have on your quality of life.
- What you and your family will need to do after you leave the hospital.
- The financial consequences of using uncovered services or out-of-network providers.
- Please tell your caregivers if you need more information about treatment choices.
- *Discussing your treatment plan.* When you enter the hospital, you sign a general consent to treatment. In some cases, such as surgery or experimental treatment, you may be asked to confirm in writing that you understand what is planned and agree to it. This process protects your right to consent to or refuse a treatment. Your doctor will explain the medical consequences of refusing recommended treatment. It also protects your right to decide if you want to participate in a research study.
- *Getting information from you.* Your caregivers need complete and correct information about your health and coverage so that they can make good decisions about your care. That includes:
- Past illnesses, surgeries or hospital stays.
- Past allergic reactions.
- Any medicines or dietary supplements (such as vitamins and herbs) that you are taking.
- Any network or admission requirements under your health plan.
- *Understanding your health care goals and values.* You may have health care goals and values or spiritual beliefs that are important to your well-being. They will be taken into account as much as possible throughout your hospital stay. Make sure your doctor, your family and your care team know your wishes.
- *Understanding who should make decisions when you cannot.* If you have signed a health care power of attorney stating who should speak for you if you become unable to make health care decisions for yourself, or a "living will" or "advance directive" that states your wishes about end-of-life care; give copies to your doctor, your family and your care team. If you or your family need

Continued

BOX 12-11

The Patient Care Partnership: Understanding Expectations, Rights and Responsibilities— cont'd

help making difficult decisions, counselors, chaplains and others are available to help.

■ **Protection of your privacy.** We respect the confidentiality of your relationship with your doctor and other caregivers, and the sensitive information about your health and health care that are part of that relationship. State and federal laws and hospital operating policies protect the privacy of your medical information. You will receive a Notice of Privacy Practices that describes the ways that we use, disclose and safeguard patient information and that explains how you can obtain a copy of information from our records about your care.

■ **Preparing you and your family for when you leave the hospital.** Your doctor works with hospital staff and professionals in your community. You and your family also play an important role in your care. The success of your treatment often depends on your efforts to follow medication, diet and therapy plans. Your family may need to help care for you at home.

You can expect us to help you identify sources of follow-up care and to let you know if our hospital has a financial interest in any referrals. As long as you agree that we can share information about your care with them,

we will coordinate our activities with your caregivers outside the hospital. You can also expect to receive information and, where possible, training about the self-care you will need when you go home.

■ **Help with your bill and filing insurance claims.** Our staff will file claims for you with health care insurers or other programs such as Medicare and Medicaid. They also will help your doctor with needed documentation. Hospital bills and insurance coverage are often confusing. If you have questions about your bill, contact our business office. If you need help understanding your insurance coverage or health plan, start with your insurance company or health benefits manager. If you do not have health coverage, we will try to help you and your family find financial help or make other arrangements. We need your help with collecting needed information and other requirements to obtain coverage or assistance.

While you are here, you will receive more detailed notices about some of the rights you have as a hospital patient and how to exercise them. We are always interested in improving. If you have questions, comments, or concerns, please contact _____.

Reprinted with permission of the American Hospital Association, copyright 2003.

force that had studied the use of interdisciplinary teams in health care. Six characteristics of successful interdisciplinary teams were identified:

■ Team members provide care to a common group of patients.
■ Team members develop common goals for performance outcomes and work together toward these goals.
■ Appropriate roles and functions are assigned to each team member.
■ Members understand and respect the roles of others.
■ All members contribute and share essential information about both tasks and the group process.
■ The team has a mechanism to ensure that plans are implemented, services are coordinated, and the performance of the team is evaluated.

The interdisciplinary medical team functions as a whole and requires the understanding and involvement of all team members. Individual tasks may lend themselves to one team member or another with specialized skills, but the final outcome is a team effort. Deciding on the diagnostic and therapeutic criteria that must be met for patients to be managed optimally is a job that typically falls to the physician.

Behaving in a professional manner in the medical environment creates trust. Trust is one of the most important factors in avoiding cases of medical professional liability. *Professionalism* means conforming to the technical or ethical standards of

a profession. It involves exhibiting courtesy, being conscientious, and conducting oneself in a businesslike manner at the workplace. Characteristics of professionalism include loyalty, dependability, courtesy, initiative, flexibility, credibility, confidentiality, and a good attitude. Professionalism is vital in the medical setting.

The Health Insurance Portability and Accountability Act of 1996

As mentioned in the earlier discussion of HIPAA, the Health Insurance Portability and Accountability Act of 1996 covers a multitude of the regulatory aspects of the health care environment. The Centers for Medicare and Medicaid Services (CMS) is responsible for implementing various, unrelated provisions of HIPAA, therefore HIPAA may mean different things to different people. For example, Title I of the act protects health insurance coverage for workers and their families when they change or lose their jobs.

Administrative Simplification. Title II, the administrative simplification provisions of the act, requires the Department of Health and Human Services to establish national standards for electronic health care transactions and national identifiers for providers, health plans, and employers. It also addresses the security and privacy of health data. Adopting these standards will improve the efficiency and effectiveness of the nation's health care system by encouraging the widespread use and exchange of electronic data in the health care industry.

Pre-existing Condition Exclusions. Under HIPAA, a group health plan or a health insurance issuer offering group health insurance coverage may impose a pre-existing condition exclusion with respect to a participant or beneficiary only under these conditions: (1) the exclusion relates to a condition for which medical advice, diagnosis, care, or treatment was recommended or received during the 6 months before the individual's enrollment date; (2) the exclusion may not last longer than 12 months (18 months for late enrollees) after an individual's enrollment date; and (3) the 12-month (or 18-month) period must be reduced by the number of days of the individual's prior creditable coverage, excluding coverage before any break in coverage of 63 days or more.

HIPAA also seeks to limit administrative costs by supporting the use of electronic transfer of information, and it establishes guidelines for preventing fraud and abuse. The privacy rules included in HIPAA have been the most discussed and debated topics with regard to this law. The massage therapist should receive in-service training about procedures relating to HIPAA requirements and how they are implemented in the specific health care environment.

Best Practice

Gradually, the world of health services appears to be changing from one in which individual doctors provide care one-on-one to a limited number of patients, to a world in which physician-led interdisciplinary teams will provide a wide array of services to populations of patients. To the fullest extent possible, the activities of teams of the future will be founded on evidence-based interventions, and their performance will be closely monitored by team members themselves as they constantly seek to improve their outcomes, as measured by clinical quality, service quality, and cost.

Knowing one's limitations and working with physician supervision, from the basis of quality medical practice, as well as effective risk management (i.e., best practices), make the massage therapist a contributing member of the health care team.

Because most patients are not at their best when visiting the physician's office, the attitude of the staff plays an important role in patients' attitude while in the office. Massage therapists need patience and understanding when working with those who are injured or ill.

Teamwork makes any job easier to complete. Helping coworkers who may be overwhelmed with duties supports the concept that they will return the favor when the situation is reversed in the future. It may not be part of your job description to straighten up the waiting room or stuff envelopes, but if you are not busy with massage-related activities, a team player helps out wherever and whenever he or she can. Never participate in gossip (if you do, others are likely to gossip about you as well; it simply is not constructive or acceptable professional behavior). Make a good attempt to get along with every employee.

Insubordination is being disobedient to any type of authority figure, usually the supervisor, and it can be grounds for immediate dismissal. When given a task, you should complete the work unless it is unlawful or unethical. If you have concerns about tasks not in your job description, speak with a supervisor. Discuss the issue and attempt to reach an agreement about the appropriateness of performing the task in the future.

First impressions are critical in the medical environment. Dress, attitude, and appearance all influence the credibility of the massage therapist (Figure 12-3). You should be neat and clean. Typically you will wear scrubs; flat, closed-toe, rubber-soled shoes; little or no jewelry; little or no makeup; short, clear, unpolished finger nails; no fragrances; and a modest hair style that is pulled away from the face. Tattoos and other visible forms of body art may be a concern, therefore make sure they can be concealed by the typical professional clothing.

Health Insurance

Reimbursement for services by health insurance companies is a common practice in health care. Currently, reliable reimbursement is one of the main obstacles to inclusion of many complementary methods, such as massage, in the health care process. This situation probably will improve as more research identifies a positive risk/benefit/cost value for massage services to justify reimbursement.

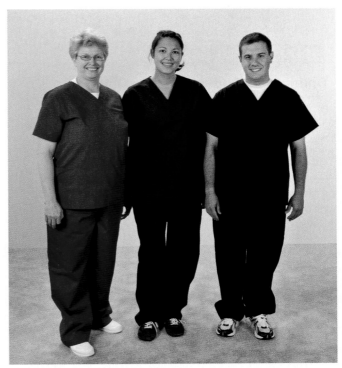

FIGURE 12-3 Professional dress for clinical massage therapists.

The infrastructure already exists for billing insurance companies for services rendered. Large facilities, such as hospitals, have designated departments to handle health insurance billing; small medical practices usually have a person who is responsible for this process. In the typical health care setting, the massage therapist would not bill directly for services rendered; rather, the massage practitioner would be responsible for making sure all records are kept correctly and are up-to-date and for following the preauthorized treatment plan. Although some massage therapists in some areas bill directly for insurance payment, this is not a common practice. The massage therapist with a career in health care needs to understand enough about health insurance and reimbursement to support the specialist in this area (i.e., the insurance biller and coder) (Box 12-12).

Health insurance is a type of third-party payer system. This means that the consumer (or his employer) pays for the insurance, and when medical expenses occur, the costs are billed to the insurance company, which pays them according to the consumer's (or the employer's) specific coverage plan. Numerous third-party payers base reimbursements on what is referred to as the *allowable charge;* what constitutes the allowable charge has been the subject of considerable debate and jockeying by managed care organizations, health insurance companies, and the government.

Health insurance is available to people in many ways. They can buy individual policies, but most get health insurance by being a member of a group, which pools resources to buy health insurance. Examples of groups that provide health insurance are businesses, which may offer health insurance as a job benefit; Chambers of Commerce, where small business owners can get coverage; and, for the massage profession, professional associations, such as the American Massage Therapy Association (AMTA) or the Associated Bodywork and Massage Professionals (ABMP).

Insurance policies have many coverage options, from minimal coverage to maximal coverage that includes independent nursing facilities, and some are including alternative and complementary care coverage. Because the cost of health insurance is rising quickly, growing numbers of people do not have insurance and therefore do not receive some types of necessary medical care. Some countries have government-based health care, and others have combined processes. In the United States, for example, many people have some type of private insurance, and certain at-risk populations, such as the elderly and poor, are eligible for Medicare and Medicaid, which are government programs.

Health care has changed tremendously in recent years, and the cost of quality health care has skyrocketed. Efforts have been made in both the public and private sectors to introduce various health care reforms to contain these costs. Health care reform has had little success on a national level; however, state legislatures are beginning to pass laws that have brought improvement.

Managed care is a broad term used to describe a variety of health plans developed to provide health care services at lower costs. There is a lot of confusion as to what managed care entails. Managed care has had both positive and negative effects on health care delivery.

Workers' compensation covers employees who are injured or who become ill as a result of accidents or adverse conditions in the workplace. Disability programs reimburse individuals for monetary losses incurred as a result of an inability to work for reasons other than those covered under workers' compensation. Automobile insurance coverage operates in many different ways, has different requirements, and may or may not cover personal injury.

The entire health insurance system is in crisis. Fortunately, a major advantage of employment in the health care environment is that the responsibility for billing falls to the gatekeeper, and you are paid a salary or fee for each massage, regardless of reimbursement. The massage therapist's responsibility is to maintain appropriate records to justify insurance reimbursement and to follow the preauthorized treatment plans as presented by the supervisory health care professional.

Record Keeping (Documentation)

Record keeping in various medical settings is extremely important (Figure 12-4). It is a skill that needs to be practiced and perfected. Massage therapy training often is lax in this area, therefore massage therapists who want a career in health care need to pay additional attention to it. (NOTE: Also see Chapters 3 and 10.)

Record keeping is the recording of relevant data. The word *documentation* can be used to describe the record keeping process.

BOX 12-12

Billing and Coding Responsibilities

- Assign Current Procedural Terminology (CPT) when required for facility and professional fee billing.
- Assign CPT for services and procedures and HCPCS billing codes for medical equipment and devices, with appropriate modifiers, when required for facility and professional fee billing and statistical indices.
- Assign codes to each diagnosis (ICD9CM) and identify and code the providers who ordered or provided services (ICD-9-CM Codes/Diagnostic) in each healthcare encounter as required for facility and professional fee billing.
- Assemble the patient's health information by making sure that initial medical charts are complete, including the member ID number and group number to verify eligibility of benefits.
- Follow federal and state regulations governing the assignment of any of the above codes for reimbursement.
- Work with insurance companies on issues such as prior approval and medical necessity to ensure payment.

Welcome

Thank you for selecting our health care team! To help us meet all your health care needs, please fill out this form completely in ink. If you have any questions or need assistance, please ask us - we will be happy to help.

Patient Information (CONFIDENTIAL)

Patient #_____

Soc. Sec. #_____

Date _____

Name_____ Birth date _____ Home phone _____

Address_____ City _____ State_____ Zip_____

Check appropriate box: ☐ Minor ☐ Single ☐ Married ☐ Divorced ☐ Widowed ☐ Separated

If student, name of school/college _____ City _____ State__ ☐ Full time ☐ Part time

Patient's or parent's employer _____ Work phone _____

Business address _____ City _____ State_____ Zip_____

Spouse or parent's name _____ Employer_____ Work phone _____

Whom may we thank for referring you?_____

Person to contact in case of emergency_____ Phone _____

Responsible Party

Name of person responsible for this account _____ Relationship to patient _____

Address_____ Home phone _____

Driver's license #_____ Birth date _____ Financial institution_____

Employer_____ Work phone_____ SSN#_____

Is this person currently a patient in our office? ☐ Yes ☐ No

Insurance Information

Name of insured _____ Relationship to patient _____

Birth date _____ Social Security #_____ Date employed_____

Name of employer_____ Union or local #_____ Work phone _____

Address of employer_____ City _____ State_____ Zip_____

Insurance company_____ Group #_____ Policy/ID #_____

Ins. co. address_____ City _____ State _____ Zip_____

How much is your deductible? _____ How much have you used?_____ Max. annual benefit _____

DO YOU HAVE ANY ADDITIONAL INSURANCE? ☐ Yes ☐ No   IF YES, COMPLETE THE FOLLOWING:

Name of insured _____ Relationship to patient _____

Birth date _____ Social Security #_____ Date employed_____

Name of employer_____ Union or local #_____ Work phone _____

Address of employer_____ City _____ State_____ Zip_____

Insurance company_____ Group #_____ Policy/ID #_____

Ins. co. address_____ City _____ State _____ Zip_____

How much is your deductible? _____ How much have you used?_____ Max. annual benefit _____

I authorize release of any information concerning my (or my child's) health care, advice and treatment provided for the purpose of evaluating and administering claims for insurance benefits. I also hereby authorize payment of insurance benefits otherwise payable to me directly to the doctor.

X_____

Signature of patient or parent if minor   Date_____

FIGURE 12-4 Some examples of record-keeping forms. (From Young AP, Proctor DB: *Kinn's the medical assistant: an applied learning approach,* ed 10, St. Louis, 2007, Saunders.)   *Continued*

PART A — PRESENT HEALTH HISTORY (continued)

IV. GENERAL HEALTH, ATTITUDE AND HABITS (continued)

Have you recently had any changes in your: If yes, please explain:

Marital status?   No ___ Yes ___
Job or work?   No ___ Yes ___
Residence?   No ___ Yes ___
Financial status?   No ___ Yes ___
Are you having any legal problems
or trouble with the law?   No ___ Yes ___

PART B — PAST HISTORY

I. FAMILY HEALTH

Please give the following information about your immediate family:

Relationship	Age, If Living	Age At Death	State of Health Or Cause of Death
Father			
Mother			
Brothers and Sisters			
Spouse			
Children			

Have any **blood relatives** had any of the following illnesses? If so, indicate relationship (mother, brother, etc.)

Illness	Family Members
Asthma	
Diabetes	
Cancer	
Blood Disease	
Glaucoma	
Epilepsy	
Rheumatoid Arthritis	
Tuberculosis	
Gout	
High Blood Pressure	
Heart Disease	
Mental Problems	
Suicide	

II. HOSPITALIZATIONS, SURGERIES

Please list all times you have been hospitali

Year	Operatio

III. ILLNESS AND MEDICAL PROBLE

Please mark with an (X) any of the following
If you are not certain when an illness started,

Illness	(X)
Eye or eye lid infection	
Glaucoma	
Other eye problems	
Ear Trouble	
Deafness or decreased hearing	
Thyroid trouble	
Strep throat	
Bronchitis	
Emphysema	
Pneumonia	
Allergies, asthma or hay fever	
Tuberculosis	
Other lung problems	
High blood pressure	
Heart attack	
High cholesterol	
Arteriosclerosis (Hardening of arteries)	
Heart murmur	
Other heart condition	
Stomach/duodenal ulcer	
Diverticulosis	
Colitis	
Other bowel problem	
Hepatitis	
Liver trouble	
Gallbladder trouble	

Page 2   © 1979, 1983 Bibbero Systems Int
(REV. 6/92)

C O N F I D E N T I A L

PART C — BODY SYSTEMS REVIEW

MEN: Please answer questions 1 through 12, then skip to question 18.
WOMEN: Please start on question 6.

N ONLY

Have you had or do you have
prostate trouble? .... No ___ Yes ___
Do you have any sexual problems
or with impotency? .... No ___ Yes ___
Have you ever had sores or
lesions on your penis? .... No ___ Yes ___
Have you ever had any discharge
from your penis? .... No ___ Yes ___
Do you ever have pain, lumps
or swelling in your testicles? .... No ___ Yes ___
ck here if you wish to discuss any special problems with the doctor.

	Rarely/ Never	Occasionally	Frequently
Is it sometimes hard to start your urine flow?			

(many rows with checkboxes)

the doctor ....

	Rarely/ Never	Occasionally	Frequently

No ___ Yes ___
No ___ Yes ___

No ___ Yes ___
No ___ Yes ___

No ___ Yes ___
No ___ Yes ___
No ___ Yes ___
No ___ Yes ___

No ___ Yes, Traveled in:

Measles ___	Smallpox ___
Mumps ___	Tetanus ___
Polio ___	Typhoid ___

No ___ Yes ___ Date ___
Neg ___ Pos ___
Pos ___

RN THIS PAGE   19-711-4   5/83   Page 3

C O N F I D E N T I A L

Chart No. ___

ANDRUS/CLINI-REC® HEALTH HISTORY QUESTIONNAIRE

Identification Information   Today's Date ___

Name ___   Date of Birth ___
Occupation ___   Marital Status ___

PART A — PRESENT HEALTH HISTORY

I. CURRENT MEDICAL PROBLEMS

Please list the medical problems for which you came to see the doctor. About when did they begin?

Problems	Date Began

What concerns you most about these problems?

If you are being treated for any other illnesses or medical problems by another physician, please describe the problems and write the name of the physician or medical facility treating you.

Illness or Medical Problem	Physician or Medical Facility	City

II. MEDICATIONS

Please list all medications you are now taking, including those you buy without a doctor's prescription (such as aspirin, cold tablets or vitamin supplements).

III. ALLERGIES AND SENSITIVITIES

List anything that you are allergic to such as certain foods, medications, dust, chemicals, or soaps, household items, pollens, bee stings, etc., and indicate how each affects you.

Allergic To:	Effect	Allergic To:	Effect

IV. GENERAL HEALTH, ATTITUDE AND HABITS

How is your overall health now? .... Health now: Poor ___ Fair ___ Good ___ Excellent ___
How has it been most of your life? .... Health has been Poor ___ Fair ___ Good ___ Excellent ___
In the past year:
  Has your **appetite** changed? .... Appetite: Decreased ___ Increased ___ Stayed same ___
  Has your **weight** changed? .... Weight: Lost ___ lbs. Gained ___ lbs. No change ___
  Are you **thirsty** much of the time? .... Thirsty: No ___ Yes ___
  Has your overall 'pep' changed? .... Pep: Decreased ___ Increased ___ Stayed same ___
Do you usually have **trouble sleeping**? ...... Trouble sleeping: No ___ Yes ___
How much do you **exercise**? .... Exercise: Little or none ___ Less than I need ___ All I need ___
Do you **smoke**? .... Smokes: No ___ Yes ___ If yes, how many years? ___
How many each day? .... ___ Cigarettes ___ Cigars ___ Pipesfull
Have you ever **smoked**? .... Smoked   No ___ Yes ___ If yes, how many years? ___
How many each day? .... ___ Cigarettes ___ Cigars ___ Pipesfull
Do you **drink alcoholic beverages**? .... Alcohol: No ___ Yes ___ I drink ___ Beers ___ Glasses of Wine
                                                              ___ Drinks of hard liquor - per day
Have you ever had a problem with alcohol? ...... Prior problem: No ___ Yes ___
How much **coffee** or tea do you usually drink? . Coffee/Tea: ___ cups of coffee or tea a day.
Do you regularly wear **seatbelts**? .... Seatbelts: No ___ Yes ___

DO YOU:	Rarely/ Never	Occasionally	Frequently	DO YOU:	Rarely/ Never	Occasionally	Frequently
Feel nervous?				Ever feel like committing suicide?			
Feel depressed?				Feel bored with your life?			
Find it hard to make decisions?				Use marijuana?			
Lose your temper?				Use "hard drugs"?			
Worry a lot?				Do you want to talk to the doctor about a personal matter? No ___ Yes ___			
Tire easily?							
Have trouble relaxing?							
Have any sexual problems?							

Created and Developed by "Medical Economics" Professional Systems
Copyright © 1979, 1983 Bibbero Systems International, Inc.   STOCK NO. 19-711-4   5/83   Page 1

C O N F I D E N T I A L

FIGURE 12-4, cont'd

There are nine characteristics of quality health data:

- *Validity* refers to the accuracy of the information.
- *Reliability* means that others can count on the information to be accurate, and medical decisions can be made based on the information.
- *Completeness* means that the information is available in its entirety.
- *Recognizability* means that the data can be understood by those who use them.
- *Timeliness* means that the information is the latest available about a patient or treatment.
- *Relevance* refers to the usefulness of the information.
- *Accessibility* means that the information is easily available to the provider when it is needed.
- *Security* encompasses the effort to keep unauthorized people from accessing the information.
- *Legality* refers to the correctness of the information and its authentication by the health care provider.

The following general guidelines can help practitioners create a credible patient record.

- Each page of the record should identify the patient by name, hospital or clinic, private physician, and clinical record number.
- Each entry in the record should include the date and time the entry was made, as well as the signature and credential of the individual making the entry.
- No blank spaces should be left between entries.
- All entries should be written in ink or produced on a printer or typewriter.
- The record must not be altered in any way. Erasures, use of correction fluid, and marked-out areas are not appropriate.
- Errors should be corrected in a manner that allows the reader to see and understand the error. The following procedure is recommended:
  1. A single line is drawn through the error, maintaining the legibility of the previous entry.
  2. The correct information is inserted.
  3. The correction is dated and initialed.
  4. If there is not enough room to make the correction legibly at the error, a note is made indicating where the corrected entry can be found, and the reference is dated and initialed. The correct information is entered in the proper chronologic order for the date the error was discovered and corrected.
- All information should be recorded as soon as possible. Memories can fade, and important facts can be omitted.
- Abbreviations should be used sparingly and should include only those that have been approved by the organization; an abbreviation code should be included on the document. Otherwise, a single abbreviation can have different meanings, which can be misleading.
- Health care providers must write legibly. It is embarrassing, and can be expensive, when caregivers cannot read their own entries in court. Because the patient record is used by so many other clinicians in providing care, it is important to the quality of care that the record be legible.

- All entries must be consistent with one another. The assessment must agree with the diagnostic testing, or an explanation must be given as to why it does not.
- Entries should be factual accounts. Criticisms of the patient or a colleague should never be included. Records that blame or belittle others can be damning evidence in a lawsuit.
- All information given to the patient before any procedures should be recorded. This ensures and verifies that the patient was properly informed of the benefits and risks before the person consented to the procedure.
- Telephone contacts with the patient should be entered in the record immediately.
  - Some method of organizing entries must be used (e.g., the SOAP format [see Chapter 3]) to ensure that they are comprehensive and reflect the thought process used when decisions are made about the patient's care.

If these rules are followed, the record will be accurate, timely, specific, objective, concise, consistent, comprehensive, logical, and legible and will reflect the thought processes of the health care providers.

The Computer-Based Patient Record and the Electronic Health Record

The paper medical record is fast becoming a thing of the past. A paper record is difficult to access, often lacks information, must be kept in a single location, and is available only for a single user at a time. Over the past three decades, significant strides have been made in automating the record-keeping process. Technology has improved, allowing the design and implementation of electronic record-keeping systems that are easy to use. Automated record-keeping systems have many different names, such as *computer-based patient record (CPR), electronic health record (HER), computerized medical record,* and *electronic record.* Massage therapists must become competent with the electronic record-keeping system in use where they work. For all these systems, the thought process is the same, and the data record is the same. The massage practitioner may need to jot paper notes while working with the patient, but eventually the notes must be entered into the electronic system (Figure 12-5).

Patient health care records are confidential. Most health care providers, and certainly hospitals, have policies and procedures governing the release of any information about a patient. Massage therapists must be aware of those policies. Most health care providers have established policies and procedures that incorporate the HIPAA requirements.

All states have laws about which diseases, conditions, and events must be reported to appropriate agencies. These may include births, deaths, gunshot wounds, communicable diseases, and evidence of child abuse. If massage therapists are confronted with any such incidents in the health care setting, they should report the situation to the supervisor, who will deal with it. Massage therapists should ask their supervisors if the therapist should expect to encounter any specific reportable circumstances. When reporting is required by law,

FIGURE 12-5 Electronic record examples.

FIGURE 12-5, cont'd

confidentiality is no longer an issue. However, the format of the report may or may not include the identity of the patient, therefore the therapist should make sure to ask about the proper method of reporting. Reporting such incidents to anyone other than the responsible agency is a breach of confidentiality.

Massage Career in Health Care

Career development for massage therapists in the health care system is in its infancy. The two main obstacles are a lack of appropriately trained massage therapists and the inability to obtain health insurance reimbursement.

Hopefully, a dedicated group of massage professionals will commit to the training necessary to perform well in the health care environment. The financial issues are more of a concern, but the trends point to health care coverage that will allow health care organizations and professionals to provide massage therapy. Health insurance currently covers massage if the practitioner is supervised by an approved gatekeeper, if the procedure is billed correctly, and if treatment is provided in the appropriate environment. As previously mentioned, in some instances massage therapists may participate in specific insurance networks that allow direct billing. However, this situation is not common in a health care environment such as a hospital or physician's office.

As in any job search, networking and contacting employers directly are the two best methods of finding a job. Networking involves developing a group of individuals who can assist you in finding employment. This group may include coworkers, relatives, or friends who provide leads to potential employers. Contacting employers directly includes taking resumés to specific offices and/or setting appointments to gain knowledge about the facility before using that knowledge during the job search. Make sure your resumé is free of errors. Be sure everything is spelled correctly, but do not rely solely on the computer's spell-check feature. Proofread the document (and have someone else who is knowledgeable proofread it) to catch errors that may have been overlooked. Salary expectations should never be stated on the resumé, nor should a photograph be included. Do not include personal information, such as height and weight.

Employers in the health care setting have some basic expectations. They want an employee who is well trained, has a good appearance, and looks as if he or she fits into the medical profession. A massage therapist must also be dependable and have the skills to do the job for which he or she was hired.

Employers look for three types of skill strengths: job skills, self-management skills, and transferable skills. *Job skills* are the skills needed to perform the job (e.g., the ability to give a beneficial massage based on outcomes). *Self-management skills* usually are personality based; they include honesty, dependability, a sense of humor, tolerance, and flexibility, to name just a few. *Transferable skills* are skills that can be taken from one job to another or used on any job. Examples include the ability to maintain appropriate records, to communicate effectively, and to lead and manage individuals.

The way in which massage therapy will be provided in the health care setting is evolving. Therefore volunteering in various settings can both create awareness of the benefits of massage and put you in a position to be noticed by potential employers. Volunteer opportunities are available in most hospitals, cancer centers, hospices, and other facilities. You can also volunteer to work with medical staff (i.e., doctors, nurses, and others). Massage therapists in private practice can gain the respect of the medical community by following the guidelines in this text, and networking with health care professionals can result in referrals.

Compatibility of Massage and Health Care

The extensive list of professionals who make up the health care staff is incredible. Increased specialization is driven both by increases in available information and by advances in technology. It is almost impossible to be a generalist anymore in any field; there is just too much to know.

How do current massage education and credentialing compare with the education and credentialing of those who work in the health care system? This is a good question. Where in the hierarchy does massage fit in? Who will be the supervisors? Is it possible to justify massage as a beneficial modality in the health care system? What will be the extent of responsibility and accountability? Based on a comparison of the most typical massage education programs in the United States, an associate's degree in massage has little availability, although this situation is improving. Even fewer opportunities exist to obtain a bachelor's degree in massage therapy. Some in the massage profession do not believe that a degree is necessary. This is a valid viewpoint, because some health care staff members (e.g., emergency medical technicians [EMTs]) obtain certification rather than a degree.

As mentioned previously, entry level education (500 to 750 contact hours) is the most commonly pursued massage education. This level of education can be combined with specialized clinical massage training, such as that delivered in a minimum of 250 contact hours plus clinical experience of a minimum of an additional 250 hours, resulting in a total of about 1,200 contact hours. This number of contact hours can be compared to about 36 credit hours, typical of 1 year of college (three terms of 12 credits each). The comparable educational level in health care would be a certified technician, nondegreed but vocationally trained. Future educational requirements for clinically based massage may rise to the associate's degree level.

What does this mean for the massage therapist working in the health care setting? The simple answer is status, responsibilities, and pay comparable to that of others at this level of professional development. This implies that massage therapists will recognize their comparative level of training and abide by their limited scope of practice, maintaining humility and a cooperative attitude and respecting other professionals who have much more extensive training and responsibilities. To get respect, we must first give it.

Pay Scales for Therapeutic Massage in the Health Care Environment

Concrete data that compare similar training levels and degrees of responsibility limited to a highly focused medical intervention should provide at least a basis for determining how massage therapists will fit into the health care system. Consider the EMT; the responsibilities of an EMT are to:

- Respond to an emergency call, assesses the situation, obtain a basic medical history, perform a physical examination of the patient, and provide emergency medical care at the scene and during transit to the hospital
- Use medical equipment to treat patients and ascertain the extent of their injuries or illness
- Communicate with the medical facility receiving the patient about the patient's condition, status, and arrival time
- Have a high school diploma, successfully complete EMT training, register with the EMT national registry, obtain licensure from the state emergency medical services (EMS) authority, and have 2 to 4 years of related experience

- Be familiar with standard concepts, practices, and procedures in a particular field
- Rely on experience and judgment to plan and accomplish goals and perform a variety of tasks
- Work under the supervision of a manager

The annual salary for an EMT can range from $23,000 to $30,000.

A comparison of educational requirements for health professionals (Bureau of Labor Statistics http://www.bls.gov/) shows that those who provide direct, hands-on care to patients usually have an associate's degree. Health professions that have training programs similar to those for massage include phlebotomist, certified nurse aide, dental assistant, EMT, and occupational therapy assistant. Based on these data, the annual entry-level salary for massage therapy will range from $22,000 to $30,000. In addition, typical benefits packages, including health care, are offered. If a massage therapist has an associate's degree or higher, previous health care experience, or is dually trained (e.g., is a licensed practical nurse [LPN]), the pay rate may be as high as $35,000 a year (Box 12-13).

BOX 12-13

Professional Perspective of Massage in Healthcare

The owner and director of the College of Integrative Healthcare in Oceanside, California, Dr. Randy Snyder, gives his perspective on the role of massage in health care.

As we continue to move through a new century, it is interesting to look back on the progress the massage profession has made and ponder about what lies ahead. I would not hesitate to say that as of this date, the profession is poised for rapid growth. As our country struggles with a health care crisis based on problems that focus on quality, affordability, and access to health care, our profession continues to define its place in mainstream health care. The United States in particular faces many health care challenges, since we are the only major industrialized nation without universal access to medical care. On the other hand, universal access to care does not guarantee access to massage therapy services. Nor does it create automatic acceptance of our services in mainstream health care settings. This book is one step closer to helping close the administrative and clinical gaps that currently block increased utilization of massage services and greater recognition of massage therapy in the health care community.

Health care today remains a fragmented delivery system with a lack of coordinated care. Expenses continue to skyrocket, with health care premium rates growing much higher than general inflation. Iatrogenic events, or health care–caused injury or illness, are at an all-time high. As massage therapists, we might think we are immune to these events, but the truth is, we must learn to look at these issues if we want to be part of the bigger picture. The new paradigm in health care will demand safer, cost-effective, and more accessible care, no matter who is providing it. Consider this: when looking at the three main complementary provider services, that is, acupuncture, chiropractic, and massage, massage appears to be the safest, most medically integrated, and most popular

service! I would say the profession is off to a great start, but the work is hardly just beginning.

Part of our future will depend on how well our services compare with and complement existing complementary therapies and medical care. All health care providers are being held to a higher level of accountability. This means we must accept the challenge to provide and to prove that we offer effective care that has measurable clinical and cost benefits. Our care must be evidence based and supported by the current research literature. Anecdotal stories of miraculous cures will no longer replace published literature based on high-quality research. As health care adopts technology to improve record keeping and other administrative tasks, we must learn to adopt these tools for better business and clinical efficiency.

Many factors move a profession toward maturity. Some of these are licensure, accreditation, and third-party reimbursement. Currently, the profession has 40 licensed states with legislative initiatives toward licensing in several others. Accreditation by the Commission On Massage Therapy Accreditation (COMTA) and other major accrediting agencies, although still a voluntary process that represents a small number of schools, continues to grow. The profession continues to work toward improved regulation and licensure portability. The Massage Research Foundation sponsored the first United States massage research conference in September, 2005, and drew more than 180 attendees. Financing for the conference was partly sponsored by a grant from the National Center of Complementary and Alternative Medicine, a division of the National Institutes of Health. The National Certification Board of Therapeutic Massage and Bodywork (NCBTMB) now allows 300 hours of distance education out of the 500 hours of required training. The state of Florida is running a pilot project examining the effects of including massage therapy with their Medicaid program. This government program has previously

Continued

BOX 12-13

Professional Perspective of Massage in Healthcare—cont'd

excluded massage therapy in all states. These and many more are signs of an emerging profession whose growth and development will accelerate in the coming years. As our profession grows alongside traditional health care, we will have further exposure to and opportunities with third-party reimbursement. This is the main reimbursement source for health care that will open accessibility to massage therapy services for patients who could not afford or were unaware of your services in the past. Also, this will expand the marketability of massage therapy and exposure to the value of massage therapy services, which will grow the existing demand for your services.

There is currently an increased trend in health care to move more services into the purview of vocationally trained individuals. Some of the reasons include greater cost effectiveness and greater access to larger pools of trained individuals. This will help the profession in many ways, as massage therapists are one of the few vocationally trained professionals in the complementary and alternative health care arena. Your services will continue to grow in demand, and your skills will continually need to be updated and enhanced to accommodate this growth. Health care will become a team approach, requiring you to work and communicate more effectively in a variety of environments and under the supervision of other healthcare professionals. You will have opportunities you never expected if you expand your knowledge and thinking and become a lifelong learner!

I work as a case manager for an insurance company and have reviewed many treatment plans submitted by massage therapists. Although managed care is new to most massage therapists, it is not new to most healthcare providers. There are several things you must know.

First, realize that most insurance companies have resources that allow you to access information about clinical reasoning and treatment planning. These resources are generally provided through an operations manual or by electronic access via a CD or the Internet. Often we tend to overlook this because we want to speed through the process as easily as possible. This often hinders our ability to work adequately within the system and can cause frustration. Think of it this way: if you're going to play the game, you need to learn the rules.

It is important to have certain information presented through medical records or insurance forms that give the patient's complaints and medical history. The frequency and duration of complaints, as well as the mechanism of injury, if available, should be described. This is usually recorded on a patient intake form by the patient and includes biographical information such as name, address, date of birth, and so forth. In addition, you will need to provide assessment information in the form of postural evaluation, gait, and palpation. These findings can be further broken down into graded information (mild, moderate, severe) with regard to range of motion, tenderness, muscle tone, and trigger points. Although it is not necessary to have all this information recorded for every complaint, you should provide enough findings to adequately evaluate all complaints. If you intend to treat something, you need assessment findings that justify the treatment plan, and are reasonable based on the magnitude of the complaints. Once you have assessed the patient, your treatment frequency and duration should be based on the particular needs of the patient, taking all historical and assessment information into consideration. This information should include any historical information about comorbidities (e.g., diabetes, fibromyalgia, and so on) that might influence how the patient responds to care. It is not necessary to have a physician's referral with all insurance companies, but referral and comanagement to or from another health care professional must be recorded when indicated. All these things have to do with the accountability factors in health care that other health care professionals must adhere to. The documentation should support and justify your treatment request in a rational manner based on the available evidence-based literature and/or consensus of the profession. If someone else is going to pay the bill, they have the right and obligation to review this information. In fact, it goes farther than that. It is also based on health and safety concerns for which the insurance company is held accountable by regulators and accreditation agencies

Think, learn, and grow. Don't just graduate and remain stagnant. In this day and age, you will never succeed in any profession unless you stay actively involved in professional development.

THERAPEUTIC MASSAGE IN THE SPORTS AND FITNESS ENVIRONMENT

 12-2

SECTION OBJECTIVES

Using the information presented in this section, the student will be able to perform the following:

- Provide massage in various environments and in the context of typical sports schedules
- Adjust massage to respect the habitual behavior of the athlete
- Use simple, safe applications of adjunct therapies to support the massage outcome related to common sports and performance sports injuries

---

It is encouraging to see that more and more sports, fitness, and rehabilitation professionals are turning to massage as part of the treatment or management of various conditions. Unfortunately, many misconceptions, inaccurate information, and even dangerous methods are being passed off as sports massage.

Clients of sports and fitness massage represent a range of different needs. Some clients are undergoing physical rehabilitation that requires an exercise program (e.g., cardiovascular and cardiorespiratory rehabilitation, physical therapy for an orthopedic injury). Other clients are taking up exercise as part of a comprehensive fitness and wellness program, including weight management. Still other clients are recreational athletes or competitive athletes, both amateur and professional.

Many practitioners of massage (some legitimate and some not) who are interested in "sports massage" want to work with professional athletes. The reality is, those jobs are rare, and tending to professional athletes requires a lot of time, travel, and flexibility. There are not that many professional or Olympic athletes around. The National Basketball Association (NBA) has fewer than 400 players, and the National Football League (NFL) has fewer than 2,500. The other team sports fall somewhere between those numbers. Individual professional athletes, such as tennis players, golfers, and bowlers, are also a small community. Most massage therapists will serve the high school, collegiate, amateur, or semiprofessional athlete and, even more, those undergoing rehabilitation or striving to maintain fitness. A common misconception is that professional athletes make millions and millions of dollars; the truth is, only a few make it into that category. Most make far less, and amateurs generate no athletic income at all. Therefore justifying the cost benefit of therapeutic massage, compared with the expense and regularity of use, is an ongoing issue. More commonly, sports fitness and rehabilitation cost money, often lots of it. If a person is going to use massage regularly, the fees have to be manageable.

First off, there is no such thing as "sports massage"—only the appropriate massage application for each client. If the client is a runner; bowler; swimmer; surfer; golfer; or baseball, basketball, football, or soccer player, or a "civilian" who has just finished a treadmill stress test, that is an important factor to consider as part of the treatment plan. The immediacy and intensity of the athlete's world demand an integrated body/mind/spirit approach delivered by well-trained massage professionals who have obtained training beyond the entry-level program.

Additional demands are placed on professionals who work with athletes or in physical rehabilitation because of the extraordinary circumstances of these clients. The environment of competitive sports or physical rehabilitation makes for "bigger than life" moments. There is the drama of win or lose, the trauma of injury, and the career-determining or even life or death situations of surgery and rehabilitation. Working in the sports and fitness environment can be like a roller coaster ride, but with a lot of monotony between the highs and the lows. Obviously, massage therapists in this field must be highly skilled in the massage applications appropriate for the particular type of sport or fitness activity. What is not so obvious is that they also must have the characteristics of motivation, maturity, reliability, compassion, tenacity, tolerance, stamina, flexibility, commitment, faith, hope, perseverance, humbleness, self-esteem, and little need for personal glory, as well as the ability to work behind the scenes, to improvise, and, above all, to think and problem solve.

Common Goals and Outcomes for Massage in Sports and Fitness

Two primary goals of sports massage are to assist the athlete in achieving and maintaining peak performance and to support the healing of injuries. Any massage professional should be able to recognize common sports injuries and should refer the athlete to the appropriate medical professional. Once a diagnosis has been made and the rehabilitation plan developed, the massage professional can support the

athlete with general massage application and appropriate methods to enhance the healing process.

Many factors contribute to mechanical injuries or trauma in sports. In sports, *trauma* is defined as a physical injury or wound sustained in a sport that was produced by an external or internal force. Healing mechanisms manifest as the inflammatory response and resolution of the inflammatory response. The different tissues heal at different rates. For example, skin heals quickly, whereas ligaments heal slowly. Stress can influence healing by slowing the repair process. Sleep and proper nutrition are necessary for proper healing.

Types of Sports Massage

In the past, massage for athletes has been categorized by when it is given and the reasons for the massage. Some of those categories are discussed in the next paragraphs. However, if outcome-based goals are used, these categories become irrelevant. If massage is used to assist pre-exercise warm-up, it should focus on those goals. As with "sports massage," there really is no such thing as a "pre-event massage"; the same goes for massage that focuses on supporting the recovery process after competition (the so-called postevent massage).

Dealing with the terminology as it is currently used, some categories of sports massage are the pre-event (or warm-up) massage; the intercompetition massage; the remedial, medical, or orthopedic massage; the recovery massage; the postevent (or maintenance) massage; and the promotion (or event) massage.

Pre-event (Warm-up) Massage

The pre-event, or warm-up, massage is a stimulating, superficial, fast-paced, rhythmic massage that lasts 10 to 15 minutes. The emphasis is on the muscles used in the sporting event, and the goal is to help the athlete feel that his or her body is perfect physically. Uncomfortable techniques should be avoided. The pre-event massage is given in addition to the physical warm-up; it is not a substitute. This style of massage can be used from 3 days before the event until just before the event. Massage techniques that require recovery time or are painful are strictly contraindicated. The massage therapist should focus on enhancing circulation and should be very careful not to overwork any area. The sports pre-event massage should be general, nonspecific, light, and warming. Neither friction nor deep, heavy strokes should be used; this is a pain-free massage. Preferably, only massage therapists who work on a continual basis with a particular athlete should give the person a pre-event massage.

Intercompetition Massage

Intercompetition massage, given during breaks in the sports event, concentrates on the muscles being used or those about to be used. The techniques are short, light, and focused. It is suggested that only massage therapists familiar with a particular athlete provide intercompetition massage.

Recovery massage focuses primarily on athletes who want to recover from a strenuous workout or competition and who have no injuries. The method used to help an athlete recover from a workout or competition is similar to a generally focused, full-body massage and incorporates methods that support a return to homeostasis.

Remedial, Rehabilitative, Medical, and Orthopedic Massage

Terminology can be confusing; the terms *remedial massage, rehabilitative massage, medical massage,* and *orthopedic massage* are all interrelated. Remedial massage is used for minor to moderate injuries. Methods used in remedial massage include all those presented in this text. Rehabilitative massage is used for more severe injuries or as part of the postsurgical intervention plan; if the injury or surgery is related to bones or joints, this type of massage can be considered orthopedic massage. The massage methods used in rehabilitation vary. Immediately after injury or surgery, the techniques used generally are more nonspecific and focus on reducing stress and promoting healing. Attention is given to the entire body while the area of injury or surgery heals. If immobility, use of crutches, or changes in posture or gait are factors during recovery, compensation patterns are likely to develop. Massage can manage these compensation patterns while the physician, physical therapist, and trainer focus on the injured area. During active rehabilitation, massage can become part of the total treatment plan for recovery, when supervised by an appropriately qualified professional.

Promotional (Event) Massage

Promotional massages usually are given at events for amateur athletes. The massages are offered as a public service to provide educational information about massage. It is important to have written documentation of informed consent from each person who wants to receive a massage at these events (Box 12-14). One way to do this is to provide an informed consent statement on the top of a sign-in sheet and have each participant read and sign it before receiving the massage. Each participant should be given a short brochure or pamphlet explaining the benefits, contraindications, and cautions for sports massage. If the organizer of the event allows it, the brochure could include contact information to allow participating athletes to get in touch with the massage professional at a later date.

The sports event massage is quick paced and lasts about 15 minutes. In this type of public, promotional environment, following a sports massage routine is important. The use of lubricants is optional, and the massage practitioner may choose not to use them because of the risk of allergic reaction, staining of an athlete's uniform, or other unforeseen factors.

It is important to watch for swelling that may indicate a sprain, strain, or stress fracture; if any of these are noted, the athlete should be referred to the medical tent for immediate evaluation. It also is important to watch for evidence of thermoregulatory disruption, such as symptoms of hypothermia or hyperthermia; if these are noted, the massage therapist should refer the individual immediately but without using any diagnostic terms or unduly alarming the person.

If a massage professional is doing promotional work at a sports event and is working with many unfamiliar athletes, the best course is to do postevent massage, because the effects of any neurologic disorganization caused by the massage are not significant.

BOX 12-14

Sample Informed Consent Form for Use at Sporting Events

Name: _____

Sporting event: _____

Date: _____

I have received, read, and understand informational literature concerning the general benefits of massage and the contraindications for massage. I have disclosed to the massage practitioner any condition I have that would be contraindicated for massage. Other than to determine contraindications, I understand that no specific needs assessment will be performed. The qualifications of the massage practitioner and reporting measures for misconduct have been disclosed to me.

I understand that the massage given here is for the purpose of stress reduction. I understand that massage practitioners do not diagnose illness or disease, perform any spinal manipulations, or prescribe any medical treatments. I acknowledge that massage is not a substitute for medical examination or diagnosis, and it is recommended that I see a health care provider for those services.

I understand that an event sports massage is limited to providing a general, nonspecific massage approach using standard massage methods but does not include any methods to address specifically soft tissue structure or function.

Participant's signature: _____   Date: _____

Participant's signature: _____   Date: _____

Participant's signature: _____   Date: _____

No connective tissue work, intense stretching, trigger point work, or other invasive work should be done with an athlete at a sporting event. The massage should be superficial and supportive and should be focused more on enhancing circulation.

The Sports Massage Team

Often a group of massage professionals and supervised students work an event as a team. A team leader who is familiar with the sport usually is in charge at the sporting event. All the participating massage practitioners follow a similar routine. Remember, each member of a sports massage team represents the entire massage profession. Ethical, professional behavior is essential. This is the reason the permission of the organizer is required if you intend to put contact information on a brochure about massage that you distribute at such an event. The textbook, *Sports and Exercise Massage: Comprehensive Care in Athletics, Fitness, and Rehabilitation,* by Sandy Fritz (Mosby, 2006) provides comprehensive information about working in this environment (Box 12-15).

SPECIAL POPULATIONS

The first part of this chapter dealt with where massage is provided. This part of the chapter focuses on the people (and animals) receiving massage. In this section we examine ways massage professionals can show respect for and help those who need special consideration, and we provide information on ways to accommodate those who need a specific massage environment. The intent is to help massage professionals focus the benefits of therapeutic massage for clients with specific needs. Each section offers a general description of the special situation, the application for massage, and directions for obtaining further training and information. Individuals (and/or animals) can be seen in any of the previously described environments: spas, the health care environment, and the sports and fitness environment. The following special populations or circumstances are considered in this part of the chapter (the topics are presented in alphabetical order for ease of reference):

- Animal massage
- Athletes
- Breast massage
- Children
- Chronically ill individuals
- The elderly
- Infants
- On site massage
- Physically challenged individuals
  - Visual impairment
  - Speech impairment
  - Hearing impairment
  - Mobility impairment
  - Size (height and weight)
  - Burns
  - Amputation
- Psychologically challenged individuals
  - Addictions
  - Chemical imbalances of the brain
  - Developmental disabilities
  - Learning disorders
  - Psychiatric disorders
  - Post-traumatic stress disorder/abuse
- Pregnant women
- The terminally ill

The basic skills presented in this textbook seldom change when applied in special situations and unique environments, such as a cruise ship, day or destination spa, hospital, extended living facility, hospice, business office, or baseball field. Gliding and kneading for a person (or animal) with special needs is still gliding and kneading. The difference is in the recipient of the treatment and the way the treatment is done. Working with special populations requires additional knowledge about the specific situations or conditions addressed. The practitioner also must keep in mind the effects of any training protocols, developmental stages, medical treatments, accommodations (e.g., barrier-free access), or counseling in conjunction with the therapeutic massage.

In the exploration of each situation, it is important always to see the individual as a person first, with the special need as only a secondary consideration. There are no visually impaired, hearing impaired, sick, or abused people; there are people who have visual or hearing impairments, who deal with various illnesses, or who have been abused. For example, athletes are just people expected to maintain peak performance. Basic

---

BOX 12-15

Athletic Training

The Board of Certification of the National Athletic Trainers Association has established six performance domains, based on the 1999 Role Delineation Study:

- Prevention of athletic injuries
- Recognition, evaluation, and assessment of injuries
- Immediate care of injuries
- Treatment, rehabilitation, and reconditioning of athletic injuries
- Health care administration
- Professional development and responsibility

Education competencies established by the Education Council are:

- Acute care of injury and illness
- Assessment and evaluation
- General medical conditions and disabilities
- Health care administration
- Nutritional aspects of injury and illness
- Pharmacologic aspects of injury and illness
- Professional development and responsibility
- Psychosocial intervention and referral
- Risk management and injury prevention
- Therapeutic exercise
- Therapeutic modalities

massage skills are sufficient to serve all people because they promote general health and increase well-being. Certainly specific rehabilitative massage requires additional education, but the most common application of therapeutic massage, in conjunction with special situations, is general, nonspecific support, which is within the training levels presented in this text.

It is the massage professional's responsibility to learn as much as possible about the client's situation and the environment in which the massage is provided. If working with tennis players, the therapist should learn about tennis; if working with survivors of abuse, the therapist should learn about abuse; if the work is in pain management, the therapist needs to understand pain and its treatment protocols; if working with children with attention deficient disorder (ADD), the massage therapist must understand ADD and its treatment protocols. If working with a family dog, the massage therapist needs to understand dogs. Unique environments present challenges. Providing massage in a posh spa is different from working with a marathon runner lying on the ground, a football player in an athletic training room, a dancer backstage at the ballet, a client in a pain clinic, or a horse in a stall. Using the clinical reasoning model, the massage professional can develop intervention plans and justifications for the benefits of therapeutic massage as part of a comprehensive care program regardless of the circumstances.

The best way to obtain information about a client's special needs is to ask the person directly. It is important to understand clearly the action plans required for various environments. It is necessary to expand skills and knowledge in response to real practice challenges. There is no way a school or textbook can prepare you for every conceivable situation you may encounter in professional practice. Various research avenues are available, and the Internet is an especially wonderful source of information. When the practitioner understands the client's particular situation, the physiologic effects of massage that provide the most benefit can be identified and intervention plans can be developed (Box 12-16).

BOX 12-16

Use of the Clinical Reasoning Model to Determine Self-Study Needs, Develop a Treatment Plan, and Justify the Efficacy of Massage Therapy

The following example shows how the massage therapist can use the clinical reasoning model effectively in approaching a particular condition.

Example: Therapeutic massage for children with attention deficit disorder

1. Gather facts to identify and define the situation.

Key questions:

What is the problem?

What are the facts?

Attention deficit disorder (ADD) is primarily an organic condition that tends to have a genetic manifestation. It is characterized by the inability to sustain focused attention, a condition called *distractibility* or *inattention.* Often one or more of the following also are present: free association to many thoughts, impulsivity, moodiness, anxiety, withdrawn or spaced-out behavior (more prevalent in females), propensity to high-stimulation activities and behavior, bad temper, impatience, poor impulse control, and hyperactivity (in attention deficit/hyperactivity disorder [ADHD]).

ADD tends to be a biochemical disorder of dopamine, norepinephrine, and serotonin imbalance. Stimulant medication is used to normalize the neurochemical imbalance. Stimulant medication increases sympathetic arousal, which can lead to side effects of appetite suppression, digestive upset, headache, and sleep difficulties.

Massage affects the neurochemicals involved in ADD by increasing dopamine and serotonin levels and increasing the norepinephrine level during the first 15 minutes. Massage inhibits sympathetic arousal if it lasts approximately 30 minutes or longer and acts as a form of sensory stimulation.

2. Brainstorm possible solutions.

Key question:

What might I do? or What if . . . ?

If massage stimulates the same neurochemicals as the medications, it might be possible to lower the dosage of medication. Because it stimulates sympathetic arousal, massage may support effective use of medication at a lower dosage. Mild cases of ADD might be controlled with massage and similar methods.

Because massage can also inhibit sympathetic arousal, it may alleviate some of the side effects of the medication, allowing the use of a higher dosage if necessary. It may also reduce generalized stress in both child and parent.

Possible interventions include the following:

- Self-help methods
  - A simple hand massage routine
  - Complicated finger tapping exercises to provide sensory stimulation
  - Progressive relaxation
  - A breathing pattern consisting of a short inhalation through the nose and a long exhalation through the mouth
  - Training methods such as blowing up a balloon, blowing through a flute, and blowing bubbles
  - Stimulation of acupressure points
  - Entrainment mechanisms (e.g., rhythmic rocking)
- Professional massage
  - Full-body, broad-based compression for 30 to 45 minutes
  - Shiatsu technique
  - Chair massage for 15 to 30 minutes
- Massage methods taught to parents
  - Compression
  - Slow-stroke massage
  - Assisted progressive relaxation
  - Rocking

BOX 12-16

Use of the Clinical Reasoning Model to Determine Self-Study Needs, Develop a Treatment Plan, and Justify the Efficacy of Massage Therapy—cont'd

3. Evaluate possible interventions logically and objectively; look at both sides and pros and cons.

Key question:

What *would* happen if . . . ?

Headaches and stomachaches could be helped the most by massage interventions. The interventions could help reduce stress symptoms and off-task behavior, although not every child would respond to the same type of intervention.

Medication could be used effectively, although the dosage would need to be monitored.

Parental involvement is necessary because the physiologic benefits of the methods are most effective if reinforced daily. However, parental participation could be minimal and inconsistent.

The child would usually relax with a very firm pressure. Light pressure would usually stimulate and agitate. Disrobing would be problematic.

Drawbacks to this program include cost, parental consistency, and time factors. Also, children under age 10 may not be old enough to learn self-help methods.

4. Evaluate the effect on the people involved.

Key question:

How would each person involved feel?

The child would enjoy the interventions, although a great deal of energy would be needed to keep such children focused.

Appreciation of these children is necessary to work effectively.

These children become bored and inattentive when required to do repetitive tasks.

5. Develop an intervention plan and justification statements.

Bodywork methods clearly have much to offer in the management of behavioral difficulties and the stress faced by children with ADD/ADHD. Many interventions could be used, such as teaching self-help methods, clinical sessions, and parental teaching and coaching.

Massage methods provided over the clothing would be emphasized to avoid the need for lubricant and disrobing. The longer 30- to 45-minute session for stress management and relaxation would be recommended for the clinical sessions. The shorter 15-minute massage would be helpful in focusing attention for task concentration, such as doing homework. This 15-minute session could be taught to the parent.

Self-help methods could be taught to older children. A simplified version of the soothing massage could be taught to parents to encourage effective sleep and provide a calming effect. Parents could benefit from the same massage methods for stress management.

Consistent self-massage by the child and massage by the parent to provide various forms of sensory stimulation are necessary to achieve benefits. Continuing education and encouragement for the parents, who are also stressed, are important. A supportive coaching role can be provided to complement the bodywork interventions.

Massage can be a wonderful way to reduce stress, promote well-being, and provide a respite from the daily challenges faced by those with special needs. Being able to respond successfully and provide massage in any setting or environment, such as the rushed and hectic setting of an airport or the sacred space of the deathbed, expands your client base and ability to serve.

ANIMAL MASSAGE

SECTION OBJECTIVES

Using the information presented in this section, the student will be able to perform the following:

- Identify the difference between massage, grooming, and petting
- Explain the benefits of massage both for well animals and for those receiving veterinary care
- Adapt a massage based on outcomes and the animal's size and species
- List necessary components of specific animal massage education

Just as with humans, massage for animals is a complementary therapy that encourages the animal's own healing and wellness processes. Therapeutic massage works in animals for the very same reasons, already described, that it does in humans.

Massage is more than petting. Petting is less focused and much more general than massage. Petting animals is pleasurable and beneficial to both the animal and the person. However, massage is a deliberate, focused technique of touching. It is the manipulation of soft tissue to promote well-being at both a physical and an emotional level. The desired effect for an individual animal can be achieved by applying various mechanical forces to different areas of the body. Each animal is assessed and treated as an individual. What works for one animal might not be right for the next. Determining factors include species, age, size, activity level, injuries, and medications. Assessment identifies target areas, contraindications, and outcomes. The history is based on information from the person responsible for the animal's well-being (Figure 12-6).

The specialist in the health care of animals is the veterinarian. Methods such as massage should never be substituted for proper veterinary care. The American Veterinary Medical Association (AVMA) has offered the following guidelines for massage therapy in conjunction with medical care:

Massage therapy on nonhuman animals should be performed by a licensed veterinarian with education in massage therapy or, where in accordance with state veterinary practice acts, by a graduate of an accredited massage school who has been educated in nonhuman animal massage therapy. When performed

FIGURE 12-6 A, Greeting the animal. **B,** Use a gentle, confident touch. **C,** Pay attention to body language. **D,** Secure, confident handling is important.

by a nonveterinarian, massage therapy should be performed under the supervision of or referral by a licensed veterinarian who is providing concurrent care.

Just as humans do, animals respond to the wellness benefits of massage. With animals, just as with infants and young children, body language is an important communication process. Animals generally are very good communicators if you take the time to observe and to learn how they communicate with you.

The various methods used for human massage are also used for animal massage. The anatomy and physiology of animals are very similar to human anatomy and physiology. However, before working with a particular species, the massage therapist should review the anatomy unique to that species.

As with children and their parents, massage therapists who work with animals are likely to find themselves in the role of teacher. They often must demonstrate massage techniques and instruct the caretaker in their use for the specific animal. The massage therapist must be confident and comfortable with the particular animal, or the massage application will be stressful for both the massage therapist and the animal. An excellent resource for understanding animal behavior is *Animals in Translation: Using the Mysteries of Autism to Decode Animal Behavior,* by Temple Grandin and Catherine Johnson (Scribner, 2004).

Communication

Animals tend to interpret our movements and gestures just as if we were one of them. For example, if a person approaches an unfamiliar dog tied to a post, then looks at the dog and reaches down to pet it on top of the head, the intention of the gesture is greeting and friendliness. To the dog, however, the direct eye contact and reaching down from above are threatening because this is what dogs do to each other to threaten a stranger. The dog that is being petted on the head may become unnecessarily frightened or might even become aggressive to the well-meaning stranger. Common sense dictates that we do not assume that animals understand our words and gestures the way we mean them. This is especially true for unfamiliar animals. Animals that we live with may learn that our stares and petting are not threats, but the unfamiliar animal may not know this.

The fact that different species of animals may interpret our behavior in very different ways makes it difficult to always know the proper way to act. For example, to dogs, standing and facing them head on can be threatening, whereas for cattle, turning your side to them can be threatening.

Some good rules for dealing with unfamiliar animals include the following:

- Do not approach or reach for an unfamiliar animal.
- Quick movements toward an animal can be frightening or threatening to the animal.

FIGURE 12-7 Performing animal massage. **A,** Take a history. **B,** Interact. **C,** Assess. **D,** Perform massage. **E,** Move joints (toys okay). **F,** Enjoy the interaction.

- Do not stick out a hand for an animal to smell.
- Direct eye contact is threatening to many species of animals.
- Standing over most animals is threatening to them.
- Speaking loudly or sharply to animals can be frightening.
- Dogs may interpret deep voices as growls.

The best advice is to become familiar with the gestures and signals of the animals you are going to massage. Do not risk interacting with the animal if you are uncertain how it will respond. Just as with infants and children, it is important to approach animals at their level. For small animals (dogs and cats), sit down on the floor and wait for the animal to approach you. For large animals (horses), stand still, look down. and wait for the animal to approach you. Rely on the human caregiver to comfort the animal and stay by its side. Never force an interaction (Figure 12-7).*

Massage Benefits for Animals

Typical outcomes for animal massage are support, bonding, stress reduction, relaxation and pleasure, pain relief, and

*Proper Etiquette With Animals, Daniel Estep, Ph.D. and Suzanne Hetts, Ph.D. www.AnimalBehaviorAssociates.com Copyright ABA, Inc. Retrieved April 2006

increased performance. Massage can enhance muscle function and efficiency and reduce recovery time from injury or sore muscles. Many veterinarians and respected research scientists believe that massage can assist the body in the healing process. Massage has been proven to increase health and vitality. It can be used in conjunction with prescribed veterinary care and to augment that care.

Animals That Benefit from Massage

Working Animals

Dogs. Guide dogs; service dogs; police dogs; search and rescue dogs; dogs used to detect drugs, explosives, and evidence of arson; sled dogs; and other dogs that work for humans endure tremendous physical performance stress. Massage can ease the strain of the demands placed on them.

Horses. Massage can be beneficial for police horses; horses that pull sightseeing carts in resort areas; racehorses; horses used to teach people to ride; pleasure horses that may have erratic riding schedules; horses involved in competitions such as jumping, dressage, and endurance; horses that work farms and ranches; and horses involved in therapeutic riding programs. These animals benefit from the stress reduction and physical comfort provided by massage.

Various Animals

Various animals involved in entertainment and education are good subjects for massage. These animals are typically transported in confining cages and moved into unfamiliar locations. Massage can ease the stiffness caused by confinement, as well as performance stress.

Athletic Animals

Animal athletes that compete in races and in agility, obedience, and field trials, as well as other such activities, need to be kept in peak condition. Regular massage can increase range of motion, lengthen stride, and improve overall muscle tone. Incorporating massage into the training regimen can also reduce the risk of injuries.

Older Animals

Geriatric animals can benefit from massage in many ways. It can reduce the pain and tension caused by arthritis and other joint and bone conditions. Massage is also good for animals who are less active because of advanced age.

Infant and Adolescent Animals

Massage can alleviate the discomfort often caused by rapid growth of bones and muscles. It can also calm and focus the excitable, active adolescent. Massage can reduce the risk of injury that frequently results from rowdy play, jumping, rolling, wrestling, and generally being adventurous.

Shy or Recently Adopted Animals

Massage can reduce the stress and anxiety experienced by animals adjusting to new homes. It can also help shy or mistrustful animals to accept human touch and build confidence.

Animals Recovering from Injury or Undergoing Postoperative Rehabilitation

Massage administered in cooperation with the animal's veterinarian can reduce recovery time, support fluid movement, prevent problems caused by muscle atrophy and adhesion, and ease the transition back to normal levels of activity (Box 12-17).

Human Benefit

Animal massage bestows some very important benefits on the person doing the massage. Teaching those who are anxious, lonely, or depressed to massage animals can be a productive aspect of the person's treatment and care. Research has shown that when stroking an animal, people relax and their blood pressure drops.

Pain Management

A major outcome for animal massage is pain management. Animals' behavior changes in response to pain, particularly persistent pain. The changes that occur depend on the degree of pain, the animal's tolerance of it, the animal's species, the situation in which the pain occurs, the animal's stress level, and a variety of other factors. Acute pain may produce an aversive reaction in an animal. A normally compliant, friendly animal may attempt to bite a person who is causing it pain, or the animal may try to flee from the cause of the pain.

BOX 12-17

Massage Benefits for Animals

- Improve circulation, increasing the supply of blood and nutrients to muscles and bone
- Aid the elimination of wastes and toxins from the body
- Increase flexibility and function of the joints
- Help maintain posture and body balance
- Stimulate metabolism, aiding weight loss
- Improve muscle tone
- Enhance range of motion and gait function
- Promote a healthy skin and coat
- Help age-related problems and assist in recovery from injury or surgery
- Help reduce muscle atrophy resulting from inactivity or disuse
- Relieve muscle tension, soreness, and spasms
- Aid in the elimination and prevention of muscular adhesions and connective tissue changes
- Shorten the time required for rehabilitation of soft tissue injuries
- Reduce chronic pain and discomfort caused by arthritis, hip dysplasia, and other conditions
- Calm hyperactive, anxious, and nervous animals
- Counteract the effects of stress and anxiety
- Build trust and acceptance of being touched
- Support bonding

Chronic or long-term pain (e.g., arthritis) is likely to produce more subtle behavioral changes. Animals, just like people, react to pain through coping mechanisms that are both internal and external. Descending pathways from the brain to the spinal cord inhibit neuronal activity and reduce the sensation of pain. In addition, compounds are released that have opioid effects (e.g., endorphins and encephalin).

Animals in pain often withdraw from their social group, choosing instead to remain alone, to be less active, and to be less responsive to external stimuli. Persistent pain sometimes causes an animal to traumatize the area that hurts, typically by excessively scratching, rubbing, biting, or licking the site. This behavior may actually be an attempt at pain management through counterirritation. Abnormal postures, such as a hunched back or a tiptoe gait, may also point to pain. Food and water intake often is altered when an animal is in pain, regardless of the source of the pain.

Grooming is an important activity for animals, and failure to groom is an early sign of pain. The hair or fur may be standing up rather than lying down smooth. It may be dull rather than shiny, and it may be matted or clumped, particularly around the face and mouth and the anal and genital openings.

Pain Behavior in Animals That Are Commonly Massaged (Figure 12-8)

Dogs. Dogs in pain generally appear quieter, less alert, and withdrawn. Their body movements are stiff, and they are unwilling to move. A dog in severe pain may lie still or adopt an abnormal posture to minimize discomfort. In less severe pain states, the dog may appear restless, because the immediate response to acute but low-intensity pain may be an increased alertness. Shivering and increased respirations with panting may be seen. Spontaneous barking is unlikely; the dog is more likely to whimper or howl, especially if left unattended, and it may growl without apparent provocation. A dog may lick or scratch at painful areas of its body, and the tail is often between the legs. Penile protrusion and frequent urination also may occur. A dog in pain may have an anxious look, and it may seek a cold surface on which to lie. When handled, the dog may be abnormally apprehensive or aggressive.

Cats. Cats in pain generally are quiet and have an apprehensive facial expression. The forehead may appear creased. The cat may cry or yowl, and it may growl and hiss if approached

FIGURE 12-8 Examples of animals most likely to be pet massage clients.

or made to move. Cats in pain have a tendency to hide or to separate from other cats. The posture usually becomes stiff and abnormal, varying with the site of the pain. A cat with head pain may keep its head tilted. If the pain is generalized in the thorax and abdomen, the cat may be crouched or hunched. With thoracic pain alone, the head, neck, and body may be extended. With abdominal or back pain, the cat may lie on its side with the back arched. If the animal is standing or walking, the back is arched and the gait is stilted. Incessant licking is sometimes associated with localized pain. Pain in one limb usually results in limping or holding up of the affected limb.

A cat in severe pain may show demented behavior and make desperate attempts to escape. Touching or palpating a painful area may produce an instant and violent reaction. The animal may pant, and the pulse rate may be increased and the pupils dilated. A cat in chronic pain may have an ungroomed appearance and may show a marked change from its normal behavior. The limbs are tucked, the head and neck are hunched, the ears are flattened, and the animal utters a distinctive cry or hissing and spitting sound. Cats in pain show fear of being handled and may cringe.

Horses. Periods of restlessness are typically observed in horses experiencing pain or distress. Food is held in the mouth uneaten. The horse exhibits an anxious appearance, with dilated pupils and glassy eyes; other signs include increased respiration and pulse rate, flared nostrils, profuse sweating, and a rigid stance. With prolonged pain, the animal's behavior may change from restlessness to depression, with the head lowered. With pain associated with skeletal damage, the limbs may be held in unusual positions, the head and neck are "fixed," and the horse may be reluctant to move. Pain-induced tachycardia may be seen.

With abdominal pain, a horse may look at, bite, or kick its abdomen; it may get up and lie down frequently, walk in circles, or roll. When near collapse, the horse may stand very quietly, rigid and unmoving. Horses in pain generally show a reluctance to be handled.

Birds. Birds in pain may show escape reactions with vocalization and excessive movement. Head movements increase in extent and frequency. The heart and respiratory rates also may increase. Prolonged pain results in inactivity, with a drooping, miserable appearance. The eyes may be partly closed, the wings held flat against the body, and the neck retracted. When the bird is handled, the escape reaction may be replaced by a state of immobility. Birds with limb pain avoid using the affected limb and "guard" it to prevent extension.

Table 12-1 summarizes the signs of pain. It is presented as a checklist of possibilities rather than a complete description.

Pain Medication for Animals

Opioid Agonists. Opioids used in veterinary medicine include morphine, meperidine, fentanyl, oxymorphone, etorphine (M99), and carfentanil. They are all effective analgesics that work through the central nervous system.

TABLE 12-1

Signs of Pain in Animals

Characteristic	Sign
Protecting injured part (e.g., limb, abdomen)	Commonly seen; animal may be reluctant to move the part
Vocalizing	Especially if forced to move
Respiration	Increased rate; breathing may be shallow
Attitude	May be depressed and unresponsive to stimuli
Food and water intake	Usually decreased
Urination and defecation	Reduced volume and frequency
Appearance	Unkempt, piloerection, reduced self-care
Eyes	May be sunken, occasional discharge

Implications for Massage. The side effects of the opioid antagonists in animals are similar to those in humans. These medications can depress the central nervous system and affect breathing and levels of consciousness. It is important to observe for these effects and immediately report them to the veterinarian.

Nonsteroidal Antiinflammatory Drugs. Nonsteroidal antiinflammatory drugs (NSAIDs) produce analgesia by reducing inflammation and peripheral sensitization. They typically do not act on the central nervous system, as do opiates. Side effects of NSAIDs include interference with platelet function, anticoagulative action, kidney function, and gastric ulcers. Cats metabolize NSAIDs slowly, and toxicity can quickly occur, therefore these pain medications are not typically used in cats. NSAIDs commonly used in dogs are aspirin, naproxen, meclofenamic acid, flunixin, phenylbutazone, dipyrone, and piroxicam.

Implications for Massage. The side effects of NSAIDs are similar to those seen in humans: altered pain perception and a tendency for increased bleeding and bruising, which would influence the amount of compressive force delivered during massage. Kidney failure is a serious condition. Signs of kidney failure include decreased appetite, increased water consumption and urination, increased sleeping, lethargy, itching, and a change in the smell of the breath. If these behaviors are noticed, the animal should be immediately referred to the veterinarian for emergency care.

Local Anesthetics. Pain relief can be obtained by using local anesthetics, which can be injected around specific nerve trunks that supply a surgical or injury site, or infiltrated into the muscular and subcutaneous tissue layers around the area.

Implication for Massage. Do not massage over the area where local injections are given.

Topical Analgesics. Various ointments that act as counterirritants can be used for local pain. It is important to make sure that the ingredients are nontoxic, because animals typically lick areas that are painful.

Implications for Massage. Massage can be used to apply the ointment and to enhance its action through the use of tactile stimulation to increase the counterirritant effects.

Rehabilitative Massage

Rehabilitation therapy is any measure taken to restore maximum function after an injury or illness as well as after surgery. Conditions for which rehabilitative massage may be used include the following:

- Arthritis
- Hip dysphasia
- Fractured limb (after repair)
- Cruciate ligament injury
- Intervertebral disk disease
- Muscle sprains and strains
- Scar tissue management after surgery

Rehabilitative massage for an animal should be supervised by the veterinarian and/or an experienced animal handler as part of a total treatment program.

Providing Massage for Animals

Formal training for animal massage is varied, and opinions on the correct methods are inconsistent. A massage student who is interested in obtaining specific education in animal massage should thoroughly investigate any provider of animal massage training to make sure the individual is qualified to teach. Massage therapists who want to work with animals should obtain training in animal grooming, animal training, or some sort of veterinary assistant education. You must understand the anatomy, physiology, and behavior of each species you intend to work with. Learning grooming procedures, especially for large animals, such as horses, provides the necessary skills for safety, sequence, and flow for the massage, which would follow grooming patterns and some animal behavior. The massage professional providing massage must not be tentative or afraid of the animal and must work with each animal client with confidence and respect while continually being aware of subtle communication from the animal. Animals generally have an excellent sense of smell. Avoid using any scented products.

The methods of massage application presented in this text can all be adapted to animals; there are no unique modalities. Animals comprise a population, just as do infants, the elderly, and athletes. Animals can be babies, toddlers, adolescents, parents, middle aged, and elderly. Each of these life stages presents unique circumstance that must be considered. In general, recommendations for humans can be translated to animals. For example, baby animals and baby humans act similarly, except that animals go through the stages much faster. They may be babies for only a few weeks, and then become rambunctious toddlers, and then independent adolescents. Nursing mothers can be very protective of their babies, and elderly animals have most of the characteristics of human elders.

Humans become very attached to their animal companions. Pets are part of the family, and the massage therapist who works with animals must be able to communicate and respect the human as much as the animal. People sometimes have requirements for their pets (e.g., clothing or "hair styles") that are not particularly important to the animal. Humans can become quite eccentric about their animal companions, and these eccentricities must be respected unless they present a danger to the animal. If they do pose a danger to the animal, education about animal safety and health is important, and referral to the veterinarian may be necessary.

History and Assessment

A history and assessment are required for an animal just as they are for a human client. The massage therapist should obtain the following information from the animal's caretaker:

1. The animal's name
2. Any medical problems
3. Is the animal used to being handled?
4. Does the animal bite?
5. Is the animal easily frightened?

The massage therapist should meet the animal and become familiar with it and its human companion. Once the animal feels comfortable with the massage therapist, the next step is a visual and physical assessment to make sure the animal does not have any open wounds or sores that would be a contraindication to massage or require referral to a veterinarian.

Massage therapists need to be alert for problems that can be indicated by body temperature, texture of the skin and muscle fibers, tenderness of certain areas, and tension. The outcome for massage needs to be determined and a treatment plan established.

Massage Application

The qualities of touch previously described in this textbook also apply to massage for animals.

Pressure. Just as with humans, it is important to be sure that the pressure applied is effective in achieving the determined outcomes but does not cause unnecessary pain or tissue damage. Animals do not like to be poked, prodded, and dug on. The animals with which I have worked did not have a problem communicating when the pressure was inappropriate. Animals can vocalize, attempt to move away, and nip (not bite). If the pressure is appropriately intense, the animal typically vocalizes but does not attempt to move away from the pressure and may even lean into it.

Pressure (applied compressive force) varies with the size of the animal. A pet ferret does not need as much pressure as a horse.

Drag. Hair, fur, and feathers make it difficult to apply drag to the skin surface. The superficial fascia and deeper tissues can be worked by lifting the skin (which may be quite loose) and then using various mechanical forces to move the tissues into ease and bind.

Direction. The direction of massage application, which is similar to that in human massage, varies according to the desired outcome (e.g., fluid movement or changes in muscle motor tone).

Duration. The duration of a massage depends on the animal's acceptance and condition. The first session typically is an introductory meeting to allow the massage practitioner to become more familiar with the animal, to learn about its history, and to help the animal build trust and an acceptance of being touched. The first session lasts about 1 hour; the massage itself lasts 15 to 20 minutes, depending on the animal. Some animals accept a 60-minute, full-body massage at the first session, and others may take multiple sessions to learn to enjoy massage. The massage therapist works with the specific needs of each animal and teaches the person responsible for care how to perform the massage.

Frequency. Therapeutic massage can be given daily for 10 to 30 minutes for healthy animals. If a disease or injury is involved, massage of different areas of the body every other day is recommended. However the needs of each animal vary. For animals as well as people, a weekly massage provided as part of a well-balanced maintenance plan is recommended.

Specifics of Massage Application

Each species has unique behaviors, anatomy, and physiology. The massage therapist needs to consider the nature of the animal species when developing the massage approach. The following are brief explanations of species specifics; further research is needed to work with a particular species (Figure 12-9).

Dogs. Dogs come in many different sizes, and the intensity of mechanical forces applied during massage must be adjusted accordingly. Dogs are very domesticated, and most, but not all, of the innate wild behavior has been bred out of them. Dogs are pack animals and display pack behavior. They can be very protective of their caregivers and become aggressive if they perceive that their caregiver is threatened. Some breeds are more aggressive and protective than others. Unless conditioned otherwise, dogs are eager to interact with humans. Once acclimated, they love massage and are cooperative in the process.

Pet Pigs. Pigs come in a variety of sizes, and some breeds have become pets. Pigs are very intelligent and make good human companions if the human has the proper commitment and facilities to care for them. Pigs can act very much like dogs, and the interaction and massage are very similar.

Cats. Domesticated cats typically do not vary in size as much as dogs, therefore fewer adjustments are required in the intensity of mechanical force. However, cats are much more independent than dogs and retain more of their wild instincts. Forcing a cat to do something against its instincts is very difficult. Some people have exotic large cats as pets. These cats

FIGURE 12-9 **A,** Canine musculature. **B,** Equine musculature. (From Christenson DE: *Veterinary medical terminology,* ed 2, St. Louis, 2009, Saunders.)

retain most of their wild instincts, and unless you are specially trained to handle big cats, it is best not to massage them.

Birds. Birds can be surprisingly interactive and affectionate, especially birds that have a long life span, such as parrots. Birds are social and enjoy being touched and being close to their human. However, they can become very possessive and territorial. The bite of a parrot can be very serious.

Birds have more porous bones, which supports flight, and pressure levels must be adjusted. In most domesticated birds the flight feathers have been clipped to limit the bird's ability to fly. Birds are extremely smart and have been shown to solve problems and plan. Some species can be taught to vocalize and are excellent mimics. They may only need to hear something once to be able to repeat it, so watch what you say if you work with talking birds. Massage for birds is not as common as for dogs and cats but is appropriate. The feathers are a bit more difficult to work with than fur or hair.

Rodents, Rabbits, and Ferrets. Rodents, rabbits, and ferrets are popular pets and enjoy human touch if conditioned to the pleasure of it when babies. These animals are also very social and are very intelligent. Size varies tremendously, from tiny mice and hamsters to guinea pigs and giant rabbits. Rabbits and ferrets can be litter trained and are good companions for adolescents and adults; like cats, they can live indoors their entire life. With the increase in apartment dwelling by humans, these pets are becoming more common. Just as with all animals (including us), these animals go through various life stages, and massage needs to be adjusted based on outcomes.

Horses. Massage for horses, or equine massage, is very popular. Like dogs, horses have a long historical relationship with humans. They just recently have taken on a companion role more than a work role in humans' lives. Because horses are large animals, the potential for harm to the massage therapist is greater. The following suggestions are important when massaging a horse (or any large animal):

- Do not jump around or move suddenly, do not wear shiny or noisy jewelry or strongly scented products, and do not behave nervously around horses. All of these result in a nervous horse that is unsafe to work around.
- Wear hard-toed shoes or boots when working around horses. One of the most common horse-related injuries is having a foot stepped on.
- Always let the horse know what you intend to do. Quick, sudden movements startle horses and should be avoided.
- Keep all equipment away from the work area unless it is being used at the moment. This prevents the horse from stepping on it, playing with it, or chewing on it; it also prevents the massage therapist from accidentally tripping over it.
- Start massaging on the left side of the neck and work toward the rear of the horse. Then repeat on the right side. This pattern follows the standard grooming process for horses. Areas that have few muscles and bones near the surface, such as the face, legs and hips, should be massaged carefully and gently. Stand near the horse during the massage and use fluid, rhythmic movements, not quick, jerky movements that are likely to startle the animal.
- When changing sides, either walk far enough away to avoid getting kicked or stay close to the horse's rear quarter with a hand on the rump, to break the momentum of the kick. Never step over the lead rope or crossties. This puts you in a very dangerous position should the horse panic and pull back on the rope. Never crawl under the horse's belly. Even the most docile horse can spook and step on you.
- Be aware that some horses are ticklish and may become fidgety. During fly season, particularly, a horse often thrusts its hind leg forward to chase flies from the abdomen; therefore, it is wise to keep your head and body out of striking range when working in that area.
- When massaging the legs, bend at the hips or remain in a squat position. Do not sit on the ground or rest one or both knees on the ground. These are committed positions, which mean once in them, it takes longer than a split second to get out of them. In committed positions, if the horse should become frightened, the time it would take you to move away from scrambling hooves and the chance of becoming seriously injured are increased. It always helps to have your free hand resting on the horse's body while working on the legs; this way you can feel the muscles tense up and be warned that the horse is about to panic.

Cows, Goats, Sheep, and Other Farm Animals. Each of these species, as well as each individual animal, has a set of behaviors and a personality that need to be respected. Small differences in anatomy need to be understood, and the massage therapist must study the specific anatomy of each animal with which they work. These animals typically serve the human population in a way different from a pet, although any of these creatures can be socialized and become companions. As mentioned, pigs are especially social and intelligent and are often pets.

These animals usually supply food or products for human use, such as eggs, milk, wool, and meat. If the animal is raised for meat consumption, eventually it will be slaughtered. This text does not take a position on whether this is correct, nor does it present a judgment on how animals serve humans. Instead, the position is that all creatures should be treated with respect and provided safe and healthy living conditions. Regardless of how the animal serves humans, it is our responsibility to serve them as well by making sure that all creatures are treated humanely. This is important not only for farm animals but also for laboratory animals. Again, the book by Temple Grandin and Catherine Johnson, mentioned previously, is strongly recommended. Massage is nurturing and calming, regardless of the situation, be it daily milking, wool shearing, or other interactions with these creatures that, by serving humans, make humans' lives better.

Body of Knowledge for Animal Massage

Before providing massage to any animal on a professional basis, the massage therapist should obtain additional training in the following areas (Proficiency Exercise 12-1).

- Animal behavior and handling: Animal behavior, handling, breed characteristics, developmental periods, proper socialization, basic health routines, disease prevention, and animal communication
- Training tools: Clickers, collars, leashes, housetraining aids, chewing deterrents, interactive toys, and safety devices
- Anatomy and physiology specific to the animal: Anatomic terms, the musculoskeletal system, and comparative anatomy and physiology
- Kinesiology and biomechanics: Joint movements, physical structures, and gait
- Massage training: Continuing education as an aspect of massage education above entry-level requirements in a qualified and valid education program
- Pathology: Animal health, common ailments, and emergency care

See the Evolve Web site on animal massage research articels.

 PROFICIENCY EXERCISE 12-1

1. *Discuss with a groomer or veterinary technician what it is like to work with animals.*
2. *Spend time at the local Humane Society or animal rescue shelter and massage the animals to support socialization.*

ATHLETES

(Author's note: The author's knowledge base in this area has been acquired through her extensive work with professional football and basketball teams, along with individual athletes.)

SECTION OBJECTIVES

Using the information presented in this section, the student will be able to perform the following:

- List the experts in the care and training of athletes
- Identify common athletic injuries
- Explain the three types of restorative sports massage
- Explain the concept of event sports massage
- List the necessary components of additional sports massage training

An athlete is a person who participates in sports as either an amateur or a professional. Athletes require precise use of their bodies. The athlete trains the nervous system and muscles to perform in a specific way. Often the activity involves repetitive use of one group of muscles more than others, which may result in hypertrophy; changes in strength and movement patterns; connective tissue formation; and compensation patterns in the rest of the body. These factors contribute to the soft tissue difficulties that often develop in athletes. Fitness (see Chapter 13) is necessary for everyone's wellness, but the physical activity of an athlete goes beyond fitness; it is performance based.

Massage can be very beneficial for athletes if the professional performing the massage understands the biomechanics required by the sport. If the specific biomechanics are not understood, massage can impair optimal function in the athletic performance. Because of the intense physical activity involved in sports, an athlete may be more prone to injury.

The experts for athletes are sports medicine physicians, physical therapists, athletic trainers, exercise physiologists, and sports psychologists (Box 12-16). It is especially important for athletes to work under the direction of these professionals to ensure proper sports form and training protocols. The professional athlete is more likely to have access to these professionals. Amateur athletes may not have the financial resources to hire training personnel and can incur injury from inappropriate training protocols. With athletes, the psychological state is crucial to performance; often the competition is won in the mind. State-dependent memory, as described in the previous section, applies to athletes as well, especially if an injury has occurred during competition.

Athletes depend on the effects of training and the resulting neurologic response for precise functioning. This is especially important before competition. Without the proper training and experience, massage therapists can easily disorganize the neurologic responses if they do not understand the patterns required for efficient functioning in the sport. The effect is temporary, and unless the athlete is going to compete within 24 hours, it usually is not significant. However, if the massage is given just before competition, the results could be devastating. Any type of massage before a competition must be given carefully.

If a massage professional plans to work with an athlete on a continuing basis, it is important that the practitioner come to know the athlete and become part of the entire training experience.

Common Sports Injuries

massage professionals working with athletes should be able to recognize common sports injuries and should refer the athlete to the appropriate medical professional. The massage therapist adapts the massage application using appropriate methods to enhance the healing process once a diagnosis has been made and the rehabilitation plan developed.

Many factors contribute to mechanical injuries or trauma in sports. In sports, *trauma* is defined as a physical injury or wound sustained in a sport that was produced by an external or internal force. Healing mechanisms manifest as the inflammatory response and resolution of the inflammatory response. The different tissues heal at different rates. Skin heals quickly, whereas ligaments heal slowly. Stress can influence healing by slowing the repair process (Table 12-2). Sleep and proper nutrition are necessary for proper healing.

Massage that focuses on enhancing circulation (see Chapter 11) is appropriate, as are the other methods presented in Chapters 9 and 11, except for deep transverse friction, specific myofascial release, and extensive trigger point work. Medications, particularly analgesics for pain and antiinflammatory drugs, are commonly used, and the effects of these drugs must be considered (see Appendix C). Pain medication reduces pain perception so that the athlete can continue to perform before healing is complete. This interferes with successful healing. Antiinflammatory drugs may slow the healing process, particularly connective tissue healing.

Understanding sports injuries and massage application requires a knowledge of tissue susceptibility to trauma and the mechanical forces involved.

Tissues have relative abilities to resist a particular load. A *load* can be one or a group of outside or internal forces acting on the body. A *force* can be defined as a push or pull. The resistance to a load is called *mechanical stress*, and the internal response is a *deformation*, or change in dimensions. Deformation is also defined as a mechanical strain. The stronger the tissue, the greater magnitude of load it can withstand.

All human tissues have viscous and elastic properties, allowing for deformation. Tissue such as bone is brittle and has fewer viscoelastic properties than soft tissue, such as muscle. The loads (forces) applied to bone and soft tissues that can cause injury are tension, compression, bend, shear, and torsion. When tissue is deformed to the extent that its elasticity is almost fully exceeded, a yield point has been reached. When the yield point has been exceeded, mechanical failure occurs, resulting in tissue damage.

These same forces are applied therapeutically during massage to encourage tissue repair. Care needs to be taken not to superimpose extensive force that may increase the injury. It also is important to use the type of force that offers the most therapeutic value. In general, during the stage 1 acute and

TABLE 12-2

Stages of Tissue Healing and Appropriate Massage Interventions

	Stage 1 (Acute): Inflammatory Reaction	Stage 2 (Subacute): Repair and Healing	Stage 3 (Chronic): Maturation and Remodeling
Characteristics	Vascular changes Inflammatory exudate Clot formation Phagocytosis, neutralization of irritants Early fibroblastic activity	Growth of capillary beds into area Collagen formation Granulation tissue Fragile, easily injured tissue	Maturation and remodeling of scar Contracture of scar tissue Alignment of collagen along lines of stress forces (tensegrity)
Clinical signs	Inflammation Pain before tissue resistance	Decreased inflammation Pain during tissue resistance	Absence of inflammation Pain after tissue resistance
Massage intervention	(3 to 7 days after injury) Main goal: Protection Control and support effects of inflammation PRICE treatment (protection, rest, ice, compression, and elevation) Promote healing and prevent compensation patterns Passive movement midrange General massage and lymphatic drainage with caution Support for rest with full-body massage	(14 to 21 days after injury) Main goal: Controlled motion Promote development of mobile scar Cautious and controlled soft tissue mobilization of scar tissue along fiber direction toward injury Active and passive, open- and closed-chain range of motion (midrange) Support for healing with full-body massage	(3 to 12 months after injury) Main goal: Return to function Increase strength and alignment of scar tissue Cross-fiber friction of scar tissue coupled with directional stroking along lines of tension away from injury Progressive stretching and active and resisted range of motion (full range) Support for rehabilitation activities with full-body massage

Massage Approach During Healing

Acute Phase
- Manage pain
- Support sleep

Subacute Phase (Early)
- Manage pain
- Support sleep
- Manage edema
- Manage compensation patterns

Subacute Phase (Later)
- Manage pain
- Support sleep
- Manage edema

- Manage compensation patterns
- Support rehabilitative activity
- Support mobile scar development
- Support tissue regeneration process

Remodeling Phase
- Support rehabilitation activity
- Encourage appropriate scar tissue development
- Manage adhesions
- Restore firing patterns, gait reflexes, and neuromuscular responses
- Eliminate reversible compensation patterns
- Manage irreversible compensation patterns
- Restore tissue pliability

From Fritz S: *Sports and exercise massage: comprehensive care in fitness, athletics, and rehabilitation,* St Louis, 2006, Mosby.

stage 2 subacute phases, the massage therapist should not use the same force as that which loaded the tissue and produced the injury. For example, if a sprain occurs from a torsion load, then kneading, which applies a torsion force, may not be the best choice until healing is progressing and stability has been restored in the area. For old injuries that have not healed in the best way possible, the massage therapist, during the massage, may need to carefully introduce the same force that caused the injury to achieve results.

Skin Injuries

Numerous mechanical forces can adversely affect the skin's integrity, such as friction (rubbing), scraping, compression (pressure), tearing, cutting, and penetration.

Wounds are classified according to the mechanical force that caused them:

- *Friction blister:* Continuous rubbing over the surface of the skin causes a collection of fluid below or within the epidermal layer; this is called a *blister.*
- *Abrasions:* Abrasions commonly arise from conditions in which the skin is scraped against a rough surface. The epidermis and dermis are worn away, exposing numerous blood capillaries.
- *Skin bruise:* When a blow compresses or crushes the skin surface and causes bleeding under the skin, the condition is identified as a *bruise,* or *contusion.*
- *Laceration:* A laceration is a wound in which the flesh has been irregularly torn.
- *Skin avulsion:* Skin torn by the same mechanism as a laceration, to the extent that tissue is completely ripped from its source, is an avulsion.
- *Incision wound:* An incision is a wound in which the skin has been sharply cut.

■ *Puncture wound:* A puncture is a wound caused when a sharp object penetrates the skin.

Skin injuries are a regional contraindication to massage. Sanitation is essential, and care must be taken to prevent infection.

Muscle Injuries

Overexertion Muscle Problems. Overexertion is a problem that arises in physical conditioning and training. Even though the pattern of gradually overloading the body is the best way to achieve ultimate success, many athletes and training personnel still believe the old adage, "no pain, no gain."

Overtraining is reflected by muscle soreness, decreased joint flexibility, and general fatigue 24 hours after activity. Four specific indicators of possible overexertion are acute muscle soreness, delayed onset muscle soreness, muscle stiffness, and muscle cramps and spasms.

Acute Muscle Soreness. Overexertion in strenuous muscular exercise often results in muscular pain. At one time or another, most people have experienced muscle soreness, usually as a result of some physical activity to which the person is unaccustomed. The older a person gets, the more easily muscle soreness seems to develop. Acute muscle soreness accompanies fatigue. This muscle pain is transient and occurs during and immediately after exercise. It is caused by a lack of oxygen to the muscles and the buildup of metabolic waste from anaerobic functions. This type of soreness dissipates as oxygen is restored and metabolic waste is removed from muscle tissue.

Delayed Onset Muscle Soreness. Delayed onset muscle soreness becomes most intense after 24 to 48 hours and then gradually subsides, so that the muscle becomes symptom free after 3 or 4 days. This type of pain is described as a syndrome of delayed muscle pain leading to increased muscle tension, swelling, stiffness, and resistance to stretching. Delayed onset muscle soreness is thought to result from several possible causes. It may arise from very small tears (microtrauma) in the muscle tissue, which result in an inflammatory process and seem to be more likely with eccentric or isometric contractions. Delayed onset muscle soreness may also arise from disruption of the connective tissue that holds muscle tendon fibers together. Another contributor is increased interstitial fluid, which results in pressure on pain-sensitive structures.

Muscle soreness can be prevented by beginning an exercise at a moderate level and gradually increasing the intensity of the exercise over time. Treatment of muscle soreness usually involves general massage with a focus on lymphatic drainage. Muscle soreness can be treated with ice applied within the first 48 to 72 hours. Antiinflammatory drugs should be avoided, if possible, because they delay healing.

Muscle Stiffness. Muscle stiffness does not produce pain. It occurs when a group of muscles has been worked hard for a long period. The fluids that collect in the muscles during and after exercise are absorbed into the bloodstream slowly. As a result, the muscles become swollen, shorter, and thicker and therefore resist stretching. Light exercise, lymphatic drainage–type massage, and passive mobilization help reduce stiffness. Stiffness also results with decreased pliability of connective tissue. This occurs when the ground substance thickens as part of an enzyme process that occurs during sympathetic dominance. Massage to restore connective tissue pliability (slow, sustained compression and kneading) plus hydration helps reduce the stiffness.

Muscle Cramps and Spasms. Muscle cramps and spasms can lead to muscle and tendon injuries. A *cramp* is a painful, involuntary contraction of a skeletal muscle or muscle group. Cramps often occur as a result of lack of water or other electrolytes, muscle fatigue, or interruption of the appropriate neurologic interaction between opposing muscles. A *spasm* is a reflex reaction caused by trauma of the musculoskeletal system. The two types of cramps and spasms are the clonic type, with alternating involuntary muscular contraction and relaxation in quick succession, and the tonic type, with rigid muscle contraction that lasts a period of time.

Cramps can be temporarily reduced with firm pressure on the belly of the cramping muscle. Cramps and spasms respond to proper hydration and rest.[4]

Muscle Guarding. When an injury occurs, the muscles that surround the injured area contract in an effort to splint the area, thus minimizing pain by limiting movement. Quite often this splinting is incorrectly referred to as a muscle spasm; however, *muscle guarding* is a more appropriate term for the involuntary muscle contractions that occur in response to pain after musculoskeletal injury. Muscle guarding is appropriate during the acute and subacute healing processes (see Table 12-2), and massage application should not attempt to reduce it.

Contusion. A *bruise,* or *contusion,* arises from a sudden traumatic blow to the body. Contusions can range from superficial injuries to injuries involving deep tissue compression and hemorrhage (Figure 12-10). NOTE: A brain contusion is a *concussion;* this is a serious condition. If bruises are seen in the muscles of the head and neck, caution and referral are necessary.

FIGURE 12-10 A contusion.

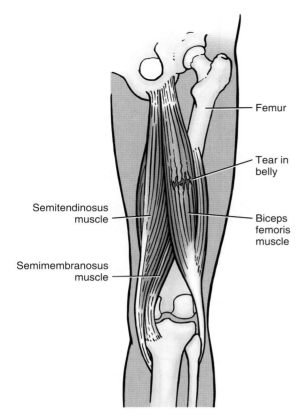

FIGURE 12-11 Muscle strain. This muscle strain is located in the biceps femoris muscle of the hamstring group (in this case, a tear in the midportion of the belly of the muscle).

A contusion can penetrate to the skeletal structures, causing a bone bruise. The extent to which an athlete may be hampered by this condition depends on the location of the bruise and the force of the blow. The speed with which a contusion heals, as with all soft tissue injuries, depends on the extent of tissue damage and internal bleeding. Caution is necessary when providing massage over contusions. Compressive force and depth of pressure need to be modified to prevent further injury. Lymphatic drainage–type applications are usually appropriate.

Strain. A *strain* is a stretch, tear, or rip in the muscle or adjacent tissue, such as the fascia or muscle tendons (Figure 12-11). The cause of muscle strain frequently is not clear. Often a strain is produced by an abnormal muscular contraction during reciprocal coordination of the agonist and antagonist muscles. Possible explanations for the muscle imbalance may be a mineral imbalance caused by profuse sweating, the collection of fatigue metabolites in the muscle itself, or a strength imbalance between agonist and antagonist muscles. Synergistic dominance of firing patterns is also crucial.

A strain may range from a tiny separation of connective tissue and muscle fibers to a complete tendinous avulsion or muscle rupture (grade 1, grade 2, or grade 3). The resulting pathology is similar to that of a contusion or sprain, with capillary or blood vessel hemorrhage. The three types of strain are:

■ *Grade 1 (mild) strain:* Local pain, which is increased by tension of the muscle, and minor loss of strength; mild swelling and local tenderness

■ *Grade 2 (moderate) strain:* Similar to a mild strain but with moderate signs and symptoms and impaired muscle function

■ *Grade 3 (severe) strain:* Severe signs and symptoms, with loss of muscle function and, commonly, a palpable defect in the muscle

The muscles with the highest incidence of strain in sports are the hamstring group, the spinalis group of the back, the deltoid, and the rotator cuff group of the shoulder. Muscle strain usually causes muscle guarding. The guarding should not be reduced by massage, because it protects the area from further injury. Gentle massage over the area to encourage circulation and lymphatic drainage can support healing. During the acute and subacute phases, the soft tissue should be massaged in the direction of the fibers and crowded toward the site of the injury to promote reconnection of the ends of the separated fibers. Depth of pressure, duration, and intensity all need to be adjusted during the healing phase. Once the acute phase of healing is complete, the methods that support mobile scar formation can be introduced, including moving the tissue away from the injury site and massaging across the fibers.

Tendon Injuries. The tendon contains wavy, parallel, collagenous fibers that are organized in bundles surrounded by a gelatinous material that reduces friction. A tendon attaches a muscle to a bone and concentrates a pulling force in a limited area. Tendons can produce and maintain a pull of 8,700 to 18,000 pounds per square inch. When a tendon is loaded by tension, the wavy collagenous fibers straighten in the direction of the load; when the tension is released, the collagen returns to its original wavy shape. In tendons, collagen fibers break if the physiologic limits are exceeded. A breaking point is reached after a 6% to 8% increase in length. Because a tendon usually is double the strength of the muscle it serves, tears most commonly occur in the muscle belly, musculotendinous junction, or bony attachment.

Tendon injuries usually progress slowly over a long period. Often repeated acute injuries can lead to a chronic condition. Constant irritation caused by poor performance techniques or constant stress beyond physiologic limits eventually can result in a chronic condition. These injuries often are attributed to overuse microtrauma.

Repeated microtrauma can evolve into chronic muscle strain that resorbs collagen fibers and eventually weakens the tendon or other connective tissue structures. Collagen resorption occurs in the early period of sports conditioning. During resorption, collagenous tissues are weakened and susceptible to injury, therefore a gradually paced conditioning program and early mobilization in the rehabilitation process are necessary.

Chronic muscle injuries represent a low-grade inflammatory process with a proliferation of fibroblasts and scarring. Chronic injury can result if the acute injury is improperly managed or if the athlete is allowed to return to activity before healing is complete. The sports massage professional should be especially knowledgeable about five chronic muscle conditions: myositis/fasciitis, tendinitis, tenosynovitis, muscle atrophy, and muscle contracture.

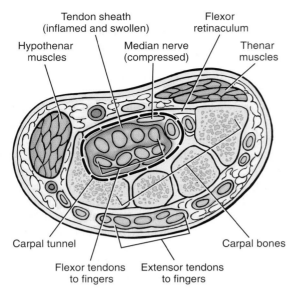

FIGURE 12-12 Tenosynovitis and carpal tunnel syndrome.

FIGURE 12-13 A sprain was the mechanism of injury to the lateral ligament complex of this ankle.

Myositis/Fasciitis. In general, the term *myositis* means inflammation of muscle tissue. More specifically, it can be considered a fibrositis, or connective tissue inflammation. Fascia that supports and separates muscle can also become chronically inflamed after injury. A typical example of this condition is plantar fasciitis.

Tendinitis. *Tendinitis* is marked by a gradual onset and diffuse tenderness caused by repeated microtrauma, as well as degenerative changes. Obvious signs of tendinitis are swelling and pain.

Tenosynovitis. *Tenosynovitis* is inflammation of the synovial sheath surrounding a tendon. In the acute stage, rapid onset of pain, articular crepitus, and diffuse swelling are seen. In chronic tenosynovitis, the tendons become locally thickened, and pain and articular crepitus are present during movement (Figure 12-12).

Muscle Atrophy and Muscle Contracture. Two complications of muscle and tendon conditions are atrophy and contracture. *Muscle atrophy* is the wasting away of muscle tissue. Its main cause in athletes is immobilization of a body part, inactivity, or loss of nerve stimulation. *Muscle contracture* is an abnormal shortening of muscle tissue, marked by considerable resistance to passive stretching. A contracture is associated with a joint that, because of muscle injury, has developed unyielding and resistant scar tissue. The type of massage depends on whether inflammation or fibrosis is present. Inflammation can be caused by the rubbing of short structures, and massage should focus on restoring normal length to the muscles in the area. Therapeutic exercise to strengthen muscles that have been inhibited is necessary. If tissue has become fibrotic, connective tissue methods are used to restore pliability.

Synovial Joint Injuries

The major injuries affecting the synovial joints are sprains, subluxations, and dislocations. Sprains are among the most common and disabling injuries seen in sports. A *sprain* is a traumatic twisting of the joint that results in stretching or complete tearing of the stabilizing connective tissues (Figure 12-13). Ligaments, the articular capsule, and the synovial membrane all are injured.

A sprain causes the effusion of blood and synovial fluid into the joint cavity, producing joint swelling, a local temperature increase, pain or point tenderness, and skin discoloration. Ligaments and capsules, like tendons, can experience forces that completely rupture them or that produce an avulsion fracture. Ligaments and joint capsules heal slowly because of their relatively poor blood supply; however, they are plentifully supplied with nerves, and injury to these structures often causes a great deal of pain.

Like muscle strains, sprains are classified into one of three grades according to the extent of injury:

- *Grade 1 (mild) sprain:* Some pain, minimum loss of function, mild point tenderness, little or no swelling, and no abnormal motion when tested
- *Grade 2 (moderate) sprain:* Pain, moderate loss of function, swelling, and in some cases slight to moderate instability
- *Grade 3 (severe) sprain:* Extreme pain, major loss of function, severe instability, tenderness, and swelling; may also represent a subluxation

The joints most vulnerable to sprains in sports are the ankles, knees, and shoulders. Sprains occur less often to the wrists and elbows. Distinguishing between joint sprains and tendon or muscle strains often is difficult, therefore the massage professional should expect the worst possible condition and manage it accordingly. Repeated joint twisting eventually can result in chronic inflammation, degeneration, and arthritis. Once the proper diagnosis has been made, the massage therapist can provide general full-body massage to reduce compensation patterns from changes in gait function and posture. In addition, lymphatic drainage massage can manage swelling outside the joint capsule. Massage methods that support circulation enhance healing, and hyperstimulation and counterirritation methods reduce pain. Care must be taken not to disrupt the healing tissue in the acute phase. Once the inflammation has diminished, mobilization of the soft tissue promotes mobile scar formation. The duration and intensity of massage increase as healing progresses. Ligaments can take 3 to 6 months or longer to heal fully.

Acute Synovitis. The synovial membrane of a joint can be acutely injured by a contusion or sprain. Irritation of the membrane causes fluid production to increase, and swelling occurs in the capsule. The result is joint pain during motion, along with skin sensitivity from pressure at certain points. In a few days, with proper care, the excess fluid is absorbed and the swelling and pain diminish. This condition is best managed by the athletic trainer.

Dislocations and Diastasis. Dislocations are second to fractures in terms of disabling the athlete. The fingers and the shoulder joint have the highest incidence of dislocation. Dislocations result primarily from forces that cause the joint to go beyond its normal anatomic limits. The two classes of dislocations are subluxations and luxations. *Subluxations* are partial dislocations in which two articulating bones are separated incompletely. *Luxations* are complete dislocations, or a total disunion of bone apposition between the articulating surfaces.

There are two types of diastases: a disjointing of two bones parallel to each another (e.g., the radius and ulna or the tibia and fibula); and the rupture of a "solid" joint, such as the symphysis pubis. A diastasis commonly occurs with a fracture.

Several factors are important in recognizing dislocations:
- Limb function is lost. The athlete usually complains of having fallen or of having received a severe blow to a particular joint and then suddenly being unable to move that part.
- Deformity is almost always apparent. Because the deformity often can be obscured by heavy musculature, it is important that the injured site be evaluated by the appropriate medical professional.
- Swelling and point tenderness are immediately present.

As with fractures, x-ray examination of the dislocation sometimes is the only absolute diagnostic measure.

First-time dislocations or joint separations may result in a rupture of the stabilizing ligamentous and tendinous tissues surrounding the joint and in avulsion, or pulling away of the tissues from the bone. The trauma often is so violent that small chips of bone are torn away with the supporting structures, or the force may separate growth epiphyses or cause a complete fracture of the neck in long bones. These possibilities indicate the importance of administering complete and thorough medical attention to first-time dislocations. It has often been said, "Once a dislocation, always a dislocation." In some cases this statement is true, because once a joint has been either subluxated or completely luxated, the connective tissues that stabilize the joint and hold it in correct alignment are stretched to such an extent that the joint is extremely vulnerable to subsequent dislocations. Chronic, recurring dislocations may occur without severe pain because of the somewhat slack condition of the stabilizing tissues. The massage practitioner needs to be aware of any history of dislocation. Increased muscle tension and connective tissue formation may occur around the dislocated joint as an appropriate stabilization process. Care must be taken to maintain joint stability while supporting mobility.

Chronic Joint Injuries. Like other chronic physical injuries or problems that arise from sports participation, chronic synovial joint injuries stem from microtrauma and overuse. The two major categories in which they fall are osteochondrosis and traumatic arthritis (*osteoarthritis,* or inflammation of surrounding soft tissues, such as the bursal capsule and the synovium). A major cause of chronic joint injury is failure of the muscles to control or limit deceleration during eccentric function. Athletes can avoid such injuries by avoiding chronic fatigue, by not training when tired, and by wearing protective gear to enhance active absorption of impact forces.

Traumatic arthritis usually is the result of accumulated microtrauma. With repeated trauma to the articular joint surfaces, the bone and synovium thicken, and pain, muscle spasm, and articular *crepitus* (grating on movement) occur. Joint wear leading to arthritis can come from repeated sprains that leave a joint with weakened ligaments. Misalignment of the musculoskeletal structure, which stresses joints, can be a factor, or arthritis can arise from an irregular joint surface or be caused by repeated articular chondral injuries. Loose bodies that have been dislodged from the articular surface can also irritate the joint and produce arthritis. Athletes with joint injuries that are improperly immobilized or who are allowed to return to activity before proper healing has occurred eventually may be afflicted with arthritis. Massage applications for chronic joint injury involve palliative care to control pain.

Bursitis. A bursa is a fluid-filled sac that is found in places where friction might occur in body tissues. Bursae provide protection between tendons and bones, between tendons and ligaments, and between other structures where friction occurs. Sudden irritation can cause acute bursitis. Overuse of muscles or tendons, as well as constant external compression or trauma, can result in chronic bursitis. The signs and symptoms of bursitis include swelling, pain, and some loss of function. Repeated trauma may lead to calcific deposits and degeneration of the internal lining of the bursa. Bursitis in the knee, elbow, and shoulder is common among athletes. Massage can be used to lengthen the shortened structures, reducing friction. Ice applications and rehabilitative exercise are indicated. Short-term use of antiinflammatory medication may be helpful. Steroid injections at the site are a common treatment. Massage is contraindicated in the area of steroid injection until the medication has been fully absorbed by the body. Five to 7 days is a safe waiting period, after which massage may be resumed.

Capsulitis and Synovitis. With repeated joint sprains or microtrauma, a chronic inflammatory condition called *capsulitis* may develop. *Synovitis* is a condition that usually is associated with capsulitis. Acute synovitis can occur, but a chronic condition arises with repeated joint injury or with joint injury that is improperly managed. Chronic synovitis involves active joint congestion with edema. As with the synovial lining of the bursa, the synovium of a joint can undergo degenerative tissue changes. Several movements may be restricted, and joint noises may be heard, such as grinding or creaking. Massage focuses on pain management and on supporting mobility without causing irritation.

Bone Injuries

Because of its viscoelastic properties, bone can bend slightly. However, bone generally is brittle and a poor shock absorber because of its mineral content. This brittleness increases under tension forces more than under compression forces. Bone trauma generally can be classified as periostitis, acute bone fractures, and stress fractures.

Periostitis. Inflammation of the periosteum can be caused by various types of sports trauma, but the main cause is a contusion. Periostitis often appears as rigidity of the skin over the injured area. The condition can occur as an acute episode or can become chronic. Lymphatic drainage–type massage is indicated.

Acute Bone Fractures. A bone fracture can be a partial or a complete interruption of the bone's continuity. It can occur without external exposure or can extend through the skin, creating an external wound (open fracture). As a result of normal remodeling, a bone may become vulnerable to fracture during the first few weeks of intense physical activity or training. Weight-bearing bones undergo bone resorption and become weaker before they become stronger. Fractures also can result from direct trauma; that is, the bone breaks directly at the site where a force is applied. A fracture that occurs some distance from the point where force is applied is called an *indirect fracture*. A sudden, violent muscle contraction or repetitive abnormal stress to a bone also can cause a fracture. Fractures are one of the most serious hazards of sports and should be routinely suspected in musculoskeletal injuries.

Stress Fractures. The exact cause of stress fractures is unknown, but a number of possibilities are likely: an overload caused by muscle contraction; altered stress distribution in the bone as a result of muscle fatigue; a change in the ground traction force (e.g., moving from a wood surface to a grass surface); or rhythmically repetitive stress.

Early detection of a stress fracture may be difficult. Because of their frequency in a wide range of sports, stress fractures always must be suspected in susceptible body areas that fail to respond to the usual management. The major signs of a stress fracture are swelling, focal tenderness, and pain. In the early stages of the fracture, the athlete complains of pain when active but not at rest. Later, the pain is constant and becomes more intense at night. Percussion (i.e., light tapping on the

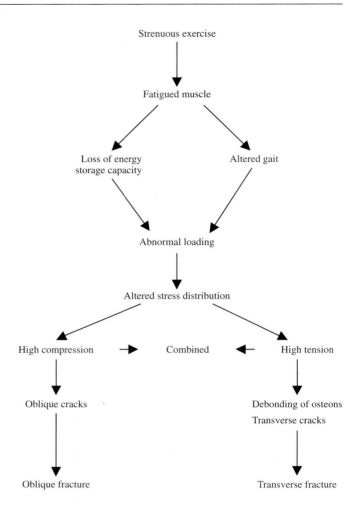

Sport	Location of Most Common Stress Fractures
Running	Tibia (distal), fibula, metatarsals
Basketball	Tarsal navicular, tibia (midshaft)
Football	Metatarsals, first metatarsophalangeal sesamoids
Dancing	Metatarsal (base), tibia (midshaft)
Recruits	Metatarsal (distal shaft), calcaneus, tibia (proximal)

FIGURE 12-14 A, The sequence of events leading to stress fractures. Loss of the muscle's energy storage capacity (fatigue) leads to microscopic bone failure (stress fracture). **B,** Locations of sport-specific stress fractures. (**A** modified from Malone et al: *Orthopedic and sport physical therapy,* ed 3, St Louis, 1997, Mosby; **B** modified from Miller et al: *Review of sports medicine and arthroscopy,* ed 2, Philadelphia, 2002, WB Saunders.)

bone at a site other than the suspected fracture) produces pain at the fracture site. The most common sites of stress fractures are the tibia, fibula, metatarsal shaft, calcaneus, femur, lumbar vertebrae, ribs, and humerus (Figure 12-14).

The management of stress fractures varies with the individual athlete, the injury site, and the extent of injury. Stress fractures that occur on the concave side of bone heal more rapidly and are managed more easily than those on the convex side. Stress fractures on the convex side can quickly produce a complete fracture. The massage practitioner needs to be aware of the potential for stress fractures and refer the athlete if necessary. The main massage approach during fracture healing is support for the whole body with general massage and methods to reduce compensation from changes in gait and reduced activity.

Nerve Injuries

The two main forces that cause major nerve injury are compression and tension. As with injuries to other tissues in the body, nerve injury may be acute or chronic. Any number of traumatic experiences that directly affect nerves can also produce a variety of sensory responses, including pain. For example, sudden stretching or pinching of a nerve can produce both muscle weakness and a sharp, burning pain that radiates down a limb. Neuritis, a chronic nerve problem, can be caused by a variety of forces that usually have been repeated or continued for a long period. Symptoms of neuritis can range from minor nerve problems to paralysis.

Pain that is felt at a point in the body other than its actual origin is known as *referred pain*. A potential cause of referred pain is a trigger point, which occurs in the muscular system. Massage applications for nerve injuries are palliative to reduce pain. If the nerve is impinged by short muscles and fascia, massage can be used to restore normal length and reduce pressure on the nerve.

Microtrauma and Overuse Syndromes

Injuries that occur as a result of abnormal and repetitive stress and microtrauma fall into a class known as *overuse and repetitive stress injuries,* which have certain identifiable syndromes. Such stress injuries frequently result in either limitation or curtailment of sports performance. Most of these injuries in athletes are directly related to the dynamics of running, throwing, or jumping. The injuries may result from constant and repetitive stress placed on bones, joints, or soft tissues; from forcing a joint into an extreme range of motion; or from prolonged strenuous activity. Overuse and repetitive stress injuries may be relatively minor, yet they still can be disabling. General massage is used to manage pain and edema, to restore mobility, and to normalize gait and firing patterns. Rest is important in the treatment of microtrauma and overuse conditions. Massage methods that create parasympathetic dominance help support restorative sleep.

Postural Changes

Postural deviations often are a major underlying cause of sports injuries. Postural malalignment may arise from unilateral (one side of the body) muscle and soft tissue asymmetries or bony asymmetries. As a result, the athlete engages in poor mechanics of movement (pathomechanics). Many sports activities, such as weight lifting, are unilateral and thus lead to asymmetries in body development. For example, a consistent pattern of knee injury may be related to asymmetries in the pelvis and legs (short leg syndrome) or reduced mobility of the ankles. A number of postural conditions are genuine hazards for athletes, making them prone to specific injuries. Some of the more important conditions are foot, ankle, and leg anomalies; spinal anomalies; and various stress syndromes. Unfortunately, not much in the form of remedial work is usually performed. As a result, an injury often becomes chronic, sometimes to the point that the athlete must stop participating in a sport. When possible, the massage professional should try to reverse faulty postural conditions through therapy, working under the direction of an athletic trainer, orthopedist, or other qualified medical professional.

Heat Illnesses

Exercising in a hot, humid environment can cause various forms of heat illness, including heat rash, heat syncope, heat cramps, heat exhaustion, and heatstroke.

Heat Rash. Heat rash, also called prickly heat, is a benign condition associated with a red, raised rash that is accompanied by sensations of prickling and tingling during sweating. It usually occurs when the skin is continuously wet with unevaporated sweat. The rash generally is localized to areas of the body covered with clothing. Massage is regionally contraindicated.

Heat Syncope. *Heat syncope,* or heat collapse, is associated with rapid physical fatigue during overexposure to heat. It is usually caused by standing in heat for long periods or by not being accustomed to exercising in the heat. It is caused by peripheral vasodilation of superficial vessels, hypotension, or a pooling of blood in the extremities, which results in dizziness, fainting, and nausea. Heat syncope is quickly relieved by laying the athlete down in a cool environment and replacing fluids.

Heat Cramps. *Heat cramps* are extremely painful muscle spasms that occur most commonly in the calf and abdomen, although any muscle can be involved. The occurrence of heat cramps is related to excessive loss of water and several electrolytes or ions (sodium, chloride, potassium, magnesium, and calcium), which are essential elements in muscle contraction. Profuse sweating results in the loss of large amounts of water and small amounts of electrolytes, which destroys the balance in concentration of these elements in the body. This imbalance ultimately results in painful muscle contractions and cramps. The person most likely to develop heat cramps is one who is in fairly good condition but simply overexerts in the heat.

Heat cramps can be prevented by adequate replacement of sodium, chloride, potassium, magnesium, calcium, and, most important, water. Ingestion of salt tablets is not recommended. Sodium can be replaced by simply salting food a bit more heavily; bananas are particularly high in potassium; and calcium is present in green, leafy vegetables, milk, cheese, and dairy products. The immediate treatment for heat cramps is ingestion of large amounts of water with electrolytes added and mild stretching, with ice massage of the muscle in spasm. An athlete who experiences heat cramps generally is not able to return to practice or competition that day, because cramping is likely to recur. Massage is contraindicated and will not relieve heat cramps. Rest and hydration are indicated.

Heat Exhaustion. *Heat exhaustion* results from inadequate replacement of fluids lost through sweating. Clinically, the victim of heat exhaustion collapses and has profuse sweating, pale skin, a mildly elevated temperature (102° F), dizziness, hyperventilation, and a rapid pulse.

It sometimes is possible to spot athletes who are having problems with heat exhaustion. They may begin to develop heat cramps. They may become disoriented and light-headed, and their physical performance will not be up to their usual standards. In general, people in poor physical condition who attempt to exercise in the heat are most likely to suffer from heat exhaustion.

Immediate treatment of heat exhaustion requires ingestion and eventually intravenous replacement of large amounts of water. Massage is contraindicated.

Heatstroke. Unlike heat cramps and heat exhaustion, *heatstroke* is a serious, life-threatening emergency. The specific cause of heatstroke is unknown. It is characterized clinically by sudden collapse with loss of consciousness; flushed, hot skin with less sweating than would be seen with heat exhaustion; shallow breathing; a rapid, strong pulse; and, most important, a core temperature of 106° F or higher. In the heatstroke victim, the body's thermoregulatory mechanism has broken down because of an excessively high body temperature; the body loses the ability to dissipate heat through sweating.

Heatstroke can occur suddenly and without warning. The athlete usually does not experience signs of heat cramps or heat exhaustion. The possibility of death from heatstroke can be reduced significantly if the body temperature is lowered to normal within 45 minutes. The longer the body temperature is elevated to 106° F or higher, the higher the mortality rate. Death is imminent if the body's core temperature rises to 107° F (41.7° C) or higher.

Every first aid effort should be directed toward lowering the body temperature. Get the athlete into a cool environment, strip off all clothing, sponge the person down with cool water, and fan the individual with a towel. Do not immerse the athlete in cold water. It is imperative that the victim be transported to a hospital as quickly as possible. Do not wait for an ambulance; transport the victim in whatever vehicle happens to be available. The replacement of fluid is not critical in initial first aid. Massage is contraindicated.

Hypothermia

Cold weather is a common condition in many outdoor sports in which the sport itself does not require heavy protective clothing; consequently, the weather becomes a pertinent factor in the athlete's susceptibility to injury. In most instances, the activity itself enables the athlete to increase the metabolic rate sufficiently to function normally and dissipate the resulting heat and perspiration through the usual physiologic mechanisms. If an athlete fails to warm up sufficiently or becomes chilled because of relative inactivity for varying periods, the individual is more prone to injury.

Dampness or wetness further increases the risk of hypothermia. An air temperature of 50° F is relatively comfortable, but water at the same temperature is intolerable. The combination of cold, wind, and dampness creates an environment that easily predisposes the athlete to hypothermia.

A relatively small drop in the body's core temperature can induce shivering sufficient to materially affect an athlete's neuromuscular coordination and performance. Shivering stops when the body temperature drops below 85° to 90° F (29.4° to 32.2° C). Death is imminent if the core temperature drops to 77° to 85° F (25° to 29.4° C). Treatment involves warming and drying the athlete.

Ongoing Care of the Athlete

For athletes, regular massage allows the body to function with less restriction and accelerates recovery time. There are no specific protocols for massage targeting athletes. The basic massage process presented in Chapter 9, coupled with appropriate assessment procedures (see Chapter 10) with the addition of various aspects of fluid movement, connective tissue application, and trigger point therapy (see Chapter 11) is combined to address the needs of this population.

Athletes in training have reduced adaptive capacity. Therefore, observe the following rules:

- *Do not* overmassage.
- *Do not* cause tissue damage.
- *Do not* assume that athletes require an aggressive approach.
- *Do* consider all aspects of the individual who is an athlete and provide massage to the individual, not to an athlete.

Most athletes require varying depths of pressure, from light to very deep, therefore effective body mechanics on the part of the massage practitioner are essential. Working with athletes can be very demanding. Their schedules may be erratic, and their bodies change almost daily in response to training, competition, or injury. Athletes can become dependent on massage, therefore commitment by the massage professional is necessary. Many specialized training programs for sports massage are available. Massage professionals who intend to work with athletes must obtain additional training. Such training should include the physiologic and psychological functions of an athlete; overuse and repetitive use syndromes; the biomechanics of specific sports; the use of cryotherapy, ice massage, and other hydrotherapy methods; injury repair and rehabilitation; and education in training regimens.[4] The text, *Sports and Exercise Massage: Comprehensive Care in Athletics, Fitness, and Rehabilitation (Mosby's Massage Career Development)*, by Sandy Fritz (Mosby, 2006) covers these areas (Proficiency Exercise 12-2).

BREAST MASSAGE

SECTION OBJECTIVES

Using the information presented in this section, the student will be able to perform the following:

- Determine when breast massage is appropriate
- Consider ethical principles in deciding when breast massage is performed

NOTE: Massage of the female breast is a controversial issue. A conservative approach is taken in this textbook. Although a

PROFICIENCY EXERCISE 12-2

1. *Look through professional journals and send for information about three advanced sports massage training sessions.*
2. *Contact a university with a sports team and speak with the athletic trainer. Find out how massage might be used to enhance athletic performance.*
3. *Contact a local exercise club or physical therapy department and talk with the exercise physiologist about how massage could enhance the work being done.*
4. *Volunteer to work at a sponsored sports massage event held by your school or local professional massage organization.*
5. *With your classmates, organize a sports massage event for a local sporting function.*
6. *Obtain a catalog from a university that offers degrees in athletic training or exercise physiology. List the classes required to earn these degrees.*

body area is not a population, the topic needs to be addressed, and this appears to be the best location in this book.

Breast massage can be appropriate for certain conditions, such as fibrosis and the development of scar tissue after surgery (surgery for breast cancer is the most common cause of such scar tissue). Surgery for breast cancer may involve either removal of only the cancerous tissue or a mastectomy. Often reconstructive surgery is performed. The massage practitioner must attend to contraindications and cautions in connection with treatments given after surgery. For example, radiation over the area can weaken the bones, predisposing them to fracture.

Breast implants are another consideration. Care must be taken to apply gentle pressure over the implants while still addressing the connective tissue changes that can occur when implants are used.

Breast reduction surgery is performed for both cosmetic and health reasons. The same attention to scar tissue development and healing is taken as with other surgical procedures.

As for any surgery or area of healing, specific massage to the area is not provided during the acute phase. After the initial healing is complete and the attending physician has approved treatment, gentle massage that mobilizes the tissue around the surgical area can be performed. After 4 weeks, if healing is progressing well, the scar itself can be gently massaged. The most common method used is a very gentle form of skin rolling. After 3 months, myofascial methods can be used.

When the therapist works with existing scar tissue, the work progresses slowly and deliberately. Most scar tissue tends to be less pliable than the surrounding tissue. It also tends to shorten and pull. Breast surgery can result in a pulling forward of the shoulder and discomfort from taut, long tissue in the midback.

Myofascial methods (see Chapter 11) are effective for managing scar tissue. More generalized massage manipulations,

such as gliding, kneading, and compression, prepare the tissue for more specific work.

If breast massage for a specific condition is deemed appropriate by a health care professional and the client is referred to the massage professional, the following measures are recommended:

- Work with specific written informed consent for breast massage.
- Work with another professional in the room, much as a male gynecologist has a female nurse present during examinations. If this is not possible, male therapists should refer a female client to a female therapist.
- Use careful draping. Do not expose the entire breast unless absolutely necessary. Do not expose both breasts.
- Work gently, professionally, and confidently.
- Avoid the nipple area.

Ethical Considerations in Breast Massage

The ethical principles discussed in Chapter 2 serve as the basis for decision making regarding the appropriateness of breast massage for either men or women. The massage professional should particularly consider the following:

- *Proportionality:* The benefit must outweigh the burden of treatment.
- *Nonmaleficence:* The practitioner must do no harm and must prevent harm from occurring.
- *Beneficence:* The treatment must contribute to the client's well-being.

Anatomically the breast is part of the integumentary system. It becomes a functional part of the female reproductive system only during lactation. In both men and women, the breast is considered an erogenous zone. An *erogenous zone* is an area of the body where sexual tension concentrates and can be relieved through stimulation. Other erogenous zones are the mouth, genitals, and anus. These areas usually have some sort of erectile tissue that engorges with blood when stimulated. In the breast, the nipple constitutes this erectile tissue. The controversy over the appropriateness of massage of the female breast centers on the breast as an erogenous area.

Soft tissue under the breast tissue can be accessed effectively by placing the client in the side-lying position, in which the breast tissue falls away from the chest wall toward the table. In the supine position the breast tissue usually falls to the side, allowing massage over the sternum and intercostal area. These two positions provide adequate access to the soft tissue of the chest wall. For this reason, there is no reason to massage through the breast tissue proper to reach these areas (Figure 12-15).

Breast examination and the teaching of breast self-examination are adequately undertaken by other health care professionals. It is not necessary for the massage professional to provide such services.

Breast massage as part of a general massage serves no specific physiologic purpose that cannot be achieved in ways other than breast massage; therefore the concerns may outweigh the benefit (Proficiency Exercise 12-3).

FIGURE 12-15 Methods for providing massage around the breast.

CHILDREN

12-3

SECTION OBJECTIVES

Using the information presented in this section, the student will be able to perform the following:

- Apply general massage methods to ease growing pains
- Train family members in massage techniques for use at home

Providing massage services for children is not much different from providing massage for adults. For the purposes of this textbook, children are people ranging from 3 to 18 years of age. Children love physical contact. It is interesting that the horsing around and wrestling that occur during play look a lot like massage. Because children and adolescents may have shorter attention spans than adults, a 30-minute massage usually is sufficient.

From age 3 to puberty, physical growth is seen mostly in height. At adolescence, growth in height accelerates under the influence of increased hormone levels, and sexual maturation occurs. Both physical and emotional growing pains are common. Physical growing pains occur because the long bones grow more rapidly than the muscle tissue, resulting in a pull on the periosteum, or connective tissue bone covering, which is a very pain-sensitive structure. Massage can help by gently lengthening the muscles, stretching the connective tissue, and providing symptomatic relief of pain through the effects of counterirritation, hyperstimulation analgesia, gait control, and release of endorphins (Figure 12-16).

Adolescents live in bodies that are changing every second. Hormone levels fluctuate constantly, and mood swings occur regularly. Growth is accelerated, and natural sleep-wake patterns often are disrupted. It is not uncommon for a teenager to be up all night and want to sleep all day. Massage may help an adolescent become more comfortable with this ever-changing body. It certainly helps with physical growing pains. Use special caution when working with adolescent boys. The reflexive physical sexual response is sensitive, and almost anything can trigger an erection. The therapist should be sensitive to this by not using a smooth sheet over the groin area when working with male adolescents. Instead, keep the sheet bunched in this area to disguise any physical response to the massage.

It also is important that the practitioner never work with children or adolescents unless a parent or guardian is present. Part of the massage time can be used to teach the parent or guardian some massage methods to help the child and to teach the child some massage methods for use on the parent. Massage provides a structured approach to safe touch. It may help families stay connected during both good and difficult times (Figure 12-17) (Proficiency Exercise 12-4).

PROFICIENCY EXERCISE 12-3

Investigate the surgical procedure for breast cancer, breast augmentation with implants, or breast reduction. Write an intervention plan and justification statement for the use of therapeutic massage. Use the model in Box 12-14 as an example.

Example: Therapeutic massage for _____

1. Gather facts to identify and define the situation.

Key questions:
What is the problem?
What are the facts?

2. Brainstorm possible solutions.

Key question:
What might I do? or What if . . . ?

3. Evaluate possible interventions logically and objectively; look at both sides and at the pros and cons.

Key question:
What would happen if . . . ?

4. Evaluate the effect on the people involved.

Key question:
How would each person involved feel?

5. Develop an intervention plan and justification statements.

FIGURE 12-16 Massage for children.

PROFICIENCY EXERCISE 12-4

1. *Give massages to three children or adolescents of various ages. Make sure the parent or guardian is present.*
2. *On separate sheets of paper, develop a one-page handout with five massage techniques that families can share.*

CHRONIC ILLNESS

SECTION OBJECTIVES

Using the information presented in this section, the student will be able to perform the following:

- Explain the basic etiology of chronic illness
- Explain the difference between acute illness and chronic illness
- Develop realistic expectations for working with people who have a chronic illness

Chronic illness is defined as a disease, injury, or syndrome that shows either little change or slow progression. **Acute illness** or injury is a short-term condition that resolves through normal healing processes and, if necessary, supportive medical care. Compared with chronic illness, acute conditions can be dealt with relatively easily, because healing produces measurable results. Dealing with chronic illness is difficult for the person who has it, for the physician and the health care team, and for the massage therapist. In many situations little can be done except to make day-to-day living with the illness more tolerable. Healing is an option in some situations, but even then total recovery is a long process that requires work, commitment, and support.

The dynamics of family relationships, work situations, emotions, and coping skills play an important role in the etiology of a chronic illness. Chronic illness affects every aspect of a person's life and the lives of those around him or her. An entire family's dynamic functioning pattern may be set up around a chronically ill family member. Shifting chronic illness patterns, therefore, may be difficult. Entire relationship dynamics may change if the chronically ill individual improves. Personal and professional responsibilities that the client has been able to avoid because of the illness must be addressed if chronic conditions improve. Benefit gained from chronic illness is called *secondary gain.* This process may be subconscious and therefore difficult for the client to recognize or change. The dynamics required to support chronic illness patterns reach far beyond the physiology of the disease, and professional counseling may be required.

Working with chronic illness does not often produce measurable improvements. More often a slowed deterioration or, at best, stabilization is seen. For this reason, the treatment of chronic illness does not easily fit into the current medical system, which is geared mostly toward acute and traumatic care.

Long-term debilitating diseases such as Parkinson's disease, multiple sclerosis, systemic lupus erythematosus, rheumatoid arthritis, fibromyalgia, chronic fatigue syndrome, asymptomatic HIV infection, AIDS, and disk problems that cause back pain respond well to the short-term symptomatic relief massage provides. Massage also can reduce general stress, helping the individual to cope better with the condition.

Chronic illness follows an uneven cycle, with good and bad periods. On good days the person may overexert herself and deplete an already weakened energy source. The immune system may be compromised, making the person with a chronic illness more susceptible to infections such as colds and influenza. Because most chronic illness patterns have good days and bad days, the intensity of massage sessions must be geared to the client's condition that day. When symptoms are more active, the better course may be to give massages more often for shorter periods.

One approach to rehabilitating chronically ill individuals is a hardening or toughening program. **Hardiness** is the physical and mental ability to withstand external stressors. Individuals with chronic illnesses often reduce their activity levels, isolate themselves, and become less hardy. Massage, hydrotherapy, specially designed hardening programs, and exercise can increase a person's hardiness.

People with chronic illnesses usually are under a physician's care and may be taking medications. The massage practitioner must work closely with these medical professionals to understand the effects of the various treatments and medications. Appendix C presents some guidelines for determining the interplay of massage with various medications.

Mind/body approaches, behavior modification, relaxation techniques, spiritual healing, and other types of interventions and alternatives are helpful to those with chronic illnesses. All these approaches tend to empower the client, rallying the powerful internal resources that human beings have. It is important not to discount a method that a person may use for self-help. The only caution about alternative interventions is that some of those offering such services do not have the client's greatest good as their top priority. Instead, they prey

FIGURE 12-17 Massage for children and adolescents. **A,** Most kids prefer to keep their clothes on and like a mat. **B,** Interact with parent or guardian (not in picture). **C,** Maintain focus on child. **D,** Continue to connect with parent or guardian and explain massage methods. **E, F,** Relax and nurture and remember to teach parent or guardian.

on the misery of the chronically ill. These people usually offer cures, charge high fees for treatment sessions, require frequent sessions, and try to convince the client that their way is the only way, making the client dependent on them. This type of behavior is unethical.

The massage professional who wants to work with the chronically ill must have realistic expectations. Instead of developing a massage approach to bring about a cure for the illness, which is out of the scope of massage practice anyway, the focus should be on helping the client feel better for a little while. Although this can get very frustrating for the massage practitioner, we can see that our work has value if we remember that we may be the only ones who provide this type of care, that not getting worse is an improvement, that some people need their illness to cope, and that massage eases their suffering in the illness pattern.

A clinical reasoning process is necessary to make appropriate decisions as to the type of care most beneficial for a client with a chronic illness (see Chapter 5). Treatment plans revolve around therapeutic change, condition management, or palliative care. Because of the nature of chronic illness, the emotional factors involved, and possible secondary gain, the treatment most often chosen is condition management, with palliative care provided during acute episodes of the illness. This recommendation does not mean that an actual therapeutic change plan is not possible; it simply is not as common.

The massage therapist's expectations must be realistic, and the therapist must remain professionally detached from the actual outcomes for the client with a chronic illness while maintaining a compassionate connection. Often the client's present situation is the best that can be achieved under the existing circumstances. If each pattern presented by a client is seen as a solution, it is easier to understand why approaches that relieve the symptoms and support healing often are met with resistance.

For example, a client with a chronic fatigue syndrome pattern consumes four or five cups of coffee after noon and finds that she cannot sleep at night because caffeine is known to disturb sleep. Massage has been ineffective in supporting sleep. The client will not stop drinking coffee in the afternoon because she cannot function at work if she does. So what do you do? There is no easy answer, and survival mechanisms reinforce short-term solutions even if the behaviors create long-term problems.

Often additional training is required just to understand chronic illness patterns, the effects of the medications involved, and the skill necessary to work in conjunction with other health care professionals. As with athletes, massage therapists who work with people with a chronic illness should understand as much as possible about the illness. By using this information and conferring with the physician and other health professionals involved in the client's care, the massage practitioner can integrate the effects of massage into the comprehensive treatment plan, helping the client achieve the highest quality of life possible.

A resourceful goal for working with people with chronic illness is helping a client rediscover the fact that each person is in charge of his or her own life, and the illness is not. The illness may have been allowed to take over the person's life and personal power. "Healing" may be the act of reasserting control over one's life, not getting rid of the disease. The benefits of massage may provide enough relief to enable the client to find the necessary inner resources for dealing constructively with the effects of chronic illness, enhancing the client's quality of life and the lives of those around him or her (Proficiency Exercise 12-5).

(Author's note: I speak from personal experience; I continue to learn from an endocrine condition and a compressed disk in my lower back.)

THE ELDERLY 12-4

SECTION OBJECTIVES

Using the information presented in this section, the student will be able to perform the following:

* Provide a rationale for the benefits of massage for the elderly
* Understand the need for fee and time adjustments when working with the elderly

In the industrialized societies, the fastest growing segments of the population are those over age 80. People in their advanced years can benefit greatly from massage. Although the massage methods are no different, elderly individuals do present spe-

---

PROFICIENCY EXERCISE 12-5

1. *Choose one chronic illness and investigate it thoroughly.*
2. *Develop an educational brochure explaining the benefits of massage as part of a plan for coping with the chronic illness you have investigated. Share the brochure with fellow students.*

---

cific concerns, and appropriate adjustments are required in massage application.

The age range for the category "elderly" is considered to be 70 years of age and older. However, some 60-year-olds have the problems of the aged, and some 85-year-olds are in better physiologic condition than some 60-year-olds. Because of this, the wiser course with people over age 60 is to consider the physiologic condition rather than the chronologic age.

The aging process is normal. Muscle tissue diminishes, as do fat and connective tissue. Connective tissue in general is affected during the aging process. It becomes less pliable, reproduces more slowly, and forms fibrotic tissue more easily. Bones are not as flexible and are more prone to breaking. Joints are worn, and osteoarthritis is common. The skin is thinner, circulation is not as efficient, and fluid in the soft tissue is reduced. Medications may be prescribed to control blood pressure and other conditions.

The body tends to collapse a bit during aging. The spaces provided for the nerves are reduced, and bones and soft tissue structures can put pressure on the nerves, resulting in sciatica and thoracic outlet syndrome. Feet hurt because the intricate joint structure of the foot has broken down. Circulation to the extremities is diminished, often resulting in a burning pain. These conditions are not life-threatening, but they surely can cause a person to feel miserable. If only temporarily, massage can help ease the discomfort of these conditions.

Many elderly people take several medications. The elderly also are more sensitive to the dosage level of medication and less able to self-regulate homeostatic processes. The massage professional must be attentive to the physiologic interactions between the effects of massage and the medications. Regular massage may allow reduction of the dosages of some medications.

Elderly people often are depressed. This frequently is a chemical depression as well as a situational condition. Massage stimulates neurochemicals that can lift mild depression temporarily. Dementia conditions, such as Alzheimer's disease, have shown temporary improvement after massage. Wandering behavior has decreased, and an increased awareness of the current environment has been observed.

Dehydration, lack of appetite, and weight loss can be problems with advanced age, but the parasympathetic stimulation produced by massage can increase appetite and improve digestion for elderly clients. Proper hydration is very important. Sleep also can be improved. Many elderly people have periods of insomnia or disrupted sleep patterns. Improved sleep supports restorative mechanisms and increases vitality.

Many elderly people are alone. Their spouses have passed away, and their families are busy with their own lives. We all

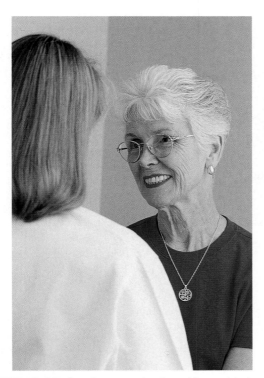

FIGURE 12-18 Good communication with an elderly patient. (From Seidel HM et al: *Mosby's guide to physical examination,* ed 5, St Louis, 2003, Mosby.)

need to be touched. If a person is not physically and emotionally stimulated, neurologic function begins to deteriorate. The interaction with a massage therapist can provide both physical and emotional stimulation for the elderly. If nothing else, the physical contact with another human being provides sensory stimulation, with beneficial results (Figure 12-18).

Because the elderly often are alone or isolated in extended care facilities and have a limited income, the massage therapist should take into consideration not only the fees charged but also the amount of time spent with the elderly client. Many elderly people want to talk. This social interaction may be just as important as the physical interaction of the massage. If the massage professional listens attentively, much can be learned from the elderly, who have many years of experience to share. The time should be given willingly. However, professional boundaries need to be maintained. When the massage practitioner tells an elderly person how much time can be spent, most respect the time boundary.

If a person does not have adequate cognitive functioning skills, as in cases of dementia caused either by the aging process or by medications taken for other conditions, she will be unable to give informed consent for the massage. The guardian, physician, or other health care professional must intervene to give the necessary permission.

As in the previous discussions, massage practitioners who plan to work with elderly individuals may need more training to learn about their special needs. In most cases a general massage session using the skills presented in this text and an attentive, caring attitude are sufficient for interacting professionally with the elderly (Figure 12-19) (Proficiency Exercise 12-6).

 PROFICIENCY EXERCISE 12-6

1. *Volunteer to give massages at a local senior citizens center for at least 4 weeks or a total of 32 hours.*
2. *Contact a local nursing home and ask if there is a resident who has few visitors and who would appreciate receiving a massage. Commit to a minimum of two massages per month for 6 months.*

INFANTS 12-5

SECTION OBJECTIVES

Using the information presented in this section, the student will be able to perform the following:

- Explain the importance of the first year of life
- Explain the importance of organized sensory stimulation for infants
- Teach parents to massage their babies
- Understand the importance of a confident touch when working with infants

Most authorities designate babies from birth to 18 months of age as infants. For the purposes of this textbook, the classification is expanded to 3 years of age because infants are still developing neurologically until that time. One or both parents must provide informed consent for the massage and must be present during any professional interaction with the infant.

Compared with other mammals, human infants are born about halfway through the gestation period, while the head is still small enough to pass through the birth canal. Otherwise, babies would stay in the safe haven of the womb at least another year. The womb is a much safer place to be unless the pregnant mother uses tobacco, drugs, alcohol, or other chemicals that cross the placental barrier, or if she does not provide adequate nutrition and care for herself and thus her baby.

Protection, nutrition, connection, bonding, stimulation, and soothing acceptance are crucial for human infants. Infants are born with a need for sociability, along with the more basic needs for food, shelter, and so forth. The people of most cultures massage their infants. Although this practice has been almost lost in the westernized world, it is being revived. Research by Dr. Tiffany Field and her associates shows that premature infants who have been massaged fare much better than those who have not. Massage provides an organized, logical approach to sensory stimulation, which is important for infants because part of their growth is learning to sort and organize sensory stimulation.

As mentioned, physiologically the infant's growth pattern is not complete until 3 years of age (Figure 12-20). By 12 months of age (when, if our heads were not so big, a child would just have been born), the infant can move independently from place to place but still is utterly dependent on the protection of a parent or family group. Two-year-olds are still babies. Three-year-olds are quite different in both function and body form. By the time a child can control bladder and bowel functions reliably (about age 3), cognitive functions are better able to be organized. Now is the time to work on learning the meaning of "no," picking up toys, and sharing, and the infant is ready to pass into childhood.

FIGURE 12-19 Massage procedure for an elderly individual. **A,** Drape the client for modesty and warmth. **B,** Interact appropriately with the client. **C,** Be cautious but confident in providing the massage. **D,** Respectfully move underclothing. **E,** Maintain secure draping. **F,** Use broad-based contact and be cautious about depth of pressure and degree of drag. **G,** Be vigilant in observing the client's reactions and adapt the massage as appropriate. **H,** The side-lying position often is most comfortable for elderly clients.

FIGURE 12-19, cont'd **I,** Assess range of motion carefully; never force movement. **J,** Stretch cautiously; pin and stretch methods increase tension on tissue while protecting joints. **K,** Abdominal massage supports digestive and elimination functions. **L,** Gentle oscillation (shaking and rocking) is effective for supporting joint function. **M,** If necessary, assist the client in getting off the massage table and donning clothing. **N,** Professional hugs initiated by the client are okay.

Understanding the limitations of these walking infants is important. How many 2-year-olds have been spanked for not sharing toys or putting toys away, when physically and developmentally they are incapable of understanding the concept? Touch then becomes negative in connotation. Lots of hurts happen at this age. The parents' expectations often are too high, resulting in frustration on the part of both parents and child. These wonderful and challenging twos are a great time to take time out and give the baby a massage. If the child is

approached appropriately, this experience can be calming for both the parent and the child, and touch then becomes a very positive experience.

When working with anyone, the massage professional needs to "meet" the person where he or she is at that moment. This is most important when working with infants. A fussy baby or a 2-year-old in a tantrum is caught up in the physiologic process. It takes time for both the nervous and endocrine systems to calm down. When verbal skills are not

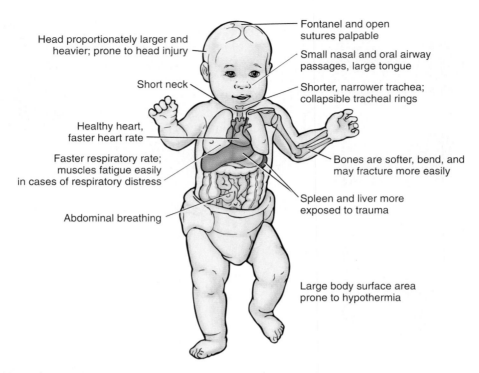

Head proportionately larger and heavier; prone to head injury

Short neck

Healthy heart, faster heart rate

Faster respiratory rate; muscles fatigue easily in cases of respiratory distress

Abdominal breathing

Fontanel and open sutures palpable

Small nasal and oral airway passages, large tongue

Shorter, narrower trachea; collapsible tracheal rings

Bones are softer, bend, and may fracture more easily

Spleen and liver more exposed to trauma

Large body surface area prone to hypothermia

FIGURE 12-20 The unique anatomic and physiologic features of infants and young children.

sufficient to express the problem, crying may be a way to burn off internal agitation that has built up through the day. A parent or massage practitioner who expects the infant to settle into the massage immediately may be disappointed. Relaxing takes time. Repetitive long strokes and rhythmic movement of the limbs can initiate a calming response in an infant (Figure 12-21). Bilateral (on both sides) pressure is calming. Swaddling provides this type of consistent, even pressure that reduces neural activity. If the baby stiffens with the massage, the tactile stimulation most likely is too intense, too light, uneven, or painful. The infant nervous system is very sensitive. Confining the massage to the feet or rhythmic rocking may be preferable to stroking for infants who seem highly tactile sensitive. When just the right combination of methods is found, the infant will respond calmly to the touch.

It is appropriate to teach parents to massage their own babies. Massage may be especially helpful for parents who have trouble bonding with their infants. Bonding is the attachment process that occurs between parent and child. Although bonding is considered primarily an emotional response, it is theorized that some biochemical and hormonal interaction may support the process. The hormone oxytocin is present in both the mother and the father and may be a factor in the bonding process. Massage, through skin stimulation, increases the oxytocin level.

Other than in a hospital-type setting, the massage practitioner is unlikely to develop a clientele of infants. But teaching infant massage can be an exciting career addition. Classes and various books and videos are available to help the massage therapist develop infant massage classes for caregivers. Learning massage is an excellent way for parents to become confident with their touch. In well-baby care, a shorter massage of 15 to 30 minutes is sufficient. A confident touch is important;

babies can detect nervousness immediately. To them this is not a "safe" touch, and they will not respond and may even try to withdraw. The parents may then feel rejected by the infant.

Infants born to mothers addicted to drugs and alcohol have a nervous system that is especially challenged (Figure 12-22). Research is underway to determine whether the gentle, organized, tactile approaches of massage can help these special babies. The initial findings are promising. Babies, especially babies of drug-addicted mothers, sometimes are abandoned, and hospitals place these infants in what is called a *boarder nursery*. A hospital may be open to the volunteer efforts of a massage therapist, which could provide a great learning experience for both the massage professional and the hospital staff.

Remember, each baby is different. "Listen" to these little bodies, structure the massage to best meet the baby's needs, and the baby will respond with a purity that fills your heart (Proficiency Exercise 12-7).

ON SITE MASSAGE

SECTION OBJECTIVE

Using the information presented in this section, the student will be able to perform the following:

* Conduct himself or herself appropriately while providing on site massage.

 PROFICIENCY EXERCISE 12-7

1. *Using professional journals, investigate resources for learning more about infant massage.*
2. *Find a litter of puppies or kittens and massage these "babies."*

FIGURE 12-21 Well baby massage. **A,** Use a firm, confident touch. **B,** Massage and move the baby's limbs. **C,** Teach the caregiver or parent how to massage the baby. **D,** The baby can be massaged in a number of different positions.

Chapter 8 described the logistical concerns of on site massage, such as where to set up for the massage and issues of privacy. Because many people wish to have massage in their home or office, this environment deserves further discussion.

A basic premise of massage is that it is a service-based professional interaction between the client and the practitioner. A person may want massage services in their location for a number of reasons, including convenience and time efficiency, privacy, or inability to travel to the therapist's office. Many people who live a high-profile life, such as prominent political or business people, entertainers, and professional athletes, especially appreciate the convenience and privacy of massage in their home or in some cases where they work. The massage professional usually charges a premium for travel and for setup at the location. Many clients who have the financial resources will be willing to purchase a massage table and other equipment and create a permanent massage area.

Providing massage in a client's home presents the most challenges. As mentioned in Chapter 8, certain logistical issues, such as the location of the massage area, are relatively easy to manage. Of more concern are the professional interaction challenges in a client's home or office space. It is important to move efficiently into and out of the area without disrupting the natural rhythm of the environment. It is important to respect the client's environment. Examples include removing shoes to protect the carpet and carrying special rubber-soled shoes to wear during the massage or wiping up

water splashes in the restroom after washing your hands. It is important to make sure the massage equipment and lubricants do not damage the client's floors or walls. Place a sheet on the floor under the massage table to protect the flooring.

Work or family members and pets can present challenges. The issues of tolerance and flexibility must be considered. How would you respond if a young child wanted to help you with the massage or if the client's cat insisted on being on the massage table during the massage? Are you able to remain centered and focused on the massage while the client watches television or talks on the phone? What is your responsibility to other family members, friends, or coworkers of the client as far as conversation or questions are concerned? What if a family member also wants a massage?

Confidentiality is extremely important. When you are in someone's private environment, you become privy to all sorts of information, from their housekeeping skills to their tastes in decorating. You may see mail or reading material casually left on the table or overhear phone calls and private conversations.

The intimacy of the environment makes it more difficult to maintain professional boundaries and time management without seeming distant and hurried. It takes longer to enter and exit the on site environment, not just because of the equipment setup and breakdown, but also because of the need to be respectful of the area and polite. This needs to be considered when scheduling so that plenty of time is allowed to

FIGURE 12-22 Massage for an ill or injured infant. **A,** Assess the infant and explain to the parent or caregiver what you intend to do. Always follow the treatment plan provided by the physician. **B,** Take the time to connect with the baby. **C,** Move the baby confidently, securely, and safely. **D,** Position the infant carefully. **E,** Teach the parent or caregiver how to massage the baby. **F,** Show care and concern for the baby and also for the parent or caregiver.

provide the on site massage service and get to the next appointment without rushing.

The personal safety of the massage professional is a concern, because the on site massage environment has fewer safeguards than an office setting. It is necessary to be cautious (see Box 2-15). Get to know the client ahead of time, make sure someone always knows where you are, and check in with that person often. Always carry a cell phone with you.

On site massage service is a viable and very appropriate business option. With attention to the special circumstances and challenges, both the client and the massage practitioner can achieve successful outcomes (Proficiency Exercise 12-8).

PHYSICALLY CHALLENGED INDIVIDUALS

SECTION OBJECTIVES

Using the information presented in this section, the student will be able to perform the following:

- Communicate more effectively with people who have a physical disability
- Adjust the massage environment to better support those with physical disabilities
- Become aware of subtle discrimination

PROFICIENCY EXERCISE 12-8

Based on the information in this section, evaluate your own home or business location for challenges that would arise if you wanted to provide on site massage.

According to the guidelines of the Americans with Disabilities Act, a physical disability or impairment is any physiologic disorder, condition, cosmetic disfigurement, or anatomic loss that affects one or more of the following body systems: neurologic, musculoskeletal, special sense organ, respiratory (including speech organs), cardiovascular, reproductive, digestive, genitourinary, hemic and lymphatic, skin, and endocrine. Extremes in size and extensive burns also may be considered physical impairments.[6]

People with physical impairments can benefit from massage for all the same reasons that any other individual can. The client's body may develop compensation patterns in response to the disability. For instance, a person in a wheelchair could have increased neck and shoulder tension from moving the chair. In addition, dealing with a physical impairment daily can make routine functions more stressful. The following sections present guidelines that may help the therapist provide services for these clients. A person with a disability should be treated the same as anyone else. The right of individuals to choose the kind of help they need must be respected.

A therapist must never presume to know, understand, or anticipate a client's need. *It is important to ask!* A concerned therapist does not try to pretend that the disability does not exist, but rather responds professionally. The disability affects only a small part of the whole person. After the client has provided the necessary information about the disability, the therapist should accept the impairment as part of how the person functions.

Personal Awareness

People who are not physically challenged may be uncomfortable around those who are. This discomfort comes from not knowing what to do or say, from being afraid of the person's disability, or from various other causes.

Often the disability is put first rather than the person. If the disability is first in the massage therapist's mind, the person is not. Lack of knowledge is a huge contributing factor to this form of subtle discrimination. Overcompensation and patronization by the person who is not disabled make normal communication difficult. The massage professional is responsible for acting professionally and communicating effectively with all clients, including those who have disabilities. Not understanding how to interact effectively is not an excuse, because the best source of information is the person with the impairment. Ask your client to explain his or her limitations; what assistance, if any, might be needed; and how that assistance should be given if requested.

The practitioner should use good judgment when deciding whether to ask if assistance is needed and then should wait until the person accepts the offer before providing assistance. The client can give the best directions on how to proceed. For example, in offering assistance, it may be best to say, "If you need any assistance, I am glad to help. Tell me what you need." If the offer is declined, no offense should be taken. If the person is abrupt, it may be that this question has been asked many times already but not in such a pleasant or respectful manner.

If another person is present, all remarks should be directed to the client and not to the companion. Talking to the companion rather than the client is very degrading; it occurs when the therapist is more comfortable with the able-bodied companion and therefore finds it easier to address that person.

Sometimes we are uncomfortable and cannot move beyond these feelings. The client will sense our discomfort. Simple disclosure allows communication and understanding. For example, when working with a severely burned client, I found that the texture of the skin was difficult for me to massage. It unsettled me. The client was also very much disfigured. He could sense my discomfort but did not understand the source and assumed it was from his appearance, which was not a factor. Because he was familiar with people's reaction to his appearance, the client asked me about the cause of my discomfort. Simple disclosure and the understanding that resulted helped me to deal more effectively with the tactile difficulties I was having and helped the client to understand the source of my feelings. This was a valuable lesson in the importance of simply, professionally, and honestly using disclosure as described in Chapter 2. It often is difficult to communicate these types of feelings and difficult for professionals to accept their personal limitations. Sometimes referral to a practitioner who is not affected by a particular situation is the best choice for both the massage professional and the client.

Supporting Clients with a Visual Impairment

Many people with a visual impairment have some type of sight. Comparatively few people have no vision at all. When assisting a client with a visual impairment, the therapist should never push or pull on the person. Instead, if guiding is necessary, the therapist should stand just in front and a bit to the left of the client, who can then touch the therapist's right elbow when following.

Useful directions should also be given to a person with a visual impairment. If asked where something is, the therapist should not point and say "over there." Instead, terms such as *left, right, about 10 steps,* and so on are much easier to follow. It is not necessary to speak more loudly to individuals with a visual impairment; they usually can hear just fine.

The therapist should begin the conversation by using the client's name so that the person is aware of being addressed. The therapist then should state his name; he should not touch the client until the person is aware of his presence in the room.

If a person with a visual impairment places anything anywhere, it should not be moved. If a door is opened, the direc-

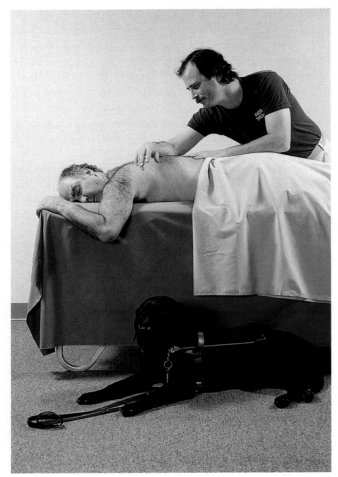

FIGURE 12-23 A guide dog trained to lie quietly by the massage table.

tion of the opening (toward or away from the person) and the location of the hinges (left or right) should be explained. It is best to let the client open the door in order to become better oriented to its position.

If a service dog is harnessed and working, be it a guide dog for someone with a visual impairment or any other support service, the therapist must not pet, feed, or in any other way interact with the dog. This distracts the dog and makes its job difficult. It must become very tiresome for a person with a service dog to be stopped repeatedly and asked if someone can pet the dog (Figure 12-23).

Supporting Clients with a Speech Impairment

Understanding a person with a speech problem can be difficult. The therapist should ask the person to repeat anything that was unclear until it is understood and then should repeat what was said so that the person can clarify if necessary. If the therapist cannot understand what is being said, the client should be informed of this. If necessary, a notepad can be used to put communication in writing. Although having an accent

is not a speech impairment, it can make communication difficult. Not speaking the same language also hinders communication.

Supporting Clients with a Hearing Impairment

To gain the attention of a client with a hearing impairment, the therapist should lightly tap the person once on the shoulder or discreetly wave a hand. If no interpreter is present, all talking should be done in a normal tone and rhythm of speech.

If a client can lip read, it is important that the massage therapist always face the person and not cover her own mouth when talking. A normal voice tone and speed should be used. If the therapist normally speaks quickly, the speed should be slowed a bit. If necessary, a notepad can be used to put communication in writing.

Hearing aids amplify sound; they do not make sound clearer. Reducing background noise helps the hearing impaired to hear better. With this in mind, it may be wise to ask before using any music during the massage session. Getting too close to a hearing aid can make it squeal, therefore take care when massaging near the ears.

Supporting Clients with a Mobility Impairment

There are many types of mobility impairment and many reasons for it. Just because a person is paralyzed does not mean that a particular area has no feeling. Furthermore, just because a person uses a wheelchair does not mean that the person is paralyzed.

When speaking to a client in a wheelchair, the therapist should do so from eye level. Looking up strains the client's neck. The process obviously requires the massage therapist to sit down.

A wheelchair must never be pushed unless the person in the chair gives permission. The individual also will give directions for pushing the wheelchair over barriers.

When a client must be transferred from a wheelchair to the massage table (Figure 12-24, *A*), the client can give the best directions on how to proceed. A transfer to a mat on the floor may be easier to accomplish, in which case the massage should be given there. The most efficient transfer is a lateral transfer to a table that is the same height as the wheelchair (Figure 12-24, *B*). This entails a shift in body mechanics by the massage therapist to accommodate a lower table.

Special care must be taken in giving a massage to a person with paralysis because normal feedback mechanisms are not functioning. Clients with catheters or other equipment must instruct the therapist in the handling of the devices. In most cases the catheter can be ignored.

If the client has undergone amputation and uses a prosthesis, he or she may or may not want the device removed during the massage. Ask permission before massaging the amputated area. If the client is comfortable with this, massage can be especially beneficial if a prosthesis is used. Although no scientific validation is available, professional experience has shown

FIGURE 12-24 A, A transfer from a wheelchair to the massage table. **B,** A low table that allows a lateral transfer is best.

that massage strokes carried the full length of the amputated limb seem to feel good to the client.

Supporting Clients with a Size Impairment

If the client is short, a stool may be needed to help him or her reach the massage table, clothing hangers, or restroom fixtures. The massage professional should casually sit down to establish eye contact with the client so that the person does not have to look up, which strains the neck.

A very large person may not trust the massage table and may be more comfortable on a floor mat. Getting up and down from the floor may be difficult. Sometimes seated massage is the better option. Ask the client what is preferable. If the practitioner is nervous about doing the massage on the massage table, the client must be told (disclosure), because the therapist's anxiety will affect the quality of the massage.

Supporting Clients with Burns and Disfigurements

People who have been burned may face an assortment of challenges ranging from impaired mobility to disfigurement. As burns heal, scar tissue replaces functional epithelial tissue. All the functions of the skin are compromised, including excretion, sensation, and protection. Scar tissue tends to contract and pull, which can make the area of the healed burn feel shortened or tight. Severe contractures sometimes develop and must be treated medically. Myofascial release, craniosacral therapy, and other connective tissue techniques can soften and gently stretch connective tissue. Massage of this type may reduce the effect of this shrinkage somewhat. Professionals who want to serve clients who have been burned need additional training in these methods.

Many disfigurements tend to draw our attention because the mind is designed to notice differences. Although many disfigurements do not limit function in any way, they can create social difficulties. Attempting not to notice a disfigurement usually fails. The client recognizes that the situation exists and has various levels of comfort with the condition. Honest communication is effective in redirecting the attention from the disfigurement to the person over time. The practitioner might offer a simple statement such as, "I can't help but notice (the particular disfigurement). I'm not uncomfortable, but the difference naturally draws my attention. Please be patient with me until I become more familiar with you."

Barrier-Free Access

All massage facilities must be barrier free. Commercial buildings usually are required by law to have barrier-free access and elevators, as well as restroom facilities accessible to individuals with a handicap (Proficiency Exercises 12-9 and 12-10).

PSYCHOLOGICALLY CHALLENGED INDIVIDUALS

SECTION OBJECTIVES

Using the information presented in this section, the student will be able to perform the following:

- Understand the importance of verifying informed consent when working with individuals who have a psychological disability
- Structure a massage to support other psychological interventions

PROFICIENCY EXERCISE 12-9

1. *Obtain a course catalog from a college and compare your current massage education with the curriculum required for a nurse, a physical therapy assistant, an occupational therapist, a respiratory therapist, or other similar health care professional.*
2. *Discuss with a physician, chiropractor, physical therapist, or psychologist the skills he or she would want to see in a massage professional who would work with the person in the professional setting.*

PROFICIENCY EXERCISE 12-10

Contact your local building department and speak with the person in charge of the barrier-free code requirements. Find out the requirements and the reason for each.

The Americans with Disabilities Act defines mental impairment as any mental or psychological disorder, such as mental retardation (developmental disabilities), organic brain syndrome, emotional or mental illness, and specific learning disabilities.[3] The conditions considered in this section include:

- Addictions
- Chemical imbalances in the brain
- Developmental disabilities
- Learning disorders
- Psychiatric disorders
- Post-traumatic stress disorder

The actual massage approach is no different when the therapist works with psychologically challenged individuals. The important factor is the person receiving the massage. Practitioners who want to work with clients with psychological challenges need additional training to be able to understand the physiology and psychology of the various disorders and the challenges these clients face. An understanding of psychotropic pharmacology is important, because massage and these medications affect the body in similar ways. This type of work should be supervised closely by a psychologist or psychiatrist.

At times we are all challenged psychologically. It is important to understand how our minds work and the interaction that constitutes the mind/body connection. It is now well excepted in the scientific community that there is a link joining the mind, the body, and the spirit with health and well being. A dedicated student of massage will seriously consider taking some psychology courses at a community college or other educational center and will keep up-to-date on new research findings. Massage will continue to have a very important place in mind/body medicine and treatments, along with other forms of mental health services.

The Importance of Informed Consent

Informed consent is an important concern when working with clients influenced by drugs (both prescribed and not), internal chemical imbalances, and developmental disabilities. Special care must be taken to ensure that the client is able to provide informed consent. When doubt exists, the massage should not be given.

Addictions

Individuals withdrawing from chemical and alcohol addictions may find that massage helps reduce stress levels. The type of chemical to which the person is addicted determines the types of stressful experiences incurred. The massage therapist assesses the client to decide whether the massage could calm an anxious client or give a boost to a depressed client. Heavy connective tissue massage should be avoided during withdrawal phases. Toxins released from this type of massage may overtax a system already burdened with withdrawal detoxification.

Chemical Imbalances in the Brain

Certain types of mental disability arise from an imbalance of brain chemicals. Hyperactivity, ADD, bipolar (manic-depressive) disorder, schizophrenia, seasonal affective disorder, obsessive-compulsive disorder, and clinical depression are just a few brain chemical disorders.

Medication is important in helping these individuals. The massage professional should never make the client feel guilty for taking medication or suggest that medication is not necessary. Medication must be monitored carefully by a physician, with the smallest effective dosage given to avoid side effects. Massage cannot replace medication, but the client who receives regular massage may be able to reduce the dosage and duration in some situations. In other situations the side effects of certain medications can be managed with massage. It is very important to work with the client's physician and chart the client's response to the massage carefully.

Developmental Disabilities

Massage for those with developmental disabilities has the same effect as for everyone else. Care must be taken to communicate at the client's level of understanding but not below functioning level. Adults with developmental disabilities are not children and should not be treated as such. Developmentally disabled people may become frustrated and anxious during a day of challenges. Life is more difficult for them to manage. If accepted by these clients, massage is soothing, calming, and beneficial; but remember, not everyone likes to be touched, and the individual's needs must be respected.

Autism is believed to be a developmental disorder characterized by impaired social interaction and communication and a restricted repertoire of interests. Contrary to popular belief, most children and adults with autism do want to be touched. A very reliable, structured touch with firm, consistent pressure usually is preferred. Massage applied in a very deliberate way within the client's comfort level has been shown to increase social interaction somewhat and reduce anxiety.

Learning Disorders

Difficulties with processing sensory input, which occurs in some learning disorders, may be helped by the organized, systematic, sensory stimulation of massage. Having a learning difficulty is stressful. *(Author's note: I have dyslexia, as well as an inner ear dysfunction that makes hand-eye coordination difficult. Thank goodness for assistants, computers, spell checkers, and editors!)* Life is more difficult when one is dealing with any special situation. Stress from dealing with the environment aggravates the learning difficulty. Self-esteem is hard to maintain when a person has been made to feel stupid in school because he or she could not write, spell, or read. People with learning disabilities are not stupid, they just need to learn differently. Massage helps reduce their stress, thereby facilitating learning and enabling them to feel more positive about themselves.

Psychiatric Disorders

Psychiatric disorders such as anxiety, panic, depression, and eating disorders interplay in a combination of autonomic nervous system functions and hormone neurotransmitters, neuropeptides, and other brain chemicals.

Anxiety is an uneasy feeling usually connected with increased sympathetic arousal responses. Panic is an intense, sudden, and overwhelming fear or feeling of anxiety that produces terror and immediate physiologic change that results in paralyzed immobility or senseless, hysterical behavior. A panic attack is an episode of acute anxiety that occurs at unpredictable times with feelings of intense apprehension or terror. It may be accompanied by a feeling of shortness of breath that leads to hyperventilation, dizziness, sweating, trembling, and chest pain or heart palpitations. Most symptoms can be directly related to overactivation of the sympathetic autonomic nervous system.

Depression is characterized by a decrease in vital functional activity; mood disturbances of exaggerated emptiness, hopelessness, and melancholy; or unbridled periods of high energy with no purpose or outcome.

Anxiety and depressive disorders are commonly seen with fatigue and pain syndromes. Pain and fatigue syndromes are multicausal and often chronic, nonproductive patterns that interfere with well-being, activities of daily living, and productivity. Some such syndromes are fibromyalgia, chronic fatigue syndrome, infection with the Epstein-Barr virus, sympathetic reflex dystrophy, headache, arthritis, chronic cancer pain, neuropathy, low back syndrome, idiopathic pain, somatization disorder, and intractable pain syndrome. Acute pain, as well as acute "episodes" of chronic conditions, can be factors in these syndromes. Panic behavior, phobias, and the sense of impending doom, along with a sense of being overwhelmed and/or hopelessness, are common with these conditions. Mood swings, breathing pattern disorders, sleep disturbance, concentration difficulties, memory disturbances, outbursts of anger, fatigue, and changes in habits of daily living, appetite, and activity levels are symptoms of these conditions and syndromes.

Eating disorders involve mood disorders, physiologic responses to food, and control issues. They are complicated situations that usually require professional intervention. The job of the massage therapist is to be aware of a possibility of an eating disorder and to refer the client. Any substantial weight loss must be referred to a physician. Individuals who have anorexia nervosa (a starving disorder) lose a great deal of weight. It is more difficult to recognize bulimia, which involves binge eating and purging by vomiting and laxatives. The teeth and gums are affected by the stomach acids, and the massage professional may notice this. Referral should be made

because of symptoms, not because the therapist is attempting to diagnose the disorder.

A *breathing pattern disorder* often is a significant underlying factor with anxiety and panic. Massage can normalize the breathing muscles, which must be done to correct a breathing pattern dysfunction.

Because acute pain and chronic pain are managed somewhat differently, it is important to distinguish between the two. Intervention for acute pain is less invasive and focuses on supporting a current healing process. Chronic pain is managed with either symptom relief or a more aggressive rehabilitation approach that incorporates a therapeutic change process.

With clients with psychiatric disorders, the most common approach is general stress reduction massage. This type of massage may take the edge off the mood through the influence of massage on the autonomic nervous system. The type of massage given can be adjusted to be a little more stimulating or a little more relaxing. The key is to begin where the person is at the time of the massage. Someone who is anxious initially may resist long, slow strokes and instead may do better with a strategy that begins with active joint movement, postisometric relaxation, lengthening and stretching, and rapid compression, and then gradually shifts into a calming, rocking massage with long, slow strokes. The person who is a little depressed may not initially want to join in with an active participation massage. Instead, the work might begin with rocking and long, slow strokes and end with stimulating active joint movement, rapid compression, and tapotement.

Massage affects the brain chemicals by encouraging the release of serotonin, dopamine, and the endorphins, which alter mood. It also affects the release of various hormones that influence mood. Massage has a strong normalizing effect on the autonomic nervous system and can support other interventions for psychiatric disorders.

Post-traumatic Stress Disorder

Post-traumatic stress disorder (PTSD) is the re-experiencing of flashback memory, as well as state-dependent memory, somatization, anxiety, irritability, sleep disturbance, concentration difficulties, times of melancholy or depression, grief, fear, worry, anger, and avoidance behavior. Excessive stress can manifest as a number of disorders, such as cardiovascular problems, including hypertension; digestive difficulties, including heartburn, ulcer, and bowel syndromes; respiratory illness; susceptibility to bacterial and viral illnesses; endocrine dysfunction, particularly adrenal or thyroid dysfunction; delayed or diminished cellular repair; sleep disorders; and breathing pattern disorders, to mention just a few. Post-traumatic stress disorder can have long-term effects.

Trauma occurs as a result of physical injury by violent or disruptive action or by a toxic substance or as a result of psychic injury caused by a short-term or long-term severe emotional shock. Of special concern are military personnel who have experienced trauma.

Because therapeutic massage is effective in normalizing the effects or physiologic manifestations of stress on the body, it can be an effective tool in the management of or recovery from post-traumatic stress disorder.

Adrenaline is the key to solidifying events into memory. If adrenaline is blocked through the use of the medication propranolol, memory is impaired. Apparently when traumatic events occur, adrenaline is secreted. The more adrenaline and the longer the exposure to the elevated levels, the stronger the memory. Post-traumatic stress disorder may be a manifestation of memories that were encoded in the presence of increased and sustained adrenaline exposure. These memories are literally too strong. If the adrenaline levels are reduced as soon as possible after a traumatic event, lingering post-traumatic stress symptoms are not as permanent. Therapeutic massage can influence adrenaline levels by reducing sympathetic dominance and supporting parasympathetic dominance.

Researchers, including Tiffany Field of the University of Miami School of Medicine's Touch Research Institute, have found that massage is effective in calming individuals with PSTD. The military is investigating the use of multiple interventions, including massage, to treat military personnel exposed to trauma. The drug propranolol can be used to weaken old memories. Old memory patterns are recalled, and the medication (which interferes with adrenaline) is administered. The memory is not lost, it is just reduced in intensity. The implications are vast, and it will be interesting to watch advancing treatment of this debilitating condition. In the meantime, therapeutic massage appears to provide benefit. (*Author's note: Through years of professional experience, I have been privileged to support many people as they become less affected by distressful memories when they receive regular massages. Often clients would discuss the events while receiving a massage. All I had to do was listen and massage.*)

Abuse

People who have experienced various forms of **abuse** usually experience PTSD. Words synonymous with *abuse* include *exploit, misuse, prostitute, batter, mishandle, mistreat, molest, ravish, violate, harass, condemn, persecute, torment, belittle, ridicule, insult, offend, neglect, ignore, berate, criticize, defile, desecrate, dishonor, attack, reject,* and *pervert.* Words that have the opposite meaning are *honor, respect, consider, regard, protect, defend, preserve, praise, value, safeguard, shelter, sustain, support, tolerate, appreciate, approve, recognize, understand,* and *accept.*

When people are abused, whatever the form of abuse, they must learn to survive as best they can at the time of the abuse. These survival mechanisms take many forms, such as dissociation, hypervigilance, aggressive behavior, learning to "disappear," low self-esteem, and withdrawal. As mentioned, PTSD is common. These patterns may generalize into many life situations.

If the abuse happens to a young child, the victim's coping mechanisms develop around a twisted reality. The younger the child, the more difficult effective survival will be, and possibly the more magnified the inappropriate survival mechanisms that develop. The older we are, the more inner resources we have to support effective coping.

People most often think of abuse as physical or sexual torture. It is safer to consider the acts of the "monster" or sociopath than to recognize the subtler abuses we all have experienced. Most abusers are members of the family (including siblings) or friends. Mixed signals can be very devastating; those who have experienced both abuse and support from the same person have difficulty with trust and esteem. Guilt is common and secrecy the norm.

Subtler forms of mistreatment, especially emotional abuse, are also common. The effects of the abuse should not be judged by their intensity or context. Children or adults who have been deceived or belittled have had their trust violated and their personal power taken away, just as has a person who was raped. Abuse removes a person's self-empowerment, no matter what the means. The severity of the results depends on the frequency of the abuse, whether someone was able to validate the victim's self-worth, whether the victim received help in coping at the time, and inherent inner resources.

Trauma, State-Dependent Memory, and Dissociative Behavior

The body remembers trauma in some way. The technical term for this is **state-dependent memory**. This type of memory is encoded in the brain in a manner that includes the position, emotion, and chemicals, as well as the nervous system activation and all other combined physiologic effects that influence the internal functions, at the time the experience occurred. Later, when the physical and emotional states change, the memory of the incident may be vague or forgotten.

State-dependent memory functions in all life experiences. When a person gets ready to hit a baseball or drive a car, the individual assumes the appropriate position and the body remembers what is required. In a traumatic experience, this mechanism locks in all the factors that coincide with the experience. In the future, this repressed memory may be triggered by any one of the sensations or physiologic factors involved in the state-dependent memory. For example, the sense of smell often triggers a memory. With massage, the pressure, location of the touch, and position or movement of the client may trigger the client's memory.

The myelinization of nerves and the development of the nervous system continue from birth to about 3 years of age. During this period memories are transient and spotty and may be stored in the memory centers in scattered ways. During the first year of life, the senses of touch, sound, smell, taste, and vision are functioning and in some ways are keener than they are in the adult. However, the processing, storage, and retrieval of all this information are not keenly developed. Trauma and sustained abuse are particularly devastating when they occur during this crucial time of learning about the world and of dependence on a caregiver to meet not only basic needs (e.g., food, clothes) but also the need for connection, bonding, and love. Physical, sexual, or emotional abuse at this time is recorded by the body but is not always understood, coped with, or remembered in detail.

A person who experiences trauma during the formative years may have difficulty sorting it all out in adulthood. The memories may be spotty or piecemeal, or only one of the sensations (e.g., smell, touch, position) may be encoded in the memory. It is important not to discount this memory pattern simply because all the pieces do not fit together to form a whole picture. It may be affirming to know that all the pieces do not have to fit together for the person to have enough information to resolve and integrate past experiences and develop more resourceful behavior for the present and future.

Sexual abuse in an older child often is laden with mixed signals, role confusion, and secrecy. Role confusion occurs when the child takes on the duties or family function of one of the parents. Because the child is older, memories may be clear or, because of state-dependent memory patterns, they may be clouded or shut off and separated. The perpetrator may develop a relationship with the child and then use the child to meet the adult's or older adolescent's sexual and emotional needs. Again, feelings, emotions, relationship roles, coping styles, and behavior all shift somehow to put the abuse into a context that can be endured.

Physical abuse (e.g., beatings, neglect) and emotional abuse (e.g., criticism, unrealistic expectations, brain washing, indoctrination) demand survival as well. How many times have we been expected to do something that we did not have the skill, physical ability, or knowledge to accomplish and were belittled after trying our very best? This type of trauma riddles the self-esteem with holes.

Some life experiences that may affect a person in a manner similar to deliberate abuse are illness, medical procedures, hospitalization, accidents, or other trauma, such as that experienced by military personnel or victims of natural disasters, such as Hurricane Katrina. For example, this process is common in the training and development of athletes, dancers, and musicians. Developing these skills is difficult and often physically painful. The success of the individual's coping skills depends on the type of support received during and soon after the traumatic event, as well as the dynamics surrounding the situation. A child who attempts to hide the pain during a medical procedure so as not to upset the parents is being denied full emotional and physical expression in the situation. If the medical staff does not explain the procedure so that the child comprehends or if the child is too young to understand, this, too, may become a difficult situation to integrate into a person's life experiences. If a parent or support person is physically separated from or emotionally unavailable to a child or adult during a crucial time, this can have a lasting effect.

Abuse of an adult, such as occurs with rape, violent crime, stalking, spouse beating, and abuse of the elderly, must also be considered. Typically, adults feel powerless in the situation and may feel as though the abuse is deserved or that they somehow did something to cause it. If elderly individuals are also mentally impaired, such as with Alzheimer's disease, they may become childlike in their reasoning and survival mechanisms. Those who have experienced upheaval in their environment, war-torn areas, or areas of disaster can develop feelings of powerlessness and devastation even when the person is no longer in the environment and is now safe.

The touch of the massage therapist may remind the body of the trauma. As the body remembers, it may somehow resolve and integrate the experience. Often the client does not remember the details or recall who, what, where, when, or how. Instead, a vague uneasiness, or **dissociation** (i.e., detachment, discontentedness, separation, isolation), develops. One mechanism for surviving physical, sexual, and emotional trauma is to "leave the body" and therefore not feel the abuse or to believe that the abuse is happening to someone else.

Many types of appropriate dissociative coping mechanisms are valuable in times of performance, demand, emergency, or survival. This is sometimes called *entering the zone* or *zoning out*. However, if the pattern of dissociation becomes repetitive and generalized, coping becomes strained. One way to relearn appropriate touch is through giving and receiving massage.

The massage professional should be aware of a client dissociating during a massage. It is not our job to change the dissociative pattern by reminding the client to remain aware of his or her body unless the client specifically requests it. More specialized training is required to deal effectively with all the ramifications of a client's shift in coping style. This frequently involves professional counseling.

The massage practitioner should never shift a coping mechanism for a client or imply guilt for using it when it still serves a purpose. It takes time to learn to cope differently. Most of the time people dissociate from sensation in order to avoid feeling pain. The timing and situation must be just right for the person to be able to focus the energy necessary to "feel" again. The process must happen gently, at the client's pace, and must never be hurried. The client leads, and the therapist follows that lead. As this happens, the practitioner can begin to recognize the pattern of the dissociation and the massage techniques or positions that seem to trigger the pattern. With this information the therapist can alter the approach to the massage, providing the client with the opportunity to stay with the body more easily.

For example, if the therapist notices that every time the client's left knee is bent the client's body becomes unresponsive, the eyes become distant, or the breathing shifts, it is best to work with the knee in a different position. Also, rather than moving the client, the practitioner can have the client move himself into the position, which is more empowering for the individual. Over time, it becomes easier to notice these little steps, which will reacquaint the client with his body.

Some people who have been traumatized may also self-abuse, which can take many forms, such as a destructive lifestyle, addictive processes, and self-inflicted trauma. It may seem hard to understand, but self-abuse may be calming for the person. Endorphins and other chemicals are released during self-abuse. The mechanisms of counterirritation and hyperstimulation analgesia come into play. The massage professional may notice bruises, cuts, burns, or other injuries on the client's body. In a professional manner, the practitioner should bring these areas to the client's attention and note them in the client's record. Acknowledging an injured area to a person who abuses herself may cause the person to feel guilty or ashamed, tell a cover story, or ignore the question.

Occasionally a client demands or requests very deep massage when the soft tissue condition does not indicate the need for this type of invasive work. Self-abuse mechanisms may be involved in this situation. It is important not to become involved in a situation that perpetuates an abuse pattern. The therapist needs to trust his or her intuition about appropriate care but should not force the client to face the situation by confronting the person with the possibility of self-abuse mechanisms. The decision to deal actively with an abusive history requires commitment and time from the client. Professional help and/or support groups often are needed. Also, some individuals do not want to recover their memories of abuse; this is a valid response for these clients. The practitioner must not suggest that a client was abused or that the client needs to deal with his or her situation. Our job is to honor, respect, consider, regard, protect, defend, preserve, praise, value, safeguard, shelter, sustain, support, tolerate, appreciate, approve, recognize, understand, and accept, and never to harm.

Boundaries are very important. Review the importance of respect for personal boundaries (see Chapter 2).

Listening and believing what the body and the client say are significant. The client may personalize the nurturing touch of the therapist (transference) and may want to involve the therapist in the experience. Referral for appropriate counseling is important. When a person is actively exploring personal trauma and its results, it is important that the massage therapist not take on the client's problems (countertransference).

Re-enactment and Integration: Dealing with Flashbacks

Re-enactment means reliving the event as though it were happening again right now. **Integration** involves remembering the event, yet being able to remain in the present moment, with an awareness of the difference between then and now, to bring some sort of resolution to the event.

Re-enactment does not necessarily provide the awareness and understanding necessary to integrate the physical response and emotional feelings into the client's experience in an empowering way. Instead, with re-enactment the client repeats an abusive pattern and feels disempowered and lost. The massage professional must be aware of the potential for harm to a client by deliberately triggering a reenactment response. Without the additional and necessary support of qualified counselors and other support personnel to provide for an integration process, a re-enactment is undesirable.

If a client should respond during the massage by crying, shaking, becoming ticklish, agitated, or fearful, or demonstrating another emotional pattern, it is important for the massage professional to be quiet and let the person experience the emotion. If needed, provide tissues in an unobtrusive way. Changes in breathing are common. For example, the client may cough, hold the breath, increase the breathing rate, or yawn. It is wise during these situations to avoid telling the client how to breathe. Breathing patterns are usually directly linked to experiences. Unless a client has high blood pressure and is holding the breath, the massage therapist should only observe the breathing and identify changes. In some instances it is best to continue to massage the area in the same way as that which triggered the response but to slow down, allowing the body to integrate the information. The client should be

asked no questions other than "Do you want me to continue?" The practitioner should be calm and accepting of the response and should never try to encourage or stop the response.

It is important not to interfere with the person's experience by interjecting suggestions. At other times it is appropriate to stop the massage and wait for the response to dissipate. It is important for the therapist to stay connected with the client but distanced from the client's experience. The emotional experience belongs to the client, not to the practitioner, who works as a support in a quiet, simple way. When the emotional response has dissipated, the massage can be continued. If the client asks what happened, a simple explanation based on state-dependent memory is sufficient. Similar explanations, as previously mentioned, help the client understand what happened. A client who seems unsettled and needs additional help coping should be referred to a qualified counselor.

Confidence, respect, and trust are necessary to provide the type of massage that enhances the well-being of those who have been or are being traumatized. Always remember that confidentiality is a sacred trust; the therapist does not talk about clients or any experience with clients to anyone else.

Working with those who have been traumatized is rewarding, but it can be very difficult. Additional training is needed to serve clients who have a history of trauma. The actual techniques of massage are no different, but an understanding of coping mechanisms and somatic (body) memories requires additional study. Bodywork in some form may be a valuable tool for some individuals who want to resolve these issues, whereas for others it is not the best choice. Effective decision-making skills and support and supervision by qualified professionals determine the appropriateness of massage interventions for this population (Proficiency Exercises 12-11 and 12-12).

PREGNANCY 12-7

SECTION OBJECTIVES

Using the information presented in this section, the student will be able to perform the following:

- Explain the importance of prenatal care
- Describe the three basic stages of pregnancy
- Design a general massage session to meet the needs of a pregnant woman
- Teach a support person basic massage methods to use during labor

Pregnancy is not an illness; it is a natural event. Early prenatal care provided by qualified health care professionals is very important for pregnant women. Prenatal care is needed to ensure that proper nutrition is provided for the mother, that the pregnancy is progressing normally, and to identify any potential problems early. If a woman is planning to become pregnant, she should improve and maintain her health for about 6 months beforehand. This means eliminating all alcohol, drugs, and nicotine, normalizing her weight, developing a moderate exercise program, and eating a nutritious diet. These activities help prepare the best environment for the baby's growth. Smoking, alcohol, and drug use are very dangerous to the unborn child. Excessive stress also is dangerous

PROFICIENCY EXERCISE 12-11

Based on the information presented in this section, choose one psychological challenge and write an intervention plan and justification statement for the use of therapeutic massage. Use the model in Box 12-14 as an example.

STUDENT NOTE: *Here is the clinical reasoning process again. If you have been practicing by doing the exercises in the beginning of this chapter, you should be starting to understand the process.*

Example: Therapeutic massage for _____

1. **Gather facts to identify and define the situation.**

   Key questions:
   What is the problem?
   What are the facts?

2. **Brainstorm possible solutions.**

   Key question:
   What might I do? or What if . . . ?

3. **Evaluate possible interventions logically and objectively; look at both sides and the pros and cons.**

   Key question:
   What would happen if . . . ?

4. **Evaluate the effect on the people involved.**

   Key question:
   How would each person involved feel?

5. **Develop an intervention plan and justification statements.**

PROFICIENCY EXERCISE 12-12

1. *Find and read three books that deal with surviving trauma, or research PubMed on the Internet (www. pubmedcentral.nih.gov) for the treatment of trauma.*
2. *Visit a safe house or shelter for abused women and talk with the volunteers who work there.*
3. *Contact the child protection agency in your community and obtain information on recognizing child abuse and reporting suspected cases.*
4. *Investigate methods used by the military to help soldiers.*
5. *In the space provided, describe an incident in which you felt abused. Also describe an incident in which you feel you abused someone.*

I felt abused when:

I abused someone when:

AUTHOR'S NOTE: Years of working with a clinical psychologist contributed to the experience acquired in this area.

to the developing infant and can be the cause of miscarriage and inability to conceive.

Pregnancy is divided into three distinct segments: the first, second, and third trimesters. A pregnant woman undergoes extensive physical and emotional changes during each of these stages.

First Trimester

During the first 3 months (the first trimester), the woman's body must adjust to tremendous hormonal changes, which are likely to cause mood swings. This is also a very vulnerable time for the developing baby. Positioning is not a concern unless the breasts are tender. Deep work on the abdomen is avoided so as not to disrupt the attachment of the baby to the uterine wall. Surface stroking can be pleasurable to the client.

The following changes are common during the first trimester:

■ *Nausea,* or the sensation of feeling sick, and vomiting are commonly referred to as *morning sickness.* Morning sickness tends to be most severe in the early morning but can occur in the evening and may last all day and night. Symptoms usually diminish by the tenth week of pregnancy and usually are gone by the end of 14 weeks. Only rarely does this last through the entire pregnancy.

■ *Frequent urination* occurs because of the presence of the hormone progesterone, which causes relaxation of the smooth muscle of the bladder. This tendency diminishes by the second trimester.

■ *Constipation* occurs because the hormone progesterone causes relaxation of the smooth muscle of the large intestine. This results in slow movement of the fecal matter through the system, as well as increased water absorption from the colon. Constipation may continue throughout the pregnancy. Mechanical pressure from the enlarging uterus contributes to the problem.

■ *Blood pressure* often falls in early pregnancy, specifically the diastolic pressure. This is also the result of the presence of progesterone, which relaxes the muscular wall of the blood vessels. The expectant mother may be fatigued and may feel lightheaded or faint, especially during prolonged standing. Blood pressure usually returns to normal during the fourteenth week of pregnancy.

■ *Breast changes* begin during this stage, including a sense of increased fullness, tenderness, and heightened sensitivity. These changes may continue throughout the pregnancy.

■ *Musculoskeletal changes* are caused by the influence of estrogen, progesterone, and relaxin. Relaxin is produced as early as 2 weeks into the pregnancy and is at its highest levels in the first trimester; it then falls 20% and remains at that level until labor. Relaxin affects the composition of collagen in the joint capsules, ligaments, and fascia to allow greater elasticity. This enables more movement in the joints and creates more yield in the abdomen. Although all joints are affected, the most vulnerable are those of the pelvis, such as the symphysis pubis and sacroiliac joint, and those that bear weight, such as the ankle and the joints of the foot.

■ *Taste and smell* are altered in the early stages of the pregnancy. Certain smells and foods become disagreeable to the woman.

Massage given during the first trimester is general wellness massage, which may help balance the mother's physiologic responses.

Second Trimester

The second trimester usually brings a leveling of the hormones, and the woman feels better. During this time she may start to "show" and feel the first movements of the baby. If the pregnancy was planned, this is a joyful time. If not, the physical evidence of the growing baby may cause additional stress for the mother.

Toward the end of the second trimester, the connective tissue, under the influence of relaxin, begins to soften to allow the pelvis to spread. Common considerations during the second trimester include the following:

■ *Joint "sloppiness"* develops because of the softening of the connective tissue, and the muscles of the legs, gluteals, and hip flexors must provide joint stabilization and tension; as a result, pain can develop. Overstretching must be avoided.

■ *Carpal tunnel syndrome,* caused by fluid retention, is common among pregnant women and may be perpetuated even after the birth as a result of caring for the infant.

■ *Edema* is common at any time during the pregnancy as a result of the retention of fluid. As the pregnancy advances, edema of the legs occurs in up to 40% of women. The mechanical obstruction created by the uterus and its contents causes an increase in venous pressure distally, resulting in edema. Although edema may be caused by excessive weight gain, it may also be a symptom of pre-eclampsia. In the latter case, the midwife or physician should be informed.

- *Pre-eclampsia* is a very serious complication that requires medical attention. The diagnosis of pre-eclampsia is made when the patient has an elevated blood pressure, generalized edema, and a high concentration of protein in the urine. Some common elements that may predispose women to pre-eclampsia are:
    - First pregnancy
    - Multiple pregnancy
    - Chronic hypertension or long-term hypertension
    - Chronic renal disease
    - Malnutrition
    - Diabetes
- *Supine hypotension* occurs as the fetus grows and compresses the aorta and inferior vena cava against the lumbar spine. This may cause the woman to feel faint when she is lying on her back.
- *Shortness of breath* is also common. This is the result of a combination of mechanical changes in the thorax and the position of the diaphragm and physiologic changes.

During massage in the second trimester, support for the abdomen is important. The side-lying position is most comfortable, and lying on the left side produces the least amount of abdominal congestion for the expanding uterus. The therapist need not be extensively concerned with position as long as the expectant mother is comfortable.

Be attentive for strain in the back muscles during positioning. Keep the head in alignment with the spine. Using a support so that the shoulder lies comfortably and does not fall forward or toward the ear is helpful. Support between the knees helps keep the hips in the neutral position and relieves stress in this area. A support under the top arm may also be comfortable Allow the client to change position often. As in the first trimester, deep work on the abdomen must be avoided.

Third Trimester

During the last (third) trimester, the weight of the growing baby, the postural shifts, and the movement of the internal organs may cause discomfort for the pregnant woman. Because many of the internal organs are pushed up and back, the diaphragm does not work as efficiently. The mother uses her neck and shoulder muscles to breathe, possibly causing discomfort or thoracic outlet symptoms. Breathing pattern disorders may develop. Massage offers temporary relief of these symptoms.

About 2 weeks before birth (in the first pregnancy), the baby turns head down and drops into the birth canal. This provides more space for the diaphragm to work and breathing becomes easier, but pressure on the bladder causes frequent urination. Impingement on lymph vessels may cause the legs and feet to swell. Edema or fluid accumulation may be a symptom of more serious complications, and the client should be referred to a physician immediately if these are noted. The low back may ache from the postural shift. The breasts have enlarged in preparation for lactation. A woman may not feel very attractive at this point and most likely is not very comfortable physically. Fatigue and sleep disturbances may result. Massage is gentle, supports comfort, and assists circulation. If a comfortable position cannot be found, allow the client to change position often and use the restroom as needed. General massage may help the woman feel better for a little while and support comfortable sleep.

Disorders of Pregnancy

Although pregnancy and delivery are considered normal physiologic functions, problems can occur. Early recognition and referral are important. Warning signs of a pregnancy at risk that require immediate referral include the following:
- Vaginal bleeding
- Severe, continuous abdominal pain
- Breaking of water (rupture of membranes)
- Pre-eclampsia, edema, dizziness, elevated blood pressure, severe headache
- Fever, frequent and painful urination (may indicate a urinary tract infection)
- Excessive vomiting of such severity and frequency that no food or fluids can be retained
- Excessive itching (occasionally may suggest a liver or kidney dysfunction [cholestasis])

Labor

Labor occurs as the baby moves down the birth canal before birth. Education and birthing classes are important, especially for first pregnancies. It may be appropriate to teach the woman's support person some massage techniques before the onset of labor. Massage given by the support person helps that person to feel useful and involved with the pregnancy and birthing process. Massage of the lower back and stroking of the abdomen may provide comfort and a point of focus during labor. Massaging the feet often is helpful. Massage can relax the body and divert the attention of the nervous system, thereby providing distraction during early labor. Labor proceeds easier and faster if the woman is relaxed and works with her body.

During a phase of labor called *transition,* the woman often does not want to be touched. Transition occurs just before the second stage of labor, with the actual movement of the baby down the birth canal. The contractions at this time are very hard and have not yet been replaced by the urge to push. After delivery, massage may help the woman's body return to normal, it may reduce the stress of taking care of a new baby, and it may give the client some time to take care of herself.

Recommendations for Massage During Pregnancy

Unless specific circumstances or complications are involved, massage for pregnant women should be a general massage

(Figure 12-25). Do not massage vigorously or extremely deeply, do not overstretch, and do not massage the abdomen other than with superficial stroking. Avoid massage on the inside of the ankle, because a reflex point in that area can stimulate uterine contractions (this area is located on the spleen meridian). Watch for fever, edema, varicose veins, and severe mood swings. After birth, postpartum depression can become a serious problem for some women. Refer a client with these conditions to her physician immediately.

In some cases pregnancy is not a joyous event, as in an unwanted pregnancy. The practitioner must not try to convince the woman that she really does want the baby or try to change her mood. The client must be supported with caring, quiet touch, and listening.

Interrupted pregnancies are also difficult. Whether the cause is spontaneous abortion in the first 3 months, induced abortion, or miscarriage, an interrupted pregnancy is a strain on a woman's body and emotional well-being. If a client has

FIGURE 12-25 Prenatal massage. **A,** Explain the procedures for prenatal massage. **B,** Place the client in the side-lying position and use bolsters for support (most of the massage is done on the left and right sides). **C,** Frequently check in with the mother-to-be. **D,** Gentle massage and rocking of the abdomen are comforting to both the mother and the baby. **E,** Proceed with the general massage. **F,** All massage manipulations are appropriate as long as they are comforting.

FIGURE 12-25, cont'd G, Massage of the back is comforting. **H,** Rhythmic, gentle compression around the ribs aids breathing. The supine position may be used if the woman is comfortable and well bolstered. **I,** Take care around tender breasts. Massage of the shoulders, neck, head, and face is comforting. **J,** Foot massage is pleasurable and can easily be taught to the baby's father or the mother's support partner. **K,** Low back compression is beneficial during pregnancy and labor. **L,** A useful massage position during pregnancy and labor.

had an interrupted pregnancy, watch for emotional changes at what would have been the projected time of birth. Extra caring and support are helpful then.

The massage professional must have permission from the physician or licensed midwife to work with a woman during pregnancy. Giving a general massage to a pregnant woman can be a very rewarding experience, one that allows the massage professional to watch the miracle of life develop (Proficiency Exercise 12-13).

 PROFICIENCY EXERCISE 12-13

1. *Contact your local hospital or other agency offering childbirth classes. Ask if it would be possible to attend as an observer.*
2. *Locate a pregnant dog, cat, or horse. While giving the animal a massage, gently palpate the abdomen.*

PROFICIENCY EXERCISE 12-14

1. *Plan your funeral. List all plans and details regarding final arrangements.*
2. *Talk with an attorney about living wills.*
3. *Volunteer to provide massage for hospice staff members. Spend a minimum of 32 hours.*
4. *In the space provided, write about how you wish to be taken care of when it is your time to die. How much intervention do you want? Do you want to die in a hospital or at home? When do you want hospice services?*

TERMINAL ILLNESS, END OF LIFE CARE, AND HOSPICE CARE

SECTION OBJECTIVES

Using the information presented in this section, the student will be able to perform the following:

- Obtain additional information about the process of dying
- Explain the importance of comfort measures

When nothing further can be done to prolong life, care focuses more on comfort measures. The experts in terminal illness are the dedicated hospice nurses and staff members who treat death with dignity. It has been said that the staff members of hospices are midwives to the dying.

To work successfully with those dealing with a terminal illness, the massage practitioner must be aware of his or her personal feelings about death. Massage professionals who want to work with clients during this very important, challenging, and special time of life are strongly encouraged to become hospice volunteers and to take the training that hospices offer.

No one knows when a person is going to die. However, two very powerful psychological forces influence living and dying: hope and the will to live. Attitudes about death vary. Adults usually have more fears about death than children do. They fear pain, suffering, dying alone, the invasion of privacy, loneliness, and separation from family and loved ones. They worry about who will care for and support those left behind. Elderly people usually have fewer of these fears than younger adults. They may be more accepting that death will occur and have had more experience with dying and death. Many have lost family members and friends. Some welcome death as freedom from pain, suffering, and disability.

Dr. Elisabeth Kübler-Ross has written about death, and her works have much to offer. Bernie Siegal's books also are excellent. Massage professionals interested in working with the terminally ill would benefit from reading their works.

Massage has much to offer in comfort measures for the terminally ill. Being bedridden and immobile is painful. Massage can distract the sensory perception and provide temporary comfort measures. It provides continued human contact and can give caregivers something useful, rewarding, and positive to do for their loved one who is dying.

Massage can become an important stress reduction method and a means of support for family members and caregivers. Caring for someone who is terminally ill can be very stressful. The support person may need to receive massage simply to have someone take care of him or her for an hour. Teaching simple massage methods to the caregivers provides them with a means of meaningful and structured interaction with their loved one, as well as a means of connecting with and supporting each other.

The massage professional should be an integral part of the team that works to make this time of passage as gentle as possible. This means that once the decision to work with someone who is terminally ill has been made, it is important to stay with the process until the client dies, if possible. The therapist probably will grow to care for the person and will mourn and grieve when death comes.

As always, it remains the client's choice as to what is wanted, and he or she must give informed consent. The client who is dying needs to retain as much personal empowerment as possible. It should not be discouraging if all that is done during a massage session is to stroke a client's hands. At this time, especially, it is crucial to "listen" and "allow" (Proficiency Exercise 12-14).

evolve

12-1 Find internet links to various spas around the world.

12-2 Log on to the Evolve Website for a demonstration of computer-based record keeping.

12-3 Find links to research on benefits of animal massage.

12-4 Log on to the Evolve Website to read about hospice care.

Don't forget to study for your certification and licensure exams! Review questions for this chapter are located on Evolve.

■ ■ ■   SUMMARY

The three main career tracks for therapeutic massage serve various populations and environments. The environment in which massage is offered (i.e., the various types of spas, health care settings, and sports and fitness facilities, as well as on site massage) can serve all the groups discussed: an athlete in a rehabilitation center, a person dying at home, and pet massage offered as part of the grooming process. The combinations are endless; the massage is similar, but unique to the client based on outcomes.

Respect is important in any interaction with another person or with an animal. In all situations, remember to see and address the person first and then to accommodate the individual's special needs by offering assistance and following the directions provided by the client. Massage therapists who want to focus their professional skills to best meet a client's specific needs will seek out training and information pertinent to the client's therapeutic needs. Often the knowledge required to provide massage to many populations becomes too extensive, and specialization becomes necessary. When this is the case, such as when a massage professional obtains additional training for pregnancy, labor, and delivery massage, the information is integrated into the fundamentals of massage, and the additional training focuses on the application of the massage fundamentals for the special situation.

The wise professional recognizes when less intervention is more appropriate. Considerable learning, great skill, and patiently developed empathy are required to therapeutically hold a person's hand.

REFERENCES

1. http://finewaters.com/water_wellness/American_Healingwaters.asp
2. http://www.medicalspaassociation.org/guidelines.htm
3. http://dayspafyi.com/day-spa-treatments.html
4. Arnheim DD, Prentice WE: *Principles of athletic training: a competency based approach*, ed 12, Boston, 2005, McGraw-Hill Higher Education.
5. Benjamin PJ, Lamp SP: *Understanding sports massage*, ed 2, Champaign, Ill, 2004, Human Kinetics.
6. McGladre Y, Pullen R: *The Americans with Disabilities Act (rev)*, New York, 1994, Panel Publishers.

BIBLIOGRAPHY

American Psychiatric Association: *Diagnostic and statistical.*

American Veterinary Medical Association: Colloquium on recognition and alleviation of animal pain and distress, *J Am Vet Med Assoc* 191:1184, 1987.

Association of Veterinary Teachers and Research Workers (Working Party): Guidelines for the recognition and assessment of pain in animals, *Vet Rec* 118:334, 1986.

Australian Council for the Care of Animals in Research and Teaching (ACCART): Proceedings of the animal pain conference, *ACCART Newsletter* 3:11, 1990.

Bateson P: Assessment of pain in animals, *Anim Behav* 42:827, 1991.

Canadian Council on Animal Care (CCAC): Ottawa, Ontario, CCAC, 1984. Accessed April, 2006, at www.ccac.ca/en/CCAC_Programs/ETCC/Module09/06.html

Corydon V, Clark G: *ADHD throughout the life span*, Las Vegas, 1997, Random Clark Publications.

Gentle MJ: Pain in birds, *Animal Welfare* 1:235, 1992.

Horacek HJ Jr: Brainstorms: understanding and treating the emotional storms of attention deficit/hyperactivity disorder from childhood through adulthood, New Jersey, 2000, Aronson.

Short CE, Van Poznak A, editors: *Animal pain*, New York, 1992, Churchill Livingstone.

Silverman J: How much is enough? *Lab Animal* 20:20, 1991.

Wall PD: Defining pain in animals. In Short CE, Van Poznak A, editors: *Animal pain*, New York, 1992, Churchill Livingstone.

RESOURCES

The Day Spa Association
310 17th Street, Union City, New Jersey 07087
Phone: 201-865-2065 Fax: 201-865-3961
Web site: dayspaassociation.org
The Medical Spa Association 520 23rd Street, Union City, New Jersey 07087
Phone: 201-865-2065; Fax: 201-865-3961

International Spa Association
Lexington, Kentucky
Phone: 1-888-651-ISPA Fax: 1-859-226-4445
experienceispa.com

This Web site contains comprehensive information about the Library, the scope of its collections, and how to use its services. There is a range of catalogues for different types of material, thousands of images and hundreds of sound samples.

The British Library
St Pancras
96 Euston Road
London
NW1 2DB
http://www.bl.uk/TheBritishLibrary

Workbook Section

Answers for the Workbook Section for Chapter 12 are provided on p. 774.

■ ■ ■ SHORT ANSWER

1. What are the three main career tracks in massage? Compare and contrast their similarities and differences.

2. What is the single most important factor in effective communication with individuals who have special needs?

3. What special massage skills are needed to work with people who have special needs?

4. What is the best source of information about any special situation?

5. What factors must be considered when massaging animals?

6. What is the importance of state-dependent memory in working with people who may have a history of trauma?

7. What responses might the massage practitioner receive when pointing out an area of injury to a client who self-abuses?

8. How should a massage practitioner respond if a client experiences an emotional response during the massage?

9. Why is massage beneficial for athletes?

10. What is restorative massage for athletes?

11. What type of massage is provided at sports events?

12. What adjustment to a massage session may be required when working with children?

13. Why do children like massage?

14. What is a major benefit of massage for children and adolescents?

15. Why is it important to teach parents and children some basic massage methods to share with each other?

16. Who gives informed consent for massage for individuals under 18 years of age?

17. What is a realistic goal for the massage professional when working with people who have a chronic illness?

18. What is the importance of hardiness and how does massage encourage it?

_____

_____

_____

19. Why is close supervision by the physician or another health professional important when the massage professional is working with people who have a chronic illness?

_____

_____

_____

20. What can the massage therapist learn from working with the elderly?

_____

_____

_____

21. What special physical conditions are common among the elderly?

_____

_____

_____

22. Are special skills required for working with the elderly?

_____

_____

_____

23. Why is massage beneficial for infants?

_____

_____

_____

24. Who is the best person to massage a baby?

_____

_____

_____

25. What key elements are important when massaging an infant?

_____

_____

_____

26. What are the unique concerns of massage professionals who work in the medical environment or with people receiving home health care?

_____

_____

_____

27. What important points should the massage professional remember when working with clients who have a physical disability?

_____

_____

_____

28. When working with people who have an emotional or a developmental disability, the massage therapist must keep in mind what important factor?

_____

_____

_____

29. How can massage be beneficial for withdrawal from addiction, for learning disabilities, and for developmental disabilities?

_____

_____

_____

30. Are special massage skills required for working with pregnant women? Explain.

_____

_____

_____

31. What part can teaching massage to the expectant father or other support person play?

_____

_____

_____

32. What can the massage therapist learn from providing massage for a person who is dying?

_____

_____

_____

33. What is the best source of information about working with the dying?

_____

_____

_____

34. What can massage offer to someone who is dying?

_____

_____

_____

Workbook Section—cont'd

■ ■ ■ PROBLEM-SOLVING EXERCISES

1. You are working at an organized sporting event as a volunteer for the local sports massage team. You notice that one of the other team members is doing deep invasive work on one of the clients. What should you do?

_____

_____

_____

_____

2. A client begins to shake and to breathe very deeply during the massage. What do you do?

_____

_____

_____

_____

3. An elderly client wants you to stay after the massage and have a cup of coffee. What do you do?

_____

_____

_____

_____

_____

4. A young father is having trouble holding his newborn baby. What can you do?

_____

_____

_____

_____

5. A client with a speech difficulty needs to provide informed consent. How could this be accomplished?

_____

_____

_____

_____

6. A client is near death. She does not want a full massage but needs to be touched. What can you do?

_____

_____

_____

_____

■ ■ ■ ASSESS YOUR COMPETENCIES

Now that you have studied this chapter, you should be able to:

1. Identify the three main career tracks based on the massage setting: spas, sports and fitness, and health care.

2. Develop a massage environment to best serve individuals with special needs.

3. Demonstrate the communication skills that are important for working with a client with special needs.

4. Gather information on additional training to help you better serve clients with special needs.

On a separate sheet of paper, write a short summary of the content of this chapter based on the competencies listed above. When writing this paper, assume you are speaking to someone—a client, prospective employer, co-worker, or other interested person. Write the paper as if you were having a conversation and explaining the importance of the information and skills to professional massage development.

Next, in small student discussion groups, share the papers and compare and contrast how the information was presented. Discuss the content, looking for similarities, differences, potential misunderstanding of the information, and clear and concise methods of description.

■ ■ ■ PROFESSIONAL APPLICATION EXERCISES

You are asked to give a presentation to a group of nurses at a local hospital. They are looking for ways to use massage in various outpatient situations. They need a general explanation of ways massage would be beneficial for many different conditions. What major points would you make during the talk?

■ ■ ■ RESEARCH FOR FURTHER STUDY

A major approach in massage is generalized, nonspecific, body-supportive care. This approach does not seek to intervene, but rather tries to provide support and to nurture health. Brainstorm the various applications for massage in special needs situations and then do some research to find sources that support some of the concepts.

Wellness Education

CHAPTER OBJECTIVES

After completing this chapter, the student will be able to perform the following:

- Identify the basic components of a wellness program
- Locate resources to develop a wellness program
- Develop a personal wellness program
- Provide general wellness guidelines to clients

CHAPTER OUTLINE

STRESS

WELLNESS COMPONENTS
    Communication
    Demands
    Loss
    Seeking Help
    Intuition
    Body
    Mind
    Spirit

SUMMARY

KEY TERMS

Aerobic exercise
Challenge
Commitment
Control
Deep inspiration
Defensive measures
Denial
Endurance
Fitness
Forced expiration
Forced inspiration
Overload principle
Quiet expiration
Quiet inspiration
Stressors
Training stimulus threshold

This chapter teaches the massage professional about the general concepts of wellness. Massage is an important part of any wellness program because it restores body balance and provides a connection with other human beings. As such, it is necessary that the massage professional understand the components of "wellness." With this information the professional can explain to clients how massage fits into the overall wellness picture. It is impossible to define a step-by-step process that provides for wellness, because each person is an individual, who needs to develop a personal plan according to the general concepts of wellness. It is important to read this chapter with your heart and soul as well as with your mind.

Wellness programs can be built around the following factors:

The body
- Nutrition
- Light and dark exposure
- Sleep
- Breathing
- Physical fitness
- Sensory stimulation

The mind
- Relationships with oneself and others
- Communication
- Beliefs
- Intellectual stimulation

The spirit
- Sense of purpose
- Connection
- Faith

- Hope
- Love

We are considered well when the body, mind, and spirit are in ideal balance.

We are not well when imbalance exists and balance cannot be restored.

In the words of a renowned nutrition scientist, Professor Jeffrey Bland, many people are "vertically ill."[1] Such people are not sick enough to lie down, but they are certainly not well. More than just the type of stress is involved in this condition; it is the amount of stress that accumulates until the breakdown begins. It is only a matter of time before physical health, the mind, or the quality of life simply falls apart under the accumulation of multiple stressors.

Everyone would benefit by developing a personal wellness plan. Just as in designing a massage, there is no right way or wrong way to formulate this plan. However, by following a few basic guidelines, each of us can discover what works for us as individuals, and that is the best plan. Massage practitioners need to remember that as wonderful as massage is, it addresses only a part of the person. Wellness is about the whole person. The empathetic massage professional realizes that during a client's search for wellness, the time spent with the massage practitioner provides focused attention, acceptance, and effective listening, which are as important as the massage methods used.

This chapter examines the basic guidelines necessary for building a wellness program. It provides enough information to give some direction in the development and implementation of a wellness plan. As with massage, often the simpler the program is, the better it is. We are supposed to be well. Our bodies will recognize the best process. Wellness has a domino effect. Simple alterations in lifestyle create a chain reaction throughout a person's entire life. Therefore people need to commit to only a few carefully planned lifestyle changes and then allow the rest of the pieces of their lives to fall into place.

Resistance usually occurs when an adjustment is necessary. Initially we may resist change, which can come from our own bodies or coping patterns, or from family and friends who interact with us. Remember, if our behavior changes, the people around us will have to change as well. Changes should be made slowly, if possible, to allow the "pieces" (your own body, family, friends, or coworkers) to comment, complain, support, and resist; but do not give in and quit. Persist with the wellness program and give your body, family, and friends time to get used to your new lifestyle.

Making a change to wellness takes determination. Letting go of behavioral patterns is difficult. It is very hard to do this alone, therefore relationships with those who are supportive and believe in us (e.g., support groups, professional therapy) are helpful. The massage professional can be an important support person for the client making wellness changes.

STRESS

Stress is our response to any demand on the body or mind to respond, adapt, or alter. It is a state of readiness to survive, one that requires hypervigilance by the body and mind. A person's emotional reaction to stress may be the difference between positive action and destructive breakdown, especially if many of the stressors seem beyond control.[1] According to Dr. Hans Selye, an expert on stress:

> The ancient Greek philosophers clearly recognized that, with regard to human conduct, the most important, but perhaps also the most difficult, thing was "to know thyself." It takes great courage even just to attempt this honestly. Yet it is well worth the effort and humiliation, because most of our tensions and frustrations stem from compulsive needs to act the role of someone we are not.[2]

Before any wellness program can be developed, a person needs to at least "explore thyself." The next step is to analyze and explore the stressors that we all encounter in our daily lives. The three major elements of stress are the stressor itself, defensive measures, and mechanisms for surrender.

Stressors are any internal perceptions or external stimuli that demand a change in the body. The **defensive measures** are the ways our bodies defend against the stressor, such as the production of antibodies and white blood cells or behavioral and emotional defenses. Sometimes defending is not the best way to deal with stress. It is important and resourceful to know when to quit, or surrender. Hormonal and nervous stimuli encourage the body to retreat and ignore stressors. On an emotional level this sometimes is called **denial**, which can be an important method of coping with stress.[2]

It has long been known that mental excitement and physical stressors cause an initial exhilaration followed by a secondary phase of depression. A law of physics states that for every action, there is an equal and opposite reaction. Certain chemical compounds, such as the hormones produced during the acute alarm reaction phase of the general adaptation syndrome (see Chapter 4), are able first to key up the body for action and then to cause depression (Box 13-1). Both effects may have great protective value for the body. It is necessary to be keyed up for peak accomplishment, but it is equally important to relax and restore in the secondary phase of depression. This prevents us from carrying on too long at top speed. As Selye has written:

> The fact is that a person can be intoxicated with his own stress hormones. I venture to say that this sort of drunkenness has caused much more harm to society than the alcoholic kind. We are on our guard against external toxicants, but hormones are parts of our bodies; it takes more wisdom to recognize and overcome the foe which fights from within. In all our actions throughout the day, we must consciously look for signs of being keyed up too much, and we must learn to stop in time. To watch our critical stress level is just as important as to watch our critical quota of cocktails. More so. Intoxication by stress is sometimes unavoidable and usually insidious. You can quit alcohol and, even if you do take some, at least you can count the glasses; but it is impossible to avoid stress as long as you live, and your conscious thoughts often cannot gauge its alarm signals accurately. Curiously, the pituitary is a much better judge of stress than the intellect. Yet, you can learn to recognize the danger signals fairly well if you know what to look for.[2]

Depending on our conditioning and genetic makeup, we all respond differently to general stress. As a whole, each

BOX 13-1

Common Stress Responses

- General irritability, hyperexcitation, or depression
- Pounding heart
- Dry throat and mouth
- Impulsive behavior and emotional instability
- Overpowering urge to cry, run, or hide
- Inability to concentrate
- Weakness or dizziness
- Fatigue
- Tension and extreme alertness
- Trembling and nervous tics
- Intermittent anxiety
- Tendency to be easily startled
- High-pitched, nervous laughter
- Stuttering and other speech difficulties
- Grinding the teeth
- Insomnia
- Inability to sit still or physically relax

- Sweating
- Frequent need to urinate
- Diarrhea, indigestion, queasiness, and vomiting
- Migraine and other tension headaches
- Premenstrual tension or missed menstrual cycles
- Pain in the neck or lower back
- Loss of appetite or excessive appetite
- Increased use of chemicals, including tobacco, caffeine, and alcohol
- Nightmares
- Neurotic behavior
- Psychosis
- Proneness to accidents

These signs of stress result from fluctuations in the autonomic nervous system and resulting shifts in endogenous chemicals.

person tends to respond consistently, with one set of signs, in individualized patterns caused by the malfunctioning of whatever happens to be the most vulnerable part in his or her physiology (genetic weak link). When warning signs appear, it is time to stop, change the activity, and divert the body's attention to something else.

If proportionately too much stress occurs in any physical or emotional area of the body, the energy needs to be diverted to a different area. If a person is thinking too much, then he or she should use the larger muscles of the body (e.g., gardening, taking a brisk walk). If too much exercise is causing stress, balance can be restored by reading a novel, watching a movie, or listening to soft music. If too much stress occurs in the body as a whole, rest is required. If we do not rest of our own accord, the body may become ill so that we rest for awhile.

WELLNESS COMPONENTS

Wellness training requires an extensive amount of information about diet, exercise, lifestyle, and behavior patterns. It is important to consult those with experience to obtain that information. Do not depend on only one information source. Talk with two, three, or four "experts" and read three or four books on each topic before making decisions about what could be done to benefit or improve your wellness. Remember, only a few symptoms combine to create a huge array of illness and disease patterns. Fortunately, a combination of only a few lifestyle changes is required to redirect a disease pattern toward a more resourceful and healing pattern.

When developing a wellness program, consider your mental and physical history. Our sense of self in relation to others is also important. If this connection with others is not respected and nurtured, the wholeness of our life is strained. This strain may interfere with our spiritual, emotional, and physical health.

Many of us have been sick, or at the very least vertically ill. It may take extraordinary effort to reverse these situations. That is when we realize maybe we should have taken better care of ourselves in the first place. Taking care of ourselves is what wellness and massage are all about.

Communication

People are not designed to be alone, therefore we must be able to communicate effectively with each other. If we do not communicate effectively with others and with ourselves, our energy is confused and our responses scattered. Communication is one of the biggest problems for humans because it is so subjective. It is very difficult to be truly objective; knowing this is an important part of wellness. Wellness requires assuming responsibility for our communication. Chapter 2 provides guidelines for communication in the professional world, but these same skills enhance communication in all personal interactions.

Demands

Today, many of the demands placed on us are outside the design of the body: too much information, too much to know, too much to do, too many responsibilities, and too many places to be. Our lives have become hurried, marked by a constant battle for time. There are too many options with too many choices, and it all costs too much.

Wellness often revolves around simplification of a person's lifestyle. Simplification requires choices, boundaries, discipline, and "letting go" in many dimensions.

Loss

Sometimes an event in life removes some part of us. It could be a body part, a body function, a relationship, a member of our family, or a job. Loss heals through grieving. Grief is a physiologic response that includes stimulation of the sympathetic autonomic nervous system. The emotional response is first alarm, then disbelief and denial, progressing to anger and guilt. This process continues toward finding a source of comfort and finally adjusting to the loss. To heal, we need to reconstruct that part or learn to live resourcefully without it.

Seeking Help

Many professionals can help us with specific therapeutic interventions as the wellness program is developed. Doctors, counselors, other health care providers, educators, and religious and spiritual advisors all play an important part in helping us become well again or maintain our wellness. Ultimately, each of us must do the work and take responsibility for who, what, and where we are, but it is important to use the help that is available. For example, if a person has a large tumor and a surgeon can safely remove it, the doctor's help will give the body a head start on healing.

Intuition

A balance exists between intuition and research in wellness. In developing a wellness program, it is important to consider these two very important sources of information. Hippocrates advised, "Do no harm." A wellness program relies on adherence to this advice, in addition to a balance between what science knows and *what we know we need*. A wellness program needs to change as we change. When an effective wellness program is carried out, a person looks forward to getting back to living life to the fullest and, at the appropriate time, to dying with dignity (Proficiency Exercise 13-1).

Body

Our bodies are our dwelling places in this life. They are the most concrete aspects of our being. The care of our bodies is an important part of any wellness program. Areas that require attention in a wellness program to support the body include nutrition, breathing, exercise and stretching, relaxation, sleep, and feelings.

Nutrition

According to the National Cancer Institute, poor nutrition is the reason 3 of 4 people develop a disease or illness. Given these statistics, it is clear that good nutrition means more than just choosing certain foods; it is about wanting to live a life

without the complications of disease and illness. Therefore people need to educate themselves about why whole foods are the best food choice. Figure 13-1 breaks down into very simple form what constitutes a good food choice and what is a bad food choice, as well as the possible pathologic outcomes for each of the bad food categories.

National Institutes of Health (NIH) sponsors two databases, one through the Office of Dietary Supplements (see http://dietary-supplements.info.nih.gov/) and the National Center for Complementary and Alternative Medicine (NCCAM) (see http://www.nccam.nih.gov/). Both provide unbiased information on the safety and effectiveness of supplements. However, neither site contains as much detailed or easily accessible information as the Consumer Reports database (see http://www.consumerreportsmedicalguide.org/), which allows consumers to check which natural medicines might be effective for specific health problems.

Proper nutrition is easy to explain. However, because of our fast-paced lifestyle, people do not always follow recommendations. This is because nutrition involves more than just eating. Eating affects the mood, mood influences feelings, and behavior supports feelings. Food, therefore, becomes an emotional issue.

The basics of balanced nutrition are explained in the Department of Agriculture's new guide to good eating. The new recommendations have reconfigured the original four food groups into a six-section pyramid (see http://www. mypyramid.gov). The Food Pyramid suggests a diet high in vegetables, grains, legumes, and fruit. The protein requirement from animal sources has been reduced, and dairy needs are moderate to small. For any animal products, naturally raised, and hormone-free products are best.

Although fat and sugar requirements in the diet are minimal, human beings have a strong urge for sweets and fats. This instinctive craving contributes to most dietary problems. In the early days of human existence, these two substances were difficult to find. Humans had to have a deep instinctual desire to fight the bees for their honey and the animals for their fat or to gather fatty seeds. Today these substances are abundantly available, but our primitive nature still acts as though we need to store up for a future famine. Nonetheless, people often find that if they detox themselves from sugar, the urge for sweets goes away.

An ideal diet is low in saturated fats; it includes oils such as olive oil and eliminates all trans fats. The bulk of calories in the Food Pyramid come from complex carbohydrates. Some nutritional experts suggest that diets should be higher in protein and lower in carbohydrates. There seem to be many expert opinions on proper diets. Regardless, cycles of high and low blood sugar are produced by unbalanced diets, aggravated by improper spacing between meals, and promoted by substances such as coffee, alcohol, and soft drinks. These fluids stimulate the production of adrenaline, which forces the release of sugar into the bloodstream. The body then releases insulin to lower the sugar level again.

Drinking enough pure water is very important to a wellness program. Because our bodies are more than 70% water (Box 13-2 and Table 13-1), most diets recommend that a person

PROFICIENCY EXERCISE 13-1

Begin to build a library about wellness. Take inventory of the books and magazines you already have. Categorize them and commit to adding one new book at least every 3 months. Explore your public library and the Internet to become familiar with the wellness resources they offer.

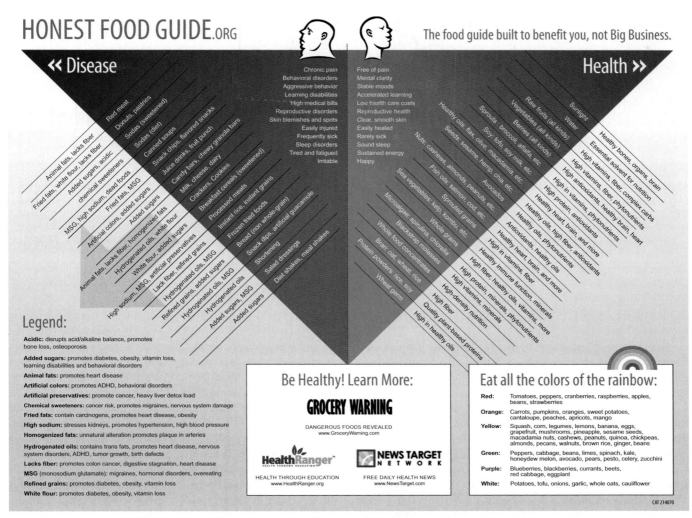

FIGURE 13-1 Honest food guide. (Courtesy Mike Adams at www.truthpublishing.com)

BOX 13-2

Functions of Water in the Human Body

- Provides a medium for chemical reactions
- Plays a crucial role in regulating chemical and bioelectric distributions within cells
- Transports substances such as hormones and nutrients
- Aids oxygen transport from the lungs to body cells
- Aids carbon dioxide transport from body cells to the lungs
- Dilutes toxic substances and waste products and transports them to the kidneys and liver
- Distributes heat around the body

From Fritz S: *Mosby's essential sciences for therapeutic massage: anatomy, physiology, biomechanics, and pathology,* ed 3, St Louis, 2009, Mosby.

TABLE 13-1

Water Composition of Body Tissues

Tissue	Water Composition (%)
Blood	83.0
Kidneys	82.7
Heart	79.2
Lungs	79.0
Spleen	75.8
Muscle	75.6
Brain	74.8
Intestine	74.5
Skin	72.0
Liver	68.3
Skeleton	22.0
Adipose tissue	10.0

From Fritz S: *Mosby's essential sciences for therapeutic massage: anatomy, physiology, biomechanics, and pathology,* ed 3, St Louis, 2009, Mosby.

FIGURE 13-2 Tests for dehydration. **A,** Hydrated skin. **B,** Dehydrated skin.

drink at least 64 ounces of water per day for efficient body function (Figure 13-2).

Adequate fiber and water in the diet promote bladder and bowel habits that support wellness. Eating on a regular schedule is important to support body rhythms that in turn support wellness (Figure 13-3).

Nutritional Supplements. Many people take nutritional supplements. Experts disagree on the value of all vitamins, but many recommend a quality multivitamin. Food sources of vitamins and minerals are compromised by depleted soil and artificial fertilizers and tainted by pesticides and other chemicals. Nutritional value also is compromised by long-term storage and preservation. Obtaining optimal nutritional value from the food we eat is difficult without extraordinary attention to our diet, which requires time, dedication, and discipline.

Supplementation is a plausible answer to this problem. The only recommendation offered is that the closer a supplement is to a "real food," the better the body will be able to use it. Supplements usually are best taken with food to enhance absorption.

evolve Herbs, which are very powerful substances, should not be used as nutritional supplements or medicines without knowledge of their effects (Proficiency Exercise 13-2). See the Evolve Web site for a comprehensive list of various nutritional supplements and herbs.

General Dietary Recommendations. A healthy diet consists of appropriate portions of healthy fats, such as olive, grapeseed, and flaxseed oils, and healthy carbohydrates (whole grain foods), such as whole wheat bread, oatmeal, and brown rice. Vegetables and fruits should be eaten in abundance. The diet includes moderate amounts of healthy sources of protein such as nuts, legumes, fish, poultry, lean meat, eggs, and dairy. A healthy diet minimizes the consumption of fatty red meat; refined grains, including white bread, white rice, and white pasta; and sugar. It eliminates foods made with trans fats, which eliminates as much fast food and prepared food as possible. A high-quality multiple vitamin that breaks down quickly in the digestive system is suggested for most people.

Fruits and vegetables reduce the risk of cardiovascular disease. Folic acid and potassium appear to contribute to this effect, which has been seen in several epidemiologic studies. Inadequate consumption of folic acid also is responsible for higher risks of serious birth defects, and a low intake of lutein, a pigment in green, leafy vegetables, has been associated with greater risks of cataracts and degeneration of the retina. Fruits and vegetables also are the primary source of many vitamins needed for good health; if these foods are eaten raw, the nutrients are not diminished, such as occurs with cooking or processing. Only a few vegetables provide better nutrient absorption when cooked.

High consumption of red meat has been associated with an increased risk of coronary artery disease, probably because of meat's high saturated fat content. Excessive consumption of fatty red meat also increases the risk of type 2 diabetes and colon cancer, can aggravate the inflammatory response, and increases pain sensitivity. The elevated risk of colon cancer may be partly related to the carcinogens produced during cooking and the chemicals found in processed meats such as salami and bologna.

Poultry and fish have less saturated fat and more unsaturated fat than red meat. Fish also is a rich source of the essential omega-3 fatty acids. Eggs do not appear to increase the risk of heart disease (except among diabetics), probably because the effects of a slightly higher cholesterol level are counterbalanced by other nutritional benefits, especially with eggs from chickens fed special vegetarian diets to increase nutritional value.

PROFICIENCY EXERCISE 13-2

Keep a food diary for 2 days. If your diet is not well balanced, decide what it would take to develop a plan that cuts saturated fat and sugar intake and increases water intake to recommended levels.

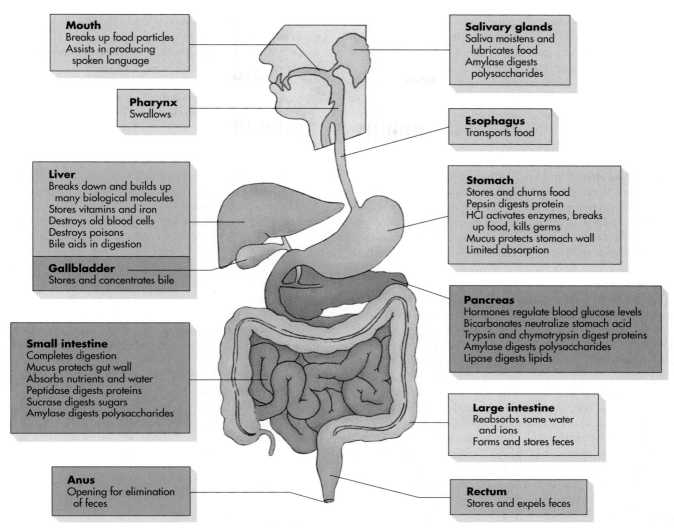

FIGURE 13-3 Summary of digestive function. (From Thibodeau GA, Patton KT: *Anatomy and physiology,* ed 5, St Louis, 2003, Mosby.)

Many people have avoided nuts because of their high fat content, but the fat in nuts, including peanuts, is mainly unsaturated, and walnuts in particular are a good source of omega-3 fatty acids. Also, people who eat nuts are actually less likely to be obese. Perhaps because nuts are more satisfying, eating them seems to significantly reduce the intake of other foods.

People need to eat clean, fresh food as much as possible. Organic foods and free-range and hormone-free meat, poultry, and fish are becoming easier to obtain. Even though the cost is higher, the value is usually worth the investment.

An important aspect of health maintenance is the management of inflammation, therefore eating a diet targeted to reduce inflammation is prudent. An antiinflammatory diet follows the recommendations just provided (Box 13-3). Foods especially high in antioxidants also are valuable.

Main Food Groups

Proteins. Proteins are large, high-molecular-weight substances that contain carbon, hydrogen, oxygen, and nitrogen

---

BOX 13-3

Guidelines for an Antiinflammatory Diet

- Eat fruits, vegetables, whole grains, omega-3 eggs, fish, chicken, yogurt (unsweetened) with live cultures, extra virgin olive oil, and flaxseed oil.
- Avoid dairy (except yogurt), pork, beef, processed meat, refined grains and sugar, artificial food, and most fats and oils, especially hydrogenated oils.
- Foods and herbs (e.g., ginger, turmeric, cumin, pineapple, and papaya) are especially valuable for controlling inflammation.

From Fritz S: *Sports and exercise massage: comprehensive care in fitness, athletics, and rehabilitation,* St Louis, 2006, Mosby.

and smaller amounts of other elements. Proteins break down into amino acids, which the body then absorbs. The body uses 24 amino acids to meet its metabolic requirements. Most can be manufactured in the liver from other amino acids, but eight cannot. These eight, called *essential amino acids,* are phenylalanine, valine, threonine, leucine, isoleucine, methionine, tryptophan, and lysine. In addition, histidine and arginine are required for growth and development. Dietary proteins include animal products and bean and grain combinations.

Proteins are the chief structural components of the body. Enzymes, some hormones, muscle tissue, and a substantial proportion of chromosomes are proteins. Proteins are essential components of the cell membrane. Important compounds such as epinephrine and acetylcholine are derived from amino acids.

Carbohydrates. The basic components of carbohydrates are carbon, hydrogen, and oxygen in definite proportions. Complex carbohydrates are long chains of glucose molecules found in brown rice, vegetables, and so on. Animal starch, or glycogen, is the storage form of glucose in the liver and muscles. Starch is digested in the mouth and small intestine and breaks down into monosaccharides and disaccharides, which are sugars or simple carbohydrates.

Glucose is the main fuel for the manufacture of adenosine triphosphate in the cell. The liver converts sugars to glucose.

Fats. Fats, or triglycerides, break down into fatty acids and glycerol. A *fatty acid* is a molecule consisting of a chain of carbons with no double bonds (saturated) or several double bonds (unsaturated). The unsaturated fats most closely resemble body fat and are more easily assimilated and used. Saturation (the addition of hydrogen molecules) makes fat a solid and less desirable in the diet. Linoleic acid is an example of a fatty acid that is essential to human nutrition. In addition to serving as a reservoir of stored energy, fats are essential components of many hormones, the cell membrane, and the myelin sheath of the nerve fibers. Dietary fats are found in nuts, seeds, oils, and animal products.

evolve **Vitamins.** Vitamins are growth factors needed in small amounts for daily body metabolism. They are classified as fat soluble or water soluble. Many vitamins act as enzyme activators (coenzymes). The fat-soluble vitamins are more toxic because excess amounts are stored in the fat tissue and are not excreted readily. Water-soluble vitamins are absorbed and excreted more easily. See the vitamin chart on the Evolve Web site.

Minerals. There are two kinds of minerals: **macrominerals** and **trace minerals.** The body needs larger amounts of macrominerals than trace minerals. The macromineral group is made up of calcium, phosphorus, magnesium, sodium, potassium, chloride, and sulfur. The body needs trace minerals, but just a tiny bit of each one. Trace minerals includes iron, manganese, copper, iodine, zinc, cobalt, fluoride, and selenium.

Metabolic Rate. The metabolic rate is the rate of energy release. The basal metabolic rate (BMR) is not the minimum metabolic rate and does not indicate the smallest amount of energy that must be expended to sustain life. The BMR is the smallest energy expenditure that can sustain life and also maintain the waking state and a normal body temperature in a comfortably warm environment. It is the rate of energy expenditure under basal conditions; that is, when the individual is (1) awake but lying down and not moving; (2) in a comfortably warm environment; and (3) 18 to 23 hours have passed since the last meal.

The BMR is not the same for all individuals because of the following factors:

- *Size:* The BMR is calculated from an individual's height and weight. A large individual has more surface area (and a higher BMR) than a small individual.
- *Gender:* Men oxidize their food approximately 5% to 7% faster than women. Therefore even if a man and a woman are the same size, the man has a higher BMR. This gender difference probably results from the difference in the proportion of body fat determined by sex hormones. Women tend to have a higher percentage of body fat (and thus a lower total lean mass) than men. Fat tissue is less metabolically active than lean tissue, such as muscle.
- *Age:* The younger the individual, the higher the BMR for a given size and sex.
- *Thyroid hormones:* Thyroid hormones (triiodothyronine [T_3] and thyroxine [T_4]) stimulate basal metabolism. Without a normal amount of these hormones in the blood, the body cannot maintain a normal BMR.
- *Body temperature:* An increase in body temperature increases the BMR. A decrease in body temperature (hypothermia) has the opposite effect.
- *Drugs:* Stimulants increase the BMR, and depressants reduce the BMR.
- *Other factors:* Other factors, such as emotions, pregnancy, and lactation (milk production), also influence basal metabolism.

Breathing

Breathing provides us with air—a very essential nutrient. Breathing patterns are a direct link to altering autonomic nervous system patterns, which in turn affect mood, feelings, and behavior. Almost every meditation or relaxation system uses breathing patterns. Other ways to modulate breathing are through singing and chanting.

Proper breathing is important, yet most of us do not breathe efficiently. For many the air quality is poor. The rest of us may be in too big a hurry to breathe deeply. Slow, deep breathing takes time. The simple bellows breathing mechanism is a bodywide coordination of muscle contraction and relaxation. A good way to recognize the full-body effect of breathing is to do the following activity:

1. Tighten your feet by gripping the floor with your toes. Take a deep breath and feel what happens.
2. Relax your feet and again notice what happens.
3. Tighten the gluteal muscles and take a deep breath. Then relax the muscles and take another deep breath, again noting what happens.

This exercise should demonstrate that breathing involves more muscles than just the diaphragm and the intercostals.

The shoulders should not move during normal relaxed breathing. The accessory muscles of respiration in the neck area should be activated only when a demand exists for increased oxygen and increased physical activity. If the accessory muscles activate without an increase in physical activity,

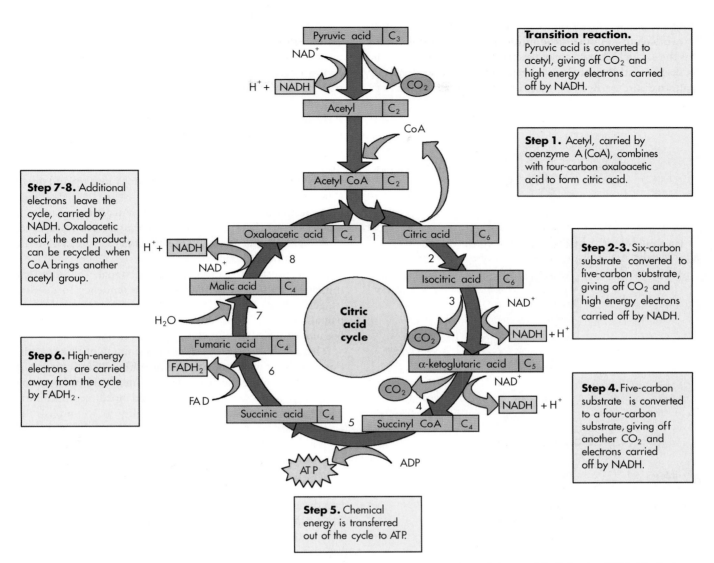

FIGURE 13-4 The Krebs cycle. (From Thibodeau GA, Patton KT: *Anatomy and physiology,* ed 6, St Louis, 2007, Mosby.)

the body resorts to the sympathetic dominance breathing pattern. If the person does not balance the oxygen and carbon dioxide levels through increased activity levels, breathing dysfunction (hyperventilation) occurs in the extreme. Breathing pattern disorders can perpetuate anxiety states and many disturbing physical symptoms (see Box 4-4).

The accessory muscles of respiration (e.g., the scalenes, sternocleidomastoid, serratus posterior superior, levator scapulae, rhomboids, abdominals, and quadratus lumborum) may be constantly activated for breathing when forced inhalation and expiration are not needed (Figure 13-5). This will result in dysfunctional muscle patterns. Often shortening in the quadratus lumborum or shoulder pain is not identified as an inefficient breathing pattern during assessment by the massage professional.

Phases of Breathing. Breathing comprises three phases of *inspiration* (bringing air into the body) and two phases of *expiration* (moving air out of the body). **Quiet inspiration** takes place when an individual is resting or sitting quietly. The diaphragm and external intercostals are the prime movers. As **deep inspiration** occurs, the actions of quiet inspiration are intensified. When people need more oxygen, they breathe harder. Any muscles that can pull the ribs up are called into action. **Forced inspiration** occurs when an individual is working very hard and needs a great deal of oxygen. Not only are the muscles of quiet and deep inspiration working, but also the muscles that stabilize and/or elevate the shoulder girdle to elevate the ribs directly or indirectly.

Quiet expiration is mostly a passive action. It occurs through relaxation of the external intercostals and the elastic recoil of the thoracic wall and tissue of the lungs and bronchi, with gravity pulling the rib cage down from its elevated position. Essentially no muscle action is involved. **Forced expiration** brings in muscles that can pull down the ribs and muscles to compress the abdomen, forcing the diaphragm upward.

Normal breathing consists of a shorter inhale in relation to a longer exhale. The ratio of inhale time to exhale time is one count inhale to two to four counts exhale. The ideal pattern is two to four counts for the inhale and at least eight counts for the exhale. The reverse of this pattern, in which the exhale is shorter and the inhale is longer, is the basis for breathing pattern disorders. Bodywork and breathing retraining methods seek to restore normal breathing.

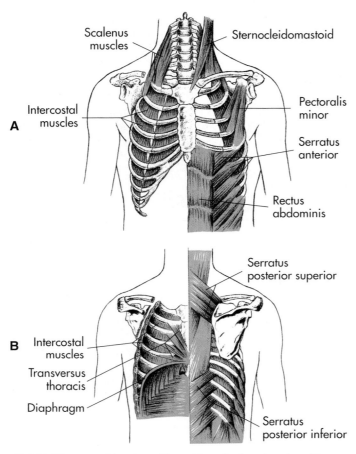

FIGURE 13-5 Muscles of breathing. **A**, Anterior view. **B**, Posterior view. (From Seidel HM et al: *Mosby's guide to physical examination,* ed 5, St Louis, 2003, Mosby.)

Some people may wonder why tightening the feet interferes with breathing. It seems to be a chain reaction between prime mover and antagonist muscle patterns. For the abdominals to contract to compress the abdominal cavity, their antagonist patterns have to relax all the way up and down the body.[3,4]

Massage to Support Breathing Function. Consider breathing mechanisms during the assessment. One way to determine whether a client uses the accessory muscles for relaxed breathing is to place your hands on the person's shoulders while he or she breathes; the shoulders should not move up and down (Figure 13-6).

Another method to detect the use of accessory muscles is to observe the client; if the accessory muscles are being used, movement is concentrated in the upper chest instead of in the lower ribs and abdomen.

If the breathing pattern is dysfunctional, the accessory muscles show increased tension and a tendency to develop trigger points. These conditions can be identified through palpation. Also, connective tissue changes are common, because breathing dysfunction often is chronic.

Therapeutic massage can normalize many of these conditions and support more effective breathing. Breathing well is very difficult if the mechanical components are not working efficiently. Many who have attempted breathing retraining have become frustrated by their inability to accomplish the pattern. They may be more successful after the body and the mechanism of breathing have become more normal. The breathing retraining program presented in Box 13-4 can be taught to clients. The box can be photocopied and used as a handout. Three common activities can help normalize a breathing pattern: yelling, crying, and laughing, because all three support an extended exhale. Each of these activities is sustained for 3 to 5 minutes, and they can be valuable in any breathing retraining program (Proficiency Exercise 13-3).

Physical Fitness

Our bodies are designed for purposeful movement toward a goal, such as gathering food for the day or running for safety.

FIGURE 13-6 Methods for performing a breathing assessment. Place hands on upper trapezius area (supine, **A;** seated, **B**) and monitor for movement. No movement should occur during relaxed breathing.

Our bodies still function as though this were the reality, but we do not need to work as hard to gather our food in the grocery store, and seldom do we really have to run or fight for our lives.

Exercise and stretching programs are important parts of any wellness program because they provide the activity our body was designed to have. Now we run in place and ride stationary bikes. Exercise has become an essential purpose unto itself. Fitness programs need to be appropriate; it is important to modify exercise systems and stretching programs to fit the individual. Many resources are available for studying exercise and stretching programs.

Frequent 5-minute stretches and breathing breaks should be built into everyone's day, especially those who spend prolonged periods in static positions. Such breaks may increase productivity, and people may feel less fatigue at the end of a busy day.

Any exercise and stretching program must begin slowly. Activity levels can be increased gradually each week. It takes

about 7 to 8 weeks for those new to movement to reach a level of comfort. More activities may be added slowly once the body has adapted (Proficiency Exercise 13-4).

Therapeutic Exercise

Fitness is a general term used to describe the ability to perform physical work. Performing physical work requires cardiorespiratory functioning, muscular strength and endurance, and musculoskeletal flexibility. To become physically fit, individuals must participate regularly in some form of physical activity that challenges all large muscle groups and the cardiorespiratory system and promotes postural balance.

Deconditioning

Deconditioning occurs with prolonged bed rest, and its effects are frequently seen in someone who has had an extended illness. Deconditioning is marked by a decrease in maximal oxygen consumption, cardiac output, and muscular strength,

---

BOX 13-4

Breathing Exercises

The following breathing exercises should be taught to clients who lift their shoulders during quiet and deep inspiration. (The exercises are presented in an instructional form that addresses the client. See p. 612 for photos.)

Exercise 1 (Figure A)
1. Sit in a relaxed position.
2. Place your hands in your lap and interlace the fingers.
3. Firmly press your fingers and thumbs into the tops of your hands.
4. Hold this position as long as possible without discomfort as you breathe normally.

Exercise 2 (Figure B)
1. Place your hands behind your head.
2. Point your elbows up and back.
3. Hold this position as long as it is comfortable while breathing normally.

Exercise 3 (Figure C)
1. Sit in a relaxed, upright position in a chair with arms.
2. Place your arms on the arms of the chair.
3. Firmly press the part of your forearms that is closest to the elbow into the arms of the chair.
4. Hold this position as long as it is comfortable and breathe normally.

Exercise 4 (Figure D)
1. Interlace your fingers behind your back.
2. Pull your shoulder blades together.
3. Hold this position as long as possible while breathing normally.

These exercises inhibit the accessory breathing muscles. Essentially, in these positions the client cannot use the accessory muscles to breathe, and the intercostal muscles and diaphragm are supported in breathing function. Clients should do these exercises as often as possible throughout the day. They should try to accumulate 30 minutes of exercise per 24-hour period.

Stretch to Open the Chest Wall (Figure E)
1. Stand facing a corner. Your arms are in line with your shoulders and spread out on the two walls that form the corner.
2. Firmly press your arms into the walls for a count of five.
3. Relax your arms and allow your body to fall gently into the corner to stretch the soft tissue of the chest. Hold this position for 10 to 30 seconds.
4. Move your fingers up the wall until you feel resistance. Then repeat the entire sequence, beginning with step 1.

Exercises for Controlled Breathing
1. Lift your chin into the air and relax your shoulders.
2. Slowly exhale through your mouth, similar to blowing out a candle, and at the same time pull in your abdomen. Then exhale until you have expelled as much air as possible without straining.
3. At the bottom of the breath (i.e., when no further air can be exhaled without strain), stop breathing. This is different from holding your breath, which requires effort. Remain in this resting phase for 3 to 5 seconds.
4. Before inhaling, relax all muscles, drop your chin to your chest, and keep your shoulders relaxed.
5. Inhale slowly through your nose until your lungs are comfortably full, allowing your abdomen to expand.
6. Stop breathing for 3 to 5 seconds. Then repeat the entire sequence, beginning with step 1.

The exhalation should take two to four times as long as the inhalation.

Many additional resources are available for retraining breathing patterns. Find one that is comfortable and use it regularly. An recommended resource is Leon Chaitow's Breathing Pattern Disorder (Chaitow L, Bradley D, Gilbert C. (2002). *Multidisciplinary approaches to breathing pattern disorders*. Edinburgh, Churchill Livingstone).

Continued

BOX 13-4

Breathing Exercises—cont'd

PROFICIENCY EXERCISE 13-3

1. *This exercise helps you understand how normalizing breathing affects the entire body. Begin by doing a simple physical assessment: move yourself into forward trunk flexion, side-bending lateral trunk flexion, trunk extension, neck flexion, extension, and lateral flexion. Identify the areas of your body that seem most restricted. Now yell or howl as loud as you can for 1 minute. Next, pretend to cry and sob for 1 minute. Finally, belly laugh as hard and as long as you can.*

Now perform the simple physical assessment again. In the space provided, describe the results.

2. *Develop a "how to breathe" handout to give to clients. Include at least three different breathing patterns.*

 PROFICIENCY EXERCISE 13-4

Locate an exercise and stretching program taught by a qualified instructor at your local community center or health club (Eastern examples include tai chi, martial arts, and yoga; Western examples include spinning, dance, aerobics, and swimming); or, as an alternative, purchase an exercise and stretching video. Participate in the program for 6 weeks, monitoring all movements for correctness and comfort.

which occurs very rapidly. These effects are also seen, although possibly to a lesser degree, in an individual who has spent some time on bed rest without any accompanying disease process and in an individual who is sedentary because of lifestyle or increasing age.

Endurance is a measure of fitness. It is the ability to work for prolonged periods and the ability to resist fatigue. It includes muscular endurance and cardiovascular endurance. Muscular endurance refers to the ability of an isolated muscle group to perform repeated contractions over a period of time; cardiovascular endurance refers to the ability to perform large muscle dynamic exercise, such as walking, swimming, or biking, for long periods.

Aerobic Exercise Training

Aerobic exercise training is an exercise program that focuses on increasing fitness and endurance. A training response requires exercise of sufficient intensity, duration, and frequency to produce both cardiovascular and muscular adaptation in a person's endurance. This is different from training for a particular sport or event, by which the individual improves in the exercise task used for training and may not improve in other tasks or in whole body conditioning.

Adaptation

Adaptation results in increased efficiency of body function and represents a variety of neurologic, physical, and biochemical changes in the cardiovascular, neuromuscular, and myofascial systems. Performance increases as a result of these changes, and these systems adapt to the training stimulus over time. Significant changes in fitness can be measured in 10 to 12 weeks.

A person with a low level of fitness will have more potential to improve than one who has a high level of fitness. This is reflected in the training stimulus threshold, or the stimulus that elicits a training response. The higher the initial level of fitness, the greater the intensity of exercise needed to elicit a significant change.

Energy Expenditure

Energy is expended by individuals engaging in physical activity. Activities can be categorized as light or heavy by determining the energy cost. Most daily activities are light activity and are aerobic (oxygen based) because they require little power but occur over prolonged periods. Heavy work usually requires energy supplied by both the aerobic and anaerobic systems (non–oxygen based).

Physiologic Response to Aerobic Exercise

The rapid increase in energy requirements during exercise requires equally rapid circulatory adjustments. The adjustments are essential to meet the increased need for oxygen and nutrients; to remove the end products of metabolism, such as carbon dioxide and lactic acid; and to dissipate excess heat. The shift in body metabolism occurs through a coordinated activity of all the systems of the body: neuromuscular, respiratory, cardiovascular, metabolic, and hormonal.

Effective endurance training must produce a conditioning or cardiovascular response. Conditioning depends on three critical elements of exercise: intensity, duration, and frequency.

Intensity. Intensity of exercise is based on the overload principle. The overload principle is a stress on an organism that is greater than the one regularly encountered during everyday life. To improve cardiovascular and muscular endurance, an overload must be applied to these systems. The exercise intensity load must be just above the training stimulus threshold for adaptation to occur. Once adaptation to a given load has occurred, the training intensity (exercise load) must be increased for the individual to achieve further improvement. Increasing intensity too quickly can result in injury. Training stimulus thresholds vary, depending on the individual's health, level of activity, age, and gender.

Duration. The optimal duration of exercise for cardiovascular conditioning depends on the total work done, the intensity and frequency of the exercise, and the person's fitness level. Generally speaking, the greater the intensity of the exercise, the shorter the duration needed for adaptation. The lower the intensity of the exercise, the longer the duration needed. A 20- to 30-minute session at 70% of the maximum heart rate generally is optimal. When the intensity is below the heart rate threshold, a 45-minute continuous exercise period may provide the appropriate overload. With high-intensity exercise, 10- to 15-minute exercise periods are adequate. Three 5-minute daily periods may be effective in someone who is deconditioned. Exercising for longer than 45 to 60 minutes increases the risk of musculoskeletal injury and soreness, and the risk does not justify the benefit.

Frequency. The optimum frequency for fitness training generally is three to four times a week. Frequency varies, depending on the person's health and age. If training is done at low intensity, greater frequency may be beneficial. A frequency of two times a week does not generally evoke cardiovascular changes, although individuals who are deconditioned initially may benefit from a program of that frequency. As frequency increases beyond the optimal range, the risk of musculoskeletal injury and soreness increases. For individuals who are in good general health, exercising 30 to 45 minutes at least three times a week appears to protect against coronary heart disease.

Maintaining Fitness

The frequency or duration of physical activity required to maintain a certain level of aerobic fitness is less than that required to improve it. The beneficial effects of exercise training are reversible. The process of deconditioning occurs rapidly when a person stops exercising. After only 2 weeks of reduced activity, significant reductions in work capacity can be measured, and improvements can be lost within several months.

The Exercise Program

An appropriate exercise program can result in higher levels of fitness for a healthy individual, slow the decrease in functional capacity of the elderly, and recondition those who have been ill or who have chronic disease or a sedentary lifestyle. The three components of an exercise program are (1) the warm-up, (2) aerobic exercise, and (3) the cool-down.

The Warm-Up. The purpose of the warm-up period is to enhance the numerous physiologic adjustments that must take place before physical activity. Physiologically, a time lag exists between the onset of activity and the adjustments the body must make to meet the physical requirements.

A warm-up raises the muscle temperature. The higher temperature increases the efficiency of muscular contraction by reducing connective tissue viscosity and increasing the rate of nerve conduction. More oxygen is extracted from hemoglobin at higher muscle temperatures, which supports the aerobic process. Dilation of constricted capillaries, resulting in increased circulation, increases oxygen delivery to the active muscles and minimizes oxygen deficit and the formation of lactic acid. Venous return also increases. Adaptation in the

sensitivity of the neural respiratory center increases the respiratory rate.

Warm-up activities include rhythmic movement of the large muscles of the body. An increasingly brisk walk is an excellent warm-up activity.

Aerobic Exercise. The aerobic exercise period is the conditioning part of the exercise program. Attention to the intensity, frequency, and duration determines the effectiveness of the program. In choosing a specific method of training, the exerciser's main consideration is intensity; it should:
- Be sufficient to stimulate increased cardiac output
- Enhance local circulation
- Increase aerobic metabolism within the appropriate muscle groups
- Not cause injury
- Be weight bearing, to support bone health
- Exceed the threshold level, to allow adaptation
- Not evoke fatigue symptoms

In aerobic exercise, submaximal, rhythmic, repetitive, dynamic exercise of large muscle groups is emphasized. The four types of training that condition the aerobic system are continuous, interval, circuit, and circuit-interval methods.

Continuous Training. This type of training involves a submaximal energy requirement sustained throughout the exercise period. Once the steady state is achieved, the muscle obtains energy by means of aerobic metabolism. Stress is placed primarily on the slow-twitch muscle fibers. The activity can be prolonged for 20 to 60 minutes without exhausting the oxygen transport system. The work rate is increased progressively as training improvements are achieved; overload can be accomplished by increasing the exercise duration. In a healthy individual, continuous training is the most effective way to improve endurance. Brisk walking and swimming laps are excellent examples of continuous training.

Interval Training. In this type of exercise program, the exercise period is interspersed with relief or rest intervals. Interval training is generally less demanding than continuous training. In a healthy individual, interval training tends to improve strength and power more than endurance. The relief interval is either a rest relief (passive recovery) or a work relief (active recovery), and it ranges in duration from a few seconds to several minutes. Work recovery involves continuing the exercise but at a reduced level from the work period. During the relief period, a portion of the muscular stores of adenosine triphosphate (ATP), the source of energy for muscle, as well as the oxygen associated with myoglobin, both of which were depleted during the work period, are replenished by the aerobic system.

The longer and more intense the work interval, the more the aerobic system is stressed. With a short work interval, the duration of the rest interval is critical if the aerobic system is to be stressed. A rest interval equal to one-and-a-half times the work interval allows the succeeding exercise interval to begin before recovery is complete and stresses the aerobic system. An example would be a 5-minute work interval followed by a 7-minute rest interval.

A significant amount of high-intensity exercise can be achieved with interval or intermittent work if the work-relief intervals are spaced appropriately. An example would be lap swimming with rest periods or race walking or sprinting short distances with slower periods of walking interspersed.

Circuit Training. Circuit training uses a series of exercise activities. At the end of the last activity, the individual starts from the beginning and again moves through the circuit. The series of activities is repeated several times. Several exercise modes can be used involving large and small muscle groups and a mix of static or dynamic effort. Use of circuit training can improve strength and endurance by stressing both the aerobic and anaerobic systems. Often a combination of aerobic activities and weight training is included in the exercise program. Core training that strengthens the postural muscles of the torso can be included in circuit training. Activities using various sizes of exercise balls promote postural balance and core strength.

Circuit-Interval Training. A combination of circuit and interval training is effective because of the interaction of aerobic and anaerobic production of ATP. In addition to the aerobic and anaerobic systems being stressed by the various activities, the relief interval allows a delay in the need for anaerobic processes and the production of lactic acid, because the rest period allows the blood oxygen levels to replenish.

The Cool-Down. A cool-down period is necessary after the aerobic exercise period. The cool-down period prevents pooling of the blood in the extremities because the exerciser continues to use the muscles to maintain venous return. The cool-down enhances the recovery period through oxidation of metabolic waste and replacement of the energy stores and prevents myocardial ischemia, arrhythmias, or other cardiovascular conditions.

The characteristics of the cool-down period are similar to those of the warm-up period. Total body exercises, such as calisthenics or brisk walking, that decrease in intensity are appropriate. The cool-down period should last 5 to 10 minutes and should be followed by a flexibility regimen.

Physiologic Changes That Occur with Exercise

Changes in the cardiovascular and respiratory systems, as well as changes in muscle metabolism, occur with endurance training. These changes happen at rest and with exercise. It is important to note that all of the following training effects cannot result from one training program. A regular regimen of exercise with a variety of activities is necessary to achieve and maintain fitness.

Cardiovascular Changes. Changes at rest involve a reduction in the resting pulse rate with a decrease in sympathetic dominance and lower levels of norepinephrine and epinephrine. Parasympathetic restoration mechanisms increase, and a decrease in blood pressure can occur. Blood volume and hemoglobin often increase, which facilitates the oxygen delivery capacity of the system.

Changes during exercise include an increase in the pulse rate and a decrease in norepinephrine and epinephrine. Cardiac function increases, as does extraction of oxygen by the working muscle.

Respiratory Changes. Changes at rest include larger lung volumes as a result of improved pulmonary function. Changes during exercise occur as a result of a larger diffusion capacity in the lungs because of the larger lung volumes and a greater alveolar-capillary surface area. Breathing is deeper and more efficient.

Metabolic Changes. Muscle hypertrophy and increased capillary density are observed at rest and during exercise after endurance training. Also, the number and size of mitochondria increase significantly, which increases the capacity to generate ATP aerobically. The rate of depletion of muscle glycogen decreases, and blood lactate levels during submaximal work are lower because of an increased capacity to mobilize and oxidize fat, as well as an increase in fat-mobilizing and metabolizing enzymes.

Other System Changes. Changes in other systems that occur with exercise training include a decrease in body fat, blood cholesterol, and triglyceride levels and an increase in heat acclimatization and the breaking strength of bones, ligaments, and tendons.

Flexibility

Flexibility is the ability to move a single joint or series of joints through a normal, unrestricted, pain-free range of motion. Flexibility depends on the extensibility of muscle tissue, which allows muscles that cross a joint to relax, lengthen, and yield to a stretch force. The arthrokinematics of the moving joint, as well as the ability of connective tissues associated with the joint to deform, also affect joint range of motion and an individual's overall flexibility.

Dynamic flexibility refers to the active range of motion of a joint. This aspect of flexibility depends on the degree to which a joint can be moved by a muscle contraction and the amount of tissue resistance met during the active movement. *Passive flexibility,* the degree to which a joint can be passively moved through the available range of motion, depends on the extensibility of muscles and connective tissues that cross and surround a joint. Passive flexibility is a prerequisite for but does not ensure dynamic flexibility.

Muscle tissue and fascial shortening cause a change in the length-tension relationship of the muscle. As the muscle shortens, it is no longer able to produce peak tension. The result is a muscle that is weak but short and tight. Loss of flexibility, for whatever reason, can also cause pain arising from muscle, connective tissue, or the periosteum. This also reduces muscle strength.

Stretching

Stretching is a general term used to describe any therapeutic technique designed to lengthen (elongate) shortened soft tissue, particularly connective tissue structures, to increase range of motion. The end result is increased flexibility.

Passive stretching involves an external force, applied either manually or mechanically, that lengthens the shortened tissues while the person is relaxed. Active inhibition uses various muscle energy methods in which the person participates in the stretching maneuver to inhibit tonus in a tight muscle.

The soft tissues that can restrict joint motion are muscles, connective tissue, and skin. When stretching methods are applied to these soft tissues, the velocity, intensity, and duration of the stretch force, as well as the temperature of the soft tissues, all affect the response of the different types of soft tissues.

Muscle is composed primarily of contractile tissue but is attached to and interwoven with noncontractile tissue, such as tendon and fascia. The connective tissue framework in muscle, not the active contractile components, is the primary source of resistance to passive elongation of muscle.

Contractile Elements of Muscle. Individual muscles are composed of many muscle fibers. A single muscle fiber is made up of many myofibrils. A myofibril is composed of sarcomeres, which lie in series. The sarcomere is the contractile unit of the myofibril and is composed of overlapping cross-bridges of actin and myosin. The sarcomere gives a muscle its ability to contract and relax. When a muscle contracts, the actin-myosin filaments slide together and the muscle shortens. When a muscle relaxes, the cross-bridges slide apart slightly, and the muscle returns to its resting length. If the muscle is inappropriately short, it will not return to its resting length and therefore loses the ability to contract effectively.

One of the main elements of a flexibility program is a controlled, sustained load on the muscles and connective tissue components that does not strain the joint structure. Many types of flexibility programs are available. Yoga is an excellent example. When a muscle is passively stretched, initial lengthening occurs in the neuromuscular component and tension rises sharply. After a point, mechanical disruption of the cross-bridges of actin and myosin occurs as the filaments slide apart and the sarcomeres abruptly lengthen (sarcomere give). Various applications of muscle energy methods support this process. When the stretch force is released, the individual sarcomeres return to their resting length.

The tendency of muscle to return to its resting length after short-term stretch is called *elasticity* (although this process is more appropriately called *lengthening* with stretching specifically targeting the connective tissue structures). The increase in connective tissue pliability and length is called *plasticity*. Massage is an excellent way to support flexibility programs, especially if the methods used address both the elasticity and pliability of the soft tissue.

Appropriate exercise is necessary for wellness. Because the components of an exercise program can be accomplished in many ways, a person can engage in many activities that support health. One day you might walk for about an hour, and the next day you might strengthen the core muscles with activities on exercise balls or a movement program, such as tai chi. Yoga supports flexibility. Climbing stairs is a great exercise. When the body gets the movement it needs, relaxation activities are more effective (Figure 13-7).

Relaxation

Relaxation methods initiate a parasympathetic response. Because muscle tension patterns are habitual, most successful relaxation methods combine the movements of moving, stretching, tensing, and then releasing the muscles (progressive relaxation). The heart and breathing rates are synchronized (entrainment) while the individual focuses on a quiet or neutral topic, event, or picture *(visualization)*. Slow, rhythmic music can be a beneficial component of a relaxation program. Most meditation and deliberate relaxation processes are built around this pattern. The focus of relaxation is to quiet the physical body, not to create a spiritual experience; however, many prayer systems use similar patterns, which are beneficial for relaxation as well.

Almost any type of pleasurable, simple, repetitive activity that requires focused attention induces the relaxation response. Gardening, needlepoint, knitting, playing music, and watching fish in an aquarium or birds at a bird feeder are all forms of relaxation if there is no need to achieve, compete, or produce results in a specific period. Knitting a sweater for pleasure and having to finish one in a week are two different activities. Relaxation takes time, and when something is urgent, it usually interferes with the ability to relax.

Mindfulness is a concept of relaxation. Being mindful is similar to the centering or focusing methods presented in Chapter 8. Mindfulness is being attentive to the moment, secure that we have learned from and then have let go of the past, and that we are planning for the future without worry. A human "doing" is not mindful. Mindfulness is about a human "being."

Just as tension patterns are habitual, relaxation can become a habit. Typically, it takes 8 to 10 weeks of consistent reinforcement to build a habit pattern. Unlike exercise, which can be varied to prevent boredom, a relaxation sequence needs to be the same each time to reinforce the conditioned response to the habit structure. It is important to use the same location, music, time of day, smells (such as essential oils), colors, posi-

FIGURE 13-7 Client self-stretching.

tion, and breathing pattern in the sequence. Any of the components of the relaxation program can soon become triggers to relaxation.

A person should experiment with relaxation methods until the right program is found, then consistently use it every day for at least 15 minutes. (It takes this long for the physiology to make a shift from an aroused state to a relaxed one.) Many audiocassette programs provide progressive relaxation and self-hypnosis and pull together all the components of a relaxation program. This type of resource can be very useful (Proficiency Exercise 13-5). Self-massage can also support relaxation. Many more examples of self-help massage can be found on the Evolve Web site; these can be printed and given to clients (Figure 13-8).

FIGURE 13-8 Self-massage. **A,** Teaching self-massage to a client. **B,** Products for use in self-massage. **C,** Self-muscle energy technique method using resistance band (resembles a tire's inner tube).

PROFICIENCY EXERCISE 13-5

In the space provided, design a daily 15-minute relaxation program especially for you.

Sleep

Restorative sleep is necessary for wellness. Lack of quality sleep is becoming a major health concern. Many people do not get enough sleep. An absolute minimum of 6 hours of uninterrupted sleep is necessary, and most people require 8 to 9 hours.

Many things can interrupt sleep, such as pain that repeatedly awakens the person, external random noise (e.g., traffic noise), tending to infants and children, varied work schedules, a restless or snoring bed partner (including pets!), sinus or other respiratory difficulties (e.g., coughing), and urinary frequency. The list of possible interruptions is endless. Regardless of the perpetuating factors, sleep is compromised and the deep sleep stage is seldom achieved.

Others have disrupted sleep patterns because of insomnia, sleep apnea, hormone fluctuations, high cortisol (stress hormone) levels, medications, and stimulant intake, such as caffeine. Again, quality sleep is sacrificed.

Light/dark cycles regulate sleep patterns. For effective sleep we need adequate exposure to daylight, which stimulates serotonin. We also need adequate exposure to darkness. With the advent of artificial lighting, we have spent less and less time in the dark, which disturbs sleep. Absence of light supports the release of melatonin, a pineal gland hormone that is involved with the sleep pattern.

During sleep the body renews, repairs, and generally restores itself. Growth hormone is an important factor in this process, with more than half of its daily secretions taking place during sleep. If the deeper stages of sleep are not sustained, the body's restorative mechanisms are compromised. Sleep disturbances are a major factor in many chronic fatigue and pain syndromes.

Sleep, especially during dreaming, is when we seem to repair, sort, and restore emotionally. Dreaming is still a mystery, but research indicates that it is essential for emotional well-being. Methods to support effective sleep are presented in Box 13-5 (Proficiency Exercise 13-6).

Feelings

Feelings are the body's interpretation of emotions. They occur as a response to the effect of hormones, neurotransmitters, and other endogenous chemicals. People use chemical substances such as food, nicotine, alcohol, and drugs to create feelings.

Behaviors such as the need to create crises, eating disorders, accident proneness, hypervigilance, panic, illness, and codependent relationships generate feelings. Behaviors such as gentle care giving, giving presents, and appreciating beauty generate feelings of compassion, nurturing, and belonging.

Often if a person's physiology can be changed, his or her feelings can also be changed. The easiest way to change the physiology is to move, as in exercising or breathing.

A massage also changes the physiology. This is perhaps why massage "feels" so good. Being touched in a resourceful way supports wellness. Sensory stimulation is essential for the body to thrive. Many people are deprived of touch, and many adults exchange touch only in the context of a sexual relationship. Touch is essential for wellness. Touching generates and expresses feelings. The power of touch was explored in the very beginning of this text.

When feelings are unresourceful, an opposing response must be activated to restore a balance. For example, if you are weighed down with too much thinking, moving around and pulling some weeds in the garden creates a balance. If you feel angry, find a way to laugh. If you feel down, help someone. If you feel anxious and alone, get a hug or a massage (Proficiency Exercise 13-7).

Mind

The mind is the part of us that reasons, understands, remembers, thinks, and adapts. It coordinates the conscious and subconscious parts of us that influence and direct mental and physical behavior. The mind processes what we believe. We can change our mind (beliefs) fairly quickly, although habitual belief patterns are difficult to overcome. Belief changes need to be supported over time to be reflected in lifestyle and wellness programs. The body responds to mind changes, but more time may be required for the effects of that response to manifest in the organic form of the body's anatomy and physiology. Patience is required to objectively identify body changes in response to mind changes. This interaction between mind and body is the basis for current approaches to mind/body medicine. The mind involves emotions, behavior, self-concept, and coping.

Emotions

Emotions are feelings driven by thoughts. They lead to actions that represent the consequences of how we think and what we do. What we think and feel and how we live are all inextricably linked.

The immune system is controlled directly by the mind. The science of psychoneuroimmunology has clearly established that unresolved emotions and thought patterns of hate, fear, anger, and jealousy reduce the efficiency of the body's defenses.[1]

In 1975, Dr. Robert Adder conditioned rats to dislike sweetened water by injecting them with a chemical to make them feel ill whenever they drank it. After the injections stopped for some time, some rats began dying. On investigation, Adder found that the chemical he had used was a suppressor of immune function. The rats not only had become

BOX 13-5

Supporting Restorative Sleep

Therapeutic massage supports restorative sleep in the following ways:

- It reduces the activity of the sympathetic autonomic nervous system and also cortisol levels.
- It promotes parasympathetic autonomic nervous system dominance.
- It relieves or reduces pain and discomfort that may interrupt sleep.

Self-help measures for supporting restorative sleep include the following:

- Maintain a regular sleep/wake cycle. Get up and go to bed at the same time every day, including days off.
- Get at least 30 minutes of daylight exposure by being outside or placing yourself in front of an open window.
- Exercise moderately on a regular basis but do not exercise aerobically 4 hours before sleeping.
- Reduce stimulant intake substantially and ingest no stimulants 10 hours before sleeping. If you go to bed at 11 PM, do not drink colas or coffee after 1 PM.
- Concentrate protein food intake 6 hours before going to sleep. Eat carbohydrates after this time. Do not eat a heavy meal before going to bed. Do not go to bed hungry. Eat a small snack of complex carbohydrates without sugar with some dairy product (e.g., yogurt) 30 minutes before bed if hungry. Although a protein, turkey is high in tryptophan, which encourages sleep. A small turkey sandwich is a possible bedtime snack.
- Stretch gently 1 hour before retiring. A slow, rhythmic pattern is best.
- Get into the dark or soft lighting (only enough light for safe movement) 1 hour before bedtime. Stretching in the dim light is an excellent way to begin the winding down process to prepare for sleep.
- Develop a bedtime ritual that you follow consistently. The ritual should begin 30 minutes before going to bed. Make sure to stay in dim lighting. This ritual should be 15 minutes long. It can include hygiene (e.g., washing up and brushing your teeth) but should not consist of full body application of water, because both hot and cold application can stimulate the body. (A warm bath 1 hour before sleep is relaxing.) Meditating or reading something that is gentle and can be finished in 5 or 10 minutes may be helpful. Listening to soft and gentle music is soothing. Various aromas are considered relaxing and are available in such forms as scented candles, incense, and essential oil diffusers. Drinking a cup of relaxing herbal tea is soothing. Meditate, pray, and review your day in a thankful way. After you develop this ritual, it needs to be reinforced. Do it the same way every night. Eventually the ritual will signal the body into a sleep pattern.
- When drowsiness occurs, immediately relax into sleep. The drowsy pattern lasts only about 15 minutes and then a new body rhythm cycle begins, which lasts about 90 minutes.
- If you miss the sleep window, continue with calm activities until the sense of drowsiness again occurs. Then go to bed.
- Sleep in the dark. Especially, do not sleep with the television on.
- Get up at the same time in the morning regardless of when you went to bed.
- Avoid long naps. A short 15- to 30-minute nap usually is all right for midday fatigue.

 PROFICIENCY EXERCISE 13-6

In the space provided, analyze your personal sleep pattern using the information in this section. Identify three activities that support restorative sleep and three activities that can be improved.

My current sleep pattern is as follows:

Three current activities that support sleep are the following:

1.

2.

3.

Three activities that could improve sleep are the following:

1.

2.

3.

PROFICIENCY EXERCISE 13-7

Honestly identify two personal behaviors that have a repetitive pattern, one resourceful and one unresourceful. What feelings are generated by these behaviors? For the unresourceful behavior, identify one alternative resourceful behavior to generate similar feelings.

Example

Resourceful behavior: **Watching uplifting human interest movies**
Feelings: Empowerment, security, connectedness
Unresourceful behavior: **Overeating at night**
Feelings: Being connected, fulfilled, cared for
Replacement behavior: **Playing with my dog**

Your Turn

1. Resourceful behavior: _____

   Feelings: _____

   Unresourceful behavior: _____

   Feelings: _____

   Replacement behavior: _____

2. Resourceful behavior: _____

   Feelings: _____

   Unresourceful behavior: _____

   Feelings: _____

   Replacement behavior: _____

conditioned to feeling ill whenever they drank sweet water, they also were mimicking the chemical's other effects and depressing their immune systems. This ability to depress the immune function was proof of nervous system control over the immune system. Many subsequent tests have confirmed this finding in human beings.[1]

As human beings, we *learn* to be helpless, to be addictive, and to have low self-esteem. We learn to hate. The important point to remember is that if we learned the maladaptive behavior in the first place, we can also learn a more resourceful behavior to use instead.

Emotions can be very powerful. If used resourcefully, they can provide us with the empowerment to reach our goals. Many good things have come from an emotion turned into resourceful behavior.

Wellness encompasses a full range of emotion. Some of us pride ourselves on not feeling certain emotions, but if we can experience an emotion in a resourceful way, it is not healthy to deny its expression. For example, if something as powerful as anger is turned inward, it does not lead to positive outcomes. However, if expressed resourcefully, to the person or situations involved, then a sense of resolution takes place and we can get on with our lives, free of the anger.

Wellness comes from using the emotion instead of the emotion using us. Used resourcefully, emotions can provide the motivation to achieve wellness; used unresourcefully, they can make us ill and can be destructive to those who share our lives.

Sometimes we need someone, such as a daughter, who loves us in spite of ourselves to put our emotions and resulting behavior into perspective (Proficiency Exercise 13-8).

Behavior

Behavior is what we do in response to feelings, to trigger thoughts and feelings, and occasionally to avoid feelings. Resourceful behavior results in feeling good about what has happened. Unresourceful behavior still results in a good

 PROFICIENCY EXERCISE 13-8

List any emotions that gave you the motivation to complete this educational program in therapeutic massage.

feeling (or we would not do it), but often we feel bad about what happened, and/or others feel bad.

Addictive behavior can take many forms. A person who is addicted to food, drugs, alcohol, exercise, pain, crisis, or loss will develop a lifestyle that both protects and supports the substance or behavior of choice. Addictions require a great deal of time and energy. Addictive behavior throws the balance of wellness off course. It takes hard work and lots of support to change an addictive behavior. Sometimes a less damaging addiction is replaced by a more damaging one, and vice versa.[1] A person may alter a food habit by creating an exercise dependency. Whichever is the more damaging addiction needs to be evaluated. Behavior changes that are at least steps in the resourceful direction should not be discouraged. To truly alter behavior, a person must evaluate his or her sense of self (Proficiency Exercise 13-9).

Self-Concept

What we think about ourselves and how we talk to ourselves are very important contributors to wellness. Some people do not have a positive self-concept.

Most of us want a purpose and a sense of achievement, success, and self-confidence. This is achievable when we stop

PROFICIENCY EXERCISE 13-9

List three addictive behaviors. For each, list three alternative behaviors that are less damaging yet may generate similar feelings.

Addictive behavior: _____

Alternative behavior: _____

1.

2.

3.

Addictive behavior: _____

Alternative behavior: _____

1.

2.

3.

Addictive behavior: _____

Alternative behavior: _____

1.

2.

3.

 PROFICIENCY EXERCISE 13-10

Clean up two "messes," one you made in someone else's life, and one someone made in your life. Notice how your self-concept blossoms.

important and needed service and its benefits often cannot be measured objectively. As with any type of preventive activity, it is difficult to know what did not happen because someone took preventive measures.

When we have developed a healthy relationship with ourselves, we can also develop and sustain healthy relationships with others. Supportive relationships are important to wellness. If a relationship continues to generate messes in your life, maybe it is not a resourceful relationship. This does not mean that effort and concern are not required for family and friends or even concern for a population more globally. What is important is that we are empowered in a relationship and free to give and receive with a balance of energy exchanged. Sometimes one gives more and other times one receives more, but the total outcome is mutual support for one another's highest good that supports wellness (Proficiency Exercise 13-10).

Coping

Wellness is the ability to live each day and be able to say we did our jobs well, as we enter sleep with a thankful heart. How we lived that day is the coping part, and sometimes the simplest things can make a difference.

One day, when things were going particularly poorly in an office, a 5-year-old boy walked through the office. He stopped and said, "Good morning, everybody. Have you noticed that the sun is shining today?" It was a better day for all after that.

Resourceful coping consists of commitment, control, and challenge. **Commitment** is the ability and willingness to be involved in what is happening around us, to have a purpose for being. This purpose is more than what we do; it is how we serve. It is possible to serve in many ways. A career in massage can be a path of service or just a job. Purpose and service have nothing to do with the task. Picking up garbage is as much a service as is being a doctor. Cleaning house, cutting hair, building houses, and packing cartons can all be paths of service. The commitment to support wellness contributes to the greater good.

Control is characterized by the belief that we can influence events by the way we feel, think, and act. This is internal control, not external control. Internal control involves adjusting ourselves to the situation and looking for ways to respond resourcefully. Those who exert external control attempt to control circumstances and people. It is impossible to control the weather, most circumstances, and most people. Relying on external control is a poor coping mechanism.

The eternal wisdom in the saying, "Grant me the serenity to accept the things I cannot change, the courage to change the things I can, and the wisdom to know the difference," speaks to self-concept and internal versus external control.

comparing ourselves with one another. Instead, wellness involves reaching out to others for support and information.

Rather than basing their personal value on an external standard, healthy people develop internal standards of self-worth. We need to own both our successes and our mistakes and attempt to correct the mistakes. It is healthy to "clean up our own messes." Putting relationships and mistakes back in order can resolve issues and allow energy to be used in more beneficial ways.

It is also healthy to clean up a mess that someone else may have left. Often the person or situation that created the disorder does not, or will not, assume responsibility for it. If we wait for it to be cleaned up, we may have to live with the mess for a long time. Part of wellness is eliminating physical, mental, and spiritual disarray and clutter that we no longer need, regardless of who is responsible. As adults, it is also our responsibility to be proactive and disallow preventable messes. Sometimes we have to be very assertive with other people about what we will and will not allow in our space. Some messes, such as natural disasters, are not created by anyone. When people unite in communities to clean up these messes, wellness is supported.

Another threat to wellness is misjudging our worth. Everyone is good at something; no one is good at everything. Measure success and self-worth by how good you feel about your accomplishments, instead of by money or fame. Especially with massage, an inner sense of accomplishment is important. Massage is a quiet, unpretentious profession. It does not usually receive a lot of public glory. Massage is an

PROFICIENCY EXERCISE 13-11

In the space provided, take inventory of yourself to see what coping mechanisms you have. List three effective coping mechanisms and three that are not as effective. Choose one of these ineffective coping mechanisms and develop a plan to change it.

Effective coping mechanisms:

1.

2.

3.

Ineffective coping mechanisms:

1.

2.

3.

Plan for change of one ineffective coping mechanism:

 PROFICIENCY EXERCISE 13-12

On a separate sheet of paper, write a poem, story, or song or draw a picture about your source of faith. This piece of art is just for you, so do not be concerned that anyone else will see it.

 PROFICIENCY EXERCISE 13-13

Complete the following sentence 10 different ways.

I hope

I hope

I hope

I hope

I hope

I hope

I hope

I hope

I hope

I hope

Living each day as a challenge, filled with things to learn, skills to practice, tasks to be accomplished, and obstacles to overcome, supports wellness. Beginning each day with the affirmations of "I greet the day and all that it holds" may generate an attitude of challenge. Those who see change as a challenge cope much better than those who do not. Using available resourceful coping mechanisms to cope with change in life allows the individual to welcome changes as leading to personal development.

Poor stress-coping skills in the form of attempted external control and unproductive emotions such as unresolved anger suppress our immune systems and predispose us to infection and poor health. It is the individual's response to the stress that determines the effect on immunity, not the stress itself.[1] Wellness includes learning more efficient ways to cope with life, through counseling and behavior modification programs if needed.

To improve coping skills, pay attention to people who cope well and ask them to share how they cope. Attending seminars and reading books on effective coping, assertiveness, and development of internal control provide additional resources. Professional counseling can be helpful. Remember, we learned the coping mechanisms we currently have, and we can learn even better ways to cope (Proficiency Exercise 13-11).

Spirit

Our spirit is the part of us that transcends. Our spiritual selves "know our truth." Spiritual wellness consists of faith, hope, and love.

Faith

Faith is the ability to believe, trust, and know certain things that science cannot prove. Faith is the strength of wellness and involves the expression of that connecting strength each day through faith in ourselves, our partners, our families, and humanity as a whole. Faith is essential to wellness (Proficiency Exercise 13-12).

Hope

Hope is the belief, assurance, conviction, and confidence that our future will somehow be okay. It is the belief that the choices we make now will be the most resourceful choices as we create our future. Without hope, no sense of continuity exists. Temple Grandin, an admirable woman with autism, said, "I like to hope that even if there is no personal afterlife, some energy impression (of me) is left in the universe. I do not want my thoughts to die with me"[5] (Proficiency Exercise 13-13).

Love

Love has no concrete explanation. Love is a prerequisite for wholeness, and wholeness is necessary for wellness. This is not romantic love; it is bigger, stronger, more empowering, and mightier. It is quiet, gentle, forgiving, and nonjudgmental.

A teenage boy was struggling to put these most important issues into perspective. He came to his mother and said, "I have figured out the meaning of life." Wondering this herself, she asked her son what he had discovered. The son replied, "When I play my music and I feel great and those who listen to me feel great, then I have shared my love, and my power gets bigger and so does theirs. But if I play my music, and only I feel great and those who listen feel bad and weak, then I have taken their power, and this is evil. This is the meaning of life." This type of love celebrates the irrepressible process of life. This is the love of wellness (Proficiency Exercise 13-14).

PROFICIENCY EXERCISE 13-14

During a learning experience, one or two people may emerge who teach us more than we expected to learn. Often the learning has nothing to do with the courses we are studying. This is a love sharing. Go to those who have shared their love with you and say "Thank you."

■ ■ ■ **SUMMARY**

Wellness comprises more than the components discussed in this chapter. Wellness is living life in a simple, gentle, respectful way for ourselves, with others, and in the environment. Wellness is the result of the healing that takes place on multiple levels when we take care of ourselves, which then extends to caring for others and the planet in general. A competent massage professional practices self-care and educates clients about the basic components of wellness. This chapter has addressed methods for managing the physical, emotional, and spiritual stress in our lives.

Someone once said, "When half the world is receiving a massage and the other half is giving a massage, we shall have peace." Wellness is peace within and sharing that peace in simple ways. Sharing this peace consistently with respect and compassion can support the wellness of us all, and with faith, hope, and love provide peace for our world.

evolve

13-1 Additional wellness and nutritional guidelines are available on the Evolve Web site.

13-2 Find comprehensive vitamin and mineral charts on the Evolve Web site.

Don't forget to study for your certification and licensure exams! Review questions for this chapter are located on Evolve.

REFERENCES

1. Chaitow L: *The body/mind purification program,* New York, 1991, Fireside.
2. Selye H: *The stress of life,* ed 2, New York, 1978, McGraw-Hill.
3. Kisner C, Colby LA: *Therapeutic exercise: foundations and techniques,* ed 5, Philadelphia, 2007, FA Davis.
4. Lippert L: *Clinical kinesiology and anatomy,* ed 4, Portland, Ore, 2006, The Author.

Workbook Section

Answers for the Workbook Section for Chapter 13 are provided on p. 775.

■ ■ ■ SHORT ANSWER

1. What are the basic components of a wellness program?

_____

_____

_____

2. List common stress responses.

_____

_____

_____

3. How are communication, demands, loss, seeking help, and intuition interrelated?

_____

_____

_____

4. List the components of a balanced diet.

_____

_____

_____

5. List the steps for efficient, relaxed breathing.

_____

_____

_____

6. What are the main components of a physical fitness exercise program?

_____

_____

_____

7. What are the main components of an exercise program?

_____

_____

_____

8. List the changes that occur with exercise.

_____

_____

_____

9. Define flexibility and stretching.

_____

_____

_____

10. Explain how entrainment and mindfulness support relaxation.

_____

_____

_____

11. Explain the interrelationship of self-concept, behavior, and emotions.

_____

_____

_____

12. How can spiritual fitness support resourceful coping?

_____

_____

_____

■ ■ ■ ASSESS YOUR COMPETENCIES

Now that you have studied this chapter, you should be able to:

1. Identify the basic components of a wellness program.

2. Locate resources to develop a wellness program.

3. Develop a personal wellness program.

4. Provide general wellness guidelines to clients.

On a separate sheet of paper, write a short summary of the content of this chapter based on the competencies listed above. When writing this paper, assume you are speaking to someone—a client, prospective employer, co-worker, or other interested person. Write the paper as if you were having a conversation and explaining the importance of the information and skills to professional massage development.

Next, in small student discussion groups, share the papers and compare and contrast how the information was presented. Discuss the content, looking for similarities, differences, potential misunderstanding of the information, and clear and concise methods of description.

CHAPTER 14

Business Considerations for a Career in Therapeutic Massage

CHAPTER OBJECTIVES

After completing this chapter, the student will be able to perform the following:

- Determine his or her personal motivation for pursuing a career in therapeutic massage
- List the pros and cons of independent and employee status
- Develop skills to achieve employee success
- Identify the responsibilities of business ownership
- Develop a 5-year career plan
- Design a marketing strategy and advertising materials for a massage business
- Negotiate rental and employment contracts
- Develop a business management and record-keeping system
- Make an informed choice about career paths

CHAPTER OUTLINE

MOTIVATION
Seeking Help

BURNOUT

THE RESUMÉ
Developing a Resumé

THE INTERVIEW
Dressing for Success
Closing the Interview

SELF-EMPLOYMENT OR EMPLOYMENT BY OTHERS
Advantages and Disadvantages of Self-Employment
Advantages and Disadvantages of Employment by Others

CLIENT RETENTION
Developing a Client-Practitioner Agreement and Policy Statement

REIMBURSEMENT
Comparing Self-Employment and Employee Incomes

THE BUSINESS/CAREER PLAN
The Goal-Setting Plan

THE BUSINESS STRUCTURE
Start-up Costs
Self-Employment

THE TARGET MARKET
Marketing

MANAGEMENT
Obtaining Licenses
Choosing a Business Location
Determining the Legal Structure of the Business
Registering the Name of the Business
Registering for Tax Purposes
Arranging for Insurance
Opening Business Banking Accounts
Setting Up Investments
Keeping Records: the Paper Trail
Hallmarks of a Successful Employee

SUMMARY

KEY TERMS

Burnout
Career
Employee
Job
Marketing
Motivation
Self-employed
Start-up costs

onsider the difference between a career and a job. A **career** is commonly defined as a chosen pursuit, a life work. A **job** is a regular activity performed for payment.

Therapeutic massage can be either a job or a career. Which do you want? The answer to that question will determine in large part how you proceed with your professional development. This text in general, and this chapter in particular, views therapeutic massage as a career. A career can evolve whether you are self-employed or you work for someone else. If you choose to work for someone else, your employer will take care of most of the nuts and bolts of developing and managing a business. You, as an employee, can concentrate on being an excellent massage therapist and supporting the business by being an excellent employee. If you choose to be self-employed, you must be an excellent massage therapist and also able to manage all business-related responsibilities.

evolve This chapter presents specific information for individuals who want to develop a massage business, but it does not attempt to be a course in small business management. The information presented here is unique to therapeutic massage. It is sufficient to guide the student toward additional learning opportunities and to generate classroom discussion (Box 14-1). This chapter takes the position that the nuts and bolts of business are no different for massage than for any other professional service business. Detailed information on topics such as marketing methods, financial record keeping, and tax requirements can be found in business textbooks and on the Internet. Resources on the business aspects of massage therapy also are available, and professional organizations often provide business information. The Evolve Web site provides additional information.

Success depends on the following elements:
- Intention—what are the goals?
- Intuition—following inner guidance
- Inspiration—the ideas that manifest the dream

These three areas, like body, mind, and spirit, provide the foundation for success.

BOX 14-1

Business Experience

To substantiate the validity of the business information in this chapter, a brief business profile of the author is presented:
- Certificate in bookkeeping
- 30+ years as a massage practitioner
- 12 years in full-time private practice (30 to 40 clients a week)
- 18 years in part-time practice (10 to 20 clients a week)
- Professional practice locations: health club, on site (private homes, small businesses, and corporations), chiropractor's office, full-service day spa, private country club, home office, various sports, National Football League (NFL) team, amateur athletes, and professional athletes
- 6 years of professional practice with a psychologist in private practice
- Owner of a massage therapy school (director and instructor for 21 years)
- Employer of 39 associates
- Owner and manager of three commercial properties for 15 years
- Master's degree in Organizational Management and Leadership

Business-wise, for this author "been there, done that" fits, and the experience gained over these many years has resulted in a realistic knowledge of a career in therapeutic massage.

MOTIVATION

SECTION OBJECTIVES

Using the information presented in this section, the student will be able to perform the following:

- Understand the importance of motivation in successfully developing a career
- Determine a suitable client base for an individual massage therapist
- Explore personal strengths and weaknesses that would aid or impede the development of a successful career
- Develop a personal application of methods to prevent burnout

To succeed at anything, a person must be motivated. Motivation is an internal drive that provides the energy to do what is needed to accomplish a goal. One of the primary reasons businesses fail is lack of drive and motivation on the part of the owners. Without the motivation to stick to the commitment, people give up during difficult times. This is especially true of small businesses with single owners, a category that includes most singly owned massage businesses.

Motivation begins with knowing what you want. Plans must be developed, but the massage professional must be willing to change them if a strategy is not working. If success is the goal, quitting cannot be an option. The following are some important points:
- *Know thyself.* No one should persist with something that goes against his or her core values, no matter how successful the process may be for someone else.
- *Follow your dream.* Success flows from desire and motivation. Desire and motivation are the driving forces for the dreams that come from deep within us to bring us joy and healing. Hard times and hard work are part of the process of building a new career. If we follow our dreams and live our purpose, the hard work provides a rewarding, intrinsic sense of satisfaction.
- *Accept that experience is the best teacher.* We learn from our mistakes as well as from our successes. Implementing plans is the only way to find out whether they work. It may become obvious over time that another approach is more advantageous, but being afraid to make mistakes will limit you as a professional.
- *Ask "What's in it for me?"* To succeed in any endeavor, we need to recognize the benefits to be gained from the process. This is an important consideration in any decision. It is not a selfish attitude; rather, it is a smart approach. People will not put energy into something that does not give them satisfaction. This concept applies to money as well. Business is business, and earning money is part of any successful business operation. However, money itself is a poor source of motivation. Motivation is a deeper-felt sense that comes from the heart and soul.
- *Recognize that self-concept matters.* People have ideas about who they should be, and these often conflict with what we have been told and believe that we are. Self-esteem is very important for career success. Trying to live up to others' expectations is a bad practice. A successful career is built on who we are, not on what others want us to be. Develop your ability to use all aspects of yourself to the best advantage.

- *Believe in your product.* Understand and be able to explain the benefits of therapeutic massage. It is most acceptable to explain the benefits of massage in terms of physiologic responses that all people share. Explanations of this type are easy for most people to understand.
- *Provide a quality product.* The massage practitioner must be a skilled technician. Clients pay for the benefits they experience from massage. Client retention is based on your ability to continue to produce those benefits. To be truly successful the practitioner must put the person, not his or her condition, first. People seek caring, nurturing, and nonjudgmental touch as much as technical skill.

Seeking Help

The practitioner brings more than his or her massage skills to a career in therapeutic massage. Each professional also brings personal strengths and weaknesses, successes and failures, and experiences and learning. It is important to use all our strengths. It is even more important to recognize the areas in which we are not as strong, because these limitations influence our business activities in a negative way.

Business owners are wise to hire help for areas in which they may be weak. They need a diverse group of people to serve as consultants, such as a lawyer, an accountant, a skilled bookkeeper, an advertising and marketing consultant, and an adviser for business planning. Consulting these resource people need not be expensive. The local Chamber of Commerce and the Small Business Administration (SBA) offer free services. The SBA supports an organization of retired business people known as the Service Corps of Retired Executives (SCORE). The members of this organization want to help others succeed. It is essential that the massage professional talk to many people and listen to their experiences, both those that were successful and those that involved mistakes. This core information, along with the fundamentals of therapeutic massage, lays the foundation for a successful practice.

Although experts, authorities, and mentors are helpful, no single individual has all the answers or knows the whole truth. Each of us must find his or her own answers. Truth is personal, empowering, and freeing. Many motivational audio programs, books, and speakers are available that can be used for inspiration.* The following overlapping themes, which can be found in most of these sources, are the kernels of truth:

- Whatever we believe—with emotion and feeling—becomes our reality.
- What we do with confidence can become our self-fulfilling prophecy.
- We attract into our lives that which harmonizes with our dominant thoughts.

BURNOUT

When a person is burned out, motivation is lost. Burnout occurs when you use up your energy faster than you can replenish it. For massage therapists this means taking better

care of others than of ourselves. Burnout can be a problem in most service professions. Taking care of others is a big job. If we do not take care of ourselves also, we soon have nothing to give others or ourselves. Each of us must take care of our physical needs, such as resting, eating well, getting regular massages, and paying attention to our emotional needs. Surround yourself with people who believe in you. Take care of your spiritual needs, which connect the value of what you want to accomplish with a much higher purpose. Follow the wellness guidelines presented in Chapter 13.

The actual practice of massage is simple, repetitious touch, which sometimes can get boring. It is important to keep yourself excited about the benefits of such simple applications of touch. One of the best ways to do this is to continue your education. Classes make you think and bring you together with other massage professionals. These are good opportunities to share and learn together. State-licensed massage schools and professional organizations are the best sources for massage education. Efficient body mechanics is essential to prevent physical burnout (see Chapter 7).

It also is important to get away from massage for a bit. The massage professional occasionally should take classes or vacations that have nothing to do with massage or muscles. If you commit to saving your earnings from one massage a week, you will have $500 to $1,000 a year to spend on continuing education and vacations. You deserve it. Take care of yourself, and let others take care of you. Take a vacation, and burnout will be less of a problem.

After a person begins to live life—including his or her career life—*on purpose,* the energy to develop the career focus will be available. Living on purpose is the key to motivation. It means drawing strength from knowing that what we have to offer is valuable. When the massage practitioner truly believes this, he or she can begin developing a business structure or seek rewarding employment (Proficiency Exercise 14-1).

THE RESUMÉ

A *resumé* is a compilation of professional and personal data about a person. Before we can develop a business plan and set goals or apply for employment in massage, it is important to find out who we are. A good resumé becomes part of the promotional materials we use when self-employed and is necessary to apply for a job in the massage field. The resumé should list not only massage experience but also other work experience. This is very important. We are the sum total of all our experiences, and we bring that knowledge base into all work and business situations.

Some think that effective communication is one of the most important skills an employee can have. To communicate effectively at the job interview, you can research the company, the setting, and the position for which you are applying. This is a very good way to prepare for the interview.

Many professional resources are available to help you develop your resumé. Contact the local Chamber of Commerce or a nearby library branch to locate such assistance. Internet sites also can help with resumé development (Proficiency Exercise 14-2).

---

*Brian Tracy is one of my favorite motivational speakers and was a keynote speaker at an AMTA convention.

PROFICIENCY EXERCISE 14-1

In the space below, explore your beliefs to find motivation for developing your career in therapeutic massage.

1. Answer the following questions:

What do I believe—
about therapeutic massage as a professional service:

about my abilities as a massage professional:

about myself as a person:

about my future clients:

2. Complete the following statement five times:

I feel confident about

I feel confident about

I feel confident about

I feel confident about

I feel confident about

3. Complete the following statement five times:

A dominant thought that influences my life is

A dominant thought that influences my life is

A dominant thought that influences my life is

A dominant thought that influences my life is

A dominant thought that influences my life is

PROFICIENCY EXERCISE 14-2

Helpful Internet Web sites for writing a resumé include www. michworks.org, www.hotjobs.com, www.monster.com, www. careerbuilder.com.
1. *Draft your resumé. A sample resumé is shown in Box 14-2. Many computer word processing programs offer a resumé template with resumé options.*
2. *Contact your local community college, library, or public service organization and attend a class in resumé writing.*

A resumé should list information about present and past employment in this order: dates of employment, companies, titles held, and job functions. It also should list when and where you received your education. The resumé should include highlights of the scope and depth of your experience and your responsibilities at each position. It describes the knowledge you have gained and developed throughout your career that relates to the position for which you are applying; this information, in turn, prompts the interviewer to ask questions.

A cover letter for your resumé is like an introduction to the hiring company. It tells them who you are, the position for which you are applying, how you found out about the position, and a brief explanation of why they should call you for an interview. In writing the cover letter, use action verbs that are descriptive and concrete, that really sell your experience,

skills, and abilities. The cover letter should be one half to three fourths of a page in length.

Developing a Resumé

The main heading of the resumé highlights your name and provides the contact information on one line, followed by empty space (Box 14-2). Your name could be shown in a different, larger, or bold font that will make the name on the resumé stand out. Use the same name on your references page, cover letters, and thank you letters. By creating a professional-looking letterhead, you offer a consistent image to the hiring manager (Proficiency Exercise 14-2).

Section headings are assigned to different areas of the resumé (e.g., experience, education, extracurricular activities).

A resumé can be written in many different ways. Most begin by summarizing the applicant's qualifications that pertain to the position. This section should be put at the beginning of the resumé, right under the space left after the name and contact information. The summary of your qualifications should be confined to three high-impact statements that quantify your accomplishments:

- The first statement should highlight your years of experience in the profession and industry.
- The second statement should identify the areas of expertise you want to emphasize.
- The third statement should identify personal attributes that are important to the role and the company.

BOX 14-2

Sample Resumé

NAME
Street address:
City, State ZIP code:
Phone:
e-mail address:
Career Objectives: To provide relaxation and stress reduction massage as well as illness and injury assistance.
(Student note: Put your job experience in chronologic order, starting from the most current job.)

EXPERIENCE

Student Intern   2006-2007   Detroit, MI
- Performed massage therapy assessment prior to starting massage.
- Gathered information to quickly develop a massage plan.
- Accurately and efficiently completed all paperwork.
- Developed goals to assist clients with quality of life concerns.
- Performed massage therapy methods to effectively achieve client goals and outcomes.

Nurse's Aide   2005-2006   Saginaw, MI
- Assisted nurses with patient care, including taking temperatures, blood pressure, and other duties.
- Completed client notes as directed by nurse or doctor.

EDUCATION

2006-2007 Health Enrichment Center, Inc.   Lapeer, MI

(Student note: Depending on the amount of space left on the page, you can list other things about yourself: interests, highlights of qualifications, hobbies, extracurricular activities, and so on.)

HIGHLIGHTS OF QUALIFICATION
Massage practitioner at student clinic Detroit VA Hospital, Hospice [and so on]

INTERESTS
Little League coaching assistant, playing softball and volleyball.

Other options that can be added to this section include a summary of your expertise, career highlights, professional achievements, and so on.

evolve The Evolve Web site presents an example of another resumé and lists additional Web sites where resumé help can be found. Microsoft provides templates for resumés, cover letters, and professional documents in some word processing programs.

THE INTERVIEW

The interview allows the employer to get to know the person applying for the position. It also allows the applicant to ask questions about the company and the available position, building on the information he or she accumulated to prepare for the interview. Through the interview process, the employer develops a good sense of the applicant's communication skills, which are demonstrated when the applicant answers questions, provides feedback on possible situations, and asks questions about the position and company. A lack of conversation by the applicant could lead the interviewer to think that the applicant has a lack of interest. Also, the applicant should write down the interviewer's answers to questions about the position and the company for future reference; this is another way of showing the employer that the applicant truly wants the position.

The applicant's attire and shoes should be neat and clean, conservative, and appropriate for the job, even if a uniform is usually worn. The applicant should bring a uniform and massage supplies to the interview in case the interviewer wants a demonstration massage.

Dressing for Success

For both men and women, attention to the details of one's appearance is crucial to the success of an interview. The following tips can help you present a professional appearance:
- Wear clean and polished, conservative dress shoes.
- Wear a well-groomed hairstyle.
- Make sure your fingernails are clean and trimmed.
- Wear no or minimal cologne or perfume.
- Make sure no body piercings or tattoos are visible other than conservative ear piercings.
- Make sure you have well-brushed teeth and fresh breath.
- Do not have gum, candy, or other objects in your mouth.
- Wear minimal jewelry.
- Make sure you do not have any body odor.
- If performing a massage as part of the interview, bring an appropriate uniform to the interview and change before giving the massage.

When the interviewer asks questions, make eye contact when you answer and be confident. The following are just a few questions that could be asked, for which you need to prepare answers:

- What do you consider to be your greatest strengths and weaknesses?
- Describe a time when you were faced with problems or stresses at work that tested your coping skills. What did you do?
- How do you deal with competition? Are you a competitive person?
- What would you consider an ideal work environment?
- What are your long-range career objectives, and what steps have you taken toward obtaining them?
- How well do you work with people? Do you prefer working alone or as part of a team?
- What do you think are the qualities of an effective leader?
- What do you do when people disagree with you. How do you manage conflict

Closing the Interview

Have an idea of what you would say when leaving the interview. Make sure you state the skills you have that would make this job a definite fit for you and the reasons your strengths make you right for the position. You may want to ask the interviewer if you could send some references or set up an appointment to give the person a massage. Asking when the decision will be made reinforces your desire for the position, and verifying how you should contact the employer to follow up (phone or e-mail) shows that you are considerate and polite. Finally, shake hands with the interviewer as you make a parting comment, such as, "Thank you very much for taking the time to speak with me about the [massage] position. I look forward to speaking with you again soon."

SELF-EMPLOYMENT OR EMPLOYMENT BY OTHERS

SECTION OBJECTIVES

Using the information presented in this section, the student will be able to perform the following:

- Develop the skills required for self-employment
- Develop a mission statement to use as the basis for a business plan
- Develop business goals
- Develop a personal start-up cost worksheet

This chapter does what generic business texts cannot do; it shares the experience of walking the career path in therapeutic massage, both as an employee and as a professional who is self-employed. Throughout the text, you have been encouraged to ask questions, to use clinical reasoning as a problem-solving method, and to challenge information. You have been urged to seek authoritative sources carefully and to compare information from many different experts. It is no different in the business world.

Successful self-employment requires an entrepreneurial spirit. An *entrepreneur* is a person who organizes, operates, and assumes the risk of a business venture. Not everyone is cut out for self-employment. The hours are long, and 100% commitment is required. Self-employed people must be self-starters with a broad range of professional and business skills. Some people think that self-employed individuals get to be their own boss—not so; instead of one or two bosses, every client becomes the boss. Besides an entrepreneurial spirit, self-employment requires a deep internal commitment. During the latter part of this century, therapeutic massage has been provided primarily by self-employed massage professionals. The entrepreneurial spirit runs high in the massage/bodywork profession, but times are changing. The profession has seen a steady increase in jobs and career opportunities in the more traditional employee market, in which the massage practitioner goes to work for an individual or a company at an hourly wage or salary.

More employment opportunities are opening up for massage professionals in the personal service industry and the medical establishment. The most rapid expansion of employment opportunities is occurring in the spa setting and in the health care system. Massage professionals are working for physicians, physical therapists, mental health professionals, and other health care professionals.

The service industry is growing as well. The concepts of the *destination spa,* which provides for extended visits, and the *day spa,* a place in the local area where people can "get away" for a day of pampering and massage, are very popular. The spa industry is a major source of employment for massage professionals. Full-service cosmetology businesses offer employment opportunities as well.

The fitness industry is another source of employment. Many health clubs offer the services of a massage professional. The recreation industry (e.g., hotels, cruise ships, retreats, resort centers) also is an active employer of massage practitioners.

The independent massage therapy clinic offers opportunities for employment when the owner or manager of the clinic handles all business responsibilities and hires massage practitioners to do the work. Franchises and business chains are spreading quickly and also offer employment options.

You can be either self-employed or an employee, and you can either have a career or hold a job in massage. Do not think that you must be self-employed to have a career. Each of these two options has its advantages and disadvantages, and only you can decide what is an advantage and what is a disadvantage. For example, one person may feel that the independent decision making involved in self-employment is an advantage, whereas a person who has difficulty coming up with independent ideas would consider this a disadvantage.

The key is "know thyself." If you have the commitment, drive, skill, and discipline necessary for self-employment and are willing to make the 100% commitment (and more) that it takes to build and maintain a massage therapy practice, self-employment may be the best option for you. Questions a professional must ask himself or herself are: How disciplined am I? Do I wait until the last minute to do a job? Am I on time, or do I usually run late? Do I keep myself organized? The very skills that make a wonderful massage therapist—intuition, sensitivity, an ability to respond to the moment—can be a source of difficulty in meeting the business requirements of planning ahead, keeping bills paid on time, carefully planning business strategy, and staying in one place long enough to carry out the business plan. If you do not have either the self-discipline or the skills necessary for self-employment, employee status may be the better choice.

Experience supports this observation: Many excellent massage professionals are inherently poor at business management. The intuition, spontaneous feelings, and people orientation of those entering the profession do not necessarily work in harmony with the logical, impersonal, structured nature of business. Individuals who want to develop a career in massage frequently are gentle, intuitive people who may find the concepts of developing and enforcing policy statements and determining fee structures difficult. Many people have difficulty with the discipline and organization required to manage a small business. It is difficult to watch excellent massage professionals fail in their effort to serve the public because they did not recognize that they would do far better in an employee situation. It is equally disturbing to see those with the entrepreneurial spirit constrained in the structure of someone else's business dream.

Technical business information often seems alien to the student of therapeutic massage. This chapter shares information about business issues. It is important that the student understand the steps involved in setting up and managing a small business. These issues are not contrary to the service orientation and the gentle, caring attitude necessary for a practitioner of therapeutic massage. Rather, careful attention to these concerns is part of the responsibility of the massage professional.

Whether a massage practitioner is self-employed or an employee, an understanding of business practices related to the massage profession is important. Therapeutic massage is the same as any other business. It is important to market the product—your skills as a massage practitioner—and attend to the record keeping and financial commitments required to run a business (Box 14-3).

To earn $25,000 of net income, a self-employed massage therapist must generate about $50,000 of gross income. Based on 50 weeks of work per year and 20 massage clients per week at $50 per client, the gross receipts are $50,000 per year. Fifty percent will be spent on overhead costs, including rent, advertising, linens, supplies, phone, mailings, and postage. It also is important to remember that the self-employed massage therapist must consider *real time*, which is the amount of time actually put into the business. At a minimum, for every hour spent giving a massage, at least 1 hour will be spent on business work such as records, clean up, advertising, and marketing. Remember, self-employed people never really leave their business.

When all factors are considered, the earnings end up being about the same whether the practitioner is an hourly wage employee or the owner of his or her business.

BOX 14-3

Building a Business: Applying the Pregnancy and Child-Rearing Metaphor

Consider your education in therapeutic massage as a pregnancy. It takes time for the baby to grow until it has developed enough to survive in an unprotected environment. It is the same with going to school to learn therapeutic massage. The time will come for the baby (the professional practice) to be born. This is a natural process, but it is not without its struggles and hard work. Graduation, the birth from school, comes for the student as well. Everyone is excited about the baby, but soon the parents (the massage practitioner) realize that for about 2 years, this new little life will require constant care, hard work, attention to detail, and very long, focused hours. The 2-year-old child seeks independence, but constant supervision is necessary until the child is about 5 years old. At age 5 the child has learned many lessons and can begin some self-care as the parents supervise from a little farther away. Each year after that, the child becomes more independent, although attention from the parents is still necessary, just as it is with a new business.

A professional should plan to give a new business 2 years of constant attention to enable it to develop strong roots from which to grow. It will take about 5 years before attention to the business can be eased and small portions of it entrusted to another supervising person for short periods. Yet, careful attention and participation will always be required if a business is to remain successful. Building a business is hard work that in time reaps rewards.

Advantages and Disadvantages of Self-Employment

The advantages of self-employment should be considered. For example, the business income could be increased by subletting the office space (make sure any rental agreement allows for this). Likewise, after the first few years the advertising and marketing expenses decline because you have established a repeat business with clients who return regularly for massage, and net income increases. Some feel that self-employment offers more freedom to self-direct the business structure, as well as flexibility in scheduling work hours and long-term financial security. Disadvantages include numerous responsibilities both for business concerns and for client services, isolation, lack of peer support and supervision if working alone, and inability to leave the business for any length of time. Income can vary, and no group benefits are available, such as insurance packages or paid vacations. Membership in professional associations can offset the benefits issue because group insurance programs are available through them.

Advantages and Disadvantages of Employment by Others

Employees who have established long-term relationships with their employers often get pay increases. Over a 5-year period the massage practitioner could start at the low end ($9 per hour) and work up to $20 per hour. When choosing a career option, consider that as a therapeutic massage employee, you are not responsible for any of the business concerns and can focus most of your professional energy on client services. Employee status usually involves working with other professionals in some way, creating an environment of support and mentoring. Some businesses may offer benefits and paid vacations. Income usually is stable.

The disadvantages of being an employee might include adherence to business rules and regulations, less flexibility in work scheduling, and having to share a work space.

Currently, more employment options are available, and this likely will become the dominant career status, especially in the spa and health care settings (Box 14-4).

Many massage professionals underestimate the value of their service, whereas others overestimate themselves. When

---

BOX 14-4

U.S. Department of Labor: Occupational Outlook for Massage Therapists

Significant Points
- Employment is expected to grow faster than average over the 2008-2014 period as more people learn about the benefits of massage therapy.
- Many states require formal training licensing or national certification for the practice of massage therapy.
- This occupation has a large number of part-time and self-employed workers.

Nature of the Work
Many physicians have been recommending massage therapy for years. The medical benefits of "friction" were first documented in Western culture by the Greek physician Hippocrates around 400 BC. Today, massage therapy is being used as a means of treating painful ailments, decompressing tired and overworked muscles, reducing stress, rehabilitating sports injuries, and promoting general health. This is accomplished by manipulating a client's soft tissues to improve the body's circulation and remove waste products from the muscles.

Although massage therapy is done for medical benefit, a massage can be given simply to relax or rejuvenate the person being massaged. It is important to note that this type of massage is not intended for a medical purpose and provides medical value only through general stress reduction and increased energy levels. Massage therapy, on the other hand, is practiced by thoroughly trained individuals who provide specialized care with their client's medical health in mind.

Massage therapists can specialize in more than 80 different types, or modalities, of massage. Swedish massage, deep tissue massage, reflexology, acupressure, sports massage, and neuromuscular massage are just a few of the many approaches to massage therapy. Most massage therapists specialize in several modalities, which require different techniques. Some use exaggerated strokes ranging the length of a body part, whereas others use quick, percussion-like strokes with a cupped or closed hand. A massage can last as long as 2 hours or only 5 or 10 minutes. Usually, the type of massage a therapist gives depends on the client's needs and physical condition. For example, the techniques used for elderly clients would not be used for athletes, and the approaches used for clients with injuries would not be appropriate for clients seeking relaxation. Some forms of massage are given solely to one type of client (e.g., prenatal massage and infant massage).

Massage therapists work by appointment. Before beginning a massage therapy session, the therapist conducts an informal interview with the client to find out about the person's medical history and desired results from the massage. This gives the therapist a chance to discuss which techniques could be beneficial to the client and which could be harmful.

Because massage therapists tend to specialize in only a few areas of massage, customers often are referred to or seek a therapist with a certain type of massage in mind. Based on the person's goals, ailments, medical history, and stress- or pain-related problem areas, the massage therapist will determine whether a massage would be harmful and, if not, will move forward with the session while concentrating on any areas of particular discomfort to the client. While giving the massage, the therapist alters the approach or concentrates on a particular area as necessary.

Many modalities involve the use of massage oils, lotions, or creams to massage and rub the client's muscles. Most massage therapists, particularly those who are self-employed, supply their own table or chair, sheets, pillows, and body lotions or oils. For most massage modalities, clients undress or wear loose clothing and are covered with a sheet or blanket. The therapist exposes only the body part that currently is being massaged. Some types of massage are done without oils or lotions and are performed with the client fully clothed.

Massage can be a delicate issue for some clients, and those clients may indicate that they are comfortable with contact only in specified areas. For this reason, and also because of general purpose business risks, about half of all massage therapists have liability insurance, through either a professional association or some other insurance carrier.

Massage therapists must develop a rapport with their clients if repeat customers are to be secured. Because those who seek a therapist tend to make regular visits, developing a loyal clientele is an important part of becoming successful.

Working Conditions
Massage therapists work in an array of settings, both private and public, including private offices, studios, hospitals, nursing homes, fitness centers, sports medicine facilities, airports, and shopping malls. Some massage therapists also travel to clients' homes or offices to provide a massage. It is not uncommon for full-time massage therapists to divide their time among several different settings, depending on the clients and locations scheduled.

Most massage therapists give massages in dimly lit settings. The use of candles, incense, or both is not uncommon. Ambient or other calm, soothing music often is played. The dim lighting, smells, and background noise are meant to put clients at ease. On the other hand, when visiting a client's office, a massage therapist may not have those amenities. The working conditions depend heavily on a therapist's location and what the client wants.

Continued

BOX 14-4

U.S. Department of Labor: Occupational Outlook for Massage Therapists—cont'd

Because massage is physically demanding, massage therapists can succumb to injury if the proper technique is not used. Repetitive motion problems and fatigue from standing for extended periods are most common. This risk can be limited by the use of good technique, proper spacing between sessions, exercise, and in many cases by regular massage for the therapists themselves.

Because of the physical nature of the work and the time needed between sessions, massage therapists typically give massages less than 40 hours per week. Therapists who give massages anywhere from 15 to 30 hours per week usually consider themselves to be full-time workers.

Training, Other Qualifications, and Advancement

Training standards and requirements for massage therapists vary greatly by state and locality. In 2004, 33 states and the District of Columbia had laws regulating massage therapy in some way. Most of the boards governing massage therapy in these states require practicing massage therapists to complete a formal education program and pass the national certification examination or a state exam. Some state regulations require that therapists keep up on their knowledge and technique through continuing education. It is best to check information on licensing, certification, and accreditation on a state-by-state basis.

There are roughly 1,300 massage therapy postsecondary schools, college programs, and training programs throughout the country. Massage therapy programs generally cover subjects such as anatomy, physiology (the study of organs and tissues), kinesiology (the study of motion and body mechanics), business practices, and ethics, as well as hands-on practice of massage techniques. Most formal training programs require an application and some require an in-person interview. Training programs may concentrate on certain massage modalities. Several programs also provide alumni services, such as postgraduate job placement and continuing education services. Both full- and part-time programs are available.

These programs vary in accreditation. Massage therapy training programs are generally accredited by a state board or other accrediting agency. Of the many massage therapy programs in the country, about 300 are accredited by a state board or Department of Education–certified accrediting agency. In states that regulate massage therapy, graduation from an approved school or training program is usually required to practice massage therapy.

After completion of a training program, many massage therapists opt to take the national certification examination for therapeutic massage and bodywork. This exam is administered by the National Certification Board for Therapeutic Massage and Bodywork (NCBTMB), which has eligibility requirements of its own. Several states require that a massage therapist pass this test in order to practice massage therapy. In states that require massage therapy program accreditation, an exam candidate must graduate from a state-licensed training institute with at least 500 hours of training or submit a portfolio of training experience for NCBTMB review; in locations that do not require accredited training programs, this is unnecessary. After the applicant is approved for testing, the

applicant may schedule a test time at a local testing center. Tests are available 6 or 7 days a week, depending on the test site, and are entirely computer based with multiple choice questions. The exam covers six areas of content: general knowledge of the body systems; detailed knowledge of anatomy, physiology, and kinesiology; pathology; therapeutic massage assessment; therapeutic massage application; professional standards and ethics; and business and legal practices.

When a therapist passes the national certification exam for therapeutic massage and bodywork, he or she can use the recognized national credential: Nationally Certified in Therapeutic Massage and Bodywork (NCTMB). The credential must be renewed every 4 years. To remain certified, a therapist must perform at least 200 hours of therapeutic massage during the 4-year period and complete a minimum of 48 credit hours of continuing education. In 2005, the NCBTMB introduced a new national certification test and corresponding professional credential. These are the national certification exam for therapeutic massage and the Nationally Certified in Therapeutic Massage (NCTM) credential. The new test covers the same topics as the traditional national certification exam but covers fewer modalities of massage therapy. Recognition of this new national certification varies by state.

Many of the national, state, and local requirements coincide. States that require the national credential also require accredited training programs to comply with NCBTMB standards of training. Professional associations require that a professional member graduate from a training program that meets NCBTMB standards, have a state license, and/or have national certification from the NCBTMB. Actual requirements differ on a state-by-state basis.

Because of the nature of massage therapy, opportunities for advancement are limited. However, with increased experience and an expanding client base, therapists have opportunities to increase client fees and thus income. Both strong communication skills and a friendly, empathetic personality are extremely helpful qualities for fostering a trusting relationship with clients and, in turn, expanding the client base. Massage therapists who are well organized and have an entrepreneurial spirit may even go into business for themselves. Self-employed massage therapists with a large client base have the highest earnings.

Employment

Massage therapists held about 97,000 jobs in 2004. About two-thirds were self-employed. Of those self-employed, most owned their own business, and the rest worked as independent contractors. Others found employment in salons and spas; the offices of physicians and chiropractors; fitness and recreational sports centers; and hotels. About three-quarters of all massage therapists worked part-time or had variable schedules, although as mentioned earlier, many massage therapists who work 15 to 30 hours per week consider themselves to be full-time workers.

Job Outlook

Employment for massage therapists is expected to increase faster than average over the period from 2004 to 2014 as more

BOX 14-4

U.S. Department of Labor: Occupational Outlook for Massage Therapists—cont'd

people learn about the benefits of massage therapy. In states that regulate massage therapy, therapists who complete formal training programs and pass the national certification exam are likely to have very good job opportunities. Because referrals are a very important source of work for massage therapists, networking will increase the number of job opportunities. Joining a state or local chapter of a professional association can also help build strong contacts and further increase the likelihood of steady work.

Massage is an increasingly popular technique for relaxation and stress reduction. As workplaces try to distinguish themselves as employee friendly, providing professional, in-office, seated massages for employees is becoming a popular on-the-job benefit.

Increased interest in alternative medicine and holistic healing will mean increased opportunities for those skilled in massage therapy. Health care providers and medical insurance companies are beginning to recognize massage therapy as a legitimate treatment and preventive measure for several types of injuries and illnesses. The health care industry is using massage therapy more often as a supplement to conventional medical techniques for ailments such as muscle problems, some illnesses and diseases, and stress-related health problems. Massage therapy's growing acceptance as a medical tool, particularly by the medical provider and insurance industries, will greatly increase employment opportunities.

Older people in nursing homes or assisted living homes are also reaping benefits from massage, such as increased energy levels and reduced health problems. The demand for massage therapy should grow among older age groups, because they increasingly enjoy longer, more active lives. Also, the 55 and older age group is projected to be the fastest growing segment of the U.S. population over the next decade. Currently, demand for massage therapy is greatest among young adults, who are likely to continue to enjoy the benefits of massage therapy as they age.

Earnings
The median hourly earning of massage therapists, including gratuities earned, was $15.36 in May, 2004. The middle 50% earned between $9.78 and $23.82. The lowest 10% earned less than $7.16, and the highest 10% earned more than $32.21. Generally, massage therapists earn 15% to 20% of their income as gratuities. However, tipping is not common for those who work in a hospital or other clinical setting.

Sources of Additional Information
(Links to non–Bureau of Labor Statistics [BLS] Internet sites are provided for convenience and do not constitute an endorsement.)

General information on becoming a massage therapist is available from state regulatory boards.

For more information on becoming a massage therapist, contact:

- Associated Bodywork and Massage Professionals, 1271 Sugarbush Dr., Evergreen, CO 80439. Web site: http://www.abmp.com
- American Massage Therapy Association, 500 Davis St., Suite 900, Evanston, IL 60201. Web site: http://www.amtamassage.org

For a directory of schools providing accredited massage therapy training programs, contact:

- Commission on Massage Therapy Accreditation, 1007 Church St., Suite 302, Evanston, IL 60201. Web site: http://www.comta.org
- Accrediting Commission of Career Schools and Colleges of Technology, 2101 Wilson Blvd., Suite 302, Arlington, VA 22201. Web site: http://www.accsct.org

Information on national testing and national certification is available from the National Certification Board for Therapeutic Massage and Bodywork, 1901 S. Meyers Rd., Suite 240, Oakbrook Terrace, IL 60181. Web site: http://www.ncbtmb.com

Modified from the Bureau of Labor Statistics, US Department of Labor: *Occupational outlook handbook, 2006-07*, Massage Therapists. Accessed March 1, 2007, at http://www.bls.gov/oco/ocos295.htm

---

you are thinking about money and how much to charge for a service or what your wage or salary should be, it is important to realize that people usually live according to an equal exchange for services rendered or for goods received; this is called the *equity hypothesis*. It is important to charge what a massage is worth in time value. If the fee is too high, the professional does not support those stable weekly and biweekly clients who are the mainstays of a massage practitioner's client retention. However, if fees or wages are too low, the career will not generate enough income to support the practitioner.

CLIENT RETENTION

The key to building a successful massage practice is developing a client base that maintains a regular appointment schedule. Development of a regular client base is possible with therapeu-

tic massage because massage benefits wear off if massage is not continued; also, the benefits of massage are cumulative and better sustained with regular appointments. Clients will commit to a regular schedule of massage if they have measurable benefits, if they understand the physiologic reasons for the results of massage, and if they experience a safe, professional, and ethical massage environment. (This point was thoroughly explained in Chapters 2, 4, and 5.) Client education based on this information is necessary for retention.

Clients who maintain a regular appointment schedule typically have quantifiable and qualifiable goals that they want to achieve. Long-term treatment or care plans are important for these clients. If the massage practitioner does not have the skill base to help the client achieve these goals, the client will not be satisfied and will not return for massage. Proper marketing is important as well. Clients should be asked to reschedule appointments and should be reminded of their appointment schedule by telephone or e-mail. Literature should be available that explains the benefits of regular massages. If retention is a problem and clients do not reschedule massage sessions, the massage practitioner needs to evaluate his or her professional interaction with those clients.

REIMBURSEMENT

Another concern for the client is how much the massage will cost. Setting fees and using incentives are great marketing tools. When you are trying to decide how much to charge for massage services, it is helpful to investigate what other massage practitioners within a 1-hour radius of your business location are charging. Consider setting your fees in the midrange of current fees in the area.

Incentives and coupons can be offered to generate interest in the business (Figure 14-1), but attempting to undercut the competition by charging very low fees usually is unwise. The range for massage fees usually is as follows: 30 minutes, $25 to $30; a full hour, $40 to $60 (Box 14-5). For sessions under 30 minutes, the common charge is $1 per minute. These fees represent the current national average and can vary up or down, depending on the location. Typically, fees in urban areas are higher, and those in rural areas are lower.

FIGURE 14-1 Sample coupons and gift certificates.

Another way to determine the fees appropriate for your area or target market is to calculate the average hourly wage of the people in your target market and multiply that by three (up to a maximum hourly fee, which usually is $75). For example, if the employees of ABC Packing Company make $9 per hour, the fee for a 1-hour massage would be $27. If the target market is business professionals with an average hourly wage of $25, the fee could be $75. The justification for this structure is that people may understand the value of working 3 hours a week to provide self-care.

Wages for massage professionals can be hourly, salary, or percentage based as long as the minimum wage requirement per hour worked is paid to the employee. Wages per hour vary widely for massage professionals and depend on location and experience. The average pay range is $9 to $20 per hour (see the Bureau of Labor Statistics at http://www.bls.gov). When setting fees for clients, consider how much you would be willing to pay for a nonspecialized massage.

It is important to review fees yearly. A good time is at the end of the year when taxes are filed (this usually happens in April, so May is a good time to raise rates). Clients should be notified at least 30 days in advance of any price changes. Also, having a full schedule of clients for 3 months is an indicator that a rate increase might be considered.

Comparing Self-Employment and Employee Incomes

If you intend to be self-employed, plan on spending half the gross income of your business (all income generated by business activities) on overhead expenses and setting aside one third of the net income (gross income minus business expenses) to pay income taxes. Consider these costs for the employer situation because they are the business owner's responsibility.

Always remember that each hour spent doing massage requires at least 1 hour of business management time. Giving 20 1-hour massage sessions is at least 40 hours of work if a person is self-employed.

The half-hour massage is the most expensive per minute for the client because of the linen usage and necessary paper costs. Doing a half-hour massage costs as much as doing an hour massage. The hour massage and the hour-and-a-half massage are more cost-effective for generating income.

For an on site massage session, the practitioner travels to the client's home or business, and travel and setup time must be figured into the fee. Because the therapist is already organized to do massage, other sessions at the same location can be provided at the regular rate. If a person is housebound for health reasons, the massage therapist commonly takes this into consideration when setting the fee. The massage professional who has only an on site business saves on rental and utility costs, which may influence the on site fee structure. Remember that time is money, and it takes longer to do an on site massage than one in the office.

If the practitioner sets a fee of $40 to $50 an hour for the packing company workers, these clients are unlikely to be able to afford weekly massage sessions, but regular every-other-

BOX 14-5

Typical Fee Schedule and Analysis of Income

$\frac{1}{2}$ hour	$25 to $30
1 hour	$50 to $60
1$\frac{1}{2}$ hours	$60 to $75
On site 1-hour massage	$80 to $100 (special circumstances may reduce or increase this fee)

The pricing structure for rural areas is somewhat lower than for urban areas.

It is essential to consider *real time* when calculating income. There is always time between massage sessions:

45 minutes to do a $\frac{1}{2}$-hour massage

1 hour and 15 minutes to do a 1-hour massage

1 hour and 45 minutes to do a 1$\frac{1}{2}$-hour massage

3 hours to do a 1-hour on site massage

Now consider the actual amount of money generated per hour, figured on low-end fees:

Two $\frac{1}{2}$-hour massages can be done in 1$\frac{1}{2}$ hours: Income generated = $50 ($33 per hour)

It takes 2$\frac{1}{2}$ hours to do two 1-hour massages: Income generated = $80 (about $32 per hour)

It takes 3$\frac{1}{2}$ hours to do two 1$\frac{1}{2}$-hour massages: Income generated = $110 ($33 per hour)

It takes 3 hours to do an on site 1-hour massage: Income generated = $80 ($27 per hour)

Note: Remember that the income per hour is estimated gross income; all expenses must be paid before the net income is determined. Typically 50% of gross goes to overhead, therefore the net would be one half the amount indicated; an average of about $15 per hour will be income eligible for taxes. Also, an additional 10 to 12 hours of real time are required to maintain a business, pay bills, clean the facility, and handle paperwork.

---

week appointments are possible. If the $50 fee is set for the business professional group, weekly appointments are more likely.

Many therapeutic massage professionals or businesses give a discount to clients who schedule regular visits. This can be done in a variety of ways. One possibility is a package of massages for which the client pays in advance. For example, a client may pay for 10 massage sessions in advance with a $5 discount for each massage. The package deal for the $50 session would be 10 massages for $450 rather than $500. Another option is to give a $5 discount to anyone who books a weekly appointment.

Hourly Wage Employment

An increasingly common practice is to hire massage professionals at an hourly wage. A beginning wage is $8 to $10 per hour. According to the U.S. Bureau of Labor Statistics, the average yearly net income for a full-time massage professional is $20,000 to $35,000. This is about $10 to $15 per hour based on a 40-hour workweek. Remember that income taxes must be paid on this amount. When practitioners work for an hourly wage, they usually are paid for the time spent at the job location, regardless of whether massage is given. Sometimes an agreed-on salary is offered instead of an hourly wage. Those who work for a salary often are paid on the basis of completion of certain tasks rather than the number of hours worked. A salary structure for therapeutic massage might be $400 per week based on completion of 20 massage sessions per pay period. An hourly wage may seem like less than a self-employed practitioner earns, but overall the actual amount in the therapist's pocket is about the same.

THE BUSINESS/CAREER PLAN

Whether you intend to be self-employed or to approach a massage career as an employee, it is important to have a plan.

To make the plan workable, the professional needs to know where he or she is in the present, what his or her path has been, and what he or she has learned from accumulated experiences. When this information has become available, future plans can be made.

One career plan option is to move gradually into a new massage career by working at it part time while letting the business grow slowly (keeping your full-time job). Another option is to commit to the new massage business full time. If the practitioner chooses to do this and is self-employed, he or she will need to have enough money saved up to meet basic needs for about a year.

Either path is acceptable. You need to decide what fits for you. This is the type of information that becomes formalized when you develop a career/business plan.

In all business planning, the important thing is to find and fill a need. What is the massage need that you, as a practitioner, are willing to fill? The answer to this question becomes the basis of your mission statement. A *mission statement* expresses the intent of the business plan. To develop a mission statement, you must answer this question: What will be the main focus of my business?

An example of a mission statement might be:

My business mission is to serve the blue-collar labor population in my area by providing therapeutic massage and self-help education at a reasonable cost, with flexible appointment hours, and at an easily accessible location.

Development of your formal business plan begins while you are still in school. Education in the skills needed to carry out the mission statement is the first step of the business plan. Another part of the business plan is the development of a financial plan to support the educational process and the first year of business, a time when income may be low. While in school, students should use the expertise of teachers and other students to explore career options (Proficiency Exercise 14-3 and 14-4).

The Goal-Setting Plan

When the "big picture" concepts of the career/business plan are in place, smaller steps to implement the plans are identified. These are goals. Goals are important because they provide direction and landmarks for achievement (Box 14-6).

Goals may change over time. Goal setting can be compared to taking a trip. To stay fresh and alert during a trip, a person must stop and rest. If these stops are planned ahead of time, the journey seems shorter. The journey to a successful business is similar when attainable goals are placed along the way.

When you plan for a trip, it is important that you identify any obstacles that may be encountered. What are your financial and personal resources? It is the same with a business. Review the support available from others. Be willing to learn along the way.

Basic survival skills promote self-sufficiency in business as well as in life. A good question to ask is, "What is the worst possible thing that could happen as a result of this decision?"

Think ahead to possible solutions should the worst happen and try to determine whether you could survive that experience. What would be gained? It is important to take calculated risks. If these risks are small and entered into slowly, you can change strategies if need be (Proficiency Exercise 14-5).

The clinical reasoning model used throughout this text is an invaluable tool for setting attainable goals (Box 14-7).

THE BUSINESS STRUCTURE

SECTION OBJECTIVES

Using the information presented in this section, the student will be able to perform the following:

- Negotiate lease agreements based on a flat fee or on a percentage of gross receipts
- Determine average start-up costs, overhead expenses, and yearly income
- Apply business structure concepts to either self-employment or employment by others

Business is business. If you are self-employed, all business responsibilities fall on your shoulders, including all costs. If

PROFICIENCY EXERCISE 14-3

1. *Investigate the fee structure for massage therapy in your area.*
2. *After you have determined the average fee in your area, decide how many massage sessions per month you could afford. What could you afford to pay for a massage session twice a month?*
3. *On a piece of paper, develop a sample incentive plan. Explain how you would track the discounts.*

PROFICIENCY EXERCISE 14-4

Pretend that you are a successful massage practitioner 5 years from now. You have been asked to return to your massage school and speak to the business class about how you succeeded in your business. Talk into a tape recorder for 30 minutes as though you were addressing the class. Play back the tape and write down the steps you took that led to a successful business. Use these steps to develop an outline for a business plan. Then meet in groups of four students and share your outlines with one another.

BOX 14-6

Guidelines for Setting Goals

1. State your goals in the present tense. Act as though your goal has already been achieved. Make sure you are the main character. Use the pronouns *I, me,* and *my.*
2. Make sure your goals are realistic and attainable. Can you achieve these goals from your own resources with little help from others? If the activity of a specific person is necessary to achieve your goal, rethink it. What other people may be able to be part of the goal? Avoid depending on only one other person.
3. Speak positively. Avoid words such as *should, would, could, try,* and *never.*
4. Set target deadlines for yourself; they will give you something to work toward.
5. Make sure your goals are small steps toward your ultimate plan. For example, graduating from school is too big to be a goal; it is more like a mission statement. Completing all the exercises in this chapter within 4 weeks is an attainable goal.

PROFICIENCY EXERCISE 14-5

Picture yourself 5 years from now enjoying a successful massage therapy business. A new student comes to you and asks how you achieved your success. You begin to tell the story of the past 5 years and all the steps it took to get where you are now. All the steps you list are possible goals. When you begin by visualizing the end result, all you have to do is identify the probable steps that got you there. In the space provided, write down two professional goals that you identified.

Goal 1

Goal 2

BOX 14-7

Using the Clinical Reasoning Model to Set Goals

1. **Gather facts to identify and define the situation. (This can be the mission statement.)**

   Key questions:

   What is the desired outcome?

   What are the facts?

   My business mission is to serve the blue-collar labor population in my area by providing therapeutic massage and self-help education at a reasonable cost, with flexible appointment hours and at an easily accessible location.

   I will need a group of people for a client base.

2. **Brainstorm possible goals.**

   Key questions:

   What might I do?

   What if . . . ?

   What are the possibilities?

   What does my intuition suggest?

   What if I contact the XYZ manufacturing plant as a potential population?

   What if I contact the ABC packing company as a potential population?

3. **Evaluate each possible goal identified in step 2 logically and objectively; look at both the pros and the cons.**

   Key questions:

   What would happen if . . . ? (Insert each brainstormed idea from step 2.)

   What are the costs, resources needed, and time involved?

   What are the logical cause and effect of each possibility identified?

   What are the pros and cons of each goal suggested?

   What are the consequences of not acting?

   What are the consequences of acting?

   What would happen if I contacted the XYZ manufacturing plant?

   - *I would need a massage room on site.*
   - *Travel time to work would be 45 minutes.*
   - *Pro: This plant has 300 employees, a large potential client base.*
   - *Con: This plant has a history of striking.*

   What would happen if I contacted the ABC packing company?

   - *I could work at my existing office site.*
   - *I am 15 minutes from work on foot.*
   - *Pro: This company is in a growth phase.*
   - *Con: This company has only 50 employees.*

4. **Evaluate the effect of each possible goal on the people involved.**

   Key questions:

   How would each person involved feel if . . . ? (Insert each brainstormed idea from step 2.)

   For each goal, what would be the impact on the people involved: client, practitioner, and other professionals working with the client?

   How does each person involved feel about the possible goals?

   Does a feeling of cooperation and agreement exist among all parties involved?

   How might people feel if I contact the XYZ manufacturing plant?

   - *This company is quite traditional. The president is sometimes resistant to change. I am socially acquainted with the plant manager, and he might like the idea.*

   How might people feel if I contact the ABC packing company?

   - *This company is very progressive in terms of human resources. I have a personality conflict with one of the vice presidents but have a good rapport with the other members of the human resources board.*

5. **Choose a goal and develop an implementation plan after carefully processing steps 1 through 4.**

   Based on this process, I believe the most attainable goal is to contact the ABC packing company.

6. **Implement the plan and set a date for re-evaluation.**

   Implementation plans are step-by-step procedures that detail what must be done to achieve the goals; these procedures can be considered subgoals.

   Steps for implementing the goal of contacting the ABC packing company:

   - *Develop a presentation packet (1 week)*
   - *Send a letter of inquiry (tomorrow)*
   - *Make an appointment for an interview (2 weeks)*

---

you are an employee, it is important that you appreciate what is required of your employer.

Start-Up Costs

Start-up costs are the initial expenses required to begin a business. In addition to these start-up costs, you should have a minimum cash reserve equal to the amount of money needed to cover basic business and personal living expenses for 6 months to 1 year. Many people begin a business without these cash reserves and do fine. Others give up the business venture because they do not have enough money to pay bills. This situation forces them to find other jobs. Keeping a cash reserve

allows you to focus on developing your business with less financial worry (Proficiency Exercise 14-6). If you intend to look for employment, it is important that you determine whether the business is stable and well planned; otherwise, you may lose your position if your employer goes out of business.

In giving a massage, the student is taught to keep it simple and to go slowly. The same ideas apply to business. A person beginning a massage business does not need a suite of offices. For self-employed individuals, the least expensive way to do business is to develop an on site massage business for private homes or offices and have the business office in your home.

PROFICIENCY EXERCISE 14-6

1. *Talk with three massage practitioners and ask them what it cost to start their massage businesses.*
2. *Use professional massage publications and other resources to complete a sample start-up cost worksheet.*

Starting small, with the bare essentials, keeps start-up costs at about $4,000. A basic portable table should not cost more than $500. Business cards and a simple brochure are needed, as are client-practitioner statements, policy and procedure booklets, receipt books, and client information forms. The total cost for these is about $500. It is a good idea to have a separate telephone and answering system, which together cost about $300. Membership in one of the professional organizations also provides liability insurance; the membership and insurance usually cost less than $300. Linens and supplies should cost about $300, and opening a bank account, plus miscellaneous expenses, takes about $500. An expenditure of $1,000 for initial advertising is reasonable.

Renting a small office can push up the start-up cost to about $6,000. This includes the expenses detailed above plus office costs, such as rent (about $1,000, because renting office space often requires payment of the first and last months' rent up front) and office furniture and utility hook-ups (another $1,000).

Self-Employment

The self-employed massage professional typically becomes affiliated with an established business (e.g., a health club, chiropractor, or full-service cosmetology business) by renting a room in that business establishment. It is important to make sure that any agreement of this type is written in contractual form and reviewed by an attorney (Figure 14-2).

Agreement, made this _____ day of _____, 20__, by and between_____, Massage Therapist, DBA, Cantonville, Maryland, and _____.

Whereas, _____ Massage Therapist, DBA, is a massage therapist and an independent contractor wishing to use the facilities and services of _____ at _____ for the express purpose of the rendition of therapeutic massage services or activities related to massage therapy.

TERMS OF AGREEMENT
1. Fee for a 1-hour therapeutic massage is $55. Massage Therapist receives 75% of massage fees and _____ receives 25%. The same percentage applies regardless of the cost of the massage.
2. Fees may be adjusted only on agreement by both parties.
3. This contract is in effect through March 31. At that time either party may cancel or modify the agreement. A new contract will be issued from April 1.

The following facilities and services will be provided by the chiropractor for the massage therapist:

A. Storage for all massage supplies
B. Use of the facility and its services, i.e., telephone, bathroom, microwave, refrigerator
C. Booking and confirmation of all massage therapy appointments
D. All collection of money, whether cash or insurance
E. A room for the massage therapist to use in the rendition of therapeutic massage services or activities related to massage therapy, and _____ also furnishes electricity, heat, and cleaning for this room
F. Promotion of therapeutic massage as an enhancement to chiropractic care

The massage therapist will abide by the following conditions:

A. Bring all necessary supplies associated with therapy
B. Launder all sheets
C. Pay any and all own costs associated with being an independent contractor, i.e., liability insurance and professional membership
D. Control own hours and schedule
E. Not be held accountable for any expenses incurred by facilities or services not included in this agreement
F. Keep all tips
G. Keep all client information confidential
H. Work at facility by appointment only
I. Reconcile all accounts and pay proper percentage to chiropractor at the end of each month

Cancellation of use of facilities and services is to be in writing, giving at least 30 days' notice, thereafter releasing each party from all financial and legal obligations with the other.

Having read the terms of this agreement, _____ does hereby agree to terms and by signing does agree to use _____ facilities and services to begin on _____.

_____   _____
Date: _____   Date: _____

FIGURE 14-2 Sample facilities and services agreement written in contract form.

A pitfall in this type of arrangement develops when the owner or manager of the business wants the massage practitioner to function as an employee but, for payment and tax purposes, to be classified as self-employed. With this arrangement, the business owner does not have to pay matching payroll taxes or benefits. For true self-employment status, it is important to realize that the professional essentially is renting space from the owner. The massage business is completely independent in the way business is conducted. The business owner cannot direct the massage practitioner regarding what hours to work, what kind of work to do, or what to wear.

Facility Rental

The owner of the existing business can be paid in one of two ways. One arrangement is to pay the owner a percentage of every massage performed. This percentage varies from 10% to 50% (the average is 30%). With this arrangement, the business owner profits from every massage done and may be more likely to support your business with word-of-mouth advertising and referrals. The two businesses also commonly advertise together.

Under the other type of agreement, the practitioner pays the owner a monthly rent. Rental fees vary depending on the business location and the area of the country. Giving a range is difficult, but most rooms in established businesses can be rented for $200 to $600 per month. One formula for figuring rent involves calculating the percentage of the total square footage of the space. For example, let's say that the room you want to rent is 12 feet by 12 feet, or 144 square feet. The business occupies 2,000 square feet. The 12 by 12 room is about 7% of the total available space. The owner pays $2,800 per month for rent ($14 per square foot); 7% of $2,800 is $196. The business owner needs to make some money to apply the business principle of making a reasonable profit. A 50% return is normal; 50% of $196 is $98. The rent for the space would be $196 plus $98, or $294 per month.

The better choice at first may be to pay a percentage for each massage. If the practitioner has a slow week or gives very few massages, he or she is not obligated to pay a monthly bill. As the business builds, the practitioner commonly ends up paying more per month with a percentage agreement than with a flat fee. If a mutually beneficial relationship is desired, a compromise can be negotiated, such as an upper limit cap on monthly rent. This is the type of information that must be included in a written legal agreement, or contract.

THE TARGET MARKET

SECTION OBJECTIVES

Using the information presented in this section, the student will be able to perform the following:

- Develop a word-of-mouth marketing plan
- Develop an informational brochure, business card, and media story
- Design a fee structure for therapeutic massage services
- Determine whether third-party insurance reimbursement is available or appropriate for the practice of therapeutic massage

In developing a business, it is important to know the market. Many opportunities are open for the massage business, ranging from the service approaches of stress reduction massage to the allied health opportunities of working in clinical settings. The future for massage is bright. Research has provided the long-awaited verification of the benefits of massage. Educational standards continue to improve, and the profession is becoming standardized and formalized. These developments should achieve a broader acceptance of therapeutic massage and bodywork methods. As a result, more people will consider using massage as part of a health maintenance program.

Massage probably will assume a larger role in corporate stress reduction programs. Athletes will use the services of a massage practitioner more often. Pain control clinics will see its value. Both elderly and young persons can benefit from the nurturing touch of the massage therapist. Opportunities for the development of the massage business will be even greater after people understand the benefits of massage. The need for consistently well-trained practitioners will increase.

There is no typical massage business. Successful massage professionals can be found practicing in many different formats. Massage professionals may be full-time employees of a chiropractor or may work part time out of their homes. A business could be developed entirely at one location or in three or four locations. A massage therapist may work one day at a local manufacturing business for the employees and the next day may do home (on site) visits for local business people. The third day could be spent teaching a self-help massage class for the local community education program. On the fourth day, the therapist may see clients at a full-service cosmetology establishment in the morning and, that evening, provide on site massage for a local support group dealing with stress.

With all the available possibilities, the massage practitioner is wise to narrow the focus to one, two, or three specific markets to keep advertising and promotional activities manageable. Answering the following questions begins the process of narrowing and developing a target market for a therapeutic massage business:

- Where do you plan to work?
- What potential client groups or populations are available within a half-hour drive of the location?
- What type of massage or bodywork do you enjoy giving?
- What group or type of people do you want to help most?
- How are you going to reach those potential clients?
- When do you want to be available to do massage?

By the fifth year of business, the practitioner usually has established a solid focus, a narrow target market, and a consistent clientele (Proficiency Exercise 14-7).

Marketing

Marketing encompasses the advertising and other promotional activities required to sell a product or service. Advertising is a must when starting a new business, and many forms of advertising are very costly. For massage, some types of advertising work better than others.

PROFICIENCY EXERCISE 14-7

Locate the phone numbers of all the service clubs (e.g., Rotary International) in your community (the local phone book often lists these organizations). Send a short letter of introduction to three of the organizations offering to do a 30-minute presentation about therapeutic massage for the group. Follow up with phone calls. Arrange to do a presentation (as a student) for the group.

Word of mouth is the best advertising. Meeting people and talking with them is far more effective than placing an ad in a newspaper. Having satisfied clients who tell other potential clients about you is even better. In the beginning, the massage practitioner must talk with many people to develop a client base. Building a business takes time. It is important not to become discouraged, because if you want to succeed, quitting is not an option.

evolve 14-2   The massage practitioner should persist in handing out business cards and brochures and giving demonstrations until the clients are found. Placing an ad and then sitting in an office waiting for clients to call does not work. Success comes by arranging to speak at service clubs and churches in the area or by volunteering to work at races and local events. Businesses may want to offer a stress management class. Local school districts often have adult education classes, and short classes that teach simple massage routines are popular. Charitable organizations often have auctions, which are wonderful opportunities to give away gift certificates for massage. The Evolve Web site presents an interactive activity for creating a business card.

Being visible in the community helps to generate business. A regular base clientele of about 100 is sufficient to support a thriving therapeutic massage business. Some clients will have weekly standing appointments, others biweekly appointments, and the rest will visit monthly or occasionally. It may be necessary to talk to 2,000 people to find 100 clients.

The main marketing obstacles for personal service wellness massage are (1) convincing the public that regular massage is beneficial to a lifestyle program that focuses on managing stress and striving for wellness and (2) helping would-be clients justify the fees for massage. A wellness massage business is built on clients who receive therapeutic massage regularly. Clients who get a massage on a weekly, bimonthly, or monthly basis are the mainstay of a personal service massage business. A successful business of this type depends on quality; consistent, personal attention to the client; and affordable fees. Clients who are happy with the work are the best source of word-of-mouth advertising.

The Brochure

evolve

The brochure is the primary tool for educating the public and potential clients about the services offered. It should give specific information about the following (Proficiency Exercise 14-8):

PROFICIENCY EXERCISE 14-8

1. *Locate three different professional brochures. Evaluate them against the criteria listed in this section.*
2. *Develop a sample professional brochure for your future business.*

1. *The nature of the services offered.* The brochure should explain clearly that therapeutic massage is a general health service. It should state that no specific treatment of any kind is given for pre-existing physical or mental problems. It also should make clear that all specific problems of a medical, structural, psychological, or dietary nature will be referred to the appropriate licensed professional. Written permission and supervision by the medical professional or other licensed health professional will be required in order for the massage practitioner to work with any conditions that fall within that specific scope of practice.

2. *A description of the services offered.* The brochure should give a simple explanation of the process of a massage. It should include a full description of the types of services offered and the procedures followed in rendering those services. It should explain that the client may remain dressed and will always be properly draped. It should clearly state that the client may stop the session at any time and may choose not to have any area of the body touched or to have any particular technique used.

3. *The qualifications of the practitioner.* The massage professional's credentials, documenting his or her education, training, and experience, should be outlined in a manner that allows potential clients to verify the practitioner's competence. A valid organization that issues the credentials, such as a school or continuing education provider, must have a record of the practitioner having completed the course.

4. *The client's financial and time investment.* The brochure must provide a realistic statement of costs and fees. It should emphasize that the effects of massage are temporary and that massage is best used as a maintenance system. The brochure should state that the massage practitioner will teach self-help to the client if requested. It also should make clear that the best results from massage are maintained when treatment is given on a weekly or biweekly basis, and that therapeutic massage, when used only occasionally, provides only temporary effects.

5. *The client's role in health care.* The brochure should address the importance of the client's responsibility for his or her personal health care. It is important that the client realize that the massage practitioner is a facilitator in the wellness process.

The Media

Local newspapers often run stories about new and unusual businesses. A word of caution about newspapers: the massage professional should write the story in order to avoid embarrassing mistakes. Including a black and white photograph of the professional giving a massage is a great idea. It is also beneficial to provide the writer with copies of other good news stories about therapeutic massage.

Media advertising (newspaper, radio, and television) is very expensive and not the best idea initially. The clientele developed most likely will be located within a 30-mile radius of the business location. A direct mailing to a specific area is more effective than newspaper advertising. Also, Web sites and Internet advertising are rapidly expanding the advertising medium.

Before advertising in the Yellow Pages of the telephone book, which also is very expensive, the massage professional must be sure that the business location will not change for at least a year. The advertisement will be locked in for a year after the phone book has been distributed, and the contract must be paid even if the business moves.

A much more cost-effective method is to use media advertising the way automotive companies do: a group of massage professionals in the area can advertise together. When the cost is split, newspaper, radio, Internet, and television advertising (which is expensive for one person) becomes affordable. Whenever a cooperative venture such as group advertising is formed, the professionals involved *must get the agreement in writing with the help of an attorney.* Never make oral contracts or agreements.

When you develop any written material or advertising, make sure you provide potential clients with the answers to these basic questions:

- Who? (You)
- What? (Therapeutic massage)
- Where? (Address and phone number)
- When? (Appointment times)
- How? (They can reach you by phone, e-mail, or Web page)

evolve This information also should be provided on your business card. The card should be simple and direct and should not list all your credentials. It is convenient to put the information about the next appointment date on the back of the card (Proficiency Exercise 14-9). See the Evolve Web site for more examples.

Insurance or Third-Party Reimbursement

As was explained in Chapter 2, insurance companies do not usually pay for wellness-oriented, personal service therapeutic massage. The paperwork requirements for collecting insurance are extensive. Most massage professionals are unable to bill the insurance company directly for reimbursement. The managed care system is affecting the ability to bill insurance directly and is reducing the number of health care providers who can bill directly. On the other hand, some insurance companies are covering massage and providing programs in which massage providers who meet certain criteria are eligible to be listed in their members' directories. The insurance company prenegotiates a discounted fee with the massage therapist for its clients. The clients pay the massage professional the discounted fee. No billing is required. The return

---

PROFICIENCY EXERCISE 14-9

1. *Locate three stories about new businesses in your area on the Internet or in the newspaper. Cut or print them out.*
2. *Write a newspaper story about yourself. Include your picture.*
3. *Obtain three current, positive Web, magazine, or newspaper articles about therapeutic massage.*
4. *Design a small advertisement for your future massage business that is suitable for the Yellow Pages. Call an ad representative from your local telephone company and find out how much it would cost to run the ad.*
5. *Design a piece of direct mail advertising for your future massage business. Locate a direct mail advertising source and find out how much the ad would cost and the expected rate of return on this type of advertising investment.*
6. *Contact your local newspaper and ask an ad representative to help you design a display ad for your future massage business. Find out how much it would cost to run the ad. Repeat with Internet advertising.*
7. *In the space provided, design the front and back of a business card.*

for the discount is the appearance of approval by the insurance company and the marketing and advertising received in the member publications.

If the massage therapist is an employee of a licensed medical professional or of a managed care corporation with access to insurance billing codes and is working under direct supervision, the massage services may be available for billing. In this situation the massage therapist receives an hourly wage or salary. The burden of collecting from the insurance company falls on the physician, chiropractor, physical therapist, dentist, psychiatrist, or corporate entity, not on the massage practitioner. However, the massage practitioner needs to be able to perform effective assessments, write appropriate treatment plans, and maintain charts.

Occasionally a client can collect from the insurance company by providing a prescription for massage from the physician and a receipt showing payment, the diagnostic code from the physician, and a description of the procedure. It is important to have the insurance company preapprove payment for therapeutic massage. This is done by having the client contact the insurance company before any massage begins. Documentation on the benefits of massage, the physician's prescription, and any other information required by the insurance company are presented for review. This usually is the client's responsibility. Based on this information, the insurance company determines whether the client will be reimbursed for the massage services and notifies the client in writing of the decision. The client pays the massage professional directly, and the massage professional provides the receipt with the physician's diagnostic code, the procedure used, and the duration of the session. Responsibility for collecting insurance reimbursement falls to the client.

A good deal of controversy exists about the advisability of dealing with insurance companies. Some massage professionals seem to do well with insurance reimbursement. Workers' compensation and smaller insurance companies are more apt to pay. Therapists who choose to deal with insurance companies, however, must be very careful. Many massage practitioners have been unable to collect insurance payments due and have lost a considerable amount of money. It remains to be seen what effect the managed health care system will have on independent health care professionals, including massage practitioners.

Personal service massage is not likely to fall under the accepted coverage of current or future health care plans. However, the possibility exists that future insurance coverage will be available for preventive health care. Some managed care systems are currently investigating various options for extending some limited coverage in this area.

Massage is a wonderful addition to any wellness program. If insurance coverage becomes available in this realm, it probably still will fall under the medical umbrella and will not be easily accessible to the independent massage practitioner.

The current widespread lack of health insurance coverage for therapeutic massage services should not discourage the new massage professional. Many health care professionals are discouraged and frustrated with the health insurance system and the limits it places on their attempts to provide their

---

PROFICIENCY EXERCISE 14-10

1. Contact a local chiropractor, physical therapist, mental health professional, or physician's office and talk with the billing clerk about the paperwork involved in insurance reimbursement. Ask how much the insurance company covers for various treatments.
2. Call your personal health insurance company and ask whether massage therapy is covered, what the requirements are for receiving coverage, and how much is reimbursed for a massage session.

---

patients with quality care. Some professionals are even beginning to refuse to participate in health insurance programs; they have begun to adjust their fee schedule and are returning to a cash-for-services system.

Employment will become available for those who wish to work in the medical system, those who wish to have access to health insurance reimbursement, and those who want to be independent business people providing massage services outside the medical establishment on a cash-for-services basis. It is beneficial for both the client and the therapist to have options, and as the future unfolds, all of these career opportunities will continue to develop.

Remember, payment by the client for services rendered is the most dependable income base (Proficiency Exercise 14-10).

MANAGEMENT

SECTION OBJECTIVES

Using the information presented in this section, the student will be able to perform the following:

- Use a step-by-step procedure to set up business management practices
- Set up business files
- Develop the paper trail required for business records

Management consists of all the activities required to maintain a business, particularly record keeping and financial disbursement. The KISS principle (keep it simple and specific) is an excellent concept to help organize the details of business practices. Of course, a business operation can be set up in many ways. A business consultant and an attorney usually are the best advisers. The simplest business arrangement, the sole proprietorship, is detailed in this textbook. The steps in setting up this arrangement are as follows:

1. Obtain all necessary licenses.
2. Choose a business location.
3. Determine the legal structure of the business.
4. Register the name of the business.
5. Register for tax purposes.
6. Arrange for insurance.
7. Open business banking accounts.
8. Set up investments.
9. Keep records.
10. Develop a client-practitioner agreement and policy statement.

Obtaining Licenses

Massage professionals usually deal with two distinct types of licenses: professional and business. A professional license shows that you have achieved the skills to practice your profession. It may be issued by the state or by a local governmental body (see Chapter 2) and may be required for all who practice massage. With massage, difficulties occasionally arise with local licensing if state licensing is not in place. If this problem is encountered, it is important to organize a group of massage professionals and other supporters in the local community and work to change any local control that does not support massage as a profession.

evolve If a state licenses massage practitioners, the professional usually must show proof of a certain level of education and pass some sort of licensing test. The best way to find out about licensing in any state is to contact the Department of Licensing and Regulation in the state capital. Usually the licensing department for massage is in the Occupational License Department. This agency can provide the necessary information. Most states now license massage therapists or are in the process of developing licensure. See the Evolve Web site for a list of states that license massage therapists.

A business license, which is obtained from the local government, allows that governmental body to regulate the type and location of business operations. If a profession is licensed, the professional may need to show a copy of the license to obtain a business license. Any required forms should be filled out carefully.

Choosing a Business Location

When deciding where to locate your business, remember that each community has specific zoning regulations. These regulations protect the investment of those who own property. Without zoning, someone could put a junkyard next to a home. Usually the zoning that a massage business requires is general office or commercial zoning. Because of difficulties with local ordinance control of massage establishments, some restrictions may apply to locations for a massage business. To obtain this information, the practitioner should visit local government offices and ask to see the zoning ordinances.

A permit or business license may be needed. It is important that the business owner develop a good working relationship with government officials. These officials usually have a sincere concern for their communities, and the massage professional must respect this. Occasionally these officials need to be educated about therapeutic massage. As with a massage, go slowly and be gentle and understanding.

Difficulty with massage parlor ordinances has diminished substantially over the past 5 years, but the problem still exists. Hopefully, growing public awareness about therapeutic massage eventually will resolve this problem.

Determining the Legal Structure of the Business

A *sole proprietorship* (one-owner business) is the simplest way to set up a business. Partnerships and corporations are complicated business structures, and the need for them should be discussed with an attorney. This chapter is structured around the sole proprietorship.

Registering the Name of the Business

Registering the name of your business is known as obtaining a *DBA* (i.e., *doing business as* _____). When choosing a business name, the public's interpretation must be considered. One person chose *BODY-WORKS* and received calls about automotive body repair. The fee to register the name of your business is about $20, and it usually is done at the county clerk's office. The clerk will check to see whether anyone else in the county is using the name and then issue the DBA. This document may be needed to open a business checking account.

Registering for Tax Purposes

Federal, state, and local taxes must be paid. A sales tax identification number may also be needed. Information about federal taxes can be provided by the Internal Revenue Service (IRS) at 1-800-829-1040. State tax information can be obtained from the Department of the Treasury in any state. Information about local taxes can be obtained from both the county and local government offices. The IRS has many publications and counseling services that help explain the payment of business taxes. The business owner is strongly urged to seek the advice of a business attorney or certified public accountant regarding tax requirements.

One third of the gross income of a business usually is needed to cover various taxes. This money must be set aside every month and left untouched. One of the biggest problems new business owners have is nonpayment of taxes because the tax money was spent on overhead expenses. The best protection is to pay the government first, because the penalties are high and tax laws are difficult. A professional tax preparer can help a great deal with management of your taxes.

Arranging for Insurance

All massage practitioners need professional liability insurance, often called *malpractice insurance*. The term *malpractice* refers to professional negligence or maleficence. *Negligence* is an unintentional wrong. A negligent person fails to act in a reasonable and careful manner and consequently causes harm. *Maleficence* is causing deliberate harm. Clients expect a certain level of professional education, standards of practice, and responsibility for conduct. Unfortunately, in the highly litigious climate of today's world, the best protection against a lawsuit is insurance. Insurance reduces the risk of having a liability claim filed against you personally. To advertise this, however, only invites a lawsuit. Accurate, comprehensive records are the next best protection; anything that seems even slightly important must be documented.

evolve The best place to obtain liability insurance is through the professional organizations. Those that have been in existence for many years are the Associated Bodywork and Massage Professionals (ABMP) and the American Massage Therapy Association (AMTA). Other professional organizations for massage and bodywork professionals have been established, and careful investigation into their insurance plans is recommended. The insurance costs usually are part of the dues structure of these organizations, an arrangement that makes insurance available at a reasonable cost. Obtaining insurance from private companies is very expensive.

Premise liability insurance also is needed; this is often called "trip and fall" insurance. It can be obtained through professional organizations or from a local insurance agent. Because home business offices are not covered under a homeowner's policy, additional coverage in the form of a business rider is needed. The insurance agent also can discuss fire and damage insurance on equipment.

The more complicated a business, the more comprehensive the insurance coverage must be. Sale of products requires *product liability insurance. Independent contractor liability insurance* protects the contractor against third-party claims from hired independent contractors, and so on. The insurance agent and the insurance representative of the professional organization can provide additional information.

Opening Business Banking Accounts

A business account can be opened at a local bank. The DBA usually is required to use a business name. All income from the business is deposited in the business account, which serves as a record of gross income. All expenses are paid from this checking account, which provides a record of business deductions. What is left over is called the *net income*.

If the massage professional is disciplined enough to pay off a charge card every month, a business credit card is a good idea. The monthly statement is a good record of business expenses.

Taxes are paid quarterly on the net income. A wise professional will contact a good bookkeeper or accountant to help set up the payment schedule for taxes.

After all business expenses and taxes have been covered, the massage professional may write himself or herself a paycheck (called a *draw check*). This money should be deposited in a personal account, and personal expenses can be paid from this account. *Personal and business money must not be mixed.*

Setting Up Investments

All massage professionals, whether self-employed or employed by others, should set up an individual retirement plan. After taxes are paid, 10% of income could be invested in a long-term growth investment. A local bank or insurance company may have access to stable mutual funds. Individual retirement accounts (IRAs) also are available. Some employers offer investment plans. Money can be invested in compound interest-bearing accounts in many ways. This takes discipline, but

we inevitably get older, and planning for that time now is important.

Another investment to consider is giving away one massage per week to someone who really needs it. What is given out truly does come back tenfold. Remember the equity hypothesis. This person always has something to return to the massage professional. Maybe it is only a smile of appreciation, which can be worth more than gold.

Keeping Records: the Paper Trail

All business receipts must be saved and filed. Copies of all important documents should be stored in a location other than that of the originals. Everything must be dated, and no oral contracts should be made. Information should be organized monthly on a spreadsheet so that when it is time for the tax preparer to do the business and personal taxes, everything can be verified. This so-called paper trail is very important for a properly run business, and it must be established.

Comprehensive client files must be kept in order (see Chapter 3). Payment records also are kept in the client files. Note whether payment was made by cash, credit card, or check. If a check is used, note the check number. If cash is paid, note the receipt number. If a monthly billing system is used, post the date the bill was sent and the date the check was received, along with the check number. Any credit card information should be taken and recorded. Records must be kept current. If you must use professional liability insurance or if you are billed by a client's insurance company, the first thing the company will request is the client's records.

Anyone who wants to manage his or her own business is advised to take some classes in small business management at a community college or to attend workshops offered by the local Chamber of Commerce. *For the self-employed, the need to keep accurate records is unavoidable.* Many commercial record-keeping systems are available. A wise course is to choose one and use it consistently. All massage professionals, whether employees or self-employed, must keep accurate, comprehensive client files. The success of your professional life depends on it. The current trend toward electronic data storage and various types of user friendly software supports this option.

Developing a Client-Practitioner Agreement and Policy Statement

It is essential to have the client read a client-practitioner agreement and policy statement, as presented in Chapter 2. This is the document in which you set forth the professional rules for the client. People usually do quite well with information presented to them in a clear, concise, up-front way. The potential for conflict increases if the rules are not understood and agreed upon or if they are changed too often in midstream. The client-practitioner agreement and policy statement prevents conflicts by clearly stating all policies. This agreement is more comprehensive than the brochure (discussed later in the chapter) and becomes part of the informed consent process, but it is not protection against a lawsuit. It does have value in that it can do the following:

- Clarify for the client the nature of the service rendered
- Help protect against unwarranted and unrealistic expectations on the part of the client
- Serve the practitioner as a constant reinforcement of the scope and limits of his or her practice within acceptable legal parameters
- Serve as a valuable factual tool if required in court action

The agreement or policy statement should be presented in simple, easily understood language. It gives the practitioner an opportunity to define his or her practice. The practitioner-client agreement is of little value if it does not accurately describe the type of service offered to the public (Proficiency Exercise 14-11).

PROFICIENCY EXERCISE 14-11

Using the information in this section and the following outline, develop a checklist for your personal business management plan. The first item is done as an example to get you started.

1. *Obtain licenses*
   - Check with the state about license requirements
   - Obtain a copy of licensing forms
   - Complete forms and return
   - Check with local government about licensing requirements for:
     - Business license
       a. Obtain copy of licensing forms
       b. Complete forms and return
     - Professional practice license or ordinance
       a. Obtain copy of licensing forms
       b. Complete forms and return

2. *Choose a business location*

3. *Establish the legal structure of the business*

4. *Register the name of the business*

5. *Register for tax purposes*

6. *Arrange for insurance*

7. *Open business banking accounts*

8. *Set up investments*

Continued

PROFICIENCY EXERCISE 14-11—cont'd

9. *Keep records: the paper trail*

10. *Develop a client-practitioner agreement and policy statement*

evolve

Hallmarks of a Successful Employee

If after reading about the responsibility of owning and managing a business, you decide that you are better suited to achieving success as an employee, commit to being an excellent employee. See the Evolve Web site for links to important information on employee success.

Many employers complain about the quality and commitment of their employees. The massage/bodywork industry is no different. If you choose to be an employee, the information in this text should help you understand the commitment and responsibility required of an employer to create an environment that allows you to pursue your career as a massage professional free of business responsibilities. As an employee, keep in mind the "Do's" and "Don'ts" listed in Box 14-8 (Proficiency Exercise 14-12).

In applying for a therapeutic massage position, you must submit a resumé and a personal list of career expectations for the job. It is important to understand the job description, the hours that will be spent on the job, and obligations to the employer—and it is vital to get all this in writing, along with any special arrangement that may be made. This document should be signed and dated by all parties involved so that everyone has an original copy. The job interview may include performing a massage session as a skills test.

Author's note: Box 14-9 contains important information. Besides serving as good guidelines for job seekers, the bulleted items can be considered characteristics that employers find valuable. Those same characteristics help both employers and the self-employed to create a successful career. Some work hand-in-hand and are very widely found. Just because you do not have all of them or most of them doesn't mean you won't be successful. Some are learned. Keeping constantly aware of the purpose of the business can help those who are willing and eager to learn to acquire some of these valued characteristics. Because of our own uniqueness, we may not have as many of those employability skills as other coworkers, and we may be outperformed in certain areas. However, this should not cause you to doubt your self-worth and the value you have for your employer and your clients. I, myself, have a form of dyslexia, but my accomplishments go far beyond what some would think are the limits for a person with dyslexia. The sky's the limit as long as you believe and have inspiration. Any aspiration can be achieved and any obstacle overcome.

BOX 14-8

Employee "Do's" and "Don'ts"

Don't
- Gossip
- Complain without providing a viable solution
- Be dishonest
- Behave unethically
- Behave irresponsibly

Do
- Get to work on time
- Look and act like a professional
- Be consistent and accurate with recording requirements of the business
- Be courteous and supportive
- Be assertive and communicate openly with your employer
- Develop a sense of commitment and loyalty to your employer
- Take your responsibilities seriously
- Improve your skills
- Own your mistakes and correct them
- Be willing to extend yourself in the short term for everyone's long-term gain
- Be a team player
- Be flexible and creative
- Use problem-solving skills to resolve potential conflict
- Commit to the job

 PROFICIENCY EXERCISE 14-12

Develop your personal lists of pros and cons for self-employment and employee status.

Self-Employment

Pros	Cons

Employee Status

Pros	Cons

BOX 14-9

Eight Keys to Employability

1. Personal Values
Valued workers:
- Are honest.
- Have good self-esteem and a positive self-image.
- Have personal and career goals.
- Demonstrate emotional stability.
- Exhibit a good attitude.
- Are self-motivated.
- Do not limit themselves.

2. Problem-Solving and Decision-Making Skills
Valued workers:
- Are flexible.
- Are creative and innovative.
- Can adapt to changing demands of a job.
- Can reason and make objective decisions.
- Can keep their mind on several parts of a job at a time.

3. Relations with Other People
Valued workers:
- Work well with peers.
- Accept authority and supervision.
- Accept constructive criticism.
- Are team members.
- Are friendly.
- Are consistent in their relations with people.
- Are cooperative.
- Accept assignments pleasantly.
- Are tactful.
- Accept all types of people.
- Respect the property of other people.
- Have leadership qualities.

4. Communication Skills
Valued workers:
- Ask relevant questions.
- Seek help when needed.
- Notify supervisors of absences and the reason for the absences.
- Clearly express themselves when talking.
- Listen actively and communicate comprehension

5. Task-Related Skills
Valued workers:
- Complete work on time.

- Can follow directions.
- Are not distracting or distractible.
- Work neatly and leave work environment clean and orderly.
- Care for equipment and materials.
- Are accurate.
- Constantly improve their performance.

6. Maturity
Valued workers:
- Work well without supervision.
- Are reliable and dependable.
- Accept responsibility.
- Don't let their personal problems interfere with their work.
- Are willing to perform extra work and work overtime.
- Are always prepared for work.
- Show pride in their work.
- Show initiative.
- Remain calm and self-controlled.
- Accept responsibility for their own behavior including mistakes and successes.
- Demonstrate maturity.
- Evaluate their own work accurately.
- Are patient and tolerate.
- Use time wisely.
- Are assertive when necessary.
- Show self-confidence.

7. Health and Safety Habits
Valued workers:
- Observe safety and sanitation rules.
- Practice good personal hygiene.
- Dress appropriately and are well groomed.
- Are in good health.
- Practice stress management

8. Commitment to the Job
Valued workers:
- Are punctual and have good attendance records.
- Observe all organization policies.
- Consider work more than a job.
- Are interested and enthusiastic
- Obtain relevant continuing education

Modified from TTG Consultants www.ttgconsultants.com
Courtesy David Bowman. Bowman is the Chairman of TTG Consultants/Lincolnshire, a Los Angeles-based, full-service human resource consulting firm with 200 offices worldwide.

evolve

14-1 Complete an interactive business card and brochure exercise.

14-2 To help you in your job search, several examples of brochures and resumés are presented on the Evolve Web site.

Don't forget to study for your certification and licensure exams! Review questions for this chapter are located on Evolve.

■ ■ ■ SUMMARY

This chapter is full of details, regulations, requirements, obligations, paperwork, and responsibilities. Someone once said that the job is not complete until the paperwork is done. Be sure to do the paperwork, and use professional help in business where necessary. Success takes time and does not usually happen overnight. Persistence, flexibility, and determination are your keys to a successful business practice. Keep your goals realistic and keep your professional dreams before you to fuel your motivation to strive for success. Define success not only by the amount of money you make, but also by the value obtained from providing professional therapeutic massage services. Take care of yourself to avoid professional burnout so that you can continue to serve your clients in this wonderful and needed profession.

Both self-employment and working for someone else are viable avenues for success. Each has its pros and cons. It is important to make good decisions about what is best for you. Initially, commitment to being an excellent employee can provide you with valuable experience without all the additional responsibilities of maintaining a business structure. Whatever path you choose, commit to excellence.

Workbook Section

Answers for the Workbook Section for Chapter 14 are provided on p. 776.

■ ■ ■ SHORT ANSWER

1. Why is motivation so important in building a massage business?

_____

_____

_____

2. Why is it important for a massage professional to explore individual strengths and weaknesses when developing a business?

_____

_____

_____

3. What is burnout and how can it be prevented?

_____

_____

_____

4. Why is it important to develop a good resumé?

_____

_____

_____

5. What is a business plan?

_____

_____

_____

6. What are start-up costs?

_____

_____

_____

7. What are the most effective marketing and advertising strategies?

_____

_____

_____

8. What is the importance of a brochure?

_____

_____

_____

9. How do you set fees?

_____

_____

_____

10. What is real time?

_____

_____

_____

11. What are the prospects of obtaining medical insurance reimbursement for personal service massage?

_____

_____

_____

12. What are the three main types of business opportunities available for the massage professional?

_____

_____

_____

13. What is the KISS principle and why is it important?

_____

_____

_____

14. What types of insurance does the massage professional need?

_____

_____

_____

15. What is the importance of the paper trail?

_____

_____

_____

16. Why is the client-practitioner agreement and policy statement so important?

_____

_____

_____

17. Why does everyone, including employees, need to understand business operations?

_____

_____

_____

Workbook Section—cont'd

■ ■ ■ ADDITIONAL ACTIVITY

In developing a client-practitioner agreement and policy statement, you need to be specific about certain areas of information. For each of the sections presented, put in the information that a client needs to know. When you are done, you will have a comprehensive outline to use in creating a booklet.

Use Box 2-6 in the text as a guideline for the information needed. For example, the text says to explain the type of work you provide. You are to list therapeutic massage, reflexology, or whatever it is that you do.

Some of the answers for this section are samples you can use to compare your responses; others are a reiteration of the information that you will need to detail.

■ ■ ■ CLIENT-PRACTITIONER AGREEMENT AND POLICY STATEMENT

All entries should be specific as to the following items.

1. The nature of the service offered:

a. _____

b. _____

c. _____

d. _____

2. Description of the service offered:

a. _____

b. _____

c. _____

d. _____

3. Qualifications of the practitioner:

a. _____

b. _____

4. Client financial and time investment:

a. _____

b. _____

c. _____

d. _____

e. _____

5. Role of the client in health care:

a. _____

b. _____

6. Types of service:

a. _____

b. _____

c. _____

d. _____

e. _____

7. Training and experience:

a. _____

b. _____

c. _____

d. _____

e. _____

8. Appointment policies:

a. _____

b. _____

c. _____

d. _____

e. _____

9. Client and practitioner expectations and informed consent:

a. _____

b. _____

c. _____

d. _____

e. _____

f. _____

g. _____

h. _____

i. _____

10. Fees:

a. _____

b. _____

c. _____

d. _____

e. _____

f. _____

g. _____

h. _____

i. _____

11. Sexual appropriateness:

a. _____

b. _____

12. Recourse policy:

a. _____

b. _____

■ ■ ■ PROBLEM-SOLVING EXERCISES

1. Tom is notified that a client is unhappy with his massage fees and is considering finding another massage professional with lower fees. What steps can Tom take to support his fee structure?

_____

_____

_____

_____

2. Marilyn is having a meeting with a client who she feels may have difficulty understanding the scope of practice of massage. How can she use the client-practitioner agreement and policy statement booklet to help establish professional boundaries and obtain informed consent?

_____

_____

_____

_____

3. Calculate real time required to learn massage. Include actual class time, travel time, homework time, and so on.

_____

_____

_____

_____

4. After graduation Terry begins a private massage practice. Business begins to build slowly but then levels off. Word-of-mouth advertising is not working as well as expected. What steps can Terry take to boost business?

_____

_____

_____

_____

Workbook Section—cont'd

■■■ ASSESS YOUR COMPETENCIES

Now that you have studied this chapter, you should be able to:

1. Determine your personal motivation for pursing a career in therapeutic massage.

2. List the pros and cons of self-employed and employee status.

3. Develop a 5-year business plan.

4. Design a marketing strategy and advertising materials for a massage business.

5. Negotiate rental and employment contracts.

6. Develop a business management and record-keeping system.

7. Pretend you have been asked to present a short course on business practices. Develop a course outline based on this content. Compare with other students in small groups.

■■■ PROFESSIONAL APPLICATION EXERCISES

1. A client calls about receiving a massage. You speak with her on the phone and offer to send her your client policies and procedures booklet. Two weeks later you still have not heard from the prospective client. You make a follow-up telephone call, and the client has specific questions about certain aspects of the policy booklet. This client tells you that a previous massage therapist did not have all these rules. What would you do?

_____
_____
_____
_____

2. Motivation statement: In the space below, list three things that have motivated you to become a massage practitioner.

_____
_____
_____
_____

3. Define the following concepts as they relate directly to you:

_____
_____
_____
_____

Know thyself: _____

Follow your dream: _____

Whatever we believe with emotion and feeling becomes our reality: _____
_____

Believe in your product: _____

Provide a quality product: _____

4. Develop a personal application of methods to prevent burnout. Call it The Burnout Plan or give it some other clever name. List one idea for each of these areas:

_____
_____
_____
_____

Care of physical needs: _____

Support person: _____

Care of spiritual needs: _____

Continuing education: _____

Get-away time: _____

5. The business structure of therapeutic massage takes many forms. Working as a massage employee is different from working as a self-employed massage professional. Choose which approach you plan to pursue and list those areas of the chapter that most directly pertain to your professional development plan.

_____
_____
_____
_____

6. List five business goals. Use the five recommendations for goal setting presented in Box 14-6 as a guide:

1. State goals in the present tense.

2. Make sure your goals are realistic and attainable.

3. Speak positively.

4. Set target deadlines for yourself.

5. Make sure your goals are small steps toward your ultimate plan.

For each goal, circle any portion that meets the first recommendation.

Underline any portion that meets the second recommendation.

Put a box around any portion that meets the third recommendation.

Double underline any portion that meets the fourth recommendation.

Double circle any portion that meets the fifth recommendation.

Example:

I will (1,3) complete this exercise (2,5) within the next 30 minutes (4).

■ ■ ■ **RESEARCH FOR FURTHER STUDY**

1. Compare the business procedures outlined in the text to those of another business operation; identify both similarities and differences in those procedures.

_____

_____

_____

_____

2. The statement "business is business" applies to massage. List resources in your area for further business education, such as community college courses, the Chamber of Commerce, and so forth.

_____

_____

_____

_____

CHAPTER 15

Case Studies

CHAPTER OBJECTIVES

After completing this chapter, the student will be able to perform the following:

- Use clinical reasoning to integrate the information from science studies and this text to complete a comprehensive history, assessment, and care/treatment plan
- Write comprehensive case studies
- Analyze care/treatment plans and offer and justify alternate approaches to care

CHAPTER OUTLINE

This chapter integrates the information from this textbook and your science studies. The recommended textbook for anatomy, physiology, pathology, and kinesiology is *Mosby's Essential Sciences for Therapeutic Massage,* although other texts can be used successfully. Competency in therapeutic massage practice is reflected both in a solid understanding of the content of your science studies and an ability to devise ways to put the information into practical application with individual clients. DVD 1 at the back of this book contains three additional video case studies showing pre-treatment interviews through assessment and session.

The following 20 case studies cover the most common outcome goals of clients. These cases cover at least 80% of the common conditions seen by massage professionals in day and destination spas and in wellness, health, fitness, sports, and medical settings. If you carefully study the process of clinical reasoning exemplified in these cases, you should be able to address almost all other conditions you encounter in your professional practice.

Each case study is presented in the following format:
- Case narrative
- Assessment
- Clinical reasoning
- Treatment plan development

The cases present an integrated approach to goal-oriented and outcome-based individual client care. Each case study attempts to describe real situations with complicating factors in addition to the main issues. Seldom can you use massage to enhance athletic performance or manage low back pain without having to consider other factors, such as coexisting conditions, work activities, stress tolerance, medications, and client compliance. If the client cannot justify the cost or does not show up for regular appointments, even the best treatment plan is meaningless.

The massage work environment is also a factor; massage on a cruise ship is different from massage in a rehabilitation center.

Skills and knowledge are factors as well. What a massage professional with 2 years of experience and an entry level education is able to accomplish is far different from what a professional with 15 years of experience and hundreds of hours of advanced education can achieve.

The varying situations of clients make writing massage protocol recommendations for individual conditions almost impossible. For example, the pathology related to irritable bowel syndrome (IBS) is understood in terms of signs and symptoms; however, the issue becomes how that generic information relates to an individual client who seeks help through massage, especially in light of the multiple influences in a client's life. Therefore recommendations for massage for IBS are very limited; although the information may help a massage professional begin to think about how best to serve an individual client, this is only the beginning. The treatment plan for massage must address each client's entire set of circumstances, not just a single condition the person may have.

These case studies are within the knowledge of a student who has sufficient education to cover the content of this text, along with the recommended science text, and who is able to use clinical reasoning to determine practical applications. The treatment plans have been developed accordingly. Based on many years of professional experience, the author has found that the recommendations provided in the case studies have a good expectation of meeting realistic goals for clients. Covering all the possible situations a client may present is impossible. Each case study has a primary goal, with numerous influences that make clinical reasoning and decision making the only effective ways to evaluate and develop appropriate massage treatment plans.

Research is necessary with every new client. If the client has a diagnosed condition, it is important to look up information about that medical condition and any treatment being done for it. For example, if a client has been burned (as in one of the case studies), the massage professional needs to understand the different categories of burns, the types of scar development, the treatments used to support burn healing, the expected changes in the tissue even after healing, and other related factors.

This type of research begins during the interview with the client, because he or she has useful knowledge, and continues in the fact-gathering portion of the clinical reasoning process. This text and *Mosby's Essential Sciences for Therapeutic Massage* provide information on the most common conditions encountered by massage professionals and serve as important places to begin the research process. In addition to textbooks, medical dictionaries, texts on pharmacology and pathology, and the Internet have been used to gather pertinent information to support appropriate treatment plan development.

For example, a client might come in for massage to reduce aching caused by playing tennis. The client requests massage that has sufficient depth of pressure and drag to address the second, third, and fourth layers of muscle tissue and to increase the pliability of the connective tissue ground substance. If muscle aching were the only condition detected, those methods would be appropriate. However, this same client is taking an anticoagulant medication because of a heart condition—and all of a sudden the entire treatment plan changes. The question becomes, how does the massage professional meet the main goal of the client—reduction of deep muscle aching—without causing bruising or other complications arising from the heart condition and the medication taken to treat it? To further complicate the issue, the client wants only a 30-minute massage. Treatment plan development is not easy! To competently serve the client, the massage professional needs to understand tennis, the training effects that support tennis playing, performance-connected muscle soreness, anticoagulant medication (how and when it is used and the effects and side effects), the client's heart condition and any therapies besides medication that are being used to treat it, and any other pertinent facts. All this information influences the types of massage applications chosen and assists with the decisions on how deep or superficial, how fast or slow, how rhythmic, or how frequent the massage application should be.

The case studies attempt to give examples of ways to meet common but complicated massage client goals in the context of the bigger picture. As you study each case, evaluate it to see whether a variation of the recommended treatment plan might be effective. Also, consider all the other conditions that would benefit from a similar treatment plan. For example, one of the cases discusses a client with asthma; however, a similar massage process would be appropriate for someone with emphysema or chronic bronchitis. Another case describes a client with burn scars, yet surgical scars also are often seen. Yet another case describes a general palliative care massage for a man on vacation. Similar considerations are given to a person who is recovering from surgery or receiving hospice care. The case that presents bone fragility caused by radiation treatment for breast cancer describes a massage application that also is appropriate for an individual with osteoporosis.

When you study the cases, identify the main goal and all the conditions and complicating factors. Identify the overlapping issues that alter the treatment process or the superimposed cautions for massage application. Brainstorm about what you agree with in the presented treatment plan and what you might do differently. Dissect the assessment processes. With the physical assessment information, actually put yourself in the positions described and experience what they feel like. Relate those postures and sensations to the goals of the client and the recommendations for massage application.

CASE 1 GENERALIZED STRESS AND ANXIETY WITH BREATHING PATTERN DISORDER SYMPTOMS

Note: Generalized stress and anxiety with breathing pattern disorder symptoms is the most common stress condition seen by the massage therapist. This condition also is common in pain and fatigue syndromes and in post-traumatic stress disorder.

The client is a 37-year-old male. Friends and the client's primary care physician recommended massage to help him deal with stress-induced physical symptoms. Three weeks ago he had a complete physical because he was required to purchase a life insurance policy to cover the mortgage on a new home. The family had outgrown their smaller home with the recent birth of their third child. Although the physical indicated that all signs were within normal parameters, the man's blood pressure was slightly elevated. It was recommended that he see his family doctor, who did not find anything medically out of the norm but who did notice that the client was impatient and irritable. The client told the doctor that he was not sleeping well and said that he was experiencing some heartburn about once a week, occasional constipation, and neck and shoulder stiffness. He had also gained 10 pounds since his last visit 2 years ago. The doctor felt that stress was the main cause of the man's problems and suggested that he exercise more often, reduce the caffeine in his diet, and lose some of the extra weight. In addition, therapeutic massage was suggested for the muscle stiffness and for relaxation.

The client's administrative assistant, in the advertising firm where he had just been hired to head up a new product promotion deal, gave him the number for the massage practitioner he sees at the local fitness center. The client thought it was convenient to have both the exercise environment and ready access to massage in the same location because he was working 60 hours or more per week and time was a problem.

The client arrives for his first visit. He has never had a massage before, and he is visibly nervous and in a hurry. The massage professional introduces himself and explains that the first massage visit is primarily an initial assessment process that will take 90 minutes. The cost of the first session is $75. Each massage session after the initial session will last 60 minutes, and the cost will be $55 per session. The client states that he understands the arrangements and agrees to the assessment and treatment plan process.

ASSESSMENT

Observation

The massage professional observes the way the client moves about the office, how he breathes, and the rate of his speech. It is evident that the client is feeling rushed, because he looks at his watch many times during the interview and the massage and makes it clear that he has to be at an appointment by 4 PM. The client's shoulders move up and down during breathing. The inhale-to-exhale ratio indicates that the client routinely inhales longer than he exhales. He seems to swallow air when he talks, and he belches a couple of times during the interview. He chews gum, rolls his shoulders back, and often attempts to stretch his neck to the left. He also pulls at his right shoulder and neck area with his left hand. His eyes dart about when he talks, his voice is a bit too loud for the environment, and he cannot sit in the chair for longer than a few minutes without fidgeting or getting up and walking around. When he does sit still, his fists are clenched. He smiles often

and jokes about being stressed. His weight is proportional to his height, although he has early evidence of a middle-age "pot belly." He is right-handed. The client seems a bit uneasy with the idea of a male giving him a massage.

Interview and Goals

The interview process consists of casual conversation supported by a client information form. The client information form and conversation indicate that the client is 37 years old, married, and an advertising executive and that he recently had moved to the city from a small town. The client has three children, ages 9, 6, and 8 months. He has a family history of maturity-onset diabetes, hypertension, and stroke. He has not had any symptoms other than slightly higher than normal blood pressure. He had one surgery as a child for appendicitis. He ran track in high school and college but has not exercised regularly since then. Occasionally he enjoys playing basketball and racquetball but has not found a new group of people with whom to play since moving to the city. He occasionally takes aspirin for a headache and Tums for heartburn. He does not take any vitamins or herbs. He drinks coffee and cola beverages. He does not smoke. He was in a car accident 3 years ago and suffered a mild whiplash-type injury. He has difficulty falling asleep at night. His wife tells him that he tosses and turns in his sleep and grinds his teeth. Currently, he feels tired in the morning, and he gets only about 5 hours of sleep a night. The baby still wakes up at night, and he gets up with the child every other night. When asked about his stress load, he lists the new job, the large mortgage, and the fact that he is now concerned about his health. He says that he has always been a bit high-strung. He also discloses that he is worrying a lot. The long hours required at the new job are making his wife angry, because he is not keeping up with his tasks at home as he did before they moved. He sits at a desk, is on the phone a lot, and has to attend and run business meetings twice a week.

To allow the client to become more comfortable with the idea of a male therapist, the benefits of massage are explained in relation to therapeutic goals rather than relaxation and pleasurable sensation.

The client's main goals for the massage are to sleep better, to be more relaxed and less irritable, to lower his blood pressure, and to reduce the stiffness in his neck and shoulder.

Physical Assessment

Posture

Right shoulder is high and anteriorly rotated. Head is slightly forward, and lumbar curve is slightly flattened. Right leg is moderately externally rotated, and right arm is slightly internally rotated. Left knee is hyperextended.

Gait

Stride and arm swing are shortened on the right, and client rolls to the outside of the left foot during the heel strike and toe-off phase.

Range of Motion

Lateral bending of the neck to the left is reduced to 30 degrees. Rotation is equal on both sides but painful during the last few degrees when rotation is to the right. External rotation of the right arm is limited to 75 degrees and internal rotation of the right hip to 40 degrees. Trunk extension is limited to 15 degrees. Eversion of the left foot is slightly limited. Ribs are resistant to being sprung, more so on the left, indicating rigidity in the thorax.

Palpation

Near Touch. Upper shoulder on the right is warm.

Skin. Skin on the right shoulder, pectoralis bilaterally, lateral ribs, neck, and lumbar region has damp areas that redden when stroked. Skin of upper chest bilaterally, right shoulder, and entire lumbar region is taut. Tissue is restricted inferiorly and diagonally to the left on chest and produces a smaller skin fold in lumbar area on the left.

Superficial Connective Tissue. Neck tissue shows mild edema and a sensation of bogginess, as well as a bind resistance to movement toward the left. Connective tissues of the lumbar area and both of the lateral legs palpate shortened and thick. Surgical scar on the abdomen appears bound to underlying structures when moved.

Vessels and Lymph Nodes. No palpable differences.

Muscles. Lumbar and posterior thorax muscles in the second layer are tight but long. Pectoralis major on the right is short. Occipital base muscles are painful to moderate pressure. Abdominals and gluteus maximus are soft and reduced in tone. Hamstrings are short bilaterally. Gastrocnemius and soleus on the left are tight and short. Deep lateral hip rotators on the right are tight and short. Subscapularis on the right is short, and infraspinatus is tight but long. Anterior serratus palpates bilaterally as tender, with tender points corresponding to damp, red areas on the skin. Pectoralis minor on the right is short. Psoas is short bilaterally. Muscles of mastication are tight and short.

Tendons. Subscapular tendon on the right is tender to moderate pressure.

Deep Fascia. Lumbar dorsal fascia, iliotibial band, and abdominal fascia are thick and have reduced pliability.

Ligaments. No apparent changes.

Joints. No observable changes, but some heat, edema, and pain with moderate palpation pressure are noted in the right glenohumeral joint.

Bones. No apparent changes.

Abdominal Viscera. Abdomen is generally soft. Some rigidity is present in the large intestine at the splenic flexure.

Body Rhythms. Heart rate fluctuates from 65 to 80 beats per minute. Breathing rhythm is fast and uneven and does not appear entrained to heart rhythm. Peripheral circulation is good and even. Craniosacral rhythm is fast and uneven, similar to breathing pattern.

Muscle Testing

Strength

Pectoralis muscles and adductors muscles test strong, with inhibition in the gluteus medius, which tests weak. Muscles that retract the scapula are weak. Gluteus maximus bilaterally tests weak.

Neurologic Balance

Antagonists to pectoralis and internal shoulder rotators are inhibited. Abdominals and gluteus are inhibited.

Gait

Shoulder and hip flexors on the right are not inhibited in the normal reflex pattern. When arm flexors are activated, hip flexors do not inhibit as they should.

INTERPRETATION AND TREATMENT PLAN DEVELOPMENT

Clinical Reasoning

What Are the Facts?

The main contributing factors are generalized stress with episodes of anxiety and breathing pattern disorder symptoms. (These conditions are discussed in Chapters 4, 5, and 13 of this text.) To work effectively with a client who has these conditions, the massage professional must research them. The general experience of stress is sympathetic dominance in the autonomic nervous system when fight-or-flight or fear mechanisms are detrimental instead of beneficial. When the energy is rallied for these high-activity demands but the body stays still, such as with this client, the physiologic activity manifests internally, resulting in the symptoms of increased heart rate, high blood pressure, digestive disturbances, and changes in breathing. The muscles also assume either the flight or attack position, but movement does not occur, therefore generalized tension builds. When the respiratory mechanism is functioning with auxiliary breathing muscles, oxygen intake may exceed the physical demand, and sympathetic arousal occurs. A vicious cycle begins, with internal and external stimuli increasing sympathetic arousal, which increases breathing and muscle tension, which in turn increases sympathetic arousal. Anxiety with an increase in vigilance (looking for what is wrong) perpetuates. Mood is altered, and physical symptoms manifest in a strange collection of seemingly unrelated symptoms. Because a breathing pattern disorder is a functional process (i.e., the activity is normal but occurs at inappropriate times) no diagnosable pathology is present. The most common and measurable symptom is elevated blood pressure, which fluctuates situationally, unlike with primary hypertension, in which the blood pressure is constantly high. Because physical distress symptoms are present but medical tests indicate nothing wrong, people become frustrated. Management of a breathing pattern disorder requires that the individual make lifestyle changes. However, because of the stress syndrome and the sympathetic activation, people often look for causal factors outside themselves and can become irritable and restless. This is a very common pattern presented by many clients seeking massage.

For this client, stress is professional, personal, and financial. Time urgency is apparent. The client is generally in good health. He has mildly elevated blood pressure that is not being treated medically. There is evidence of sympathetic autonomic nervous system arousal, constipation, heartburn, disrupted sleep, and upper chest breathing, and a history of high-pressure jobs. The client talks fast and is restless, admits to being irritable, grinds his teeth at night, and chews gum during the day. This physiologic state is supported by an intake of caffeine. Assessment indicates shortening and tenderness in the auxiliary breathing muscles, with the beginning of second-degree functional stress in both the posture (stability) and phasic (movement) muscles.

What Are the Possibilities Both in Function and Dysfunction and the Massage Intervention Options?

The client seems to display breathing pattern disorder symptoms in response to sustained sympathetic arousal. The client has sufficient postural distortion to interfere with the mechanics of breathing, which would cause the symptoms and perpetuate the increase in sympathetic activity.

The client's activity levels are not in balance with the level of sympathetic nervous system arousal. Increased aerobic exercise with a stretching program would be appropriate.

The client is clearly stressed and has some mild anxiety. Causal factors could be the physical changes in posture resulting from extended sitting and talking on the phone, the decrease in physical activity, or the buildup of internal pressure from work and family. If this is primarily a cognitive problem, referral to a psychologist is indicated. If the indication is more physical, massage and exercise would be helpful. It is likely that all elements are involved.

Possibilities:

1. The massage intervention can be structured to deal with the postural alterations and the shortening in muscle and connective tissue structures that are causing the breathing dysfunction.
2. Massage would support a moderate exercise program by managing postexercise muscle soreness.
3. The client should experience some benefit; however, it is likely that some sort of cognitive or psychological intervention is needed. A combination of the two approaches would be most satisfactory.

What Are the Logical Outcomes of Each Possible Intervention Option?

Massage application should reduce the sympathetic arousal, but the effect would be temporary. Adding exercise and stretching would prolong the effects of massage. The breathing function would improve, and the breathing pattern disorder symptoms should diminish, but these results also would be temporary. The client would need to change his stress perception or reduce the stress load for symptom reversal. Massage application could help manage the physical stress response if lifestyle changes are deemed impossible at this time or if counseling is avoided. Massage would have to be given often—twice a week at minimum—to be effective.

Cost and time commitments would be required for all interventions. Massage alone twice a week would require 4 hours of total time commitment (massage and travel time), and the cost would be $110 per week. The financial burden for this client is not a concern for a short-term intervention process, but the time commitment is. If the client seeks counseling, massage could be reduced to once a week. The time would be about the same, but the cost would be higher for the counseling appointments. Some of the cost for counseling would be deferred by insurance reimbursement.

What Is the Impact on the People Involved for Each Massage Intervention Option?

The massage therapist is familiar with dealing with these conditions because the fitness center is affiliated with the local hospital's wellness and prevention program. The physician is favorable. The wife is a bit resistant, because the increase in exercise and massage further reduces the client's time at home. If his mood improves, she would be more supportive. The client is supportive of exercise and willing to try massage but is resistant to any type of counseling.

DECISION MAKING AND TREATMENT PLAN DEVELOPMENT

Quantifiable Goals

1. Reduce shortening of breathing muscles by 75%
2. Reduce postural distortion by 50% and increase range of motion in restricted areas by 75%
3. Increase connective tissue pliability by reducing bind in short areas by 75%
4. Reduce edema in shoulder by 90%
5. Normalize blood pressure to appropriate range (120-130/80-85)

Qualifiable Goals

The distressful stress symptoms will diminish, resulting in improved sleep and reduced irritability at work and at home. The client will have a more relaxed demeanor, resulting in improved relationships at work and home.

The goal is to calm the sympathetic autonomic nervous system and introduce a normal balance between the parasympathetic and sympathetic functions. When this is achieved, the client's sleep should improve as a result of a drop in cortisol levels, and tossing and turning should diminish because muscle tension will have lessened. The teeth grinding and need to chew gum during the day should decline, which would reduce the strain in the mastication and neck muscles. Breathing should move from an upper chest breathing pattern to more normal diaphragmatic breathing, with the inhale phase being shorter than the exhale phase in a ratio of 1:4. As the auxiliary breathing muscles relax, posture improves, and air swallowing declines, the belching and heartburn should improve. The neck and shoulder stiffness should diminish when these muscles are no longer used for breathing. Mood should also improve.

Appointments would be scheduled in the evening so that the client could go home and go to bed.

Treatment Regimen

This is a therapeutic change process in the short term with realistic expectations of a condition management treatment program for the long term.

It is decided that the client will join the lunchtime basketball game for local businessmen 3 days a week. He will commit to a massage twice a week for 6 weeks and then re-evaluate, hoping to reduce the massage frequency to once a week.

A general full-body massage session will be used, with a depth of pressure sufficient to elicit the relaxation response and generate an increase in endorphins and serotonin. All massage manipulations will be used except friction and tapotement, because friction causes pain, and tapotement is generally a stimulating method. The rhythm will be slow and even, meeting the client's body rhythms and then slowing over the course of the session. The direction of massage will be primarily toward the heart but with changes as necessary to address the connective tissue bind. Lymphatic drainage methods will be used on the right shoulder. Muscle energy methods will be used, especially to address the eye and neck reflexes and to lengthen all short muscles identified during the assessment.

Because the major tension is in the neck and shoulders, having the client roll his eyes in large circles or his head in small circles while broad-based compression is applied to the tender areas, especially the occipital base muscles, will be helpful. Kneading and skin rolling with myofascial techniques, coupled with lymphatic drainage, will increase pliability in the areas of thick and short connective tissues. Active trigger points in muscles will be addressed with the least invasive measures possible in order to reduce the guarding response and pain behaviors, because pain increases sympathetic arousal. Positional release will be the primary choice and will be applied to the indicated areas in the serratus anterior and intercostal muscles.

Muscles that are inhibited will be encouraged to function through the use of limited tapotement (i.e., not so much as to arouse the nervous system) at the origin and insertion of these muscles.

Range-of-motion methods will focus on reducing the internal rotation of the right arm and the external rotation of the left leg. The integrated muscle energy methods will be the primary application combining these patterns so that the muscle imbalances can be treated in sequence. The abdominal massage sequence will ease constipation.

Teaching the client simple breathing and relaxation exercises, as described in Chapter 13, is appropriate.

CASE 2 MUSCLE TENSION HEADACHE

A 26-year-old female is in good health except for frequent headaches that radiate pain from the back of her skull around her ears and over her eyes. Migraine and cluster headaches have been ruled out. The diagnosis is muscle tension headaches. Because common over-the-counter analgesics such as aspirin and acetaminophen bother her stomach, she is seeking an alternative to manage the pain. Because no medical reason has been found for the headaches, they are assumed to be related to stress. They do not follow any cyclic pattern. A relationship to the menstrual cycle has not been indicated.

The client has a temporary job as a waitress while she finishes college. She spends a lot of time sitting, reading, and working at the computer. She notices increased tension in her neck, shoulders, and lower back when she has to spend a lot of time with her studies. She swims three times a week for exercise and was a cheerleader in high school. She is careful with her diet. She has a moderate intake of caffeine and alcohol, and she smokes. She is not under any medical care.

She has tried chiropractic care, with limited success, and often experiences a headache right after an adjustment. She has heard that massage can help these types of headaches. The client has completed an informed consent process and has agreed to treatment.

ASSESSMENT

Observation

The client is nearsighted and wears glasses. She repositions her glasses often, and she squints in the bright light. She is very polite and soft-spoken. She appears frustrated and tired of the inconvenience of the headaches. She is neatly groomed and very organized; she provides a list of all the treatments that have been tried for the headaches, including a food diary and schedules attempting to identify the cause of the headaches. Her weight is normal for her height. She has long, thick hair that she wears in a ponytail.

Interview and Goals

The client's history reveals that she has had headaches for as long as she can remember. She has a headache severe enough to interfere with daily activities about 10 days out of a month. The headaches last about 12 hours, and the pain is a 7 on a scale of 1 to 10 (1 being slight, 10 being extreme). She does not remember any injury or surgery or any childhood diseases other than the normal ones. She had the headaches before cheerleading. She generally ignores the headaches, but they are becoming draining. The family history provides no insight. There is a family history of cancer. She wore braces for 3 years and recently had them removed. She has worn glasses and has had long hair since her early teens. She admits to being a perfectionist.

Her goals for the massage are to reduce the frequency and intensity of the headaches.

Physical Assessment

Posture

No obvious postural asymmetry.

Gait

No obvious gait distortions.

Range of Motion

Slightly limited in all directions in the neck with moderate reduction of capital flexion. Temporomandibular joint (TMJ) opens only to two fingers' width (three is normal).

Palpation

Near Touch. Neck near the occipital base and the lower back are warm.

Skin. All areas are normal except for goose bumps and dampness at the occipital base and lower back. Tissue texture is symmetric and normal. Unable to lift a skin fold over the entire length of the spinal column.

Superficial Connective Tissue. Superior and inferior binding of connective tissue is present at the occipital base, sacrum, forehead, and calves.

Vessels and Lymph Nodes. Normal

Muscles. Tender points are noted in the masseter, frontalis, temporalis, and occipital base muscles. Moderate pressure on these points results in pain that mimics the headaches. Neck extensors are short and tight. Surface muscle tone seems generally high. Calf muscles are tight and short bilaterally.

Tendons. Normal

Deep Fascia. Fascia from the skull to the sacrum binds. Scalp is tightly bound to the skull.

Ligaments. Normal

Joints. TMJ palpates tender to mild pressure and has reduced range of motion.

Bones. Normal

Abdominal Viscera. Normal

Body Rhythms. Rhythmic but fast

Muscle Testing

Strength

Normal except that head and neck extensors are overly strong. Head and neck flexors are inhibited.

Neurologic Balance

Tonic neck reflexes and eye-righting reflexes are overactive, consequently limb and back extensors do not inhibit when client looks down toward navel.

Gait

Normal except that head seems to be held stiffly when client walks.

INTERPRETATION AND TREATMENT PLAN DEVELOPMENT

Clinical Reasoning

What Are the Facts?

Muscle tension headaches are a common and recurring problem for many people. They are benign, although all other causes of headaches need to be ruled out. The headaches occur because muscle and connective tissue exerts pressure on the nerves and blood vessels in the face, skull, neck, and shoulders. Trigger point activity that refers pain into the headache pain pattern is common. Individuals who are light sensitive and/or who have visual problems that result in squinting are prone to muscle tension headaches. Heavy headgear or hair that is heavy or styled tightly against the skull presses on pain-sensitive structures. Stress that causes sympathetic arousal, resulting in the attack posture, is a common contributor to muscle tension headaches. Pain of any type can cause the muscles of the head, neck, and face to tighten and can perpetuate muscle tension headaches; in this way, a vicious cycle develops. Headaches often "layer," so that even if a migraine is the primary headache type, the pain of the migraine causes an accompanying muscle tension headache.

Postural strain, such as sitting at a computer or driving, or static positions, such as reading a book, result in muscle tension and pressure on pain-sensitive structures, causing a muscle tension headache. Postural strain that attempts to keep the eyes level affects the righting and ocular pelvic reflexes of the neck, eyes, and trunk. Head, neck, and torso flexors should facilitate and head, neck and torso extensors inhibit when the eyes and head move down toward the midline of the body; the process should reverse when the eyes and head move up, as in looking at the ceiling. Looking right and rotating right cause the muscles on the right to contract concentrically and the muscles on the left to be inhibited and in eccentric function, and vice versa for the left side.

Upper chest breathing is often a contributing factor, because the auxiliary breathing muscles can cause headaches if they are tense or short or have trigger points.

Low back tension and lower leg tension are also common and need to be addressed in conjunction with the more obvious muscle tension pattern near the head. Connective tissue bind from the occipital base to the sacrum can fix the head, putting pressure on pain-sensitive structures. Poor air quality and noisy environments with uneven or fluctuating lighting can cause headaches. Smoking often contributes to muscle tension headaches.

A muscle tension headache is usually a functional condition, and no obvious pathologic condition can be diagnosed. With the client in this case, no pathologic reason has been found for the headaches. However, stress is implicated; the client is a self-admitted perfectionist, which supports the stress diagnosis. Shortening of the fascial connection between the skull, occipital base, and sacrum is present. The muscles of the base of the skull and the face, as well as the muscles of mastication, are tender to moderate pressure and reproduce headache pain. The head and neck extensors are short, as are the calf muscles.

What Are the Possibilities Both in Function and Dysfunction and the Massage Intervention Options?

Eye strain, the weight and position of the glasses, and the heavy hair in a ponytail all may be contributing causal factors. Eye strain from extended sitting, coupled with the stress of studying, could be contributing to the low back and calf tension.

The clenched jaw and tight arms and legs are components of the attack posture. This posture is part of the sympathetic response and could be part of the symptoms. The noisy environment of the restaurant where the client works could be making the situation worse. Smoking is also a contributing factor. Muscle tension probably is interfering with circulation. No one significant factor appears to be causing the headache pattern; rather, the cause may be the cumulative effect of many small contributing factors, which would explain the random pattern of occurrence. If stress and strain reach a certain level, the headache occurs, such as when the client wears a tight ponytail, has to read in bright light, smokes more than normal, or is stressed by a tight work schedule or a school paper due. The cumulative effect is a headache.

Possibilities:
1. Massage and a stretching program, such as yoga, would be helpful.
2. The heavy hair, eye strain, and ill-fitting glasses may be causes, and referral to the client's optometrist is prudent. A different hair style would reduce the weight and strain on the scalp and the muscles in that area.

What Are the Logical Outcomes of Each Possible Intervention Option?

Some soft tissue factors make muscle tension headaches likely, and these can be addressed with massage. If the muscle tension is reduced and the connective tissue bind is normalized (conditions noted in the assessment), more external stress may be required to cause the headaches.

Yoga-type activity would provide stress reduction, help retrain breathing, stretch short muscles, and introduce pliability to the binding connective tissue structures.

A change in glasses to improve the client's eyesight may diminish a causal factor, as might a new hair style.

Cost and time are issues. The client is on a limited budget and very busy. Weekly massage sessions would be the minimum required for measurable results.

What Is the Impact on the People Involved for Each Massage Intervention Option?

The client does not want to cut her hair but is willing to make her ponytail less tight. She will see the optometrist for a checkup. She is not interested in yoga. She will get massages and seems excited about the possibilities for improvement. She is concerned about finances and can afford only two massage sessions a month.

DECISION MAKING AND TREATMENT PLAN DEVELOPMENT

Quantifiable Goals

1. Reduce headache pain by 75%
2. Reduce frequency and duration of headaches by 50%

Qualifiable Goal

The headaches will decline in number, reducing interference with the client's daily life activities.

Treatment Regimen

Therapeutic Change/Condition Management

The massage sessions will be standard 60-minute appointments at $40 per session, every other week, with time allocated to teach the client self-massage methods. Full-body relaxation massage, using sufficient depth of pressure to increase serotonin and endorphins and produce a parasympathetic effect, will be the main intervention. The primary methods will be compression, gliding, and kneading. Myofascial methods will be used on the areas of connective tissue bind, primarily in the occipital and lumbar areas. The short calf muscles will be addressed with muscle energy methods to lengthen the muscles. The trigger point areas that refer into the headache pain pattern will be addressed with positional release methods, if possible, and with tense-and-relax or reciprocal inhibition and lengthening if necessary. The pulsed muscle energy or integrated muscle energy method will be used for areas more resistant to lengthening. Trigger point areas that do not respond to the more conservative methods will be addressed with direct compression and stretching of the local tissue, which will be achieved by introducing bending and torsion forces into the affected soft tissue structure. Massage of the face, scalp, and neck is necessary.

The client will be taught self-positional release on the areas of trigger point activity. She will be shown how to apply muscle energy methods, particularly using the position of the eyes or the head to activate a tensing or inhibition of muscles. The main self-help method demonstrated will be to move the soft tissue area restricted by shortened muscles in the position of the tension and then to roll the eyes in slow circles. With this technique, the muscles will move into a facilitated and inhibited neurologic pattern. The area then will be gently stretched when the breath is exhaled.

Breathing exercises, as described in Chapter 13, will also be taught as self-help.

CASE 3 GENERALIZED PAIN SYNDROME: SUBCLINICAL FIBROMYALGIA

The client is a 46-year-old female. She is experiencing generalized muscle and joint aching. She has had symptoms for 5 years, but this past year has been the most difficult. The pain is not constant and fluctuates in intensity and duration. Bad days are beginning to outnumber good days. Medical testing has not revealed any pathologic condition. She has seen a rheumatologist and does not quite fit the profile for fibromyalgia syndrome, although she has many of the symptoms and some of the history. Over-the-counter pain medication upsets her stomach.

The client had a severe bout of flu and pneumonia 8 years ago. She works as an administrative assistant for a demanding boss. She has a random work schedule that often involves working into the evening. She has been with the company for 15 years and worked her way up to her current position. She enjoys the challenges of her job. She has been divorced for 7 years and has two children, who are both in college. Her finances are stable. She is 25 pounds overweight and does not exercise. She does not smoke. She is susceptible to upper respiratory infections. Her sleep and eating cycles are erratic. She was active in community playhouse musicals for many years but has not been participating for the past 12 months because of job demands. She still sings in a community choir.

Her last physical was 6 weeks ago. She is within normal parameters on all tests except thyroid function; her thyroid-stimulating hormones were a bit elevated, indicating that there may be a thyroid hormone deficiency. Currently she is not being treated with medication, but she will be retested in 6 months. She is menopausal but still has an occasional menstrual cycle marked by sporadic, heavy bleeding. She is not undergoing hormone replacement therapy at this time. She has mild stress and urinary incontinence. The excess weight is a concern, as is her bone density to some degree. A bone scan indicated some bone loss but not sufficient for a diagnosis of osteoporosis. Her cholesterol level is a bit high but still in the normal range.

Her physician recommended an exercise and weight loss program and referred her to the affiliated fitness center, where she saw a brochure for therapeutic massage.

ASSESSMENT

Observation

The client is restless, changes position often, and sighs frequently. Movement in the shoulders is noted during normal relaxed breathing. She is neatly groomed and wears high heels. She has a pleasant, even speaking voice. She provides extensive detail in answering all questions. She asks many questions, looking for specific answers. She looks bloated, with indications of swelling in the extremities, and she is more apple shaped than pear shaped.

Interview and Goals

The client does not drink much water; she usually drinks tea or juice. Her client information form shows a family history of autoimmune problems. She has a sister with multiple sclerosis, and her grandmother had lupus. The client had one vaginal birth, and the other child was born by emergency cesarean section because of a breech presentation. She takes a multivitamin but no other medications. She has tried Vioxx for pain, but it did not help. She indicates that she is stressed but not overwhelmed. She gets a cold every year in the fall, has intestinal gas, and has chronic pain in her muscles and joints. She is restless more than fatigued. She does not participate in exercise and says that she really hates it. She has always been clumsy. She enjoys singing. On the 1 to 10 pain scale (1 being slight, 10 being extreme), she indicates that her pain is usually a 6 with episodes of 8.

Her goals for the massage are to manage the pain and to relax.

Physical Assessment

Posture

Mild lordosis is present, likely functional from the wearing of high heels. Protruding abdomen, moderate forward head position, and elevated and winged scapula on the left are noted. Shoulders are bilaterally rounded forward, with both arms internally rotated. Legs are externally rotated, more so on the right. Calves are short, and most of the body weight is carried on the balls of the feet.

Gait

Counterbalancing movement of the arms is awkward and reduced. Hips move up and down instead of in a rotational pattern. Most movement occurs at the hips, and client has a short stride. Weight is carried on the ball of the foot, with little heel strike.

Range of Motion

Client is stiff, and her movements are awkward. External rotation and horizontal abduction of the arms are limited by 25%, and dorsiflexion is reduced by 50% bilaterally. Muscle guarding is apparent during passive range of motion, and the client cannot let the body areas go limp.

Palpation

Near Touch. No unusual areas noted.

Skin. Skin feels dry and pliability is reduced, with binding; skin will not easily lift in a skin fold throughout the body, more so in the lumbar area. Skin shows a reddening, histamine response with light stroking. The effect is most apparent in fleshy areas and less apparent around the joints.

Superficial Connective Tissue. Generally feels boggy and shows nonpitting edema. Edema is more apparent in the legs, which show slight pitting.

Vessels and Lymph Nodes. Normal

Muscles. Surface layer muscles generally feel soft and nonresilient. Abdominals and gluteus maximus bilaterally are flaccid and long. Second and third layers of muscles (stabilizers and fixators) are short, but client is intolerant of moderate pressure and tenses surface muscle layer so that palpation is difficult. Client is deconditioned as a result of a sedentary lifestyle. Postural muscles (layer three) in lumbar and cervical regions are short. Calves are short, with connective tissue changes resulting in fibrosis, increased tissue density, and ropiness. Muscles of the forearm are tender to moderate-pressure palpation, probably from computer work.

Tendons. Tender points activated by moderate pressure are common in musculotendinous regions bodywide.

Deep Fascia. Occipital and cervical fascia, lumbar dorsal fascia, and plantar fasciae are short and bind in all directions.

Ligaments. Joint structure generally is stiff.

Joints. End-feel of joints is stiff and binding. Client guards all range of motion and cannot relax to allow passive range of motion. Light palpation over sacroiliac (SI) and sternoclavicular joints is surprisingly painful.

Bones. Palpation is normal, but caution is indicated because of loss of bone density.

Abdominal Viscera. Difficult to palpate. Surface of abdomen is lumpy. Deeper palpation is uncomfortable to client.

Body Rhythms. Slightly slow and sluggish. Rhythms seem out of sync with each other. Breathing is labored.

Muscle Testing

Strength

Client resists muscle testing, indicating that it hurts to maintain the testing positions. She attempts to cooperate but feels everything is weak and sore. Calves and pectoralis muscles are too strong, with inhibition in antagonist patterns.

Neurologic Balance and Gait

Unable to perform.

INTERPRETATION AND TREATMENT PLAN DEVELOPMENT

Clinical Reasoning

What Are the Facts?

A strain on the adaptive capacity of the body can manifest as pain syndromes. Generalized pain syndromes are multicausal, and good medical care is required to rule out serious underlying causes. Once a diagnosis of chronic pain syndrome has been made, pain medication and muscle relaxers are often prescribed; however, these are not very successful for long-term treatment. Symptoms that go undiagnosed are especially difficult to treat. In this case the client has not been diagnosed with fibromyalgia, but she displays many of the symptoms. Fibromyalgia is a condition characterized by aching and pain in the muscles, tendons, and joints all over the body but especially along the spine. Measurable changes in body chemistry and function occur in some people who have fibromyalgia, and these changes may be responsible for certain symptoms. However, fibromyalgia is not associated with muscle, nerve, or joint injury; inadequate muscle repair; or any serious bodily damage or disease. Also, people who have fibromyalgia are not at greater risk for any other musculoskeletal disease.

The pain of fibromyalgia usually seems worse when a person is trying to relax and is less noticeable during busy activities or exercise. Other symptoms are often associated with the pain, including sleep disturbance, depression, daytime tiredness and headaches, alternating diarrhea and constipation, numbness and tingling in the hands and feet, feelings of weakness, memory difficulties, and dizziness.

The exact cause of fibromyalgia is unknown. However, many theories attempt to explain why people develop fibromyalgia. Stress contributes to the onset of the condition. Other possible causes include conscious or subconscious tension, disordered sleep, abnormal production of pain-related chemicals in the nervous system, deficient production of growth hormone, a lower pain threshold, a heightened perception of pain, and tenderness in certain areas, such as the upper back and forearms.

The onset of fibromyalgia occurs when the stress in a person's life is prominent. Stress often results in disturbed sleep patterns, a lack of restful sleep, and disruption of the production of chemicals necessary to control or regulate pain. Physical and emotional factors may also contribute to the onset of fibromyalgia. For example, a physical illness (e.g., an infection) can cause changes in body chemistry that lead to pain and sleeplessness.

This case describes a typical history pattern of fibromyalgia, including a bad bout of flu and the accumulation of internal and external stressors over many years. Cumulative trauma and age-related changes, deconditioning from lack of exercise, and a reduction in hardiness are contributing factors.

Hormone changes are common. Irregular sleep and eating patterns disrupt the body's sleep/wake cycle. The pain is usually the aching, somatic type. Often any increase in activity results in increased pain over the next 48 hours. This increases the likelihood that the client will remain inactive, which contributes to the problem.

What Are the Possibilities Both in Function and Dysfunction and the Massage Intervention Options?

The client may be slowly deteriorating toward full-blown fibromyalgia. Thyroid deficiency or menopausal symptoms also may be present.

Possibilities:

1. General constitutional massage may be helpful, with caution regarding the intensity because the pain can be aggravated by massage that is too aggressive.
2. Application of reflexology and polarity would be appropriate and would have little likelihood of increasing the current symptoms.
3. Lymphatic drainage massage is indicated, and light pressure and rhythmic application are appropriate. The deeper muscles that are short and the connective tissue changes should be addressed once pain tolerance has increased and the client can tolerate deeper pressure.
4. An exercise program was recommended by the physician. Hydrotherapy, with a focus on alternating hot and cold applications, is supported both for relaxation and for hardening. Mineral salt soaks can alleviate some edema and aching. Massage would be needed regularly, at least once a week.

What Are the Logical Outcomes of Each Possible Intervention Option?

Exercise and massage, with the integration of reflexology and polarity, may increase the pain symptoms in the short term. Hydrotherapy application of alternating hot and cold with mineral salt soaks would be well tolerated if introduced gradually. Massage is less likely to cause discomfort if given carefully. The client is able to schedule the time and has the finances.

What Is the Impact on the People Involved for Each Massage Intervention Option?

The client is not supportive of exercise, and compliance does not seem likely. She is lonely and indicates that the idea of massage and how it feels is comforting to her. She says she would do hydrotherapy but does not like to be cold.

The massage professional realizes that the client has implicated boundary issues and that this is a long-term professional commitment. Without some exercise, the condition will not improve. The client needs to be encouraged to work with a medical exercise professional to support compliance with an exercise program.

DECISION MAKING AND TREATMENT PLAN DEVELOPMENT

Quantifiable Goals

1. Reduce aching pain from a 6 to a 4 on a 1 to 10 pain scale
2. Reduce constant aching to intermediate aching with more good days per week (4 good and 3 bad)

Qualifiable Goals

The client will be able to perform daily living and work activities more efficiently and participate in a moderate exercise program without intensifying the current symptoms.

Treatment Regimen

Condition management will be pursued, with moderate applications effecting therapeutic change in a three-stage treatment plan.

Some clear soft tissue dysfunctions must be addressed. The lordosis, forward head, rounded shoulders with internally rotated arms, and immobile pelvis with externally rotated legs strain the adaptive mechanisms. This posture puts extreme pressure on the SI joints and neck stabilizers and restricts the mobility of the thorax, resulting in shallow, upper chest breathing. The shortened calf muscles and plantar fasciae, the result of wearing high heels for so many years, have bodywide implications. Reduced lymphatic movement, strain caused by maintenance of posture, control of postural sway, and restricted breathing all were indicated in the assessment. All these factors must be addressed, but caution is necessary. This client, although not sick, seems to have reached the end of her adaptive capacity. Therapeutic change must be introduced very gradually. Slowing the degeneration and managing the current symptoms are initially most important. Attempting too many adaptations likely would make matters worse.

The three phases of the treatment plan are as follows:

- *Phase One:* The first stage will focus on general relaxation and hyperstimulation analgesia for pain control. The duration of the massage will not exceed 45 minutes. The massage will be rhythmic and repetitive, using primarily gliding and kneading, with pressure and depth that the client identifies as pleasurable. Parasympathetic activation and an increase in serotonin are the goals, therefore the massage will have a compressive quality but will not cause pain. Lymphatic drainage and circulation enhancement are appropriate. Simple polarity methods will be used to comfort the client and support relaxation. Foot massage, with reflexology points in mind, will have a more intense quality, bordering on "good hurt," in an attempt to encourage endorphins and other endogenous pain-killing chemical activity, as well as hyperstimulation analgesia and counterirritation. Localization of this type of intensity to the feet prevents any other delayed muscle soreness from developing. The client will be encouraged to drink water; take hot, relaxing Epsom salt baths; and be consistent with the mild water aerobics program set up by the exercise physiologist. This phase could last 12 weeks.

■ *Phase Two:* Massage pressure and depth will increase to address the short muscles and introduce the concept of "good hurt" into the areas that are short and tight in the second and third layer of muscles. Myofascial methods will address the areas of connective tissue bind. Muscle energy, primarily positional release, will be used on tender points identified by the deeper massage. Foot massage of sufficient pressure and intensity to cause a "good hurt" will continue. The client should be only mildly sore the next day and only in a couple of areas. The exercise program will be supported by a focus on water aerobics and mild training with light weights. Self-help will include a splash of cold water after a warm bath and daily cool water foot soaks. The temperature of the foot baths should be decreased to cold within a 2-week period. This phase could last up to 12 weeks.

■ *Phase Three:* The goal now is to introduce small, incremental structural and functional shifts to the postural distortion. The massage quality will increase in depth of pressure and drag to address the connective tissue bind in the deeper postural muscle layers and the underlying muscle tension. The massage will remain relaxing, rhythmic, and pleasurable but will take on the quality of an adjunct to the exercise program. Muscle energy methods, particularly the integrated methods, can address bodywide muscle interaction patterns. More aggressive connective tissue methods to restore pliability will be introduced with muscle energy methods and muscle lengthening, but this must be coupled with strengthening of the weakened and inhibited muscle patterns. Trigger point activity, particularly in the muscle belly of concentrically short muscles, can be gradually addressed one area per session. Alternating hot and cold showers, beginning with hot and ending with cold, should replace the baths and soaks. This phase will last 12 to 24 weeks.

The entire process could take 1 year.

If the client does not maintain an exercise program, condition management would be more appropriate treatment and would level out at the first phase as the long-term plan. After 6 months the less invasive applications described in phase two could be introduced to see how the client responds. Without a corresponding exercise program, phase three would be too aggressive.

CASE 4 NECK AND SHOULDER PAIN WITH LIMITED RANGE OF MOTION

The client is a 34-year-old male. He is experiencing radiating pain into his left scapula and upper deltoid and down his left arm to the elbow. The pain was sudden in onset. The pain quality is aching and throbbing. It grows worse as the day progresses and is interfering with his sleep because he cannot find a comfortable position. He also complains of a stiff neck, especially if he tries to turn his head to the right. This has been occurring for about 6 months. He was referred to chiropractic

care by his medical doctor. The chiropractor has had limited success and suspects muscle involvement. Heat provides temporary relief, and cold makes the condition worse. Aspirin helps, as do muscle relaxers, but medications are not the best long-term solution.

The client is a truck driver. He is right-handed but drives primarily with his left hand. Three years ago he took a hard fall while riding his mountain bike. He suffered a mild concussion and remembers that his neck was stiff for about a month. He had an upper respiratory infection and a severe cough a month before the current pain symptoms began.

He is in good health, active, and exercises regularly. He eats a moderate diet and does not abuse caffeine or alcohol. He does not smoke. He is single, financially stable, and available for appointments on a regular basis.

The massage professional shares the office with the referring chiropractor.

ASSESSMENT

Observation

Client frequently rubbed the left side of his neck, left shoulder, and upper arm in a line pattern that followed the brachial plexus distribution. He is frustrated with his situation but seemed happy in general. He joked about his condition and that it was an excuse to get a massage.

Interview and Goals

Nothing out of the ordinary is seen on the client information form other than the information given in the case. Referral information from the chiropractor indicates generalized soft tissue restriction in the neck and shoulder area. In answering a question, the client says that he was on vacation in Mexico for 3 weeks before he got the cold and cough. The cough lasted for a week, and he used over-the-counter cough suppressants. For years the client has ridden a bike at least three times a week for 10 miles. The head injury from his fall was considered minor and was not treated other than with the initial evaluation. He was told the neck stiffness was normal for this type of injury and would dissipate, which it did. He looks over his left shoulder while backing up the truck he drives. He cannot remember doing anything unusual, but he woke up with the stiffness in his neck and pain in his shoulder. He thinks he "slept funny."

The client's goal is to get a massage for a few weeks, but he wants only the neck and shoulder pain addressed. He understands that full-body massage is necessary to address localized problems successfully, but he says that nothing else bothers him. He intends to keep seeing the chiropractor.

Physical Assessment

Posture

Basically symmetric with minor rotation of the head to the left. Right leg is moderately externally rotated. Lumbar curve is flat. Chin juts forward with corresponding tilt of the head back and a slight forward head position.

Gait

Head is held stiffly during walking. Arm and leg swing appears normal. Weight is carried on outside of right foot instead of evenly distributed between both feet.

Range of Motion

Right rotation and lateral flexion of the head are limited by 15%. Internal rotation of the right leg is limited by 10%.

Palpation

Near Touch. Client flinched before the neck area on the left was actually touched. Heat is noted in the area.

Skin. Surface is damp with goose bumps from the base of the head to midarm on the left. When rubbed, the area shows increased reddening and itching from histamine response. Resilience is reduced over the area of skin surfaces that are damp and red. Most superficial connective tissue binds in the caudal and diagonal directions to the right. Bilateral bind is seen on the chest from the superior to midsternal area and to the shoulder.

Superficial Connective Tissue. Skin folds between the scapulae are uneven, with the left side more restricted. Connective tissue bind in all directions exists in the right lumbar area.

Vessels and Lymph Nodes. Normal

Muscles. The neck extensors, particularly at the occipital base, and the arm horizontal adductors are short. Scalenes on the left are short, with trigger point activity and typical referred pain patterns into the symptom area. All serratus muscles are tight, with the anterior serratus short (concentric) and the posterior superior and inferior serrati long (eccentric). Eccentric muscles display attachment trigger points, and concentric muscles exhibit muscle belly trigger points. Calf muscles are short.

Tendons. Mild tenderness in response to moderate pressure is seen at the subscapular and pectoralis major arm attachments bilaterally.

Deep Fascia. Mild caudal binding (tissue moves up but binds when moving down) occurs in all superficial fascial regions: thorax, abdomen, lumbar area, iliotibial band, calves, and plantar fasciae.

Ligaments. Normal

Joints. Functional range-of-motion limitations are seen where short muscles reduce extension, horizontal abduction, and internal rotation. No specific joint problems are identified.

Bones. Normal

Abdominal Viscera. Normal

Body Rhythms. Breathing rhythm is fast in relation to other rhythms. Client has a tendency for upper chest breathing.

Muscle Testing

Strength

Muscles identified as short tested overly strong, with an exaggerated contraction response. Client had difficulty applying a gradual increase in pressure against resistance and instead responded by quickly jerking and pushing with full strength. These same muscles would not inhibit when the antagonists were contracted. Weakness was noted in the neck flexors. Movement of the eyes downward did not increase neck flexor strength, as would be expected. Movement of the eyes upward, as in looking over the head, increased flexor weakness and significantly increased tension in the neck extensors. Shoulder and hip firing patterns show synergistic dominance.

Gait

Opposite hip flexor and extensor patterns did not inhibit as expected (when the right hip flexors were activated, the left did not inhibit but maintained strength, and vice versa). Arm and leg patterns also were out of sync, with flexion bilaterally and lack of inhibition regardless of direct activation of antagonist or expected inhibition pattern in gait. The hip flexors on the same side, when activated, would be expected to inhibit the arm flexors (i.e., left inhibits left and right inhibits right), but this did not occur. Arm flexors stayed activated and tested strong regardless of the muscle pattern activated.

INTERPRETATION AND TREATMENT PLAN DEVELOPMENT

Clinical Reasoning

What Are the Facts?

Neck and shoulder stiffness and pain are among the most common complaints a massage professional encounters. These can have many causal factors. Postural distortion from a rotated or elevated shoulder girdle is common. This condition is often a compensation pattern that develops in response to postural distortion somewhere else in the body. Because the eyes must be positioned forward and level with the horizontal plane, muscle tone, firing patterns, and joint functions commonly shift in this region. To correct this, the entire body pattern needs to be addressed. A common cause of the problem is eye strain, especially combined with a static seated position, such as occurs with desk and computer work or extended periods of driving. Distorted sleep patterns, often coupled with nasal congestion, add to the situation. Upper chest breathing, such as is found with breathing pattern disorders, almost always involves neck and shoulder compensation. A forward head position strains the neck and shoulder structure. The brachial plexus and cervical plexus are often impinged, because the space through which these nerves travel is crowded, and any increase in muscle tension, changes in the joint position in the area, shortening of the connective tissue, or increases in fluid may result in pressure on nerves and blood vessels. The scalene and pectoralis minor muscles often are involved. (*Note:* Muscle aching gets worse as the day goes on. Joint pain is worse in the morning, gets better during the day, and then increases as the body fatigues.)

The client is young and generally in good health. He has a history of head trauma, along with occupational and recreational activities that have resulted in postural distortion. The anterior flexors and adductors are shortened, and the posterior extensors are inhibited, long, and locked into an eccentric contraction pattern. The generalized connective tissue binding is consistent with repetitive use and the activities that require static positions. Trigger point referred pain patterns are consistent with the symptoms.

What Are the Possibilities Both in Function and Dysfunction and the Massage Intervention Options?

Repetitive strain should be suspected with the static position of truck driving (i.e., looking left and arm positions that shorten the brachial space). The effects of biking also should be considered, given its static position of arms forward, torso bent forward with back rounded, and head forward and extended at the occipital base. Calf shortening and general fascial shortening, attributable to the client's occupational and recreational activities, may be other factors.

Both biking and driving have the arms forward and in a bent forward position with the trunk flexed; this would disrupt gait reflexes over time.

The client displays the typical muscle patterns of a person who has had an extended cough (serratus involvement).

An ongoing adaptive process over the past few years likely has finally caught up with the client, and the coughing bout probably further shortened the muscles that surround the brachial nerve plexus. Soft tissue impingement has likely irritated the brachial plexus on the left.

The head trauma and resulting stiff neck may have caused an adaptive process that has deteriorated, resulting in nerve pain in the symptom area. A trigger point referral pain pattern in the scalenes is implicated.

In situations like this, all the stated possibilities probably are involved in the pattern.

Possibilities:

1. Massage intervention would need to reduce trigger point activity in all identified areas and increase the pliability of all binding and short connective tissue structures.
2. Muscle energy methods and massage manipulations to lengthen shortened muscles, plus exercise and stretching activities that balance the repetitive posture of driving and biking, should be introduced.
3. Yoga would be a valid option.

What Are the Logical Outcomes of Each Possible Intervention Option?

Massage and a stretching program would be effective in reducing symptoms.

What seems like a simple problem is actually quite complex, and effective intervention would take longer than the client indicates he is willing to commit in time. Because the situation is likely a cumulative adaptive process, the condition may become worse before it improves.

What Is the Impact on the People Involved for Each Massage Intervention Option?

The client resists the complexity of the situation, believing it is a localized issue, and does not want long-term intervention.

He is not interested in yoga but would read a book about stretching and incorporate some of the stretches.

DECISION MAKING AND TREATMENT PLAN DEVELOPMENT

Quantifiable Goals

1. Restore normal resting length to concentrically contracted short muscles
2. Increase right rotation and lateral flexion of the head by 10%
3. Increase external rotation of the right leg by 10%
4. Reverse connective tissue bind

Qualifiable Goals

The client will be able to use his arm and turn his head without pain during normal daily work and recreational activities.

Treatment Regimen

Therapeutic Change

The treatment plan will consist of 12 weekly sessions. Each session will include a generalized massage with a myofascial drag component, coupled with muscle energy and trigger point approaches to lengthen the short muscles that are directly contributing to the brachial plexus impingement. This will include the lateral neck flexors on the left and the horizontal arm adductors and internal arm rotators bilaterally. Six weekly sessions will be scheduled, and the results will then be evaluated. Gait reflex and firing patterns will be monitored to identify any improvement. Self-help stretching education will be presented to the client. With the client's permission, information will be provided to the chiropractor on massage intervention methods for long-term chiropractic support.

CASE 5 GENERALIZED LOW BACK PAIN WITH LIMITED RANGE OF MOTION

The female client is 28 years old. She is a cashier and bagger at a large grocery store chain and has been on the job for 1 year. She is 40 pounds overweight, with fat distribution primarily in the breasts and abdomen. She has been experiencing low back pain for a few years. The pain is sporadic but worse during her menstrual period, which is also marked by moderately severe menstrual cramps. Since she started working at the store, the menstrual cramps have grown steadily worse. A general physical indicated no apparent pathologic condition. A physical examination ruled out disk and nerve problems and indicated muscle tension and strain. The client's excess weight is the probable cause. Muscle relaxants were prescribed, to be taken as needed. Lately the client has been taking the medication daily in the evening. The pain worsens as the day goes on; it is relieved initially when she lies down but becomes worse if she lies or sits still for an extended period. This supports the diagnosis of muscle tension.

On her doctor's recommendation, she started a walking program. Her diet is generally good, but she eats too much food in relation to her lack of physical activity; she has been reducing portions to support gradual weight loss. She was referred to a physical therapist, who designed a rehabilitation exercise program and recommended massage intervention under the physical therapist's supervision. The massage therapist is an employee of the physical therapist.

ASSESSMENT

Observation

The client is restless; she is in and out of her chair during the entire interview because she is unable to sit for longer than about 10 minutes before her back begins to hurt. Each time she gets up, she places her hands on her knees and pushes herself up. She places her hands behind her back and rubs the lumbar area frequently. When she stands, she distributes her weight evenly on both feet, locks the knees back, and crosses her arms across her chest. She then paces, putting her hand on her left hip. She sighs, as if movement is labored. She also appears to be retaining fluid. Her face is strained. Her manner is pleasant, but her conversation is peppered with negatives and frustration.

Interview and Goals

The history indicates that the client has worked as a cashier since high school and is a student studying computer science. She either stands at the counter, moving groceries and packing bags, or sits in class or at the computer. She has always been a bit overweight, as are her mother and father. She has never been active, and the only sports activity she enjoys is bowling. Nothing unusual shows up on the history form other than painful menstrual cramps, use of muscle relaxants, and typical childhood diseases. A sharp pain occurs in her back when she coughs or sneezes. Rolling over in bed is uncomfortable. When asked to place her hands on the pain area, she presses across the lumbar area as she moves the pelvis into anterior and posterior rotation. She also specifically points at the sacroiliac (SI) joints. She is single and has a small circle of friends. Her parents and sister live in the next town. She is in a bowling league in the winter.

The client's goals for the massage are to reduce her low back dysfunction substantially and to increase her general well-being.

Physical Assessment

Posture

Moderate lordosis, slight kyphosis, and an increased cervical curve with a forward head and a tendency for hyperextended knees are seen. Posture is bilaterally symmetric from the anterior and posterior views. Postural distortion is most apparent when client is viewed from the side.

Gait

Client walks stiff legged, with little movement at the SI joints. Contralateral arm swing is minimal.

Range of Motion

Trunk flexion in the lumbar area is restricted, and most forward movement occurs at the hips; it is limited by short hamstrings. Muscle spasm pain limits side bending of the torso to 20 degrees bilaterally. Rotation at lumbar area is limited to the right.

Palpation

Near Touch. Heat is noted in the lumbar area.

Skin. Damp areas are noted in the lumbar area lateral to the spine near the sides of the body, and the skin is generally tight in the areas where symptoms occur. The fingernails have some horizontal ridges and hangnails. Adherence of the skin with binding is palpated in the lumbar area, more lateral and adjacent to the iliac crest.

Superficial Connective Tissue. Bogginess and a mild tendency for surface edema are noted.

Vessels and Lymph Nodes. Normal

Muscles. Abdominals and gluteus maximus are long, weak, and flaccid. Neck flexors, latissimus dorsi, psoas, hamstrings, quadratus lumborum, and all calf muscles are short.

Tendons. Musculotendinous junction of the hamstrings is tender at the ischial hamstring attachment and taut at the knee attachment.

Deep Fascia. Lumbar dorsal fascia is short and binding, with influence extending up into the cranial base and along the lateral aspect of the legs and bottoms of both feet. The abdominal fascia is loose, nonelastic, and nonresilient.

Ligaments. Reduced pliability is noted around the SI joint.

Joints. SI joint is restricted bilaterally; the knees are hyperextended. Lumbar vertebrae seem compressed. Symphysis pubis is up-slipped on the left with a bilateral anterior pelvic rotation, more so on the right.

Bones. Normal

Abdominal Viscera. Abdomen is soft with no palpable abnormalities.

Body Rhythms. Fast with mild dysrhythmia

Muscle Testing

Strength

Difficult to access because client experiences pain in low back during testing. Abdominals and gluteus maximus are weak, back extensors are too strong, and psoas bilaterally appears weak.

Neurologic Balance

Difficult to test because client experiences pain. Generally client seems deconditioned.

Gait

Muscle interaction pattern has shifted from the normal opposite arm/leg flexor/flexor-extensor/extensor facilitation pattern to a same-side arm/leg flexor and arm/leg extensor pattern. As a result, the contralateral arm swing has been lost, and a substantially reduced, same-side arm swing pattern is noted. Gluteus maximus does not fire in the normal sequence. Hamstrings fire first during leg extension.

INTERPRETATION AND TREATMENT PLAN DEVELOPMENT
Clinical Reasoning

What Are the Facts?

Low back pain in the absence of disk dysfunction is very common in both males and females. Causal factors vary, but common elements exist. Client histories include either standing or sitting in static positions, coupled with upper torso twisting or some sort of trauma, such as a car accident or strain during lifting or pushing. Medication is not very effective in the management of low back pain. Some sort of pelvic rotation distortion usually is present, as well as an upper body compensation pattern of a rotated shoulder girdle, altered head position, or change in the thoracic or cervical spinal curvature. Sternoclavicular joint dysfunction is often seen with SI joint dysfunction.

The three most common causes of low back pain are:

- Muscle/connective tissue shortening with some nerve entrapment.
- Trigger point activity in the psoas, quadratus lumborum, and hamstrings, which causes a more generalized, aching pain with painful spasm on sudden movement or coughing and sneezing. This pattern is aggravated by any type of static position, including prolonged lying down, and often results in restless activity, such as changing positions frequently.
- SI joint dysfunction, which has a more localized pain pattern. The pain normally gets worse as the day progresses and eases when the person lies down.

The three forms are often found in conjunction, which further complicates the issue.

The client in this case fits the profile of combined muscle, connective tissue, and SI joint dysfunction. She does not like exercise and movement, especially because walking is labored and awkward. She stands, twists, and lifts weight with her arms as she bags groceries, which puts strain on her low back. She is overweight, with the "apple type" fat distribution that shifts the center of gravity forward, requiring the back extensors to work harder to maintain an upright posture.

She has menstrual cramping, and the low back pain is worse during menstruation. This makes sense, because psoas tightening is common during menstruation. Stress tends to lower pain tolerance and increase muscle tension. The ridges in her nails and the hangnails indicate both long-term and current stress influence. The physical therapist has instituted a rehabilitation exercise program, and the client is following a walking program. Medication has not been identified as a long-term option.

What Are the Possibilities Both in Function and Dysfunction and the Massage Intervention Options?

The client has common symptoms of general low back pain with SI joint involvement. Her job activities are common causes of activities that can aggravate an existing situation. In her case, the job seems to be aggravating the symptoms, which range from occasional and bearable to constant and distressing.

She could likely be helped by mobilization of the SI joint, with recommendations provided to the physical therapist.

Because of the edema, some subclinical kidney dysfunction may be present that would result in low back aching: the patient should be referred for diagnosis of this condition. Menstrual difficulties are part of the history and might be an underlying factor.

Stress levels are increased and are likely contributing to the increase in pain perception. Chronic pain is disempowering emotionally and draining on the neurochemical functions of the body. All the endogenous opioids, such as endorphins and serotonin, and other mood-elevating neurochemicals may be insufficient for the current demands in her life, and the results of this insufficiency are sporadic mood difficulties and increased pain perception. Referral to the physician with a recommendation for counseling and possible trial of one of the serotonin-modulating medicines is prudent.

The client's generally inactive lifestyle has resulted in deconditioning and a predisposition to muscle aching. This, combined with her excess weight and the abdominal fat distribution, is likely a main causal factor.

Possibilities:

1. General massage can be provided with a focus on restoring pliability to shortened connective tissue structures and reducing trigger points activated in the short muscles, accompanied by muscle energy methods to lengthen the short muscle groups and restore normal firing patterns.
2. Lymphatic drainage massage is indicated to manage the edema.

3. Reflexology may be effective, especially when combined with full-body massage, because it is well tolerated and the client shows shortening of the plantar fasciae.
4. Stress levels could be managed with massage and some sort of gentle movement activity, such as walking and/or yoga.
5. Aromatherapy is an option in conjunction with massage and as a self-help measure.

Recommendations are indicated for increased intake of water, fresh fruits, and vegetables, as well as mineral salt soaking baths, to support normal fluid balance in the interstitial space; this would reduce the edema. A combined, multidisciplinary approach offers the greatest likelihood of sustained benefit.

What Are the Logical Outcomes of Each Possible Intervention Option?

Cost is a factor in all the massage applications. Time is limited, as is the client's stamina. Too much intervention would tend to overwhelm her, and compliance would decrease. She is already seeing a physical therapist and walking.

Massage may provide the most benefit, with little energy requirement from the client. Aromatherapy and hydrotherapy are self-maintaining and pleasant and have low cost and time factors.

What Is the Impact on the People Involved for Each Massage Intervention Option?

The client likes the massage, mineral salt bath, and aromatherapy ideas but is resistant to yoga. She seems a bit desperate, and the massage therapist will have to monitor boundary issues, as well as maintain a supportive relationship with other caregivers.

DECISION MAKING AND TREATMENT PLAN DEVELOPMENT

Quantifiable Goals

1. Increase mobility of the lumbar region by 75%
2. Reduce pain-affected days by 50%
3. Restore normal gait and firing patterns

Qualifiable Goals

The client will be able to perform work and school activities without limitations caused by low back pain 5 of 7 days a week. She will experience less fatigue when walking.

Treatment Regimen

Condition management will be pursued, with moderate expectations of therapeutic change.

A 1-hour massage will be provided twice a week for the first 4 weeks or until improvement is noted and indicated by reduced pain perception and an increased range of motion. The frequency then will be reduced to once a week. This may be the maintenance schedule, because ongoing massage inter-

vention is probably in order to maintain a stable condition after physical therapy is complete.

The massage will consist of full-body application with reflexology and lymphatic drainage.

The focus is to increase mood-elevating chemicals with a broad-based, deep but not painful, compressive force and rhythmic application. Once the stress levels have dropped, the decreased pliability of shortened connective tissue structures can be addressed with myofascial methods. Reduction of trigger point activity in the short muscles is indicated, using positional release and direct pressure. Trigger point work will be combined with muscle energy methods and lengthening for the short muscle groups.

The client will be referred to an aromatherapist for consultation and recommendation regarding essential oils to be used during the massage and for self-application.

The client will be taught self-help measures, including hydrotherapy consisting of soaking baths, heat on the aching muscles, and cold on the joint pain. The client will be taught self foot massage and how to use softballs, baseballs, and foam rollers to massage painful areas in her back.

Close contact with the physical therapist will be necessary to achieve effective treatment for the client. The client will also be referred to her physician for recommendations regarding counseling and medication for mood regulation.

CASE 6 ATHLETIC DELAYED ONSET MUSCLE SORENESS

The client is a 22-year-old rookie cornerback professional football player. It is the second week of training camp, and the weather is hot and humid. He reports to the trainer that he aches all over and has some cramping in his hamstrings and calves. The leg cramping goes away with increased hydration and ingestion of electrolytes. He has been referred to the team massage therapist for management of delayed onset muscle soreness. The training staff has been diligent about keeping all players hydrated, and ice baths are available. The client has been regularly soaking his legs in the ice water tubs. The team's warm-up includes stretching activities. The training regimen includes various running and sprinting segments, position-dependent drills, and strength and conditioning with a weight-lifting program. Maximum performance is required to secure a position on the team, and the competition is fierce. During the past 5 days, the team has been practicing in full equipment for the morning practice and in pads, helmet, and shorts for the afternoon practice. The client does not want the massage during the afternoon break because he is afraid it will affect his afternoon practice, therefore he is requesting evening sessions after team meetings.

ASSESSMENT

Observation

The client is emotionally pumped but seems fatigued. His movements are generally a bit stiff. He keeps trying to stretch out while talking. He shows upper chest breathing, he is talking fast, and the exhale is shorter than the inhale. His phasic (movement) muscles appear bulked up.

Interview and Goals

When asked how well he is sleeping, he reports that he is tossing and turning and cannot get comfortable. He also reports a 5-pound weight gain and an increase in thigh, arm, and chest measurements. His history indicates a grade 2 groin pull on the right the last year of college. It healed well but continues to get stiff. He has to keep the area stretched out or he feels the pulling. He has been playing football since high school. Nothing unusual is disclosed in the history form except a recent tendency for constipation. On a pain scale of 1 to 10, he says he feels like a 12.

His goals for the massage are to reduce the aching and stiff feelings and to enhance his athletic performance. The trainer's goal is management of delayed onset muscle soreness.

Physical Assessment

Posture

Appropriate for football positional demands.

Gait

Slightly reduced stride on the right.

Range of Motion

Abduction of the right leg is reduced by 10% compared with the left leg and has a binding end-feel. Elbow and knee flexion bilaterally are reduced slightly because of soft tissue approximation (muscle tissue bumping into itself).

Palpation

Near Touch. Client generally is giving off heat.

Skin. Generally taut and damp with axillae, feet, and hand sweating. Binding at clavicles; may interfere with lymph flow. Tissue in general feels dense but boggy.

Superficial Connective Tissue. Dense

Vessels and Lymph Nodes. Difficult to palpate because they seem buried in tissue.

Muscles. Muscle tone is appropriate for training effect. General tone is increased from client's first visit a month ago, indicating a response to training effects during training camp. Gluteus maximus is short and tight.

Tendons. General tenderness at musculotendinous junction in the phasic (movement) muscles of the arms and legs.

Deep Fascia. Mild binding during both superior and inferior movement in the sheath that runs from the cranial base to the sacrum and continues down the iliotibial band into the calves.

Bind also is noted in the abdominal muscles and the pectoralis fasciae.

Ligaments. Normal

Joints. Aching increased with traction, indicating a soft tissue problem as a primary causal factor.

Bones. Normal

Abdominal Viscera. Abdominal muscle development makes palpation difficult; appears normal, with some fullness over the descending colon.

Body Rhythms. Fast upper chest breathing pattern.

Muscle Testing

Strength

All muscles test strong, but excessive synergistic recruitment is evident.

Neurologic Balance

Generalized hypersensitivity, evidenced by a fast, jerky contraction pattern and inability to contract muscles slowly.

Gait

Normal, but inhibition pattern for the arms is slow to engage (it takes a few seconds for muscles to let go).

INTERPRETATION AND TREATMENT PLAN DEVELOPMENT

Clinical Reasoning

What Are the Facts?

Delayed onset muscle soreness is a complicated response to increased physical and muscular activity demands. It can be local or generalized, depending on the activity. Although the term *delayed onset muscle soreness* indicates a muscle problem, the situation more likely involves the circulatory, lymph, and autonomic nervous systems and breathing functions. Simple delayed onset muscle soreness in local areas results when a muscle moves repetitively in eccentric contractions. This is common in any type of weight-training program intended to bulk up, or create hypertrophy, in muscles. Inflammation occurs and possibly some microtearing of muscle fibers. Inflammatory mediators (primarily histamine), which are released during physical activity, increase capillary permeability; as a result, interstitial fluid accumulates, causing simple edema. The increased fluid pressure in the tissue stimulates pain receptors, making the person feel stiff and achy.

Metabolic byproduct (not lactic acid) buildup from exercise irritates nerve endings as well. Increased muscle tone can result in pressure on lymphatic vessels, interfering with the normal lymphatic flow and further stressing the lymphatic system. In addition, increased sympathetic arousal, which is part of athletic function, especially in contact sports, increases arterial pressure and blood flow. If the normal expansion in the capillary bed of the muscle is restricted because of increased muscle tension and connective tissue thickening, more plasma flows out of the capillaries but cannot return, requiring the lymphatic system to handle the increased interstitial fluid volume. When the body is in a sympathetic state, the ground substance of the connective tissue thickens to provide more resistance to impact. This process should reverse itself when arousal diminishes and parasympathetic dominance takes over, but often with athletes the arousal levels do not reverse and the connective tissue remains thicker, placing pressure on pain receptors and contributing to stiffness. The combination of fluid pressure and connective tissue thickening makes the tissue feel taut and dense. More complex patterns result with sustained sympathetic arousal. Upper chest breathing patterns and a tendency for breathing pattern disorders are common and perpetuate the underlying sympathetic arousal.

Management of this condition requires the reduction of any muscle tension interfering with circulation and lymphatic flow, mechanical drainage of interstitial fluid, support for arterial and venous circulation, reduction of the sympathetic arousal pattern, and an increase in ground substance pliability. The process must be accomplished without adding any inflammation to the tissues. Frictioning and any other methods that would cause tissue damage are contraindicated.

The delayed onset muscle soreness seen in planned training programs is to be expected. Each sport, or in this case, football position, places specific demands on certain movement patterns. It is essential that massage applications support the training effect and not interfere with it. Although symmetry in form is ideal, specific sport demand causes hypertrophy in certain muscle groups, and bodywide compensation occurs during a normal training regimen. This has to be considered during the assessment and the application of massage.

This particular client/player has symptoms of combined delayed onset muscle soreness and sustained sympathetic arousal. His breathing is appropriate to training activity but is not reversing during down time, therefore his sleep is disturbed and he is constipated. Tissues are filled with fluid, and thickened ground substance makes the tissue feel dense. Connective tissue binding exists in the back and the groin, especially on the right, and in the chest in the area of the right and left lymphatic ducts. Reduced abdominal movement, resulting from the upper chest breathing and the overdeveloped abdominal muscles (primarily the rectus abdominis), does not support movement of the lymph in the abdominal cavity. The muscle strength, with synergistic recruitment and slow response to inhibition patterns, can be attributed to overtraining and sympathetic arousal.

What Are the Possibilities Both in Function and Dysfunction and the Massage Intervention Options?

The client probably is excited about being in professional football and trying to prove himself in camp. He may have some anxiety about making the team, because competition is fierce for his position. This all contributes to the sympathetic arousal. He may be overtraining, especially in the weight room, because he is quickly bulking up.

The training regimen in general is a cause of a delayed onset muscle soreness pattern and stress. The weight of equipment worn during practice (about 20 pounds) is a new strain on the system, and adjusting to it can increase soft tissue soreness. Needing to learn all the plays in the playbook can add to the stress.

Possibilities:

In combination with the athletic trainer's support and proper hydration, massage can be focused to achieve the following:

1. Reduce the sympathetic arousal
2. Soften the connective tissue ground substance
3. Increase lymphatic flow

Stretching could be increased and weight training intensity reduced to more appropriate levels.

What Are the Logical Outcomes of Each Possible Intervention Option?

The massage will likely help but needs to be done in the evening before the client goes to bed. This will make scheduling difficult.

The player must stay hydrated, and increased urine production may awaken him at night, interfering with sleep.

If the massage intervention is too intense, he may be sluggish the next day and his performance will be compromised.

Sleep would improve, which would reduce the recovery time. Reflexes should be more appropriate, and coordination and timing should improve, which supports performance.

What Is the Impact on the People Involved for Each Massage Intervention Option?

Training personnel referred the client, therefore they are supportive. The position coach does not like rookies "babied" and feels that the client should "tough it out" a bit and not look like a whiner. The player has had massage before and liked it but is worried about anything that could affect his performance. The massage therapist feels that it is important to deal with the situation but does not enjoy beginning massage at 9:30 PM. The player is likely to respond to the nurturing and to notice a reduction in anxiety.

DECISION MAKING AND TREATMENT PLAN DEVELOPMENT

Quantifiable Goals

1. Reduce pain sensation to a tolerable 5 (on a scale of 1 to 10)
2. Ease feelings of stiffness by 50%
3. Normalize breathing

Qualifiable Goals

The player will be able to perform at or near optimum levels and will be able to participate in all training activities without excessive soreness.

Treatment Regimen

Condition Management

Daily massage will be given for 5 days just before bed for 45 minutes. The frequency then will be reduced to two times per week. Lymphatic drainage and circulation enhancement massage with rhythmic, broad-based compression deep enough to spread muscle fibers in all muscle layers and to increase serotonin and endogenous opiate (endorphin) availability will be provided. Application of all methods should not create any inflammation or alter the training effect. The focus will be on reducing sympathetic arousal and normalizing muscle tension, reflex patterns, and fluid dynamics in the body. Limited use of myofascial release in the binding tissue of the back, groin, and chest, along with controlled used of kneading, primarily to squeeze out the capillary beds and soften the ground substance, is appropriate. Abdominal massage to encourage peristalsis, with a specific focus on the large intestines to move fecal matter, is indicated. Breathing, muscle tone, firing pattern, reflexes, and sleep patterns will be monitored as indicators that the player is responding to massage.

CASE 7 THIRD TRIMESTER PREGNANCY

The client is 34 years old and in the eighth month of her second pregnancy. She has a 9-year-old son. The pregnancy has progressed normally, and the client has had the usual minor complaints of nausea, swelling in the ankles, low back ache, and shoulder and neck pain. She has noticed that her breathing has become more labored in the past 2 weeks. She feels pressure on her bladder, but bowel function is normal. She has been receiving massage on and off during the pregnancy. Now that her posture is changing with the increase in the size of the baby, she is more uncomfortable and wants to begin a more frequent and regular schedule of massage until the baby is born. She lives in the country, and the weather has been snowy and icy. Because she feels clumsy and is concerned about falling, she has been staying home and would prefer on site massage sessions.

ASSESSMENT

Observation

The client's movement is awkward, and she often places her hands on the lumbar area for support. She breathes with her neck and shoulder muscles and is at times short of breath. The baby looks as if he or she has taken up all available abdominal space and is still being carried high in the abdomen.

Interview and Goals

The baby has a normal activity level and has not settled into the head-down position. Nothing on the history form indicates problems with the pregnancy or cautions for massage. The client takes a prenatal vitamin but no other medications.

Her obstetrician is an osteopath who supports massage. The doctor did some joint manipulation earlier in the pregnancy but would prefer that other methods be used until after the baby's birth.

The client's goals for the massage are to be more comfortable in general, to reduce the edema, to sleep better, and to ease the muscle and joint aching in both her low back and neck. She realizes that the effects of massage are temporary, but at this point, even a few hours of relief would be welcome.

Physical Assessment

Posture

Functional lordosis as a result of the pregnancy.

Gait

Normal contralateral gait pattern is evident, but the increased weight in the front, coupled with the change in the center of gravity, makes movement awkward and labored.

Range of Motion

Forward flexion of the trunk is limited by the pregnancy. Lateral bending is limited in both directions and is linked to the client feeling as if she is losing her balance. Range of motion in the ankles and wrists is mildly limited by the edema. Lateral flexion of the head is reduced to 30 degrees bilaterally.

Palpation

Near Touch. Increased heat is noted in the upper shoulders. Over the abdomen there is a sense of an increase in the density of the air, and the baby moves during this palpation.

Skin. Skin is generally dry and a bit flaky but shows no abnormal color changes. It is slightly rough, and stretch marks are present in the lower abdomen. The skin is mobile over the connective tissue except in areas of edema. Hair is a bit dry, and some has fallen out.

Superficial Connective Tissue. Pliable and resilient.

Vessels and Lymph Nodes. Normal

Muscles. Neck and shoulder muscles that function as breathing muscles are short, as are the back extensors.

Tendons. Tenderness at abdominal attachments.

Deep Fascia. Normal for this stage of pregnancy; abdominal fascia is stretched.

Ligaments. General laxity, normal for this stage of pregnancy.

Joints. Joint play is increased in all major joints. Symphysis pubis is up-slipped on the right. SI joint is mobile but compressed, as are the lumbar vertebrae. Rib movement is restricted by the baby.

Bones. Normal

Abdominal Viscera. Unable to palpate

Body Rhythms. Even and slightly slow. Breathing is labored and occasionally out of sync with the other body rhythms. Pulse points are even in the legs.

Muscle Testing

Not performed.

INTERPRETATION AND TREATMENT PLAN DEVELOPMENT

Clinical Reasoning

What Are the Facts?

Normal pregnancy is a healthy state, with caution implicated for massage. In the first trimester, the main concern is not to overstress the mother in any way that would interfere with normal development of the baby. Deep abdominal massage is avoided, as are any invasive and painful massage or bodywork approaches.

Consideration is necessary for the hormonal changes that may result in increased sensitivity to odors or mood changes. Breasts enlarge and are tender, and fatigue is common. During the second trimester, the hormonal changes result in connective tissue changes, and joint stability may become somewhat loose. The abdomen begins to expand, and lying on the stomach is uncomfortable unless support is provided. The body's response to hormonal changes evens out. In the third trimester, strain is put on the postural muscles because the center of gravity shifts forward. Pressure from the growing baby compresses the abdominal contents; this interferes with normal diaphragmatic breathing and can increase the urgency or frequency of urination. Edema is common in the ankles and wrists. Getting comfortable becomes difficult. Backaches and neck and shoulder aching are common. Backache results from the shift in the center of gravity and from the intraabdominal pressure; neck and shoulder pain arises from the use of accessory muscles for breathing. The breasts continue to change and enlarge, preparing for lactation. All these conditions reverse themselves over time after the baby's birth. Management and comfort care (palliation) are the goals at this stage of pregnancy.

This client shows the normal third trimester adaptations of the body.

What Are the Possibilities Both in Function and Dysfunction and the Massage Intervention Options?

The SI joint pain and lumbar area aching are likely caused by the functional lordosis and joint laxity. The short shoulder and neck muscles are attributable to the use of accessory breathing muscles. The mild edema in the ankles and wrists is common in the third trimester because of the increased strain on the lymphatic system and because some of the lymph pathways are obstructed by the baby and by postural shifts. *Possibilities:*

1. Full-body massage can provide hyperstimulation analgesia to reduce the aching. It also can lengthen the shortened neck and shoulder muscles and assist in movement of the lymphatics, with caution.
2. Caution is indicated with stretching and joint movement, because hypermobility is noted in the joints. The up-slipped symphysis pubis is consistent with the posture shifts and compression of the SI joints; this condition increases the sensation of pelvic instability.
3. Because the client's obstetrician is an osteopath, referral for manipulation of the SI joints and symphysis pubis could bring short-term relief. This could be continued until the baby has been born and the pelvis stabilizes.

What Are the Logical Outcomes of Each Possible Intervention Option?

The client wants massage at home, therefore the cost is higher to cover travel and set-up time. Her husband and son can be taught basic massage methods so that they can help during the final weeks of pregnancy.

Positioning on the side will require alteration of some massage applications and can strain the massage practitioner's body mechanics somewhat, because the ideal positioning for leaning uphill in some areas may not be available. The side-lying position is generally supportive and is effective for body mechanics. Additional bolsters are necessary.

What Is the Impact on the People Involved for Each Massage Intervention Option?

The massage therapist is supportive of home visits for a short time.

DECISION MAKING AND TREATMENT PLAN DEVELOPMENT

Quantifiable Goal

Increase comfort levels, as self-reported by the client

Qualifiable Goals

The client will be supported, her stress will be reduced in the final stages of pregnancy, and she will be prepared for effective delivery.

Treatment Regimen

Palliative Care/Some Condition Management

Full-body massage will be provided twice a week for 1 hour at an in-home rate of $50 per hour plus a $30 travel and set-up fee. The massage position will be altered to side-lying, with the client lying primarily on the left side as long as she is comfortable.

Pressure will be broad based and applied to a depth that is comfortable, and the focus will be on supporting the circulation but not specifically on performing full-body lymphatic drainage. Broad-based compression will be used for the short muscles of the neck, shoulders, and upper chest while the client moves her head or arm in circles to relax the accessory breathing muscles. Gentle traction of the SI joint and lumbar vertebrae to ease compression will be incorporated into the general massage session. Full-body rhythmic massage will create counterirritation and hyperstimulation analgesia, reducing the perception of discomfort for a short time.

Note: For these massages, special attention should be given to atmosphere, such as soft music and lighting, with a parasympathetic focus. Scentless massage lubrication should be used, because the client is sensitive to odors. It is important to entrain the body rhythms of the mother and baby. Care must be taken to match but not superimpose any rhythm patterns. Gentle, soothing, circular stroking of the abdomen can increase the pliability of the stretched skin in the area. Foot massage is comforting and balancing. Pressure on the inside of the ankle and up the calf should be avoided. If the client's breasts are aching, she can be taught a circular gliding massage technique for the breast area.

CASE 8 PREMENSTRUAL SYNDROME

The client is a 29-year-old female who has been diagnosed with premenstrual syndrome (PMS). After ovulation she is increasingly irritable and anxious. She experiences general swelling and some bloating. Often, but not always, she gets a migraine headache about a week before her menstrual period. She craves chocolate and carbohydrates. Her weight is within normal range for her height, but she can increase half a clothing size during the menstrual period. She is single and has a 5-year-old child. She works as an administrative assistant. She has a stable income, but the days off work and the mood fluctuations during her premenstrual period are beginning to disturb her employer. She recently joined a PMS support group. She takes ibuprofen as needed for pain, and she is taking a multivitamin and additional B vitamins. She is weaning herself off coffee by switching to green tea, which also has caffeine but not as much as coffee. On weekends she rides her bike and roller-blades for exercise. She has not changed her diet. Currently, she is 3 days past ovulation and just beginning to experience symptoms. Her workplace is near the massage professional's office.

ASSESSMENT

Observation

The client is clearly distressed about her mood swings, as indicated by her emphatic voice tone and her facial expression. She appears bloated.

Interview and Goals

The history form indicates that the client has migraine headaches and that she uses a barrier method for birth control. She has had one pregnancy. She severely sprained her right ankle 3 years ago. She experiences digestive bloat and low back ache just before her period. She appears fatigued, and she says she suffers from sleep difficulties and nervous tension the second half of her menstrual cycle. She falls asleep but wakes up frequently and cannot get back to sleep.

The client is intent on management of the premenstrual syndrome and indicates that her goals for the massage are to focus on and deal with the fluid retention and chemical imbalance that accompany PMS.

Physical Assessment

Posture

Posture is symmetric, with the shoulders slightly rolled forward. Weight is dispersed to the inside of the right foot, and the right knee is mildly hyperextended.

Gait

Normal except for flat-foot loading, in which the weight is on the inside rather than the outside of the right foot.

Range of Motion

Within normal range except for moderate hypermobility in the right ankle.

Palpation

Near Touch. No perceivable abnormality.

Skin. Oily and smooth with binding noted in the superior (cranial) direction (tissue moves down, binds when moved up) around the right ankle and upper chest.

Superficial Connective Tissue. Evidence of fluid retention, with pitting edema in the ankles.

Vessels and Lymph Nodes. Lymph node areas in the axillae display tenderness to moderate pressure.

Muscles. Trigger point activity is present in the right medial gastrocnemius.

Tendons. Right Achilles tendon is slightly short.

Deep Fascia. Sheath between the gastrocnemius and the soleus on the right seems bound together.

Ligaments. Deltoid ligament on the right ankle is unstable and lax.

Joints. Right ankle is hypermobile and has increased joint play.

Bones. Normal

Abdominal Viscera. Abdomen is boggy and moderately distended. Lower abdomen is tender to moderate pressure.

Body Rhythms. Breathing is uneven and slow, with no current evidence of upper chest breathing. Cardiac pulses are normal but changeable from 55 to 70 beats per minute without change in activity. Craniosacral undulation is reduced, which is common with static lymphatic movement.

Muscle Testing

Strength

Not performed.

Neurologic Balance

Not performed.

Gait

Normal except for the gastrocnemius and the soleus on the right, which do not inhibit when appropriate.

INTERPRETATION AND TREATMENT PLAN DEVELOPMENT

Clinical Reasoning

What Are the Facts?

Premenstrual syndrome is a collection of symptoms that include fluid retention, bloating, headache, backache, changes in balance mechanisms and coordination, food cravings, irritability, anxiety, depression, and decreased ability to concentrate. Women may experience a few or many of the symptoms, and this is changeable from cycle to cycle. All of the causal factors for premenstrual syndrome have yet to be discovered. Imbalances in serotonin and dopamine are evident. The increase in progesterone during the postovulation period supports fluid retention. Prostaglandins seem to be a factor in the pain and cramping, and aspirin and other nonsteroidal antiinflammatory drugs are often prescribed because they interfere with prostaglandin synthesis.

This client shows common premenstrual symptoms, especially bloating, fluid retention, irritability, food cravings, and headache. The symptoms are severe enough to compromise her work situation. She also has mild postural distortion and ankle hypermobility.

What Are the Possibilities Both in Function and Dysfunction and the Massage Intervention Options?

Serotonin imbalance is evidenced by the chocolate and carbohydrate cravings, and dopamine imbalance by the irritability. Because ibuprofen helps the pain and cramping, prostaglandins are likely to be involved. The progesterone increase during the postovulation period can contribute to the fluid retention, bloating, and breathing changes. The distress from the symptoms could be increasing the sympathetic fight-or-flight response, creating a self-perpetuating cycle.

Possibilities:
1. Massage would promote fluid and neurochemical balance and reduce sympathetic arousal.
2. Recommendations for meditative movement activity, such as tai chi or yoga, and referral to an herbalist and aromatherapist for evaluation are viable options.

What Are the Logical Outcomes of Each Possible Intervention Option?

Massage is cost-effective, and the closeness of the massage practitioner's office to the client's work place makes it convenient. The appointment schedule may vary, depending on the symptoms. Massage once a week is appropriate during the preovulatory phase; more frequent sessions should be scheduled during the symptom phase.

The only herbalist and aromatherapist is a 2-hour drive away, but because frequent appointments are not required, this should not be a limiting factor. These products can be expensive. A tai chi class is available through the support group.

What Is the Impact on the People Involved for Each Massage Intervention Option?

The client is motivated and indicates compliance with keeping appointments. The support group also recommends tai chi and yoga and other therapies, such as aromatherapy.

DECISION MAKING AND TREATMENT PLAN DEVELOPMENT

Quantifiable Goals

1. Reduce self-reported PMS symptoms by 50%
2. The number of days the client takes off work because of PMS symptoms will be reduced by 75%

Qualifiable Goal

The client will experience increased well-being and reduction of mood swings.

Treatment Regimen

Condition Management

Massage appointments will be made weekly until the symptoms appear and then twice weekly until the symptoms dissipate. One-hour sessions are indicated at $40 per session. The sessions will include general massage to reduce sympathetic arousal, with a broad-based compressive force that has pressure depth but that does not cause any guarding or pain. Sufficient pressure will be necessary to increase serotonin and endorphin availability. An increase in these chemicals should reduce food cravings and pain perception and hopefully level the mood fluctuations. Lymphatic drainage will be used to reduce tissue fluid. Because the pressure of superficial lymphatic drainage is very light (just moving the skin), this will be the last method used during the massage.

The client also displays compensation patterns from the ankle sprain and a rolled shoulder pattern, likely from the biking. Because these areas have no direct effect on premenstrual syndrome management and the client's goals, they will not be addressed specifically during the initial treatment plan massage, although improvement may be noted with general massage application. The ankle compensation patterns may become an issue in future sessions, and the treatment plan can be amended at that time.

CASE 9 REPETITIVE STRAIN/ OVERUSE INJURY: BURSITIS

The client is a 48-year-old man who has been diagnosed with bursitis of the left elbow. The bursa at the olecranon around the attachment of the triceps has become irritated and inflamed. The client fell and hit the elbow 6 months ago. The bursa was injured but healed with no apparent problems. The client recently began a weight-training program that includes biceps and triceps toning. He admits that he overtrained, doing both upper body and lower body exercises every day instead of following an alternate-day pattern. In addition, he used more weight than was necessary. He was given a cortisone injection at the inflamed site and is taking aspirin. He has been told to rest the area and maintain range of motion but not to lift weight with the arm. The client expresses concern about losing recently acquired muscle tone and bulking. He had become overweight and deconditioned in his early forties after being very fit in his twenties and thirties. He is determined to reclaim a fit body. He is already receiving massage on a weekly basis with the goal of managing stress and the muscle soreness caused by exercise. He is now specifically focused on reversing the bursitis.

ASSESSMENT

Observation

The client is a bit restless and impatient. Frustration is evident in his voice over what seems to him to be a delay in his training program. He rubs the sore elbow often.

Interview and Goals

The client is taking a muscle-building supplement that contains various vitamins and amino acids. He slipped on the ice and severely bruised the left elbow. It was speculated that he may have ruptured the bursa at the olecranon. The bursitis is in the acute, possibly subacute, stage. The history indicates a family tendency for cardiovascular problems, primarily arteriosclerosis. The death of a relative prompted the client to begin a diet and exercise program. His blood pressure is slightly elevated but is not being treated medically, and his doctor expects that it will fall into the normal range with weight reduction, stress management, and exercise.

Physical Assessment

Posture

Mild anterior rotation of the left shoulder and moderate anterior rotation of the left pelvis are seen. The left elbow is carried in a flexed, loose-packed position.

Gait

Client's stride is short when he moves forward on the right leg and counterbalances, with the right arm moving into extension instead of the left arm.

Range of Motion

Pain limits flexion and extension of the left elbow to 100 degrees. External rotation of the left arm is limited to 70 degrees.

Palpation

Near Touch. Area of the bursa in the left arm is warm.

Skin. Skin is damp and slightly red near the bursal inflammation. Goose bumps are seen with light skin stroking over the bursal inflammation, and skin binding at the triceps attachment.

Superficial Connective Tissue. Adherent at the triceps attachment at the elbow.

Vessels and Lymph Nodes. Normal

Muscles. Triceps and biceps are short on the left. Quadriceps are long and taut and hamstrings are short on the right. Muscle mass of biceps seems out of proportion to triceps. Internal rotators of the left arm are short, with inhibition of the external rotators. Gluteus maximus on the left is inhibited and flaccid and not firing appropriately during hypertension.

Tendons. Tendons are tender to moderate pressure at the right hamstring attachment at the pelvis and at all attachments of the left triceps.

Deep Fascia. Iliotibial band is binding in all directions on the right leg.

Ligaments. No palpable problems.

Joints. Compression of the left elbow joint does not cause additional pain, but traction does; the problem likely is in the primary soft tissue.

Bones. Normal

Abdominal Viscera. Normal

Body Rhythms. Fast, with some indication of sympathetic arousal and upper chest breathing.

Muscle Testing

Strength

Triceps on the left is inhibited, and biceps is too strong; quadriceps is inhibited and hamstring is too strong on the right. Left gluteus maximus is weak. Trigger point activity is found in these same muscle groups, with the trigger point in the belly of the short, concentrically contracted muscles and at the attachments of the inhibited, long, eccentrically contracted muscles.

Neurologic Balance

Client is unable to increase resistance gradually against pressure; he uses maximal force, and movement is abrupt and jerky. Abdominal muscles are not firing appropriately.

Gait

Gait patterns are normal, even though there is local inhibition and increased tone with individual strength testing of direct antagonist and antagonist patterns.

INTERPRETATION AND TREATMENT PLAN DEVELOPMENT

Clinical Reasoning

What Are the Facts?

Bursitis is an inflammation of the synovial fluid–filled sacs around joints, tendons, and ligaments. Bursitis develops with impact trauma, sustained compression (it is often found in the knees of carpet layers, carpenters, and others who do a lot of work on their knees), and repetitive strain. Repetitive movement causes both friction and a tendency for shortening of the muscle and connective tissue structures, which further increases the tendency for rubbing, causing inflammation. Bursitis can also occur if the position of the bones of the joint and ligament alignment change, or if the muscles pull unevenly on the joint structures.

This type of inflammation responds to applications of ice, nonsteroidal antiinflammatory drugs (e.g., aspirin) and, if necessary, localized injection of a steroid. The medication, especially aspirin, thins blood. Massage pressure needs to be altered to prevent bruising during massage. Areas where the steroid was injected must be avoided, because the medication exerts its effect on the local tissues, and massage may disperse the steroid. Recently, transdermal patches of antiinflammatory and analgesic drugs have been used successfully instead of injection, but the same cautions exist. The muscle and connective tissue elements around the inflamed bursa are usually short, and lengthening and stretching of this soft tissue are necessary. If the problem is localized and not the result of a more general postural shift, spot work may be helpful. However, as soon as the body begins to compensate for the condition, full-body effects develop, therefore even localized bursitis is best addressed in the context of full-body massage.

This client shows connective tissue shortening around the olecranon, with both the agonist and antagonist for elbow flexion short and tight on the affected side. A corresponding pattern that does not show symptoms is present in the opposite leg.

What Are the Possibilities Both in Function and Dysfunction and the Massage Intervention Options?

The previous injury may have caused some scar tissue and shortening of the triceps tendon. The rotational pattern of the shoulder and hip also increases the likelihood of the triceps rubbing at the attachment on the elbow. The short, tight muscles with trigger points may be changing the joint angle and orientation of the connecting bones, increasing the likelihood of friction at the bursa. The repetitive strain of the weight lifting for the biceps and triceps is partly causal and likely aggravating the scar tissue from the previous injury. The client admits to overtraining, and he also may be training the flexors more than the extensors of the affected elbow, setting up the muscle imbalance. Massage is indicated, and better results would be obtained if the sessions were scheduled for every other day.

Possibilities:

1. Friction and myofascial release are options in the areas of connective tissue adhesion.
2. Direct pressure combined with muscle energy methods is indicated for the trigger points in the concentrically short muscles.
3. Lengthening and stretching of the short muscles, with stimulation of the eccentric and inhibited muscles, could be effective.

What Are the Logical Outcomes of Each Possible Intervention Option?

Massage to lengthen the shortened muscles and ease the connective tissue dysfunction would reduce the tendency for rubbing. If eccentrically activated muscles are further inhibited and become longer, the situation can worsen. Connective tissue binding is at the triceps, and further complications of the situation would need to be addressed in combination with muscle stimulation of the triceps and reduction of excessive shortening of the biceps.

Massage directly over the site of the steroid injection is contraindicated for at least 7 more days, which interferes with application of scar tissue release in the area. The client is taking aspirin and therefore may bruise with direct application of compression to trigger points. Alternate methods are needed to address the trigger point problem. The client needs to ice the area frequently.

Because this is a regular client, an increase in massage frequency is a time and cost burden. The massage therapist will have to find available scheduling to accommodate the more frequent appointments.

What Is the Impact on the People Involved for Each Massage Intervention Option?

Because the client is already receiving massage, the additional appointments are acceptable as long as results are readily apparent within a month. The client's expectations are a bit unrealistic. He resists ice application.

The massage therapist is willing to accommodate the increase in the number of appointments for a short time.

DECISION MAKING AND TREATMENT PLAN DEVELOPMENT

Quantifiable Goals

1. Restore range of motion of the left elbow and arm to normal
2. Reverse any compensation caused by postural changes

Qualifiable Goals

The client will be able to resume work and moderate, appropriate exercise and weight training without causing irritation of the bursa or elbow.

Treatment Regimen

Therapeutic Change/Return to Condition Management

Full-body massage appointments will be increased from once a week to three times per week for 1 month. The focus will be on generalized massage to address the compensation patterns in the opposite leg and the rotational pattern of the shoulder and pelvis. Compression, gliding, and kneading will be applied to the short biceps and hamstrings with tense-and-relax and lengthening techniques.

Tapotement and pulsed muscle energy methods will be used after general gliding and kneading to stimulate inhibited muscles and to focus on reducing trigger point activity and lengthening short muscles. In 1 week, connective tissue work will begin on the elbow, with myofascial approaches and skin rolling used to soften the ground substance for the first four sessions of connective tissue application. No additional inflammation will be introduced.

After this application, if heat and other indicators of inflammation are reduced in the area, very controlled use of friction and bending and shearing of adhered tissue can begin. This process needs to be monitored carefully to ensure that the bursitis symptoms do not recur. Aspirin should be discontinued before the introduction of therapeutic inflammation, or the methods will not be as effective, because it is the inflammatory process that changes the connective tissue fiber structure. Depth of pressure will elicit a "good hurt" sensation, and all layers of the short and tight tissues need to be addressed, especially synergists and fixators in the deeper muscle layers.

CASE 10 JOINT SPRAIN WITH UNDERLYING HYPERMOBILITY AND LAX LIGAMENT SYNDROME

The client is a 16-year-old female cheerleader. She has been involved in dance and gymnastics since she was 5 years old. She fell during a routine and sprained both her right ankle and knee. The deltoid ligament on the lateral aspect of her right ankle received a second-degree sprain when she landed on the outside of her foot. Her leg tangled in a fellow cheerleader's leg, resulting in a grade 1 sprain of the lateral collateral ligament of the right knee. She was on crutches for a few days until she could bear weight on her foot. Appropriate first aid was administered, and follow-up medical care included external stabilization and passive and active movement without weight bearing to promote healing with pliable scar tissue formation. Weight bearing has been allowed for the past 5 days. It has been 10 days since the accident. The client's mother cleared the massage with her doctor, who supports the intervention to manage some of the compensation from using crutches and to promote healing of the injured area. The client complains of neck, shoulder, and low back stiffness and pain. Antiinflammatory and pain medications were used for the first 3 days and then withdrawn because these medications can slow healing. The client is generally in good health but has a history of various sprains and strains. This particular ankle was sprained last year. She also sprained her left wrist when she was 10 years old.

ASSESSMENT

Observation

The client is limping slightly. Discoloration is present around the ankle but not the knee. The ankle still appears swollen, but the knee looks normal. The client fidgets during the interview. Her mother is concerned but not overbearing, letting the client answer most questions and adding information where pertinent. The right ankle is wrapped with an elastic support.

Interview and Goals

The history notes multiple sprain injuries and a tendency for generalized hypermobility. The client hopes to participate in a cheerleading competition in 2 months. Her mother is more realistic, thinking it will be at least 3 months before the ankle is strong enough for competition. The client complains of being stiff all over. No unusually pertinent information is indicated on the history form.

The client's goals for the massage are to support healing of the injured ankle and knee, reduce the general stiffness, and reverse the compensation from limping and the use of crutches.

Physical Assessment

Posture

Client is not fully weight bearing on the injured leg. Her posture is very good except for a slight lordosis and hyperextension of her knees, which is common in gymnasts.

Gait

Limited by limping, pain, and a sense of instability.

Range of Motion

Client is generally hypermobile, most likely because of training effects from dance training, gymnastics, and cheerleading.

Palpation

Near Touch. Heat is detected at the ankle and knee injury sites and in the shoulders.

Skin. Drag and dampness are present in areas of heat. Bruising surrounds the area of ankle injury. Skin is smooth and pliable with no areas of bind noted.

Superficial Connective Tissue. Connective tissue is resilient. Localized swelling remains at lateral right ankle.

Vessels and Lymph Nodes. Normal

Muscles. Muscles feel elastic but generally shorter in the belly, especially the calves, hamstrings, and adductors. Trigger point activity is evident in the belly of the adductors, hamstrings, and quadriceps in the injured leg. Supraspinatus, upper trapezius, and pectoralis major and minor are short bilaterally, with tenderness in the axillae where the crutches contact. Psoas is short bilaterally. Muscles of the right leg have increased tone, most likely because of normal guarding of the injured joints. Quadratus lumborum and the gluteal group on the left are tender to moderate pressure. A very tender area near the musculotendinous junction of the lateral head of the right gastrocnemius palpates like a grade 1 muscle tear.

Tendons. Tendons in the muscles of the right leg are tender to moderate pressure.

Deep Fascia. Resilient but seem too long.

Ligaments. Generally loose.

Joints. End-feel is not identified until the joint is in hyperextension. Increased joint play is noted in major mobility joints.

Bones. Normal

Abdominal Viscera. Normal

Body Rhythms. Normal

Muscle Testing

Strength and Neurologic Balance

Muscles test normal except for those guarding the injured knee and ankle, which is expected. These muscles are displaying increased tone and are not inhibited as expected. Left quadratus lumborum is firing before tensor fasciae latae and gluteus medius.

Gait

Gait is disrupted by limping and crutches. Flexor patterns in the arms are facilitating together instead of following contralateral patterns. Flexors and extensors of the left leg do not inhibit when tested against the arms.

INTERPRETATION AND TREATMENT PLAN DEVELOPMENT

Clinical Reasoning

What Are the Facts?

Ligament sprains and muscle strains are common injuries and are diagnosed as slight (first degree), moderate (second degree), or severe (third degree). When a joint shows a sprain (i.e., rupture of some or all of the ligament fibers), there is usually accompanying muscle strain with the possibility of muscle fiber tears. It is important not to stretch muscle tears in the acute phase. Protective spasm (guarding) is intense and painful in first- and second-degree tears. If a total breach of a muscle or tendon has occurred, the person may feel very little pain. First- and second-degree injuries are more painful and have a greater tendency for swelling than a third-degree injury. When a joint is sprained, strain in the muscles that are extended during the injury is common. Spasm around the tear (tiny microtears to more severe tears) acts to approximate (bring torn fibers together to support healing), protect, and guard the area. In general, all the muscles that surround the joint increase in tone to stabilize and reduce movement. This should dissipate as the injury heals but can become chronic, limiting range of motion of the area. Ligaments begin repair immediately, and the inflammatory response is an important part of this process. Some inflammatory mediators are vasodilators, which help blood reach ligaments. This is important, because ligaments do not have a good blood supply. Muscle tears heal much easier because of the high vascular component of the tissue. It takes 3 to 6 months or longer for a grade 2 sprain to heal fully. Repeated injury contributes to ligament laxity and joint instability.

Sprains are common in people with joint hypermobility. The hypermobility can occur in only one joint that has a recurring injury or can be more general, appearing in most joints of the body. Some disorders (e.g., Marfan's syndrome) are characterized by lax connective tissue. Most ligament laxity is functional, such as an increased range of motion required in many sports or dance activities. Once the plastic range of a ligament has been increased, it does not return to the previous range but remains long and lax. Joint play is increased, and instability results.

The client fits this profile. She will likely remain hypermobile, with increased compensating muscle tone to provide stability. This situation leads to general stiffness, especially if activity is reduced. Depending on the degree of laxity, the client may find that stretching does not reduce muscle tightness, because joint end-feel and longitudinal tensile force do not occur until the joint is hyperextended or reaches an anatomic barrier.

What Are the Possibilities Both in Function and Dysfunction and the Massage Intervention Options?

The client's gait changes seem to arise from the use of crutches. Because the injury is recent and the crutches are no longer used, gait dysfunction should easily reverse with massage and general activity.

The low back pain may stem from a dermatome distribution referring back from the knee combined with postural changes from limping and the use of crutches. The tendency for low back pain may exist because the client's psoas muscles are short.

Possibilities:

1. Massage can support the healing process in the acute, subacute, and final healing stages by increasing circulation to the area, maintaining normal and appropriate muscle tone, and supporting mobile scar formation.
2. Referral for diagnosis of the suspected muscle tear is recommended.
3. Referral to a physical therapist or exercise physiologist for a sequential strengthening program for the vulnerable joints is indicated.

What Are the Logical Outcomes of Each Possible Intervention Option?

Massage intervention would need to be long term to meet the client's goals, with an incremental treatment plan for the current acute and subacute healing stages.

Cost and time are factors, and the mother or father needs to be with the client because she is a minor.

What Is the Impact on the People Involved for Each Massage Intervention Option?

The client has unrealistic healing expectations and likely will be frustrated with a 6-month intervention plan.

DECISION MAKING AND TREATMENT PLAN DEVELOPMENT

Quantifiable Goals

1. Reduce generalized stiffness by 75%
2. Reverse compensation caused by the use of crutches
3. Support circulation and scar formation in injured areas

Qualifiable Goals

The client will be able to resume normal daily activities, but not sports activities, within 2 weeks. She will be able to resume limited cheerleading activities within 6 weeks and full use of the area in 6 months.

Treatment Regimen

Condition Management/Therapeutic Change

Condition management consists of two phases. Therapeutic change is phase three.

- *Phase one: Acute phase (current).* One-hour massage will be provided three times for the first week. Full-body massage will be used to support circulation and reverse the muscle tension in the shoulders and chest caused by the use of crutches. Specific application of gliding will be used along the sprained ligament and associated strained tendons in the fiber direction of the muscle and toward the injury to help align the scar tissue. Lymphatic drainage in the swollen areas will support healing. Passive range of motion with rocking and gentle shaking to all adjacent joints will encourage mobility and healing in the injured areas. Ongoing ice application will encourage circulation as a secondary effect of the cold. The injured areas would benefit from ice application for 20 minutes two or three times a day.

- *Phase two: Subacute phase.* Ice applications will be valuable for 1 or 2 more weeks. Massage applications will be provided for full-body sessions twice a week for 6 weeks and then reduced in frequency to once a week for 3 months if healing is progressing well. Very gentle gliding across the fiber configuration of the tissue will support mobile scar formation. The intensity of gliding and cross-fiber friction on the injured tissues will gradually increase as healing continues. Trigger points and general tone in the muscles that are guarding will be addressed with muscle energy methods, lengthening, and broad-based compression. Kneading can restore the pliability of the connective tissue ground substance. The area of the gastrocnemius that may have been torn will be treated with caution. No deep pressure will be used, but localized stroking across the grain of the muscle can support mobile scar formation. Because self-stretching is not effective without moving into hyperextension patterns, the client's muscle tissue can be manually stretched and lengthened during massage with compression and kneading that introduce bending and torsion forces into the soft tissue. The psoas muscles can be lengthened with muscle energy methods.

- *Phase three: Therapeutic change.* Six months of weekly full-body massage will be provided. Once healing of the injury is complete, the underlying hypermobility can be addressed. Systematic frictioning can be applied to lax ligaments to introduce therapeutic inflammation and encourage increased connective tissue fiber formation. This will be applied to the injured lateral collateral ligament and deltoid ligament, as well as the rest of the connective tissue stabilizing units of the ankle and knee. This needs to be done in small increments, and the area should not be excessively painful the next day. Pain to the touch with moderate pressure is appropriate, but pain should not occur with movement. This is a painful intervention and needs to be done frequently. It is appropriate to teach a family member to perform the technique. Antiinflammatory drugs should not be used, nor should ice be applied to the area, because the goal is creation of controlled inflammation to encourage collagen formation. Full-body massage with direct tissue stretching should continue. At the end of the 6-month period, the frequency of massage intervention could be reduced to a maintenance schedule of every other week.

The client will be encouraged to maintain a strengthening and stretching program and to reduce exaggerated joint movements to support restabilization of the joints.

CASE 11 OSTEOARTHRITIS

The client is a 67-year-old male with osteoarthritis in both knees. The left knee is more painful. In the future he may undergo joint replacement surgery, but for now he is exploring any methods that will allow him to remain active. Currently he enjoys golf and racquetball. He does not want to use a golf cart because he enjoys the walking and knows he needs the exercise. He plays racquetball for an hour on Tuesdays and Saturdays but really suffers with knee pain between times. His condition is worst at his early morning Sunday golf game. Initially, he is very stiff, which interferes with his golf swing, but he warms up as time goes on. He uses topical capsicum cream and takes aspirin for the arthritis and for a cardiac condition. Because of the heart issue, he needs to stay active and keep his weight down. He is currently 20 pounds over what his doctors would like him to weigh. The extra weight bothers his knees. He thinks that he has gained some of the weight because the knee pain has slowed him down. He has always been active and has a history of participating in high school and college sports. He ran track and played basketball. During this time, he had various minor to moderate injuries, including knee trauma. In his words, "I would just tough it out and play anyway." To compound the problem, he was in a car accident when he was 36 and broke his left ankle. He also spent 12 years in the U.S. Marine Corps as a sergeant. He has never had massage and has the support of his physicians. He is a sales manager, is financially stable, and has a flexible schedule. Admittedly, he is skeptical about massage. He says he is not one to be fussed over and just wants the job done.

ASSESSMENT

Observation

The client is tall, 6 feet, 4 inches. He has long legs, a short torso, broad shoulders, and a bit of a pot belly. His center of gravity is high, which would place strain on the knees. He carries himself like a Marine. He is loud and gruff but seems kind underneath the facade. He seems a bit nervous about massage therapy. His shoulders move when he breathes.

Interview and Goals

The client says he aches all over but that he has lived hard and should expect to be creaky. The joint pain is worse in the morning, gets better as he moves around, and then gets worse again. He has had various and numerous joint injuries and soft tissue trauma. Four years ago his blood pressure rose, and he had angioplasty to unclog two coronary arteries. He takes aspirin to keep his blood thin and to manage the arthritis. He says that he does not seem to bruise easily. He was taking blood pressure medication but did not like the sexual side effects and insisted he go off it. The doctor agreed as long as the client could keep his blood pressure down with diet and exercise. He has done a good job of this. Nothing else of concern is indicated on the history form. He used to smoke but quit 10 years ago. He used to drink heavily but now drinks only some red wine. His sleep is restless because his knees ache. Heat application helps.

The client's goal for the massage is management of his knee pain.

Physical Assessment

Posture

Overall, client has decent postural symmetry. Cervical curve is flat. Left foot is a bit flat. Ribs are held tight and rigid.

Gait

Client walks stiffly with reduced knee flexion and extension.

Range of Motion

Range of motion in most jointed areas is in the acceptable range for mild daily activities but stiff and resisting for any exercise. The left ankle is moderately restricted in eversion and inversion.

Palpation

Near Touch. Heat is noted at the knees and between the scapulae. Client has a presence of high energy that is felt as the air pressure–type of resistance noted when the same poles of a magnet are held together.

Skin. Rough and binding almost everywhere, with edema at the knees; there is evidence of many traumas (i.e., various scars in many body areas).

Superficial Connective Tissue. Reduced pliability bodywide—almost an armorlike feel, with edema at the knees.

Vessels and Lymph Nodes. Seem normal, but ability to palpate is restricted by tissue density.

Muscles. Well developed but dense and inflexible. Trigger point activity is evident in quadriceps and gluteals. Muscles that surround the knees have increased tone and isometric contraction in both antagonist and agonist patterns. These muscles obviously are attempting to guard the knee joints.

Tendons. Tender to moderate pressure around the knees and scapular attachment.

Deep Fascia. Thick and inflexible.

Ligaments. Mild laxity at injured ankle and knees.

Joints. Most are within the normal range of motion, but crepitus is common, as is a tendency for leathery or hard end-feel. Knees hurt with compression and traction. Most other joints show resistance to traction, indicating binding. Client indicates that most joints are stiff but not painful. Most of the pain is in the knees.

Bones. Increased bony development around the area of the ankle break. Bump noted in the right clavicle (client had forgotten he had broken it falling out of a tree when he was a child).

Abdominal Viscera. Difficult to palpate because of internal abdominal fat distribution.

Body Rhythms. Strong and fast. Client breathes with his chest but does not necessarily display breathing pattern disorder symptoms other than talking loudly and mild evidence of sympathetic arousal. Pulses are even, and cranial rhythm displays a strong, even undulation.

Muscle Testing

Strength

Client pushes hard against resistance and finds it difficult to use 50% effort. No areas of weakness are noted. Client was unable to isolate a muscle pattern and continually recruited and contracted muscles in areas other than the test area during assessment.

Neurologic Balance

Antagonist balance at knees is lost. All muscles around joint have a tendency for isometric contraction with uneven pull on the knee joint. Synergistic dominance is noted with knee firing patterns.

Gait

Leg muscles do not inhibit as they should against arm activation. Eye reflex patterns do not inhibit movement (phasic) muscles when appropriate. Hip extension and abduction firing patterns are activating in unison instead of in normal sequence.

INTERPRETATION AND TREATMENT PLAN DEVELOPMENT

Clinical Reasoning

What Are the Facts?

Osteoarthritis is very common and has a number of causes. A genetic tendency to develop this condition is one factor. The most common cause is wear and tear on the joint structure, in addition to past trauma and increased weight. The pain is caused by irritation of the synovial membrane and joint capsule and by muscle spasm attempts to guard the area. Osteoarthritis has no cure, but it can be managed to improve the quality of life. Joint replacement surgery is a last option. Advances in technology have greatly improved the outcomes of this surgery.

Muscle spasm usually occurs in all the muscles that cross the joint. Because flexors, adductors, and internal rotators have more mass, when tone increases, the pull is greater from these muscles than from the extensors, abductors, and external rotators. The bone fit at the joint can be pulled out of alignment, creating further irritation in the joint capsule. Also, muscles that cross the joint pull the joint space together. This, coupled with weight bearing at the hips, knees, and ankles, reduces the joint space and increases the potential for rubbing of the bony structures, increasing the inflammation, swelling, and pain. Arthritic joints are often unstable and have a lax ligament structure. Because the client's knees are affected (closed kinetic chain—hip/knee/ankle), disruption of the knees affects the hips and ankles.

Management includes easing mechanical strain on the knee joint by normalizing the muscle tone without reducing stability and resourceful muscle guarding. Corresponding muscle shortening and weakening in the hips and ankles also must be addressed. Lymphatic drainage–type methods work well if the fluid is outside the capsule. Edema can increase stiffness and reduce range of motion. Sometimes needle aspiration is necessary if excess fluid builds up inside the capsule. Some increase in synovial fluid in the capsule can be beneficial, because an increase in hydrostatic pressure can separate the bone surfaces, easing the rubbing. Correcting posture deviation that contributes to the joint irritation may be possible in younger clients, but in older clients, especially after 75 years of age, this becomes more difficult. Pain management is supported with counterirritation and hyperstimulation analgesia applications, a reduction in sympathetic arousal, and an increase in the pain-modulating chemicals in the system, such as serotonin and enkephalins. The joints must be kept moving or the condition will worsen. Massage that incorporates passive and active joint movement is supportive for pain management, allowing the client to move with less pain. Joint tractioning can offer temporary relief. Application of hot and cold hydrotherapy to manage pain and encourage circulation is appropriate. Cold can be applied after activity, and heat can be used to warm up before activity or as a counterirritation at night to promote sleep.

This client's history and posture give strong indications of the development of osteoarthritis. His body type (long legs with upper body mass) strains the knees in general. In addition, he has used his body hard for a long time.

What Are the Possibilities Both in Function and Dysfunction and the Massage Intervention Options?

The client is still relatively young and in good health. He is motivated to change, as indicated by his previous diet and exercise alterations. The knee joints and left ankle are likely damaged beyond regeneration.

Possibilities:

1. Massage can be beneficial for management of pain, stiffness, and muscle spasm. Also, deterioration may be slowed, prolonging the time before replacement surgery is required. Generally, increasing tissue pliability and circulation, combined with management of sympathetic arousal, could help

this client. Short-term symptomatic pain relief or pain reduction is a reasonable expectation, but the massage effects will wear off, and an ongoing appointment schedule is needed.

2. Racquetball may not be the best activity, because the constant running in different directions in short bursts and the starting and stopping are hard on the knees. Swimming could be an option.

3. Gradual introduction of a conservative flexibility program would be helpful.

What Are the Logical Outcomes of Each Possible Intervention Option?

The recreational center where the client plays racquetball has a swimming pool, therefore access is convenient. There is a senior yoga class available at the recreation center as well. Massage is available at the same recreation center for convenience. Cost and scheduling are not primary concerns.

Massage has a good likelihood of successful management of conditions as long as the client has regular appointments and realizes that this is a long-term care program. Cardiac medication may alter the amount of pressure tolerated by the client. Regular reports should be sent to his doctor.

What Is the Impact on the People Involved for Each Massage Intervention Option?

Swimming does not meet the client's desire for competition. He may try anyway but will not commit. Yoga does not thrill the client, but he is willing to try it as long as the class is not full of "old fogies." He is willing to play less racquetball and more golf but says golf does not make him sweat like racquetball, and he needs something to make him sweat.

Patience is necessary for everyone. The progress from the massage will most likely be slow, and the effectiveness wears off. The massage therapist needs to realize that under the gruffness is likely an individual who is afraid and vulnerable. Awareness of and respect for boundary issues are necessary to keep the client empowered.

DECISION MAKING AND TREATMENT PLAN DEVELOPMENT

Quantifiable Goal

Reduce sensation of stiffness and pain by 50% as long as regular appointments are scheduled

Qualifiable Goal

The client will be able to participate in moderate low-impact sports exercise activities without being hindered by arthritic pain and joint stiffness.

Treatment Regimen

Condition Management

A long-term massage program is required with an initial schedule of twice a week right after racquetball. This will help reduce some of the strain on the client's knees from racquetball. Because of the client's size and the complex application of massage, $1\frac{1}{2}$-hour sessions are needed. The cost is $70 per session. The appointment schedule will be reduced to weekly as soon as improvement is noted and the client's condition stabilizes.

Full-body massage with multiple goals is needed. The fibrotic and binding connective tissue structure noticed bodywide will need to be systematically but slowly addressed. The focus is on increasing the pliability of the ground substance to reduce muscle density and fascial shortening and maintain more flexibility of the body. Effective methods could be myofascial release plus broad-based application of compression with the forearm, and possibly the knee and foot, against the tissue to compress the soft tissue and carry it away from the bone, with the client actively moving the adjacent joint. Sidelying positioning for the legs and working on a floor mat would facilitate this type of application.

The client will likely require varying degrees of pressure and depth of application. The sensation should be on the edge of "good hurt," sufficient to trigger endorphin and serotonin release but not enough to elicit guarding or bracing. Caution for bruising is indicated because of his use of aspirin. Gliding with drag can stretch the soft tissue. Until the client's muscle tone normalizes, use of active resistance for muscle energy methods may be counterproductive. Direct manipulation of the spindle cell and tendon responses or having the client make circles with his eyes and head to initiate muscle facilitation and inhibition in the limbs is likely to be more effective. Kneading can introduce shear, bending, and torsion forces to increase ground substance viscosity, especially around all the scars. The client must drink water so that the connective tissue rehydrates.

The knees can be a primary focus after muscle tone normalizes a bit. The trigger point activity can be addressed, specifically the ones in the quadriceps and gastrocnemius that refer pain into the knees. Traction of the knees can temporarily separate joint surfaces. Surface edema can be moved with lymphatic drainage.

Application of ice and heat between massage sessions will be encouraged.

CASE 12 NERVE IMPINGEMENT SYNDROME

The client is a 34-year-old female. She has been a cosmetologist for 12 years and maintains a very busy practice. The client has been self-employed for the past 4 years and has two employees. The business specializes in hair weaving and various types of braiding. She has been experiencing right arm and wrist pain for the past 2 years. She was diagnosed with carpal tunnel syndrome (median nerve impingement), but surgery is not recommended until more conservative interventions have been exhausted. There are also indications of brachial plexus impingement from a minor whiplash injury 3 years ago. Another contributing factor is the client's use of birth control pills. She is experiencing the typical symptoms of pain in the wrist and hand with numbness in the thumb and first two fingers. The muscles in the hand show no signs of atrophy. Her right arm feels heavy, and she has aching and numbness from her upper arm down into the right scapular area. Tapping the wrist makes the hand tingle, and reaching for the floor with the right hand and lateral flexing of the head to the left increase the symptoms. She wakes up at night with her arm feeling numb. Heat applications help. She takes an over-the-counter pain medication, Aleve (naproxen sodium). She was referred for massage by the physician in the pain clinic where the massage practitioner is also employed.

ASSESSMENT

Observation

The client's height and weight appear to be normal. She seems a bit swollen. She is a pleasant, energetic, and accommodating person. She draws a distinct line pattern of pain down her arm and hand and across the shoulder under the scapula.

Interview and Goals

The client information form does not indicate any contributing factors other than stress and fatigue from long working hours. She uses birth control pills. The client is "not complaining" because she has worked so hard for her business success. She rates her pain a 7 on a 1 to 10 scale. She indicates that she begins her day at a pain level of 3 and that the pain worsens as the day progresses. She can tolerate the pain in the morning but finds that by the afternoon, her capability is adversely affected.

The client's goal for the massage is to reduce the arm pain.

Physical Assessment

Posture

Right shoulder is high and anteriorly rotated. Right arm is internally rotated. Head is tilted to the right.

Gait

Arm swing is short on the right.

Range of Motion

External rotation is limited to 60 degrees. Client resists lateral flexion of the head to the left because it feels tight and makes the arm ache.

Palpation

Near Touch. Anterior triangle of the neck on the right is warm.

Skin. Dampness is noted in the upper right shoulder region, which corresponds with an area of heat. Skin is smooth and resilient. Tissue binds around the right wrist and up into the forearm.

Superficial Connective Tissue. Generally boggy.

Vessels and Lymph Nodes. Normal

Muscles. Scalenes on the right are short, and scalenes on the left are inhibited and long. Sternocleidomastoid is short and fibrotic on the left, right rhomboids are inhibited and long, anterior serratus is short on the right, right subscapularis is short, and pectoralis minor is short on the right. Wrist flexors are bilaterally short, with trigger point activity in the flexor pollicis longus, pronator teres, brachioradialis, and supraspinatus on the right.

Tendons. Tender at insertion of right flexor digitorum group bilaterally. Subscapular tendon on the right is tender to moderate pressure.

Deep Fascia. Palmar fasciae bilaterally are short. Retinaculum on the right is short, with reduced pliability compared with the left hand.

Ligaments. Retinaculum at the right wrist is thick.

Joints. Normal

Bones. Normal

Abdominal Viscera. Normal

Body Rhythms. Normal; respiratory circulation is craniosacral.

Muscle Testing

Strength

Short muscles with trigger point activity test strong but cannot sustain the resistance because of an increase in symptoms.

Neurologic Balance

Normal

Gait

Muscles in the right arm are not inhibiting appropriately.

INTERPRETATION AND TREATMENT PLAN DEVELOPMENT

Clinical Reasoning

What Are the Facts?

Nerve impingement (entrapment) syndromes are a common cause of pain. The distribution of pain depends on the nerve impinged. Impinged cervical plexus nerves usually refer pain up into the head. Brachial plexus nerve impingement refers pain into the shoulder and down the arm. Lumbar plexus impingement refers into the gluteals and groin or down the side of the leg to the knee. Sciatic nerve pain radiates down the back of the leg. The pain of individual nerve impingement, such as the median nerve in carpal tunnel syndrome, follows the distribution of the nerve. Trigger point pain patterns can follow similar distribution patterns and are a common component of nerve-type pain. The person usually has a history of trauma or repetitive strain with resulting muscle spasm. Fluid retention in vulnerable areas, such as the wrist, can be causal. This can happen with pregnancy or the use of birth control pills. Often the condition has multiple causal factors. Soft tissue impingement of nerves is the easiest of these types of syndromes to manage, and surgery should be avoided if possible because scar tissue formation after the surgery can cause future problems. If surgery is performed, scar development needs to be managed in the acute, subacute, and remodeling stages. Bony impingement usually requires referral to a chiropractor, an osteopath, a physical therapist or, in extreme cases, a surgeon. Tight muscles, both concentric and isometric (short) and eccentric (long), can press on nerves. Connective tissue shortening and adhesions are common causes of impingement. Women are somewhat more vulnerable to impingement syndromes such as carpal tunnel syndrome.

This client has multiple causal factors. Her job and increased demands for her service are increasing the amount of repetitive strain in the affected area. The whiplash injury can predispose the scalenes and other muscles of the neck and shoulder girdle to shortening. She is also retaining fluid, likely from the birth control pills.

What Are the Possibilities Both in Function and Dysfunction and the Massage Intervention Options?

The client probably has brachial plexus impingement, as well as trigger point activity that is referring into the wrist area. Edema at the wrists is adding to the impingement. The connective tissue at the carpal tunnel is also thick. The source of most of the symptoms is unclear.

Possibilities:

1. Massage intervention would need to address each area: short, spasming muscles; trigger points in the belly of the muscles; short, thick connective tissue; and edema.
2. Spot work is possible but usually unsuccessful, because areas of compensation, although not currently noticed, are likely developing. The client indicates that she is stressed, therefore full-body massage is most beneficial.
3. The client would benefit from a moderate exercise and flexibility program.

What Are the Logical Outcomes of Each Possible Intervention Option?

Massage is likely to reduce symptoms and prevent the condition from getting worse. It at least would slow the deterioration. Long-term care is probable.

Time is the biggest issue. Also, repetitive strain injury benefits from rest, which the client cannot easily do because of work demands. Early morning weekday appointments are available, and this is the best time for the client.

Because the massage therapist is an employee of the pain clinic, the clinic may be able to receive some reimbursement from the client's insurance company for the acute care. Insurance probably will not pay for maintenance massage care.

What Is the Impact on the People Involved for Each Massage Intervention Option?

The client is compliant but unwilling to reduce her work schedule. She says she will begin a regular stretching program, but compliance seems unlikely because of time constraints.

DECISION MAKING AND TREATMENT PLAN DEVELOPMENT

Quantifiable Goal

Reduce pain to level 3 on a 1 to 10 pain scale without pain increasing throughout the work day

Qualifiable Goal

The client will be able to work a 40-hour week without limiting pain.

Treatment Regimen

Therapeutic Change/Condition Management

A 1-hour full-body massage with a lymphatic drainage component will be given twice a week. Methods to increase natural pain-modulating mechanisms (e.g., endorphins and serotonin) and to support the parasympathetic process for stress management are appropriate.

Acute-phase treatment will proceed as follows:

- Short muscles will be addressed with general massage and muscle energy and lengthening methods. All layers of muscles will be worked, because synergists and fixators are involved. Inhibited antagonists will be stimulated.
- Trigger point activity that refers symptoms in short muscles will be addressed with positional release or integrated muscle energy methods and lengthening. The results will be evaluated before connective tissue methods are introduced.
- Self-help methods will be taught to the client. Pulsed muscle energy and lengthening for short muscles and positional release for more active trigger points will be demonstrated.

This phase could take 6 weeks.

After the acute phase, connective tissue methods will be introduced to restore pliability to the thick fascial areas of the right forearm and wrist. Careful use of friction to create therapeutic inflammation is necessary. Monitoring will ensure that the methods do not aggravate the symptoms.

The client will be observed for posture improvement and the development of symptoms in the areas of compensation, such as the low back. Should such symptoms develop, she will be reassessed for short muscle imbalance and connective tissue shortening. Also, trigger points that refer to areas experiencing symptoms will be identified and treated.

When the client's condition is stable, appointments will be reduced to a maintenance schedule of once a week.

CASE 13 GENERAL RELAXATION

The client is a 44-year-old male who is on a vacation cruise. He has a high-stress job and has personal relationship problems. He will be on the cruise for 2 weeks and would like to schedule four massage sessions (two each week). Although he knows he has numerous minor musculoskeletal issues, he is not interested in addressing any of them. His goal is relaxation and pampering. He has no contraindications for relaxation massage.

ASSESSMENT

Observation

The client appears fatigued and frazzled. His weight appears normal for his height, and he looks moderately physically fit.

Interview and Goals

The client does not state anything on the client information form that would indicate contraindications. He indicates that he is stressed and that he gets an occasional tension headache. He takes no medication, although he takes a daily general multivitamin.

He wants general massage with firm pressure that does not hurt. He does not want to participate; in fact, he hopes that he falls asleep.

When asked what type of relaxation sensation he would like and his goal for the massage, he replies that he wants to feel loose, sleepy, and calm.

Physical Assessment

Note: The client did not want to participate in an extensive physical assessment process. Assessment information is gathered during the general observation and the first massage.

Posture

Slight forward head position and hyperextended knees when standing in symmetric stance.

Gait

Somewhat rigid.

Range of Motion

Within normal range.

Palpation

Near Touch. Skin is warm; client has a slight sunburn.

Skin. Skin is normal. Binding is seen in the lumbar and occipital base areas. Client has extensive body hair.

Superficial Connective Tissue. Fibrotic at iliotibial band bilaterally.

Vessels and Lymph Nodes. Normal

Muscles. Muscle tissue is dense. Hamstrings are short, and abdominals are long and weak.

Tendons. Normal

Deep Fascia. Plantar and lumbar fasciae are short.

Ligaments. Normal

Joints. Knee flexion bilaterally is limited by 10 degrees.

Bones. Normal

Abdominal Viscera. Normal

Body Rhythms. Upper chest breathing pattern.

Muscle Testing

Not performed.

INTERPRETATION AND TREATMENT PLAN DEVELOPMENT

Clinical Reasoning

What Are the Facts?

This case falls into the category of palliative care. The focus is on relaxation in a vacation environment, but similar treatment plans would be indicated for individuals having surgery before and after the procedure, acute care, and for care of the terminally ill.

Relaxation and pleasurable sensation are important functions of therapeutic massage. Massage is used to balance the autonomic nervous system functions and usually provides support for a reduction in sympathetic arousal, as well as the potential for a more parasympathetic balance. Relaxation can mean different things to different people. For most clients, relaxation is an experience of parasympathetic dominance with serotonin, dynorphin, enkephalin, and endorphin responses. For those who would like to be alert but relaxed, the focus must be on stimulating norepinephrine and dopamine production. It is important to determine what the client means by "being relaxed." Asking questions that help the client clarify his or her interpretation of the relaxation experience can provide information on what the physiologic outcomes should be.

Entrainment is an important aspect of relaxation because it coordinates body rhythms. Soft, rhythmic music and indirect lighting can be helpful in achieving a parasympathetic result. Aromatherapy is an advanced intervention requiring specialized training, but simple, safe application of some common essential oils is said to be calming. Lavender is one of the most calming. Various applications of heat are also comforting. A warm hot water bottle at the feet or behind the neck is pleasurable.

What Are the Possibilities Both in Function and Dysfunction and the Massage Intervention Options?

The client has numerous areas of short and long muscles actively coupled with connective tissue dysfunction, but addressing these areas would not meet the client's goal. The upper chest breathing pattern could be addressed because that should result in a calming effect.

Possibilities:

1. The massage practitioner can offer the client a selection of aromas and music, and he could pick the ones he prefers.
2. Warm compresses can be placed over the client's eyes, and a warm pack can be provided for his feet. An alternative would be a warm foot bath before the massage.

What Are the Logical Outcomes of Each Possible Intervention Option?

Because of his sunburn, the client may not want the hot water application.

He may be allergic to the volatile oils in the essential oils.

The massage environment must be quiet, and the massage professional must limit conversation so that the client can fall asleep if he wishes and is not required to engage in conversation.

What Is the Impact on the People Involved for Each Massage Intervention Option?

The massage professional must remain focused on the client's goal and not address the other musculoskeletal issues identified.

DECISION MAKING AND TREATMENT PLAN DEVELOPMENT

Quantifiable Goal

Induce the relaxation response and support parasympathetic dominance, indicated by slowing of breathing and client self-reports

Qualifiable Goal

The client will feel relaxed, sleepy, and calm.

Treatment Regimen

Palliative Care

A full-body massage will be given with gliding, kneading, compression, and rocking for 90 minutes, with a rhythmic approach used to match the music selected by the client. The pressure level will be moderate to deep but will not elicit discomfort. Sufficient nonirritating lubricant will be used to prevent pulling of the body hair or irritation of the sunburn. The client will be offered a warm, damp towel to remove the lubricant after the massage. The massage professional can do this for the client as a way of gently waking him up after the massage. A massage focused on the feet, hands, head, and face

sends the most signals into the central nervous system for relaxation. Attention to the thorax, shoulders, neck, and midback muscles provides inhibition and lengthening of the auxiliary breathing muscles to support relaxed breathing. The client will be positioned in the prone, side-lying, and supine positions, and he will be moved unobtrusively. The scent selected will be placed in a diffuser or mist bottle to prevent any skin irritation.

The massage practitioner will stay focused and calm, intent on creating a quiet space with empathy and compassion, no expectations, and no interruptions for the client.

CASE 14 SLEEP DISTURBANCE

The client is a 52-year-old female. She is menopausal, and among other changes, she is experiencing sleep problems. Her uterus was removed when she was 46, but she still has her ovaries. She is mildly hypertensive but is not taking medication for it. She is taking a low-dose hormone replacement (estradiol) and uses a topical progesterone cream. The estrogen and progesterone, plus the addition of soy to her diet and vitamin E supplementation, have controlled her hot flashes. However, she is still moody and restless. She is considering returning to school to advance her career options. Currently, she works part-time as a nurse. She is 15 pounds above her ideal weight. She is active; she plays golf and tennis and bowls. For the past 6 months she has been on a very-low-fat diet and has lost 12 pounds. She is married and has two grown children and one in high school. She is satisfied with her personal and professional life most of the time. There is some tension with her 16-year-old daughter.

She loves coffee. She quit smoking 9 years ago, after her 68-year-old father died of lung cancer. Her mother is living but has osteoporosis, which is interfering with her quality of life.

She has minor aching in her knee joints and is generally stiff in the morning but loosens up with a hot shower and some stretching. She has had an occasional massage while on vacation but has never had massage that focused on a specific outcome goal. She became aware of the benefits of massage in a book she was reading about managing menopause.

ASSESSMENT

Observation

The client's appearance is appropriate for her age. She has some wrinkling, which is explained by the smoking and by the greater susceptibility of Caucasian skin to sun damage. She colors her hair, therefore the color and texture will not provide reliable information on stress response. She is a bit overweight, with fat distribution in the lower abdominal area, which is typical for menopause. The fat helps convert body chemicals to estrogen-like substances, replacing the estrogen production of the ovaries. The fat appears to be between the abdominal wall and the skin, which is of much less concern than fat distribution in the abdominal cavity, which is an indication of stress and increased cortisol secretion, with implications for cardiovascular problems. Her mood seems even, although she is a bit intense in her conversation. She yawns and sniffs frequently, which may indicate a tendency for a breathing pattern disorder.

Interview and Goals

The client information form indicates that she uses reading glasses; has minor sinus congestion, especially in the fall; and has urge incontinence, which causes a need to urinate frequently, including at night. She has a tendency to bloat and has the aching knees and generalized morning stiffness previously mentioned. She has had three pregnancies and a hysterectomy. She has mild hypertension and is fatigued from lack of sustained sleep. When questioned, she reports that just as she is falling asleep, she has to get up to urinate. Then she has difficulty falling asleep again. During the night she either just wakes up and then feels the urge to use the restroom, or bladder pressure wakes her up. She feels as if she is up and down all night. In an attempt to reduce bladder frequency, she has restricted her fluid intake. She is also having some vivid dreams with the themes of running, looking for things, or trying to find people in a crowd.

She is undergoing hormone replacement therapy and takes a multivitamin supplement for menopausal women that includes some herbs, particularly black cohosh, gingko biloba, and extra vitamin E. She also takes a calcium/magnesium supplement. She had her appendix and tonsils out as a child. She is involved with various sports for leisure and exercise.

Her main goal for the massage is to sleep better. After being educated about the effects of massage on mood-regulating neurochemicals and the morning stiffness and joint aching in her knees, she has become interested in addressing these goals as well. However, she is mainly concerned about the sleep quality and will base her evaluation of the effectiveness of the massage on this outcome.

Physical Assessment

Posture

Generally symmetric, but the shoulders are held a bit high and bilaterally rotate forward; this is so slight at this time that no compensation pattern is noted in any other body area.

Gait

Normal

Range of Motion

Knees are restricted in flexion, and range of motion is reduced by 10%. External rotation of both shoulders results in a minor reduction in mobility.

Palpation

Near Touch. Slightly increased heat in the upper thorax.

Skin. Surface texture is dry; hair is brittle; nails are well formed, but cuticles are dry and cracked. Elasticity is reduced

in upper thorax around clavicles and at sacrum and on the bottoms of the feet. Skin is somewhat tight against the subcutaneous layer and does not lift easily.

Superficial Connective Tissue. Generally reduced pliability, with indications of minor dehydration (pinched skin fold holds its shape longer than normal).

Vessels and Lymph Nodes. Normal

Muscles. No obvious neuromuscular issues or trigger point activity.

Tendons. Normal

Deep Fascia. Short and binding.

Ligaments. Slightly dense.

Joints. Minor stiffness with soft but binding (leathery) end-feel. Knees are moderately painful with both compression and traction.

Bones. Normal with reservations; family history indicates possible tendency for osteoporosis.

Abdominal Viscera. Moderate bloat.

Body Rhythms. Breathing is a bit irregular and has an upper chest quality. Heart rate has moments of increased rhythm. Cranial rhythm seems inhibited (sluggish lymphatic movement is likely responsible).

Muscle Testing

Strength
Normal

Neurologic Balance
Normal

Gait
Normal

INTERPRETATION AND TREATMENT PLAN DEVELOPMENT

Clinical Reasoning

What Are the Facts?

The client is menopausal and has typical manifestations of that stage of life; she is taking measures to manage the uncomfortable mood and circulatory changes. She has a family history of osteoporosis and cancer, and she herself has a history of smoking.

Menopause is a normal process that begins as a woman's hormonal patterns change and ovarian production and menstruation cease. Changes in urinary and sleep patterns are common. The urinary stress and urge incontinence can be related to changes in membranes in the urinary tract in response to reduced estrogen levels. Sleep changes are related to urinary urge, hot flashes, and changes in the serotonin level in relation to the estrogen level.

Breathing function is mechanically altered with the connective tissue changes, causing an upper chest breathing pattern; this results in oxygen levels in the blood that support sympathetic nervous system arousal.

Connective tissue changes and dry skin indicate mild dehydration and insufficient dietary fat intake. Estrogen also helps tissues maintain proper hydration, and with a reduction in estrogen, connective tissue ground substance does not hydrate as easily.

Evidence of osteoarthritis is present in the client's knees (pain on compression), and soft tissue involvement (pain on traction) is noted.

What Are the Possibilities Both in Function and Dysfunction and the Massage Intervention Options?

The client may be predisposing herself to connective tissue changes by restricting water and an appropriate healthy fat intake. She is doing this because of the weight gain and urinary urge. The reduction in estrogens may have altered the serotonin balance; this affects the production of melatonin, which controls aspects of the sleep cycle. Also, the bladder urgency is disturbing her sleep.

Breathing changes may be increasing the tendency for sympathetic dominance with increased cortisol levels; these higher levels would interfere with deep sleep and contribute to the type of dreams the client is having.

Possibilities:

1. A general full-body massage is indicated, with deep but not painful compression to encourage parasympathetic dominance and to support levels of serotonin, endorphins, dynorphins, and enkephalins for mood and sleep. This massage approach, coupled with a drag quality to increase the pliability of the superficial connective tissue, should address the client's major and minor concerns, including the knee pain. The mechanics of breathing must be addressed as well, but the major anatomic reason for upper chest breathing seems to be connective tissue binding with sympathetic arousal.
2. The client needs to increase her intake of fluids and essential fatty acids (e.g., olive oil) to support proper tissue hydration and hormone and neurotransmitter function.
3. She should be referred to her doctor for the urinary urgency. However, reducing cortisol levels and supporting deep sleep should help with the nighttime urgency.
4. A slow stretching program with a meditative quality would be helpful.

What Are the Logical Outcomes of Each Possible Intervention Option?

The massage should result in management of the conditions of concern. Regular ongoing appointments are required, and this creates a time and cost burden for the client. Referral to the doctor is necessary to rule out more serious reasons for the urinary problem, which requires time and money.

Increasing fluid may temporarily aggravate the urinary stress. The stretching program may temporarily increase stiffness if the client is too aggressive, but moderate stretching would help maintain relaxation, joint mobility, and connective tissue pliability.

The client is self-seeking massage, and this type of client often is the most compliant in terms of keeping appointments and following through with self-help education.

What Is the Impact on the People Involved for Each Massage Intervention Option?

The massage professional needs to be committed to a regular appointment schedule.

Some emotional undertones to the client's case, especially the restlessness, wanting to return to school, and tension with her daughter, may surface during the sessions. The massage professional must maintain appropriate boundaries and make the appropriate referrals. The client likely does not realize the emotional nature of the situation and may be confused if these issues surface. Redirection to the massage process and the referral will be helpful.

DECISION MAKING AND TREATMENT PLAN DEVELOPMENT

Quantifiable Goals

1. Improve sleep quality, as self-reported by client
2. Balance mood and physical stress levels, as self-reported by client
3. Reverse upper chest breathing pattern, as measured by therapist

Qualifiable Goals

The client will be less fatigued and stiff, which will allow her to perform her desired daily exercise activities.

Treatment Regimen

Condition Management

A weekly 1-hour massage will be provided on an open-ended, ongoing basis. The cost will be $50, and every tenth massage will be free.

The massage methods used will include gliding with moderate to deep but not painful pressure to increase the levels of serotonin and other mood-regulating neurochemicals and to reduce sympathetic arousal. Gliding also will be done with sufficient drag to cause connective tissue creep in binding areas and to increase viscosity in areas that show reduced pliability. Kneading also will be done, with localized use of skin rolling at the thorax and sacrum to increase connective tissue water binding. Rhythmic rocking with entrainment to the client's selected soft, slow music will encourage parasympathetic dominance. The range of motion of the knees and shoulders will be normalized with muscle energy methods and lengthening. Binding connective tissue will be stretched by means of bending and torsion forces applied with compression and kneading.

The client will be taught breathing exercises as presented in Chapter 13 of this textbook. The information in Chapter 13 also will be used to teach her methods of maintaining a supportive sleep cycle.

She will be educated in the importance of drinking water and of appropriate fat intake and will be referred to her physician and nutritionist for confirmation of this information for her specific needs, as well as for diagnosis of the bladder urgency.

She will be referred to a slow stretching program, such as yoga, to address the connective tissue stiffness and to support sleep and relaxation.

CASE 15 CIRCULATION IMPAIRMENT

The client is a 57-year-old male with type 2 diabetes mellitus. He is non-insulin-dependent at this point and is taking an oral hypoglycemic medication that stimulates the secretion of insulin. He is 40 pounds overweight, and part of his diabetic management is weight loss. He lost 25 pounds initially but has not lost any weight in 3 months. His exercise is closely monitored to minimize blood sugar fluctuations. He walks and uses a rowing machine. He has begun to notice some impaired circulation in his legs and some burning in his feet. He reports that he has developed minor symptoms of vascular insufficiency and diabetic neuropathy, a common complication of diabetes. His doctors are exploring all options to manage the condition. The nurse on the diabetic management team has recommended massage, because recent studies have shown benefit both in supporting circulation and in more optimal insulin regulation. The client is willing to try anything that can help, and because the massage therapist is affiliated with the medical team, he feels confident that the nurse who is responsible for the management of his program will supervise the process.

The client is in a long-term relationship and has a good support system.

ASSESSMENT

The following information was provided by the medical team:

The client is a 57-year-old male with moderate type 2 diabetes mellitus. He is being treated with Glucotrol, diet, exercise, and education in diabetes and stress management. Renal function is good. Recent developments include vascular impairment and diabetic neuropathy in the feet. The massage prescription is for stress reduction with secondary support for peripheral circulation. The frequency and duration are two times per week for 1 hour per session.

(*Note:* This is an example of responding to a massage prescription. The goals for the massage are determined by the physician. The assessment that follows is to determine how best to meet those goals and respond to the treatment plan provided.)

Observation

The client is visibly nervous and fidgety. He prefers to stand to complete the intake process. He wrings his hands often and regularly sighs deeply. The client's excess weight is carried in his abdomen and gluteal area.

Interview and Goals

The client reports that he has never had a massage. He is ticklish and is concerned about taking off his clothing. He was in a car accident 10 years ago and had a whiplash injury and a concussion. He experiences aching after exercise. Other than the diabetes, he is in good health. He works as a maintenance supervisor and trouble-shooter for a local manufacturing firm. He used to drink beer, but alcohol is no longer part of his diet. He also quit smoking 3 years ago. He still misses smoking, especially the morning coffee and cigarette, but he is determined to do whatever it takes to manage the diabetes. His mother died of complications of the same disease.

He understands that the goal for the massage is to help him relax, which will help regulate insulin levels. Additional outcomes would be to increase circulation and reduce the numbing and prickling sensation in his feet caused by the neuropathy.

Physical Assessment

Posture

Moderate lumbar lordosis and forward head position.

Gait

Clumsy, with a flat-foot landing on his feet rather than the normal heel strike–toe off pattern.

Range of Motion

Trunk flexion is inhibited by the abdominal fat mass. Plantar flexion and dorsiflexion are decreased by 20% bilaterally.

Palpation

Near Touch. No noticeable difference.

Skin. Normal except for a bluish cast in the feet. Lower extremities are cool. Binding is present in the lumbar area and at the base of the neck. Palpable fat layer is present under the skin, with excessive accumulation in the abdomen and gluteals.

Superficial Connective Tissue. Bind in the lumbar area, thorax, and calves.

Vessels and Lymph Nodes. Lymph circulation appears normal, but pulses are weaker in the feet, and vessels seem constricted.

Muscles. Somewhat decreased in tone overall, with evidence of the exercise effect increasing muscle tone in the legs and arms but not in the abdomen or gluteal region.

Tendons. Right Achilles tendon is nonpliable.

Deep Fascia. Binding in the lumbar and anterior thoracic sheaths and nonresilience in the abdomen. Plantar fasciae are short bilaterally.

Ligaments. Normal

Joints. No evidence of arthritis or pain on compression or traction. Lumbar curve is exaggerated. Knees and feet ache.

Bones. Normal

Abdominal Viscera. Difficult to palpate because of internal and external fat distribution.

Body Rhythms. Slow, uneven breathing rate.

Muscle Testing

Not performed.

INTERPRETATION AND TREATMENT PLAN DEVELOPMENT

Clinical Reasoning

What Are the Facts?

Diabetes is caused by impaired release of insulin by the pancreas, by inadequate or abnormal insulin receptors on the cells, or by destruction of insulin before it can become active. Type 2 diabetes is a maturity onset form often found in adults who are overweight, especially if a family history of the disease is a factor. Diabetes symptoms include increased thirst and appetite. The high blood glucose levels have detrimental effects on most body systems; these effects include impaired eyesight, neuropathy, impaired circulation, a tendency for thrombosis and emboli, and diminished resistance to infection. Wounds heal slowly, and kidney function is strained. The individual also is susceptible to atherosclerosis. All this must be taken into account when massage is applied.

The client in this case has impaired peripheral circulation with neuropathy in the lower legs. Kidney function is normal. The client has no history of blood clots. He is taking medication that has common side effects of diarrhea, dizziness, fatigue, headache, heartburn, loss of appetite, upset stomach, sun sensitivity, vomiting, and weakness. Serious side effects of medication that require referral include blood disorders, breathing difficulties, dark urine, itching, jaundice, light-colored stools, low blood sugar, muscle cramps, rash, sore throat, fever, tightening in the hands and feet, and unusual bleeding or bruising. The massage practitioner needs to pay particular attention to dizziness, weakness, breathing, jaundice, itching, and symptoms of low blood sugar (besides dizziness and weakness, these include pallor, a rapid heart rate, and excessive sweating). Diabetic clients should always have their medications with them, and fruit juice or another quick-acting carbohydrate should be available. Muscle cramps, rash, and bruising also need to be considered. Cautions and accommodations are necessary. The skin can become thin and fragile in areas of impaired circulation.

This client is also anxious, indicating sympathetic dominance. He is ticklish and uncertain about taking off his clothes. He is overweight and experiences muscle aches after exercise. His knees bother him. He was in a car accident that injured his neck. He has fascial shortening in the feet, lumbar area, and thorax.

What Are the Possibilities Both in Function and Dysfunction and the Massage Intervention Options?

The possibilities for intervention are limited by the treatment plan provided by the physician. The physician has ordered relaxation massage and support for peripheral circulation with a schedule of biweekly 1-hour sessions.

Of more concern is how to follow the treatment plan when the client is ticklish and nervous about taking his clothes off. The client could be introduced to massage through use of a seated massage format over the clothing until he is more comfortable and then could be transferred to the more traditional massage on the table with draping.

What Are the Logical Outcomes of Each Possible Intervention Option?

The chair massage over the clothing would address the issue of the client not wanting to take off his clothes. However, this type of massage may not provide enough relaxation response to support the goals of the physician. Also, addressing the problem of impaired circulation in the legs would be more difficult.

Tickling can be managed by using more pressure. Because the client's skin is in good shape and he has no history of thrombosis or embolism, broad-based compression would be a good method.

What Is the Impact on the People Involved for Each Massage Intervention Option?

The client would be more comfortable with the chair massage initially, and over time he would be able to move from the chair to the table. Once he realizes that he enjoys the massage and is not being tickled, he should relax.

DECISION MAKING AND TREATMENT PLAN DEVELOPMENT

Quantifiable Goals

As determined by the physician.

Qualifiable Goals

As determined by the physician.

Treatment Regimen

In accordance with treatment orders, the client will be given a 1-hour massage twice a week. The fees will be billed through the physician's office. Massage intervention will begin in the chair, with education provided about the effects of massage. Demonstration of the type of massage used to prevent tickling will be included, and draping methods also will be demonstrated.

While the client is using the seated position, the main focus of the massage will be to reduce sympathetic dominance and support normal breathing. Compression will be applied over the clothing, with shaking and rhythmic rocking of the arms and wrists and passive and active range of motion of the neck.

Once the client's apprehension about getting on the table and taking off his clothing has eased, a general full-body massage will be used to promote parasympathetic dominance. The connective tissue shortening will be addressed with myofascial release, always with an awareness of skin fragility. With the increase in connective tissue pliability, circulation and breathing should improve. The short, tight calf muscles will be addressed with slow gliding strokes, accompanied by monitoring for bruising. The calf muscle must have sufficient contractile capacity to promote circulation.

Circulation in the lower extremities will be encouraged with general full-body massage, with compression over the arteries moving proximal to distal. Caution will be used so that any evidence of thrombosis can be detected.

Addressing any areas of discomfort related to past injury or causes other than the diabetes will be cleared with the physician before the treatment plan is altered.

Recommendations to the physician will include massage application to reduce postexercise aching, which will support compliance with the exercise program; alteration of the exercise program to include some resistance exercises targeting the gluteal and abdominal areas; and normalization of the posture to support optimum energy expenditure. There is also evidence of an altered upper chest breathing pattern; because this perpetuates sympathetic arousal, it would be beneficial to address the problem by having the client participate in a breathing retraining program.

CASE 16 FATIGUE CAUSED BY CANCER TREATMENT

The client is a 46-year-old female with early detected, stage I breast cancer. The cancer was detected by mammography 12 months ago. She had a lumpectomy and radiation therapy. The outcome looks good. She is currently undergoing treatment with tamoxifen.

Two years ago the client married for the first time. She has not had children, and she does not plan to have any. She managed a branch bank for many years but retired from that job and is seeking a more meaningful career.

She loves restoring antiques and hopes to pursue this as both a hobby and a money-making enterprise. Although money is a concern for her, life is more of an issue, and she is willing to commit both time and resources to those things that increase the quality of her life. She heard about massage at a support group meeting and was intrigued by the studies that showed that massage supports the immune function and helps with the anxiety and depression that can accompany the diagnosis and treatment of cancer. She is also involved with a yoga class through the support group. This is her first formal exercise program, and she is enjoying it. Although she is sore, it feels beneficial. She is a bit overweight, and although weight loss is not a goal, she hopes to become more fit.

Her main concern is fatigue. After a year of focusing on treatment, she wants to get on with her life, but the fatigue keeps her motivation suppressed. She experienced fatigue during radiation treatment but expected to resume her normal energy level once treatment was over. In addition to the benefits mentioned in the studies, she hopes that massage will help her regain her energy. All medical test results, including those from thyroid and bone density tests, are within normal parameters. Her doctor is very supportive of massage but wants to speak to the massage practitioner before sessions begin to review the proposed treatment plan.

ASSESSMENT

Observation

The client is soft spoken but direct and does not avoid eye contact or difficult topics. Her body motions seem slow, and she appears tired. Her body fat is evenly distributed.

Interview and Goals

Information from the client history form indicates that there is a slight family history of breast cancer but not in her immediate family. She has always been a bit overweight. She had her first menstrual period at 10 years of age, and she still has regular menstrual periods. She has taken birth control pills on and off for years. Birth control is not an issue at this point, because her husband has had a vasectomy. She gets an occasional headache but nothing significant. She has had the normal childhood illnesses. She feels as if she is not sleeping deeply.

Her goal for the massage is an improved energy level.

Physical Assessment

Posture

Concave upper chest and bilaterally internally rotated arms. Slight kyphosis. Jutting chin with slight forward head position. Flattened lumbar curve with bilateral posterior pelvic rotation. Left knee is hyperextended.

Gait

Weight is carried on the heels, with shortened stride and arm swing.

Range of Motion

Capital and cervical flexion combined allow only 10 degrees of motion. External rotation of arms is limited to 75 degrees.

Abduction and extension of shoulders are limited to 20 degrees. Trunk extension at lumbar region is limited to 15 degrees. Hip extension is limited to 20 degrees and dorsiflexion to 15 degrees.

Palpation

Near Touch. Energy field seems uneven and erratic.

Skin. Skin is dry and shows obvious effects of radiation in treatment area. Two large moles are present on left shoulder. Bind is present in the thorax between the scapulae and in the lumbar area. Bind also is noted in the hamstrings and calves. Connective tissue seems dense in the lumbar area and hamstrings but thin in the thorax and abdomen.

Superficial Connective Tissue. Scar tissue at the surgical site is pliable, with a small area of bind near the axilla.

Vessels and Lymph Nodes. Normal, although caution is indicated in the left axilla adjacent to the treatment area.

Muscles. Occipital base, arm external rotator and adductor, and hamstring muscles are short. Gluteal group and abdominals are weak and almost flaccid. Calves are short.

Tendons. Pain reported on palpation of the subscapular tendon bilaterally. Achilles tendons are short.

Deep Fascia. Nonpliable and short in the cervical and lumbar areas and in the plantar fasciae. Abdominal fascia is nonresilient.

Ligaments. Normal

Joints. Minor pain with direct compression over the SI joints. Joints of the foot seem immobile.

Bones. Probable fragility over the radiation site.

Abdominal Viscera. Abdomen is soft and has no detectable masses or abnormalities.

Body Rhythms. Uneven and erratic; client feels out of sync with herself. Rhythms fluctuate often.

Muscle Testing

Strength

General muscle strength is fair, with excessive tone in calves and occipital base muscles.

Neurologic Balance

Normal

Gait

Normal contralateral pattern but labored. Gluteus maximus does not fire effectively.

INTERPRETATION AND TREATMENT PLAN DEVELOPMENT

Clinical Reasoning

What Are the Facts?

The client has received successful treatment for breast cancer. The causes of breast cancer are not fully known. However, health and medical researchers have identified a number of risk factors that increase a woman's chances of getting breast cancer. Risk factors are not necessarily causes of breast cancer, but they are associated with an increased risk of developing the disease. It is important to note that some women have many risk factors but do not develop breast cancer, whereas other women have few or no risk factors but do get the disease. Being a woman is the number one risk factor for breast cancer. (*Note:* Males do get breast cancer as well.) For this reason, it is important for females to perform regular breast self-examinations, have clinical breast examinations, and have routine mammograms to detect any problems at an early stage. Massage therapists need to understand the risk factors for cancer in general and in this case for breast cancer specifically.

Factors that can be controlled include the following:

- Having more than one alcoholic drink per day
- Taking birth control pills for 5 years or longer (slightly increases the risk of breast cancer)
- Not getting regular exercise
- Currently using or having recently used some forms of hormone replacement therapy for 10 years or longer (may slightly increase the risk of breast cancer)
- Being overweight or gaining weight as an adult
- Being exposed to large amounts of radiation (e.g., having frequent spinal x-rays during scoliosis treatment)

Factors that cannot be controlled include the following:

- Aging
- Having a mother, daughter, or sister who has had breast cancer
- Having the mutated breast cancer genes *BRCA-1* or *BRCA-2*
- Having had breast cancer
- Being young (under 12 years of age) at the time of the first menstrual period, starting menopause later than usual (over 55 years of age), never being pregnant, or having the first child after 30 years of age

Breast cancer can recur at anytime, but many recurrences happen within the first 2 years after diagnosis. Breast cancer may recur locally within the breast or chest area, in areas adjacent to the breast (underarm lymph nodes), or at distant locations (metastatic type). The most common sites for metastatic breast cancer are the lungs, liver, bones, and brain.

This client is 1 year postdiagnosis and has multiple risk factors for cancer development. She is currently taking tamoxifen. The most common side effect of the medication is hot flashes similar to those experienced during menopause. Tamoxifen may induce menopause in a woman who is close to menopause; however, it rarely does in young women. Other common side effects are vaginal dryness, irregular periods, and weight gain.

The surgical procedure used for breast cancer depends on the stage of the disease, the type of tumor, the woman's age and general health, her preference, and the physician's recommendation. Surgery is a form of local treatment for breast cancer, as opposed to systemic treatment that involves the entire body, such as chemotherapy. Studies have shown that most women with early-stage disease (stage I or stage II) who are treated with breast conservation measures (procedures that preserve the breast) and irradiation have the same survival rate as women treated with mastectomy.

This client had a lumpectomy, which is appropriate treatment for her stage of cancer, and underwent radiation therapy. Radiation therapy uses high-energy x-rays to destroy cancer cells in the treated area (local treatment). It is most often used with breast-conserving surgery but may also be recommended after a mastectomy for women who have four or more lymph nodes that test positive for cancer cells. The purpose is to destroy any cancer cells that may be left after breast surgery. Radiation therapy may also be used palliatively to relieve symptoms, shrink tumors, and reduce pressure, bleeding, pain, or other symptoms of advanced cancer.

Cancer cells grow and divide rapidly, and they are very sensitive to the effects of radiation. Normal cells grow and divide less rapidly and recover more fully from the effects of radiation. The side effects of radiation are the result of temporary damage to the normal cells. It is important to remember that the side effects of radiation are directly related to the dose and the area treated. Common side effects include:

- *Local skin reactions:* Itching, redness, or dryness and scaling of the skin. The degree of skin reaction is very individualized. Skin irritation continues for approximately 2 weeks after the end of treatment. Healing then begins.
- *Fatigue:* This resolves gradually after treatment.

The client in this case also has a stage 2 postural distortion; this indicates functional stress that is causing a nonoptimal movement pattern characterized by fatigue with moderate activity.

What Are the Possibilities Both in Function and Dysfunction and the Massage Intervention Options?

The main goal for the massage is management of the fatigue, which could be residual from the radiation treatment and the stress of the past year. The medication also could be causing fatigue or an interrupted sleep pattern. Another factor that is contributing to the fatigue might be the postural changes that make movement labored and tiring, especially so since the client began a moderate exercise program.

Possibilities:

1. Massage could act as a stress management method, supporting effective sleep patterns and restoring a more normal movement pattern. This massage approach would be a general constitutional approach with specific but cautious focus on the postural distortion.

2. Because the client's body rhythms seem out of sync, a rhythmic focus and approach to massage with music she enjoys could support entrainment.

3. The short muscles and connective tissue could be addressed with various massage, muscle energy, lengthening, and stretching methods.

What Are the Logical Outcomes of Each Possible Intervention Option?

The general massage, focused on quieting the stress response and supporting sleep and well-being, would help with the cancer recovery process in general but would not specifically address the postural changes that may be contributing to the fatigue. The approach should bring about some entrainment to disordered body rhythms.

A more aggressive massage approach to increase range of motion and make movement in general easier may be too aggressive this soon after cancer treatment.

What Is the Impact on the People Involved for Each Massage Intervention Option?

The doctor supports a more moderate approach that begins with the general massage and introduces the shift in muscle tension and posture gradually.

The client wants to address the problem more aggressively.

The massage therapist agrees with the slower, more cautious approach recommended by the doctor.

DECISION MAKING AND TREATMENT PLAN DEVELOPMENT

Quantifiable Goal

Increase restorative sleep by 80% as reported by client

Qualifiable Goals

The client will be able to participate in reasonable daily activities without fatigue.

Treatment Regimen

Condition Management

One-hour massage sessions will be given on a weekly basis at the massage office for $40 per session.

General full-body massage with sufficient pressure to increase serotonin levels will be given. The application will feel comfortably intense but not painful. The main methods will include variations in the depth, drag, direction, speed, and rhythm of gliding strokes. Caution will need to be observed over the irradiated site, where a decrease in pressure over the bony structure is appropriate. Rhythmic rocking and gentle shaking of the joints of the extremities will support relaxation and may increase range of motion. The two moles will be watched for changes, and any changes in the breast or axillae will be referred immediately. Gentle myofascial release methods, primarily skin stretching, can be used over the areas of connective tissue bind. Caution is required over the irradiated skin because of sensitivity and likely skin changes arising from the treatment.

The massage application will be rhythmic and relaxing. Polarity and reflexology concepts can be incorporated into the massage to support the process. Music of the client's choice that is soothing and has a rhythm of about 60 beats per minute can be used. Entrainment will be supported.

Once the client shows positive, sustained results from the methods described, positional release and pulsed muscle energy methods and lengthening can be introduced to address the postural distortion. Because the client is taking yoga classes, some postural change should occur that the massage can support. Heavy connective tissue work and invasive methods that introduce any sort of inflammation will be avoided. Any major change in the treatment plan will be approved by the physician.

CASE 17 BREATHING DISORDER: ASTHMA

The client is a 14-year-old male. His parents are exploring support care to help him manage his asthma. Massage therapy was suggested to help with stress and with relaxation of the breathing muscles. The young man is not so sure about the massage therapy. He does not want to take off his clothes, and he does not want his parents in the room watching. He thinks he is doing fine with the medications, but there has been some indication that he has been overusing his inhaler. The medical team would like him to try relaxation methods before they try adjusting his medication. The client has been managing his asthma since he was 6 years old. Asthmatic triggers include smoke, perfumes, dust allergy, and exercise. The client has just entered high school and wants to be involved in sports. He shows a talent for golf and is frustrated when his breathing problems interfere with his game.

The client uses a combined medication program that includes Singulair and Ventolin. He does well on the medication, and side effects are minimal. When using the inhaler, he occasionally gets a headache or stomachache, a racing heart, and feels agitated.

ASSESSMENT

Observation

The client slouches in the chair and looks disgusted. He fidgets. The parents are a bit overpowering and do not let the client speak for himself.

The use of auxiliary breathing muscles is evident. The client is a bit short for his age but appears normal in adolescent development. He is right-handed.

Interview and Goals

In addition to asthma, the client information form indicates headaches and a digestive disturbance (nausea) that is related to the medication he is taking. The client broke his left collarbone 5 years ago. He has typical adolescent stress and difficulty falling asleep. He is allergic to dust, and his asthma is triggered by sensitivity to scent and smoke. He has some acne on his back, chest, and face.

He takes a multivitamin daily.

He does not want to talk about massage for the asthma, but as a goal, he is interested in a sports massage application for enhancing his golf game.

Physical Assessment

Posture

Slight kyphosis (common in asthma). Slight anterior rotation and elevation of the left shoulder with a lateral head tilt to the left.

Gait

Normal; arm swing is a bit short bilaterally.

Range of Motion

Arm extension and external rotation are slightly limited bilaterally, more so on the left.

Palpation

(Palpation examination was limited because client would not take off his clothes.)

Near Touch. Heat is evident in the upper chest and shoulder.

Skin. Normal (as identified on the arm). Bruise is noted on the right forearm.

Superficial Connective Tissue. Unable to assess.

Vessels and Lymph Nodes. Unable to assess.

Muscles. Breathing muscles are short, tight, and tender to moderate palpation. Tender points in the intercostals and anterior serratus are very sensitive to pressure. Trigger point activity is evident in the sternocleidomastoid muscles.

Tendons. Subscapularis and supraspinatus tendons bilaterally are tender to moderate pressure. Muscle attachments at the occipital base are tender to moderate pressure.

Deep Fascia. Short in the cervical area; unable to assess other areas.

Ligaments. Appear normal.

Joints. Acromial clavicular and sternal clavicular joints on the left are tender to compressive force. Facet joints of the upper ribs are fixed and rigid.

Bones. Healing of broken clavicle noted.

Abdominal Viscera. Unable to assess.

Body Rhythms. Breathing is strained, particularly the exhale phase; strain was exaggerated when parents were speaking for client.

Muscle Testing

Strength

Left arm extensors are weak. Rhomboids are weak. Pectoralis major is overly strong and would not inhibit.

Neurologic Balance

Reactive muscle twitching occurs with light touch on neck and chest. Shoulder muscles misfire.

Gait

Left arm extensors do not hold when facilitated by the left hip flexors.

INTERPRETATION AND TREATMENT PLAN DEVELOPMENT

Clinical Reasoning

What Are the Facts?

Asthma is a lung disease that affects 12 million to 15 million Americans, including approximately 10% to 12% of children under age 18. Asthma is a disease of the bronchial tubes characterized by tightening of these airways. It is one of the chronic obstructive pulmonary diseases (others are chronic bronchitis and emphysema.) Common symptoms include shortness of breath, coughing, wheezing, and tightening in the chest.

When a person breathes, air is taken into the body through the nose and then passes through the windpipe into the bronchial tubes. At the end of the tubes are tiny air sacs, called *alveoli,* that deliver oxygen to the blood. These air sacs also collect unusable carbon dioxide, which is exhaled from the body. During normal breathing, the bands of muscle that surround the airways are relaxed, and air moves freely. In people with asthma, allergy-causing substances and environmental triggers, such as smoke and scents, cause the bands of muscle surrounding the airways to tighten, and air cannot move freely. Less air causes a person to feel short of breath, and the air moving through the tightened airways causes a whistling sound known as *wheezing.*

Asthma can be controlled but not cured. It is not commonly fatal, but it can become life-threatening if it is not treated or controlled. Medications are used to prevent and control asthma symptoms, to reduce the number and severity of asthma episodes, and to improve airflow. The two main types of asthma medications are antiinflammatories and bronchodilators.

Antiinflammatory Drugs. Antiinflammatory drugs are the most important class of treatment medications for most people with asthma, because these drugs prevent asthma attacks on an ongoing basis. Antiinflammatory medications reduce swelling and mucus production in the airways. As a result, the airways are less sensitive and less likely to react to triggers.

These medications must be taken daily and may need to be taken for several weeks before they begin to control the asthma. Treatment with antiinflammatories leads to fewer symptoms, better airflow, less sensitive airways, less airway damage, and fewer asthma attacks. However, these medications have side effects.

The three main types of antiinflammatory medications are corticosteroids (oral and inhaled), mast cell stabilizers, and leukotriene modifiers.

Corticosteroids (Oral). Oral forms of corticosteroids are used to relieve severe asthma attacks. These drugs are always used with other medications either to control sudden, severe asthma attacks or to treat long-term, hard to control asthma. Oral corticosteroids take 3 hours to begin working and work best after 6 to 12 hours. Sometimes corticosteroids are taken in high doses for a few days (called a steroid burst). They may also be given in a low dose daily or every other day for long-term control.

Side Effects. Long-term use can cause acne, weight gain, mood or behavior changes, upset stomach, bone loss, eye changes, and slowing of growth. These side effects rarely occur with short-term steroid bursts.

Oral Corticosteroid Medications. Methylprednisolone (Medrol), prednisone (Apo-Prednisone, Deltasone), prednisolone (Prelone, Pediapred).

Inhaled Corticosteroid Medications. Beclomethasone (Vanceril, Beclovent), budesonide (Pulmicort Turbohaler, Pulmicort Respules), flunisolide (AeroBid), fluticasone (Flovent and Flovent Rotadisk), triamcinolone (Azmacort).

Mast Cell Stabilizers. Mast cell stabilizers are available only in inhaled forms. They prevent asthma symptoms, especially in asthmatic children or children with allergies, and in people with exercise-induced asthma. Mast cell stabilizers need to be taken two to four times a day, and they require 3 to 4 weeks to begin working. Intal can be used 30 minutes before exercise to prevent exercise-induced symptoms.

Side Effects. These medications are very safe and have few side effects. Tilade can cause dry throat and may have a bad taste.

Mast Cell Stabilizer Inhalers. Cromolyn sodium (Intal), nedocromil sodium (Tilade).

Leukotriene Modifiers. Leukotriene modifiers work by blocking the actions of leukotrienes. Leukotrienes are chemicals that occur naturally in the body and that cause tightening of airway muscles and production of mucus and fluid. Studies have shown that these medications are helpful in improving airflow and reducing asthma symptoms. They are taken as pills one to four times a day and have been shown to reduce the need for other asthma medications.

Side Effects. The most common side effects are headache and nausea.

Leukotriene Modifier Medications. Zafirlukast (Accolate), montelukast (Singulair).

Bronchodilators. Bronchodilators relieve the symptoms of asthma by relaxing the muscle bands that tighten around the airways. This action rapidly opens the airways, letting more air in and out of the lungs, thereby improving breathing. Bronchodilators also help clear mucus from the lungs. As the airways open, the mucus moves more freely and can be coughed out more easily. The two main types of bronchodilators are beta$_2$-agonists (short- and long-acting forms) and anticholinergics.

Beta$_2$-Agonists. Short-acting beta$_2$-agonists are rescue medications that relieve asthma symptoms very quickly. They work within 20 minutes and last 4 to 6 hours. They are also the medications to use 15 to 20 minutes before exercise to prevent exercise-induced symptoms. The inhaled forms are best for treating sudden and severe or new asthma symptoms. The long-acting forms of beta$_2$-agonists are used for better control—not for relief—of asthma. These drugs take longer to begin to work, but the benefits last longer, up to 12 hours.

Side Effects. Nervous or shaky feelings, overexcitement or hyperactivity, increased heart rate, and, in rare cases, upset stomach or trouble sleeping.

Beta$_2$-Agonist Medications. *Short-acting forms:* Albuterol (Proventil, Ventolin), bitolterol (Tornalate), levalbuterol (Xopenex), metaproterenol (Alupent), pirbuterol (Maxair), terbutaline (Brethaire, Brethine). *Long-acting forms:* Albuterol (Proventil Repetabs, Volmax), formoterol (Foradil Aerolizer), salmeterol (Serevent, Serevent Diskus).

Anticholinergics. The anticholinergic drug ipratropium bromide (Atrovent) is available only in the inhaled form. Alone, it has no effect on asthma symptoms, therefore it is most often used with a short-acting beta$_2$-agonist to relieve sudden and severe or new symptoms. It is a reliever medication, but it takes at least 60 minutes to begin working. It has a small role in asthma treatment.

Side Effects. Side effects usually are minor; dry throat is the most common. If the medication gets in the eyes, it may cause blurred vision for a short time.

Anticholinergic Medication. Ipratropium bromide (Atrovent).

Theophylline. Theophylline is available in oral or injectable form. It is long-acting and prevents asthma attacks. It is used for difficult to control or severe asthma. It must be taken daily, and doses cannot be missed. Blood tests are required to monitor therapy.

Side Effects. Side effects include nausea, vomiting, diarrhea, stomachache, headache, rapid or irregular heartbeat, muscle cramps, jittery or nervous feelings, and hyperactivity. These symptoms may be a sign of too much medication, therefore blood levels need to be checked regularly. Certain medications, such as antibiotics containing erythromycin and seizure and ulcer medications, can interfere with the action of theophylline. Cigarette smoke and viral illnesses also can change the way the body responds to theophylline.

Theophylline Medications. Theophylline (Uniphyl, Theo-Dur, Slo-Bid, Theo-24).

Over-the-Counter Medications. The most common over-the-counter asthma medications are Primatene Mist and Bronkaid.

They both contain the drug epinephrine, which works like a bronchodilator and relaxes the muscles around the airways. They work for about 20 to 30 minutes, providing short-term relief of asthma symptoms. They do not control asthma symptoms or prevent asthma attacks. Also, people with high blood pressure, diabetes, thyroid disease, or heart disease should not take them.

Current case: The client is not interested in massage for the asthma but will discuss massage for his golf game. The restriction in arm mobility and the rotated and elevated shoulder are implicated as disturbing the golf swing.

What Are the Possibilities Both in Function and Dysfunction and the Massage Intervention Options?

The client has compensated for labored breathing since he was 6 years old. This has likely resulted in the postural shift and muscle tenderness identified during the assessment.

Playing golf may be straining the compensation patterns, making his breathing seem more labored. However, golf is a good sport choice because the activity can be controlled and calming, as long as the performance remains relaxed and competition stays within reason.

Possibilities:

1. A stretching program may be as beneficial as massage and may be more comfortable for the client. It is common for adolescents to be very body aware and to assert their need for privacy and independence. The client may be embarrassed about the acne.

2. The initial suggestion for the massage would be for the client to experience a massage over the clothing in a seated position in the massage chair. Because he is a minor, the parents must be present for supervision; however, this could be accomplished by leaving the treatment room door open and having the parents seated just outside the door. Massage could then progress to a mat and still be done over the clothing.

3. Massage on a weekly basis has shown benefit for those with asthma. As the client becomes more comfortable, additional methods could be used. The palpation assessment could be completed when the client has become tolerant of his skin being touched.

What Are the Logical Outcomes of Each Possible Intervention Option?

Medication side effects of headache and gastrointestinal distress could be reduced by the massage. Medication influence on the sympathetic autonomic nervous system may reduce the parasympathetic influence of the massage, reducing the benefits.

A stretching program may not address some of the shortening in the auxiliary breathing muscles that are most affected by the asthma.

What Is the Impact on the People Involved for Each Massage Intervention Option?

The client will accept massage better if he notices improvement in his golf game. If concrete benefits are seen, his compliance should increase.

The massage professional is uncomfortable talking the client into massage but confident that a focus on golf improvement would also gain beneficial results for the asthma.

The massage professional is also uncomfortable with the overbearing parents and would have to establish appropriate working boundaries that respect the client's and the parents' rights.

The client is resistant.

The parents are frustrated.

The medical team is very supportive.

DECISION MAKING AND TREATMENT PLAN DEVELOPMENT

Quantifiable Goal

To manage the side effects of medications and reduce sympathetic dominance

Qualifiable Goal

The client should be able to increase his performance in sports.

Treatment Regimen

Condition Management

A series of 10 weekly, 45-minute sessions of massage that begin in the chair over the clothing and focus on the respiratory function and golf swing will be provided. Broad-based compression, shaking, rocking, tapotement, vibration, range of motion (both active and passive), and various forms of muscle energy methods will be used to effectively lengthen short areas in both muscles and connective tissue. Positional release can be used on the tender points identified during assessment and can be taught to the client. Initially the focus will be on the upper body and arms, but gradually it will be extended to a more full-body approach if the client becomes willing.

A referral will be made to a flexibility program, an option that may be more comfortable for the client and that suggests that he choose the intervention he feels is most beneficial. The methods suggested for the massage sessions could be demonstrated on one of the parents so that the client can observe and become more comfortable with the process.

One of the parents must be present during the massage, and he or she can observe quietly from the open door during the session. All questions will be addressed before or after the session, but during the session the interaction must be between the client and the massage practitioner unless the client indicates otherwise.

The client and parents will monitor the effects of massage on both the asthma and the golf game and will report to the massage practitioner each session.

The golf pro where the client practices has indicated a willingness to work with helping people understand the benefits of massage and a flexibility program for good golf play.

A referral for a meeting with the golf pro is appropriate.

A report will be sent monthly to the client's doctor.

CASE 18 SEASONAL AFFECTIVE DISORDER (SAD)

The client is a 32-year-old female. She is married and has two children, 6 and 9 years old. She is a teacher but has chosen to stay home while her children are young. She has been diagnosed with a form of depression called seasonal affective disorder (SAD). She experiences moderate symptoms, including an increased appetite and a carbohydrate craving, and she gains about 20 pounds every winter. She loses some of the weight in the summer, but over the years she has become overweight. She wants to be alone and has lost all interest in sex. She is fatigued, she says she feels as if she weighs 1,000 pounds, and she cannot get enough sleep. She does not want to do anything but manages to drag herself though the day to meet her major responsibilities. She has a hard time remembering details and is impatient with unexpected demands on her time. Her muscles ache, and she continually has a dull headache.

No cause has been found for the symptoms. She feels better in the spring and summer and loves to be outside, but as the winter approaches, her depression increases. She grew up in Alabama, and the family moved to Michigan 5 years ago for a business opportunity. She loves the area in the spring, summer, and fall but does not like the cold, dreary winters.

She is taking Prozac, a selective serotonin uptake inhibitor, and has recently begun using light therapy. Both seem to help. She has read that massage can have a positive effect on depression. She loves massage and has treated herself to massage when on vacation. A holistic health center with a massage clinic just opened in her hometown, and the rates are affordable with a package plan. Her doctor is supportive, especially if massage will help her be more compliant with an outdoor walking program. She is interested in complementary methods, especially aromatherapy and homeopathy.

ASSESSMENT

Observation

The client appears fatigued and has circles under her eyes. She carries the excess weight in her hips. She wants to sit down immediately when she enters the office, and when she gets up from the chair, she appears to have to exert an extraordinary amount of effort. Her demeanor is pleasant, but she seems to have to work at it. She does not offer information but does respond to questions.

Interview and Goals

The client history form indicates that she has headaches, wears contact lenses, has bouts of diarrhea, uses birth control pills, and has some abdominal bloating when she eats ice cream (likely a dairy sensitivity). Muscle aching is described as all over the body, with more stiffness than pain. She has had two pregnancies and one miscarriage. There is a history of heart problems on her father's side of the family. She is fatigued and depressed and has periods of anxiety. Even though she sleeps more than 10 hours a day, she feels as if that is not enough and that she is not rested in the morning. She has been attempting to lose weight with a low-fat diet. She fell down some stairs a few years ago. She was shaken up and had a slight concussion but was fine in a few days.

The client's goals for the massage are to reduce her depressive symptoms and to support her efforts at relaxation and exercise.

Physical Assessment

Posture

Generally bilaterally symmetric with no obvious postural distortions.

Gait

Slow and labored with reduced arm swing.

Range of Motion

Within normal range but guarded at the end-range.

Palpation

Near Touch. Body dissemination of energy seems low. The sense of same magnetic poles placed together is absent.

Skin. Normal but dry. Hair is dry, and fingers have hangnails.

Superficial Connective Tissue. Very slight bogginess.

Vessels and Lymph Nodes. Normal

Muscles. Normal; no obvious tender areas or shortened muscles.

Tendons. Normal

Deep Fascia. Mild bind in the plantar fasciae.

Ligaments. Normal

Joints. End-feel is normal and soft, but client seems to guard and stiffen before physiologic end-range of joint movement is reached.

Bones. Normal

Abdominal Viscera. Soft with evidence of gas.

Body Rhythms. Entrainment seems off. Breathing is slow, with an even inhale-to-exhale ratio and some sighing. Heat rate is within normal range, but pulses are hard to feel. Full-body undulation (craniosacral or lymphatic, depending on the structure) is difficult to palpate.

Muscle Testing

Strength

Muscles test strong, but client exerts extraordinary effort during assessment.

Neurologic Balance

Client does not want to sustain pressure against resistance. She says she is tired. Gluteus maximus firing is off. Synergistic dominance is evident.

Gait

Shoulder and hip flexors on the opposite side inhibit instead of facilitate, whereas on the same side, they facilitate. Normal gaiting reflexes appear to be reversed. When client looks down, extensors twitch and flexors and adductors are inhibited rather than facilitated. When client looks up over her head, flexors and adductors inhibit as appropriate.

INTERPRETATION AND TREATMENT PLAN DEVELOPMENT

Clinical Reasoning

What Are the Facts?

Temporary depression is a normal reaction to loss, life's struggles, or injured self-esteem. However, feelings of sadness that become hopeless and intense, last for long periods, and prevent a person from leading his or her everyday life are not normal. A mental illness left untreated can worsen, lasting for years and causing untold suffering, and can possibly even lead to suicide. It is important for massage professionals to recognize the signs of depression and refer appropriately. These signs and symptoms include the following:
- Sadness (lingering)
- Loss of energy
- Feelings of hopelessness or worthlessness
- Loss of enjoyment of things that were once pleasurable
- Difficulty concentrating
- Uncontrollable crying
- Difficulty making decisions
- Irritability
- Increased need for sleep
- Insomnia or excessive sleep
- Unexplained aches and pains
- Stomachache and digestive problems
- Decreased sex drive
- Sexual problems
- Headache
- Change in appetite, causing weight loss or gain
- Thoughts of death or suicide
- Attempt at suicide

Suicide is an emergency situation that requires immediate intervention. Symptoms include the following:
- Talking about suicide (killing one's self)
- Always talking or thinking about death

- Making comments about being hopeless, helpless, or worthless
- Saying things such as, "It would be better if I wasn't here" or "I want out."
- Depression (deep sadness, loss of interest, trouble sleeping and eating) that gets worse
- A sudden switch from being very sad to being very calm or appearing to be happy
- Having a "death wish"; tempting fate by taking risks that could lead to death, such as driving through red lights
- Losing interest in things one used to care about
- No longer visiting or calling people one cares about
- Putting affairs in order, tying up loose ends, changing a will

Types of Depression. Sometimes physical problems can cause depression. Other times, symptoms of depression are part of a more complex psychiatric problem. There are several different types of depression: (1) major depressive disorder, (2) dysthymia, (3) seasonal affective disorder, and (4) bipolar disorder.

Major Depressive Disorder. An individual with major depression, or major depressive disorder, feels a profound and constant sense of hopelessness and despair while experiencing a depressed mood most of the day.

Major depression is marked by a combination of symptoms that interfere with the ability to work, study, sleep, eat, and enjoy once pleasurable activities. Major depression may occur only once but more commonly occurs several times in a lifetime.

In the United States approximately 10% of people suffer from major depression at any one time, and 20% to 25% suffer a major depressive episode at some point in their lives. Most people associate depression with adults, but it also occurs in children and the elderly, two groups in which it often is misdiagnosed or goes undiagnosed and untreated.

Approximately twice as many women as men suffer from depression. This is partly because of hormonal changes that occur throughout a woman's life, during menstruation, pregnancy, miscarriage, and menopause. Other contributing factors include increased responsibilities in both professional and home lives, such as balancing work while taking care of a household, raising a child alone, or even caring for an aging parent. However, depression in men may also be underreported.

Roughly 25% of people who are admitted to the hospital for a major depressive episode suffer from depression with psychosis. In addition to the symptoms of depression, psychotic depression includes some features of psychosis, such as hallucinations (seeing or hearing things that are not really there) or delusions (irrational thoughts and fears). Although people with other mental illnesses, such as schizophrenia, also experience these symptoms, individuals suffering from major depressive episodes usually are aware that these thoughts are not true. They may be ashamed or embarrassed and may try to hide them, sometimes making this type of depression difficult to diagnose.

Symptoms of a Major Depressive Episode. The symptoms of a major depressive episode include the following:

- Anxiety
- Agitation
- Depressed mood most of the day
- Fatigue/no energy
- Insomnia/hypersomnia
- Physical immobility
- Constipation
- Intellectual impairment
- Psychosis

Dysthymia. Dysthymia, sometimes referred to as chronic depression, is a less severe form of depression, but the depressive symptoms linger for a long time, perhaps even years. Those who suffer from dysthymia are usually able to function relatively normally but seem consistently unhappy.

People with dysthymia commonly experience major depression at the same time; they swing into a major depressive episode and then back to a more mild state of dysthymia. This has been called *double depression.*

Symptoms of Dysthymia. The symptoms of dysthymia include the following:

- Difficulty sleeping
- Low self-esteem
- Feelings of hopelessness
- Loss of energy or fatigue
- Difficulty concentrating, thinking, or making decisions
- Changes in appetite
- Observable mental and physical sluggishness

Seasonal Affective Disorder. Seasonal depression, called *seasonal affective disorder,* or SAD, is a depression that occurs each year at the same time, usually starting in the fall or winter and ending in the spring or early summer. It is more than just "the winter blues" or "cabin fever." A rare form of SAD known as *summer depression* begins in late spring or early summer and ends in the fall.

People who suffer from SAD have many of the common signs of depression: sadness, irritability, loss of interest in their usual activities, withdrawal from social activities, and inability to concentrate (Box 15-1). Symptoms of winter SAD differ from symptoms of summer SAD.

Symptoms of Winter SAD. The symptoms of winter SAD include the seasonal occurrence of the following:

- Fatigue
- Increased need for sleep
- Decreased levels of energy
- Weight gain
- Increased appetite
- Difficulty concentrating
- Increased desire to be alone

Symptoms of Summer SAD. The symptoms of summer SAD include the seasonal occurrence of the following:

- Weight loss
- Trouble sleeping
- Decreased appetite

In the United States, 4% to 6% of the population suffers from SAD, and 10% to 20% may suffer from a milder form of winter blues. Three-fourths of the sufferers are women, most of whom are in their twenties, thirties, or forties. Although SAD is most common during these ages, it also can

BOX 15-1

Symptoms of Seasonal Affective Disorder (SAD)*

- *Anxiety:* Tension, inability to tolerate stress, phobias
- *Social problems:* Irritability, loss of pleasure in being with others and a desire to avoid contact, which could even turn into unwillingness to leave the home or bed
- *Loss of libido:* Decreased interest in sex
- *Sleep problems:* Tendency to sleep for longer periods; sleep is restless and less satisfying
- *Mood swings:* In the spring, when SAD lifts, some sufferers experience a dramatic swing in mood and a short period of hypomania, a sudden surge of energy and enthusiasm that brings problems of its own
- *Menstrual difficulties:* During the winter, premenstrual tension may be worse than in other seasons, causing irritability, sleep problems, appetite changes, and a low energy level
- *Hopelessness:* Feelings of desperation and hopelessness, which sometimes lead to overdependence on relationships, work, or home
- *Excessive eating and drinking:* Carbohydrates, alcohol, and coffee
- *Increased sensitivity to pain:* Headaches, muscle and joint pain
- *Other physical ailments:* Constipation, diarrhea, heart palpitations

*Not all people with SAD have these symptoms.

occur in children and adolescents. Older adults are less likely to experience SAD. The illness is more commonly seen in people who live at high latitudes (geographic locations farther north or south of the equator), where seasonal changes are more extreme.

Bipolar Disorder. Bipolar disorder, or *manic-depressive disease,* is a mental illness that causes people to have severe high and low moods. People with this type of depression swing from feeling overly happy and joyful (or irritable) to feeling very sad. Because of the highs and the lows—or two poles of mood—the condition is referred to as *bipolar depression.* Between episodes of mood swings, the person may experience normal moods.

The word *manic* describes a specific period when the person feels overly excited and confident. These feelings can quickly turn to confusion, irritability, anger, and even rage. The word *depressive* describes the periods when the person feels very sad or depressed. Because the depressive episode is similar to that of major depression, people with bipolar depression sometimes are incorrectly diagnosed as having major depression. The severity of the depressive and manic phases can differ from person to person and in the same person at different times.

During manic periods, people with bipolar disorder may:
- Be overly happy, hopeful, and excited
- Change suddenly from being joyful to being angry and hostile

- Behave in strange ways and have odd beliefs
- Become restless
- Talk rapidly or feel pressure to keep talking
- Have a lot of energy and need less sleep
- Believe they have many skills and powers and can do anything
- Make grand plans
- Show poor judgment, such as deciding to quit a job or spend excessive amounts of money
- Appear headstrong, annoying, or demanding
- Become easily distracted
- Abuse drugs and alcohol
- Have a higher sex drive

Some people can become psychotic, seeing and hearing things that are not there and holding false beliefs from which they cannot be swayed. In many instances they see themselves as having superhuman skills and powers.

During depressive periods, people with bipolar disorder may:
- Feel empty, sad, or hopeless
- Feel guilty, worthless, or helpless
- Cry often
- Lose interest in things they usually enjoy, including sex
- Be unable to think clearly, make decisions, or remember things
- Sleep poorly
- Lose or gain weight
- Have low energy
- Abuse drugs and alcohol
- Complain of headaches, stomachaches, and other pains
- Become focused on death
- Attempt suicide

The dramatic and rapidly changing mood swings from highs to lows do not follow a set pattern, and depression does not always follow manic phases. Also, a person with bipolar disorder may experience the same mood state several times before suddenly experiencing the opposite mood. Mood swings or episodes can occur over a period of weeks, months, and sometimes even years. Bipolar disorder is a long-term illness that requires management throughout a person's life.

According to the National Institutes of Mental Health, more than 2 million American adults experience bipolar disorder. Bipolar disorder usually begins in early adulthood, appearing before age 35. Children and adolescents, however, can develop this disease in more severe forms and in combination with attention deficit/hyperactivity disorder (ADHD). Some studies have indicated that bipolar depression is genetically inherited, occurring more commonly within families.

Although bipolar disorder occurs equally in women and men, women with bipolar disorder have been found to switch moods more quickly; this is called *rapid cycling.* Variations in sex hormone levels and thyroid activity, together with the tendency to be prescribed antidepressants, may contribute to the more rapid cycling seen in women. Women may also experience more periods of depression than men.

An estimated 60% of all people with bipolar disorder have drug or alcohol dependence. The disease has also been shown to occur frequently in people with seasonal depression and certain anxiety disorders, such as post-traumatic stress disorder (PTSD).

Medications for Depression. Examples of safe, effective medications commonly prescribed for depression or depression-related problems are listed in Table 15-1.

The type of medication prescribed depends on the symptoms, the presence of other medical conditions, interactions with other medications, the cost of the prescribed treatments, and the potential side effects. Selective serotonin reuptake inhibitors (SSRIs) and tricyclic antidepressants (TCAs) are two widely prescribed types of antidepressant medications.

Some common side effects of SSRIs include the following:

- Agitation
- Nausea or vomiting
- Diarrhea
- Sexual problems, including low sex drive or inability to have an orgasm
- Dizziness
- Headaches
- Insomnia
- Increased anxiety
- Exhaustion

Some common side effects of TCAs include the following:

- Dry mouth
- Blurred vision
- Increased fatigue and sleepiness
- Weight gain
- Muscle twitching (tremors)
- Hand shaking
- Constipation
- Bladder problems
- Dizziness
- Increased heart rate

TABLE 15-1

Medications Used to Treat Depression and Related Disorders

Type	Generic Name	Brand Name	Condition Treated
Selective serotonin reuptake inhibitors (SSRIs)	Citalopram Fluoxetine Fluvoxamine Paroxetine Sertraline	Celexa Prozac Luvox Paxil Zoloft	Depression (Serotonin is a brain chemical thought to affect mood states, especially depression. SSRIs help increase the amount of serotonin to level the patient's mood.)
Tricyclic antidepressants (TCAs)	Amitriptyline Clomipramine Desipramine Doxepin Imipramine Nortriptyline Protriptyline Trimipramine	Elavil Anafranil Norpramin Sinequan Tofranil Pamelor Vivactil Surmontil	Depression (Clomipramine is used to treat obsessive-compulsive disorder.)
Monoamine oxidase inhibitors (MAOIs)	Isocarboxazid Phenelzine Tranylcypromine	Marplan Nardil Parnate	Depression (MAOIs increase the concentration of chemicals in particular regions of the brain that aid communication between nerves. MAOIs usually are prescribed for people with severe depression.)
Azapirone	Buspirone	BuSpar	Generalized anxiety
Benzodiazepines	Alprazolam Diazepam Lorazepam	Xanax Valium Ativan	Premenstrual syndrome, panic disorder
Lithium	Lithium carbonate Lithium citrate	Lithane Cibalith-S	Bipolar disorder, recurrent depression
Mood-stabilizing anticonvulsants	Carbamazepine Gabapentin Lamotrigine Valproate	Tegretol Neurontin Lamictal Depakote	Bipolar disorder
Other medications	Amoxapine Bupropion Maprotiline Mirtazapine Nefazodone Trazodone Venlafaxine	Asendin Wellbutrin Ludiomil Remeron Serzone Desyrel Effexor	Depression

To achieve effectiveness and to prevent a relapse of depression, medications generally are prescribed for 6 to 12 months for people treated for first-time depression. These medications usually must be taken regularly for at least 4 to 8 weeks before their full benefit takes effect.

Current case: The client in this case is taking Prozac. The side effects of Prozac, an SSRI, can include the following:

- Agitation
- Nausea or vomiting
- Diarrhea
- Sexual problems, including low sex drive or inability to have an orgasm
- Dizziness
- Headaches
- Insomnia
- Increased anxiety
- Exhaustion

The client's gait reflex patterns are disrupted. Also, she is restricting her fat intake.

What Are the Possibilities Both in Function and Dysfunction and the Massage Intervention Options?

The client might not have enough fat in her diet. There is evidence of lactose intolerance with the gas and bloating. Referral to her doctor with a recommendation that she see a nutritionist would be wise.

The client's fall could have disrupted her normal gait patterns. Although not causal to the SAD, walking reflexes are nonoptimal and require increased energy expenditure, which is contributing to the fatigue. Working to re-establish a normal gait may be helpful. A wobble board and large gym ball activities could support massage, and if improvement is not noted with general intervention, referral to an exercise physiologist would be indicated.

Although medication seems to help, some of the symptoms indicate side effects of the medication, and referral back to the physician for re-evaluation of the medication and dosage would be prudent.

Possibilities:

1. General constitutional massage has been shown to help those with various types of depression. Massage with sufficient pressure affects the serotonin and dopamine levels, and both neurotransmitters are implicated in SAD.
2. The normal gait reflex patterns can be stimulated with massage, which may make walking less fatiguing.
3. The client could be referred to the clinic's aromatherapist and homeopath but not until approval is obtained from her physician.

What Are the Logical Outcomes of Each Possible Intervention Option?

Referral to the physician for further evaluation seems a cautious and prudent choice to clarify the client's symptom pattern. This does involve time and cost factors, as do referrals to other professionals. Introducing too many interventions at one time can be confusing as to what is having beneficial or detrimental effects.

Working with the gait reflexes is a simple and safe intervention during the massage, but the consequences of the fall could be more complicated, and specific protocols for retraining the walking pattern would need to be provided by a specialist, such as an exercise physiologist.

General, nonspecific massage is likely to provide quick, observable benefits but might not be sustaining if underlying factors exist that need to be determined. The cost for massage is reasonable, and the location is convenient.

Gym balls and wobble boards are easy to locate and inexpensive. The wobble board would require a person to spot during use to prevent falling. The exercise gym ball is safe to use alone.

What Is the Impact on the People Involved for Each Massage Intervention Option?

The client likes massage and is interested in homeopathy and aromatherapy. She is open to returning to her physician for further evaluation. The physician is supportive of massage but not of homeopathy.

The massage practitioner feels confident providing the massage but feels there are unidentified factors that need to be resolved.

DECISION MAKING AND TREATMENT PLAN DEVELOPMENT

Quantifiable Goals

1. 50% improvement in gait
2. Support body's natural defenses against depression

Qualifiable Goal

The client will be able to exercise without pain and fatigue.

Treatment Regimen

The client will be referred back to her physician with the proposed treatment plan for massage and the following recommendations:

- The client may benefit from a nutritional evaluation. Medication side effects concur with the symptoms described on the client history form, and re-evaluation of the medication type or dosage may be indicated. The medication dose should be monitored, because massage does increase available levels of serotonin. Gait seems disrupted, and further evaluation from a physical therapist or exercise physiologist may be beneficial. Referral to the aromatherapist is recommended because the client has expressed an interest in this complementary method.
- The client will receive a weekly 1-hour massage, and the schedule will be increased to twice a week if her symptoms worsen. The massage will be a general full-body approach with sufficient pressure for the client to feel the intensity of the session but with no pain or guarding. A general intervention to improve gait patterns will be to have the client roll her eyes in large, slow circles while the legs and

arms are massaged. After six sessions of the general massage, pulsed muscle energy methods for the arm and opposite leg flexors will be introduced to encourage normal facilitation patterns.

- The client could benefit from a daily session of bouncing and stretching on a large exercise gym ball.

CASE 19 SPORTS PERFORMANCE ENHANCEMENT

The client is a 22-year-old female who is a competitive marathon runner. She is currently training for a marathon. She is determined to commit herself to the best performance possible. As an amateur athlete, she coordinates her own training program. She works with a running coach. She had a first-degree ankle sprain 2 years ago, experiences generalized cramping if she overtrains, and has had one experience of shin splints. These symptoms improve when she drinks enough water or sports drinks and stretches. She occasionally gets side stitches. She is a student of the sport and is constantly studying the effects of diet and training protocols to enhance her performance. She is interested in incorporating massage into her program to support recovery and flexibility and to reduce the potential for injury.

Four years ago, she lost her left leg below the knee in an automobile accident. She has rehabilitated successfully and has been fitted with a running prosthesis, as well as a prosthesis for general use. She is on a mission to prove to herself and others that she can accomplish this task.

She is a college student studying exercise science and athletic training. Finances are secure as a result of an insurance settlement from the accident. She has determined that she can afford $150 per month to pay for massage and wants the maximum benefit from the investment.

ASSESSMENT

Observation

The client is a slim, muscular, fit female. Unless she is carefully observed, there is little evidence of the amputation. The client does not attempt to conceal the prosthesis and speaks freely about the accident. She is more concerned about total body performance than the loss of the leg.

Interview and Goals

The client information form indicates minor muscle pain related to training. She experiences mild episodes of phantom pain, usually in response to an increase in training. The pain is managed with rest, massage of the stump, and stretching. Her calf gets tight, she had shin splints in her right leg 8 months ago, and she sprained her right ankle 2 years ago.

She has occasional fatigue and restless sleep if she overtrains or experiences the phantom pain. She has athlete's foot and is currently being treated for that. She takes performance-based supplements in a well-balanced formula.

The client's goal for massage is support for a training regimen to enhance performance and help prevent injury.

Physical Assessment

Posture

Symmetric except for highly developed thigh muscles, with increased development on the left and a slightly elevated iliac crest on the left.

Gait

Normal with the prosthesis except for increased arm swing on the right. She indicates that she has experienced extensive rehabilitation to support normal gait after the amputation.

Range of Motion

Normal

Palpation

Near Touch. Energy sensation off the body is high and even. Heat is present at the amputation site.

Skin. Damp areas are noted at the amputation site and on the medial calf on the right. There are no areas of inflammation, abrasion, or skin irritation from the prosthesis. Skin is smooth and resilient. Small area of bind is noted just under the right clavicle in the chest.

Superficial Connective Tissue. Small bind and increased tissue density in the legs.

Vessels and Lymph Nodes. Normal

Muscles. Normal with hypertrophy in the legs. Decreased pliability with slight increase in density and shortening of the hamstrings. Tenderness and pain radiate to three areas on the stump, two in the vastus lateralis and one in the vastus medialis, indicating trigger point activity.

Tendons. Normal except for some shortening in the right Achilles tendon.

Deep Fascia. Plantar fascia is slightly short on the right.

Ligaments. Normal

Joints. No evidence of inappropriate end-feel or bind. Slight decrease in dorsiflexion on the right.

Bones. Normal

Abdominal Viscera. Normal

Body Rhythms. Normal

Muscle Testing

Strength

Normal

Neurologic Balance

Normal

Gait

Higher degrees of facilitation between extensors and flexors on the right arm and left leg seem to be appropriate compensation for amputation.

INTERPRETATION AND TREATMENT PLAN DEVELOPMENT

Clinical Reasoning

What Are the Facts?

An understanding of the basic physical concepts involved in exercise and training protocols is important to a massage professional who works with athletes in conditioning, performance enhancement, and injury rehabilitation. To increase a sustainable power output, the athlete must follow a carefully designed training program that will improve the individual's ability to (1) produce metabolic energy by both aerobic and anaerobic means; (2) sustain aerobic energy production at high levels before lactic acid accumulates excessively in the blood; (3) recruit more of the efficient slow-twitch muscle fibers in muscle groups used in competition; and (4) become more skillful by recruiting fewer nonessential muscle fibers during competition. Careful attention to maintaining a sufficient intake of fluids and carbohydrates before, during, and after strenuous competition and training sessions is also important.

Physical exercise and sports performance are made possible by forces developed by the voluntary muscles acting through the lever and tensegrity systems of the muscle and skeletal systems. During the performance of sports skills, the recruitment of motor units for the purpose of developing force between the bony attachments of muscles may or may not result in shortening of the muscle and drawing together of the attachments (concentric). When the muscle is lengthened by external forces, muscle activation does not cause shortening but instead resists the lengthening (eccentric) to maintain coordinated muscles. When muscle tension increases and no movement results, stability increases as a result of isometric contraction.

Another objective of the muscle activation, especially in submaximal force development, is to selectively recruit an appropriate pool of motor units so that the movement is controlled. This may result in a shortening of the muscle, in the maintenance of a particular length (as in the stabilization of body parts), or in a controlled lengthening of the muscle as the distance between the bony attachments is increased.

The interaction of muscle force development and the prevailing external forces results in muscle actions that produce *static exercise* (no movement about the related joints) or *dynamic exercise* (involving either an increase or decrease in joint angles). Static exercise of activated muscle is traditionally referred to as *isometric*. Force is developed, but because there is no movement, no work is performed. All other muscle actions involve movement and are termed *dynamic*.

Human activity seldom involves pure forms of isolated concentric, eccentric, or isometric actions. This is because the body segments are periodically subjected to impact forces, as in running or jumping, or because some external force, such as gravity, causes the muscle to lengthen. In many situations the muscles first act eccentrically, and a concentric action follows immediately.

The energy of physical exercise can be considered in terms of the potential energy of the biochemical substances used for muscular actions (essentially adenosine triphosphate [ATP], carbohydrate, and fat) and the actual release of this energy. Performance in a sport can be analyzed according to its dependency on aerobic metabolism (involving glycolysis with lactic acid formation) or anaerobic metabolism, which depends on the high-energy ATP as the major source of energy. Running a marathon requires more than 10,000 repetitions of the running steps and a continuous supply of energy via metabolic mechanisms dependent on the availability of oxygen (aerobic metabolism).

At the onset of a training season, the athlete should establish a solid aerobic training foundation by training at relatively low intensities for long durations. This helps develop a greater blood volume and improves both the ability of the heart to pump blood and the network of capillaries in the trained muscles. These cardiovascular adaptations result in improved delivery of oxygen to the muscles and enhanced ability of the muscles to sustain high rates of aerobic energy production.

For the bulk of the athlete's training, the specific muscle groups involved in the competitive event should be overloaded, and the athlete should train at a pace or intensity similar to that used in competition. Metabolic adaptations to this type of training are likely to enhance the muscles' ability to use fat for energy and to spare muscle glycogen, resulting in less lactic acid production and less accumulation of lactic acid in the blood at a given pace or intensity. This means that the athlete's lactate threshold will be increased so that aerobic energy production can be sustained longer and at a greater rate than was possible before training.

The athlete should get adequate rest—approximately 24 hours between exhaustive training sessions—to allow for total replenishment of depleted glycogen stores in the muscles before the next training session. Otherwise, the quality of the next training session may be compromised because the athlete's muscles will be easily depleted of one of their main fuels. In addition, training intensity and duration should be gradually reduced during the week before a competitive event so that the athlete's energy reserves are fully loaded before competition.

The athlete should drink plenty of fluids and maintain electrolyte balance before, during, and after exercise to avoid becoming dehydrated. Dehydration can lead to a diminished ability to deliver oxygen to the muscles, heat cramps, heat exhaustion, and even heatstroke, all of which can impair muscular energy production and, in the case of heatstroke, could even be fatal.

On a daily basis the athlete should consume a diet high in carbohydrate, about 8 g of carbohydrate per kilogram of body weight (or about 4 g per pound). This ensures that the muscles can store extra glycogen and may help sustain energy production during competition.

The athlete should obtain the technical advice of competent coaches or trainers who can explain how movement patterns should be altered so that the athlete can become more skillful. Often the coach can rely on personal experience and observation to make critical improvements in an athlete's technique.

The athlete must repeat the appropriate movement patterns in a skillful manner many thousands of times during practice so that the nervous system learns to perform the movement correctly every time throughout the entire duration of competition. There is no substitute for training.

Shin splints, side stitches, plantar fasciitis, muscle cramps, muscle strains, dehydration, and hyponatremia can quickly make running a painful experience

Shin Splints. One of the most common running injuries is medial tibial stress syndrome, or *shin splints*. This is an inflammation of the tendons along the inside of the shinbone. Shin splints result when too much stress is put on tired calf muscles, as occurs with running on hard surfaces. Changing surfaces (from hard to soft) also tends to aggravate the calf muscles. The symptoms of shin splints include aching, throbbing, or tenderness of the shin. Pain is felt when the inflamed area is pressed. The best preventive measure is to stretch the calf muscles. Proper warm up and stretching before a run helps develop flexibility, which is a key factor in avoiding shin splints.

Side Stitches. Cramping of the abdomen or side is called a *side stitch*. There are several theories as to what causes this pain: a spasm or cramp in the diaphragm muscle, diminished blood flow as a result of excessive muscle contraction and dehydration, and/or micronutrient imbalances. As with shin splints, the best preventive measures are to stretch and increase flexibility and to drink plenty of fluids, such as sports drinks. One way to ease the pain is to ease the running pace. When the cramping begins, the athlete should slow down and place the arms above the head until the pain subsides. With an acute attack, temporary relief can be obtained by gently massaging the painful area.

Plantar Fasciitis. *Plantar fasciitis* is inflammation at the attachment of the small muscles and the arch of the foot into the heel bone. It is the most common problem of the foot among both runners and nonrunners. This pain can be sharp, occurring on the bottom of the foot in the midheel area. Plantar fasciitis can be caused by a number of things, such as high arches or flat feet. Worn-out or ill-fitting footwear can lead to plantar fasciitis. As with any injury, prevention is the key. A thorough warm-up and stretching of the plantar fascia can help prevent this ailment. Good running shoes are also vital, as is choosing running locations with a comfortable ground surface, such as a cinder track. Treatment for plantar fasciitis involves icing the foot for several minutes after the activity and rest. Stretching exercises should be increased to achieve optimum flexibility, and connective tissue massage to maintain pliability of the plantar fascia is appropriate.

Muscle Cramps. Muscle cramps can be caused by a number of factors, which can work singly or in combination, such as dehydration, elevated body temperature, and sodium loss. Repetitive muscle contractions associated with sports might also trigger cramps. The severity of the cramps can range from the common cramping that many runners experience in their calf muscles (gastrocnemius and soleus) and feet to intensely painful, whole-body cramps. The best preventive measure is to drink plenty of fluids with appropriate electrolytes, such as sodium and potassium, and to warm up properly before beginning a run. Stretching, massaging the tender area, or icing the muscle may help relieve the pain.

Muscle Strains. *Muscle strains* are tears in muscle fibers that occur in activities such as fast stretching, excessive concentric contraction, and quick shifts from concentric to eccentric activity. They are graded as minor, moderate, or severe. They also require three stages of healing: acute, subacute, and remodeling. Massage supports all the healing stages. Appropriate muscle tone, firing patterns, and pliability help prevent muscle strains.

Dehydration. All types of physical activity promote dehydration through sweat loss, which makes dehydration a primary concern for athletes. Dehydration results in premature fatigue and increases the risk of heat illness. Symptoms of dehydration include a run-down feeling, nausea, dizziness, and muscle cramping. The key to preventing dehydration is obvious but all too often ignored: drink early and often. If dehydration sets in, the athlete should reduce the intensity of the exercise or should stop completely and drink fluids with carbohydrates to prevent fatigue and promote rapid rehydration. Rest and staying in a cool area to lower the body temperature also are important.

Hyponatremia. A low blood sodium level is referred to as *hyponatremia*, a potentially deadly dilution of the blood that can occur as a result of drinking fluids that do not contain enough sodium during exercise. The condition is considered rare, but hyponatremia happens more often than people realize. When endurance athletes drink only water, they focus on replacing just the fluid component of their sweat loss and not the electrolytes. Drinking Pedialyte or sports drinks that have electrolytes, including sodium, can help prevent hyponatremia.

Recovery. *Recovery* is the process by which the athlete returns to a state of performance readiness. Recovery involves a restoration of nutrient and energy stores, a return to normal physiologic function, a reduction of muscle soreness, and the disappearance of the psychological symptoms associated with extreme fatigue (irritability, disorientation, inability to concentrate). In training, this allows the quality of the workout to be maintained while minimizing the risk of chronic fatigue, illness, and injury. In competition, it means being able to take part in the next round or event and to perform at the same or at a higher level.

To hasten recovery after exhaustive exercise, athletes should continue exercising for 10 to 20 minutes at progressively lower intensities to speed the removal of lactic acid from the muscles and blood. Gentle stretching of all major muscle groups should follow this activity.

Athletes should begin consuming fluids and carbohydrates immediately after exercise to help the body replace fluids lost in sweat and to replenish muscle glycogen stores. A small amount of protein (about 6 ounces) may accelerate protein synthesis in the muscles after exercise. Expensive protein powders and amino acid supplements are no more effective than normal foods (e.g., fish or eggs) at providing the necessary amino acids. It is important to replace both water and electrolytes (especially sodium) during and after exercise to minimize dehydration, stabilize blood volume, and prevent muscle cramps.

Athletes should warm up into any exercise activity and cool down after the activity, regardless of the duration of the exercise. Cooling down should consist of submaximum exercise followed by a gentle stretching regimen. Massage can facilitate both the warm up and cool down processes. After a hard workout, 10 to 20 minutes of gentle exercise can speed removal of lactic acid from the muscles and promote recovery. To minimize inflammation and delayed onset muscle soreness, the athlete can use lymph drainage and broad-based compressive massage, cold packs around the joints, and alternating cold and hot whirlpool baths.

Athletes generally require at least 8 to 10 hours of sleep each night to perform at their best. Getting sufficient sleep is just as important a part of training as practicing the skills of the sport, lifting weights, or improving endurance. One of the signs of overtraining is sleep difficulty. Given the time devoted to team travel and other commitments in athletics, getting the necessary rest often is difficult. Therapeutic massage supports restorative sleep.

When unsure about whether to train, athletes should use the neck-check rule. If the symptoms of illness are above the neck (e.g., mild headache, stuffed-up or runny nose, mild sore throat), the athlete can perform an easy warm up and then see if the symptoms have improved. If the symptoms are below the neck (e.g., congestion deep in the lungs, severe sore throat, fever, persistent coughing, upset stomach, aching muscles), training should be postponed until the symptoms disappear.

What Are the Possibilities Both in Function and Dysfunction and the Massage Intervention Options?

The client is in good physical condition, with minor changes that seem appropriate compensation for amputation and use of the prosthesis.

Trigger point activity in the leg with the amputation may be causing the phantom pain. An aggressive training program may be contributing to fatigue and muscle aching.
Possibilities:
1. Massage is indicated for support of sports training programs. It can facilitate fluid exchange in the muscles, manage symptoms of delayed onset muscle soreness, and maintain appropriate pliability in soft tissue structures.
2. Massage can help reduce trigger point activity in the client's left leg, support restful sleep, and encourage well-being.

What Are the Logical Outcomes of Each Possible Intervention Option?

The client has specific and realistic expectations for sports massage and goals that are achievable.

She has determined that funds are available for massage, but the frequency of massage needed to achieve the desired results might exceed her funds. Massage two to three times per week would be optimal, with more frequent intervention during intensive training periods. The client's funds support one massage per week.

The massage therapist is aware of the time commitment required to effectively serve a client with these goals.

What Is the Impact on the People Involved for Each Massage Intervention Option?

All parties involved are supportive of massage, and the massage therapist is qualified to work with this level of athletic performance.

The massage therapist is willing to commit to the time necessary to support this athlete but is concerned about feeling taken advantage of, because fee reductions may be required. The client is very independent and a bit demanding but realistic and understanding of the massage therapist's concerns.

DECISION MAKING AND TREATMENT PLAN DEVELOPMENT

Quantifiable Goals

1. Reduce episodes of phantom pain by 50%
2. Reduce postexercise aches by 50%
3. Increase sleep effectiveness to support recovery time

Qualifiable Goals

The client will be able to participate in a training program with minimal discomfort.

Treatment Regimen

The massage therapist is an instructor at a massage school. The client will receive a 1-hour massage twice a week for $150 per month and will allow students to observe and participate in the sessions as part of a sports massage internship program. The athlete will be supported at various preliminary events by the students.

The massage will be a performance-based, full-body application and will be structured to meet the daily needs of the training regimen. Ongoing contact with the coach is requested. The massage will support rather than seek to change compensation patterns in gait in response to the amputation, because overall posture and performance are good.

Trigger points will be addressed with a variety of methods, and the results will be monitored to see if the phantom pain episodes decrease. The massage will be scheduled in the evening so the client can go to bed afterward. Sleep will be supported through encouragement of parasympathetic activation.

Appropriate methods that affect the neuromuscular/connective tissue and fluid dynamics of the body will be chosen each session. The client requires various levels of pressure, from very light pressure for lymphatic drainage to deep pressure to address the muscles of stabilization in the layer closest to the bone. Care will be taken not to increase inflammation in any area.

CASE 20 SCAR TISSUE MANAGEMENT

The client is a 28-year-old male who is seeking massage for general stress management and reduction of stiffness in burn scars. He is in good health, active in a variety of outdoor activities, and concerned about maintaining the quality of his life. He is a computer technician, and he works 50 hours per week. Six years ago, while burning leaves, he was burned on his chest. He had first-, second-, and small areas of third-degree burns. He was fortunate to be treated in a major burn center and received the best of care. The scarring was managed very well. Only one area had to be grafted, and the donor site was on his thigh; scarring is present in that area as well. Although the areas with a first-degree burn healed with no scarring, the areas with a second-degree burn did scar, with what is called *hypertrophic scars*. The client feels as if these scars are causing tightness across his chest and finds the sensation a nuisance.

The client has had massage before on a random basis and found that it lessened the tightness in his chest for a short time. He has read about various forms of connective tissue massage and the effect on scars. In the context of general massage, he would like to explore the possibility of using massage to make him more comfortable. Because he just received a raise, he has $100 per month to spend for massage care.

ASSESSMENT

Observation

The client is of average height and weight. He looks fit and walks with an energetic flair. He is talkative and likes to tell jokes. He is left-handed. He sits calmly during the interview and fills out the necessary paperwork without difficulty.

Interview and Goals

The client information form indicates that the client has some numbness in the burn area. He had various childhood injuries, such as a broken wrist and sprained ankles, but he cannot remember just when it all happened. None of the injuries bother him. The burn has been his most serious injury. He was anxious for a time after the accident and had some nightmares, but that has passed. The surgeries he underwent were for the skin grafts on the third-degree burn area and for removal of skin from the donor site. He does not take medication or vitamins. His diet is adequate for a bachelor who lives with two other guys. He does drink and party on the weekends.

The client's goals for massage are general stress management and reduction of stiffness in his burn scars.

Physical Assessment

Posture

Symmetric with evidence of slight concavity of the chest. Knees are slightly hyperextended.

Gait

Normal

Range of Motion

Horizontal abduction of the arm is restricted to 80 degrees. Shoulder flexion on the left is restricted to 130 degrees.

Palpation

Near Touch. No observable problems.

Skin. Skin on the chest has areas of flat scars and areas of scar development that are somewhat rough and raised, with identifiable bands of scar tissue. Areas of pigment change are noted in the scarred region. Skin on the chest and between the scapulae on the back is binding. Skin fold cannot be lifted on burn scars. Skin fold can be lifted on the back with difficulty, and it is uncomfortable for the client.

Superficial Connective Tissue. Moderate adherence in the area of the scars on both the chest and donor area.

Vessels and Lymph Nodes. There is concern over pressure on the vessels in the chest and at the clavicle. There is no evidence of edema.

Muscles. Quadriceps are short, and rhomboids are long. Trigger point activity is noted in the supraspinatus and occipital base, but no recognizable referred pain pattern is seen.

Tendons. Normal

Deep Fascia. Pliability of the lumbar dorsal fascia and iliotibial bands is reduced.

Ligaments. Normal

Joints. Horizontal abduction of the shoulder is limited by soft tissue bind. Sternoclavicular joint on the left is restricted.

Bones. Bone changes in the right wrist indicate healing of a bone break.

Abdominal Viscera. Normal

Body Rhythms. Full expansion of the thorax is somewhat restricted during deep inhalation. Body rhythm is even, and pulses are in the normal range.

Muscle Testing

Strength

Left arm flexors are weak to moderate resistance.

Neurologic Balance

Normal

Gait

Normal

INTERPRETATION AND TREATMENT PLAN DEVELOPMENT

Clinical Reasoning

What Are the Facts?

The client has a restricted sternoclavicular joint on the left; referral to a chiropractor or osteopath is indicated. Treatment for this condition should correct the weak muscles of arm flexion.

Mild to moderate connective tissue binding is present, causing a concavity in the chest and reduction of horizontal abduction of the shoulder. The area corresponds with the burn scars. Corresponding areas of connective tissue bind are noted between the scapulae. The muscles in this area are also tight and long.

The short quadriceps muscles correspond with the hyperextension of the knees.

Trigger points do not refer a recognizable pain pattern.

Burn scars are evident, with reduced tissue pliability and some adhesion.

A burn that causes blisters is a second-degree burn. Typically this type of burn is characterized as superficial or deep.

- A *superficial second-degree burn* involves only the most superficial dermis. It manifests as blistering or sloughing of overlying skin, causing a red, painful wound. Typically, the burn blanches but shows good capillary refill. Hairs cannot be pulled out easily. Healing occurs within 14 days, usually without scarring and without requiring surgical intervention.
- A *deep second-degree burn* involves more of the dermis. It may manifest as blisters or a wound with a white or deep red base. Sensation is usually diminished, and healing takes longer than 14 days. Hypertrophic scarring occurs when the healing phase lasts longer than 2 weeks. Débriding and grafting, therefore, are recommended by 2 to 3 weeks.

Studies have shown that stretching the connective tissue with sufficient force creates an elastic response in scar tissue. The most common causes of contractures are scarring and lack of use because of immobilization or inactivity. Severe contracture in this client is not evident, but scar shortening is.

Scar tissue from burns and grafts can be sensitive, and work needs to proceed with caution to ensure that the area is not damaged by the tissue stretching.

What Are the Possibilities Both in Function and Dysfunction and the Massage Intervention Options?

The connective tissue shortening of the burn scars on the chest probably is binding and restricting both range of motion of the arm and upper chest motion.
Possibilities:

1. Massage that exerts a drag on the skin and superficial fascia could increase pliability in the area.
2. General massage on a weekly basis could support stress management, relaxation, and an active lifestyle.

What Are the Logical Outcomes of Each Possible Intervention Option?

Massage is indicated for the stated goals, but the finances allocated are insufficient to support massage on a weekly basis to address goals.

What Is the Impact on the People Involved for Each Massage Intervention Option?

The client and massage professional are both supportive of massage and the realistic outcome of the goals, but the finances are difficult. The client has to reassess priorities in terms of where he spends his money. He is willing to invest some of his weekend partying money to cover the cost of massage on a weekly basis if he sees enough value in his progress, and he is willing to commit to a 3-month, 12-session trial period.

DECISION MAKING AND TREATMENT PLAN DEVELOPMENT

Quantifiable Goals

1. Reduce stress symptoms by 75% as reported by the client
2. Increase connective tissue pliability in burn scars by 30%

Qualifiable Goals

The client should be able to perform work and daily activities with minor tension on the scar tissue and be less irritated by the tissue changes in the burn scars.

Treatment Regimen

Weekly massage will be provided at $45 per hour session. The massage will consist of myofascial techniques with sufficient drag to increase pliability of the scar tissue in the burn and donor areas. Caution will be needed to ensure that the intensity of the work is sufficient to address the connective tissue binding but does not damage the tissue in the area. The connective tissue work will be done before the general massage session, because generating a pulling sensation is likely to be intense and somewhat uncomfortable. The pressure used will exert force in the horizontal plane to stretch the area of the scars. Tensile and shear forces will be used first, then bend and torque as the tissue becomes more pliable. The intensity of the work will progress slowly.

When the skin and superficial fascia can be lifted, skin rolling methods will be introduced. The client will not have to endure this work for longer than 10 minutes, and frequent breaks will be included. Because mild inflammation will be introduced into the area, lymphatic drainage will be used to support movement of any restricted lymphatic flow away from the burned area. The client will need to drink sufficient water to support hydration of the ground substance of the connective tissue.

General massage will be given, with methods used as needed to address range of motion and stress management; these methods will be determined at each massage session. Pressure levels will need to be sufficient to stimulate an increase in serotonin and enkephalin blood levels to achieve the relaxation and stress management goals. The massage rhythm, speed, and duration will address the shift from the stress response to parasympathetic dominance. The massage will be rhythmic and will support entrainment, with sufficient pressure exerted to address the deeper layers of soft tissue without causing pain or guarding (Proficiency Exercise 15-1).

PROFICIENCY EXERCISE 15-1

Write up a case of your own using the format followed in this chapter.

■ ■ ■ SUMMARY

Each of the case studies in this chapter should challenge the student to continue to develop clinical reasoning skills and perfect assessment and technical therapeutic massage skills. More important, each case study told a story about a person who was seeking assistance. Remember, the most proficient application of massage is not competent practice until compassion, respect, and desire for the highest good of the client are the motivating intent of the massage. Each client you serve has the potential to be a great teacher if you are willing to learn. Knowledge needs experience to support your development as a therapeutic massage professional. Congratulations on your accumulation of knowledge as presented in this text. My hope is that each one who has learned from this text persists with the accumulation of knowledge and experience to serve and be served in this humble and important profession.

LIBRARY UNIVERSITY OF CHESTF

Workbook Section

■ ■ ■ **ASSESS YOUR COMPETENCIES**

Now that you have studied this chapter, you should be able to:

1. Use clinical reasoning to integrate the information from science studies and this text to complete a comprehensive history, assessment, and care/treatment plan.

2. Write comprehensive case studies.

3. Analyze care/treatment plans and offer and justify alternate approaches to care.

4. Pick out three of the case studies in this chapter and develop a treatment plan that differs from the one presented. Justify why your treatment plan is appropriate for the condition.

Final Word

Although this is the end of the textbook, it is just the beginning of your massage career. It has been quite a journey; it began with touch and continues with your ongoing evolution as a massage professional.

It will take some time to learn all the information presented in this book. In a year, after some massage experience, reread this textbook. You will be surprised what you can still learn from it, and you will be duly impressed with what you now understand. Most likely you will discover that the ability to think purposefully and use the reasoning process is your most valuable skill. When you can do this, you truly become your own best teacher.

Finishing this textbook and your course of study in therapeutic massage is an achievement. Be proud of yourself and all those who helped you in the learning process.

Your success now depends on your belief in your own ability. Nothing can stop you if you desire to achieve. Every obstacle is an opportunity to exercise your "achievement muscle." The origin of this muscle is in your faith and the insertion is in your hope. Its function is love and compassion for those you serve.

Success is the maximal use of the abilities you have. If a better way exists to do something, challenge yourself to find it, then share it with others. When in doubt, effleurage!

You never fail when you have done your best. Measure success by what really matters.

All great achievements require time, perseverance, and purpose. Go slowly, evaluate, and adapt to each change, seeing it as an opportunity for growth.

Massage creates space and substitutes one set of signals for another. Hopefully, a more resourceful set of signals frees the energy to reach for our highest potential without restriction. Massage brings an awareness of body, mind, and spirit. Pay attention to the subtleties and quiet messages of life. Let these things teach you.

Most importantly, massage touches people, and in turn, we are touched by them.

Thank you for letting me serve you through this textbook.

Works Consulted

The following works have been used by the author in the development of this text. They are listed by chapter in alphabetical order.
*Recommended reading for further study.
**Recommended companion textbook and/or reference.

CHAPTER 1

Arvedson J: *Medical gymnastics and massage in general practice,* London, 1930, JA Churchill.

Arvedson J: *The techniques, effects, and uses of Swedish medical gymnastics and massage,* London, 1931, JA Churchill.

Basmajian JV, Nyberg R: *Rational manual therapies,* Baltimore, 1993, Williams & Wilkins.

Baumgartner AJ: *Massage in athletics,* Minneapolis, 1947, Brugess.

Beard G: A history of massage technique, *Phys Ther Rev* 32:613, 1952.

Beck M: *Theory and practice of therapeutic massage,* ed 4, Clifton Park, New York, 2006, Thomas Delmar Learning, 2002, Milady.

Benjamin P: Massage therapy in the 1940s and the college of Swedish massage in Chicago, *Massage Ther Journal* 32(4):56, 1993.

Cantu RI, Grodin AJ: *Myofascial manipulation theory and clinical application,* ed 2, Gaithersburg, Md, 2001, Aspen.

*Chaitow L: *Palpation and assessment skills: assessment and diagnosis through touch,* New York, 2003, Churchill Livingstone.

Chaitow L: *Soft tissue manipulation,* Rochester, Vt, 1988, Healing Arts Press.

Colton H: *Touch therapy,* New York, 1983, Kensington.

Despard LL: *Textbook of massage and remedial gymnastics,* ed 3, New York, 1932, Oxford University Press.

Garofano JS: *Therapeutic massage and bodywork,* Stamford, Conn, 1997, Appleton & Lange.

Graham D: The history of massage, *Medical Record* (approximately) 1874.

Graham D: Massage, *Med Surg Rep* 35(10):1, 1874.

Graham D: *A treatise on massage, its history, mode of application and effects,* ed 3, Philadelphia, 1902, JB Lippincott.

Greenman PE: *Principles of manual medicine,* ed 3, Baltimore, 2003, Williams & Wilkins.

Gurevich D: Historical perspective, unpublished article, 1992.

Johnson W: *The anatriptic art and medical rubbing,* London, 1866, Simpkin, Marshall.

Kellogg JH: *The art of massage,* Battle Creek, Mich, 1929, Modern Medicine Publishing.

Kleen E: *Massage and medical gymnastics,* ed 2, New York, 1921, William Wood.

Knott M, Voss DE: *Proprioceptive neuromuscular facilitation: patterns and techniques,* ed 2, New York, 1968, Harper & Row.

Kruger L, editor: *Pain and touch: handbook of perception and cognition,* ed 2, San Diego, 2006, Academic Press.

Lederman E: *Fundamentals of manual therapy: physiology, neurology, and psychology,* ed 2, New York, 2005, Churchill Livingstone.

Lewit K: *Manipulative therapy in rehabilitation of the locomotor system,* ed 2, Oxford, 1991, Butterworth-Heinemann.

McMillian M: *Massage and therapeutic exercise,* ed 3, Philadelphia, 1932, WB Saunders.

Millenson JR: *Mind matters: psychological medicine in holistic practice,* Seattle, 1995, Eastland Press.

*Montague A: *Touching: the human significance of the skin,* ed 3, New York, 1991, Harper & Row.

Norstrom G: *Handbook of massage,* New York, 1896, The Faculty of Stockholm.

Northrup C: *Women's bodies, women's wisdom,* New York, 1994, Bantam Books.

Ornstein R, Sobel D: *The healing brain,* ed 2, New York, 1999, Malor.

Post SE: *Massage: a primer for nurses,* New York, 1891, Nightingale Publishing.

Roth M: *Handbook of the movement cure,* London, 1856, Groombridge & Sons.

Smith EWL, Clance PR, Imes S: *Touch in psychotherapy theory, research, and practice,* New York, 1998, Guilford Press.

Tappan FM: *Healing massage techniques: holistic, classic, and emerging methods,* ed 4, 2004, Prentice Hall.

Tappan FM: *Massage techniques: a case method approach,* New York, 1961, Macmillan.

Tappan FM, Benjamin PJ: *Tappan's handbook of healing massage techniques: holistic, classic, and emerging methods,* ed 4, 2004, Prentice Hall.

Taylor CF: *Theory and practice of the movement cure by the Swedish system,* Philadelphia, 1861, Lindsay & Blakiston.

Thomas Z: *Healing touch: the church's forgotten language,* Louisville, Ky, 1994, Westminster/John Knox Press.

van Why R: *History of massage and its relevance to today's practitioner,* 1992, The Bodywork Knowledgebase.

van Why R: *Lecture on the history of massage in four parts,* 1992, The Bodywork Knowledgebase.

van Why R: *Notes toward a history of massage,* ed 2, 1992, The Bodywork Knowledgebase.

CHAPTER 2

Administrative Rules of Michigan Occupational Regulations Department of Licensing and Regulation, Lansing, Mich, 1994, Michigan Department of Commerce.

American Massage Therapy Association: *American Massage Therapy Association code of ethics,* Chicago, The Association.

*Anderson KN, Anderson L, Glanze WD, editors: *Mosby's medical, nursing, and allied health dictionary,* ed 7, St Louis, 2005, Mosby.

*Ashley M: *Massage: a career at your fingertips,* ed 5, New York, 2005, Enterprise Publishing.

Bass E, Davis L: *The courage to heal: a guide for women survivors of child sexual abuse,* 1994, Perennial.

Blanchard K, Peale NV: *The power of ethical management,* 1996, William Morrow.

Clouser KD, Hufford DJ, O'Conner BB: Informed consent and alternative medicine, *Altern Ther* 2(2):76, 1996.

*Corey G, Corey MS, Callanan P: *Issues and ethics in the helping professions,* ed 6, 2006, Brooks/Cole.

Davis CM: *Patient practitioner interaction and experiential manual for developing the art of health care,* ed 3, Thorofare NJ, 1998, Slack.

Denny NW, Quadagno D: *Human sexuality,* ed 2, St Louis, 1992, Mosby.

Dubler N, Nimmons D: *Ethics on call,* New York, 1994, Harmony.

Guidelines for Core Curriculum for Massage Therapy School, Board of Directors of Masseurs, Province of Ontario: Regulated Health Professions Act and the Massage Therapy Act, Toronto, Ontario, Canada, June 1992.

Guidelines for Core Curriculum for Massage Therapy School, Board of Directors of Masseurs, Province of Ontario: Therapeutic massage curriculum guidelines, Toronto, Ontario, Canada, June 1992.

Hands On 14(3), 1998, American Massage Therapy Association.

International Myomassethics Federation: *Code of ethics*, Huntington Beach, Calif, 1993, The Federation.

In touch with the future massage therapy in the 90s: issues of professional development, Chicago, 1990, American Massage Therapy Association.

Keirsey D, Bates M: *Please understand me: temperament in leading*, Del Mar, Calif, 1996, Prometheus Nemesis.

Keirsey D, Marilyn B: *Please understand me: character and temperament types*, ed 2, Del Mar, Calif., 1984, Prometheus Nemesis.

Kohn A: Shattered innocence, *Psychology Today* February :54, 1987.

Leflet D: *HEMME approach to ethics*, Bonifay, Fla, 1995, HEMME Approach Publications.

Lyons DJB: *Planning your career in alternative medicine: a guide to degree and certificate programs in alternative health care*, New York, 1997, Avery Publishing Group.

McPartland JM: The Census Subcommittee on the Alternative Medicine Research Institute, and Teachers' Academy: census of bodyworkers and movement therapists in Vermont, USA, *J Bodywork Move Ther* 2(2):125, 1998.

Millenson JR: *Mind matters: psychological medicine in holistic practice*, Seattle, 1995, Eastland Press.

Mitchell BB: *Acupuncture and Oriental medicine laws*, Washington, DC, 1997, National Acupuncture Foundation.

National Certification Examination for Therapeutic Massage and Bodywork: *Candidate handbook*, Lansing, Mich, 1993, Psychological Corp.

Occupational Regulation Section of the Michigan Public Health Code, Articles 1, 7, 15, and 19 of Act 368 of 1978, Michigan Department of Licensing and Regulation, Lansing, Mich, 1978.

Oregon administrative rules, Board of Massage Technicians Chapter 334 Division 10 Massage Licensing, Portland, Ore, July 1991, Oregon Board of Massage Technicians.

Palmer D: Defining our profession: strategies for inventing the future of massage, *Massage Bodywork Q* Summer :28, 1993.

Pearson JC, Spitzberg BH: *Interpersonal communication: concept, components, and contexts*, ed 2, Dubuque, Iowa, 1987, WC Brown.

Sohnen-Moe C, Benjamin B: *The ethics of touch: the hands-on guide to creating a professional, safe, and enduring practice*, Philadelphia, 2004, Williams and Wilkins.

Sorrentino SA: *Mosby's textbook for nursing assistants*, ed 7, St Louis, 2007, Mosby.

State Medical Board of Ohio: 4731-1-05 Scope of Practice of Massage, January 1992.

State of Florida Massage Practice Act, Chapter 480. No. 1993.

Successful business handbook, Evergreen, Colo, 1997, Associated Bodywork and Massage Professionals.

Texas Public Health Act. 4512K, Title 71: Regulation of massage therapists and massage establishments, Chapter 141, January 1990.

**Thibodeau GA, Patton K: *The human body in health and disease*, ed 4, St Louis, 2005, Mosby.

Thomas C: *Bodywork: what type of massage to get and how to make the most of it*, New York, 1995, William Morrow.

Waites E: *Trauma and survival: post-traumatic and dissociative disorder in women*, New York, 1993, WW Norton.

Washington State: The Law Relating to Massage Therapy, 18.108 RCW, 1991.

Webster's new universal unabridged dictionary deluxe, ed 2, New York, 1983, Simon & Schuster.

Williams KM: Taking the "parlor" out of massage, *Zoning and Planning News* 7:6, 1989.

**Yates J: *A physician's guide to therapeutic massage: its physiological effects and their application to treatment*, Vancouver, BC, 1990, Massage Therapists Association of British Columbia.

CHAPTER 3

*Anderson KN, Anderson LE, Glanze WD, editors: *Mosby's medical, nursing, and allied health dictionary*, ed 7, St Louis, 2005, Mosby.

**Birmingham JJ: *Medical terminology: a self-learning text*, ed 3, St Louis, 1999, Mosby.

**Brooks ML: *Exploring medical language, a student-directed approach*, ed 6, St Louis, 2005, Mosby Lifeline.

**Fritz S, Paholsky K, Grosenbach M: *Mosby's basic science for soft tissue and movement therapies*, St Louis, 1999, Mosby.

Gunn C: *Bones and joints*, ed 4, New York, 2002, Churchill Livingstone.

*Hinkle CZ: *Fundamentals of anatomy and movement: a workbook and guide*, St Louis, 1997, Mosby.

Lillis CA: *A concise introduction to medical terminology*, ed 4, Stamford, Conn, 1997, Appleton & Lange.

Lindsay DT: *Functional human anatomy*, St Louis, 1996, Mosby.

Seeley RR, Stephens TD, Tate P: *Essentials of anatomy and physiology*, ed 6, St Louis, 2006, McGraw-Hill.

Sorrentino SA: *Mosby's textbook for nursing assistants*, ed 6, St Louis, 2004, Mosby.

Stewart J: *Clinical anatomy and pathophysiology for the health professional*, Miami, 1997, MedMaster.

**Thibodeau GA, Patton K: *The human body in health and disease*, ed 4, St Louis, 2005, Mosby.

Thibodeau GA, Patton KT: *Anatomy and physiology*, ed 6, St Louis, 2007, Mosby.

Thomas CL: *Taber's cyclopedic medical dictionary*, ed 16, Philadelphia, 1985, FA Davis.

Thompson DL: Goal-oriented SOAP charting: the search for functional outcomes, *Massage Magazine* May/June :82 1998.

*Thompson DL: *Hands heal: documentation for massage therapy*, Seattle, 1993, Thompson.

CHAPTER 4

Alcock J: *Animal behavior: an evaluatory approach*, Sunderland, Mass, 1989, Sinawer.

**Anderson LE, Glanze WD, editors: *Mosby's medical, nursing, and allied health dictionary*, ed 7, St Louis, 2005, Mosby.

Assendelft WJ, Morton SC, Yu EI et al: Spinal manipulative therapy for low back pain. A meta-analysis of effectiveness relative to other therapies, *Ann Intern Med* 138(11):871-881, 2003.

Astin JA, Ernst E: The effectiveness of spinal manipulation for the treatment of headache disorders: a systematic review of randomized clinical trials, *Cephalalgia* 22(8):617-623, 2002.

Astin JA: Why patients use alternative medicine: results of a national study, *JAMA* 279(19):1548-1553, 1998.

Baldry PE: *Acupuncture, trigger points and musculoskeletal pain*, ed 3, New York, 2005, Churchill Livingstone.

Barnes P, Powell-Griner E, McFann K, Nahin R: *Complementary and alternative medicine use among adults*: United States, 2002. CDC Advance Data Report #343, 2004.

*Basmajian JV, Nyberg R: *Rational manual therapies*, Baltimore, 1993, Williams & Wilkins.

Benford MS: Radiogenic metabolism: an alternative cellular energy source, *Med Hypoth* 56(1):33-39, 2001.

Berman JD, Straus SE: Implementing a research agenda for complementary and alternative medicine, *Ann Rev Med* 4(55):239-254, 2004.

Bullock BL, Rosendahl PP: *Pathophysiology adaptations and alteration in function*, ed 4, Philadelphia, 1996, JB Lippincott.

*Cailliet R: *Foot and ankle pain*, ed 3, Philadelphia, 1997, FA Davis.

*Cailliet R: *Hand pain and impairment*, ed 4, Philadelphia, 1994, FA Davis.

*Cailliet R: *Knee pain and disability*, ed 3, Philadelphia, 1992, FA Davis.

*Cailliet R: *Low back pain syndrome*, ed 5, Philadelphia, 1995, FA Davis.

*Cailliet R: *Neck and arm pain*, ed 3, Philadelphia, 1991, FA Davis.

*Cailliet R: *Shoulder pain*, ed 3, Philadelphia, 1991, FA Davis.

*Cailliet R: *Soft tissue pain and disability*, Philadelphia, 1996, FA Davis.

*Cantu RI, Grodin AJ: *Myofascial manipulation theory and clinical application*, Gaithersburg, Md, 1992, Aspen.

Chaitow L: *The book of natural pain relief*, New York, 1995, Harper Paperbacks.

*Chaitow L: *Modern neuromuscular techniques*, ed 2, New York, 2003, Churchill Livingstone.

*Chaitow L: *Muscle energy techniques*, ed 3, New York, 2007, Churchill Livingstone.

Chaitow L: Breathing patterns, connective tissue and soft-shelled eggs, *Naturopathy Digest*, January 2006.

Chaitow L: *Soft-tissue manipulation*, Rochester, Vt, 1988, Healing Arts Press.

Chaitow L et al: Breathing dysfunction, *J Bodywork Move Ther* 1(5):252, 1997.

Chaitow L, Fritz S: *A massage therapist's guide to understanding, locating and treating myofascial trigger points*, Edinburgh, 2007, Churchill Livingstone.

Chen KW, Turner FD: A case study of simultaneous recovery from multiple physical symptoms with medical qigong therapy, *J Altern Complem Med* 10(1):159-162, 2004.

Cherkin DC, Deyo RA, Sherman KJ et al: Characteristics of visits to licensed acupuncturists, chiropractors, massage therapists, and naturopathic physicians, *J Am Board Family Pract* 15(6):463-472, 2002.

Cherkin DC, Eisenberg D, Sherman KJ et al: Randomized trial comparing traditional Chinese medical acupuncture, therapeutic massage, and self-care education for chronic low back pain, *Arch Intern Med* 161(8):1081-1088, 2001.

Cherkin DC, Sherman KJ, Deyo RA et al: A review of the evidence for the effectiveness, safety, and cost of acupuncture, massage therapy, and spinal manipulation for back pain *Ann Intern Med* 138(11):898-906, 2003.

Chlan L: Music intervention. In Snyder M, Lindquist R, editors: *Complementary/alternative therapies in nursing*, ed 4, New York, 2001, Springer Publishing Company.

Colby LA, Kisner C: *Therapeutic exercise: foundations and techniques*, ed 5, Philadelphia, 2007, FA Davis.

Crenshaw K, Shaw N, Porterfield R: Muscle energy techniques (MET) in treatment of athletic injuries. In Chaitow L, editor: *Muscle energy techniques*, ed 3, Baltimore, 2006, Churchill Livingstone.

Dean BZ, Geiringer SR: Physiatric therapeutics. Part 5. Pain, *Arch Phys Med Rehabil* 71:S271, 1990.

Degenhardt B, Kuchera M: Update of osteopathic medical concepts and the lymphatic system, *J Am Osteopath Assoc* 96(2):97, 1996.

deGroot J, Chusid JG: *Correlative neuroanatomy*, ed 20, San Mateo, Calif, 1985, Appleton & Lange.

Diego M et al: Spinal cord patients benefits from massage therapy, *Intern J Neuroscience*, 112:133-142, 2002.

Diego M et al: Massage therapy of moderate and light pressure and vibrator effects on EEG and heart rate, *Intern J Neuroscience*, 114:31-44, 2004.

DiLima SN, Painter SJ, Johns LT, editors: *Orthopaedic patient education resource manual*, Gaithersburg, Md, 1995, Aspen.

Eisenberg DM, Davis RB, Ettner SL et al: Trends in alternative medicine use in the United States, 1990-1997: results of a follow-up national survey, *JAMA* 280(18):1569-1575, 1998.

Emoto M: Healing with water, *J Altern and Complem Med* 10(1):19-21, 2004.

Ernst E, editor. *The desktop guide to complementary and alternative medicine: an evidence-based approach*, Edinburgh, 2001, Mosby.

Ernst E, Harkness E: Spinal manipulation: a systematic review of sham-controlled, double-blind, randomized clinical trials, *J Pain Symptom Management* 22(4):879-889, 2001.

Ernst E: Distant healing–an "update" of a systematic review, *Wiener Klinische Wochenschrift* 115(7-8):241-245, 2003.

Ernst E: Manipulation of the cervical spine: a systematic review of case reports of serious adverse events, 1995-2001, *Med J Australia* 176(8):376-380, 2002.

Ernst M, Lee MHM: Sympathetic effects of manual and electrical acupuncture of the Tsusanli knee point: comparison with the Huko hand point sympathetic effects, *Exp Neurol*, 1986.

Esch T et al: Commonalities in the central nervous system's involvement with complementary medical therapies: limbic morphinergic processes, *Med Sci Monit*, Jun;10(6):MS6-17. Epub 2004 Jun 1. Charite-University Medicine Berlin, Institute for General and Family Medicine, Berlin, Germany.

Field T: Massage therapy, *Med Clin North Am* 86(1):163-171, 2002.

Field T et al: Massage therapy by parents improves early growth and development, *Infant Behav Develop* 27:435-442, 2004.

**Fritz S, Grosenbach M: *Mosby's essential sciences for therapeutic massage: anatomy, physiology, biomechanics, pathology*, ed 3, St Louis, 2009, Mosby.

Gallob R: Reiki: a supportive therapy in nursing practice and self-care for nurses, *J New York State Nurses' Assoc* 34(1):9-13, 2003.

Ganong WF: *Review of medical physiology*, ed 13, Norwalk, Conn, 1987, Appleton & Lange.

Goertz CH, Grimm RH, Svendsen K et al: Treatment of hypertension with alternative therapies (THAT) study: a randomized clinical trial, *J Hypertension* 20(10):2063-2068, 2002.

**Greenman PE: *Principles of manual medicine*, ed 3, Baltimore, 2003, Williams & Wilkins.

Gunn CC: Clinical research unit, rehabilitation clinic, *J Acupuncture* 6, 1978.

Gunn CC: *Reprints on pain, acupuncture and related subjects*, Seattle, 1992, University of Washington.

Hintz KJ, Yount GL, Kadar I et al: Bioenergy definitions and research guidelines, *Altern Ther Health Med* 9(suppl 3):A13-A30, 2003.

Hondras MA, Linde K, Jones AP: Manual therapy for asthma. Cochrane Database of Systematic Reviews. 2004;(2):CD001002. Accessed at www.cochrane.org on April 30, 2004.

Hooper J, Teresi D: *The three pound universe*, New York, 1986, Dell.

Horacek J: *Brainstorms*, Northvale, NJ, 1998, Jason Aronson.

Hymel G: *Research methods for massage and holistic therapies*, St. Louis, 2006, Mosby.

Knaster M: Tiffany Field provides proof positive, scientifically, *Massage Ther J* 37(1):84, 1998.

*Lederman E: *Fundamentals of manual therapy: physiology, neurology, and psychology*, New York, 1997, Churchill Livingstone.

Leflet DH: *HEMME approach to modalities*, Bonifay, Fla, 1996, HEMME Approach Publications.

Levin SR: Acute effects of massage on the stress response, master's thesis, Greensboro, NC, 1990, University of North Carolina.

Logani MK, Bhanushali A, Anga A et al: Combined millimeter wave and cyclophosphamide therapy of an experimental murine melanoma, *Bioelectromagnetics* 25(7):516, 2004.

Longworth J: Psychophysiological effects of slow stroke back massage in normotensive females, *Adv Nurs Sci* 44, 1982.

Lu Z: *Scientific qigong exploration*, Malvern, Pa., 1997, Amber Leaf Press.

Lund I, Yu LC, Uvnas-Moberg K et al: Repeated massage-like stimulation induces long-term effects on nociception: contribution of oxytocinergic mechanisms, *Eur J Neuroscience* 16(2):330-338, 2002.

*Manheim CJ, Lavett DK: *The myofascial release manual*, Thorofare, NJ, 1989, Slack.

Marieb E: *Human anatomy and physiology*, ed 2, Redwood City, Calif, 1992, Benjamin/Cummings Publishing.

Martiny K, Simonsen C, Lunde M et al: Decreasing TSH levels in patients with seasonal affective disorder (SAD) responding to 1 week of bright light therapy, *J Affective Disorders* 79(1-3):253-257, 2004.

McArdle WD et al: *Exercise physiology: energy nutrition and human performance,* ed 3, Philadelphia, 1991, Lea & Febiger.

McCraty R, Tiller WA, Atkinson M: Head-heart entrainment: a preliminary survey, 1995, Institute of HeartMath. Available at http://www._heartmath.org/research papers/Head/Hart/Headheart.html.

Meeker WC, Haldeman S: Chiropractic: a profession at the crossroads of mainstream and alternative medicine, *Ann Intern Med* 136(3):216-227, 2002.

Mehling WE, Hamel KA et al: Randomized, controlled trial of breath therapy for patients with chronic low-back pain, *Altern Ther Health Med* 11(4):44-52, 2005.

Milgrom LR: Vitalism, complexity and the concept of spin, *Homeopathy* 91(1):26-31, 2002.

Millenson JR: *Mind matters: psychological medicine in holistic practice,* Seattle, 1995, Eastland Press.

Morris CE, Skalak TC: Effects of static magnetic fields on microvascular tone in vivo. Abstract presented at Experimental Biology Meeting; April 2003, San Diego, California.

National Institutes of Health Consensus Panel. Acupuncture: National Institutes of Health Consensus Development Statement. National Center for Complementary and Alternative Medicine Web site.

Ni H, Simile C, Hardy AM: Utilization of complementary and alternative medicine by United States adults: results from the 1999 National Health Interview Survey, *Medical Care* 40(4):353-358, 2002.

NNIH funds massage studies, *Hands On* 9(4), 1993.

Oschman JL: *Energy medicine: the scientific basis of bioenergy therapies,* Philadelphia, 2000, Churchill Livingstone.

Oschman JL: What is healing energy? Part 3. Silent pulses, *J Bodywork Move Ther* 1(3):179, 1997.

Panov V, Kichigin V, Khaldeev G et al: Torsion fields and experiments, *J New Energy* 2:29-39, 1997.

Pickar JG: Neurophysiological effects of spinal manipulation, *Spine J* 2(5):357-371, 2002.

Proctor ML, Hing W, Johnson TC et al: Spinal manipulation for primary and secondary dysmenorrhoea, Cochrane Database of Systematic Reviews. 2004;(2):CD002119.

Reddy GK: Photobiological basis and clinical role of low-intensity lasers in biology and medicine, *J Clin Laser Med Surg* 22(2):141-150, 2004.

Russek L, Schwartz G: Energy cardiology: a dynamical energy systems approach for integrating conventional and alternative medicine advances, *J Mind-Body Health* 12(4):4-24, 1996.

Sancier KM, Holman D: Commentary: multifaceted health benefits of medical qigong, *J Altern Complem Med* 10(1):163-165, 2004.

Schleip R: Fascial plasticity—a new neurobiological explanation, *J Bodywork Movement Ther* 7(1): January 2003.

Selye H: *The healing brain: understanding stress, stress without distress,* Los Altos, Calif, ISHK Paperbacks.

*Selye H: *The stress of life,* ed 2, New York, 1978, McGraw-Hill.

Shealy NC: The neurochemical substrate of behavior, *Psychol Health Immun Dis* B 434, 1992.

Sisken BF, Walder J: Therapeutic aspects of electromagnetic fields for soft tissue healing. In Blank M, editor: *Electromagnetic fields: biological interactions and mechanisms,* Washington, DC, 1995, American Chemical Society.

Spector M: Connective tissue cells with muscle: expression of muscle action in and contraction of fibroblasts, chondrocytes, and osteoblasts. Article Accessed on http://healthcare.partners.org, Aug. 2, 2004.

Swenson R, Haldeman S: Spinal manipulative therapy for low back pain, *J Am Acad Orthopaedic Surgeons* 11(4):228-237, 2003.

Szabo I, Manning MR, Radzievsky AA et al: Low power millimeter wave irradiation exerts no harmful effect on human keratinocytes in vitro, *Bioelectromagnetics* 24(3):165-173, 2003.

Takeshige C: Mechanism of acupuncture analgesia based on animal experiments. In *Scientific bases of acupuncture,* Berlin, 1989, Springer-Verlag.

*Thibodeau GA, Patton KT: *Anatomy and physiology,* ed 6, St Louis, 2007, Mosby.

Thibodeau GA, Patton KT: *The human body in health and disease,* ed 4, St Louis, 2005, Mosby.

Thomas CL, editor: *Taber's cyclopedic medical dictionary,* ed 16, Philadelphia, 1985, FA Davis.

Timmons BH, Ley R: *Behavioral and psychological approaches to breathing disorders,* New York, 1994, Plenum Press.

Tortora GJ, Grabowski SR: *Principles of anatomy and physiology,* ed 11, New York, 2005, Wiley.

Touch research, *Int J Altern Complement Med* 11:7, 1993.

*Travell JG, Simons DG: *Myofascial pain and dysfunction: the trigger point manual,* Baltimore, 1984, Waverly.

*Travell JG, Simons DG: *Myofascial pain and dysfunction: the trigger point manual,* vol 2, the lower extremities, Baltimore, 1992, Williams & Wilkins.

Trew M, Everett T: *Human movement: an introductory text,* ed 5, New York, 2005, Churchill Livingstone.

Uvnas-Moberg K, Petersson M: Oxytocin, a mediator of anti-stress, well-being, social interaction, growth and healing, *Z Psychosom Med Psychother* 51(1):57-80, 2005. Swedish University of Agricultural Sciences, Department of Animal Physiology, PO Box 7045, S-75007 Uppsala, Sweden.

van Why R: *History of massage and its relevance to today's practitioner,* 1992 (self-published).

Wale JO: *Tidy's massage and remedial exercises,* Bristol, England, 1987, John Wright & Sons.

Winstead-Fry P, Kijek J: An integrative review and meta-analysis of therapeutic touch research, *Altern Ther Health Med* 5(6):58-67, 1999.

Work modification, work hardening, and work rehabilitation (Cassette #22), Physical Medicine Research Foundation, Third International Symposium, 1990, Vancouver, British Columbia.

Yates J: *Physiological effects of therapeutic massage and their application to treatment,* British Columbia, 1989, Massage Therapists Association.

Zimmerman J: Laying-on-of-hands healing and therapeutic touch: a testable theory, BEMI Currents, *J Bioelectromagnetics Institute* 2:8-17, 1990.

CHAPTER 5

*Anderson KN, Anderson LE, Glanze WD, editors: *Mosby's medical, nursing, and allied health dictionary,* ed 5, St Louis, 1998, Mosby.

Board of Directors of Masseurs, Province of Ontario: Ontario, Canada therapeutic massage curriculum guidelines, Toronto, Ontario, Canada, 1992, The Board.

Bulluck BL: *Pathophysiology adaptations and alterations in function,* ed 4, Philadelphia, 1996, Lippincott Williams & Wilkins.

Cailliet R: *Soft tissue pain and disability,* Philadelphia, 1996, FA Davis.

Caillet R: Low back disorders: a medical enigma, Philadelphia, 2003, Lippincott Williams & Wilkins.

*Cantu RI, Grodin AJ: *Myofascial manipulation theory and clinical application,* ed 2, Gaithersburg, Md, 2001, Aspen.

*Chaitow L: *Modern neuromuscular techniques,* New York, 2003, Churchill Livingstone.

*Chaitow L: *Muscle energy techniques,* New York, 1996, Churchill Livingstone.

Chaitow L: *Osteopathic self-treatment,* London, 1990, Thorsons.

Chaitow L: *Palpatory literacy,* London, 1991, Thorsons.

Chaitow L: *Soft-tissue manipulation,* Rochester, Vt, 1988, Healing Arts Press.

Chaitow L: Soft-tissue manipulation and neuromuscular techniques: improving palpatory literacy and treatment efficiency, Lapeer, Mich, 1991, Soft Tissue Manipulation Seminar.

Chaitow L et al: Breathing dysfunction, *J Bodywork Move Ther* 1(5):252, 1997.

Chopra D: *Restful sleep,* New York, 1994, Crowne Trade Paperbacks.

Colby LA, Kisner C: *Therapeutic exercise: foundations and techniques,* ed 5, Philadelphia, 2007, FA Davis.

Cowan P: *Staying well: advanced pain management for ACPA members,* 1994, American Chronic Pain Association.

Dean BZ, Geiringer SR: Physiatric therapeutics. Part 5. Pain, *Arch Phys Med Rehabil* 71:S271, 1990.

Degenhardt B, Kuchera M: Update of osteopathic medical concepts and the lymphatic system, *J Am Osteopath Assoc* 96(2):97, 1996.

deGroot J, Chusid JG: *Correlative neuroanatomy,* ed 20, San Mateo, Calif, 1985, Appleton & Lange.

Falvo DR: *Medical and psychosocial aspects of chronic illness and disability,* Gaithersburg, Md, 1991, Aspen.

Ganong WF: *Review of medical physiology,* ed 13, Norwalk, Conn, 1987, Appleton & Lange.

*Greenman PE: *Principles of manual medicine,* ed 3, Baltimore, 2003, Williams & Wilkins.

Hahn DB, Payne WA: *Focus on health,* ed 4, St Louis, 1999, Mosby.

Kruger L, editor: *Pain and touch,* ed 2, San Diego, 1996, Academic Press.

McCraty R, Tiller WA, Atkinson M: Head-heart entrainment: a preliminary survey. Institute of HeartMath. Available at http://www.heartmath.org/research papers/Head/Hart/ Headheart.html.

Melzack R: TP relationship to mechanisms of pain, *Arch Phys Med Rehabil* 62:114, 1981.

Nimmi ME: *Collagen,* vol 1, Boca Raton, Fla, 1988, CRC Press.

Oregon Board of Massage Technicians: *Sanitation requirements for the state of Oregon,* Portland, Ore, 1991, The Board.

Oschman JL: What is healing energy? Part 3. Silent pulses, *J Bodywork Move Ther* 1(3):179, 1997.

*Premkumar K: *Pathology A to Z: a handbook for massage therapists,* Calgary, Ontario, Canada, 1996, VanPub Books.

Scull CW: Massage: physiological basis, *Arch Phys Med* 159, 1945.

*Selye H: *The stress of life,* ed 2, New York, 1978, McGraw-Hill.

Shealy NC: The neurochemical substrate of behavior, *Psychol Health Immun Dis* B434, 1992.

*Sheridan CL, Radmacher SA: *Health psychology: challenging the biomedical model,* New York, 1992, John Wiley & Sons.

Tate P, Seeley RR, Stephens TD: *Understanding the human body,* St Louis, 1994, Mosby.

Thibodeau GA: *Structure and function of the body,* ed 13, St Louis, 2008, Mosby.

Thibodeau GA, Patton K: *The human body in health and disease,* ed 4, St Louis, 2004, Mosby.

Thomas CL, editor: *Taber's cyclopedic medical dictionary,* Philadelphia, 1985, FA Davis.

Thompson CW: *Manual of structural kinesiology,* ed 10, St Louis, 1985, Mosby.

Timms R, Connors P: *Embodying healing: integrating bodywork and psychotherapy in recovery from childhood sexual abuse,* Orwell, Vt, 1992, The Safer Society Press.

Waites EA: *Trauma and survival: post-traumatic and dissociative disorders in women,* New York, 1993, Norton.

Walton TH: Contraindications to massage therapy. I. Roadblocks on the way to consensus, *Massage Ther J* 37(2):108, 1998.

Yates J: *Physiological effects of therapeutic massage and their application to treatment,* British Columbia, Canada, 1989, Massage Therapist Association.

CHAPTER 6

Board of Directors of Masseurs, Province of Ontario: Ontario, Canada therapeutic massage curriculum guidelines, Toronto, Ontario, Canada, 1992, The Board.

Bulluck BL, Rosendahl PP: *Pathophysiology adaptations and alterations in function,* ed 3, Philadelphia, 1992, JB Lippincott.

**Fritz S, Grosenbach M: *Mosby's essential sciences for therapeutic massage: anatomy, physiology, biomechanics, and pathology,* ed 3, St Louis, 2009, Mosby.

**Hamann B: *Disease: identification, prevention and control,* St Louis, 1994, Mosby.

Newton D: *Pathology for massage therapists,* ed 2, Portland, Ore, 1995, Simran Publications.

Oregon Board of Massage Technicians: *Sanitation requirements for the state of Oregon,* Portland, Ore, 1991, The Board.

*Premkumar K: *Pathology A to Z: a handbook for massage therapists,* Calgary, Canada, Calgary, Ontario, Canada, 1996, VanPub Books.

Sorrentino SA: *Mosby's textbook for nursing assistants,* ed 6, St Louis, 2004, Mosby.

*Thibodeau GA, Patton KT: *Anatomy and physiology,* ed 6, St Louis, 2007, Mosby.

Thibodeau GA, Patton K: *The human body in health and disease,* ed 4, St Louis, 2005, Mosby.

Vardaxis NJ: *Pathology for the health sciences,* New York, 1995, Churchill Livingstone.

CHAPTER 7

Birnbaum JS: *The musculoskeletal manual,* ed 2, Philadelphia, 1986, WB Saunders.

Colby LA, Kisner C: *Therapeutic exercise: foundations and techniques,* ed 3, Philadelphia, 1996, FA Davis.

Kreighbaum E, Barthels KM: *Biomechanics: a qualitative approach for studying human movement,* ed 2, New York, 1985, Macmillan.

Norkin CC, Levangie PK: *Joint structure and function: a comprehensive analysis,* ed 2, Philadelphia, 1992, FA Davis.

Smith LK, Weiss E, Lehmkuhl L: *Brunnstrom's clinical kinesiology,* ed 5, Philadelphia, 1996, FA Davis.

Sorrentino SA: *Mosby's textbook for nursing assistants,* ed 7, St Louis, 2007, Mosby.

CHAPTER 8

DeDomenico G, Wood EC: *Beards massage,* ed 5, Philadelphia 2007, WB Saunders.

Small C: *A handbook for the holistic health practitioner,* Irving, Texas, 1983 (self-published).

Sorrentino SA: *Mosby's textbook for nursing assistants,* ed 6, St Louis, 2004, Mosby.

Tappan FM, Benjamin PJ: *Tappan's handbook of healing massage techniques: holistic, classic, and emerging methods,* ed 3, Norwalk, Conn, 1998, Appleton & Lange.

CHAPTER 9

Anderson KE, Anderson LE, Glanze D, editors: *Mosby's medical, nursing, and allied health dictionary,* ed 7, St Louis, 2005, Mosby.

Arvedson J: *Medical gymnastics and massage in general practice,* London, 1930, JA Churchill.

Arvedson J: *The techniques, effects and uses of Swedish medical gymnastics and massage,* London, 1931, JA Churchill.

Basmajian JV, editor: *Manipulation traction and massage,* ed 3, Baltimore, 1985, Williams & Wilkins.

*Basmajian JV, Nyberg R: *Rational manual therapies,* Baltimore, 1993, Williams & Wilkins.

Baumgartner AJ: *Massage in athletics,* Minneapolis, 1947, Brugess.

Beard G: A history of massage technique, *Phys Ther Rev* 32:613, 1952.

Bishop B: Vibratory stimulation, *Phys Ther* 54:1273, 1974.

Breakey BM: An overlooked therapy you can use ad lib, *Registered Nurse* July :50, 1982.

Butler DS: *Mobilization of the nervous system,* Melbourne, Australia, 1991, Churchill Livingstone.

*Cailliet R: *Soft tissue pain and disability,* Philadelphia, 1996, FA Davis.

*Calais-Germain B: *Anatomy of movement,* Seattle, 1993, Eastland Press.

Callander R: *Illustrated physiology,* ed 6, New York, 1996, Churchill Livingstone.

Carpenter IC: *A practical guide to massage,* Baltimore, 1937, William Wood.

**Chaitow L: *Modern neuromuscular techniques,* New York, 1996, Churchill Livingstone.

**Chaitow L: *Muscle energy techniques,* New York, 2007, Churchill Livingstone.

Chaitow L: *Osteopathic self-treatment,* London, 1990, Thorsons.

Chaitow L: *Palpatory literacy,* London, 1991, Thorsons.

Chaitow L: *Soft-tissue manipulation,* Rochester, Vt, 1988, Healing Arts Press.

Chaitow L: Soft tissue manipulation and neuromuscular techniques: improving palpatory literacy and treatment efficiency, Lapeer, Mich., 1991, Soft Tissue Manipulation Seminar.

Cyriax E: Some misconceptions concerning mechano-therapy, *Br J Phys Med* 92, 1938.

Cyriax J: Treatment by movement, *Br Med J,* 1944.

*Daniels L, Worthingham C: *Muscle testing techniques of manual examination,* ed 6, Philadelphia, 1995, WB Saunders.

Darian-Smith I: Touch in primates, *Ann Rev* 157, 1982.

DeDomenico G, Wood EC: *Beards massage,* ed 5, Philadelphia, 2007, WB Saunders.

DePuy CE: Remarks on the efficacy of friction in palsy and apoplexy, October 1817.

Despard LL: *Textbook of massage and remedial gymnastics,* ed 3, New York, 1932, Oxford University Press.

Eccles AS: *The practice of massage: its physiological effects and therapeutic uses,* ed 2, London, 1898, Bailliere, Tindall, & Cox.

Frank LK: Tactile communication, *Genet Psychol Monogr* 56:209, 1957.

Gammon GD, Starr I: Studies on the relief of pain by counterirritation, Philadelphia, July, 1940, Hospital of the University of Pennsylvania.

Garofano JS: *Therapeutic massage and bodywork,* Stamford, Conn, 1997, Appleton & Lange.

Grafstrom AV: *Medical gymnastics including the Schott movements,* London, 1899, Scientific Press.

Graham D: The history of massage, *Medical Record* approximately 1874.

Graham D: Massage, *Med Surg Rep* 35, 1874.

Graham D: *A treatise on massage: its history, mode of application and effects,* ed 3, Philadelphia, 1902, JB Lippincott.

*Greenman PE: *Principles of manual medicine,* ed 3, Baltimore, 2003, Williams & Wilkins.

*Hinkle CZ: *Fundamentals of anatomy and movement: a workbook and guide,* St Louis, 1997, Mosby.

*Hislop HJ, Montgomery J: *Daniel and Worthingham's muscle testing,* ed 6, Philadelphia, 1995, WB Saunders.

Hough T: *A review of Swedish gymnastics,* Boston, 1899, George Ellis.

Jensen K: *Fundamentals in massage for students of nursing,* New York, 1936, Macmillan.

Johnson W: *The antitryptic art and medical rubbing,* London, 1866, Simpkin, Marshall.

Kellogg JH: *The art of massage,* Battle Creek, Mich, 1929, Modern Medicine Publishing.

Kisner CD, Taslitz N: Connective tissue massage: influence of the introductory treatment on autonomic functions, *Phys Ther* 48:107, 1967.

Kleen E: *Massage and medical gymnastics,* ed 2, New York, 1921, William Wood.

Knapp ME: Massage, physical medicine and rehabilitation, *Postgrad Med* 192, 1968.

Knott M, Voss D: *Proprioceptive neuromuscular facilitation,* New York, 1956, Harper & Row.

Lee D: *Manual therapy for the thorax, a biomechanical approach,* Delta, British Columbia, Canada, 1994, DOPC.

Leflet DH: *HEMME approach to soft-tissue therapy,* Bonifay, Fla, 1992, HEMME Approach Publications.

*Lewit K: *Manipulative therapy in rehabilitation of the locomotor system,* ed 2, Oxford, 1991, Butterworth-Heinemann.

Lindsay DT: *Functional human anatomy,* St Louis, 1996, Mosby.

Lowe WW: *Functional assessment in massage therapy,* ed 2, Bend, Ore, 1995, Omeri.

McMillian M: *Massage and therapeutic exercise,* ed 3, Philadelphia, 1932, WB Saunders.

Melzack R: Hyperstimulation analgesia, *Clin Anesthesiol* 3:81, 1985.

Mennell J: *Physical treatment by movement, manipulation, and massage,* London, 1940, JA Churchill.

Mennell J: *The musculoskeletal system: differential diagnosis from symptoms and physical signs,* Gaithersburg, Md, 1992, Aspen.

Mulliner MR: *Mechano-therapy,* Philadelphia, 1929, Lea & Febiger.

Norkin CC, Levangie PK: *Joint structure and function,* ed 2, Philadelphia, 1992, FA Davis.

Norstrom G: *Handbook of massage,* New York, 1896, The Faculty of Stockholm.

Post SE: *Massage: a primer for nurses,* New York, 1891, Nightingale Publishing.

Roth M: *Handbook of the movement cure,* London, 1856, Groombridge & Sons.

Scull CW: Massage: physiological basis, *Arch Phys Med* 159, 1945.

Tappan FM: *Massage techniques: a case method approach,* New York, 1961, Macmillan.

*Tappan FM, Benjamin PJ: *Tappan's handbook of healing massage techniques: holistic, classic, and emerging methods,* ed 3, Norwalk, Conn, 1998, Appleton & Lange.

Taylor CF: *Theory and practice of the movement cure by the Swedish system,* Philadelphia, 1861, Lindsay & Blakiston.

Taylor GH: *An illustrated sketch of the movement cure: its principal methods and effects,* New York, 1866 (self-published).

Thibodeau GA: *Structure and function of the body,* ed 13, St Louis, 2008, Mosby.

Thibodeau GA, Patton K: *The human body in health and disease,* ed 4, St Louis, 2005, Mosby.

Travell JG, Simons DG: *Myofascial pain and dysfunction: the trigger point manual,* Baltimore, 1984, Williams & Wilkins.

Trew M, Everett T: *Human movement: an introductory text,* ed 5, New York, 2005, Churchill Livingstone.

Wall PD: Pain, itch, and vibration, *Arch Neurol* 2:365, 1960.

*Zahourek J: Myologik: an atlas of human musculature. In Clay-Zoologik Systems Kinesthetic Anatomy Maniken, vol 1-5, 1996, Zahourek Systems.

CHAPTER 10

Academy of Traditional Chinese Medicine: *An outline of Chinese acupuncture,* Peking, 1975, Foreign Language Press.

Alfaro R: *Applying nursing diagnosis and nursing process: a step-by-step guide,* ed 2, Philadelphia, 1990, JB Lippincott.

Basmajian JV, editor: *Manipulation traction and massage*, ed 3, Baltimore, 1985, Williams & Wilkins.

Basmajian JV, Nyberg R: *Rational manual therapies*, Baltimore, 1993, Williams & Wilkins.

**Bates B: *A guide to physical examination and history taking*, ed 5, Philadelphia, 1991, JB Lippincott.

**Biel A: *Trail guide to the body*, Boulder, Colo, 1997 (self-published).

Birnbaum JS: *The musculoskeletal manual*, ed 2, Philadelphia, 1986, WB Saunders.

*Cailleit R: *Foot and ankle pain*, ed 3, Philadelphia, 1997, FA Davis.

*Cailliet R: *Hand pain and impairment*, ed 4, Philadelphia, 1994, FA Davis.

*Cailliet R: *Knee pain and disability*, ed 3, Philadelphia, 1992, FA Davis.

*Cailliet R: *Low back pain syndrome*, ed 5, Philadelphia, 1995, FA Davis.

*Cailliet R: *Neck and arm pain*, ed 3, Philadelphia, 1991, FA Davis.

*Cailliet R: *Shoulder pain*, ed 3, Philadelphia, 1991, FA Davis.

*Cailliet R: *Soft tissue pain and disability*, Philadelphia, 1996, FA Davis.

*Calais-Germain B: *Anatomy of movement*, Seattle, 1993, Eastland Press.

Chaitow L: *Osteopathic self-treatment*, 1990, Thorsons Harper Collins.

Chaitow L: *Palpatory literacy*, Hammersmith, London, 1991, Thorsons Harper Collins.

Chaitow L: *Soft tissue manipulation*, Rochester, Vt, 1988, Healing Arts Press.

Clark J, editor: *The human body*, New York, 1989, Arch Cape Press.

Cohen B, Wood DL: *Structure and function of the human body*, ed 7, Baltimore, 2000, Lippincott Williams & Wilkins.

Colby LA, Kisner C: *Therapeutic exercise: foundations and techniques*, ed 5, Philadelphia, 2007, FA Davis.

**Daniels L, Worthingham C: *Muscle testing techniques of manual examination*, ed 6, Philadelphia, 1995, WB Saunders.

Daniels L, Worthingham C: *Therapeutic exercise for body alignment and function*, ed 2, Philadelphia, 1977, WB Saunders.

deGrout J, Chusid JG: *Correlative neuroanatomy*, ed 12, East Norwalk, Conn, 1985, Appleton & Lange.

**Greenman PE: *Principles of manual medicine*, ed 2, Baltimore, 1996, Williams & Wilkins.

Gunn C: *Bones and joints*, ed 5, New York, 2007, Churchill Livingstone.

Gunn CC: *Treating myofascial pain*, Seattle, 1989, Health Services Center for Educational Resources, University of Washington.

Hall-Craggs ECB: *Anatomy as a basis for clinical medicine*, Baltimore, 1985, Urban & Schwarzenberg.

*Hinkle CZ: *Fundamentals of anatomy and movement: a workbook and guide*, St Louis, 1997, Mosby.

**Hislop HJ, Montgomery J: *Daniel and Worthingham's muscle testing*, ed 8, Philadelphia, 2007, WB Saunders.

Jacobs PH, Anhalt TS: *Handbook of skin clues of systemic diseases*, ed 2, Philadelphia, 1992, Lea & Febiger.

**Kapit W, Elson M: *The anatomy coloring book*, New York, 1977, Harper Collins.

Kreighbaum E, Barthels KM: *Biomechanics: a qualitative approach for studying human movement*, ed 4, New York, 1995, Macmillan.

*Lederman E: *Fundamentals of manual therapy: physiology, neurology, and psychology*, ed 2, New York, 2005, Churchill Livingstone.

Lee D: *Manual therapy for the thorax: a biomechanical approach*, Delta, British Columbia, Canada, 1994, DOPC.

LeVay D: *Human anatomy and physiology*, Binge Suffolk, England, 1974, Hodder & Stoughton.

*Lewit K: *Manipulative therapy in rehabilitation of the locomotor system*, ed 2, Oxford, 1991, Butterworth.

*Lewit K: *Manipulative therapy in rehabilitation of the motor system*, ed 3, London, 1999, Butterworth.

**Lowe WW: *Functional assessment in massage therapy*, ed 3, Bend, Ore, 1997, Omeri.

McNaught AB, Callander R: *Illustrated physiology*, ed 6, New York, 1997, Churchill Livingstone.

Memmler RL, Wood DL: *Structure and function of the human body*, ed 3, Philadelphia, 1983, JB Lippincott.

**Mennell J: *The musculoskeletal system: differential diagnosis from symptoms and physical signs*, Gaithersburg, Md, 1992, Aspen.

Norkin CC, Levangie PK: *Joint structure and function: a comprehensive analysis*, ed 4, Philadelphia, 2005, FA Davis.

Smith LK, Lehmkuhl LD: *Brunnstrom's clinical kinesiology*, ed 5, Philadelphia, 1996, FA Davis.

Sorrentino SA: *Mosby's textbook for nursing assistants*, ed 7, St Louis, 2007, Mosby.

Sparks SM, Taylor CM: *Nursing diagnosis reference manual*, ed 2, Springhouse, Pa, 1993, Springhouse.

Tate P, Seeley RR, Stephens TD: *Understanding the human body*, St Louis, 1994, Mosby.

Thibodeau GA: *Structure and function of the body*, ed 12, St Louis, 2004, Mosby

Thibodeau GA, Patton KT: *Anatomy and physiology*, ed 3, St Louis, 1996, Mosby.

Thibodeau GA, Patton KT: *Anatomy and physiology*, ed 6, St Louis, 2007, Mosby.

Thibodeau GA, Patton KT: *The human body in health and disease*, ed 4, St Louis, 2005, Mosby.

*Timmons BH, Ronald Ley: *Behavioral and psychological approaches to breathing disorders*, New York, 1994, Plenum Press.

*Travell JG, Simons DG: *Myofascial pain and dysfunction: the trigger point manual*, vol 2, Baltimore, 1993, Williams & Wilkins.

Wale JO, editor: *Tidy's massage and remedial exercises*, ed 11, Bristol, England, 1987, John Wright & Sons.

Walther DS: *Applied kinesiology synopsis*, Pueblo, Colo, 1988, SDC Systems.

CHAPTER 11

*Baldry PE: *Acupuncture, triggers points and musculoskeletal pain*, New York, 2005, Churchill Livingstone.

Basmajian JV, editor: *Manipulation traction and massage*, ed 3, Baltimore, 1985, Williams & Wilkins.

Berube R: *Evolutionary traditions: unique approaches to lymphatic drainage and circulatory massage techniques*, Hudson, NH, 1988 (self-published).

Buchman DD: *The complete book of water therapy: 500 ways to use our oldest natural medicine*, New York, 1979, EP Dutton.

Bugaj R: The cooling analgesic and rewarming effects of ice massage on localized skin, *Phys Ther* 55:11, 1975.

*Cailliet R: *Soft tissue pain and disability*, Philadelphia, 1996, FA Davis.

*Cantu RI, Grodin AJ: *Myofascial manipulation: theory and clinical application*, Gaithersburg, Md, 1992, Aspen.

Chaitow L: Extremely light manipulative methods: time for research, *Int J Altern Complement Med* 10:12, 1992.

Chaitow L: *Soft-tissue manipulation*, Rochester, Vt, 1988, Healing Arts Press.

Chaitow L: Workshop notes, Lapeer, Mich, 1988, 1991, 1992, 1993.

*Chengnan S: *Chinese bodywork, a complete manual of Chinese therapeutic massage*, Berkeley, Calif, 1993, Pacific View Press.

Ciolek J: Cryotherapy: review of physiological effects on clinical application, *Cleveland Clin Q* 52:193, 1985.

Cohen MR: *The Chinese way to healing: many paths to wholeness*, New York, 1996, Berkeley Publishing Group.

*Connelly DM: *Traditional acupuncture: the law of five elements*, ed 2, Columbia, Md, 1994, Traditional Acupuncture Institute.

Coulter J: Interview with Hildegard Wittlinger, *J Soft Tissue Manipulation* 1:12, 1993.

Cyriax J, Coldham M: *The textbook of orthopaedic medicine treatment by manipulation massage and injection,* vol 2, ed 11, East Sussex, England, 1984, Bailliere Tindall.

Daulby M, Mathison C: *Guide to spiritual healing,* London, 1996, Brockhampton Press.

Degenhardt B, Kuchera M: Update of osteopathic medical concepts and the lymphatic system, *J Am Osteopath Assoc* 96(2):97, 1996.

Ding Li: *Acupuncture meridian theory and acupuncture points,* San Francisco, 1990, China Books & Periodicals.

Ewig J, Provost STP: *An inaugural essay on the effects of cold upon the human body,* Philadelphia, 1797, Joseph Gales.

Gold R: *Thai massage: a traditional medical technique,* ed 2, St. Louis, 2007, Mosby.

Gunn CC: *Reprints on pain, acupuncture and related subjects,* Seattle, 1992, University of Washington.

Gunn CC: *Treating myofascial pain: intramuscular stimulation (IMS) for myofascial pain syndromes of neuropathic origin,* Seattle, 1989, University of Washington Medical School.

Harris R: Edema and its treatment in massage therapy, *J Soft Tissue Manipulation* 1:4, 1993.

Hayden CA: Cyrokinetics in an early treatment program, *J Am Phys Ther Assoc* 44, 1964.

Holmes G: Hydrotherapy and spa treatment, *The Practitioner* CXLI, 1938.

Ingham ED: *Stories the feet have told,* St Petersburg, Fla, 1982, Ingham Publishing.

Johari H: *Ayurvedic massage: traditional Indian techniques for balancing body and mind,* Rochester, Vt, 1996, Healing Arts Press.

Kreighbaum E, Barthels KM: *Biomechanics: a qualitative approach for studying human movement,* ed 4, New York, 1995, Macmillan.

Leadbeater CW: *The chakras,* Wheaton, Ill, 1927, Theosophical Publishing House.

Lederman E: *Fundamentals of manual therapy: physiology, neurology, and psychology,* New York, 1997, Churchill Livingstone.

Maciocia G: *The foundations of Chinese medicine,* ed 2, New York, 2005, Churchill Livingstone.

*Manheim CJ, Lavett DK: *The myofascial release manual,* Thorofare, NJ, 1989, Slack.

*Masunaga S, Ohashi W: *Zen shiatsu: how to harmonize yin and yang for better health,* New York, 1997, Japan Publications.

*Nikola RJ: *Creatures of water: hydrotherapy textbook,* Salt Lake City, 1995, Europa Therapeutic.

*Ohashi W: *Do-it-yourself shiatsu: how to perform the ancient Japanese art of acupuncture without needles,* New York, 1976, Penguin Books.

Philips P: Polarity therapy: bodywork to address our energetic nature, *Massage Magazine* May/June :28, 1998.

Segal M: *Reflexology,* North Hollywood, Calif, 1976, Hal Leighton.

Singer E: *Fasciae of the human body and their relations to the organs they envelop,* Baltimore, 1935, Williams & Wilkins.

Tappan FM, Benjamin PJ: *Tappan's handbook of healing massage techniques: holistic, classic, and emerging methods,* ed 3, Norwalk, Conn, 1998, Appleton & Lange.

*Travell JG, Simons DG: *Myofascial pain and dysfunction: the trigger point manual,* Baltimore, 1984, Waverly Press.

*Travell JG, Simons DG: *Myofascial pain and dysfunction: the trigger point manual,* vol 2, the lower extremities, Baltimore, 1992, Williams & Wilkins.

Walther DS: *Applied kinesiology synopsis,* Pueblo, Colo, 1988, SDC Systems.

Yao JH: *Acutherapy,* Libertyville, Ill, 1984, Acutherapy Postgraduate Seminars.

CHAPTER 12

Allison TG: How to counsel patients with chronic fatigue syndrome, *Psychol Health Immun Dis* A:5, 1992.

Bandler R, Grinder J: *Patterns of the hypnotic techniques of Milton H. Erickson, MD,* vol 1, Cupertino, Calif, 1975, Meta Publications.

Bass E, Davis L: *The courage to heal: a guide for women survivors of child sexual abuse,* New York, 1988, Harper & Row.

*Benjamin PJ, Lamp CP: *Understanding sports massage,* Champaign, Ill, 1996, Human Kinetics.

Calvert R: Dolores Krieger, PhD and her therapeutic touch, *Massage* 47:56, 1994.

Cunningham AJ: The healing journey: how to organize healing efforts at the psychological, social, and spiritual levels, *Psychol Health Immun Dis* A:63, 1992.

Denny NW, Quadagno D: *Human sexuality,* ed 2, St Louis, 1992, Mosby.

Doore G, editor: *Shaman's path: healing, personal growth and empowerment,* Boston, 1988, Shambhala Publications.

Hahn DB, Payne WA: *Focus on health,* ed 2, St Louis, 1994, Mosby.

Hammerschlag CA: *The dancing healers: a doctor's journey of healing with Native Americans,* San Francisco, 1988, Harper.

Jevne R: Enhancing hope in the chronically ill, *Psychol Health Immun Dis* A:127, 1992.

Kohn A: Shattered innocence, *Psychol Today* Feb :54, 1987.

*Kubler-Ross E: *To live until we say goodbye,* Englewood Cliffs, NJ, 1978, Prentice-Hall.

Lee D: Amplifying the power of visualization techniques with neurolinguistic programming, *Psychol Health Immun Dis* A:215, 1992.

Luhman R: *The sociological outlook,* ed 8, 2007, Rowman & Littlefield.

*Meagher J, Boughton P: *Sportsmassage,* Barrytown, NY, 1990, Station Hill Press.

McArdle WD et al: *Exercise physiology: energy nutrition and human performance,* ed 3, Philadelphia, 1991, Lea & Febiger.

McGladrey, Pullen: The Americans With Disabilities Act (Rev), New York, 1994, Panel Publishers.

Northrup C: *Heal your symptoms naturally,* Potomac, Md, 1996, Phillips.

*Northrup C: *Women's bodies, women's wisdom,* New York, 1994, Bantam Books.

Pearson JC, Spitzberg BH: *Interpersonal communication: concept, components, and contexts,* ed 2, Dubuque, Iowa, 1987, William C Brown.

Perry HM, Morley JE, Coe RM: *Aging and musculoskeletal disorders,* New York, 1993, Springer.

*Selye H: *The stress of life,* ed 2, New York, 1978, McGraw-Hill.

Shaughnessy J, editor: *The roots of ritual,* Grand Rapids, Mich, 1973, William B Eerdmans.

Shealy NC: The neurochemical substrate of behavior, *Psychol Health Immun Dis* B:434, 1992.

*Sheridan CL, Radmacher SA: *Health psychology: challenging the biomedical model,* New York, 1992, John Wiley & Sons.

Siegal BS: *Peace, love and healing,* New York, 1989, Harper & Row.

Sorrentino SA: *Mosby's textbook for nursing assistants,* ed 7, St Louis, 2007, Mosby.

Tate DA: Health, hope, and healing: a survivor's perspective, *Psychol Health Immun Dis* A:304, 1992.

Tate P, Seeley RR, Stephens TD: *Understanding the human body,* St Louis, 1994, Mosby.

Thibodeau GA, Patton K: *The human body in health and disease,* ed 4, St Louis, 2005, Mosby.

Timms R, Connors P: *Embodying healing: integrating bodywork and psychotherapy in recovery from childhood sexual abuse,* Orwell, Vt, 1992, Safer Society Press.

Wade C, Tavris C: *Psychology,* ed 2, New York, 2004, Harper.

Waites E: *Trauma and survival: post-traumatic and dissociative disorder in women,* New York, 1993, WW Norton.

Work modification, work hardening and work rehabilitation, Physical Medicine Research Foundation Third International Symposium, Vancouver, British Columbia, Canada, 1990.

CHAPTER 13

*Benson H: *Timeless healing: the power and biology of belief,* New York, 1996, Scribner.

Castleman M: *Nature's cures,* Emmaus, PA, 1996, Rodale Press.

*Chaitow L: *The body/mind purification program,* New York, 1991, Fireside.

Chaitow L et al: Breathing dysfunction, *J Bodywork Move Ther* 1(5):252, 1997.

Chopra D: *Restful sleep,* New York, 1994, Crowne Trade Paperbacks.

Commings DE: *Tourette syndrome and human behavior,* Duarte, Calif, 1997, Hope Press.

**Fritz S, Grosenbach M: *Mosby's essential sciences for therapeutic massage: anatomy, physiology, biomechanics, pathology,* ed 3, St Louis, 2009, Mosby.

*Golan R: *Optimal wellness,* New York, 1995, Ballantine Books.

Hahn DB, Wayne PA: *Focus on health,* ed 2, St Louis, 1994, Mosby.

Hoffman CJ: *HEV 370 Nutrition,* ed 2, Mount Pleasant, Mich, 1996, Central Michigan University.

Lippert L: *Clinical kinesiology for physical therapist assistants,* Portland, Ore, 1991 (self-published).

Millenson JR: *Mind matters: psychological medicine in holistic practice,* Seattle, 1995, Eastland Press.

Northrup C: *Heal your symptoms naturally,* Potomac, Md, 1996, Phillips.

Ornstein R, Sobel D: *The healing brain,* New York, 1987, Simon & Schuster.

Sacks O: An anthropologist on Mars, *New Yorker,* December 27, 125:106, 1993.

*Sapolsky RM: *Why zebras don't get ulcers: a guide to stress, stress-related disease and coping,* New York, 1994, WH Freeman.

*Selye H: *The stress of life,* ed 2, New York, 1978, McGraw-Hill.

Shealy NC: The neurochemical substrate of behavior, *Psychol Health Immun Dis* vol B, 1992.

Sheridan CL, Radmacher SA: *Health psychology: challenging the biomedical model,* New York, 1992, John Wiley & Sons.

Tate P, Seeley RR, Stephens TD: *Understanding the human body,* St Louis, 1994, Mosby.

**Timmons BH, Ley R: *Behavioral and psychological approaches to breathing disorders,* New York, 1994, Plenum Press.

**Travis JW, Ryan RS: *Wellness workbook,* ed 2, Berkeley, Calif, 1998, Ten Speed Press.

**Travis JW, Ryan RS: *Wellness workbook: how to achieve enduring health and vitality,* ed 3, 2004.

Whitney EN, Rolfes SR: *Understanding nutrition,* ed 11, Minneapolis-St. Paul, Minn, 2007, West.

CHAPTER 14

Bliss E: *Getting things done,* Boulder, Colo, 1986 (cassette series).

Calano J, Salzman J: *Success shortcuts: 25 career skills you were never taught, but must know,* Chicago, Career Track Publications.

*Capo M: *The business of massage: a manual for students and professionals,* New York, 1992, Ten Plus Ten.

Jordan DM: An analysis of existing law governing licensed and unlicensed health practices, *Am Holistic Med* 1, 1979.

Ornstein R, Ehrlich P: *New world, new mind: moving toward conscious evolution,* New York, 1989, Doubleday.

**Sohnen-Moe C: *Business mastery,* ed 2, Tucson, 1991, Sohnen-Moe Associates.

Tracy B: *The psychology of achievement,* Chicago, Solana Beach, Calif, Brian Tracy Learning Symposium (cassette series).

Verbury K: *Managing the modern Michigan township,* Lansing, Mich, 1990, Community Development Publishers, Michigan State University.

GLOSSARY

Abbreviation: Shortened forms of words or phrases.

Abuse: Exploitation, misuse, mistreatment, molestation, neglect.

Acquired immunodeficiency syndrome (AIDS): A dysfunction in the body's immune system, which defends the body against disease.

Active assisted movement: Movement of a joint in which both the client and the therapist produce the motion.

Active joint movement: Movement of a joint through its range of motion by the client.

Active range of motion: Movement of a joint by the client without any type of assistance from the massage practitioner.

Active resistive movement: Movement of a joint by the client against resistance provided by the therapist.

Acupressure: Methods used to tone or sedate acupuncture points without the use of needles.

Acupuncture point: Asian term for a specific point that correlates with a neurologic motor point.

Acute: A term that describes a condition in which the signs and symptoms develop quickly, last a short time, and then disappear.

Acute illness: A short-term illness that resolves by means of the normal healing process and, if necessary, supportive medical care.

Acute pain: A symptom of a disease condition or a temporary aspect of medical treatment. Acute pain acts as a warning signal because it can activate the sympathetic nervous system. It usually is temporary, of sudden onset, and easily localized. The client frequently can describe the pain, which often subsides without treatment.

Adaptation: A response to a sensory stimulation in which nerve signaling is reduced or ceases.

Aerobic exercise training: An exercise program focused to increase fitness and endurance.

Allied health: A division of medicine in which the professional receives training in a specific area of medicine to serve as support for the physician.

Anatomic barriers: Anatomic structures determined by the shape and fit of the bones at the joint.

Antagonism: Occurs when massage produces the opposite effect, such as with medications.

Antagonists: The muscles that oppose the movement of the prime movers.

Anxiety: A feeling of uneasiness, usually connected with an increase in sympathetic arousal responses.

Applied kinesiology: Methods of evaluation and bodywork that use a specialized type of muscle testing and various forms of massage and bodywork for corrective procedures.

Approximation: The technique of pushing muscle fibers together in the belly of the muscle.

Aromatherapy: The art and science of using natural distilled extracts from aromatic plants called essential oils in healing the mind, body, and spirit.

Art: Craft, skill, technique, and talent.

Arterial circulation: Movement of oxygenated blood under pressure from the heart to the body through the arteries.

Arthrokinematic movement: Accessory movements that occur as a result of inherent laxity or joint play that exists in each joint. The joint play allows the ends of the bones to slide, roll, or spin smoothly on one another. These essential movements occur passively with movement of the joint and are not under voluntary control.

Aseptic technique: Procedures that kill or disable pathogens on surfaces to prevent transmission.

Asian approaches: Methods of bodywork that have developed from ancient Chinese methods.

Assessment: The collection and interpretation of information provided by the client, the client's family and friends, the massage practitioner, and referring medical professionals.

Asymmetric stance: The position in which the body weight is shifted from one foot to the other while standing.

Athlete: A person who participates in sports as an amateur or a professional. Athletes require precise use of their bodies.

Autonomic nervous system: The body system that regulates involuntary body functions using the sympathetic "fight-flight-fear response" and the restorative parasympathetic "relaxation response." The sympathetic and parasympathetic systems work together to maintain homeostasis through a feedback loop system.

Autoregulation: Control of homeostasis through alteration of tissue or function.

Ayurveda: A system of health and medicine that grew from East Indian roots.

Bacteria: Primitive cells that have no nuclei. Bacteria cause disease by secreting toxic substances that damage human tissues, by becoming parasites inside human cells, or by forming colonies in the body that disrupt normal function.

Balance point: The point of contact between the practitioner and client.

Beating: A form of heavy tapotement involving use of the fist.

Bending forces: A combination of compression and tension. One side of a structure is exposed to compressive forces, while the other side is exposed to tensile forces.

Benign: A term that describes the type of tumor that remains localized within the tissue from which it arose and does not undergo malignant changes. Benign tumors usually grow very slowly.

Body mechanics: Use of the body in an efficient and biomechanically correct way.

Body/mind: The interaction between thought and physiology that is connected to the limbic system, hypothalamic influence on the autonomic nervous system, and the endocrine system.

Body segment: The area of the body between joints that provides movement during walking and balance.

Body supports: Pillows, folded blankets, foam forms, or commercial products that help contour the flat surface of a massage table or mat.

Bodywork: A term that encompasses all the various forms of massage, movement, and other touch therapies.

Boundary: Personal space that exists within an arm's length perimeter. Personal emotional space is designated by morals, values, and experience.

Burnout: A condition that occurs when a person uses up energy faster than it can be restored.

Breathing pattern disorders: A complex set of behaviors that lead to overbreathing in the absence of a pathologic condition. These disorders are considered a functional syndrome because all the parts are working effectively; therefore, a specific pathologic condition does not exist.

Care or treatment plan: The plan used to achieve therapeutic goals. It outlines the agreed objectives; the frequency, duration, and number of visits; progress measurements; the date of reassessment; and massage methods to be used.

Career: A chosen pursuit; a life's work.

Carrier oils: High-quality, fresh vegetable oils that are used to dilute essential oils.

Centering: The ability to focus the mind by screening out sensation.

Certification: A voluntary credentialing process that usually requires education and testing; tests are administered either privately or by government regulatory bodies.

Chakra: Energy fields or centers of consciousness within the body.

Challenge: Living each day knowing that it is filled with things to learn, skills to practice, tasks to accomplish, and obstacles to overcome.

Chemical effects: The effects of massage produced by the release of chemical substances in the body. These substances may be released locally from the massaged tissue, or they may be hormones released into the general circulation.

Chronic: A term that describes the type of disease that develops slowly and lasts for a long time, sometimes for life.

Chronic illness: A disease, injury, or syndrome that shows little change or slow progression.

Chronic pain: Pain that persists or recurs for indefinite periods, usually for longer than 6 months. It frequently has an insidious onset, and the character and quality of the pain change over time. It frequently involves deep somatic and visceral structures. Chronic pain usually is diffuse and poorly localized.

Circulatory: Systems that depend on the pumping action of the skeletal muscle (i.e., the arterial, venous, lymphatic, respiratory, cerebrospinal fluid circulatory systems).

Client information form: A document used to obtain information from the client about health, preexisting conditions, and expectations for the massage.

Client outcome: The results desired from the massage and the massage therapist.

Client/practitioner agreement and policy statement: A detailed written explanation of all rules, expectations, and procedures for the massage.

Coalition: A group formed for a particular purpose.

Cognition: Conscious awareness and perception, reasoning, judgment, intuition, and memory.

Comfort barrier: The first point of resistance short of the client's perceiving any discomfort at the physiologic or pathologic barrier.

Commitment: The ability and willingness to be involved in what is happening around us so as to have a purpose for being.

Communicable disease: A disease caused by pathogens that are easily spread; a contagious disease.

Compensation: The process of counterbalancing a defect in body structure or function.

Compression: Pressure into the body to spread tissue against underlying structures. (This massage manipulation sometimes is classified with pétrissage.) Also, the exertion of inappropriate pressure on nerves by hard tissue (e.g., bone).

Compressive force: The amount of pressure exerted against the surface of the body in order to apply pressure to the deeper body structures; pressure directed in a particular direction.

Compressive forces: Occur when two structures are pressed together. Compressive force is a component of massage application and is described as depth of pressure.

Concentric isotonic contraction: Application of a counterforce by the massage therapist while allowing the client to move, which brings the origin and insertion of the target muscle together against the pressure.

Condition management: The use of massage methods to support clients who are unable to undergo a therapeutic change but who wish to function as effectively as possible under a set of circumstances.

Confidentiality: Respect for the privacy of information.

Conflict: An expressed struggle between at least two interdependent parties who perceive incompatible goals, scarce resources, and/or interference from the other party in achieving their goals.

Connective tissue: The most abundant tissue type in the body; it provides support, structure, space, stabilization, and scar formation.

Conservation withdrawal: A parasympathetic survival pattern that is similar to "playing possum" or hibernation.

Contamination: The process by which an object or area becomes unclean.

Contraindication: Any condition that renders a particular treatment improper or undesirable.

Control: The belief that we can influence events by the way we feel, think, and act.

Cortisol: A stress hormone produced by the adrenal glands that is released during long-term stress. An elevated level indicates increased sympathetic arousal.

Counterirritation: Superficial stimulation that relieves a deeper sensation by stimulating different sensory signals.

Counterpressure: Force applied to an area that is designed to match exactly (isometric contraction) or partly (isotonic contraction) the effort or force produced by the muscles of that area.

Countertransference: The personalization of the professional relationship by the therapist in which the practitioner is unable to separate the therapeutic relationship from personal feelings and expectations for the client.

Craniosacral and myofascial approaches: Methods of bodywork that work both reflexively and mechanically with the fascial network of the body.

Cream: A type of lubricant that is in a semisolid or solid state.

Credential: A designation earned by completing a process that verifies a certain level of expertise in a given skill.

Cross-directional stretching: Tissue stretching that pulls and twists connective tissue against its fiber direction.

Cryotherapy: Therapeutic use of ice.

Culture: The arts, beliefs, customs, institutions, and all other products of human work and thought created by a specific group of people at a particular time.

Cupping: The type of tapotement that involves the use of a cupped hand; it is often used over the thorax.

Cutaneous sensory receptors: Sensory nerves in the skin.

Database: All the information available that contributes to therapeutic interaction.

Deep inspiration: Movement of air into the body by hard breathing to meet an increased demand for oxygen. Any muscles that can pull the ribs up are called into action.

Deep transverse friction: A specific rehabilitation technique that creates therapeutic inflammation by creating a specific, controlled reinjury of tissues by applying concentrated therapeutic movement that moves the tissue against its grain over only a very small area.

Defensive measures: The means by which our bodies defend against stressors (e.g., production of antibodies and white blood cells or through behavioral or emotional means).

Denial: The ability to retreat and to ignore stressors.

Depression: A condition characterized by a decrease in vital functional activity and by mood disturbances of exaggerated emptiness, hopelessness, and melancholy or of unbridled high energy with no purpose or outcome.

Depth of pressure: Compressive stress that can be light, moderate, deep, or varied.

Dermatome: Cutaneous (skin) distribution of spinal nerve sensation.

Direction: Flow of massage strokes from the center of the body outward (centrifugal), or from the extremities inward toward the center of the body (centripetal). Direction can be circular motions; it can flow from origin to insertion of the muscle, following the muscle fibers, or can flow transverse to the tissue fibers.

Direction of ease: The position the body assumes with postural changes and muscle shortening or weakening, depending on how it has balanced against gravity.

Disclosure: Acknowledging and informing the client of any situation that interferes with or affects the professional relationship.

Disinfection: The process by which pathogens are destroyed.

Dissociation: Detachment, discontentedness, separation, isolation.

Dopamine: A neurochemical that influences motor activity involving movement (especially learned fine movement, such as hand writing), conscious selective selection (what to pay attention to), mood (in terms of inspiration), possibility, intuition, joy, and enthusiasm. If the dopamine level is low, the opposite effects are seen, such as lack of motor control, clumsiness, inability to decide what to attend to, and boredom.

Drag: The amount of pull (stretch) on the tissue (tensile stress).

Drape: Fabric used to cover the client and keep the individual warm while the massage is given.

Draping: The procedures of covering and uncovering areas of the body and turning the client during the massage.

Draping material: Coverings that provide the client with privacy and warmth. The most commonly used coverings are standard bed linens because they are large enough to cover the entire body and are easy to use for most draping procedures.

Dual role: Overlap in the scope of practice, with one professional providing support in more than one area of expertise.

Duration: The length of time a method lasts or stays in the same location.

Dysfunction: An in-between state in which one is "not healthy" but also "not sick" (i.e., experiencing disease).

Eccentric isotonic contraction: Application of a counterforce while the client moves the jointed area, which allows the origin and insertion to separate. The muscle lengthens against the pressure.

Effleurage: (Gliding stroke); horizontal strokes applied with the fingers, hand, or forearm that usually follow the fiber direction of the underlying muscle, fascial planes, or dermatome pattern.

Electrical-chemical functions: Physiologic functions of the body that rely on or produce body energy; often called Chi, Prana, and meridian energy.

Employee: A person who works for another for a wage.

Endangerment site: Any area of the body where nerves and blood vessels surface close to the skin and are not well protected by muscle or connective tissue; therefore deep, sustained pressure into these areas could damage these vessels and nerves. The kidney area is included because the kidneys are loosely suspended in fat and connective tissue, and heavy pounding is contraindicated in that area.

End-feel: The perception of the joint at the limit of its range of motion. The end-feel is either soft or hard. (See *joint end-feel*.)

Endogenous: Made in the body.

Endurance: A measure of fitness. The ability to work for prolonged periods and the ability to resist fatigue.

Energetic approaches: Methods of bodywork that work with subtle body responses.

Enkephalins and endorphins: Neurochemicals that elevate mood, support satiety (reduce hunger and cravings), and modulate pain.

Entrainment: The coordination of movements or their synchronization to a rhythm.

Entrapment: Pathologic pressure placed on a nerve or vessel by soft tissue.

Environmental contact: Contact with pathogens found in the environment in food, water, and soil and on various surfaces.

Epinephrine/adrenaline: A neurochemical that activates arousal mechanisms in the body; the activation, arousal, alertness, and alarm chemical of the fight-or-flight response and all sympathetic arousal functions and behaviors.

Essential touch: Vital, fundamental, and primary touch that is crucial to well-being.

Ethical behavior: Right and good conduct that is based on moral and cultural standards as defined by the society in which we live.

Ethical decision making: The application of ethical principles and professional skills to determine appropriate behavior and resolve ethical dilemmas.

Ethics: The science or study of morals, values, or principles, including ideals of autonomy, beneficence, and justice; principles of right and good conduct.

Exemption: A situation in which a professional is not required to comply with an existing law because of educational or professional standing.

Experiment: A method of testing a hypothesis.

Expressive touch: Touch applied to support and convey awareness and empathy for the client as a whole.

External sensory information: Stimulation from an origin exterior to the surface of the skin that is detected by the body.

Facilitation: The state of a nerve in which it is stimulated but not to the point of threshold, the point at which it transmits a nerve signal.

Fascial sheath: A flat sheet of connective tissue used for separation, stability, and muscular attachment points.

Feedback: A method of autoregulation to maintain internal homeostasis that interlinks body functions; a noninvasive, continual exchange of information between the client and the professional.

Fitness: A general term used to describe the ability to perform physical work.

Forced expiration: Movement of air out of the body, produced by activating muscles that can pull down the ribs and muscles that can compress the abdomen, forcing the diaphragm upward.

Forced inspiration: Movement of air into the body that occurs when an individual is working very hard and needs a great deal of oxygen. This involves not only the muscles of quiet and deep inspiration but also the muscles that stabilize and/or elevate the shoulder girdle in order to directly or indirectly elevate the ribs.

Frequency: The number of times a method repeats itself in a time period.

Friction: Specific circular or transverse movements that do not glide on the skin and that are focused on the underlying tissue.

Fungi: A group of simple parasitic organisms that are similar to plants but that have no chlorophyll (green pigment). Most pathogenic fungi live on tissue on or near the skin or mucous membranes.

Gait: Walking pattern.

Gate control theory: A hypothetical gating mechanism that functions at the level of the spinal cord; a "gate" through which pain impulses reach the lateral spinothalamic system. Painful impulses are transmitted by large-diameter and small-diameter nerve fibers. Stimulation of large-diameter fibers prevents the small-diameter fibers from transmitting signals. Stimulating (rubbing, massaging) large-diameter fibers helps to suppress the sensation of pain, especially sharp pain.

General adaptation syndrome: The process that calls into play the three stages of the body's response to stress (i.e., the alarm reaction, the resistance reaction, and the exhaustion reaction).

General contraindications: Factors that require a physician's evaluation to rule out serious underlying conditions before any massage is indicated. If the physician recommends massage, the physician must help develop a comprehensive treatment plan.

Gestures: The way a client touches the body while explaining a problem. These movements may indicate whether the problem is a muscle problem, a joint problem, or a visceral problem.

Gliding strokes: Applied horizontally in relation to the tissue fibers, generating a tensile force. Gliding also can be applied across fibers to create a bending force.

Goals: Desired outcomes.

Golgi tendon receptors: Receptors in the tendons that sense tension.

Growth hormone: A hormone that promotes cell division; in adults it is implicated in the repair and regeneration of tissue.

Guarding: Contraction of muscles in a splinting action, surrounding an injured area.

Hacking: A type of tapotement that alternately strikes the surface of the body with quick, snapping movements.

Hardening: A method of teaching the body to deal more effectively with stress; sometimes called *toughening*.

Hardiness: The physical and mental ability to withstand external stressors.

Healing: The restoration of well-being.

Health: Optimal functioning with freedom from disease or abnormal processes.

Heavy pressure: Compressive force that extends to the bone under the tissue.

Hepatitis: A viral inflammatory process and infection of the liver.

Histamine: A chemical produced by the body that dilates the blood vessels.

History: Information from the client about past and present medical conditions and patterns of symptoms.

Homeostasis: Dynamic equilibrium of the internal environment of the body through processes of feedback and regulation.

Hormone: A messenger chemical in the bloodstream.

Human immunodeficiency virus (HIV): The virus that appears to be responsible for AIDS.

Hydrotherapy: The use of various types of water applications and temperatures for therapy.

Hygiene: Practices and conditions that promote health and prevent disease.

Hyperstimulation analgesia: Diminishing the perception of a sensation by stimulating large-diameter nerve fibers. Some methods used are application of ice or heat, counterirritation, acupressure, acupuncture, rocking, music, and repetitive massage strokes.

Hyperventilation: Deep or rapid breathing in excess of physical demands.

Hypothesis: The starting point of research; it is based on the statement, "If this happens, then that will happen."

Impingement syndromes: Conditions that involve pathologic pressure on nerves and vessels; the two types of impingement are compression and entrapment.

Indication: A therapeutic application that promotes health or assists in a healing process.

Inflammatory response: A normal mechanism, characterized by pain, heat, redness, and swelling, that usually speeds recovery from an infection or injury.

Informed consent: Client authorization for any service from a professional based on adequate information provided by the professional. Obtaining informed consent is a consumer protection process that requires that clients have knowledge of what will occur, that their participation is voluntary, and that they are competent to give consent. Informed consent is an educational procedure that allows clients to make knowledgeable decisions about whether they want to receive a massage.

Inhibition: A decrease in or the cessation of a response or function.

Initial treatment plan: A plan that states therapeutic goals, the duration of the sessions, the number of appointments necessary to meet the agreed goals, costs, the general classification of intervention to be used, and the objective progress measurement to be used to identify attainment of goals.

Insertion: The muscle attachment point that is closest to the moving joint.

Integrated approaches: Combined methods of various forms of massage and bodywork styles.

Integration: The process of remembering an event while being able to remain in the present moment, with an awareness of the difference between then and now, to bring some sort of resolution to the event.

Intercompetition massage: Massage provided during an athletic event.

Intimacy: A tender, familiar, and understanding experience between beings.

Intuition: Knowing something by using subconscious information.

Isometric contraction: A contraction in which the effort of the muscle or group of muscles is exactly matched by a counterpressure, so that no movement occurs, only effort.

Isotonic contraction: A contraction in which the effort of the target muscle or group of muscles is partly matched by counterpressure, allowing a degree of resisted movement.

Job: A regular activity performed for payment.

Joint end-feel: The sensation felt when a normal joint is taken to its physiologic limit. (See *end-feel*.)

Joint kinesthetic receptors: Receptors in the capsules of joints that respond to pressure and to acceleration and deceleration of joint movement. The two main types of joint kinesthetic receptors are type II cutaneous mechanoreceptors and pacinian (lamellated) corpuscles.

Joint movement: The movement of the joint through its normal range of motion.

Joint play: The inherent laxity present in a joint.

Kinetic chain: The process by which each individual joint movement pattern is part of an interconnected aspect of the neurologic coordination pattern of muscle movement.

Kneading: Focused vertically and involves twisting. The main purpose of this manipulation is to lift tissue, applying bend, shear, and torsion forces.

Law: A scientific statement that is true uniformly for a whole class of natural occurrences.

Lengthening: The process in which the muscle assumes a normal resting length by means of the neuromuscular mechanism.

Leverage: Leaning with the body weight to provide pressure.

License: A type of credential required by law; licenses are used to regulate the practice of a profession to protect the public health, safety, and welfare.

Longitudinal stretching: A stretch applied along the fiber direction of the connective tissues and muscles.

Lubricant: A substance that reduces friction on the skin during massage movements.

Lymph system: A specialized component of the circulatory system, responsible for waste disposal and immune response.

Lymphatic drainage: A specific type of massage that enhances lymphatic flow.

Malignant: The type of tumor (cancer) that tends to spread to other regions of the body.

Manipulation: Skillful use of the hands in a therapeutic manner. Massage manipulations focus on the soft tissues of the body and are not to be confused with joint manipulation using a high-velocity thrust.

Manual lymph drainage: Methods of bodywork that influence lymphatic movement.

Marketing: The advertising and other promotional activities required to sell a product or service.

Massage: The scientific art and system of assessment of and manual application of certain techniques to the superficial soft tissue of skin, muscles, tendons, ligaments, and fascia and the structures that lie within the superficial tissue. The hand, foot, knee, arm, elbow, and forearm are used for the systematic external application of touch, stroking (effleurage), friction, vibration, percussion, kneading (pétrissage), stretching, compression, or passive and active joint movements within the normal physiologic range of motion. Massage includes adjunctive external applications of water, heat, and cold for the purposes of establishing and maintaining good physical condition and health by normalizing and improving muscle tone, promoting relaxation, stimulating circulation, and producing therapeutic effects on the respiratory and nervous systems and the subtle interactions among all body systems. These intended effects are accomplished through the physiologic energetic and mind/body connections in a safe, nonsexual environment that respects the client's self-determined outcome for the session.

Massage chair: A specially designed chair that allows the client to sit comfortably during the massage.

Massage environment: An area or location where a massage is given.

Massage equipment: Tables, mats, chairs, and other incidental supplies and implements used during the massage.

Massage mat: A cushioned surface that is placed on the floor.

Massage routine: The step-by-step protocol and sequence used to give a massage.

Massage table: A specially designed table that allows massage to be done with the client lying down.

Mechanical methods: Techniques that directly affect the soft tissue by normalizing the connective tissue or moving body fluids and intestinal contents.

Mechanical response: A response that is based on a structure change in the tissue. The tissue change is caused directly by application of the technique.

Mechanical touch: Touch applied with the intent of achieving a specific anatomic or physiologic outcome.

Medications: Substances prescribed to stimulate or inhibit a body process or replace a chemical in the body.

Mental impairment: Any mental or psychological disorder, such as mental retardation, developmental disabilities, organic brain syndrome, emotional or mental illness, and specific learning disabilities.

Mentoring: Career support by someone more experienced.

Metastasis: Migration of cancer cells.

Moderate pressure: Compressive pressure that extends to the muscle layer but does not press the tissue against the underlying bone.

Motivation: The internal drive that provides the energy to do what is necessary to accomplish a goal.

Motor point: The point where a motor nerve enters the muscle it innervates and causes a muscle to twitch if stimulated.

Movement cure: Term used in the nineteenth and early twentieth centuries for a system of exercise and massage manipulations focused on treating a variety of ailments.

Multiple isotonic contractions: Movement of the joint and associated muscles by the client through a full range of motion against partial resistance applied by the massage therapist.

Muscle energy techniques: Neuromuscular facilitation; specific use of active contraction in individual muscles or groups of muscles to initiate a relaxation response; activation of the proprioceptors to facilitate muscle tone, relaxation, and stretching.

Muscle spindles: Structures located primarily in the belly of the muscle that respond to both sudden and prolonged stretches.

Muscle testing procedures: An assessment process that uses muscle contraction. Strength testing is done to determine whether a muscle responds with sufficient strength to perform the required body functions. Neurologic muscle testing is designed to determine whether the neurologic interaction of the muscles is working smoothly. The third type, applied kinesiology, uses muscle strength or weakness as an indicator of body function.

Musculotendinous junction: The point where muscle fibers end and the connective tissue continues to form the tendon; a major site of injury.

Myofascial approaches: Styles of bodywork that affect the connective tissues; often called *deep tissue massage, soft tissue manipulation,* or *myofascial release.*

Myofascial release: A system of bodywork that affects the connective tissue of the body through various methods that elongate and alter the plastic component and ground matrix of the connective tissue.

Needs assessment: History taking using a client information form and physical assessment using an assessment form. The information is evaluated to develop a care plan.

Nerve impingement: Pressure against a nerve by skin, fascia, muscles, ligaments, or joints.

Neurologic muscle testing: Testing designed to determine whether the neurologic interaction of the muscles is proceeding smoothly.

Neuromuscular: A term describing the interaction between nervous system control of the muscles and the response of the muscles to the nerve signals.

Neuromuscular approaches: Methods of bodywork that influence the reflexive responses of the nervous system and its connection to muscular function.

Neuromuscular mechanism: The interplay and reflex connection between sensory and motor neurons and muscle function.

Neurotransmitter: A messenger chemical in the synapse of the nerve.

Norepinephrine/noradrenaline: A neurochemical that functions in a manner similar to epinephrine but that is more concentrated in the brain.

Occupation: A productive or creative activity that serves as a regular source of livelihood.

Oil: A type of liquid lubricant.

Open-ended question: A question that cannot be answered with a simple, one-word response.

Opportunistic invasion: Potentially pathogenic organisms are found on the skin and mucous membranes of nearly everyone that do not cause disease until they have the opportunity, such as in depressed immunity.

Origin: The attachment point of a muscle at the fixed point during movement.

Oscillation: Any effect that varies in a back-and-forth, or reciprocating, manner.

Osteokinematic movements: The movements of flexion, extension, abduction, adduction, and rotation; also known as *physiologic movements*.

Overload principle: A stress on an organism that is greater than the one regularly encountered during everyday life.

Oxytocin: A hormone that is implicated in pair or couple bonding, parental bonding, feelings of attachment, and care taking, along with its more commonly known functions in pregnancy, delivery, and lactation.

PRICE first aid–Protection, Rest, Ice, Compression, Elevation.

Pain and fatigue syndromes: Multicausal and often chronic nonproductive patterns that interfere with well-being, activities of living, and productivity.

Pain-spasm-pain cycle: Steady contraction of muscles, which causes ischemia and stimulates pain receptors in muscles. The pain, in turn, initiates more spasms.

Palliative care: Care intended to relieve or reduce the intensity of uncomfortable symptoms but that cannot effect a cure.

Palpation: Assessment through touch.

Panic: An intense, sudden, and overwhelming fear or feeling of anxiety that produces terror and immediate physiologic change resulting in immobility or senseless, hysterical behavior.

Parasympathetic autonomic nervous system: The restorative part of the autonomic nervous system. The parasympathetic response often is called *the relaxation response*.

Passive joint movement: Movement of a joint by the massage practitioner without the assistance of the client.

Passive range of motion: Movement of a joint in which the therapist, not the client, effects the motion.

Pathogenic animals: Large, multicellular organisms sometimes called metazoa. Most metazoa are worms that feed off human tissue or cause other disease processes.

Pathologic barrier: An adaptation of the physiologic barrier that allows the protective function to limit rather than support optimal functioning.

Pathology: The study of disease.

Peer support: Interaction among those involved in the same pursuit. Regular interaction with other massage practitioners creates an environment in which both technical information and dilemmas and interpersonal dilemmas can be sorted out.

Person-to-person contact: Pathogens can often be carried in the air from one person to another.

Pétrissage: Kneading; rhythmic rolling, lifting, squeezing, and wringing of soft tissue.

Phasic muscles: The muscles that move the body.

Physical assessment: Evaluation of body balance, efficient function, basic symmetry, range of motion, and ability to function.

Physical disability: Any physiologic disorder, condition, cosmetic disfigurement, or anatomic loss that affects one or more of the following body systems: neurologic, musculoskeletal, special sense organ, respiratory (including speech organs), cardiovascular, reproductive, digestive, genitourinary, hemic and lymphatic, skin, and endocrine. Extremes in size and extensive burns also may be considered physical impairments.

Physiologic barriers: The result of the limits in range of motion imposed by protective nerve and sensory functions to support optimal performance.

Piezoelectricity: The production of an electrical current by application of pressure to certain crystals such as mica, quartz, Rochelle salt, and connective tissue.

Placebo: A treatment for an illness that influences the course of the disease even if the treatment is not specifically validated.

Polarity: A holistic health practice that encompasses some of the theory base of Asian medicine and Ayurveda. Polarity is an eclectic, multifaceted system.

Positional release: A method of moving the body into the direction of ease (the way the body wants to move out of the position that causes the pain); the proprioception is taken into a state of safety and may stop signalling for protective spasm.

Positioning: Placing the body in such a way that specific joints of muscles are isolated.

Postevent massage: Massage provided after an athletic event.

Postisometric relaxation (PIR): The state that occurs after isometric contraction of a muscle; it results from the activity of minute neural reporting stations called the *Golgi tendon bodies*.

Post-traumatic stress disorder: A disorder characterized by episodes of flashback memory, state-dependent memory, somatization, anxiety, irritability, sleep disturbance, concentration difficulties, times of melancholy or depression, grief, fear, worry, anger, and avoidance behavior.

Postural muscles: Muscles that support the body against gravity.

Powder: A type of lubricant that consists of a finely ground substance.

Prefix: A word element placed at the beginning of a root word to change the meaning of the word.

Premassage activities: Any activity that is involved in preparation for a massage, including setting up the massage room, obtaining supplies, and determining the temperature of the room.

Pressure: Compressive force.

Prime movers: The muscles responsible for movement.

Principle: A basic truth or rule of conduct

Profession: An occupation that requires training and specialized study.

Professional: A person who practices a profession.

Professional touch: Skilled touch delivered to achieve a specific outcome; the recipient in some way reimburses the professional for services rendered.

Professionalism: The adherence to professional status, methods, standards, and character.

Prone: Lying face down.

Proprioceptive neuromuscular facilitation (PNF): Specific application of muscle energy techniques that uses strong contraction combined with stretching and muscular pattern retraining.

Proprioceptors: Sensory receptors that detect joint and muscle activity.

Protozoa: One-celled organisms that are larger than bacteria and can infest human fluids and cause disease by parasitizing (living off) or directly destroying cells.

Pulsed muscle energy: Procedures that involve engaging the barrier and using minute, resisted contractions (usually 20 in 10 seconds), which introduces mechanical pumping as well as PIR or RI.

Qualified: Criteria that indicate when the goal is achieved.

Quantified: Goals measured in terms of objective criteria, such as time, frequency, 1 to 10 scale, measurable increase or decrease in the ability to perform an activity, or measurable increase or decrease in a sensation, such as relaxation or pain.

Quiet expiration: Movement of air out of the body through passive action. This occurs through relaxation of the external intercostals and the elastic recoil of the thoracic wall and tissue of the lungs and bronchi, with gravity pulling the rib cage down from its elevated position.

Quiet inspiration: Movement of air into the body while resting or sitting quietly. The diaphragm and external intercostals are the prime movers.

Range of motion: Movement of joints.

Rapport: The development of a relationship based on mutual trust and harmony.

Reciprocal inhibition (RI): The effect that occurs when a muscle contracts, obliging its antagonist to relax in order to allow normal movement to take place.

Reciprocity: The exchange of privileges between governing bodies.

Recovery massage: Massage structured primarily for the uninjured athlete who wants to recover from a strenuous workout or competition.

Reenactment: Reliving an event as though it were happening at the moment.

Referral: Sending a client to a health care professional for specific diagnosis and treatment of a disease.

Referred pain: Pain felt in an area other than the source of the pain.

Reflex: An involuntary response to a stimulus. Reflexes are specific, predictable, adaptive, and purposeful. Reflexive methods work by stimulating the nervous system (sensory neurons), and tissue changes occur in response to the body's adaptation to the neural stimulation.

Reflexive methods: Massage techniques that stimulate the nervous system, the endocrine system, and the chemicals of the body.

Reflexology: A massage system directed primarily toward the feet and hands.

Refractory period: The period after a muscle contraction during which the muscle is unable to contract again.

Regional contraindications: Contraindications that relate to a specific area of the body.

Rehabilitation massage: Massage used for severe injury or as part of intervention after surgery.

Remedial massage: Massage used for minor to moderate injuries.

Resourceful compensation: Adjustments made by the body to manage a permanent or chronic dysfunction.

Resting position: The first stroke of the massage; the simple laying on of hands.

Rhythm: The regularity of application of a technique. If the method is applied at regular intervals, it is considered even or rhythmic. If it is choppy or irregular, it is considered uneven or not rhythmic.

Right of refusal: The entitlement of both the client and the professional to stop the session.

Rocking: Rhythmic movement of the body.

Root word: The part of a word that provides the fundamental meaning.

Safe touch: Secure, respectful, considerate, sensitive, responsive, sympathetic, understanding, supportive, and empathetic contact.

Sanitation: The formulation and application of measures to promote and establish conditions favorable to health, specifically public health.

Science: The intellectual process of understanding through observation, measurement, accumulation of data, and analysis of findings.

Scope of practice: The knowledge base and practice parameters of a profession.

Self-employment: To work for oneself rather than another.

Serotonin: The neurochemical that regulates mood in terms of appropriate emotions, attention to thoughts, calming, quieting, and comforting effects; it also subdues irritability and regulates drive states.

Service: An action performed for another person that results in a specific outcome.

Sexual misconduct: Any behavior that is sexually oriented in the professional setting.

Shaking: A technique in which the body area is grasped and shaken in a quick, loose movement; sometimes classified as *rhythmic mobilization*.

Shear: A sliding force in which significant friction often is created between the structures that slide against each other.

Shiatsu: An acupressure and meridian-focused bodywork system from Japan.

Side-lying: The position in which the client is lying on his or her side.

Skin rolling: A form of pétrissage that lifts skin.

Slapping: A form of tapotement that uses a flat hand.

SOAP charting: A problem-oriented method of medical record keeping; the acronym SOAP stands for subjective, objective, assessment (analysis), and plan.

Soft tissue: The skin, fascia, muscles, tendons, joint capsules, and ligaments of the body.

Somatic: Pertaining to the body.

Somatic pain: Pain that arises from stimulation of receptors in the skin (superficial somatic pain) or in skeletal muscles, joints, tendons, and fascia (deep somatic pain).

Spa treatments: Various hydrotherapy, application of preparations to the body, and massage applications found in the spa setting.

Speed: Rate of application (i.e., fast, slow, varied).

Spindle cells: Sensory receptors in the belly of the muscle that detect stretch.

Stabilization: Holding the body in a fixed position during joint movement, lengthening, and stretching.

Standard precautions: Procedures developed by the Centers for Disease Control and Prevention (CDC) to prevent the spread of contagious diseases.

Standards of practice: The principles that form specific guidelines to direct professional ethical practice and quality care, including a structure for evaluating the quality of care. Standards of practice represent an attempt to define the parameters of quality care.

Start-up costs: The initial expenses involved in starting a business.

State-dependent memory: The encoding and storing of a memory based on the effects of the autonomic nervous system and the resulting chemical levels of the body. The memory is retrievable only during a similar physiologic experience in the body.

Sterilization: The process by which all microorganisms are destroyed.

Stimulation: Excitation that activates the sensory nerves.

Strain-counterstrain: Using tender points to guide the positioning of the body into a space where the muscle tension can release on its own.

Strength testing: Testing intended to determine whether a muscle is responding with sufficient strength to perform the required body functions. Strength testing determines a muscle's force of contraction.

Stress: Any substantial change in routine or any activity that forces the body to adapt.

Stressors: Any internal perceptions or external stimuli that demand a change in the body.

Stretching: Mechanical tension applied to lengthen the myofascial unit (muscles and fascia); two types are longitudinal and cross-directional stretching.

Stroke: A technique of therapeutic massage that is applied with a movement on the surface of the body, whether superficial or deep.

Structural and postural integration approaches Methods of bodywork derived from biomechanics, postural alignment, and the importance of the connective tissue structures.

Subtle energies: Weak electrical fields that surround and run through the body.

Suffering: An overall impairment of a person's quality of life.

Suffix: A word element placed at the end of a root word to change the meaning of the word.

Superficial fascia: The connective tissue layer just under the skin.

Superficial pressure: Pressure that remains on the skin.

Supervision: Support from more experienced professionals.

Supine: The position in which the client is lying face up.

Symmetric stance: The position in which body weight is distributed equally between the feet.

Sympathetic autonomic nervous system: The energy-using part of the autonomic nervous system, the division in which the fight-or-flight response is activated.

Symptoms: The subjective abnormalities felt only by the patient.

Syndrome: A group of different signs and symptoms that usually arise from a common cause.

Synergistic: The interaction of medication and massage to stimulate the same process or effects.

System: A group of interacting elements that function as a complex whole.

Systemic massage: Massage structured to affect one body system primarily. This approach usually is used for lymphatic and circulation enhancement massage.

Tapotement: Springy blows to the body at a fast rate to create rhythmic compression of the tissue; also called *percussion*.

Tapping: A type of tapotement that uses the fingertips.

Target muscle: The muscle or groups of muscles on which the response of the methods is specifically focused.

Techniques: Methods of therapeutic massage that provide sensory stimulation or mechanical change of the soft tissue of the body.

Tendon organs: Structures found in the tendon and musculotendinous junction that respond to tension at the tendon. Articular (joint) ligaments contain receptors that are similar to tendon organs and adjust reflex inhibition of the adjacent muscle when excessive strain is placed on the joints.

Tensegrity: An architectural principle developed in 1948 by R. Buckminster Fuller. The tensegrity principle underlies geodesic domes. A tensegrity system is characterized by a continuous tensional network (tendons, ligaments, and fascial structures) connected by a discontinuous set of compressive elements, or struts (bones).

Tension forces: Occur when two ends of a structure are pulled in opposite directions (also called tensile force).

Therapeutic applications: Healing or curative powers.

Therapeutic change: Beneficial change produced by a bodywork process that results in a modification of physical form or function that can affect a client's physical, mental, and/or spiritual state.

Therapeutic relationship: The interpersonal structure and professional boundaries between professionals and the clients they serve.

Tonic vibration reflex: Reflex that tones a muscle with stimulation through vibration methods at the tendon.

Torsion: Twisting forces.

Touch: Contact with no movement.

Touch technique: The basis of soft tissue forms of bodywork methods.

Toughening/hardening: The reaction to repeated exposure to stimuli that elicit arousal responses.

Traction: Gentle pull on the joint capsule to increase the joint space.

Training stimulus threshold: The stimulus that elicits a training response.

Transference: The personalization of the professional relationship by the client.

Trauma: Physical injury caused by violent or disruptive action, toxic substances, or psychic injury resulting from a severe long- or short-term emotional shock.

Trigger point: An area of local nerve facilitation; pressure on the trigger point results in hypertonicity of a muscle bundle and referred pain patterns.

Tuberculosis (TB): An infection caused by a bacterium that usually affects the lungs but may invade other body systems.

Vibration: Fine or coarse tremulous movement that creates reflexive responses.

Viruses: Microorganisms that invade cells and insert their genetic code into the host cell's genetic code. Viruses use the host cell's nutrients and organelles to produce more virus particles.

Wellness: The efficient balance of body, mind, and spirit, all working in a harmonious way to provide quality of life.

Yang: The portion of the whole realm of function of the body, mind, and spirit in Eastern thought that corresponds with sympathetic autonomic nervous system functions.

Yin: The portion of the whole realm of function of the body, mind, and spirit in Eastern thought that corresponds with parasympathetic autonomic nervous system functions.

Indications and Contraindications to Massage

Because each situation is different, it is difficult to make recommendations on when to give a massage and when not to give one. Each situation needs to be evaluated to determine whether massage is indicated or contraindicated. The existence of contraindications does not always mean that therapeutic massage is inappropriate. What most contraindications require is caution, which may call for modification of the massage treatment and, in some cases, supervision by and cooperation with the health care team. The clinical reasoning model is a valuable tool for making decisions about contraindications. This appendix presents two models of a guideline system for determining the indications and contraindications for massage. Specific conditions, symptoms, indications, and contraindications for massage follow. Use a medical dictionary to look up unfamiliar terms.

THE ONTARIO MODEL

The following are absolute contraindications (CI) to massage (i.e., massage treatment should not be given).

General

1. Acute-stage pneumonia
2. Advanced kidney failure (modified treatment may be possible with medical consent)
3. Advanced respiratory failure (modified treatment may be possible with medical consent)
4. Diabetes with complications (e.g., gangrene, advanced heart or kidney disease, very high or unstable blood pressure)
5. Eclampsia-toxemia in pregnancy
6. Hemophilia
7. Hemorrhage
8. Liver failure (modified treatment may be possible with medical consent)
9. Postcerebrovascular accident (CVA, stroke), condition not yet stabilized
10. Postmyocardial infarction (MI, heart attack), condition not yet stabilized
11. Severe atherosclerosis
12. Severe hypertension (if unstable)
13. Shock (all types)
14. Significant fever (higher than 101° F [38.3° C])
15. Some acute conditions that require first aid or medical attention
    - Anaphylaxis
    - Appendicitis
    - CVA
    - Diabetic coma, insulin shock
    - Epileptic seizure
    - MI
    - Pneumothorax, atelectasis
    - Severe asthma attack, status asthmaticus
    - Syncope (fainting)
16. Some highly metastatic cancers not judged to be terminal
17. Systemic contagious/infectious condition

Local (Regional)

1. Acute flare-up of inflammatory arthritis (e.g., rheumatoid arthritis, systemic lupus erythematosus, ankylosing spondylitis, Reiter's syndrome); may be general CI, depending on case
2. Acute neuritis
3. Aneurysms deemed life-threatening (e.g., of the abdominal aorta); may be general CI, depending on location
4. Ectopic pregnancy
5. Esophageal varicosities (varices)
6. Frostbite
7. Local contagious condition
8. Local irritable skin condition
9. Malignancy (especially if judged unstable)
10. Open wound or sore
11. Phlebitis, phlebothrombosis, arteritis; may be general CI if located in a major circulatory channel
12. Recent burn
13. Sepsis
14. Temporal arteritis
15. Twenty-four to 48 hours after antiinflammatory treatment (target tissue and immediate vicinity)
16. Undiagnosed lump

General

The following conditions require an awareness of the possibility of adverse effects from massage therapy. Substantial treatment adaptation may be appropriate. Medical consultation often is needed.

1. Any condition of spasticity or rigidity
2. Asthma

3. Cancer (including finding appropriate relationships to other current treatments)
4. Chronic congestive heart failure
5. Chronic kidney disease
6. Client taking antiinflammatory drugs, muscle relaxants, anticoagulants, analgesics, or any other medications that alter sensation, muscle tone, standard reflex reactions, cardiovascular function, kidney or liver function, or personality
7. Coma (may be absolute CI, depending on cause)
8. Diagnosed atherosclerosis
9. Drug withdrawal
10. Emphysema
11. Epilepsy
12. Hypertension
13. Immunosuppressed client
14. Inflammatory arthritides
15. Major or abdominal surgery
16. Moderately severe or juvenile-onset diabetes
17. Multiple sclerosis
18. Osteoporosis, osteomalacia
19. Pregnancy and labor
20. Post-MI
21. Post-CVA
22. Recent head injury

Local (Regional)

1. Acute disk herniation
2. Aneurysm (may be general CI, depending on location)
3. Any acute inflammatory condition
4. Any antiinflammatory treatment site
5. Any chronic or long-standing superficial thrombosis
6. Buerger's disease (may be general CI if unstable)
7. Chronic arthritic conditions
8. Chronic abdominal or digestive disease
9. Chronic diarrhea
10. Contusion
11. Endometriosis
12. Flaccid paralysis or paresis
13. Fracture (while casted and immediately after cast removal)
14. Hernia
15. Joint instability or hypermobility
16. Kidney infection, stones
17. Mastitis
18. Minor surgery
19. Pelvic inflammatory disease
20. Pitting edema
21. Portal hypertension
22. Prolonged constipation
23. Recent abortion/vaginal birth
24. Trigeminal neuralgia

Other Important Considerations

1. Massage therapists are expected to know how and when to consult with physicians and other health professionals.

2. Most emotional or psychiatric conditions affect massage treatment. Individual decisions must be made according to case circumstances and, in many instances, medical advice. Medications may be a factor.
3. The client may be allergic to certain massage oils and creams or to cleansers or disinfectants used on sheets and tables.
4. The presence of pins, staples, or artificial joints may alter treatment indications.

   The massage therapist should be aware of the role of common chronic conditions that affect public health (e.g., cardiovascular disease, cancer, substance abuse, chronic mental diseases).

   The local health department can provide additional information on public mental health services, environmental hazards, occupational health, or various health care organizations available in the community.

THE OREGON MODEL: INDICATIONS AND CONTRAINDICATIONS BY BODY SYSTEM

This extensive list was developed by the Oregon Board of Massage. However, no specific recommendations regarding indications or contraindications for massage were made. The descriptions of the disease processes and the massage recommendations were added by this author, using a very conservative approach. If an indication for massage is not listed for a disease process, massage has no direct benefit; such cases are designated N/A. This textbook covers basic massage. Advanced training in the medical application of massage, as well as direct supervision by a physician, chiropractor, physical therapist, psychologist, dentist, podiatrist, or other health care professional, will greatly expand the application of massage in rehabilitative situations.

The Integumentary System

Assessment parameters include color (e.g., pallor, jaundice, cyanosis, erythema, mottling), texture (e.g., dry, moist, scaly), scars (normal and keloid), vascularity (e.g., dilated veins, angiomas, varicosities, ecchymoses, petechiae, purpura), temperature, rashes, lesions, nail condition, hair condition, contour, hydration, and edema.

Deviations that suggest the need for evaluation and referral include lumps or masses, rashes of unknown origin, lesions, burns, urticaria, itching of unknown origin, cyanosis, jaundice, ulcerations, multiple bruises, and petechiae.

Specific Disease Processes and Bacterial Conditions

Acne

Definition/symptoms: Inflammation of the skin affecting the sebaceous gland ducts

Indications: Massage increases systemic circulation; may assist healing

Contraindications: Regional; avoid affected area; do not use ointments that clog pores

Carbuncle

Definition/symptoms: Mass of connected boils

Indications: Massage may increase systemic circulation and may assist healing

Contraindications: Refer client to physician; regional; avoid affected area

Cellulitis

Definition/symptoms: Inflammation of subcutaneous tissue with redness and swelling

Indications: Avoid

Contraindications: Regional; may be associated with erysipelas, a contagious condition; refer client to physician

Folliculitis

Definition/symptoms: Inflammation of hair follicle

Indications: Massage may increase systemic circulation and assist healing

Contraindications: Regional; refer client to physician; avoid affected area

Furuncle (boil)

Definition/symptoms: Pus-filled cavity formed by infection of hair follicle

Indications: Massage may increase systemic circulation and assist healing

Contraindications: Regional; refer client to physician; avoid affected area

Impetigo

Definition/symptoms: Highly contagious bacterial skin infection that occurs most often in children; begins as a reddish discoloration and develops into vesicles with a yellow crust

Indications: Massage may increase systemic circulation and assist healing

Contraindications: Regional; refer client to physician; avoid affected area

Syphilis

Definition/symptoms: Primary stage: a usually painless lesion (chancre) present on exposed skin; secondary stage: begins about 2 months after chancre disappears and produces a variety of symptoms, including skin rash

Indications: N/A

Contraindications: General; rash is contagious; refer client to physician

Viral Conditions

Bell's palsy

Definition/symptoms: Infection of seventh cranial nerve; primary symptom is paralysis of facial features, including the eyelids and mouth

Indications: Relaxation massage may facilitate healing

Contraindications: Regional; refer client to physician for diagnosis

Herpes simplex

Definition/symptoms: Acute viral disease marked by groups of watery blisters on or near mucous membranes

Indications: Recurrence is stress-induced; massage may reduce stress levels

Contraindications: Regional; contagious; avoid affected area

Herpes zoster (shingles)

Definition/symptoms: Viral infection that usually affects the skin of a single dermatome; produces a red, swollen plaque that ruptures and crusts

Indications: Condition is painful; general massage may ease pain

Contraindications: Regional; avoid affected area; may need to refer client to physician

Warts

Definition/symptoms: Usually benign, excess cell growth of the skin

Indications: N/A

Contraindications: Regional; avoid affected area; contagious; may become malignant; if any changes in wart occur, refer client to physician

Fungal Conditions

Ringworm, athlete's foot, fungal infection of the nails

Definition/symptoms: Scaly and crusty cracking of the skin

Indications: Keep area dry; do not use lubricants

Contraindications: Regional; do not use lubricants near the area because fungi thrive in a moist environment

Allergic Reactions

Atopic dermatitis (eczema)

Definition/symptoms: Common inflammation of the skin marked by papules, vesicles, and crusts

Indications: Symptom of an underlying condition; refer client to physician for diagnosis

Contraindications: Regional; avoid affected area

Contact dermatitis

Definition/symptoms: Inflammation that occurs in response to contact with an external agent

Indications: Use unscented lubricants (scents often cause allergic reactions)

Contraindications: Regional; avoid affected area

Urticaria (hives)

Definition/symptoms: Red, raised lesions caused by leakage of fluid from skin and blood vessels; primary symptom is severe itching

Indications: Do not use scented products; hives may have an emotional component

Contraindications: Regional; avoid affected area

Benign Conditions

Mole
Definition/symptoms: Pigmented, fleshy growth of skin
Indications: Watch for any change in a mole; refer client to physician if a change is noted
Contraindications: Regional; avoid mole

Psoriasis
Definition/symptoms: Chronic inflammation of the skin; probably genetic; symptoms include scaly plaque and excessive growth rate of epithelial cells
Indications: May be stress-induced; massage reduces stress
Contraindications: Regional; avoid affected area

Scleroderma
Definition/symptoms: Autoimmune disease that affects blood vessels and connective tissue of the skin; primary symptom is hard, yellowish skin
Indications: N/A
Contraindications: Regional (except in systemic cases); refer client to physician

Malignant Conditions

Skin cancer
Definition/symptoms: Squamous cell carcinoma, basal cell carcinoma, melanoma, Kaposi's sarcoma
Indications: N/A
Contraindications: Watch for any change in a mole or existing skin condition; if this occurs, refer client to physician immediately

The Skeletal System, Muscular System, and Articulations

Assessment parameters include range of motion, swelling, masses, deformity, pain or tenderness, temperature, crepitus, spasm, paresthesia, pulses, skin color, paralysis, atrophy, and contracture.

Deviations that suggest the need for evaluation and referral include malalignment of an extremity, asymmetry of musculoskeletal contour, progressive or persistent pain, masses or progressive swelling, numbness and/or tingling with loss of function, diminished or absent peripheral pulses, pallor and/or coolness of one extremity, redness and/or increased temperature of one extremity, and difference in size of extremities.

Specific Disease Processes

Atonicity (flaccidity)
Definition/symptoms: Reduced ability or inability of the muscle to contract (hypotonicity)
Indications: Massage to tone; relaxation of opposing muscle groups
Contraindications: Regional; refer client to physician for diagnosis before proceeding

Contracture
Definition/symptoms: Fixed resistance to passive stretching of muscles; usually the result of fibrosis or tissue ischemia
Indications: Massage and stretch
Contraindications: Do not stretch past fixed barrier

Convulsion
Definition/symptoms: Sudden, involuntary series of muscle contractions, sometimes called a *seizure*
Indications: N/A
Contraindications: Refer client to physician immediately

Fibrillation
Definition/symptoms: A small, local contraction of muscle that is invisible under the skin; results from spontaneous, synchronous activation of single muscle cells
Indications: Massage, direct pressure
Contraindications: If continuous, refer client to physician for diagnosis

Hypertonicity
Definition/symptoms: Increased muscle tone
Indications: Massage and stretch
Contraindications: Recurrence without explanation; refer client to physician for diagnosis

Spasms (cramp)
Definition/symptoms: Sudden, painful onset of muscle contraction
Indications: Use reciprocal inhibition; push muscle belly together and slowly stretch
Contraindications: If recurring and transient, refer client to physician

Tic
Definition/symptoms: Spasmodic twitching; often occurs in the face
Indications: May be stress-induced; massage is beneficial in reducing stress
Contraindications: Refer client to physician for diagnosis to rule out underlying pathologic condition

Soft Tissue Injuries

Dislocation
Definition/symptoms: Displacement of a bone within a joint
Indications: N/A
Contraindications: Immediately refer client to physician

Sprains
Definition/symptoms: Traumatic injury of ligaments that form a skeletal joint; may involve injury (strain) of muscles or tendons
Indications: RICE (rest, ice, compression, elevation), first aid, gentle massage, and range of motion facilitate healing
Contraindications: Regional; all traumatic injuries should be evaluated by a physician

Strains
Definition/symptoms: Traumatic injury caused by over-stretching or overexertion of muscle or tendon tissue

Indications: RICE, first aid, gentle massage, and range of motion may facilitate healing

Contraindications: Regional; all traumatic injuries should be evaluated by a physician

Subluxation

Definition/symptoms: Any deviation from the normal relationship in which the articular cartilage is touching any portion of its mating cartilage

Indications: Massage may help relieve muscle spasm

Contraindications: Refer client to physician

Infectious Processes

Osteomyelitis

Definition/symptoms: Bacterial infection of the bone; symptoms include deep pain and fever

Indications: N/A

Contraindications: General; immediately refer client to physician; difficult to diagnose and treat

Inflammatory Processes

Ankylosing spondylitis

Definition/symptoms: Chronic inflammatory disease; can be progressive; usually involves the sacroiliac joint and spinal articulations; cause is unknown, appears to be genetic; if progressive, calcification of the joints and articular surfaces occurs; begins with feelings of fatigue and intermittent low back pain; synovial tissue around the involved joints becomes inflamed; heart disease also may occur

Indications: Massage may be helpful under direct supervision of a physician

Contraindications: General; refer client to physician; avoid any area of inflammation

Bursitis

Definition/symptoms: Inflammation of bursa

Indications: Massage may take pressure off joint by relaxing and normalizing surrounding musculature; ice

Contraindications: Regional; avoid affected area; work above and below jointed area

Fibromyalgia

Definition/symptoms: General disruption in connective tissue muscle component; symptoms include tender point activity; vague symptoms of pain and fatigue

Indications: Massage may be beneficial; work with physician

Contraindications: General; refer client to physician for diagnosis; do not use therapeutic inflammation methods

Gouty arthritis

Definition/symptoms: Metabolic condition in which sodium urate crystals trigger a chronic inflammatory process

Indications: Dietary adjustment necessary

Contraindications: Regional; avoid area of inflammation

Lupus erythematosus

Definition/symptoms: Chronic inflammatory disease that affects many body tissues; common symptom is a red rash on the face

Indications: Massage may be beneficial under physician's close supervision

Contraindications: General; systemic disease

Osgood-Schlatter disease

Definition/symptoms: Osteochondrosis (inflammation of bone and cartilage) of the tibial tuberosity

Indications: N/A

Contraindications: Regional; avoid affected area

Rheumatoid arthritis

Definition/symptoms: Autoimmune inflammatory joint disease characterized by synovial inflammation that spreads to other tissues

Indications: Stress responsive; massage can be helpful under medical supervision

Contraindications: General; work closely with physician

Tendinitis

Definition/symptoms: Inflammation of tendon and tendon-muscle junction

Indications: Massage may assist healing; ice

Contraindications: Regional; avoid affected area; work above and below the area

Tenosynovitis

Definition/symptoms: Inflammation of tendon sheath, usually from repetitive movement

Indications: Massage may relieve muscle hypertension and assist healing of area; ice

Contraindications: Regional; avoid affected area; work above and below the area

Compression Processes

Carpal tunnel syndrome

Definition/symptoms: Inflammation in tendon sheaths in the carpal tunnel that creates pressure on the median nerve; symptoms include weakness and tingling in the hand

Indications: Symptoms often are confused with thoracic outlet syndrome; massage is proving to be beneficial

Contraindications: Regional; refer client to physician for diagnosis

Degenerative Processes

Muscular dystrophy

Definition/symptoms: A group of muscle disorders characterized by atrophy of skeletal muscle without nerve involvement

Indications: Massage is beneficial; work closely with supervising physician

Contraindications: General

Osteoarthritis

Definition/symptoms: Degenerative joint disease of the articular cartilage; age and joint damage are risk factors

Indications: Massage is beneficial

Contraindications: Regional; avoid area of inflammation

Osteoporosis

Definition/symptoms: Loss of minerals and collagen from bone matrix, resulting in reduced volume and strength of skeletal bone

Indications: Gentle massage is beneficial; use care and caution

Contraindications: General

Abnormal Spinal Curve

Kyphosis

Definition/symptoms: Abnormal increased convexity of the thoracic spine

Indications: Massage is beneficial as part of the treatment plan

Contraindications: Regional; in severe cases proceed after obtaining physician's recommendation

Lordosis

Definition/symptoms: Abnormal increased concavity in the curvature of the lumbar spine

Indications: Massage is beneficial as part of the treatment plan

Contraindications: Regional; in severe cases proceed after obtaining physician's recommendation

Scoliosis

Definition/symptoms: Lateral curve of vertebral column

Indications: Massage is beneficial as part of the treatment plan

Contraindications: Regional; in severe cases proceed after obtaining physician's recommendation

Disordered Muscular Processes

Low back pain

Definition/symptoms: May be of many varieties: muscular, nerve entrapment, or disk problem

Indications: Massage can be beneficial as part of the treatment plan

Contraindications: Regional; important to refer client to physician to rule out serious condition of the spine or viscera

Spasmodic torticollis

Definition/symptoms: A contracted state of the cervical muscles that causes pain and rotation of the head

Indications: Massage is beneficial

Contraindications: Regional; refer client to physician for diagnosis to rule out serious disease

Temporomandibular joint (TMJ) dysfunction

Definition/symptoms: Dysfunction in the TMJ; pain and muscle contraction

Indications: Massage is beneficial; work closely with dentist and physician

Contraindications: Regional if painful

Neurologic Conditions

Assessment parameters include mental status, the presence of involuntary movements, coordination and balance, muscle tone and strength, changes in sensory perception (i.e., touch, pain, temperature, vibration, position sense, hearing, vision).

Deviations that suggest the need for evaluation and referral include inequality of pupil size; diplopia; abnormal Babinski's sign (extensor plantar response); seizures (partial or generalized); significant personality changes; changes in sensorium; progressively worsening or persistent headache; temporary loss of speech, vision, or motion; triad of fever, headache, and nuchal rigidity; vomiting; and change in pupil size with head injury.

Specific Disease Processes

Dyskinesia

Definition/symptoms: Impairment of the power of voluntary movement, resulting in fragmentary or incomplete movement and possibly pain

Indications: Massage is beneficial as part of a physician-directed treatment plan

Contraindications: General; refer client to physician for diagnosis and treatment plan

Dystonia

Definition/symptoms: Disordered, random tonicity of muscles

Indications: Massage is beneficial as part of a physician-directed treatment plan

Contraindications: General; refer client to physician for diagnosis and treatment plan

Insomnia

Definition/symptoms: Inability to sleep or interrupted sleep

Indications: Massage is beneficial

Contraindications: Regional; refer client to physician for specific diagnosis to rule out serious underlying condition

Peripheral neuropathy

Definition/symptoms: General functional disturbances and/or pathologic changes in the peripheral nervous system caused by diabetic neuropathy, ischemic neuropathy, or traumatic neuropathy; symptoms include numbness, burning, and pain

Indications: Massage is beneficial as part of the treatment plan

Contraindications: General; refer client to physician for diagnosis to determine underlying condition

Tinnitus

Definition/symptoms: Noise in the ear; symptoms include ringing, buzzing, roaring, or clicking

Indications: N/A

Contraindications: Regional; refer client to physician for specific diagnosis

Vertigo

Definition/symptoms: Sensation of movement, not to be confused with dizziness

  Indications: N/A

  Contraindications: General; usually symptomatic of underlying condition; physician's diagnosis required

Vascular Processes

Cerebrovascular accident (CVA)

Definition/symptoms: Stroke; a disturbance in cerebral circulation; major causes include atherosclerosis (thrombosis), embolism, hypertensive intracerebral hemorrhage or ruptured saccular aneurysm; symptoms differ depending on where the disturbance in circulation occurs; general symptoms include weakness or paralysis of the arm or leg, headache, numbness, blurred or double vision, and confusion or dizziness; often only one side is affected; symptoms persist for at least 24 hours, usually much longer

  Indications: Massage may be beneficial during recovery under physician's supervision and during long-term care for continued support

  Contraindications: Refer client to physician for diagnosis

Headache

Definition/symptoms: Pain or dull ache in the head and upper neck; can have a variety of causes such as muscle tension, sinus pressure, pinched nerve, vascular disruption (e.g., migraine headache, cluster headaches), and toxins

  Indications: Massage may be beneficial

  Contraindications: Refer all clients with a persistent, severe headache to physician for specific diagnosis

Head injury

Definition/symptoms: Contusion (bump on the head); laceration (cut or break in the skin); subdural and epidural injury may produce disorientation, nausea, and uneven pupil dilation

  Indications: Immediately refer client to physician if any of the signs listed above are noted

  Contraindications: General; all traumatic injuries must be evaluated by a physician

Transient ischemic attack (TIA)

Definition/symptoms: Episodes of neurologic dysfunction that usually are of short duration (a few minutes) but may persist for 24 hours; reversible; symptom pattern is the same with each attack because the same vessel is involved; small strokes, seizures, migraine symptoms, postural hypotension, and Stokes-Allen syndrome may be misdiagnosed as TIAs

  Indications: Massage may be beneficial under physician's supervision

  Contraindications: Refer client to physician for diagnosis

Infectious Processes

Conjunctivitis

Definition/symptoms: Inflammation and/or infection of mucous membranes of the eye

  Indications: N/A

  Contraindications: Regional; refer client to physician; may be contagious; avoid affected area

Parkinson's disease

Definition/symptoms: Nervous disorder characterized by abnormally low levels of the neurotransmitter dopamine, resulting in involuntary trembling and muscle rigidity

  Indications: Massage is beneficial as part of a physician-directed treatment plan

  Contraindications: General

Poliomyelitis

Definition/symptoms: Viral infection of nerves that control skeletal muscles

  Indications: Massage is beneficial as part of a physician-directed treatment plan

  Contraindications: General

Postpolio syndrome

Definition/symptoms: Symptoms of fatigue and general muscle weakness appear years after resolution of poliomyelitis

  Indications: Massage is beneficial as part of a physician-directed treatment plan

  Contraindications: Regional; refer client to physician for specific diagnosis

Neuromuscular Processes

Multiple sclerosis

Definition/symptoms: Primary disease of the central nervous system marked by degeneration of myelin

  Indications: Massage is beneficial as part of a physician-directed treatment plan

  Contraindications: General

Spinal cord injury

Definition/symptoms: Traumatic injury or degenerative process of the spinal cord; may result from compression, cut, or tissue replacement in scarring

  Indications: Massage is beneficial as part of a physician-directed treatment plan

  Contraindications: Regional

Trigeminal neuralgia (tic douloureux)

Definition/symptoms: Compression or degeneration of fifth cranial nerve; primary symptom is recurring episodes of stabbing pain in the face

  Indications: Avoid entire area of trigeminal nerve innervation; massage may trigger pain response

  Contraindications: Regional

Miscellaneous Disorders

Seizure disorders

Definition/symptoms: Sudden bursts of abnormal neuronal activity that cause temporary changes in brain activity; may vary from mild, affecting conscious motor control or sensory perception, to severe, resulting in convulsion

  Indications: Massage may be beneficial

  Contraindications: General; follow physician's recommendation for massage

Sleep apnea

Definition/symptoms: Cessation of breathing during sleep

Indications: Stress may be a factor; massage is beneficial in reducing stress

Contraindications: Regional

Thoracic outlet syndrome

Definition/symptoms: Compression of brachial nerve plexus; primary symptom is pain that radiates to the shoulder and arm

Indications: Massage is beneficial as part of the treatment plan

Contraindications: Regional; refer client to physician for specific diagnosis

Endocrine System

Assessment parameters include fatigue, depression, changes in energy level, hyperalertness, sleep patterns, and mood. These can affect the skin, hair, and personal appearance.

Deviations that suggest the need for evaluation and referral include cold, clammy skin; numbness of fingers, toes, or mouth; rapid heartbeat, a feeling of faintness; vertigo; tremors; dyspnea (difficulty breathing); thyroid nodule; unusually warm hands and feet; and lethargy.

Specific Disease Processes

Diabetes mellitus

Definition/symptoms: Metabolic disorder; body loses the ability to oxidize carbohydrates because of faulty pancreatic activity, especially of the islets of Langerhans, which affects insulin production; symptoms include thirst, hunger, and acidosis; severe symptoms include difficulty breathing and changes in blood chemistry that lead to coma

Indications: Massage is given under supervision of the primary care physician; it is beneficial for circulation enhancement and stress reduction; exercise also is beneficial

Contraindications: General; work only under physician's supervision

Hyperglycemia

Definition/symptoms: High blood sugar, resulting from inadequate insulin in the blood; symptoms are the same as those for diabetes mellitus

Indications: See Diabetes mellitus

Contraindications: See Diabetes mellitus

Hypoglycemia

Definition/symptoms: Low blood glucose, resulting from an excess of insulin in the blood; symptoms include lightheadedness, anxiety, and forgetfulness

Indications: Dietary changes; massage is helpful and may relieve stress

Contraindications: Refer client to physician to determine the cause of low blood sugar

Hyperthyroidism

Definition/symptoms: Overproduction of thyroid hormone; can be caused by a tumor or by problems with the self-regulatory mechanism in the pituitary gland; symptoms include anxiety, bulging eyes, high metabolic rate, and nervousness

Indications: Massage is beneficial for relaxing the client

Contraindications: General; work within physician's recommendations

Hypothyroidism

Definition/symptoms: Underproduction of thyroid hormone; symptoms include sensitivity to cold, weight gain, fatigue, and dullness

Indications: Massage is beneficial for stimulating metabolic function

Contraindications: General; work within physician's recommendations

Neuropathy

Definition/symptoms: Functional disturbance or pathologic change in peripheral nervous system; symptoms include numbness, burning, and tingling pain

Indications: Massage is beneficial under medical supervision; may calm hypersensitive nerves

Contraindications: General; work under physician's direction

Cardiovascular System

Assessment parameters include skin color and appearance, respiratory rate and effort, condition of nails and nail beds (e.g., clubbing, cyanosis), pain or tenderness and points of radiation, swelling, and symmetry of chest cavity.

Deviations that suggest the need for evaluation and referral include pulse over 90 or under 60 beats per minute; dyspnea; pitting edema; distended neck veins; glossy appearance of the skin; positive Homans' sign (calf tenderness with dorsiflexion of the foot); asymmetry of limb circumference; red, warm, tender, and hard veins; edema, pain, and tenderness of extremity; clubbing of nail beds; chest pain (especially if radiating to left arm); central or peripheral cyanosis; pallor; mottling or cyanosis of a limb; stasis ulcers; and splinter hemorrhages (small red to black streaks under fingernails).

Physiologic Processes

Anemia

Definition/symptoms: Reduced red blood cell count or hemoglobin; symptoms include fatigue and pallor

Indications: Massage can be beneficial as part of the treatment plan

Contraindications: General; refer client to physician for diagnosis and proceed under physician's direction

Aneurysm

Definition/symptoms: Abnormal widening of the arterial wall; tends to form thrombi and also to burst; a pulsating bulge and pressure are felt with accompanying symptoms of pain

Indications: N/A

Contraindications: Regional; immediately refer client to physician; avoid direct heavy pressure into arterial vessels

Angina pectoris

Definition/symptoms: Chest pain caused by inadequate oxygen to heart (usually from blocked coronary arteries)

Indications: Massage is beneficial as part of a lifestyle change

Contraindications: General; massage is performed under physician's supervision

Arteriosclerosis and atherosclerosis

Definition/symptoms: Hardening of the arteries; a type of coronary heart disease; symptoms may be mild to severe; may be mistaken for other problems

Indications: Massage is beneficial as part of a lifestyle change

Contraindications: General; perform massage under physician's supervision

Congestive heart failure

Definition/symptoms: Left heart failure; inability of the left ventricle to pump effectively; one symptom is increased fluid retention

Indications: Massage is beneficial in helping diuretics remove excess fluid

Contraindications: General; must work under physician's supervision; client may have difficulty breathing in a supine position

Deep vein thrombosis

Definition/symptoms: Blood clot in deep veins; risk factor for pulmonary embolism (blood clot in the heart); often asymptomatic; symptoms may include swelling, edema, and pain described as aching and throbbing

Indications: N/A

Contraindications: Regional to general, depending on the severity of symptoms; always refer client to physician for unexplained pain; never massage over such areas

Hemophilia

Definition/symptoms: Blood clotting disorder; primary symptom is spontaneous bleeding due to inability to form clots

Indications: Extremely light energy type of massage given only under physician's direction

Contraindications: General; work only under physician's supervision

Myocardial infarction (MI)

Definition/symptoms: Death of cardiac muscle cells, usually from inadequate blood supply, often from coronary thrombosis or coronary artery disease; symptoms include severe pain in the chest or left arm, difficulty breathing, and weakness

Indications: During rehabilitation, massage can be beneficial when supervised by a physician

Contraindications: General; refer client to physician immediately

Mononucleosis

Definition/symptoms: Induced by Epstein-Barr virus; symptoms include fever, fatigue, and swollen glands

Indications: Massage is beneficial as part of the treatment plan; care must be taken with contagious conditions

Contraindications: General; refer client to physician for specific diagnosis

Phlebitis

Definition/symptoms: Inflammation of a vein; may be caused by a blood clot; symptoms include edema, stiffness, and pain; veins may streak red

Indications: N/A

Contraindications: Regional to general; see Deep vein thrombosis

Raynaud's syndrome

Definition/symptoms: Arteriospastic condition caused by vasospasms of the small cutaneous and subcutaneous arteries and arterioles; usually activated by cold but can be emotionally triggered; symptoms include skin pallor and pain

Indications: Care must be taken to avoid triggering the symptoms; interview client carefully; massage may be beneficial for stress reduction

Contraindications: Refer client to physician for specific underlying diagnosis; condition may be symptomatic of serious disorder

Syncope

Definition/symptoms: Sudden loss of strength; fainting; may be caused by a cardiac spasm resulting from closure of coronary arteries

Indications: N/A

Contraindications: General; immediately refer client to physician

Varicose veins

Definition/symptoms: Enlarged veins in which blood pools; caused by collapse of valve system; tend to form thrombi

Indications: N/A

Contraindications: Regional; avoid affected area

Lymphatic and Immune Systems

Assessment parameters include skin color and condition, evidence of eye irritation, lymph nodes, and nasal discharge/irritation.

Deviations that suggest the need for evaluation and referral include client history of chronic fatigue or recurrent physical ailments (e.g., skin, respiratory, gastrointestinal) in the absence of general illness; history of food intolerance; failure to gain weight; unexplained weight loss; rashes of unknown origin; urticaria; enlarged, tender nodes; and excessive or persistent dryness and scaliness of skin.

Specific Disease Processes

Allergy

Definition/symptoms: Hypersensitivity of immune system to relatively harmless environmental antigens; symptoms include increased mucous membrane inflammation, occasionally spastic bladder

Indications: Massage is beneficial

Contraindications: Refer client to physician for specific diagnosis

Autoimmune disease

Definition/symptoms: Disease in which the immune system attacks the body's own tissues; symptoms include inflammation, fatigue, and allergy

Indications: Massage is beneficial with physician's recommendation

Contraindications: General; refer client to physician for specific diagnosis

Chronic fatigue syndrome

Definition/symptoms: May be induced by a virus; symptoms include swollen glands, low-grade fever, muscle and joint aches, headache, and fatigue

Indications: Massage is beneficial

Contraindications: General; refer client to physician for specific diagnosis

Human immunodeficiency virus (HIV) infection

Definition/symptoms: Viral infection transmitted by means of body fluids; causes immunosuppression

Indications: Massage is beneficial with physician's recommendation; follow antiviral precautions for control of virus; 10% bleach solution; avoid body fluid contact

Contraindications: General; work with physician

Lymphedema

Definition/symptoms: Swelling of tissue caused by partial or complete blockage of lymph vessels

Indications: Massage is beneficial as part of the treatment plan and is given under the supervision of the primary care physician

Contraindications: Refer client to physician for diagnosis

The Respiratory System

Assessment parameters include the rate and pattern of respiration, chest movement, color, nodes, chest configuration, ease of chest excursions, fremitus, and pain.

Deviations that suggest the need for evaluation and referral include inspiratory flaring of the nostrils; use of accessory muscles; intercostal retractions or bulging; pursed lips on exhalation; splinting; uneven chest movement; altered tactile fremitus/crepitus (increased or decreased); cyanosis or pallor; enlarged, tender nodes; pain with breathing; and a respiratory rate over 20 respirations per minute in the absence of exertion or strong emotion.

Specific Infectious Disease Processes

Asthma

Definition/symptoms: Recurring muscle spasms in the bronchial wall accompanied by fluid retention and production of mucus; stress-specific condition

Indications: Massage is beneficial; monitor breathing closely

Contraindications: Work under direction of primary care physician

Tuberculosis

Definition/symptoms: Infectious disease caused by *Mycobacterium tuberculosis*; early stage requires testing to reveal infection; advanced cases are marked by lung destruction, coughing, fatigue, weakness, and weight loss; may be confused with bronchitis and pneumonia

Indications: Droplet transmission; contagious; be aware of sanitation

Contraindications: General; work only if physician recommends and clears for contagious condition

Upper respiratory infection (bronchitis, common cold, sinusitis, pneumonia)

Definition/symptoms: Viral or bacterial in origin; symptoms include increased production of mucus, fever, body aches, and headaches

Indications: Light massage may be beneficial to ease body ache; avoid heavy pressure; watch for contamination

Contraindications: Refer client to physician if symptoms are severe or persist longer than 2 weeks

The Gastrointestinal System

Assessment parameters include skin (see The Integumentary System, page 680); contour of abdomen (flat, rounded, concave, protuberant, distended); symmetry; observable masses; palpable masses; movement; tenderness or pain; and location and contour of umbilicus.

Deviations that suggest the need for evaluation and referral include a history of persistent or recurring nausea or vomiting; abdominal pain of unknown origin; rebound tenderness; epigastric pain that occurs 1 to 3 hours after meals; rigid or boardlike abdomen (unrelated to calisthenic exercise); persistent or increasing abdominal or epigastric pain; history of blood in stools or vomitus; difficulty swallowing; masses or nodules; enlarged, tender nodes; bulge or swelling in abdomen; change in location or inversion/eversion of umbilicus; and lesions in oral cavity or on lips or tongue.

Specific Disease Processes

Constipation

Definition/symptoms: Slow movement of bowels; hard, compacted, dry stool

Indications: Massage is beneficial; increase fiber and water consumption and moderate exercise; may be drug-related

Contraindications: Refer client to physician if severe or persistent or if a mass is felt in the large intestine

Diarrhea

Definition/symptoms: Loose bowels; excessive loss of water in stool; can be caused by a virus or bacterium or can be a symptom of other disease processes

Indications: Loose stool is not uncommon 24 hours after vigorous massage

Contraindications: Refer client to physician if symptoms persist or if dehydration is present

Flatulence

Definition/symptoms: Intestinal gas

  Indications: May be diet- or stress-related; massage may reduce stress

  Contraindications: Refer client to physician if intestinal tract is painfully distended or to rule out severe underlying condition

Halitosis

Definition/symptoms: Bad breath; may indicate digestive problems or sinus infection

  Indications: N/A

  Contraindications: Refer client to physician for specific diagnosis

Inflammatory Processes

Appendicitis

Definition/symptoms: Inflammation of the mucosal lining of the appendix, caused by trapped food or fecal matter; more common in individuals under age 25; symptoms include mild periumbilical pain, nausea, vomiting, increasing pain in the lower right quadrant, muscle spasm, and rebound tenderness

  Indications: N/A

  Contraindications: Immediately refer client to physician

Cholelithiasis and cholecystitis

  Definition/symptoms: Gallstones formed as a result of inflammation; primary symptom is severe pain in upper abdomen radiating to back and right shoulder

  Indications: N/A

  Contraindications: Immediately refer client to physician

Cirrhosis of the liver

Definition/symptoms: Chronic disease that replaces liver tissue with connective tissue; major cause is alcohol consumption; early symptoms include gas, change in bowel habits, slight weight loss, nausea in the morning, and a dull, heavy ache in the right upper quadrant of the abdomen; advanced symptoms include jaundice, peripheral edema, bleeding, and red palms

  Indications: Massage is beneficial in stress reduction and drug withdrawal

  Contraindications: Refer client to physician for diagnosis; work under physician's supervision

Colitis

Definition/symptoms: Inflammatory condition of the large intestine; one type (irritable bowel syndrome) is brought on by stress

  Indications: Painful condition; massage may be helpful in general stress and pain reduction

  Contraindications: Immediately refer client to physician; work with chronic conditions under direct supervision of physician

Crohn's disease (regional enteritis)

Definition/symptoms: Chronic relapsing inflammatory disease of the intestinal tract; symptoms include intermittent diarrhea, colicky pain in lower abdomen, fatigue, low-grade fever

  Indications: Painful condition; massage may be helpful in general stress and pain reduction

  Contraindications: Refer client to physician immediately; with chronic conditions, work under physician's direct supervision

Diverticulosis

Definition/symptoms: Formation of small pockets in the large intestine, caused by herniation of the mucosa; if pockets become inflamed, condition is called diverticulitis; symptoms include gas, diarrhea, and pain

  Indications: Diet may need adjustment to include more fiber

  Contraindications: Refer client to physician if pain or symptoms persist

Duodenal ulcer

Definition/symptoms: Ulcer caused by hyperacidity in duodenal bulb; stress-related; symptoms include burning pain that feels better after eating

  Indications: Massage is beneficial for reducing stress; lifestyle and diet changes may be necessary

  Contraindications: Refer client to physician for specific diagnosis; support physician's treatment plan

Hepatitis

Definition/symptoms: Infectious disease that has generalized effects in the body but that predominantly affects the liver; type A is common in children and in people living in institutions; it is transmitted by fecal matter, orally through contaminated food and water; usual symptoms are mild and flulike; types B and C affect all age groups and are transmitted through blood, needles, the fecal/oral route, and sexual contact

  Indications: Careful use of aseptic procedures

  Contraindications: General; refer client to physician and work only with physician's recommendation and guidelines concerning contagious condition

Gastritis

Definition/symptoms: Acute inflammation of the stomach; a common condition usually caused by irritants such as alcohol or aspirin; symptoms include pain, nausea, and belching

  Indications: Massage is beneficial because gastritis sometimes is stress related and massage may reduce stress

  Contraindications: Refer client to physician for specific diagnosis

Hernia

Definition/symptoms: Protrusion of a loop or piece of an organ or tissue through an abnormal opening; hiatal—protrusion of any structure (usually the esophagus or end of the stomach) through the hiatus of the diaphragm; inguinal—protrusion through the inguinal ring, causing swelling of the scrotum and possibly a medical emergency; umbilical—protrusion at the umbilicus; in inguinal and umbilical hernias, weakness may be felt in the abdominal wall

  Indications: N/A

  Contraindications: Refer client to physician; avoid area

Pancreatitis

Definition/symptoms: Inflammation of the pancreas; may be present with diabetes and is aggravated by consumption of alcohol; one symptom is severe abdominal pain

Indications: Painful condition; massage may be helpful in general stress and pain reduction

Contraindications: Refer client to physician immediately; with chronic conditions, work under physician's direct supervision

Stress ulcer

Definition/symptoms: Ulcer related to severe stress (e.g., trauma, burns, long-term illness); symptoms similar to those seen in gastritis

Indications: Massage is beneficial for reducing stress; lifestyle and dietary changes may be necessary

Contraindications: Refer client to physician for specific diagnosis; support physician's treatment plan

Ulcer

Definition/symptoms: Peptic ulcer—break or open sore not covered by protective mucus in the gastrointestinal wall that is exposed to pepsin and gastric juice; often caused by alcohol, pepsin, bile salts, and stress

Indications: Massage is beneficial to reduce stress levels; lifestyle and dietary changes may be necessary

Contraindications: Refer client to physician for specific diagnosis; support physician's treatment plan

The Metabolic System

Assessment parameters include eating patterns, skin, hair, nails, weight and height data, and general health status.

Deviations that suggest the need for evaluation and referral include significant underweight or overweight, evidence of nutritional deficiencies (e.g., dry hair or skin, fatigue), and respiratory problems.

Specific Disease Processes

Cystic fibrosis

Definition/symptoms: Inherited disorder that disrupts cell transport and causes exocrine glands to produce thick secretions; thick pancreatic secretions may block the pancreatic duct

Indications: Massage is beneficial with specific training to loosen mucus with percussive techniques

Contraindications: General; work under direct care of physician

Malnutrition

Definition/symptoms: Deficiency of calories in general and often in protein; malnutrition may be caused by increased nutrient demand on the body without sufficient food intake (e.g., severe burns, illness, or lack of food, especially protein); symptoms include flaking skin, brittle hair, hair loss, slow-healing sores, bruising, susceptibility to infection, and fatigue; more common in children and the elderly and with drug and alcohol abuse; be aware of eating disorders. (Note:

Malnutrition also can be caused by insufficient or improper digestion and absorption of food.)

Indications: With anorexia or bulimia, massage may be beneficial for stress reduction

Contraindications: Refer client to physician for diagnosis and treatment plan

Obesity

Definition/symptoms: Excess body fat (over 30% of normal body weight); risks of obesity include diabetes, stroke, heart attack, gallstones, and high blood pressure

Indications: Morbid obesity (over 60% of normal body fat) may cause difficulty positioning client; fluid retention, risk of blood pressure fluctuation, and interference with breathing are other possible problems; may need to alter massage position

Contraindications: Refer client for nutritional and dietary consultation

The Genitourinary System

Assessment parameters include pain (groin, periumbilical, flank, abdominal, dysuria), patterns of urination and output, urine consistency (color, concentration, or hematuria), edema (facial, ankle), weight changes, skin changes, discharge, and masses.

Deviations that suggest the need for evaluation and referral include a history of unusual vaginal, urethral, or nipple discharge; breast, penile, scrotal, or inguinal masses or lumps; genital blisters, lesions, or growths; changes in urinary frequency, output, or control or in urine characteristics; sudden weight gain, abnormal periods, edema, skin abnormalities, pain or tenderness (costovertebral angle, abdominal area, or low back), masses or lumps, and tender or enlarged nodes.

Specific Disease Processes

Breast cancer

Definition/symptoms: Abnormal, malignant tissue growth on or in the breast; most common cause of cancer in women; encourage monthly breast self-examination and regular checkups

Indications: Be aware of changes in tissue around axillary region

Contraindications: If changes are noted, refer client to physician; early diagnosis is important

Dysmenorrhea

Definition/symptoms: Painful menstruation; may be caused by endometriosis (abnormal growth and distribution of uterine lining); symptoms include heavy periods and clotting

Indications: Massage is beneficial for stress reduction and pain

Contraindications: Refer client to physician for diagnosis

Pelvic inflammatory disease

Definition/symptoms: Inflammation of the uterus, fallopian tubes, ovaries, and surrounding tissue; infection often is introduced by intercourse; symptoms include pain and tenderness in the lower abdomen, backache, pain during intercourse, heavy periods, and vaginal discharge

Indications: N/A

Contraindications: Refer client to physician for diagnosis

Premenstrual syndrome (PMS)

Definition/symptoms: Occurs approximately 1 week before onset of period; symptoms include breast tenderness and swelling, fluid retention, headache, irritability, anxiety, depression, and poor concentration

Indications: Massage is beneficial

Contraindications: Refer client to physician if symptoms are severe

Testicular cancer

Definition/symptoms: Malignant growth in testicle; usually a slow-growing lump

Indications: N/A

Contraindications: Refer client to physician immediately if he mentions such a symptom

Toxic shock syndrome

Definition/symptoms: Staphylococcal bacterial infection that can arise from the use of tampons; can be life-threatening; initial flulike symptoms with red rash; can be prevented by changing tampons several times a day. (NOTE: This condition has occurred in women who do not use tampons.)

Indications: N/A

Contraindications: Immediately refer client to physician

Urinary tract infection

Definition/symptoms: Acute pyelonephritis—inflammation of kidney and pelvis; usually occurs in women with abrupt onset of fever, chills, malaise, and back pain, also tenderness on palpation over the costovertebral region; cystitis—affects men and women, usually caused by transmission of bacteria through the urethra due to improper cleansing after bowel movement; may cause pain in lower abdomen above pubic bone and low back ache

Indications: N/A

Contraindications: Refer client to physician for diagnosis and treatment

Sexually Transmitted Diseases

Genital herpes

Definition/symptoms: Viral infection; primary symptom is blisterlike lesions

Indications: N/A

Contraindications: Refer client to physician; follow sanitation requirements

Gonorrhea

Definition/symptoms: Bacterial infection; may be asymptomatic, or symptoms may include painful urination and pus or cloudy discharge

Indications: N/A

Contraindications: Refer client to physician; contagious; follow sanitation requirements

Human immunodeficiency virus (HIV) infection

Definition/symptoms: Viral infection transmitted by blood and body fluids

Indications: Massage is beneficial with physician's recommendation; follow antiviral precautions for control of virus with 10% bleach solution; avoid body fluid contact; immediately wash area thoroughly with antiviral agent should body fluid contact occur

Contraindications: Refer client to physician for treatment; follow sanitation requirements

Syphilis

Definition/symptoms: Bacterial infection; in stage one, red sore (chancre) appears; in stage two, flulike symptoms develop; in stage three, the disease attacks the brain and nervous tissue

Indications: N/A

Contraindications: Refer client to physician; contagious; follow sanitation requirements

Psychiatric Disorders

Assessment parameters include general appearance and behavior, sensorium, mood and affect, thought content, and intellectual capacity.

Deviations that suggest the need for evaluation and referral include marked changes in posture; dress and hygiene; motor activity; speech and facial expression; lack of orientation to time, place, or person; inappropriate manifestation of anxiety, agitation, anger, euphoria, or depression; presence of hallucinations, delusions, paranoia, and illusions; changes in usual intellectual capacity; or suicidal or homicidal ideation.

Specific Disease Processes

Anxiety, depression (bipolar or manic/depressive disorders)

Definition/symptoms: All types of emotionally erratic or unusual behavior may be symptomatic; listen to conversation carefully; often symptoms are subtle and client may try to hide discomfort; symptoms may include anorexia (self-starvation); bulimia (eating and vomiting and/or laxative abuse); addictive disorders; chemical and compulsive behavior; somatization disorder; manifestation of physical pain or symptoms from emotional causes; and post-traumatic stress disorders, often associated with sexual and physical childhood abuse

Indications: Massage is beneficial under the direction of a psychiatrist or psychologist; always work within physician's or counselor's treatment parameters

Contraindications: Refer client to physician for counseling care; client often will dissociate from the body or will be hypersensitive to stimulation; the therapist must be sensitive to psychiatric issues because often the massage therapist is the first person with whom the client shares these issues; it is important to refer the client for competent counseling and psychiatric care

Skin Pathology:
Common Skin Disorders

The following photos depict commonly encountered skin disorders. Please note that skin problems may result from various causes, such as parasitic infestations; fungal, bacterial, or viral infections; reactions to substances encountered externally or taken internally; or new growths. Many skin manifestations have no known cause, and others are hereditary.

A, Basal cell carcinoma. **B,** Common warts. (From Thibodeau GA, Patton KT: *The human body in health and disease,* ed 3, St Louis, 2002, Mosby.) **C,** Contact dermatitis from shampoo. (Reprinted with permission from the American Academy of Dermatology. All rights reserved.) **D,** Contact dermatitis from shoes. (Reprinted with permission from the American Academy of Dermatology. All rights reserved.) **E,** Contact dermatitis from application of Lanacane. (From Zitelli BJ, Davis HW, editors: *Atlas of pediatric physical diagnosis,* ed 5, Philadelphia, 2007, Mosby.) **F,** Dermatitis. (From LaFleur Brooks M: *Exploring medical language: a student-directed approach,* ed 5, St Louis, 2002, Mosby.) **G,** Furuncle (boil). (From Thibodeau GA, Patton KT: *The human body in health and disease,* ed 3, St Louis, 2002, Mosby.) **H,** Herpes zoster (shingles). (From LaFleur Brooks M: *Exploring medical language: a student-directed approach,* ed 5, St Louis, 2002, Mosby.) **I,** Impetigo contagiosa. (From LaFleur Brooks M: *Exploring medical language: a student-directed approach,* ed 5, St Louis, 2002, Mosby.)

Continued

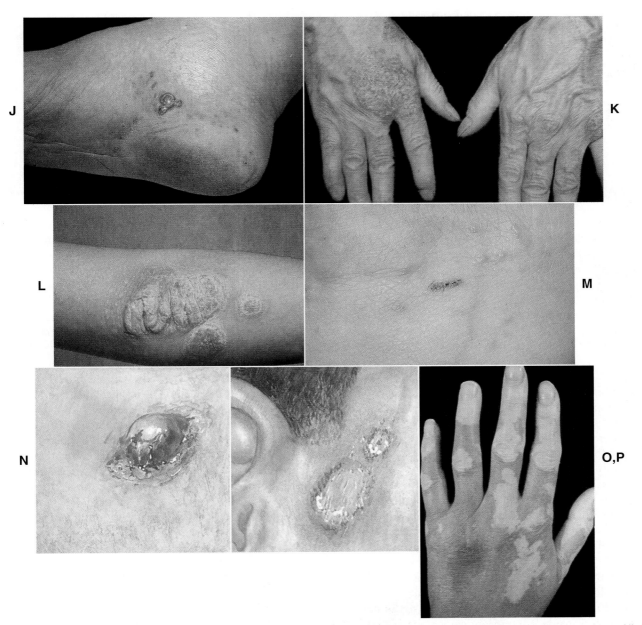

J, Kaposi's sarcoma. **K,** Nummular eczema. (Reprinted with permission from the American Academy of Dermatology. All rights reserved.) **L,** Psoriasis. (Reprinted with permission from the American Academy of Dermatology. All rights reserved.) **M,** Scabies. (From Thibodeau GA, Patton KT: *The human body in health and disease,* ed 3, St Louis, 2002, Mosby.) **N,** Squamous cell carcinoma. (From LaFleur Brooks M: *Exploring medical language: a student-directed approach,* ed 5, St Louis, 2002, Mosby.) **O,** Tinea corporis (ringworm). (From LaFleur Brooks M: *Exploring medical language: a student-directed approach,* ed 5, St Louis, 2002, Mosby.) **P,** Vitiligo. (Reprinted with permission from the American Academy of Dermatology. All rights reserved.)

Basic Pharmacology for the Massage Therapist

OVERVIEW*

Any chemical that affects the physiologic processes of a living organism can broadly be defined as a drug. The study or science of drugs is known as pharmacology. Pharmacology encompasses a variety of topics, including the following:

- Absorption
- Biochemical effects
- Biotransformation (metabolism)
- Distribution
- Drug history
- Drug origin
- Excretion
- Mechanisms of action
- Physical and chemical properties
- Physical effects
- Drug receptor mechanisms
- Therapeutic (beneficial) effects
- Toxic (harmful) effects

Pharmacology is an extensive science that incorporates several interrelated areas: pharmaceutics, pharmacokinetics, pharmacodynamics, pharmacotherapeutics, pharmacognosy, and toxicology. The various drugs discussed in each chapter of this text are described from the standpoint of one or more of these five areas.

Throughout the process of development, a drug will acquire at least three different names. The chemical name describes the drug's chemical composition and molecular structure. The generic name, or nonproprietary name, is given to the drug by the United States Adopted Names (USAN) Council. It is often much shorter and simpler than the chemical name. The generic name is used in most official drug compendiums to list drugs. The trade name, or proprietary name, is the drug's registered trademark and indicates that its commercial use is restricted to the owner of the patent for the drug. The owner is usually the manufacturer of the drug. Trade names are generally created by the manufacturer with marketability in mind. For this reason, they are usually shorter and easier to pronounce and remember than generic drug names. The patent life of a newly discovered drug molecule is normally 17 years. This is the length of time from patent approval until patent expiration. Because the research processes for new drug development normally require about 10 years, a drug manufacturer generally has the remaining 7 years for sales profits before patent expiration. A significant amount of these profits serves merely to offset the multimillion-dollar costs for research and development of the drug.

After the patent expires for a given drug, other manufacturers may legally begin to manufacturer generic drugs with the same active ingredient. At this point, the drug price usually falls substantially, which offers many patients and third-party payers the benefit of savings on the generic (vs. the original brand name) drug.

Three basic areas of pharmacology—pharmaceutics, pharmacokinetics, and pharmacodynamics—describe the relationship between the dose of a drug given to a patient and the activity of that drug in treating the patient's disorder. Pharmaceutics includes the study of how various dosage forms (e.g., injection, capsule, controlled-release tablet) influence the way in which the body metabolizes a drug and the way in which the drug affects the body. Pharmacokinetics is the study of what the body does to the drug molecules. Pharmacokinetics involves the processes of absorption, distribution, metabolism, and excretion. These four phases and their relationship to drug and drug metabolite concentrations are determined for various body sites over specified periods. The onset of action, the peak effect of a drug, and the duration of action of a drug are all part of the drug's pharmacokinetics. Pharmacodynamics, on the other hand, is the study of what the drug does to the body. Pharmacodynamics involves drug-receptor interactions. Receptor theory assumes that all drugs perform their unique actions at chemically specific receptor sites in various tissues. Receptors are usually specialized protein molecules on the outer surfaces of cells or within cells to which drug molecules bind to exert their effects. It must be noted, however, that not all mechanisms of action have been identified for all drugs. Thus, a drug may be said to have an unknown or unclear mechanism of action, even though it has observable therapeutic effects in the body.

Pharmacotherapeutics (also called therapeutics) focuses on the use of drugs and the clinical indications for administering drugs to prevent and treat diseases. It defines the principles of drug actions—the cellular processes that change in response to the presence of drug molecules. Empirical therapeutics refers to drug therapy that is effective but for which the mechanism of drug action is unknown. Rational therapeutics is drug therapy in which specific evidence has been obtained for the mechanisms of drug action. Some drug mechanisms of action are more clearly understood than others.

The study of the adverse effects of drugs and other chemicals on living systems is known as toxicology. Toxic effects are often an extension of a drug's therapeutic action. Therefore, toxicology often involves overlapping principles of both pharmacotherapy and toxicology. The study of natural (vs. synthetic) drug sources (both plants and animals) is called pharmacognosy.

In summary, pharmacology is a very dynamic science incorporating several different disciplines (as mentioned earlier). Traditionally, chemistry has been seen as the primary basis of pharmacology, but pharmacology also relies heavily on physiology and biology.

Pharmaceutics

Different drug dosage forms have different pharmaceutical properties. Dosage form design determines the rate at which drug dissolution (dissolving of solid dosage forms and their absorption [e.g., from gastrointestinal (GI) tract fluids]). A drug to be ingested orally may be taken in either a solid form (tablet, capsule, or powder) or a liquid form (solution or suspension). Oral drugs that are liquids (e.g., elixirs, syrups) are already dissolved and are usually absorbed more quickly than solid dosage forms. Enteric-coated tablets, on the other hand, have a coating that prevents them from being broken down in an acidic pH environment and therefore are not absorbed until they reach the higher (more alkaline) pH of the intestines. This pharmaceutical property results in slower dissolution and therefore slower absorption. Sometimes the size of the particles within a capsule can make different capsules containing the same drug dissolve at different rates, become absorbed at different rates, and thus have different times to onset of action. A prime example is the difference between micronized glyburide and nonmicronized glyburide. Micronized glyburide reaches a maximum concentration peak faster than does the nonmicronized formulation because of how the dosage form is pharmaceutically engineered.

A variety of dosage forms exist to provide both accurate and convenient drug delivery systems. These delivery systems are designed to achieve a desired therapeutic response with minimal adverse effects. Many dosage forms have been developed to encourage patient compliance with the medication regimen. Convenience of administration correlates strongly with medication compliance. Many of the extended-release oral dosage forms were designed with this in mind, as they often require fewer daily doses.

The specific characteristics of various dosage forms have a large impact on how and to what extent the drug is absorbed. If a drug is to work at a specific site in the body, either it must be applied directly at that site in an active form or it must have a way of getting to that site. Oral dosage forms rely on gastric and intestinal enzymes and pH environments to break the medication down into particles that are small enough to be absorbed into the circulation. Once absorbed through the mucosa of the stomach or intestines, the drug is then transported to the site of action by blood or lymph.

Many topically applied dosage forms work directly on the surface of the skin. Therefore, when the drug is applied, it is already in a dosage form that allows it to act immediately. With other topical dosage forms, the skin acts as a barrier through which the drug must pass to get into the circulation; once there, the drug is then carried to its site of action (e.g., fentanyl transdermal patch for pain).

Dosage forms that are administered via injection are called parenteral forms. They must have certain characteristics to be safe and effective. The arteries and veins that carry drugs throughout the body can easily be damaged if the drug is too concentrated or corrosive. The pH of injections must be very similar to the blood to be safely administered. Parenteral dosage forms that are injected intravenously or intraarterially are immediately placed into solution in the bloodstream and do not have to be dissolved in the body. Therefore, 100% absorption is assumed to occur immediately upon intravenous or intraarterial injection. The intraarterial route is used much less commonly than the intravenous route but is commonly used in intensive care unit and oncology care settings.

Pharmacokinetics

A particular drug's onset of action, peak effect, and duration of action are all characteristics defined by pharmacokinetics. Pharmacokinetics is the study of what actually happens to a drug from the time it is put into the body until the parent drug and all metabolites have left the body. Thus, drug absorption into, distribution and metabolism within, and excretion from a living organism represent the combined focus of pharmacokinetics.

Absorption

Absorption is the movement of a drug from its site of administration into the bloodstream for distribution to the tissues. A term used to express the extent of drug absorption is bioavailability. For example, a drug that is absorbed from the intestine must first pass through the liver before it reaches the systemic circulation. If the drug is metabolized in the liver or excreted in the bile, some of the active drug will be inactivated or diverted before it can reach the general circulation and its intended sites of action. This is known as the first-pass effect, and it reduces the bioavailability of the drug to less than 100%. Many drugs administered by mouth have a bioavailability of less than 100%, whereas drugs administered by the intravenous route are 100% bioavailable, as noted earlier. If two medications have the same bioavailability and same concentration of active ingredient, they are said to be bioequivalent (e.g., a brand-name drug and the same generic drug).

Various factors affect the rate of drug absorption. These include the presence of food or fluids ingested with the drug, the dosage formulation, the status of the absorptive surface, the rate of blood flow to the small intestine, the acidity of the stomach, and GI motility. How a drug is administered, or its route of administration, also affects the rate and extent of absorption of that drug. Although a number of dosage formulations are available for delivering medications to the body, they can all be categorized into three basic routes of administration: enteral (GI tract), parenteral, and topical. Various administration routes and their effects on absorption are examined in detail in the following sections. Drug distribution, metabolism, and excretion are then discussed.

Enteral

In enteral drug administration, the drug is absorbed into the systemic circulation through the mucosa of the stomach or small intestine. The rate of absorption of enterally administered drugs can be altered by many factors. Depending on the particular drug, it may be extensively metabolized in the liver before it reaches the systemic circulation. Normally, orally administered drugs are absorbed from the intestinal lumen into the mesenteric blood system and conveyed by the portal vein to the liver. Once the drug is in the liver, the hepatic enzyme systems metabolize it, and the remaining active ingredients are passed into the general circulation. As noted previously, this initial metabolism of a drug and its passage from the liver into the circulation is called the first-pass effect. If a large proportion of a drug is chemically processed into inactive metabolites in the liver, then a much smaller amount of drug will pass into the circulation (i.e., will be bioavailable). Such a drug is said to have a high first-pass effect (e.g., oral nitrates).

The same drug given intravenously will bypass the liver. This prevents the first-pass effect from taking place, and therefore more of the drug reaches the circulation. For this reason, parenteral doses of drugs with a high first-pass effect are often much smaller than enterally administered (oral) doses, yet they produce the same pharmacologic response.

Many factors can alter the absorption of enterally administered drugs, including acid changes within the stomach, absorption changes in the intestines, and the presence or absence of food and fluid. Various factors that affect the acidity of the stomach include the time of day; the age of the patient; and the presence and types of any medications, foods, or beverages. If food is in the stomach during the dissolution of an orally administered medication, this may interfere with the drug's dissolution and absorption and delay its transit from the stomach to the small intestine, where most drugs are absorbed. On the other hand, food may enhance the absorption of some fat-soluble drugs (depending on the fat content of the food) or drugs that are more easily broken down in an acidic environment. (Food in the stomach increases gastric acid production.)

Before orally administered drugs are passed into the portal circulation of the liver, they are absorbed in the small intestine, which has an enormous surface area. Drug absorption may be altered in patients who have had portions of the small intestine removed because of disease. Anticholinergic drugs may slow the GI transit time or the time it takes for substances in the stomach to be dissolved and absorbed into the intestines. This may allow more time for an acid-susceptible drug to be in contact with the acid in the stomach and subsequently to be broken down, which reduces drug absorption. The stomach and small intestine are highly vascularized. When blood flow to that area is decreased, absorption may also be decreased. Sepsis and exercise are examples of circumstances under which blood flow to the GI tract is often reduced. In both cases, blood tends to be routed to the heart and other vital organs. In the case of exercise, it is also routed to the skeletal muscles.

Sublingual and Buccal

Drugs administered by the sublingual route are absorbed into the highly vascularized tissue under the tongue—the oral mucosa. Sublingual nitroglycerin is an example. Sublingually administered drugs are absorbed rapidly because the area under the tongue has a large blood supply. These drugs bypass the liver and yet are systemically bioavailable. The same concepts apply for drugs administered by the buccal route (the oral mucosa between the cheek and the gum). Through these routes, drugs such as nitroglycerin are absorbed rapidly into the bloodstream and delivered to their site of action (e.g., coronary arteries).

Parenteral

For most medications, the parenteral route is the fastest route by which a drug can be absorbed, followed by the enteral and topical routes. Parenteral is a general term meaning any route of administration other than the GI tract. Most commonly it refers to injection by any method, although topical and transdermal medications can also be considered parenteral dosage forms (see later), as can sublingual and buccal medications. Intravenous injection delivers the drug directly into the circulation, where it is distributed with the blood throughout the body. An intravenous drug formulation is thus absorbed the fastest. At the other end of the spectrum are transdermal patches, intramuscular injections, and subcutaneous injections. These drug formulations are usually absorbed over a period of several hours, days, or weeks.

Drugs can be injected intradermally, subcutaneously, intraarterially, intramuscularly, intrathecally, intraarticularly, or intravenously. Medications given by the parenteral route also have the advantage of bypassing the first-pass effect of the liver. The parenteral route of administration offers an alternative route of delivery for those medications that cannot be given orally. The problems posed by acid changes in the stomach, absorption changes in the intestines (e.g., following intestinal surgery), and the presence or absence of food and fluid are no longer a concern. There are fewer obstacles to absorption with parenteral administration than with enteral administration of drugs. However, drugs that are administered by the parenteral route must still be absorbed into cells and tissues before they can exert their pharmacologic effect.

Subcutaneous, Intradermal, and Intramuscular

Parenteral injections into the fatty subcutaneous tissues under the dermal layer of skin are referred to as subcutaneous injections, whereas injections under the more superficial skin layers immediately underneath the epidermal layer of skin and into the dermal layer are known as intradermal injections. Parenteral injections given into the muscle beneath the subcutaneous fatty tissue are referred to as intramuscular injections. Muscles have a greater blood supply than does the skin; therefore, drugs injected intramuscularly are typically absorbed faster than drugs injected subcutaneously. Absorption from either of these sites may be increased by applying heat to the injection site or by massaging the site. Both increase blood flow to the area, thereby enhancing absorption. Most intramuscularly injected drugs are absorbed over several hours. However, specially formulated long-acting intramuscular dosage forms known as depot drugs are designed for slow absorption and may be absorbed over a period of several days to a few months or longer. The intramuscular corticosteroid known as methylprednisolone acetate (Kenalog injection) can provide antiinflammatory effects for several weeks. The intramuscular contraceptive medroxyprogesterone acetate (Depo-Provera) normally prevents pregnancy for 3 months per dose. The subcutaneously administered drug insulin glargine (Lantus) is a long-acting insulin product that is now in common use.

In contrast, the presence of cold, hypotension, or poor peripheral blood flow compromises the circulation, reducing drug activity by reducing drug delivery to the tissues.

Topical

Topical routes of drug administration involve the application of medications to various body surfaces. Several different topical drug delivery systems exist. Topically administered drugs can be applied to the skin, eyes, ears, nose, lungs, rectum, or vagina. As with the enteral and parenteral routes, there are benefits and drawbacks to use of the topical route of administration. Topical application delivers a more uniform amount of drug over a longer period of time, but the effects of the drug are usually slower in their onset and more prolonged in their duration of action. This can be a problem if the patient begins to experience adverse effects from the drug and a considerable amount of drug has already been absorbed into the subcutaneous or mucosal tissues. All topical routes of drug administration also avoid first-pass effects of the liver, with the exception of rectal drug administration. Because the rectum is part of the GI tract, some drug will be absorbed into the capillaries that feed the portal vein to the liver. However, some drugs will also be absorbed locally into the perirectal tissues. Therefore, rectally administered drugs are said to have a mixed first-pass and non–first-pass absorption and metabolism.

Topical ointments, gels, and creams are common types of topically administered drugs. Examples include sunscreens, antibiotics, and nitroglycerin ointment. The drawback to their use is that their systemic absorption is often erratic and unreliable. Generally, these medications are used for local effects, but some are used for systemic effects (e.g., nitroglycerin ointment for maintenance treatment of angina). Topically applied drugs can also be used in the treatment of various illnesses of the eyes, ears, and sinuses. Eye, ear, and nose drops are administered primarily for local and not systemic effects, whereas nasal sprays may be used for both (e.g., oxymetazoline for nasal sinus congestion, sumatriptan for migraine headaches). Rectally administered drugs are often given for systemic effects (e.g., antinausea, analgesia), but they are also used to treat disease within the rectum or adjacent bowel (e.g., antiinflammatory ointment for hemorrhoids, corticosteroid enemas for colitis). Vaginal medications may also be given for systemic effects (e.g., progestational hormone therapy) but are more commonly used for local effects (e.g., treatment of vaginal infection).

Transdermal

Transdermal drug delivery through adhesive drug patches is a more elaborate topical route of drug administration that is commonly used for systemic drug effects. Some examples of drugs administered by this route are fentanyl (for pain), nitroglycerin (for angina), nicotine (for smoking cessation), estrogen (for menopausal symptoms), and clonidine (for hypertension). Transdermal patches are usually designed to deliver a constant amount of drug per unit of time for a specified time period. For example, a nitroglycerin patch may deliver 0.1 or 0.2 mg of drug in a 24-hour period, whereas a fentanyl patch may deliver 25 to 100 mcg/hr of fentanyl for a 72-hour period. Transdermal drug delivery also offers the advantage of bypassing the liver and its first-pass effects. It is suitable for patients who cannot tolerate orally administered medications and in other situations provides a practical and convenient method for drug delivery. The design of the drug delivery system in a specific transdermal patch determines its duration of action.

Inhaled

Inhalation is another type of topical drug administration. Inhaled drugs are delivered to the lungs as micrometer-sized drug particles. This small drug size is necessary for the drug to be transported to the small air sacs within the lungs (alveoli). Once the small particles of drug are in the alveoli, drug absorption is fairly rapid. At this site the thin-walled pulmonary alveolus is in contact with the capillaries, where the drug can be absorbed quickly. Many pulmonary and other types of diseases can be treated with such topically applied (inhaled) drugs. Examples of inhaled drugs are pentamidine, which is used to treat Pneumocystis jirovecii (formerly Pneumocystis carinii) infections in the lung; albuterol, which is used to treat bronchial constriction in individuals with asthma; and vasopressin, which is used to treat diabetes insipidus.

Distribution

Distribution refers to the transport of a drug in the body by the bloodstream to its site of action. The areas to which the drug is distributed first are those that are most extensively supplied with blood. Areas of rapid distribution include the heart, liver, kidneys, and brain. Areas of slower distribution include muscle, skin, and fat. Once a drug enters the bloodstream (circulation), it is distributed throughout the body. At this point it is also beginning to be eliminated by the organs that metabolize and excrete drugs—primarily the liver and the kidneys. Drug molecules can be freely distributed to extravascular tissue (outside the blood vessels) to reach their site of action only if they are not bound to plasma proteins. If a drug is bound to plasma proteins, the drug-protein complex is generally too large to pass through the walls of blood capillaries into tissues. There are three primary proteins that bind to and carry drugs in the bloodstream throughout the body: albumin, α1-acid glycoprotein, and corticosteroid-binding globulin. By far the most important of these is albumin. As the most common blood protein, albumin carries the majority of protein-bound drug molecules. If a given drug binds to plasma proteins as part of its chemical attributes, then there is only a limited amount of drug that is not bound to protein. This unbound portion is pharmacologically active and is considered "free" drug, whereas "bound" drug is pharmacologically inactive. Certain conditions that cause low albumin levels, such as extensive burns, malnourished states, and negative nitrogen balance, result in the presence of a larger fraction of free (unbound and active) drug. This can raise the risk of drug toxicity.

When an individual is taking two medications that are highly protein bound, the medications may compete for binding sites on plasma proteins. Because of this competition, less of one or both of the drugs binds to the proteins. Consequently, there is more free, unbound drug. This can lead to an unpredictable drug response called a drug-drug interaction. A drug-drug interaction occurs when the presence of one drug decreases or increases the actions of another drug administered concurrently (given at the same time).

A theoretical volume, called the volume of distribution, is sometimes used to describe the various areas in which drugs may be distributed. These areas, or compartments, may be the blood (intravascular space), total body water, body fat, or other body tissues and organs. Typically a drug that is highly water soluble will have a small volume of distribution and high blood concentrations. In other words, the drug tends to stay within the blood because of its high water content. The opposite is true for drugs that are highly fat soluble. Fat-soluble drugs have a large volume of distribution and low blood concentrations. This is because they tend to be chemically repelled by the high water content of the blood and more attracted by the relatively low water content and higher fat content of the tissues. Drugs that are water soluble and highly protein bound are more strongly bound to proteins in the blood and are less likely to be absorbed into tissues. Because of this, their distribution and onset of action can be slow. Drugs that are highly lipid soluble and poorly bound to protein are more easily taken up into tissues and distributed throughout the body. They may also be reabsorbed back into the circulation from tissue.

There are some sites in the body into which it may be very difficult to distribute a drug. These sites typically either have a poor blood supply (e.g., bone) or have physiologic barriers that make it difficult for drugs to pass through (e.g., the brain due to the blood-brain barrier).

Metabolism

Metabolism is also referred to as biotransformation because it involves the biochemical alteration of a drug into an inactive metabolite, a more soluble compound, or a more potent active metabolite (as in the conversion of an inactive prodrug to its active form). Metabolism is the next step after absorption and distribution. The organ most responsible for the metabolism of drugs is the liver. Other metabolic tissues include skeletal muscle, kidneys, lungs, plasma, and intestinal mucosa.

Hepatic biotransformation involves the activity of a very large class of enzymes known as cytochrome P-450 enzymes (or simply P-450 enzymes), also known as microsomal enzymes. These enzymes control a variety of biochemical reactions that aid in the metabolism of medications and are largely targeted against lipid-soluble, nonpolar (no charge) drugs, which are typically very difficult to eliminate. These include the majority of medications. Those medications with water-soluble (polar) molecules may be more easily metabolized by simpler chemical reactions such as hydrolysis (splitting by water molecules). Drug molecules that are the metabolic targets of specific enzymes are said to be substrates of those enzymes. Specific P-450 enzymes are identified by standardized number and letter designations.

The biotransformation capabilities of the liver can vary considerably from patient to patient.

Delayed drug metabolism results in the accumulation of the drug and prolongation of the effects of or responses to the drug. Stimulating drug metabolism can thus cause diminishing pharmacologic effects. This often occurs with the repeated administration of some drugs that can stimulate the formation of new microsomal enzymes. Such drugs are said to be enzyme inducers. Conversely, many other drugs inhibit various classes of drug-metabolizing enzymes and are called enzyme inhibitors. This can lead to drug toxicity.

Excretion

Excretion is the elimination of drugs from the body. Whether they are parent compounds or active or inactive metabolites, all drugs must eventually be removed from the body. The primary organ responsible for this elimination is the kidney. Two other organs that play an important role in the excretion of drugs are the liver and the bowel. Most drugs are metabolized in the liver by various glucuronidases and by hydroxylation and acetylation. Therefore, by the time most drugs reach the kidneys, they have been extensively metabolized, and only a relatively small fraction of the original drug is excreted as the original compound. Other drugs may circumvent metabolism and reach the kidneys in their original form. Drugs that have been metabolized by the liver become more polar and water soluble. This makes their elimination by the kidneys much easier, because the urinary tract is water based. The kidneys themselves are also capable of forming glucuronides and sulfates from various drugs and their metabolites, although usually to a lesser extent than the liver.

The actual act of renal excretion is accomplished through glomerular filtration, active tubular reabsorption, and active tubular secretion. Free (unbound) water-soluble drugs and metabolites go through passive glomerular filtration, which takes place between the blood vessels of the afferent arterioles and the glomeruli. Many substances present in the nephrons go through active reabsorption at the level of the tubules, where they are taken back up into the systemic circulation and transported away from the kidney. This process is an attempt by the body to retain needed substances. Some substances may also be secreted into the nephron from the vasculature surrounding it.

The excretion of drugs by the intestines is another common route of elimination. This process is referred to as biliary excretion. Drugs that are eliminated by this route are taken up by the liver, released into the bile, and eliminated in the feces. Once certain drugs, such as fat-soluble drugs, are in the bile, they may be reabsorbed into the bloodstream, returned to the liver, and again secreted into the bile. This process is called enterohepatic recirculation. Enterohepatically recirculated drugs persist in the body for much longer periods. Less common routes of elimination are the lungs and the sweat, salivary, and mammary glands. Depending on the drug, these organs and glands can be highly effective eliminators.

Information to Help Clarify Medication Actions

A massage therapist needs to understand why a patient is taking a medication and the action of that medication to be able to determine the potential interaction of the drug with the physiologic effects of massage and the adjustments to massage that may be necessary. The following information needs to be gathered. Most of it can be found in a drug consult. The patient may be able to supply information, and supervising medical personnel also can explain the actions of medications.

- Drug name (generic name and brand name).
- Reason the patient is taking the drug.
- What does the medicine do?
- When and how is the medication taken?
- What are the possible side effects (reactions of the body to the medicine)?
- Will the medicine react with any other medicines, food, or drinks?
- Should any activities be avoided?
- Are there any signs that indicate that the medicine is working?

COMMON MEDICATIONS AND POSSIBLE IMPLICATIONS FOR MASSAGE

The information in the following sections can help the massage practitioner determine what interaction, if any, massage may have with a pharmaceutical. General categories and examples are given for each classification. This is not meant to be an exhaustive list, but rather a general guide. It is important to research any medication, vitamin, or herb a client is taking for its action in the body and possible interaction with massage.

Cardiovascular Medications

Vasodilators

Examples: Nitroglycerin, isosorbide dinitrate

Vasodilating medications cause the blood vessels to dilate (widen). Some of the antihypertensive agents lower blood pressure by dilating the arteries or veins. Other vasodilators are used in the treatment of stroke and diseases characterized by poor circulation.

Implications for massage: Massage has a mild peripheral vasodilatory effect. The action of the medications may increase the effect of the massage.

Antianginal Drugs

Examples: Isosorbide dinitrate (Dilate-SR, ISMO, Iso-Bid, Isordil, Sorbitrate, Sorbitrate-SA)

Antianginals are prescribed in cases of an insufficient supply of blood (and consequently oxygen) to the heart. These medications act by increasing the amount of oxygen that reaches the heart muscle.

Implications for massage: See implications for vasodilators.

Beta Blockers

Examples: Acebutolol, atenolol, betaxolol, bisoprolol, labetalol, metoprolol, nadolol, pindolol, propranolol, timolol

Beta-blocking medications block nerve stimulation of the heart and blood vessels, slowing the heart rate and reducing high blood pressure. They are used in the treatment of a wide range of diseases, including angina, hypertension, migraine headaches, and arrhythmias.

Implications for massage: These drugs may distort the expected effect of the massage. Caution is warranted, and the massage therapist should watch for any exaggerated effects. The client may be susceptible to cold. Massage may help with the constipation that can be a side effect of these drugs. The blood pressure–lowering effect of massage may result in dizziness after the massage. Have the client contract and relax the leg muscles for 1 to 2 minutes before getting off the massage table.

Calcium Channel Blockers

Examples: Diltiazem, nifedipine, verapamil

This group of medications is thought to prevent angina and arrhythmias by blocking or slowing calcium flow into muscle cells, which results in vasodilation (widening of the blood vessels) and greater oxygen delivery to the heart muscle.

Implications for massage: The expected effect of the massage may be distorted. Care must be taken to watch for any exaggerated effects. Massage may help with constipation. The blood pressure–lowering effect of massage may result in dizziness after the massage. Have the client contract and relax the leg muscles for 1 to 2 minutes before getting off the massage table.

Antiarrhythmics

Examples: Disopyramide, mexiletine, procainamide, propranolol, tocainide, quinidine

Antiarrhythmics are prescribed when the heart does not beat rhythmically or smoothly (a condition called *arrhythmia*).

Implications for massage: The client may complain of joint and muscle pain and swelling in the extremities that are medication related. If this occurs, refer the client to the prescribing physician. Massage may help with constipation. The client may experience dizziness after the massage. Have the client contract and relax the leg muscles for 1 to 2 minutes before getting off the massage table.

Antihypertensives and Diuretics

Examples of antihypertensives: Beta blockers, calcium channel blockers, angiotensin-converting enzyme (ACE) inhibitors (including captopril, enalapril, lisinopril, benazepril, quinapril), prazosin, terazosin, clonidine, and hydralazine

Examples of diuretics: Chlorothiazide; chlorthalidone; furosemide; hydrochlorothiazide; spironolactone chlorothiazide; hydrochlorothiazide furosemide; spironolactone, triamterene; amiloride; spironolactone and hydrochlorothiazide combination; triamterene and hydrochlorothiazide combination; amiloride and hydrochlorothiazide combination

High blood pressure, or hypertension, occurs when the pressure of the blood against the walls of the blood vessels is higher than what is considered normal; this condition eventually can cause damage to the brain, eyes, heart, and kidneys. Diuretics are used in antihypertensive therapy. Diuretics may deplete the body of potassium, and a potassium supplement or food source high in potassium may be recommended by the physician.

Implications for massage: The expected effect of the massage may be distorted. Care must be taken to watch for any exaggerated effects. Massage may help with constipation. The blood pressure–lowering effect of massage may result in dizziness after the massage. Have the client contract and relax the leg muscles for 1 to 2 minutes before getting off the massage table. The stress-reducing effect of massage may affect the dosage of these medications. Have clients monitor themselves carefully and ask their physicians to watch for a possible need to reduce the dosage or change the medication. Massage has the effect of increasing fluid movement and may enhance the diuretic effect temporarily.

Cardiac Glycosides

Examples: Digitalis, digoxin, digitoxin

Cardiac glycosides slow the heart rate but increase contraction force; they act both as heart depressants and stimulants. Their uses include regulating irregular heart rhythm, increasing the volume of blood pumped by the heart, and medicating congestive heart failure.

Implications for massage: Monitor the client's heart rate, because massage tends to slow the heart rate. If the rate falls below 50 beats per minute, stop the massage and refer the client immediately to the physician. Regular use of massage may affect the dosage of this medication. Have the client monitor the dose carefully with the physician.

Anticoagulants

Examples: Coumadin, Panwarfin, Sofarin, warfarin sodium, heparin

Anticoagulants are medications that prevent blood clotting (blood thinners). They fall into two categories: (1) heparin, which must be given by injection, therefore its use generally is restricted to hospitalized patients, and (2) oral anticoagulants, which are derivatives of the medication warfarin. Warfarin may be used in the treatment of conditions such as stroke, heart disease, and abnormal blood clotting. It also is used to prevent the movement of a clot. Warfarin acts by preventing the liver from manufacturing the proteins responsible for blood clot formation.

Implications for massage: The response to stress levels can affect the action of anticoagulants. Massage alters the body's response to stress and may interact with the dosage of this medication. Avoid any massage methods that may cause bruising, including compression, friction, tapotement, and skin rolling. Watch for bruising and report any bruising to the client. Joint swelling and aching may result from the use of these medications. Refer clients who have any joint symptoms to the physician.

Antihyperlipidemics

Examples: Cholestyramine, colestipol, lovastatin, pravastatin, clofibrate

Medications used to treat atherosclerosis act to reduce the serum levels of cholesterol and triglycerides, which form plaque on the walls of arteries. Some antihyperlipidemics bind to bile acids in the gastrointestinal tract, reducing the body's production of cholesterol.

Implications for massage: Occasional muscle pain and joint pain can occur when these medications are used. Refer clients who complain of these conditions to a physician. Massage may help constipation. Some people experience occasional dizziness. Watch clients carefully as they get up from the massage table.

Gastrointestinal Medications

Anticholinergics and Narcotics

Examples of anticholinergics: Dicyclomine (Antispas, Bentylol, Cyclobec, Dibent, Lomine)

Examples of narcotics and anticholinergics: Diphenoxylate, atropine

Anticholinergic medications slow or block nerve impulses at parasympathetic nerve endings, preventing muscle contraction and glandular secretion in the organs involved. Because these medications slow the action of the bowel by relaxing the muscles and relieving spasms, they are said to have an antispasmodic action. The also can help alleviate diarrhea.

Implications for massage: The client's response to relaxation effects may be altered as a result of alteration of parasympathetic action.

Antiulcer Medications

Examples: Cimetidine (Tagamet), Peptol, tagan, famotidine, omeprazole, ranitidine, sucralfate

These medications relieve symptoms and promote healing of gastrointestinal ulcers. The antisecretory ulcer medications work by suppressing the production of excess stomach acid. Sucralfate works by forming a chemical barrier over an exposed ulcer, protecting the ulcer from stomach acid.

Implications for massage: The stress reduction capacity of massage may enhance the effectiveness of these medications.

Hormones

A hormone is a substance produced and secreted by a gland. Hormones stimulate and regulate body functions. Most often hormone medications are used to replace naturally occurring hormones that are not being produced in amounts sufficient to regulate specific body functions. This category of medication includes oral contraceptives and certain types of medications used to combat inflammatory reactions.

Antidiabetic Medications

Examples: Tolbutamide (Glyconon, Rastinon), chlorpropamide (Diabinese), metformin (Glucophage)

The treatment of diabetes mellitus may involve the administration of insulin or oral antidiabetic medications. Glucagon is given only in emergencies (e.g., insulin shock or when blood sugar levels must be raised quickly). Oral antidiabetic medications induce the pancreas to secrete more insulin by acting on small groups of cells in the pancreas that make and store insulin. Individuals with insulin-dependent (juvenile onset, or type 1) diabetes must have their blood sugar levels controlled with injections of insulin.

Implications for massage: Changes in stress levels may affect the dosage. The client's physician should monitor the dosage if massage is used on a regular basis. Do not provide vigorous massage, because it may put undue stress on the system, requiring the blood sugar level to adjust.

Sex Hormones

Examples: Estrogens (Estradiol, Premarin, Feminone), oral contraceptives, progesterones (medroxyprogesterone [Provera]), androgens (testosterone)

Estrogens are used as replacement therapy to treat symptoms of menopause in women whose bodies are no longer producing sufficient amounts of estrogen. Medroxyprogesterone is used to treat uterine bleeding and menstrual problems. Most oral contraceptives (birth control pills) combine estrogen and progesterone, but some contain only progesterone. Testosterone stimulates cells that produce male sex characteristics, replace hormone deficiencies, stimulate red blood cells, and suppress estrogen production. Athletes sometimes take medications called *anabolic steroids* (chemicals similar to testosterone) to reduce the elimination of protein from the body, which results in an increase in muscle size. This use of these medications is dangerous; anabolic steroids can adversely affect the heart, nervous system, and kidneys.

Implications for massage: Estrogens can change the body's blood clotting ability. Watch for bruising and adjust pressures as needed. Be aware of any symptoms of blood clots and refer the patient to the physician immediately if these are noted. Estrogen and progesterone can increase fluid retention. Massage may temporarily increase fluid movement, reducing swelling. Unusual fluid retention should be referred to the prescribing physician immediately. Hormones have a widespread effect on the body and mood. Emotional states may fluctuate, and the ability to handle stress changes with the hormonal fluctuations. Massage can reduce stress levels, help even out mood, and promote a sense of well-being.

Steroids

Examples: Cortisone, prednisolone, prednisone

Examples of steroid hormone creams or ointments: Triamcinolone, hydrocortisone

Oral steroid preparations may be used to treat inflammatory diseases such as arthritis, or conditions such as poison ivy, hay fever, or insect bites. Steroids also may be applied to the skin to treat certain inflammatory skin conditions.

Implications for massage: Changes in stress levels may affect the dose. The client's physician should monitor the dosage if massage is used on a regular basis. Avoid any massage methods that may create inflammation, such as friction, skin rolling, or stretching methods that pull excessively on the tissue.

Thyroid Medications

Example: Levothyroxine (Synthroid, Levoxine)

Implications for massage: Changes in stress levels may affect the dosage. The client should monitor the dosage if massage is used on a regular basis.

Antiinfective Medications

Antibiotics

Examples: Aminoglycoside, cephalosporin, erythromycin, penicillin (including ampicillin and amoxicillin), quinolone, tetracycline

Antibiotics are used to treat a wide variety of bacterial infections. Antibiotics do not counteract viruses, such as those that cause the common cold.

Antivirals

Example: Acyclovir (Zovirax)

Antiviral medications are used to combat viral infections; however, they do not eliminate or cure viral infections.

Antifungals

Example: Nystatin

Fungal infections are treated to prevent the growth of fungi and to cure the condition.

Anthelmintics

Examples: Santonin, Spigelia, chenopodium

Anthelmintics are used to treat worm infestations.

Scabicides

Examples: Lindane, crotamiton

Scabicides are used to treat scabies.

Pediculicides

Example: Lindane

Pediculicides are used to treat lice infestations.

Implications for massage for antiinfective medications: A person who is taking an antiinfective medication is immunocompromised. Therefore it is important to avoid overstressing the system when providing massage and to take care not to expose these clients to contagious diseases, such as colds. Postpone appointments if necessary. Gastrointestinal side effects are common with these drugs. Massage may calm symptoms temporarily. Universal precautions are required when dealing with any bacterial, viral, or other condition caused by pathogens.

Antineoplastic Medications

Examples: Tamoxifen, flutamide

Antineoplastic medications are used in the treatment of cancer. Most of the medications in this category prevent the growth of rapidly dividing cells such as cancer cells. Antineoplastics are without exception extremely toxic and can cause serious side effects.

Implications for massage: Individuals undergoing chemotherapy are physiologically stressed because of the toxicity of the medications. Work gently and under the direct supervision of the client's physician.

Central Nervous System Medications

Antianxiety Drugs/Sedatives

Examples: Benzodiazepines, diazepam (Valium), clonazepam (Klonopin), alprazolam (Xanax), barbiturates, buspirone, diphenhydramine, doxepin, hydroxyzine, triazolam (Halcion)

Medications used in the treatment of anxiety, panic disorder, and insomnia selectively reduce the activity of certain chemicals in the brain.

Implications for massage: These medications generally act as CNS depressants. Massage can increase or decrease the effect of these medications, depending on whether the massage is structured to have a more stimulating or relaxing effect. The dosage of these drugs needs to be carefully monitored when they are used in conjunction with massage. The physician may be able to reduce the dosage if massage is used on a regular basis. Work in conjunction with the prescribing physician.

Antipsychotics

Examples: Phenothiazines (e.g., chlorpromazine, thioridazine), haloperidol

Major tranquilizers or antipsychotic agents usually are prescribed for patients with psychoses (certain types of mental disorders). These medications calm certain areas of the brain but permit the rest of the brain to function normally. They act as a screen that allows transmission of some nerve impulses but restricts others.

Implications for massage: These medications generally act as CNS depressants. Massage can increase or decrease the effect of these medications, depending on whether the massage is structured to have a more stimulating or relaxing effect. The dosage of these drugs needs to be carefully monitored when they are used in conjunction with massage. These medications are used to treat severe mental disorders. Work only with direct supervision from the prescribing physician. The physician may be able to lower the dosage if massage is used on a regular basis. Massage can help with constipation.

Antidepressants

Examples: Tricyclic antidepressants (amitriptyline [Amitril, Endep]), selective serotonin reuptake inhibitors (SSRIs; fluoxetine [Prozac], sertraline [Zoloft], paroxetine), tetracyclic antidepressants (maprotiline), and monoamine oxidase inhibitors (MAOIs; phenelzine)

Antidepressants are used to combat depression. They also are used as preventive therapy for migraine headaches and other types of pain, although the manner in which they help relieve pain is not clearly understood. Tricyclic antidepressants are thought to work by increasing the concentration of certain chemicals necessary for nerve transmission in the brain.

Implications for massage: Massage nonspecifically causes a shift in neurotransmitters and other brain chemicals. Massage has a stimulating effect on the CNS even when used for relaxation. The relaxation effect is a secondary result of the nervous system stimulation. Massage can increase serotonin levels. Watch carefully for any increase or decrease in the effect of the medications. Work with the supervision of the prescribing physician to adjust the dosage when massage is used as part of therapy. Massage can help with constipation.

Amphetamines

Example: Methylphenidate (Ritalin, Benzedrine)

Amphetamines or adrenergic medications are nervous system stimulants commonly used as anorectics (medications used to reduce the appetite). These medications temporarily quiet the part of the brain that causes hunger, but they also keep a person awake, speed up the heart, and raise blood pressure. After 2 to 3 weeks, these medications begin to lose their effectiveness as appetite suppressants. They also are used to treat narcolepsy. Amphetamines stimulate most people, but they have the opposite effect on hyperkinetic children and adults. When hyperkinetic children and adults take amphetamines or adrenergic medications, their level of activity is reduced. Most likely, amphetamines selectively stimulate parts of the brain that control activity.

Implications for massage: Massage nonspecifically causes a shift in neurotransmitters and other brain chemicals. Massage has a stimulating effect on the CNS even when used for relaxation. The relaxation effect is a secondary result of the nervous system stimulation. Watch carefully for any increase or decrease in the effect of the medications. Work with supervision from the prescribing physician, who may need to adjust the dosage when massage is used as part of therapy. Massage can help with constipation.

Anticonvulsants

Example: Phenobarbital (Barbita, Solfoton)

Anticonvulsants are used to control seizures and other symptoms of epilepsy. They selectively reduce excessive stimulation in the brain.

Implications for massage: Massage has a stimulating effect on the CNS even when used for relaxation. The relaxation effect is a secondary result of the nervous system stimulation. Watch carefully for any increase or decrease in the effect of the medications. Work with supervision from the prescribing physician to adjust the dosage when massage is used as part of therapy.

Antiparkinsonism Agents

Examples: Benztropine, trihexyphenidyl, levodopa, bromocriptine

Parkinson's disease is a progressive disorder that is caused by a chemical imbalance of dopamine in the brain. These medications are used to correct the chemical imbalance, thereby relieving the symptoms of the disease. Benztropine and trihexyphenidyl are also used to relieve tremors caused by other medications.

Implications for massage: Massage nonspecifically causes a shift in neurotransmitters and other brain chemicals, including dopamine. Massage has a stimulating effect on the CNS even when used for relaxation. The relaxation effect is a secondary result of the nervous system stimulation. Watch carefully for any increase or decrease in the effect of the medications. Work with supervision from the prescribing physician, who may adjust the dosage when massage is used as part of therapy. Massage can help with constipation.

Analgesics

Analgesics are used to relieve pain. They may be either narcotic or nonnarcotic. Narcotics act on the brain to cause deep analgesia and often drowsiness. Narcotics relieve pain and give the patient a feeling of well-being. They are also addictive.

A number of analgesics contain codeine or other narcotics combined with nonnarcotic analgesics (e.g., aspirin or acetaminophen). Darvon is one example. These analgesics are not as potent as pure narcotics but are frequently as effective.

Nonnarcotic pain relievers include the following:
- Salicylate (aspirin)
- Acetaminophen (relieves pain but does not reduce inflammation)
- Naproxen, piroxicam (Feldene), ketoprofen (Orudis) (inhibits prostaglandin)

Implications for massage: Massage reduces pain perception in several ways: through gate control hyperstimulation analgesia and counterirritation and by stimulating the release of pain-inhibiting or pain-modifying chemicals in the body. Massage supports analgesics and has the potential to reduce the drug dosage and the duration of treatment. Aspirin thins the blood. Watch for bruising. Pain percep-tion is inhibited when a person is taking analgesics. Feedback mechanisms for pressure and massage intensity are not accurate. Reduce the intensity of massage and avoid methods that cause inflammation. Narcotics are constipating, and massage can help with constipation. Dizziness may result with the use of these medications. Have the client relax and contract the muscles of the legs for a few minutes before getting off the table.

Antiinflammatory Medications

Antiinflammatory medications reduce the body's inflammatory response. Inflammation is the body's response to injury, and it causes swelling, pain, fever, redness, and itching. Examples of antiinflammatory medications include:
- Nonsteroidal antiinflammatory medications (NSAIDs): Examples include aspirin, fenoprofen, ibuprofen, indomethacin, naproxen, and tolmetin.
- Steroids: Adrenocorticosteroids (cortisone is also used to treat inflammatory diseases).

NOTE: Skeletal muscle relaxants often are given in combination with an antiinflammatory medication such as aspirin. However, some doctors believe that aspirin and rest are better for alleviating the pain and the inflammation of muscle strain than are skeletal muscle relaxants. When sore muscles tense, increasing muscle tone, they cause pain, inflammation, and spasm. Skeletal muscle relaxants (e.g., orphenadrine, aspirin, and caffeine combination; meprobamate and aspirin combination; and chlorzoxazone and acetaminophen combinations) can relieve pain and these symptoms.

Implications for massage: Massage therapists should not perform any techniques that create inflammation or damage tissue. Mood may be altered as well as pain perception. Feedback mechanisms for pressure and massage intensity are not accurate. The intensity of the massage should be reduced. Massage can reduce muscle spasm, reducing the need for muscle relaxants. Muscle spasm is often a protective response acting to immobilize an injured area. Use massage to reduce but not remove these protective spasms. Many of these medications are available over the counter, and the client may neglect to report their use to the massage therapist. Ask clients whether they are taking any OTC medications.

Respiratory Medications

Antitussives

Examples: Dextromethorphan, codeine

Antitussives control coughs.

Expectorants

Examples: Ammonium chloride, guaifenesin, potassium guaiacolsulfonate, and terpin hydrate

Expectorants are used to change a nonproductive cough to a productive one (one that brings up phlegm). Expectorants are supposed to increase the amount of mucus produced. However, drinking water or using a vaporizer or humidifier is probably as effective for increasing the production of mucus.

Decongestants

Examples: Ephedrine, pseudoephedrine, phenylephrine, phenylpropanolamine hydrochloride

Decongestants constrict blood vessels in the nose and sinuses to open air passages. Adrenergists (decongestants) are available as oral preparations, nose drops, and nose sprays. Oral decongestants are slow acting but do not interfere with the production of mucus or the movement of the cilia (special hairlike structures) of the respiratory tract. They can increase blood pressure, therefore they should be used cautiously by patients with high blood pressure. Topical decongestants (nose drops or sprays) provide fast relief. They do not increase blood pressure as much as oral decongestants, but they do slow cilia movement. Topical decongestants should not be used for more than a few days at a time.

Bronchodilators

Examples: Theophylline, aminophylline, albuterol, metaproterenol

Bronchodilators (agents that open the airways in the lungs) and agents that relax smooth muscle tissue, such as that found in the lungs, are used to improve breathing. Oral bronchodilators are commonly used to relieve the symptoms of asthma and emphysema. Inhalant bronchodilators act directly on the muscles of the breathing tubes.

Antihistamines

Examples: Diphenhydramine, brompheniramine, chlorpheniramine, meclizine

Histamine is a body chemical that, when released, typically causes swelling and itching. Antihistamines counteract these symptoms of allergy by blocking the effects of histamine. Antihistamines can be used for mild respiratory allergies, such as hay fever. Some types of antihistamines are also used to prevent or treat the symptoms of motion sickness.

Implications for massage for respiratory medications: Respiratory medications can reduce sweating, therefore heat hydrotherapy should be avoided. Bronchodilators are sympathomimetic and act on sympathetic nerve stimulation. Antihistamines can excite or depress the CNS. Most of these medications can cause drowsiness and anxiety. Because they act on the CNS, the expected results of the massage can be distorted. The client may be unable to relax

or may be excessively drowsy and dizzy after the massage. Many massage methods produce reddening of the skin caused by the release of histamine. The reaction may be altered and feedback may be inaccurate in clients taking antihistamines. Avoid this type of work with such clients. Codeine can cause constipation. Massage may prove beneficial. Many of these medications are available over the counter, and clients may neglect to report their use to the therapist. Make sure to ask clients if they are taking any OTC medications.

Vitamins and Minerals

Vitamins and minerals are chemical substances that are vital to the maintenance of normal body function. Many people take supplemental vitamins and minerals. A high intake of supplements, especially individual vitamins, can cause adverse reactions or may have implications for massage. The practitioner needs to investigate further to determine any suspected interaction. At this point, specific research has not been done to determine what the specific interactions might be. It is necessary to compare the effects of the vitamin and/or mineral with the type of massage application to determine whether the two together are inhibitory or synergistic. This is too comprehensive an information base to detail in this format.

Herbs

Herbs are medicinal plants. Their action is similar to that of pharmaceutical medications. Many medications are derivatives of herbs. Ask clients whether they are taking herbs, and if so, their reasons for taking them. The practitioner needs to investigate further to determine any suspected interactions. At this point, specific research has not been done to determine what the specific interactions might be. It is necessary to compare the effects of the herb with the type of massage application to determine whether the two together are inhibitory or synergistic. This is too comprehensive an information base to detail in this format.

BIBLIOGRAPHY

Consumers Guide editors: *Prescription medications,* Lincolnwood, Ill, 1995, Signet.

Corey G et al: *Issues and ethics in the helping professions,* ed 6, Belmont, Calif, 2002, Brooks/Cole.

Griffith H, Moore SW: *Complete guide to prescription and nonprescription drugs,* Los Angeles, 2002, The Body Press Division of Price Stern Sloan.

Keen J et al: *Mosby's critical care and emergency medication reference,* ed 2, St Louis, 1996, Mosby.

Mosby's drug consult, St Louis, 2004, Mosby.

Answer Key

CHAPTER 1

SHORT ANSWER

1. The skin is the largest sensory organ of the body. Many subcutaneous soft tissue structures (e.g., muscles, connective tissue), as well as visceral structures (e.g., the lungs, heart, digestive organs), project sensation to the skin. The autonomic nervous system, which regulates the visceral and chemical homeostasis of the body, is highly responsive to skin stimulation in support of well-being. Mood (the way a person feels) often is reflected in the skin, because we touch ourselves from the inside. We blush with embarrassment, flush with excitement, or pale with fear.

2. Personal space, culture and subculture, including social structure and spiritual discipline, gender, age, and life events.

3. Hostile or aggressive touch, erotic touch.

4. Socially stereotyped touch, touch that communicates information, touch technique.

5. Massage or touch as a method of healing developed from many cultural origins. This means that no one culture owns massage and that some sort of underlying, instinctive mechanism spurred the development of a type of massage in most if not all cultures on the planet.

6. Scientific research is the key to validation. Massage has been validated by the science of the day. Today we know that many of the ideas that past scientists had were incorrect. The important thing is that even though the "scientific rationale" for massage was incorrect, the benefits of massage were still real.

7. The ancient Chinese massage system consisted of kneading and rubbing down the entire body with the hands, joint movement, and traction. The ancient Chinese methods are not much different from massage today.

8. The Church was all powerful. Much of the scientific information concerning massage had been lost during this time. Massage reverted from a form of sanctioned medicine to use by the common people, many of whom held to their early traditions of healing. The Church could not explain these healing abilities, so it claimed that the power came from the devil. It is important to remember the value of objective research for validation as opposed to experiential validation, and also that practitioners of massage must not put themselves forth as "healers."

9. Ling began a recognized school to teach the methods. He did a fine job of putting much of the existing knowledge together in a usable form, but it is important to remember that much of what we consider Swedish massage came later from Mezger's work.

10. Because Ling was not trained in medicine, he did not speak the same language as the medical community of his time. Instead, he had a tendency to use poetic and mystical language that was discounted. Eventually, physicians spoke about massage with other doctors in a language that they understood, and by 1839 Ling's system had gained worldwide recognition. The importance of a common terminology is another lesson to remember as modern massage moves toward standardization.

11. Unfortunately, profit-oriented schools and educators were the major contributors to the downfall of massage. It is important to watch for this situation today.

12. Athletic or fitness massage and personal service massage have retained a small but strong following and constitute a growing market. Today, prevention, stress reduction, and health-enhancing methods are the primary avenues pursued. Massage has reasserted itself as a major contributor to personal health programs.

13. Pain research has uncovered many of the physiologic explanations for the benefits of massage.

14. Many of the massage methods currently used are a combination of structural and energetic concepts. History does repeat itself, and massage has reemerged in every age. The best results have occurred when science is advanced enough to figure out why massage works. It will be exciting to move into the future, as long as we keep in mind the lessons of the past.

MATCHING

1. j		13. m	
2. s		14. o	
3. r		15. e	
4. b		16. t	
5. i		17. f	
6. k		18. v	
7. a		19. w	
8. n		20. g	
9. q		21. y	
10. c		22. p	
11. x		23. h	
12. d		24. l	
		25. u	

TIME LINE EXERCISE

a. 2		l. 16	
b. 7		m. 17	
c. 10		n. 9	
d. 4		o. 5	
e. 1		p. 18	
f. 8		q. 3	
g. 12		r. 19	
h. 14		s. 13	
i. 11		t. 20	
j. 6		u. 22	
k. 15		v. 21	

CHAPTER 2 WORKBOOK SECTION ANSWER KEY

SHORT ANSWER

1. Ethics is the system of rules, based on morals, values, and standards of accepted conduct, that guide correct behavior.

2. The variety of massage methods makes it difficult to please all practitioners of specific approaches. It is hard to encompass all these approaches to develop a concise definition for our profession.

3. The scope of practice for therapeutic massage, when formally developed, must fit into the spaces left by these other professionals. Fortunately, the area left unfilled by other professionals is a very important space for personalized supportive wellness care. With additional training, massage therapists can become important team players and work within the scope of practice of other healthcare professionals to assist them in providing the best care for their clients.

4. To avoid such situations, massage professionals must not focus on specific treatment for specific problems, but rather provide a service that helps the client maintain or enhance good health. The massage professional also must refer the client to other healthcare professionals when appropriate.

5. The massage therapist's touch is to be safe, nonjudgmental touch. How could we ethically say that we are providing this service for a client for whom we feel dislike, disapprove, or fear?

6. If a massage professional wishes to maintain a nondiscriminatory approach but cannot best serve a particular client, simple disclosure to the client of the massage practitioner's problem allows the massage professional to best serve the needs of the client without discrimination.

7. The relationship between the massage professional and the client is based on professional trust and safety. If the client is unable to make an informed choice, the trust is broken and the touch is not safe.

8. Accountability for meeting specific requirements for professional behavior in the healthcare setting.

9. All boundary concerns could be resolved through respect for clients that equally serves our needs and theirs. We invade a person's boundaries when our needs are put above their needs.

10. If each massage professional establishes professional boundaries and these are respected by equal consideration of each person's needs in a situation, the massage professional's respect for the client and the client's understanding of professional ethics will support decision making in most such vague situations.

11. Short-lived feelings of sexual arousal that occur when a person relaxes have a physiologic basis. If the client has experienced essential touch only in a sexual situation, the client logically connects the two experiences. Education and explanation help clients understand the difference.

12. In the professional relationship, in which expectations and rules are understood clearly, clients can make an informed choice about their behavior. If the situation is vague and the rules change from week to week, the expectations between client and practitioner become unclear.

13. Massage practitioners must know what credentialing is required by law to practice massage therapy and what types of credentialing are voluntary. They also must know that credentials must be issued by verifiable sources.

14. Depending on where the massage therapist wants to practice, these legal issues to a large extent determine the requirements for starting a business.

15. The main purpose of a law is to protect the public's health, safety, and welfare.

16. Massage seems to be subdividing into wellness personal service massage and clinical massage and healthcare and sport settings. Wellness personal service massage has an entry-level educational requirement of 500 to 1000 clock hours. This is the standard in much of the United States. The clinical type of massage is most typified by the educational requirement set by the Canadian provinces of Ontario and British Columbia, which is approximately 2200 clock hours of training. This is the equivalent of the associate's degree required for medical technicians such as respiratory therapists and physical therapy assistants. Practitioners involved in clinical massage are typically supervised by a highly trained medical professional.

MATCHING

1. s	15. e
2. a	16. v
3. n	17. h
4. d	18. u
5. y	19. j
6. z	20. i
7. f	21. aa
8. q	22. t
9. b	23. k
10. c	24. l
11. g	25. m
12. p	26. r
13. w	27. x
14. o	28. bb

STANDARDS OF PRACTICE ACTIVITY

c, e, f, g, i, j, k

DETERMINING LICENSING NEEDS ACTIVITY

1. Find out if your state or province requires licensing.

2. If a licensing program exists, find out the educational requirements for sitting for the exams. If your state does not have licensing, contact the local government where you intend to work to see if a local ordinance applies.

3. Contact the state Department of Education and confirm that the school you plan to attend is licensed and in compliance with state regulations.

4. Contact the local government about zoning requirements and building codes.

5. Contact the local government and apply for any permits or business licenses required.

PROBLEM-SOLVING EXERCISES

(The numbers shown in parentheses in the answers below refer to the standards of practice list presented in Box 2-4.)

1. The client says that the massage professional told him he needed to lose weight (1); did not stop working on his feet when asked to (11); did not explain that a trigger point area could be sore the next day (10); gave him a hug at the end of the session without asking first (9); told a joke that had a sexual innuendo (18); let the drape slip while massaging the buttocks (11); talked about difficulties with her children (22); walked in to get a chart without knocking first and interrupted him getting dressed after the massage (1); said that physical therapists were bad at dealing with neck pain and that she could fix it (3, 8); and gave him no receipt for his payment (14).

2. Kathy can do any of the following:
She can ignore the situation and see if it occurs again.
After the massage, when she and Mr. Adams are in the office area, she can explain that she understands the extra stress he is under but that it is important to remember the boundaries of the therapeutic relationship. During times of loss, it is easy to personalize a professional relationship (i.e., transference).
She can acknowledge the touch when it happens and gently explain that although she understands that the massage helps with the stress and provides for professional companionship, it is important for both to remember the ethical standards of massage and the professional relationship.

3. Matt's choices are as follows:
He can thank Jeff for the offer but decline, explaining the importance of not spending time with clients outside the professional setting, even when a past acquaintance exists.
He can talk with Jeff after the massage and explain that although it's pleasant to remember school days, being a professional who provides massage services and spending social time together don't mix. He should thank Jeff for the offer but refuse it.
He can let Jeff know that if he accepts the ticket, their professional relationship will have to end, and Jeff would have to see another therapist from now on.

4. Mary's choices are as follows:
She can acknowledge to herself that her feelings are a form of countertransference and have nothing to do with the client; she then can

restore the professional boundaries and time limits of the massage and continue to see the client.

She can speak with the client about her feelings in a very brief way, explaining the difficulty with maintaining the professional relationship, and refer the client to another therapist.

She can initiate peer support by talking to an experienced therapist. Another massage professional can understand the interactions that take place in the therapy room and may be able to give her some good advice on ways to handle such a situation. This peer support system is an excellent means of preserving our professional integrity and providing encouragement and guidance for each other.

CHAPTER 3 WORKBOOK SECTION ANSWER KEY

SHORT ANSWER

1. Prefixes are placed at the beginning of the root word to change the meaning of the word. Root words contain the basic meaning of the word. A suffix is placed at the end of a word to change the meaning of the word. When translating medical terms, begin with the suffix.
2. Abbreviations are shortened forms of words or phrases. When you use abbreviations in any record keeping, including charting, provide an abbreviation key either on the forms or included in a conspicuous place in the file. Excessive use of abbreviations is discouraged.
3. Goals must be able to be quantified. This means that they are measured in terms of objective criteria. Goals need to be qualified. The question to be answered is, "How will we know when the goal is achieved?" What will the client be able to do after the goal has been reached that he or she is not able to do now?
4. Intake procedures are done once and updated periodically. Charting is ongoing after each session.
5. The four steps are the following: (1) review the facts and information collected; (2) brainstorm the possibilities; (3) consider the logical outcome of each possibility; and (4) consider the ways in which people are affected by each possibility. Decisions made from this process are reflected and recorded in the care/treatment plan.
6. S: Subjective data are recorded from the client's point of view. O: Objective data acquired from inspection, palpation, and a list of assessment procedures and interventions used during the session are recorded. A: Analysis or assessment of the subjective and objective data and an analysis of the effectiveness of the intervention and action taken are made, with a summary of the most pertinent data recorded. P: Plan, including the methodology for intervention and the progress of the sessions, is developed and recorded.
7. To maintain the integrity of client charts, make sure that any abbreviations used are universally understood, or write out the word. Use black pen or type the notes. Make sure handwritten notes are readable. Never erase or white-out a correction. Draw a single line through any error, and make the correction above or next to the error. It is important to share the charting notes with and explain them to the client regularly.

MATCHING

1. d
2. a
3. c
4. b
5. f
6. e

The first letter is the definition, and the second letter indicates whether it is a prefix (p), root word (r), or suffix (s).

1. k, p
2. a, p
3. r, s
4. h, r
5. w, r
15. q, s
16. c, s
17. i, s
18. d, s
19. n, s
28. l, r
29. jj, r
30. m, s
31. kk, p
32. t, s

6. f, p
7. g, p
8. z, r
9. cc, p
10. dd, p
11. gg, p
12. aa, p
13. b, p
14. v, r
20. e, p
21. hh, p
22. bb, p
23. ii, p
24. j, s
25. ee, s
26. nn, r
27. ff, r
33. o, s
34. ll, p
35. p, s
36. mm, r
37. x, p
38. s, p
39. y, r
40. u, r

1. g
2. h
3. o
4. c
5. i
6. d
7. k
8. m
9. q
10. n
11. j
12. a
13. b
14. p
15. l
16. f
17. e

PROBLEM-SOLVING EXERCISE

dermatitis: *derma*-skin, *itis*-inflammation
neuropathy: *neuro*-nerve, *pathy*-disease
hypothyroidism: *hypo*-less than normal, *thyroidism*-condition of the thyroid
dyspnea: *dys*-difficult, *pnea*-breathing
hemangioma: *hemi*-half, *angi*-vessel, *oma*-tumor (tumor made up of a mass of blood vessels)
polyarthritis: *poly*-many, *arthr*-joint, *itis*-inflammation
myocarditis: *myo*-muscle, *card*-heart, *itis*-inflammation
hydronephrosis: *hydro*-water, *nephr*-kidney, *osis*-condition

CHAPTER 4 WORKBOOK SECTION ANSWER KEY

SHORT ANSWER

1. Neuromuscular, connective tissue, circulation, ANS, and electrical-chemical or electrical-magnetic effects.
2. The connective tissue becomes fibrotic, and the fibrosis extends to areas surrounding the dysfunctional area.
3. Arterial flow, venous return flow, lymphatic drainage, respiration, and CSF circulation.
4. Fight, flight, and fear.
5. Relaxation response.
6. Massage may recreate state-dependent memory patterns for the client.
7. It is a protective mechanism of sensory overload caused by sustained stimulation.
8. Because of the effect on the ANS and associated functions, massage produces feelings of general well-being and comfort, allowing clients to control their own emotional state.
9. Massage has an extensive base of historical literature and current research, and it works by stimulating simple physiologic mechanisms.
10. This type of information gives the effects of the massage back to the client. Instead of a force from outside that in some mystical way exerts power over the body, this type of research shows that the effects of massage come from within the client and that massage is a great form of sensory simulation to "get the ball rolling." Many claims are made about alternative health measures; some are valid, and some are not. The effects of massage are simple and basic and require validation in order to separate fact from mere speculation.
11. In actual practice, it is impossible to divide up the wholeness of massage; this is one of the things that makes massage special. In research it is possible to study one aspect, and in the education process it is possible to study one method, but in application the

elements mingle. For example, individual ingredients make up a cookie, but they do not become the cookie until all ingredients are mixed together and a chemical reaction takes place. After the cookie is a cookie, it is almost impossible to separate the individual components.

12. Stimulation that activates the large-diameter nerve fibers wins the race to the brain and closes the "gate," so that the pain sensations are not processed. Hyperstimulation is stimulation that uses extensive or sustained sensation; counterirritation is stimulation of a different sensory fiber.

13. Tissues that can bind nerves through shortening or a shift in position are skin, fascia, muscles, ligaments, and joints. Massage can stretch the connective tissues and change the tension of muscle to relieve the pressure on a nerve.

14. Reflexes are fast, predictable, autonomic responses to a change in the environment that help maintain homeostasis. Many of the beneficial responses of massage depend on the specific stimulation of a reflex. Reflexes are important movement and protective mechanisms. Because they take priority in a sensory signal, stimulation of reflexes can result in a shift in homeostasis, and nonproductive nerve transmission pathways can be overridden.

15. Massage stimulates the secretion of certain neurotransmitters, hormones, and other endogenous chemicals, such as endorphins, and also stimulates ANS functions. The combination of endocrine and ANS functions plays a part in the body/mind phenomenon.

16. Massage can create a controlled but slightly more intense stimulus than the existing pain or stress. The increase in intensity is sufficient to trigger the release of these substances. The stimulus must last long enough to allow blood levels to rise in order for the client to feel the effects, which have a fairly long-lasting response in the body.

17. Research seems to suggest that massage stimulates proprioceptive nerve endings; releases enkephalins; stretches the musculotendinous structures to stimulate reflex mechanisms, Golgi tendon organs, and spindle receptors; and increases circulation.

18. Massage encourages circulation on a local level through compression of vessels, which changes the internal pressure and releases vasodilators, which opens the capillaries. On a systemic level, massage shifts the autonomic vascular reflexes.

19. Entrainment, piezoelectric properties of connective tissue, nervous system stimulation, and neuroendocrine responses.

MATCHING

I.

1. t	11. l
2. e	12. n
3. a	13. g
4. m	14. p
5. b	15. f
6. j	16. q
7. k	17. d
8. i	18. s
9. o	19. r
10. h	20. c

II.

1. g	8. b
2. h	9. k
3. c	10. l
4. d	11. m
5. i	12. e
6. j	13. f
7. a	14. n

III.

1. c, p	6. j, p
2. f, p	7. i, s
3. g, s	8. h, s
4. d, s	9. b, s
5. e, s	10. a, p

LABELING

A. Brain	E. Lumbar plexus
B. Cervical plexus	F. Sacral plexus
C. Spinal cord	G. Nerves
D. Brachial plexus	

PROBLEM-SOLVING EXERCISES

1. Counterirritation, hyperstimulation analgesia, release of endorphins and serotonin, toughening/hardening, and placebo effect.

2. Reduction of sympathetic arousal responses; increased ability to restore homeostasis; increased energy as a result of reduced generalized muscle tension; increased circulation, which produces a generalized increase in efficient functioning; and restoration of effective parasympathetic restorative function.

3. No specific answer; the validity of the response to the question is based on the student's ability to justify the response.

CHAPTER 5 WORKBOOK SECTION ANSWER KEY

SHORT ANSWER

1. An *indication* is a condition for which an approach would be beneficial for health enhancement, treatment of a particular disorder, or support of a treatment modality other than massage.

2. A *contraindication* is a condition for which an approach could be harmful. The following contraindications occur:
   a. General avoidance of application—Do not massage.
   b. Regional avoidance of application—Do massage, but avoid a particular area.
   c. Application with *caution,* usually requiring supervision from appropriate medical or supervising personnel—Do perform massage but carefully select the type of methods to be used, the duration of the massage, the depth and intensity of pressure, and the frequency of application.

3. Therapeutic change, condition management, and palliative care.
   Therapeutic change is a beneficial alteration produced by a bodywork process that results in a modification of physical form or function that can affect the physical, mental, and/or spiritual state of a client.
   Condition management involves the use of massage methods to support clients who are not able to undergo a therapeutic change process but wish to be as effective as possible within an existing set of circumstances.
   Palliative care is provided when the condition is most likely going to become worse and degenerative processes will continue (e.g., terminal illness, dementia). It often relates to approaches that reduce suffering. Palliative care is also considered general relaxation massage for pleasure.

4. Besides being the absence of disease, health is the optimal functioning of the body and mind.

5. Dysfunction is the in-between state of "not healthy" but also "not sick" (experiencing disease). Massage professionals serve many people at the beginning of dysfunctional patterns—when the client does not feel his or her best but is also not yet sick. It is important to monitor the

client to make sure he or she does not progress further into dysfunctional patterns. The benefits of massage are most effectively focused in assisting people to stay within the healthy range of functioning.

6. In acute conditions, homeostatic balance is recovered quickly. In chronic diseases, the body is stressed, and a fully normal state of balance may never be restored.

7. Risk factors may put a client at risk for developing a disease or injury. Sometimes signs and symptoms may be contraindications or may show a need for a referral to a physician.

8. A massage therapist may be the first to recognize the early warning signs.

9. To determine whether a massage will benefit or interfere in the process and whether a client needs to be referred to another healthcare professional.

10. The use of methods of massage to deliberately create a controlled localized area of inflammation to generate healing mechanisms.

11. Therapeutic inflammation should not be used in situations in which sleep disturbance, compromised immune function, a high stress load, or systemic or localized inflammation is already present. It also should not be used in any condition, such as fibromyalgia, that consists of impaired repair and restorative functions unless carefully supervised as part of a total treatment program. If a person is taking an antiinflammatory medication, either steroidal or nonsteroidal, the effectiveness of therapeutic inflammation is negated or reduced, and restoration mechanisms are inhibited. When these medications are present, any methods that create inflammation are to be avoided.

12. Because it is a complex, private, abstract experience.

13. For acute pain, massage can activate the parasympathetic nervous system, thereby relaxing the client. For chronic pain, a massage therapist needs to work as part of a multidisciplinary healthcare team to provide symptomatic relief of pain and to initiate hardiness. With intractable pain, massage can provide short, temporary, symptomatic relief.

14. Localized pain is confined to a specific area at the site of origin. Projected pain is a nerve pain that is continued along the nerve tract. Radiating pain is diffused around the site of origin and is not well localized. Referred pain is felt in an area distant from the site of the painful stimulus.

15. Somatic pain arises from stimulation of receptors in the skin (called deep somatic pain). Visceral pain results from stimulation of receptors in the viscera (internal organs).

16. If the client has a recurring pain pattern that resembles referred pain patterns, he or she should be referred to a physician for a more specific diagnosis.

17. When pain is referred, it is usually to a structure that developed from the same embryonic segment or dermatome as the structure in which the pain originates.

18. Phantom pain is a type of pain frequently experienced by clients who have had a limb amputated. These clients experience pain or other sensations in the area of the amputated extremity as though the limb were still there.

19. Entrapment is pressure on a nerve from soft tissue. Compression is pressure on a nerve from bony structures. Massage is often indicated for entrapment.

20. Endangerment sites are areas in which nerves and blood vessels surface close to the skin and are not well protected by muscle or connective tissue. Areas with fragile bony projections that could be broken off are also considered endangerment sites.

21. Fatigue; inflammation; lumps and tissue changes; rashes and changes in skin; edema; mood alterations (e.g., depression and anxiety); infection (local and general); changes in appetite, elimination, or sleep; bleeding and bruising; nausea, vomiting, or diarrhea; and temperature (hot [fever] or cold).

22. Have current Mosby's *GenRx, Physician's Reference*, or similar reference book and a medical dictionary.

23. The massage therapist should be able to assess the effects of the medications and discover the ways massage may interface with these effects.

24. Clients must always be referred to their personal healthcare professionals. The massage therapist should make no attempt to direct them to different healthcare professionals. If the client does not have a doctor, chiropractor, or counselor, then a list of the professionals who have been contacted and educated about therapeutic massage should be provided.

25. As a reference, this list can assist with the clinical reasoning necessary to determine the possible interactions between massage and medications and guide the development of appropriate referral and/or massage intervention.

MATCHING

1. e	14. f	26. t
2. s	15. v	27. gg
3. l	16. x	28. hh
4. r	17. dd	29. ii
5. g	18. cc	30. jj
6. k	19. b	31. h
7. d	20. c	32. l
8. w	21. bb	33. j
9. a	22. z	34. m
10. q	23. aa	35. n
11. ee	24. u	36. o
12. ff	25. kk	37. p
13. Y		

1. a, d, h
2. b, c, e, f, g

LABELING

Labels for Figure 5-6: Labels for Figure 5-7:

1. E		1.	B
2. D		2.	C
3. F		3.	E
4. H		4.	D
5. K		5.	I
6. G		6.	K
7. J		7.	H
8. A		8.	A
9. J		9.	A
10. C		10.	B
11. B		11.	F
12. I		12.	C
13. F		13.	D
		14.	J
		15.	G
		16.	L

CHAPTER 6 WORKBOOK SECTION ANSWER KEY

SHORT ANSWER

1. The massage professional represents all massage practitioners and therefore reflects the sanitary and safety practices of the massage business. If the professional's appearance does not reflect attention to hygiene and sanitation, concern may develop about the sanitation measures practiced by all massage professionals. Also, if massage

professionals are not careful, they can become the agents of disease transmission between clients. Careful hygiene limits this possibility.

2. Tobacco smoke, breath odor, body odor, incense, and perfume are some of these odors.

3. Alcohol and drug abuse, along with use of some prescription medications, affects the ability to feel and reason. The sensitivity and perception of the massage professional are altered. This definitely interferes with the ability to give the very best massage possible and could even put the client in danger.

4. Pathogenic organisms can cause disease in a client who is stressed, fatigued, injured, or weakened. Bacteria usually can be controlled with various prescription antibiotics. Today there are many resistant strains of bacteria, which makes antibiotics less effective. Viruses are not easily controlled. The few antiviral agents available only slow the reproduction of the virus. The best resistance to a virus is the body's own immune system. Fungi, protozoa, and pathogenic animals can thrive only on or in a weakened host. The massage practitioner's main focus is wellness. If a disease is present, the body will be weak. Precautions must be taken to prevent the spread of disease and avoid putting a weakened body at further risk. The massage professional must understand the mechanisms of disease to practice massage safely.

5. The skin is the main defense against the invasion of pathogens and infection. The first signs of many serious diseases manifest as skin symptoms. Because the massage practitioner observes and touches so much of the client's skin, it is important to be able to recognize the major types of skin lesions. It also is important that the massage professional prevent the spread of infection by not massaging over breaks in the skin.

6. (1) Environmental contact (e.g., food, water, soil, contaminated surfaces); (2) opportunistic invasion (when a person is weakened and the conditions are right for invasion); and (3) person-to-person contact, either through droplet transmission from direct contact or airborne particles and body fluids.

7. Sterilization kills everything, disinfection kills almost everything, antisepsis slows or stops the growth of most pathogens, and isolation separates or puts up a barrier against pathogens. Disinfection procedures using hot, soapy water and a 10% bleach solution (freshly made each day) or a commercial disinfectant are adequate for most massage situations. Disinfection procedures are used for all laundry and cleaning, and the disinfectant is allowed to air dry on surfaces.

8. Keep things clean and disinfected. Keep areas or items that are contaminated separate from clean items. The massage environment must be constructed and maintained in such a way so as to prevent the spread of disease through insects or other vermin.

9. To prevent the spread of infection through person-to-person contact or through contact with body fluids. Methods of isolation, including the use of a mask, gloves, and gown, along with disinfection and sterilization procedures, prevent the spread of communicable disease.

10. There is much confusion, misinformation, and fear about these disorders. It is the responsibility of the massage professional to stay current with new information, especially through the CDC. Massage professionals need to understand the contamination routes for hepatitis and HIV. They need to know when their own germs may pose a threat to those who are immune suppressed, including those with HIV infection or AIDS. Massage professionals need to understand that casual contact is not a transmission route for either hepatitis or HIV. If the skin is healthy, giving a massage poses no threat to the massage professional. Most of all, massage professionals who are educated enough continue to touch those who are immune suppressed, and we all need to be touched in a compassionate and healing way.

11. Careful hand washing.

12. Do not leave anyone who is at risk of falling alone in the massage therapy room. Keep all traffic areas hazard free. Provide good lighting. Regularly check all equipment for safety and make any repairs immediately.

13. Make sure all electrical equipment and wiring are in proper working order. Avoid any type of open flame. Do not allow any smoking in the facility.

14. Everyone should be skilled in first aid, CPR, and emergency care. The American Red Cross or similar organizations in other countries are best equipped to provide this training.

MATCHING

I.

1. m	9. p	16. n
2. a	10. u	17. o
3. s	11. b	18. d
4. g	12. l	19. i
5. e	13. v	20. j
6. t	14. c	21. q
7. h	15. k	22. f
8. r		

II.

1. g
2. f
3. e
4. d
5. c
6. b
7. a

PROFESSIONAL ACTIVITY

NOTE: Twenty-three suggested sanitation requirements have been listed; only 20 are required.

1. The massage therapist must clean and wash his or her hands thoroughly with an antibacterial/antiviral agent before touching each client.

2. The therapist must wear clean clothing.

3. Lockers or closets for personnel must be maintained apart from the massage room.

4. All doors and windows opening to the outside must be tight fitting and must keep out insects, rodents, or other vermin.

5. All floors must be kept clean, well maintained, and in good repair.

6. Walls and ceilings must be kept clean and well maintained.

7. Furniture must be kept clean and in good repair.

8. The room must be capable of maintaining a room air temperature of 75° F.

9. Ventilation must be adequate to remove objectionable odors.

10. Lighting fixtures must be capable of providing a minimum of 5 footcandles of light at floor level; this level of lighting must be used during cleaning.

11. All sewage and liquid waste must be disposed of in a municipal sewage system or an approved septic system.

12. The water supply must be adequate, deemed safe by the health department, and sanitary.

13. Drinking fountains of an approved type or individual paper drinking cups must be provided.

14. Every massage business must be provided with a sanitary toilet facility with an adequate supply of hot and cold running water under pressure; this facility must be conveniently located for use by employees and clients.

15. Restroom doors must be tight fitting, and restrooms must be kept clean; in good repair; and free of flies, insects, and vermin.

16. A supply of soap in a covered dispenser and single-use sanitary towels in a dispenser must be provided at each lavatory installation, along with a covered waste receptacle for proper disposal.

17. A supply of toilet paper on a dispenser must be available for each toilet installation.

18. Massage lubricants, including but not limited to oil, soap, alcohol, powders, and lotions, must be dispensed from suitable containers, which are to be used and stored so as to prevent contamination.

19. Any unused lubricant that comes into contact with the client or the massage therapist must be discarded.

20. Only freshly laundered sheets and linens are to be used.

21. All soiled (used) linens must be washed in a mechanical washing machine that provides a hot water temperature of at least 140° F, and antiviral agents must be used (e.g., 10% bleach solution [one part bleach to nine parts water]).

22. Massage tables must be covered with impervious material that is cleanable; they must be kept clean and in good repair.

23. Equipment that comes in contact with the client must be cleaned thoroughly with soap or some other suitable detergent and water, followed by adequate sanitation procedures, before use on each individual client.

PROFESSIONAL APPLICATION

1. The accident occurred on Thursday, May 1, 2—, at approximately 4:20 PM. (List your clinic name and address here.)

2. My client was receiving a massage during his weekly session. I asked that he turn from a prone position to a side-lying position. As he rolled to his side, we both heard a cracking sound. The massage table surface then partly collapsed downward. It was kept from fully giving way by the cable supports. The client was uninjured and able to climb off the table with some assistance.

   The massage table had been checked on Friday, April 25, 2—, as part of a weekly routine maintenance and safety check. No problems were found at that time.

3. I was working as the therapist. My name is (fill in your name and full address). The client was Mr. James Jackson (fill in his full name and address from your client information form). NOTE: It is always a good idea to provide phone numbers even if they are not requested.

4. The witnesses were myself and Mr. Jackson.

5. The table was model #83, "The Basic," with a retail price of $99.95. It is manufactured by Fred's Cut Rate Tables, 480 W. Shady Lane, Market Town, MV 29341. It was sold to me by Buy-Low Products of 12 Buy-Low Drive, Badtown, VN 84848.

6. The property damage was limited to the table. The top surface is split, both the wood and the vinyl covering; the outer supports are cracked; and the hinge is bent. An estimate of repair costs will be forwarded when received.

7. No one was injured in the incident.

   Note: Because the client was involved, he will be asked to provide information. You must have his written permission to provide his name, address, and telephone number because you were providing a service to him and have guaranteed confidentiality.

CHAPTER 7 WORKBOOK SECTION ANSWER KEY

SHORT ANSWER

1. To maintain good body mechanics and weight transfer, massage professionals need to be attentive to posture and balance, use the larger muscles to do the work, rely on leverage to apply the pressure, maintain a relaxed body, and avoid compressive forces on the joints.

2. Massage professionals must avoid using upper body strength to exert the pressure for massage. Tense wrists and hands also contribute to shoulder problems. These problems can be avoided if massage professionals learn to use leverage and leaning with the body weight to provide massage pressure. It is also important to avoid both pushing and the use of upper body strength and to maintain relaxed hands and wrists while giving a massage.

3. Massage professionals can protect the wrists by avoiding excessive compressive forces. Using a proper wrist angle and staying behind the massage stroke (as presented in this chapter) will protect the wrist.

4. The thumb was not meant to endure compressive force. It is designed for grasping. Avoid using the thumbs and fingers for compression. Massage professionals must learn to use the olecranon process and ulnar side of the elbow instead. When the thumb must be used, a stabilized joint position protects the thumb. Massage professionals should use the hand as a unit and rely on the forearm for many massage strokes, including most effleurage and compression.

5. Massage professionals must learn to keep their lower backs straight and avoid bending or curling at the waist while giving a massage. Core strength is important. Frequent posture shifting of the massage professional's body also helps protect the lower back, as does lifting by leaning back during stretching. The asymmetric stance presented in this chapter, along with variations using a short and tall stool, provides methods to protect the lower back. The lower back is further protected by avoiding twisting and reaching while working and keeping the point of contact with the client below the professional's waist.

6. Knee problems can be avoided by respecting the basic design of the knee and frequently shifting the weight from foot to foot. Avoid hyperextension of the knee. However, the most efficient standing position for the knee involves the normal screw-home or knee-lock position in the last 15 degrees of extension. This position provides the least compressive force on the knee capsule and the least muscular action for stability.

7. The ankle and foot are protected by an asymmetric stance, frequent position change, and sitting when possible to do massage.

8. Asymmetric standing is the most efficient standing position. The weight is shifted from one foot to the other in an energy-conserving mechanism. Symmetric standing, with the weight equal on both feet, is fatiguing and interferes with circulation. Methods to support the asymmetric stance, such as using a stool to put one foot up on, using a high stool to sit on, or putting a knee on the table, further protect the lower back and conserve energy.

9. Leaning and using the body weight focused from the abdomen as leverage

10. At the client-practitioner contact point.

11. The massage professional needs to be comfortable and dressed in loose, nonrestrictive clothing that does not interfere with movement. Before your massage day begins, warm up your body with some general aerobic activity and stretching. During the day, take stretch breaks between each massage and move all the muscles you use while giving a massage. Massage your own arms, hands, and shoulders after each massage. The massage professional should get a weekly massage. The massage table must be at a comfortable height. A stool to put a foot on is helpful. A high stool can be used to sit on while doing massage. A low stool or chair is helpful when working on the client's face, neck, and feet. If the massage professional carries a portable table, he or she must pay attention to the body mechanics used to lift and move the table. Lift the table with the knees and hips, not the waist. Do not reach for the table when moving it from the car. Avoid habitually carrying the table on only one side.

12. (a) Make sure your body is in good alignment and that your feet are in a wide base of support. The arm generating the downward pressure should be opposite the back weight-bearing leg. (b) The weight is kept

on the back leg and heel of the foot, and the client's body is in front of you. The front non–weight-bearing leg is used to modulate pressure levels and provide some stability. (c) It is important to stay behind your stroke. (d) Keep your head up. (e) Make sure that the wrists and hands are always relaxed. (f) Avoid using your fingers and thumbs. Keep kneading strokes to a minimum. Grasping is stressful on the hands and forearms. Do not use the thumb for direct pressure. (g) Do not use the triceps portion of your arm. You can damage your ulnar nerve. Use the forearm just below the elbow. (h) Positioning the client's body to enable you to lean uphill protects the shoulders. Leaning keeps the lower back relaxed. (i) Do not reach for the stroke. Keep the client close to you. (j) Never hyperextend the wrist or knees. The weight-bearing knee will move into the normal knee-lock position; this is not hyperextension, which damages the knee. Make sure the angle of the wrist is no more than 110 degrees to avoid compression of the nerves in the wrist and keep the elbows straight. (k) Change your position and method often. (l) Face the area you are working with to avoid twisting. (m) Turn your whole body when you change the direction of your movements, and shift the body weight to the back foot. (n) If using kneading, grasp the tissue and rock back to lift the tissue. Develop a rhythm of rocking forward as you compress the tissue and rocking back as you knead and pull the tissue. (o) If deep pressure is required, do not push. Instead, use counterpressure, shifting the weight on the feet as you lean back. (p) Work with smooth and even movements. (q) Allowing your body to rock and sway with the movements is important. Slow rocking keeps your strokes slow. The resulting rhythmic movement keeps your body relaxed and is comforting to the client.

13. Slowly leaning while performing the lengthening and stretching movements automatically accesses the physiologic barrier. The massage practitioner can then feel the subtle push back as the stretch reflex response signals that the muscles have stretched enough.

14. Use compression on an area and simultaneously move the joint or bone under the compression. This method creates cross-fiber friction from the inside out, using the client's bone as the mechanism moving the tissue.

PROBLEM-SOLVING ACTIVITIES

1. Most obvious would be the possibility that she is working with a tense hand and wrist, which is translating to the shoulder muscles. Also, working with the point of the elbow puts pressure on the ulnar nerve, a possible contributing factor to the numbness and tingling. The table may be too high for her to lean with leverage to provide the pressure, so she finds herself pushing with her upper body muscles, which tenses the shoulder muscles.
   Corrective actions: Using a lower massage table; learning the proper use of the forearm below the elbow.

2. It is possible that he is bending his elbow to accommodate his long arms to a tall table, thereby applying uneven pressure to the ulnar side of the wrist.
   Corrective actions: Keeping arm straight when using the palm of the hand; using forearm more, and learning to adjust pressure with width of stance and lower table

3. The long-term increased compressive force in the knee capsule from the flexed knee position coupled with the extra strain of the external rotation may be causing the pain in the right knee.
   Corrective actions: Sitting more during the massage using both a high and low stool; becoming aware of the external rotation and minimizing it; learning to allow the knee of the weight-bearing leg to extend to the normal knee-lock position to reduce compressive forces in the knee joint.

4. The table is likely to be too short, causing her to bend over while giving massage and straining the low back. The symmetric stance often causes strain to the lower back.

Corrective actions: Raising the table; using a short footstool for the front leg to provide extra stability, help keep the back straight, and support an asymmetric stance.

5. He seems to be working hard while giving massage and would conserve and increase energy by working smarter. Corrective actions: Learning to sit more while giving massage; avoiding the use of kneading and replacing it with methods that can be done with less energy using leaning methods, such as gliding and compression; limiting frictioning to areas where it is essential and then using the compression with movements methods in this chapter; ensuring that he is only providing pressure when leaning uphill and altering the position of the client to accomplish this; using the "lean and lift" method instead of the "push harder" method to increase the pressure levels if necessary; making sure his body is relaxed and the pressure comes from body weight rather than muscle strength.

CHAPTER 8 WORKBOOK SECTION ANSWER KEY

SHORT ANSWER

1. The setup of the massage area, supplies, client history and outcome, table supports for positioning, modest draping, types of lubricant, music, temperature of the massage area, and focus of the massage practitioner.

2. The massage practitioner's body, namely, the hands and forearms.

3. Always use proper body mechanics, warm up and stretch before beginning the massage, keep the hands and forearms clean and the nails carefully trimmed, and wear gloves when working outside or doing abrasive work.

4. Portable and free-standing massage tables, massage mats, massage chairs, and body supports for seated massage.

5. Simple, sturdy construction; portability if the table is to be moved often; a face cradle; adequate width and length; a washable covering; and adequate padding for comfort and firm support.

6. Structural stability, including all connectors, bolts, cables, and hinges.

7. Pillows, rolled towels, and specially cut pieces of foam are used to contour the flat surface of the massage table and provide stability and comfort.

8. Sheets, towels, or other large pieces of fabric used to cover the client during the massage to provide privacy, modesty, and warmth.

9. Cotton or cotton/polyester-blend sheets and towels and disposable linen.

10. Only white cotton sheets or towels are used to prevent possible allergic reactions.

11. All draping materials are laundered in bleach or other approved disinfecting solution. A fresh set of drapes always is used for each client.

12. Lubricants are used only to reduce friction on the skin from massage methods. Massage practitioners do not use lubricants for medicinal or cosmetic purposes.

13. Oils, creams, and powders.

14. Lubricants must be dispensed in a contamination-free manner, and they should be as natural as possible. Scents should be avoided, and powder should not be inhaled.

15. Temperature of 75° F, fresh air, designated areas for business operations and the massage session, and privacy if any clothing needs to be removed.

16. Private office or clinical setting, public setting, on-site at client's business or home, and outdoors.

17. Both the massage practitioner and the client must enjoy the music and want to listen to it. The rhythm and beat of the music must match the desired effect for the massage session.

18. The lighting must be indirect so that it does not cast a glare into the client's eyes. The practitioner also must be able to dim or reduce the intensity of the light, as well as increase it to provide visibility for cleaning the room. Practitioners never work in a dark or candle-lit room.

19. Many people are sensitive to smells and chemical scents.

20. The massage practitioner must be attentive to cigarette or other smoke odors, cold hands, keeping pets out of the massage area, and other such considerations.

21. The client may have a specific medical focus for the massage that is outside the practitioner's scope of practice, or the client may have preconceived ideas that may interfere with the acceptance of the massage.

22. Clients respond better and are less anxious if they understand such procedural details as draping, where to hang their clothes, and what types of lubricant will be used. Conditions are safer for the practitioner and client if they both understand the use of the massage equipment, such as adjusting the face cradle on a table. The client then is better able to provide informed consent for the massage session.

23. Prone, with supports under the ankles and possibly around the chest. Supine, with supports under the knees and neck. Side-lying, with supports between the knees and under the arms and head.

24. Opaque materials must be used, and only the area being massaged is undraped. Neither the genital area nor a woman's breasts are ever undraped without a physician's supervision.

25. During a typical full-body massage, the client has removed most clothing. The drape is the separation from the massage practitioner and defines the personal space of the client.

26. Contour and flat draping.

27. A chest towel is used to drape women's breasts while the larger drape is pulled back to expose the abdomen. The towel is placed over the flat sheet and stabilized, and then the larger flat sheet is pulled out.

28. Place your arms under the client's neck and knees. Lift the torso and swing the knees to the side of the table. Be sure to secure the drapes so that they do not slip.

29. Polite and courteous completion. It is difficult for some clients to conclude the massage, and they may linger before leaving. Developing a sequence that is the same at the end of each massage helps the client break the contact that was created during the massage.

30. The practitioner washes his or her hands, updates the client's records, prepares the room for the next massage, and takes a small personal break. This takes about 15 minutes and should be considered in the scheduling of the massage sessions.

PROBLEM-SOLVING EXERCISES

1. Powder or a water-based cream can be used during the massage. Compression-type massage over a clean sheet or towel can be done in these areas.

2. Switch to an over-the-clothing massage and ask the client to change into loose, nonrestrictive clothing. Turn the appointment into an educational session and teach others in the household some simple massage techniques. Do a seated massage in a private location.

CHAPTER 9   WORKBOOK SECTION ANSWER KEY

SHORT ANSWER

1. The three effects are mechanical, reflexive, and chemical. Mechanical effects in the tissue result directly from the application of the method and the forces used. Reflexive effects add sensory stimulation and cause the nervous system to respond. Chemical effects cause release of chemicals either directly at the tissue worked with or through the endocrine system and nervous system. These responses are often classified as reflexive.

2. Methods that move through the skin to the underlying tissues.

3. Methods and techniques that stay within the skin or superficial fascial layer, move the body, or add heat or cold.

4. Depth of pressure, drag, direction, speed, rhythm, frequency, and duration.

5. The body will adapt to a repetitive sensory stimulation and stop responding to the sensory input. Varying the touch quality prevents adaptation and continues to stimulate the body.

6. Regardless of when in history massage was used, it was applied to the same anatomy and physiology as it is today. Many approaches may be developed today, but they all tend to work for similar reasons.

7. Massage manipulations are based on Ling's and others' concept of passive movements. They involve the direct application of pressure or pulling of the soft tissue elements of skin, fascia, muscles, tendons, and ligaments. Massage techniques are based on gymnastics or movement-cure methods, as described by Ling, Taylor, and others. They use active involvement of the joints and movement patterns.

8. Initial contact, stillness, calling attention to an area of the body, addition of body heat, reestablishing contact.

9. With a slow, gradual, confident, secure approach, with a deliberate hesitation at the arms-length boundary, coupled with a verbal announcement that you will be touching.

10. It is applied horizontally in relation to the tissues.

11. The drag component of the heavier pressure works on a more mechanical level. It takes time for the tissues to warm and respond to the mechanical force. Going fast with a deep gliding stroke is painful, causes spasm, and is ineffective.

12. Applying lubricant, warming the area with increasing pressure, connecting one area to another, evaluation, and abdominal massage.

13. The tissue is lifted, twisted, rolled, and squeezed. The stroke functions on the vertical lifting up.

14. It involves repetitive use of the massage professional's hands and wrists, which can cause overuse injury. It is better to substitute alternative methods to warm the tissue and use pétrissage only for a specific, deliberate purpose.

15. Tissue that will not lift, edema, excessive body hair, ticklish clients.

16. Superficial applications are reflexive, especially if applied over motor nerve points and nerve tracts. Moderate applications over arteries enhance arterial blood flow. Moderate to deep applications spread spindle cells, causing the muscle to contract and thereby toning the muscle. This small toning component is good for discharging the nervous system so that the muscle can relax. Deep applications affect the connective tissue by spreading it against the underlying bony structure and releasing histamine from the surrounding tissue. Compression that enters the tissue at 90 degrees and then shifts to between 80 and 45 degrees, without slipping, will produce a drag on the tissue.

17. Avoid hyperextension of the wrist or finger joints. Avoid the use of the thumb. Do not use the tip or radial ulnar flat side of the elbow. Keep the hand and wrist relaxed when doing any work with the forearm. Change from palm to fist to forearm often.

18. At the tendon to affect the tonic vibration reflex and at motor points to stimulate nerves.

19. Shaking has a distinct snap at the end of the stroke, making the stroke irregular in its rhythm, whereas rocking is very rhythmic and regular. Shaking disrupts body rhythms, and rocking works to enhance them. Both inhibit muscle tone and relax but for different reasons.

20. Activation of the tendon reflex when applied to the tendon. This causes the muscle to contract. As soon as one muscle contracts, its antagonist is reciprocally inhibited.

21. A relaxed wrist that moves in response to contraction and relaxation at the elbow joint.

22. Friction moves superficial tissue over deeper underlying tissue. Movement on the skin is avoided to prevent friction-type burns. To prevent sliding on the skin, no lubricant is used. The movements are applied to a specific location and are transverse to the grain of the tissue or are circular.

23. 30 seconds to 10 minutes.

24. (1) No lubricant is used. The braced fingers, hand, or elbow compresses the tissue to the depth required to access the tissue to be frictioned. The massage practitioner does not slide but rather moves the tissues back and forth or around. (2) The practitioner applies compression over the area in which friction is to be used. Instead of moving the application hand, the practitioner moves the client's joint under the compression. The friction comes from the action of the underlying bone against the tissue.

25. These techniques warm the tissues, relax the nervous system, and relax and lengthen the muscles, thus reducing the need for repetitive massage manipulations.

26. (1) Joint kinesthetic receptors—position and rate of movement. (2) Spindle cells—stretch of muscle. (3) Golgi tendon organs—muscle tension at the tendon.

27. (1) Active: produced by the client. (2) Passive: produced by the massage professional.

28. The point at which motion causes a bind, catch, or pain.

29. One hand should be placed close to the joint to be moved. This hand acts both as a stabilizer and for evaluation. The other hand is placed at the distal end of the bone and is the hand that actually provides the movement.

30. Muscle lengthening, reducing spasm, strengthening weak muscles, reducing local edema, and as preparation for stretching.

31. Lengthening is a neurologic response that allows muscles to assume a normal resting length.

32. Muscle energy methods are focused on specific muscles and resultant joint function. To access the muscles for the proper contraction, the muscles must be positioned in such a way that the proximal and distal attachments are as close together as possible for contraction, whether active or passive, and lengthening (extended) with proximal and distal attachments separated.

33. Isometric: No movement, only effort.
Isotonic: Movement against resistance. There are three types:
Concentric isotonic: origin and insertion come together against resistance.
Eccentric isotonic: origin and insertion separate against resistance.
Multiple isotonic: combination of concentric and eccentric contraction against resistance for a full range of movement for a joint.

34. A muscle relaxation after a contraction.

35. When a muscle contracts, its antagonist must relax.

36. Instead of one strong contraction, small, light, rapid contractions of the muscles are used to activate the receptors and the reflexive movement.

37. The target muscle is the muscle or muscle group on which the massage practitioner is specifically focusing a particular response.

38. Usually no more than 25% of muscle strength is required. The exception to this is strengthening weak muscles. In this case, a stronger contraction or repeated contraction may be required.

39. To replace the active contraction portion of muscle energy techniques when the client cannot or does not wish to participate in the massage.

40. When specific tender points are found or if the client is in pain. It is a good method for gentle, painless release of all specific sore spots regardless of pathology (what is wrong). The tender point is the guide to the proper positioning of the client. Use a full-body approach in positioning and do not focus solely on the area around the tender point.

41. Stretching is a mechanical method that introduces forces into connective tissue to elongate and soften it.

42. To avoid protective spasm of the muscles in the area to be stretched.

43. Stretching is not used in acute situations. If the connective tissue is normal in an area and the problem is recent, only lengthening needs to be used. Stretching does need to be done in most chronic conditions.

44. Longitudinal stretching, which pulls tissue in the fiber direction, and cross-directional stretching, which pulls tissue against the fiber direction, often with a twisting component.

45. Direction of ease is the position and postural change that the body has assumed to adjust to pain, repetitive movement, or structural distortion. The massage professional must not directly pull a client out of the ease pattern but instead must increase the positioning, allowing the protective sensory receptors to "relax," and then gently coax the body into a more efficient pattern using lengthening and stretching.

46. The massage needs a base of general, broad application methods to form the structure of the massage. The methods most commonly used are effleurage/gliding stroke, compression, and rocking.

47. Stimulation of all the sensory receptors, touching all the layers and types of tissue, and moving all the major joints of the body.

48. Subtle shifts and changes in pressure, intensity, methods used, positioning, sequence, and focus allow for each massage to be different. A musical scale has only 12 notes, yet all the music comes from combinations of the notes. Massage is the same. Each client is different, and therefore each massage is different.

MATCHING

1. l	9. b	17. g	25. w
2. y	10. c	18. h	26. x
3. n	11. d	19. t	27. z
4. e	12. cc	20. u	28. aa
5. q	13. dd	21. v	29. bb
6. r	14. ee	22. i	30. m
7. s	15. ff	23. j	31. o
8. a	16. f	24. k	32. p

1. a	5. e
2. b	6. d
3. g	7. c
4. f	

1. j	10. ee	18. o	26. x
2. a	11. ff	19. p	27. w
3. q	12. gg	20. r	28. c
4. e	13. s	21. aa	29. d
5. m	14. n	22. u	30. f
6. l	15. t	23. z	31. g
7. i	16. cc	24. v	32. h
8. k	17. bb	25. y	33. b
9. dd			

PROBLEM-SOLVING EXERCISES

1. Muscle energy methods to produce lengthening, relax the muscle. Rocking of the body may relax the muscles.

2. Do compression and percussion over a towel or sheet. The resting stroke can be used, as can shaking, rocking, and all massage techniques of joint movement, muscle energy, positional release, and lengthening and stretching approaches.

3. The entire body can be accessed in the other positions of supine, side-lying, and seated.

PROFESSIONAL APPLICATION

Reduce the amount of kneading and percussion, and use it only when there is a specific purpose. Increase the muscle energy methods and lengthening.

Increase the shaking and rocking methods. He should make sure that he is centered before giving the massage and stretch his body afterward. He should check to see that he is applying strokes with the correct body mechanics and making minimal use of his hands.

CHAPTER 10 WORKBOOK SECTION ANSWER KEY

SHORT ANSWER

1. The collection and interpretation of information provided by the client, the massage practitioner, and referring medical professionals.
2. To decide whether the client should be referred to a medical professional and to gather information to be used in designing a massage that meets the individual's specific needs.
3. The client. If you watch and listen long enough, the client will tell you what is wrong and what needs to be done to restore balance.
4. The development of a relationship based on mutual trust and harmony. It is the responsibility of the massage professional to create an environment that supports rapport. This is done by following the client's lead.
5. Look for efficiency of movement, breathing patterns, and the general state of sympathetic or parasympathetic activation.
6. The way a person points and touches the body during conversation can give clues as to whether the problem is muscular, joint related, or visceral.
7. They encourage the client to discuss all situations and provide more information than questions that can be answered with "Yes" or "No."
8. To confirm the information and make sure that you understood everything that was said.
9. Thinking about what you are going to say, writing something down, interpreting information, interrupting people, finishing people's sentences, sorting through many words that express a single thought, and preconceived ideas.
10. Measurement is how we objectively quantify the client condition before and after assessment by analyzing the measurement change or lack of change is noted and appropriate adjustment in massage application is possible.
11. Heredity, disease, and habit. Habit is the easiest to adjust. Habitual patterns are occupational, recreational, and sleep related.
12. The gravitational line must fall through the axis of the weight-bearing joint. If it does not, extra effort is required of the muscles to maintain the upright position.
13. The various segments of the body must cooperate. Passive tension of ligaments, fascia, and the connective tissue elements of the muscles support the skeleton. Muscle plays a small part, through the activity of the postural muscles, by continually repositioning the body over the mechanical balance point. If the mechanical balance is disputed, the postural muscles struggle with this function.
14. This is the normal knee position of the femur as it rides back on the medial condyle and rotates medially about its vertical axis to lock the joint for the weight bearing used in standing. The design of the knee stabilizes the body in the standing position and makes that position less fatiguing.
15. A symmetric stance, with eyes focused forward and closed.
16. Bony landmarks provide markers for checking levelness and symmetry.
17. Walking is something that we do every day. If this pattern is inefficient, more energy is used than is necessary for the activity. This can translate into fatigue and possibly pain during walking.
18. It moves in an alternating-side figure-eight pattern. If the joint is limited in this very important function, the entire gait pattern is disrupted.

19. Watch for areas that move too much, as well as those that do not move during walking. It is important to consider the entire body when looking for these patterns because the activity of the arms provides a counterbalance to the legs.
20. Pain, muscle weakness, muscle shortening, limitation of joint movement, and changes in bone or soft tissue.
21. Walking is a full-body experience that demands many coordinated activities of the arms and legs, neck and trunk, and eyes and ears. Almost every joint, muscle, and bone is involved with every step taken. Walking is one of the most important survival activities. The body expends a lot of energy to walk. Full-body massage restores balance and efficiency to the walking pattern.
22. Touch assessment that differentiates between tissue textures within the same tissue types. Palpation is a way to compare tissue to tissue and check for heat and cold. Palpation is a good time to observe skin color and the state of the hair and nails.
23. The proprioceptors and mechanoreceptors of the hand receive stimulation from the tissue palpated. The brain devotes a large sensory area to the hand. The refined discriminatory sense of the hand can perceive subtle sensory shifts.
24. No. The whole body can be used to pick up sensory information. The areas most sensitive to posture shift and movement changes are the massage therapist's joints. This is because of the large concentration of positional receptors found in and around joint capsules. Therefore the hip, elbow, knee, and foot, when placed against the client, also can detect sensory data about client movement.
25. The sensory receptors in the massage practitioner's hand adapt quickly and will not respond as well to prolonged stimulation; you simply do not feel it the second time you try. Thinking about what you are feeling also interferes with perception of the sensory data. Do not think until after you have felt.
26. The skin sensory receptors are designed to detect subtle changes in heat, air pressure, and air movement. This survival mechanism becomes most sensitive at a distance of about an arm's length from the person or object.
27. We are subconsciously aware of all the sensory stimulation that we have receptor mechanisms to detect. Sensitivity, or intuition, is the ability to work with this information on a conscious level. It does not depend on extrasensory skills but rather on conscious awareness of everything.
28. Heat and cold, as well as areas of not enough or too much sensitivity to air pressure changes. Sometimes this sensation feels like the repelling action between magnets with the north poles together. There is a subtle sense of resistance or of a force field.
29. Whether the skin is damp or dry; whether there are goose bumps, moles, or surface growths; the elasticity of the skin; the surface texture; and the mobility of the skin against the superficial connective tissue.
30. This area is a spongelike layer that contains the adipose tissue. It can get waterlogged with surface edema.
31. In the superficial connective tissue; these vessels feel like soft tubes. Any changes in the superficial connective tissue affect circulation. You can feel pulses in the arteries, but if you press too hard, you lose the pulse. This may give some idea of how to locate the superficial connective tissue layer.
32. The lymph nodes can be indicators of many different conditions, from a minor local infection to a life-threatening condition. Only a physician is equipped to make that determination.
33. Skeletal muscle has a distinct, ribbed feeling created by the fiber direction. It should feel firm and resilient without feeling stringy. There are usually three and sometimes more layers to skeletal muscle, and these layers crisscross over each other and slide over one another. It is

important to feel through all the layers and assess the ability of the individual muscles to move on top of the other.

34. This is the transition area between muscle and tendons. For this reason the area is the site of the most strain and therefore the most injury. In addition, this is the area where the nerves often enter, and it is the location of the motor points that activate the muscle. Most muscle dysfunction arises at the musculotendinous junction.

35. No. Tendons are just as likely to adhere to all surrounding connective tissue. The fascial sheaths, ligaments, and other tendons, as well as bone, serve as attachment points. During palpation, it is important to be able to trace the tendon, rather than rely on the bony attachment sites shown in diagrams.

36. Deep fascial sheaths separate muscles, expand the skeleton, and provide stability. They provide grooves in which the nerves, blood, and lymph vessels lie. Deep fascial sheaths run primarily horizontally and vertically through the body. They must be pliable and distinct to serve these important functions.

37. Ligaments support and connect joints. Connection and separation of the joint is very important for posture because of the positional receptors in the joint. If the function of the ligaments is disrupted, postural distortion develops. Because of their limited blood supply, ligaments do not heal well if injured. Unless specifically trained in methods to work with ligaments, the massage therapist should avoid any direct work with them.

38. End-feel is the perception of the joint at the limit of its range of motion. It is either hard or soft. End-feel is perceived at the anatomic barrier if range of motion is unrestricted and at the physiologic barrier if the area is dysfunctional in any way.

39. Stable, supported, resilient, and unrestricted. The joint space should be able to be palpated. Much information can be obtained by palpating the joint while it is in motion.

40. With a short lever, one-jointed muscle initiates and stabilizes the joint movement. With a long lever, one-jointed muscle provides for full range of movement and power in the movement. A two-jointed muscle coordinates the movement with either the joint above or the joint below and assists the long-lever muscle.

41. Hypertonic muscles and shortened connective tissue. Usually the flexor and adductor muscles are the muscles that pull the joint out of alignment because they are approximately 30% stronger than the extensor and abductor muscles. Trauma also may push a joint out of alignment.

42. Joint dysfunction is out of the scope of practice for massage. The two ways to determine this are as follows: (1) pain on traction usually is soft tissue dysfunction; (2) pain on compression usually is joint dysfunction. If active range of motion produces pain and if passive range of motion does not, the problem usually is a soft tissue problem. If both cause pain, the problem usually is a joint problem. Always refer suspected joint problems to a physician.

43. To locate bony landmarks for comparison of symmetry.

44. Hard and spongy areas, referred pain patterns, and the location of the liver and large intestine. If any unusual areas are noted, refer the patient for diagnosis.

45. The three primary body rhythms are respiration, blood and lymph circulation, and craniosacral rhythm. These rhythms ebb and flow in an undulating fashion. The breath is particularly important. Massage tends to stabilize and even out these rhythms. The craniosacral rhythm (or lymphatic undulation) is the most subtle and requires practice to feel.

46. Strength muscle testing seeks to discover whether the muscle being tested is responding with sufficient strength and endurance. Neurologic muscle testing evaluates the ability of the nerves to respond appropriately to a signal. Applied kinesiologic muscle testing is used as a biofeedback monitor of body function.

47. With strength testing, the muscle to be isolated is placed in contraction, and the client holds it in place with a stabilizing force while the massage practitioner attempts to pull or push the muscle from its contracted position without recruiting other muscles. Strength patterns must be compared against a similar area, such as the same muscle on the other side, or against antagonist patterns. Neurologic muscle testing uses the same isolation of muscles, and the client holds the stabilizing force. The massage therapist provides a light pressure to evaluate the response of the muscle.

48. Because all muscles are linked neurologically, especially for the walking pattern, overly strong or weak muscles affect the entire pattern because they do not respond correctly to neurologic signals. Optimal contraction of firing sequences supports efficient movement.

49. Postural muscles are made up of slow-twitch red fibers that can maintain a sustained contraction; these muscles are used to keep the body balanced against gravity. When stressed, they tend to shorten. Phasic muscles are primarily used for movement and are made up of fast-twitch white fibers that contract quickly but fatigue easily. They tend to weaken in response to postural muscle shortening. A muscle can serve a dual role and have a mixed fiber configuration.

50. The body moves in segments. These areas counterbalance each other against gravity and during movement. A typical muscle imbalance pattern bounces front to back and side to side at the segments.

51. Interpretation is done after the assessment. With experience, the two are not separated. When a student is learning the process, it is easy to jump to conclusions if all the information is not gathered first. Interpretation is the process of piecing together all the information and then designing the best massage for the client.

52. Noting the client's general presence and the sequence that the client uses in gesturing and explaining. Also to be considered are symmetry of posture, efficiency of movement, tissue texture and condition, and areas that are hot or cold and overactive or underactive.

53. To provide balance by respecting current patterns and providing stimulation to encourage a more efficient function. Put simply, the purpose of the design of the massage is to cool down the hot spots, warm up the cold spots, lengthen the short areas, strengthen the weak areas, "unstick the stuck spots," and so forth.

54. All the information discussed regarding the physiologic effects of each massage method determines the methods chosen. When all is said and done, you can only push on it or pull on it, shake it, stretch it, and so on. What varies is the location of application, intensity, duration, etc. of the methods used.

55. Reassessment allows both the massage practitioner and the client to determine what was successful during the massage process. Information given before and after the massage reinforces the benefits of massage for the client.

56. Most conditions with which the massage professional deals are chronic or self-limiting problems. Symptomatic relief, combined with activity to pass the time while the body heals itself, goes a long way toward assisting clients with this type of difficulty. Massage provides the hope that the body may not always feel like this, and the physiologic effects stimulate the body to reorganize toward a more efficient pattern. This takes time, and distracting the body from the current situation for awhile is extremely helpful. Massage is simple, repetitive, and humble work. Be proud that you are studying to become part of this profession.

ADDITIONAL ACTIVITY

PROBLEM-SOLVING EXERCISES

1. In general, excessive sympathetic activation would be balanced by a relaxing massage, and excessive parasympathetic activation would be

balanced by a stimulation massage. If the client is functioning from sympathetic nervous system dominance and if relaxation methods such as rocking and slow effleurage are used initially, the work often is irritating. By beginning with a more stimulating approach and using strokes such as rapid compression, proprioceptive neuromuscular facilitation, stretching, and tapotement, the design of the massage fits the client physiologically. After some of the nervous energy has been discharged, the client is ready for the more relaxing methods.

2. A finger pointing to a specific area may suggest an acupressure or motor point hyperactivity or a joint problem. What the pointing means depends on the area indicated. Because the client is drilling into a joint, it may be wise to refer him for joint dysfunction evaluation.

3. Damp areas on the skin show that the nervous system has been activated in that area. This small amount of perspiration is part of a sympathetic activation called a facilitated segment. Surface stroking, with pressure enough to drag, elicits a red response over hyperactive areas. Deeper palpation usually elicits a tender response, such as a trigger point. The small erector pili muscles attached to each hair also are under sympathetic autonomic nervous system control. Light fingertip stroking produces goose bumps over areas of hyperactivity.

4. Pulses should be compared by feeling for a strong, even, full pumping action on both sides of the body. If differences are perceived, the client should be referred to a physician for peripheral circulation assessment. Sometimes the differences in the pulses can be attributed to soft tissue restriction of the artery, which is determined by the physician.

5. A major problem is very likely hypertonic muscles. If shortened postural muscles are found, they need to be lengthened. If shortened and weak phasic muscles are found, they first must be lengthened and stretched.

TREATMENT PLAN

Client Name: _Sue Williams_   Date: _00/00/0000_

Choose One: ✓ Original plan   Reassessment date _____

Short-term client goals:
To improve work and daily activity performance through (1) relaxation to support better sleep and (2) management of headache and arm tingling.

Long-term client goals:
Continuing stress management to manage headaches and disturbed sleep, maintain effectiveness at work, and support a healthy lifestyle.

Therapist objectives:
Normalize breathing function, reduce thoracic tension, and even stride in gait.

1) Frequency, 2) length, and 3) duration of visits:
1) _1 x per week_   2) _6 weeks_   3) _1 hour_

Progress "measurements" to be used: (Ex.—pain scale, range of motion, increased ability to perform function)
Frequency of headaches reduced by 50% and pain diminished from 8 to 4 on a scale of 1 to 10; decrease time to fall asleep by 30 minutes and increase sleep to 7 hours without interruption; reduce tingling in arms by 50%.

Dates of reassessment:
_00/00/0000_

Categories of massage methods to be used: (Ex.— relaxation, stress reduction, lymphatic, neuromuscular, connective tissue, neurochemical, etc.)
General massage, connective tissue stretching, postisometric relaxation and lengthening, entrainment rocking

Additional notes:
Client wears heels at work and spends most of the day in a seated position talking on the phone.

Client Signature: _Sue Williams_   Date: _00/00/0000_

Therapist Signature: _Robin Jones_   Date: _00/00/0000_

FIGURE 10-26 Completed physical assessment form.

SESSION NOTES
SOAP CHARTING FORM

Client Name: _Sue Williams_____   Date: _00/00/0000_____

(S)ubjective

CLIENT STATUS
• **Information from client, referral source or reference books:**
1) Current conditions/changes from last session: _____
Tingling in arm, headache 8 on 1 to 10 scale, shortness of breath, disrupted sleep.
_____

(O)bjective

2) Information from _assessment_ (physical, gait, palpation, muscle testing):
Right side tension pattern shortened chest muscles and connective tissue, weak abdominals, tight muscles in lower legs.
_____

CONTENT OF SESSION
• **Generate goal (possibilities) from analysis of information in _client status_.**
1) Goals worked on this session. (Base information on client status this session and goals previously established in Treatment Plan):
Relaxation, parasympathetic dominance, reduce shortening in right shoulder tissue.
_____

What was _done_ this session:
General massage lengthened shoulders and lower leg muscles with muscle energy methods, mild connective tissue stretching on upper chest; taught lengthening for shoulders and lower legs.
_____

(A)nalysis

RESULTS
• **Analyze results of session in relationship to what was done and how this relates to the session goals. (This is based on _cause_ and _effect_ of methods used and the effects on the persons involved).**
1) What worked/what didn't: (Based on measurable and objective post assessment)
Client reports decrease in headache (to 4 on 1 to 10 scale) and easier breathing, she feels sleepy and desires a nap. General massage with rocking entrainment seemed to be most effective. Client acknowledged the benefit of connective tissue stretching but did not enjoy the methods; will need to use the approach sparingly. Client willingly participated in muscle energy methods and found them effective.

(P)lan

PLAN: Plans for next session, what client will work on, what next massage will reassess and continue to assess:
Client will do lengthening exercises daily. Weekly sessions will continue using general massage with entrainment focus, therapist will include small amounts of connective tissue stretching and continue to use muscle energy and lengthening on the thorax to help with breathing.
_____

CLIENT COMMENTS:
Pressure was uneven at times. I prefer deep, even pressure with no poking.
_____

Time In: _____   Time Out: _____

FIGURE 10-27 Completed SOAP chart form.

Eventually, strengthening techniques and exercises will be needed. If the hypertonic phasic muscle pattern arises from repetitive use, the muscles are fatigued with muscle energy/proprioceptive neuromuscular facilitation techniques and then lengthened.

PROFESSIONAL APPLICATION

It is important to be able both to understand the assessment procedures of chiropractic and to provide the chiropractor with concise information for evaluation in the development of a total treatment plan. The ability to keep clear, concise client SOAP notes is valuable in comparing and coordinating the combined therapy.

CHAPTER 11 WORKBOOK SECTION ANSWER KEY

SHORT ANSWER

1. Each method has so much to offer, it is impossible to provide a thorough study in the few pages devoted here, when a book could be written on each topic. A higher skill level is attained with concentrated study. This chapter provides only a sample so that students can try the methods and more purposefully choose the focus of future study. An entry-level course of approximately 500 class hours is not enough class time to adequately cover these methods.

2. The effects are mainly reflexive and focus on the autonomic nervous system. The addition of heat energy or dissipation of heat from the tissue may be classified as mechanical in effect. In general, cold stimulates sympathetic responses, and heat activates parasympathetic responses. Short and long applications of hot or cold produce different results. Most short cold applications stimulate and increase circulation. Long cold applications depress and decrease circulation. A short application of heat depresses and depletes tone, whereas a long hot application results in a combined depressant and stimulant reaction.

3. Hot and cold compresses can be used. A foot bath is easy to incorporate. A bag of frozen peas makes a great ice pack. Hot water bottles are safer to use than heating pads. Water frozen in a paper cup with a stick in it makes an effective ice massage tool. Pure drinking water for clients and yourself is also an excellent hydrotherapy method.

4. The following conditions contraindicate the use of ice: vasospastic disease, cold hypersensitivity, cardiac disorder, compromised local circulation, rheumatoid conditions, an area of paralysis, and coronary artery disease. When using ice, it is important to consider the following precautions:

    Do not use frozen gel packs directly on the skin.

    Do not use cryotherapy applications for extended periods; 15-minute therapy sessions are recommended.

    Do not do exercises that cause pain after cold applications.

5. Stones should be smooth, safely placed where sanitized and care taken not to burn the skin.

6. Systemic massage entails focusing massage on a specific body system; two forms of systemic massage are lymphatic massage and circulation massage. When a massage is concentrated on a particular body system, the effects of the massage are more dramatic.

7. The massage consists of a combination of short, pumping, and active gliding strokes, followed by long surface gliding strokes, deep breathing, and passive range of motion. The direction of action is toward the drainage points. The focus of the pressure and drag is on the dermis just below the surface layer of skin and the layer of tissue just beneath the skin and above the muscles; it then may gradually increase.

8. Compression is applied over the main arteries, beginning near the heart or proximally to it and systematically moving distally, ending at the tips of the fingers or toes. The strokes are applied over the arteries and pump at a rhythm of approximately 60 beats per minute, or with the client's resting heart rate. The next step is to assist venous return flow. A combination of short gliding strokes, long gliding strokes, and joint movement is used. With venous return flow, the strokes move distal to proximal, or from the finger and toes to the heart, over the major veins. The short strokes are about 3 inches long and move the blood from valve to valve. Long strokes carry the blood through the entire vein. Passive and active joint movements help venous circulation. Placing the limb or area above the heart allows for gravity assistance.

9. The foot has many joint and reflex patterns. Sensory information about position and posture from the joint kinesthetic receptors is extensive. Sensory and motor centers of the brain devote a large area to the feet and hands. There is extensive nerve distribution to the feet and hands. The position of the foot sends a great deal of postural information through the central nervous system. Stimulation of the feet seems to activate the responses of the gate control mechanism, hyperstimulation analgesia (parasympathetic dominance). Bodywide effects are achieved by this technique. Many nerve endings in the feet and hands correlate with acupressure points, which in turn release endorphins and other endogenous chemicals when stimulated. In addition, major plexuses for the lymph system are located in the hands and feet. Compressive forces in this area stimulate lymphatic movement.

10. An excellent way to massage a foot is to apply pressure and movement systematically to the entire foot and ankle complex. The pressure stimulates the circulation, nerves, and reflexes. Moving the joints stimulates large-diameter nerve fibers, initiating hyperstimulation analgesia and joint kinesthetic receptors. The result is a shift in proprioceptive and postural reflexes. This same approach can be used to massage the hands.

11. Hand and foot massage is likely to be the most effective form of self-massage. The hands and feet have similar motor cortex distribution patterns. The stimulation of the hands during the massage does not override the sensations to the area being massaged. The hands are massaged while massaging the feet.

12. Techniques that specifically alter the configuration of the connective tissue are classified as connective tissue approaches. The methods can vary from mechanical methods, such as Cyriax's deep transverse

friction, to the very subtle approaches of craniosacral therapy. Connective tissue methods stretch, pull, drag, elongate, and move the tissue.

13. The intent of connective tissue massage is either to soften the ground substance, or plastic component, of connective tissue or to introduce small amounts of inflammation, which triggers connective tissue restructuring.

14. To use frictioning, extensive anatomic knowledge is required. Frictioning must be done very specifically, and because it introduces an inflammatory response, the effect is a controlled injury of tissue. Without the anatomic knowledge and assessment required, the precise location of an adhesion will not be known and healthy tissue may be damaged. Additional training is required to skillfully follow tissue movement to work effectively with the craniosacral system.

15. A trigger point is an area of local nerve facilitation of a muscle that can be aggravated by stress of any sort affecting the body or mind of the individual. Trigger points are small areas of hypertonicity within muscles. If these tight areas of muscle fibers are located near motor nerve points, referred pain may result from nerve stimulation. Often the area of the trigger point is the point where nerve stimulation initiates a contraction in a small sensitive bundle of muscle fibers (motor point) that in turn activates the entire muscle.

16. Using light palpation, the massage practitioner needs to notice whether the skin feels tense and whether there is resistance to gliding strokes. The skin may be slightly damp with perspiration from sympathetic facilitation. The temperature in a local area increases in acute trigger points but decreases in chronic trigger points as a result of ischemia, which is an indication of fibrotic changes within the tissues around the trigger point. Edema produces an impression of fullness and congestion within the tissues. In instances of chronic dysfunction, edema is replaced gradually with fibrotic (connective tissue) changes, and the tissue texture feels cemented. During deep palpation the massage therapist establishes contact with the deeper fibers of the soft tissues and explores them for immobility, tenderness, edema, muscle tension, and fibrotic changes. With both light and deep palpation, gliding strokes cover a region of 2 to 3 inches at a time. The trigger point is painful to pressure and refers pain to other areas.

17. The trigger point is hyperstimulated by using various methods such as compression, pushing together or apart on the spindle cells, or active contraction of the muscle. Hyperstimulation is followed by stretching of the muscle fibers containing the trigger point.

18. After treatment of a trigger point, the target (referred) area should be searched to uncover satellite or embryonic trigger points that need to be treated. Immediately afterward, the area needs to be massaged to increase local circulation. Placing a damp warm or hot towel over the region is soothing and useful. The area requires rest for a few days, with all stressful activity avoided.

19. Most acupuncture points correspond with motor points or nerve endings; meridians lie over or close to main nerve tracts; yin is parasympathetic, and yang is sympathetic.

20. A person is body, mind, and spirit. These are not separate pieces but a part of a whole. Health is achieved when harmony exists in all areas.

21. Acupuncture points usually lie in fascial divisions between muscles, near the origin and insertion. The point feels like a small hole, and pressure elicits a "nervy" feeling. Unlike a trigger point, which may be on only one side of the body, acupuncture points are bilateral (located on both sides of the body). To confirm the location of an acupuncture point, locate the point in the same place on the other side of the body.

22. To stimulate a hypoactive or "not enough energy" acupuncture point, use a short vibrating or tapping action. This method is used if the area is sluggish or if a specific body function needs stimulation. To sedate a hyperactive or "too much energy" point for pain reduction, elicit the

pain response within the point itself. Use a sustained holding pressure until the painful overenergy dissipates and the body's own painkillers are released into the bloodstream. The pressure techniques are similar to those used for trigger points, although it is not necessary to lengthen an acupuncture point after treatment.

23. Dr. Stone trained in both systems and incorporated the methods with a Western knowledge base to create an eclectic, multifaceted system.

24. Color is an aspect of the law of five elements. Incorporating it into polarity therapy can also be considered in the room environment.

25. Always dilute essential oils in appropriate carrier oil. Blend no more than three oils for massage. Use a skin patch test to determine safety. Use only safe oils in small amounts. Always ask before using essential oils.

MATCHING

1.	e	7.	k
2.	f	8.	l
3.	g	9.	h
4.	d	10.	c
5.	i	11.	b
6.	j	12.	a

1. a
2. d
3. b
4. c
5. f
6. g
7. e

LABELING

1.	U	8.	C	15.	W	22.	F
2.	B	9.	P	16.	K	23.	R
3.	BB	10.	E	17.	Z	24.	G
4.	Q	11.	N	18.	J	25.	I
5.	Y	12.	X	19.	O	26.	M
6.	A	13.	T	20.	H	27.	V
7.	L	14.	AA	21.	D	28.	S

ADDITIONAL EXERCISE

Heat 1, 3, 6, 8, 9, 10
Cold 1, 2, 5, 7, 8, 11, 12
Ice 2, 4, 7, 8, 9, 11

PROBLEM-SOLVING EXERCISES

1. Acupuncture points are bilateral. You should be able to find the same spot on the other side of the body. Trigger points usually are only on one side of the body.

2. Focus compression methods initially over the main arteries and then switch to effleurage strokes and joint movement for the major portion of the remainder of the massage.

PROFESSIONAL APPLICATION

1. Classes in trigger point therapy, deep transverse friction, myofascial release, and craniosacral therapy.

2. Answers not provided. There are a variety of solutions.

CHAPTER 12 WORKBOOK SECTION ANSWER KEY

SHORT ANSWER

1. Spa, Health Care, and Sport and Fitness. The massage delivered in all three environments are very similar based on outcomes. The spa environment does require proficiency in protocol deliver. Health care and sport and fitness are very similar even though the structure of health care enviroment may be more structured.

2. Always remember to interact with the person who has a special need. Do not allow yourself to become focused on the special situation. Consider the person first.

3. In providing wellness personal service massage, as opposed to rehabilitative massage, the skills are no different from those presented in this text. What is different is the situation presented by the client. An athlete has certain needs based on the sport, the pregnant woman based on the pregnancy, and those with a chronic illness based on the illness pattern. The massage practitioner needs additional training in the various situations and conditions to use the fundamental massage skills purposefully.

4. The client is the best source. Even if the client lacks technical knowledge about a particular illness, sport, pregnancy, disability, or emotional pattern, he or she is still the only one who really understands the effects of any situation.

5. Animals require patience, understanding their communication, and being confident.

6. The touch of the massage professional may trigger a memory pattern. Each memory, including all the sensory information, nervous system functions, and endocrine functions in play at the time of the experience, is stored in a multidimensional way. When the body state changes, the memory becomes vague and less clear. Because massage produces changes in the nervous and endocrine systems and is a source of sensory stimulation, a state that holds a memory pattern for a client could be recreated. This may help a person resolve and integrate a past experience, provided appropriate professional support is available. Often only pieces of a memory are retrieved. This is common with body memories. The massage may trigger a physiologic response, yet no visual or sequential memory is retrievable. Just because a person does not remember who, what, when, why, or how does not mean that the memory is not valid.

7. The client may discount the injury, provide a cover story, feel guilty or ashamed, or be surprised that the injury is there. It is important for the massage therapist not to press the issue and to realize that self-abuse is a coping mechanism that may calm the person. The massage therapist must not perpetuate an abuse pattern by providing invasive massage.

8. Stay connected with the client but distanced from the experience, which belongs to the client. Continue the massage methods that triggered the response if the client agrees. Ask the client if he or she would like you to continue. Slow the methods and allow the body time to integrate and resolve the body memory. Refer the client if additional coping and counseling skills are indicated.

9. Compensation patterns that may develop from any sport respond well to maintenance massage methods. In addition, recovery occurs quicker and performance is enhanced by regular massage.

10. There are three forms of restorative massage: recovery massage, which primarily focuses on the athlete who wants to recover from a strenuous workout or competition when no injury is present; remedial massage, which is used for minor to moderate injuries; and rehabilitation massage, which is used for severe injury or as part of intervention after surgery.

11. Organizing a sports massage team to provide general circulation enhancement massage is a great public education and promotional

concept. It is important to develop a simple, 15-minute routine that all massage practitioners can use. A similar concept can be used for seated neck and shoulder massage in a corporate office.

12. Children's attention spans are shorter, therefore the massage may need to take less than an hour; 15 to 30 minutes is typical.

13. Touch is important during the growing years. Massage is an organized approach to touch, and the nervous system likes to learn from it. Wrestling and horsing around, both activities that many children engage in, may provide massagelike responses.

14. Massage provides temporary relief from growing pains.

15. Massage is a great, organized, and safe way to touch. This may help families stay in touch during both difficult and good times.

16. The parent or guardian provides informed consent and must supervise the massage session.

17. It is important for the massage professional to focus on helping the client feel better for a while rather than trying to eliminate the chronic illness. Chronic illness presents a variety of problems in living. For many, "healing" is the act of taking back self-control; not getting rid of the illness, but learning to live with it in a resourceful manner. Massage can help the process by providing temporary symptomatic relief in a chronic illness.

18. Hardiness, or toughening, is the ability to physically and mentally withstand external stressors. Because of a decrease in physical activity and isolation, those with a chronic illness becomes less hardy. Massage is a gentle, organized, and controlled way to provide both physical and mental stress. It provides the client the opportunity to begin to assimilate and adjust to the sensory input in a way that increases hardiness.

19. Many people with a chronic illness are taking medication or undergoing other medical interventions. It is important for the medical professional to be able to monitor the effects of different therapies. Because massage interacts with
both the nervous and endocrine systems, it is important that massage effects be monitored as part of the entire therapeutic outcome. A reduction in medication dosage and thereby in side effects may be possible through a multidisciplinary approach to dealing with chronic illness.

20. The elderly have years of experiences to share. Patience, respect for time, and the importance of listening can be learned from the elderly.

21. Because of reduced joint space and changes in soft tissue, it is common to find nerve compression and resulting pain.

22. It is important to understand the physiology of aging and the physical changes that take place. An elderly client may take medication to control various physiologic processes, but in general, basic massage skills and an attentive, caring spirit are all that is required.

23. Massage provides an organized sensory stimulation that helps the nervous system to grow and begin to integrate information. It also provides a bonding method for parent and infant.

24. Primary caregivers gain the most from massaging the baby. The massage professional serves both the infant and the caregivers by teaching infant massage.

25. Infants instinctively know when a touch is not safe. They will not respond well to a nervous touch but depend instead on a confident touch. It is important to honor an infant's physiologic state and give him or her time to respond to the touch.

26. Supervision as part of a health care team requires tempering of independent treatment and clearing of all interventions to make sure that they coordinate with the total treatment plan. Charting is essential, as is attention to effective communication. The environment may be noisy and have interruptions and lack of privacy. The client may be taking medications or using special equipment, such as intravenous lines.

27. Ask the client to explain the disability to you, as well as any limitations and the type of assistance needed. Then pay attention to the person, not the disability.

28. Special care must be taken to ensure that the client is able to provide informed consent.

29. Any form of disability makes daily life more stressful. Massage is a great way to reduce general stress levels.

30. Fundamental massage skills are sufficient for working with pregnant women. As in the aging process, pregnancy is a normal event, not a sickness. General wellness personal service massage is indicated. Consideration must be given to positioning, and emotional swings linked to hormonal changes need to be taken into account. The abdomen is never massaged deeply, and changes such as swelling should be referred to the physician or midwife. Asian approaches sometimes indicate avoidance of the spleen meridian.

31. Massage gives that person something to do that is beneficial both as the pregnancy progresses and during labor.

32. Those who are dying are doing meaningful and serious work in going through this process. Being privileged to share in the process can teach us how to die with dignity.

33. A hospice is one of the best sources, and the massage practitioner is encouraged to support and learn from the dedicated individuals who work in hospices.

34. Massage supports other comfort measures. Physical touch can be an important link to this world. Just listening as the person puts his or her life in order and staying with the person throughout the process are important. Gentle touch and a spirit willing to connect and to mourn an inevitable loss are all that is necessary.

PROBLEM-SOLVING EXERCISES

1. This is inappropriate behavior and could injure the client. Either speak with the sports massage team leader or quietly ask to speak with the team member and remind him or her that invasive work is inappropriate and could cause harm.

2. Gently ask the client if she is comfortable and would like to continue with the massage. If she wants to end the session, do so gently and with a sense of closure. If she chooses to continue, stay general with the approach and be quietly supportive.

3. This is a judgment call. Acknowledge that the social aspect of the massage is very important, and if you choose to stay for a bit more conversation, realize that you are establishing a pattern that may need to be continued.

4. Teach him massage to provide a way to organize the touch and meet the needs of the infant.

5. The client can write the message or use other technologic means, such as a voice synthesizer, to communicate.

6. Gently stroke her hands and feet and listen to her.

PROFESSIONAL APPLICATION

- Massage is a good support for comfort care.
- Massage is good for symptomatic relief of pain.
- Massage evens the mood.
- Massage reduces general stress levels.

CHAPTER 13 WORKBOOK SECTION ANSWER KEY

SHORT ANSWER

1. Body—Nutrition, sleep, breathing, physical fitness
   Mind—Relationship, communication belief, and intellectual stimulation
   Spirit—Purpose, connection, faith, hope, and love

2. Common Stress Responses
   - General irritability, hyperexcitation, or depression
   - Pounding of the heart
   - Dryness of the throat and mouth
   - Impulsive behavior and emotional instability
   - Overpowering urge to cry, run, or hide
   - Inability to concentrate
   - Weakness or dizziness
   - Fatigue
   - Tension and extreme alertness
   - Trembling and nervous tics
   - Intermittent anxiety
   - Tendency to be easily startled
   - High-pitched, nervous laughter
   - Stuttering and other speech difficulties
   - Grinding teeth
   - Insomnia
   - Inability to sit still or physically relax
   - Sweating
   - Frequent need to urinate
   - Diarrhea, indigestion, queasiness, and vomiting
   - Migraine and other tension headaches
   - Premenstrual tension or missed menstrual cycles
   - Pain in the neck or lower back
   - Loss of or excessive appetite
   - Increased use of chemicals, including tobacco, caffeine, and alcohol
   - Nightmares
   - Neurotic behavior
   - Psychosis
   - Proneness to accidents

   The massage professional recognizes that these signs of stress result from fluctuations in the autonomic nervous system and resulting endogenous chemical shifts.

3. Intuition is often where awareness begins for the need to address wellness. As we simplify our lives and let go, then we may also need to grieve for what no longer is needed in our lives. We need to communicate these changes and feelings, and experience with others that our lives touch and ask for help.

4. Low in saturated fats, refined foods, no trans fats. High in vegetables, fruits, grains, and beans. Moderate consumption of lean protein including fish and dairy. Adequate fiber intake and water.

5.
   1. Inhale while abdomen expands
   2. Exhale as abdomen contracts
   3. Intake of air is shorter than exhale.
   4. Auxillary breathing muscles are relaxed.

6. Intensity, duration, and frequence.

7. Warming up, aerobic exercises, and cool down.

8. Cardiovascular—decrease in sympathetic ANS stress response, increase in cardiac function.
   Respiratory—More efficient breath and increase in uptake of oxygen and elimination of metabolic waste.
   Mitrocondria in cells increase. Body fat decreases—bone density increases.

9. Flexibility is the ability to move joints through a normal unrestricted, pain free range of motion. Stretch is a therapeutic modality that lengthens and softens short soft tissues and supports flexibility.

10. Mindfulness is focus on the movement and mindful focus in soft rhythms such as music or a rocking chair support entrainment resulting in parasympathetic dominance.

11. How we feel and perceive ourselves sets the stage for chemical changes that generate feelings with results in emotionally driven behavior.

Resourceful self-concept ultimately equals resourceful behavior. Dysfunctional self-concept ultimately results in dysfunctional behavior.

12. Balance in faith, hope, and love provides meaning to life, and motivates commitment, internal control, and energy to meet challenges in life.

CHAPTER 14 WORKBOOK SECTION ANSWER KEY

SHORT ANSWER

1. It takes time and commitment to build any business. The person must believe in the product or service. The massage professional must not quit when times get hard, especially during the first 2 years of the business. Motivation provides the inner strength to stay with a project long enough to succeed.

2. If we understand all aspects of ourselves, then it is easier to determine where difficulties may arise, where we will need help from others, or what other skills we may need to learn to support our weak areas. A successful business depends on maximum utilization of strengths and compensation for and understanding of weaknesses.

3. Burnout occurs when we expend more energy than we restore. It could also be described as taking care of others more than we take of ourselves. Burnout can be prevented by keeping our lives balanced. This can be achieved by getting a regular massage, taking classes, or taking a vacation.

4. A resume helps us present the professional experience, qualifications, and attributes that we bring to a business relationship.

5. Real time includes the time it takes to do a massage, as well as the time between massages and the time needed to complete the client's records. In addition, the massage professional must realize that the time spent on business record keeping and paperwork requirements will equal approximately the time spent performing actual massage.

6. Insurance companies are not focused on prevention at this time; therefore, it is unlikely that wellness personal service massage will be reimbursed by insurance in the near future. However, the medical insurance programs are changing, and prevention may become a more important consideration. Until that time, cash for services rendered is a more dependable income base. Any proposed insurance coverage must be preapproved by the insurance company before a massage is given.

7. Investigate the fees charged within a 1-hour drive of your location and set your fees midrange. To get the word out, you may have special introductory offers. It is always best to work with your fellow massage practitioners. Massage is a business of low competition because so much depends on the client-practitioner relationship. Clients continue to see you because they like you. By working together in a community, it is easier for massage professionals to educate the public about the importance of therapeutic massage.

8. A business/career plan is a map of a business's future. It provides direction, clarity of purpose, and a mechanism for setting smaller goals to achieve along the way.

9. Start-up costs comprise the amount of money it takes to begin a business. One start-up cost that often is forgotten is a reserve of money for subsidizing living expenses during the first year of business.

10. Depend most on word-of-mouth advertising and spread the word initially by making yourself visible in the community through public speaking and volunteer work. Encourage the local media (e.g., newspaper, radio) to do a story about your business. Direct mail is good. Yellow Page advertising is important after the business has been established in a location for 1 year. Form a group of massage and bodywork professionals in your community and advertise as a group in the newspaper, on the radio, internet, or even on television and share the advertising costs.

11. The brochure educates the public about your massage business in a comprehensive yet concise manner.

12. (1) Self-employment, using leased or purchased space, (2) self-employment, paying a percentage of the income from each massage instead of rent for space, and (3) employee status, earning an hourly wage or salary.

13. KISS means keep it simple and specific. If a business management system is too complicated, most people will not consistently follow through with the record keeping.

14. Without an adequate record-keeping system, we are unable to verify information, accurately report business income, keep track of clients' progress, or look back to learn from successes and mistakes in order to achieve a better business operation in the future.

15. Professional liability or malpractice insurance and premise liability insurance ("trip and fall" insurance) are crucial, and the massage professional needs this protection. Other types of insurance are available, depending on the complexity of the business.

16. This booklet, presented in a format the client can easily understand, enables the client and the therapist to set realistic expectations about what is required in the professional relationship. Thinking the details out in advance prevents many problems. The client-practitioner agreement and policy statement determines the boundaries of the professional relationship.

17. Understanding how a business works helps us appreciate the responsibilities and commitment of business owners and helps people to be better employees. We are all dealing with business concepts when we manage our personal lives. Business management is just one of those things we all need to understand.

ADDITIONAL ACTIVITY

1. The nature of the service offered:
   a. Clearly explain that therapeutic massage is a general health service.
   b. State that no specific treatment of any kind is given for preexisting physical or mental problems.
   c. Referrals will be made to the appropriate licensed professional for specific medical, structural, psychological, or dietary problems.
   d. Written permission and supervision by a medical professional or other licensed health professional will be required to work with any conditions that fall within their scope of practice.

2. Description of the service offered:
   a. Give a full description of the types of services offered and the procedures followed in rendering those services.
   b. Clients may remain dressed and will always be properly draped.
   c. The client may stop the session at any time and may choose not to have any area of the body touched or any particular techniques used.
   d. Simply explain the process of a massage.

3. Qualifications of the practitioner:
   a. List verifiable credentials documenting education, training, licensing, certifications, and experience to allow potential clients to verify for themselves the practitioner's competency.
   b. List the organization issuing the credentials, such as a school or continuing education provider.

4. Client financial and time investment:
   a. Include a realistic statement of costs and fees in the brochure.
   b. Emphasize that the effects of massage are temporary, and massage is best used as a maintenance system.
   c. Indicate that the effects of the massage session can be increased with simple exercises. The massage practitioner will teach self-help to the client if requested.
   d. The best results from massage are maintained when massage is implemented on a weekly or biweekly basis.
   e. Therapeutic massage, when used occasionally, provides only temporary effects.

5. Role of the client in healthcare:
   a. Include the importance of the client's responsibility in personal healthcare.
   b. It is important for the client to realize that the massage therapist's role is as a facilitator in the wellness process.

6. Types of service:
   a. Our clinic offers relaxation, prenatal, and sports massages.
   b. Explain what this particular style of bodywork is good for and what its limitations are.
   c. Specify if you specialize in working with any particular group (e.g., the elderly, athletes) or with specific problems, such as headaches and back pain.
   d. State whether you do not care to work with certain situations, such as pregnant women or people with certain medical conditions.
   e. Have a referral network of related professionals that you use.

7. Training and experience:
   a. Licensing information: does your state require licensing? If so, have available the facts confirming that you are licensed.
   b. State how long you have been in practice, what school you attended, if the school was approved by any professional organization, and how many classroom hours were required for graduation.
   c. Provide information about continuing education.
   d. Provide information about additional education if pertinent (e.g., that you are also an athletic trainer).
   e. Include the names of any professional organizations in which you are an active member.

8. Appointment policies:
   a. Define the length of an average session.
   b. Inform clients which days you work, your hours, and whether you do on-site work, either residential or business.
   c. Tell the client to expect that the first appointment will be longer than subsequent appointments, whether you take emergency appointments, and how often you suggest clients come for a massage session.
   d. Be clear about the cancellation policy and your policy for late appointments.
   e. Tell the client whether he or she can eat before an appointment or if physical activity should be altered or restricted before or after the session.

9. Client/practitioner expectations and informed consent:
   a. Explain in detail what happens at the first massage session (e.g., paperwork, medical history, and so on).
   b. Clients should know that they can get partly undressed or undressed down to their underclothes and that clients are covered and draped during the session.
   c. Explain the order in which you massage (face up or face down to begin), what parts of the body you work on and in what order, if you use oils, if a shower is available before or after the massage, or if bathing at home before the massage appointment is expected.
   d. Make sure the client understands whether talking is appropriate during the session and that you should be informed if anything feels uncomfortable.
   e. If you have low lighting and music is provided, the client should be comfortable with that aspect of the massage.
   f. Make clear to the client the possibility of any reactions that may be expected.
   g. Indicate that the goals for the massage session and proposed styles and massage methods will be discussed with the client before the massage and that consent must be provided for all massage procedures.

h. Inform the client that your profession has a code of ethics and indicate your policy on confidentiality.

i. If the client is in any way uncomfortable, it is permissible to be accompanied by a friend or relative.

10. Fees:

a. Fees are reviewed annually, and any increase will begin in May.

b. A sliding fee is available for retirees, those on disability, and other such individuals.

c. Cash, checks, and major credit cards are acceptable for payment.

d. Payment is expected at time of service; any arrangements for billing must be made in advance.

e. Clients are responsible for collecting from insurance companies.

f. Insurance covers our services only when the client is referred by a physician and has written preapproval from the insurance company.

g. Our fees are based on hourly rates.

h. A 20% discount is offered to all clients who purchase a series of five sessions.

i. To thank you for referring new clients to our office, we offer you a $5 discount on your next session.

11. Sexual appropriateness:

a. Sexual behavior by the therapist toward the client and the client toward the therapist is always unethical and inappropriate.

b. It is always the responsibility of the therapist or health professional to see that sexual misconduct does not occur.

12. Recourse policy:

a. If a client is unhappy or dissatisfied, a portion of the fees will be refunded.

b. If the matter is not handled in a satisfactory manner, clients can contact the Organization of Bodyworkers of Tylerville [insert your own local professional association here] to register any complaints.

PROBLEM-SOLVING EXERCISES

1. Determine fees charged by other therapists in the surrounding area. Locate information about education levels and costs comparable to this that may validate higher fees.

2. Send a booklet to clients to read before the first massage. Use the booklets as a guide for carefully thought-out policies when interviewing the client.

3. Take into account the following and then total:
Time in school
Time spent commuting to school
Time spent completing homework
Time spent doing research
Time devoted to practice

4. Terry could take the following steps to boost business:

a. Talk with current clients about their satisfaction with his service and ask whether they are referring new clients.

b. Consider offering incentives for referrals.

c. Take continuing education and advertise about his new skills.

d. Do a direct mailing with a special offer to current clients.

e. Volunteer to work at some special events.

PROFESSIONAL APPLICATION

1. Offer to have the client come in and talk with you.
Identify the areas of concern for the client, and expand on the information in the booklet.
Explain the professional aspects of informed consent.
Explain that knowledge and clarity on these aspects support the professional relationship.

Index

Page numbers with "f" denote figures; "t" tables; "b" boxes